EUROPEAN SOCIETY OF SURGICAL ONCOLOGY

U. Veronesi (Editor-in-Chief)

Surgical Oncology

A European Handbook

B. Arnesjø, I. Burn, L. Denis and F. Mazzeo (Co-Editors)

Foreword by I. Burn

With 222 Figures and 227 Tables

Springer-Verlag Berlin Heidelberg New York
London Paris Tokyo Hong Kong

Professor Dr. UMBERTO VERONESI
Direttore Generale
Istituto Nazionale per lo Studio e la Cura dei Tumori
Via Venezian, 1, 20133 Milano, Italy

Professor Dr. BO ARNESJØ
Department of Surgery, Haukeland University Hospital
University of Bergen
5021 Bergen, Norway

Professor Dr. IAN BURN
Charing Cross Hospital
Fulham Palace Road
London W6 8RF, United Kingdom

Professor Dr. LOUIS DENIS
Department of Urology
A. Z. Middelheim, Vrue Universiteit Brussel
Lindendreef 1, 2020 Antwerpen, Belgium

Professor Dr. FRANCESCO MAZZEO
Università di Napoli
Cattedra di Chirurgia Generale, II facolta'
Via Pansini, 5, 80131 Napoli, Italy

Editorial Secretariat
Scientific Secretaries: Dr. Vittorio Quagliuolo, Dr. Alberto Azzarelli
Editorial Secretary: Ms. Sheila McGrath

ISBN-13:978-3-642-72648-4 e-ISBN-13:978-3-642-72646-0
DOI: 10.1007/978-3-642-72646-0

Library of Congress Cataloging-in-Publication Data
Surgical oncology : a European handbook / U. Veronesi (editor-in-chief) ; B. Arnesjø . . . [et al.], co-editors. p. cm. Includes bibliographies and index.
ISBN-13:978-3-642-72648-4 (U.S.):1.Cancer–Surgery–Handbooks, manuals, etc. I. Veronesi, Umberto. II. Arnesjø, B. (Bo) [DNLM: 1. Neoplasms – surgery. QZ 268 S96113] RD651.S933 1989 616.99'4059 – dc20 DNLM/DLC for Library of Congress

Softcover reprint of the hardcover 1st edition 1989

2123/3145-543210 – Printed on acid-free paper

Foreword

The concept of the surgical oncologist is a strange one. Surgeons are a special breed of human beings, whose work requires a degree of pragmatism which is almost unique. Cancer would seem to be altogether too diffuse a subject to contain within the usual surgical boundaries and almost foreign to the traditional precision of surgical thinking. And yet, the responsibility for initial diagnosis and primary management of the vast majority of patients with malignant disease has always been vested in the surgeon.

For some forms of cancer, there is reason to be fairly satisfied with what has been achieved. Apart from the natural distaste of anyone to submit him- or herself to the surgeon's knife, there would seem to be little cause to seek a change of therapy. Why change a winning horse? It is true that for other forms of malignant disease, however, surgical endeavour has seen little reward in terms of cure of the disease. The analysis of such results, about which the literature is voluminous, frequently shows that ultimate failure is due to the advanced stage of the cancer at the time of first diagnosis, rather than to an integral fault of the procedure. In other words, given an earlier cancer, the same procedure will effect cure. But perhaps the argument is too facile, certainly for the patient with advanced cancer. We can never expect that all cancers will be diagnosed early enough for the surgeon, with his or her present techniques, to cure the majority. Patients will continue to present to the doctor with varying stages of malignant disease. The therapist must adapt to allow for this.

Here then lies the challenge for the surgical oncologist. Patients with cancer need to be studied before vital decisions on therapy are made. This study will be possible only if there is complete familiarity with the natural history of the disease and with the true potential of *all* available methods of treatment. Above all, knowledge must incorporate the disadvantages of these methods so as to ensure that the situation is not made worse.

Where is the knowledge to come from to enable surgeons to be more completely equipped to deal with cancer in the modern era? The "surgical oncologist" may be defined as a trained surgeon with a committed interest in the study of cancer and in the care of patients with malignant disease. Such individuals must have the opportunity and facilities to study cancer, and this is going to require some radical re-thinking in the corridors of surgical power.

Hopefully those responsible for surgical decision-making throughout the world will recognise the need for surgical oncology and will support the concept in a positive way. Trainee surgeons with a declared interest in the topic must be given the encouragement and support to pursue their interest. Their educational needs must be provided. Posts must be created in hospitals and institutes within which the surgical oncologists can ply their trade alongside other specialist oncologists. To date, this has happened only to a small degree in a few enlightened areas in the world.

Fortunately, there have been some positive moves on behalf of surgical oncology, which have at least made a start in the creation of educational facilities. Notable has been the emergence of a number of surgical oncology societies and journals. Some of these are now well established and provide a continuing exciting forum for debate and the exchange of information. Also, the last few years have seen the production of a number of text books on surgical oncology, which will undoubtedly help to foster interest in the subject.

The *European Handbook of Surgical Oncology* was spawned out of discussions which took place between members of the European Society of Surgical Oncology shortly after its formation 5 years ago. The book contains contributions from oncologists from all over Europe. It is truly comprehensive in its approach to the subject. To practise cancer surgery confidently requires a depth of knowledge about the disease which goes far beyond the simple attributes of diagnosis and dissection. This book provides that knowledge, donated by some of the most experienced oncologists of this century. It is also, notably, an international effort, which is the only logical way to deal with a disease which is a massive threat to the whole human race.

IAN BURN
President, European
Society of Surgical Oncology

Table of Contents

Treatment of Cancer of Different Organs . . . 475

List of Contributors

AARONSON, N.K.
E.O.R.T.C. Study Group
on Quality of Life
The Netherlands Cancer Institute
Plesmanlaan 121
1066 CX Amsterdam, The Netherlands

ARIAS, J.
Instituto Nacional de la Salud
Servicio de Chirurgia de
Aparato Digestivo II
Hospital 1. Octubre
Carretera de Andalucia, km 5
28041 Madrid, Spain

ARNESJØ, B.
Department of Surgery
Haukeland University Hospital
5021 Bergen, Norway

BACKLUND, E.O.
Department of Neurosurgery
University of Bergen
Haukeland Hospital
5016 Bergen, Norway

BÄCKDAHL, M.
Karolinska Hospital
10401 Stockholm 60, Sweden

BAUMEISTER, R.G.H.
Abteilung Plastische Chirurgie der
Chirurgischen Klinik und Poliklinik
Klinikum Grosshadern
Marchioninistrasse 15
8000 München 70, FRG

BERGENTZ, S.-E.
Department of Surgery
University of Lund
General Hospital
Malmö, Sweden

BERGQVIST, D.
Department of Surgery
University of Lund
General Hospital
Malmö, Sweden

BESSON, A.
Faculté de Médecine
Service de Chirurgie A du CHUV
1011 Lausanne, Switzerland

BESZNYÁK, I.
National Cancer Institute
Department of Surgery
1125 Ráth Gy. u. 7–9
Budapest, Hungary

BISCHOF-DELALOYE, A.
CHUV
Division of Nuclear Medicine
1011 Lausanne, Switzerland

BISMUTH, H.
Unité de Chirurgie Hépato-Biliaire
Hôpital Paul Brousse
94800 Villejuif, France

BLANDY, J.P.
The London Hospital Medical College
Turner Street
London E1 2AD, UK

BLOMQUIST, P.
Malmö General Hospital
Department of Surgery
University of Lund
21401 Malmö, Sweden

BLUMGART, L.H.
Klinik für Viszerale und
Transplantationschirurgie
Inselspital
3010 Bern, Switzerland

BOHMERT, H.
Abt. Plastische Chirurgie der
Chirurgischen Klinik und Poliklinik
Klinikum Grosshadern
Marchioninistrasse 15
8000 München 70, FRG

BONADONNA, G.
Istituto Nazionale per lo
Studio e la Cura dei Tumori
Divisione Oncologia Medica
Via Venezian, 1
20133 Milano, Italy

BOVEN, E.
Free University Hospital
Department of Oncology
De Boelelaan 1117
1081 HV Amsterdam, The Netherlands

BROWER, M.
University of Rochester Cancer Center
Rochester General Hospital
Department of Oncology
1425 Portland Avenue
Rochester, NY 14621, USA

BUCHEGGER, F.
Biochemistry Institute
University of Lausanne
1066 Epalinges, Switzerland

BURGER, M.M.
Friedrich-Miescher-Institut
Postfach 2543
4002 Basel, Switzerland

BURN, I.
Charing Cross Hospital
Fulham Palace Road
London W6 8RF, U.K.

BUYSE, M.
E.O.R.T.C. Data Center
Boulevard de Waterloo, 125
1000 Bruxelles, Belgium

CALAIS DA SILVA, F.
Praceta Bento Moura 2–1 Esq.
Hospital Desterro
Venda Nova
2700 Amadora, Portugal

CALLEJA, J.
Instituto Nacional de la Salud
Servicio de Chirurgia de
Aparato Digestivo II
Hospital 1. Octubre
Carretera de Andalucia, km 5
28041 Madrid, Spain

CALVO, F.A.
Department of Oncology
University Clinic Navarra
Apartado 192
31080 Pamplona, Spain

CARNEY, D.N.
Mater Misericordiae Hospital
Dublin 7, Ireland

CASCINELLI, N.
Istituto Nazionale per lo
Studio e la Cura dei Tumori
Divisione Oncologia Chirurgia B
Via G. Venezian, 1
20133 Milano, Italy

CAVALLI, F.
Ospedale San Giovanni
Oncologia Medica
6500 Bellinzona, Switzerland

CEDERMARK, B.
Karolinska Hospital
10401 Stockholm, Sweden

CLEMENTE, C.
Istituto Nazionale per lo
Studio e la Cura dei Tumori
Divisione Anatomia Patologica
Via G. Venezian, 1
20133 Milano, Italy

COSTA, A.
Istituto Nazionale per lo
Studio e la Cura dei Tumori
Divisione Oncologia Chirurgia C
Via G. Venezian, 1
20133 Milano, Italy

COSTA, J.
Faculté de Médecine
Service de Chirurgie A du CHUV
1011 Lausanne, Switzerland

DAVIES, G.C.
Department of Clinical Surgery
The Royal Infirmary
University of Edinburgh
Edinburgh EH3 9YW, UK

DE TRIBOLET, N.
Faculté de Médecine
Service de Chirurgie A du CHUV
1011 Lausanne, Switzerland

DEJACE, P.
Section of Infectious Diseases
Department of Medicine
Tulane University Medical School
1430 Tulane Avenue
New Orleans, LA 70112, USA

DELALOYE, B.
CHUV
Division of Nuclear Medicine
1011 Lausanne, Switzerland

DENIS, L.
Department of Urology
A.Z. Middelheim
Vrue Universiteit Brussel
Lindendreef 1
2020 Antwerpen, Belgium

DI RE, F.
Istituto Nazionale per lo
Studio e la Cura dei Tumori
Divisione Oncologia Chirurgica
Ginecologia
Via G. Venezian, 1
20133 Milano, Italy

DOUGLAS, P.
Faculté de Médecine
Service de Chirurgie A du CHUV
1011 Lausanne, Switzerland

DREYFUS, M.
Service de Chirurgie
Générale et Endocrinienne
Hôpital Universitaire de Hautepierre
67098 Strasbourg Cedex, France

ESCUDERO, F.
Instituto Nacional de la Salud
Servicio de Chirurgia de
Aparato Digestivo II
Hospital 1. Octubre
Carretera de Andalucia, km 5
28041 Madrid, Spain

FONTANELLI, R.
Istituto Nazionale per lo
Studio e la Cura dei Tumori
Divisione Oncologia Chirurgica
Ginecologia
Via G. Venezian, 1
20133 Milano, Italy

FORESTIERI, P.
Cattedra di Chirurgia Generale
II Divisione di Chirurgia
II Facolta', Universita' di Napoli
Via S. Pansini, 5
80131 Napoli, Italy

FOSSATI-BELLANI, F.
Istituto Nazionale per lo
Studio e la Cura dei Tumori
Divisione Oncologia Medica Pediatrica
Via Venezian, 1
20133 Milano, Italy

GALL, F.P.
Chirurgische Klinik mit Poliklinik
Universität Erlangen-Nürnberg
Maximiliansplatz
8520 Erlangen, FRG

GARCIA, I.
Instituto Nacional de la Salud
Servicio de Chirurgia de
Aparato Digestivo II
Hospital 1. Octubre
Carretera de Andalucia, km 5
28041 Madrid, Spain

GARDEN, O.J.
Department of Surgery
University of Edinburgh
Royal Infirmary
Edinburgh EH3 9YW, UK

GERBAULET, A.
Institut Gustave Roussy
Rue Camille Desmoulins
94805 Villejuif Cedex, France

GIULÌ, R.
Service de Chirurgie Digestive
Hôpital Beaujon
92110 Clichy-Paris, France

GOLDSTRAW, P.
Brompton Hospital
Fulham Road
London SW3 6HP, UK

GOMEZ, M.
Instituto Nacional de la Salud
Servicio de Chirurgia de
Aparato Digestivo II
Hospital 1. Octubre
Carretera de Andalucia, km 5
28041 Madrid, Spain

González, E.M.
Instituto Nacional de la Salud
Servicio de Chirurgia de
Aparato Digestivo II
Hospital 1. Octubre
Carretera de Andalucia, km 5
28041 Madrid, Spain

Gran, M.C.
International Agency for
Research on Cancer
Descriptive Epidemiology
150, Cours Albert Thomas
69372 Lyon Cedex 08, France

Granberg, P.-O.
Department of Surgery
Karolinska Hospital
10401 Stockholm, Sweden

Grundmann, R.
Chirurgische Universitätsklinik
Joseph-Stelzmann-Strasse 9
5000 Köln 41, FRG

Haehnel, P.
Service de Chirurgie
Générale et Endocrinienne
Hôpital Universitaire de Hautepierre
67098 Strasbourg Cedex, France

Haemmerli, G.
Institut für Pathologie
Aussenstation Universität Zürich
Birchstrasse, 95
8050 Zürich

Hall, R.R.
Department of Urology
Freeman Hospital
Freeman Road, High Heaton
Newcastle upon Tyne NE7 7DN, UK

Halvorsen, J.F.
Department of Surgery
Haukeland University Hospital
5021 Bergen, Norway

Hamberger, B.
Karolinska Hospital
10401 Stockholm 60, Sweden

Herfarth, C.
Chirurgische Universitätsklinik
Abteilung für Onkologie
Im Neuenheimer Feld 110
6900 Heidelberg, FRG

Hoekstra, H.J.
Division of Surgical Oncology
Department of Surgery
Groningen University Hospital
P.O. Box 30001
9700 RB Groningen, The Netherlands

Hohenberger, W.
Chirurgische Klinik mit Poliklinik
Universität Erlangen-Nürnberg
Maximiliansplatz
8520 Erlangen, FRG

Hultén, L.
University of Göteborg
Department of Surgery II
Sahlgrenska sjukhuset
41345 Göteborg, Sweden

Jaeck, D.
Service de Chirurgie Générale et Endocrinienne
Hôpital Universitaire de Hautepierre
67098 Strasbourg Cedex, France

Jaeger, N.
University Urological Clinic
Sigmund-Freud-Strasse 25
5300 Bonn, FRG

Jakse, G.
Department of Urology
Technische Universität
8000 München, FRG

Jiborn, H.
Malmö General Hospital
Department of Surgery
University of Lund
21401 Malmö, Sweden

Jover, J.M.
Instituto Nacional de la Salud
Servicio de Chirurgia de
Aparato Digestivo II
Hospital 1. Octubre
Carretera de Andalucia, km 5
28041 Madrid, Spain

Kehlet, H.
Surgical Department
Rigshospitalet
Afd. C 2122, Blegdamsvej 9
2100 Copenhagen, Denmark

KLASTERSKY, J.
Service de Médecine et
Laboratoire d'Investigation
Clinique H.J.Tagnon, Institut Jules
Bordet
Centre des Tumeurs de l'Université Libre
de Bruxelles
1 Rue Héger-Bordet
1000 Bruxelles, Belgium

KOTZ, R.
Allgemeines Krankenhaus der Stadt Wien
Orthopädische Universitätsklinik
9, Garnisongasse 13
1090 Wien, Austria

KULAKOWSKI, A.
Instytut Onkologii
im. Marii Sklodowskiej-Curie
ul. Wawelska 15
00-973 Warszawa, Poland

LANDA, I.
Instituto Nacional de la Salud
Servicio de Chirurgia de
Aparato Digestivo II
Hospital 1. Octubre
Carretera de Andalucia, km 5
28041 Madrid, Spain

LANDBERG, T.
Department of Oncology
Malmö General Hospital
21401 Malmö, Sweden

LÖWHAGEN, T.
Karolinska Hospital
10401 Stockholm 60, Sweden

LOTE, K.
Department of Oncology
Haukeland Sykehus
Postboks 1
5016 Haukeland, Norway

LUNDELL, G.
Karolinska Hospital
10401 Stockholm 60, Sweden

LUNDHOLM, K.
University of Göteborg
Department of Surgery I
Sahlgrenska sjukhuset
41345 Göteborg, Sweden

MACH, J.P.
Biochemistry Institute
University of Lausanne
1066 Epalinges, Switzerland

MAGUIRE, P.
Department of Psychiatry
Withington Hospital
West Didsbury
Manchester M20 8LR, UK

MATTHEIEM, W.H.
Head, Breast & Pelvic Surgical Clinic
Surgical Oncology
Free University of Brussels
Institut Jules Bordet
Bruxelles, Belgium

MAZZEO, F.
Universita' di Napoli
Cattedra di Chirurgia Generale
II facolta'
Via S.Pansini, 5
80131 Napoli, Italy

McGREGOR, I.A.
West of Scotland Regional Plastic
and Oral Surgery Unit
Canniesburn Hospital
Bearsden
Glasgow G61, 1QL, UK

METZGER, U.
Surgical Oncology
Department of Surgery
University Hospital Zürich
8091 Zürich, Switzerland

MICHEL, G.
Institut Gustave Roussy
Rue Camille Desmoulins
94805 Villejuif Cedex, France

MÖLLER, T.R.
Department of Oncology and Southern
Swedish Regional Tumor Registry
University Hospital
22185 Lund, Sweden

MOLDAWER, L.L.
Department of Surgery I
Sahlgrenska sjukhuset
University of Göteborg
41345 Göteborg, Sweden

MOZZILLO, N.
Cattedra di Chirurgia Generale
II Divisione di Chirurgia
II facolta', Universita' di Napoli
Via S. Pansini, 5
80131 Napoli, Italy

MUIR, C.S.
International Agency for
Research on Cancer
Descriptive Epidemiology
150, Cours Albert Thomas
69372 Lyon Cedex 08, France

MYKING, A.O.
Department of Pathology
Gades Institute
Haukeland University Hospital
5021 Bergen, Norway

NORTHOVER, J.M.A.
Imperial Cancer Research Fund
Colorectal Cancer Unit
St. Mark's Hospital
City Road
London, ECIV 2PS, UK

PARKER, M.C.
95, Harley Street
London W1N IDF, UK

PARKIN, D.M.
International Agency for
Research on Cancer
150, Cours Albert Thomas
69372 Lyon Cedex 08, France

PETTAVEL, J.
Faculté de Médecine
Service de Chirurgie A du CHUV
1011 Lausanne, Switzerland

PICHLMAIER, H.
Chirurgische Universitätsklinik
Joseph-Stelzmann-Strasse 9
5000 Köln 41, FRG

PINEDO, H.M.
Free University Hospital
Department of Oncology
De Boelelaan 1117
1081 HV Amsterdam, The Netherlands

PIZZOCARO, G.
Istituto Nazionale per lo
Studio e la Cura dei Tumori
Divisione di Oncologia Chirurgica
Urologica
Via G. Venezian, 1
20133 Milano, Italy

PLASCHKES, J.
Department of Pediatric Surgery
University Children's Hospital
Inselspital, Freiburgstrasse
3010 Bern, Switzerland

RILKE, F.
Istituto Nazionale per lo
Studio e la Cura dei Tumori
Divisione Anatomia Pathologica
Via G. Venezian, 1
20133 Milano, Italy

ROBERTS, P.J.
IV Department of Surgery
University of Helsinki
Kaserngatan 11-13
00130 Helsinki 13, Finland

RÜMKE, P.
The Netherlands Cancer Institute
Antoni van Leeuwenhoek Huis
Immunology and Internal Medicine
Plesmanlaan 121
1066 CX Amsterdam, The Netherlands

SARGENT, N.S.E.
Friedrich-Miescher-Institut
Postfach 2543
4002 Basel, Switzerland

SAVARY, M.
Faculté de Médecine
Service de Chirurgie A du CHUV
1011 Lausanne, Switzerland

SBANOTTO, A.
Istituto Nazionale per lo
Studio e la Cura dei Tumori
Divisione di Terapia del Dolore e Cure
Palliative
Via Venezian, 1
20133 Milano, Italy

SCHEININ, T.M.
IV Department of Surgery
University of Helsinki
Kaserngatan 11-13
00130 Helsinki 13, Finland

SCHERSTÉN, T.
Department of Surgery I
Sahlgrenska sjukhuset
University of Göteborg
41345 Göteborg, Sweden

SCHLAG, P.
Chirurgische Universitätsklinik
Abteilung für Onkologie
Im Neuenheimer Feld 110
6900 Heidelberg, FRG

SCHRÖDER, F.H.
Erasmus University Hospital
P.O. Box 1738
3000 DR Rotterdam, The Netherlands

SNOW, G.B.
Department of Otolaryngology/
Head and Neck Surgery
Free University Hospital
De Boelelaan 1117
1081 HV Amsterdam, The Netherlands

SOLHEIM, K.
Surgical Department
University of Oslo
Ulleval Hospital
Kirkeveien 166
0407 Oslo 4, Norway

SØREIDE, O.
Department of Surgery
National Hospital
University of Oslo
Oslo, Norway

SPINELLI, P.
Istituto Nazionale per lo
Studio e la Cura dei Tumori
Divisione di Endoscopia
Via G. Venezian, 1
20133 Milano, Italy

STADIL, F.
Surgical Department
Rigshospitalet
Afd. C 2122, Blegdamsvej 9
2100 Copenhagen, Denmark

STAQUET, M.
E.O.R.T.C. Data Center
Boulevard de Waterloo, 125
1000 Bruxelles, Belgium

STRÄULI, P.
Institut für Pathologie
Abteilung für Krebsforschung
Aussenstation Universität Zürich
Birchstrasse 95
8050 Zürich, Switzerland

TAGNON, H.J.
University of Brussels
Institut Jules Bordet
Boulevard de Waterloo, 125
1000 Bruxelles, Belgium

THOMSON, J.P.S.
Imperial Cancer Research Fund
Colorectal Cancer Unit
St. Mark's Hospital
City Road
London, ECIV 2PS, UK

TRAPEZNIKOV, N.N.
Institute of Experimental & Clinical
Oncology
USSR Academy of Medical Sciences
Kashirskoye shosse, 6
M-115478 Moscow, U.S.S.R.

TUBIANA, M.
Institut Gustave Roussy
Rue Camille Desmoulins
94805 Villejuif Cedex, France

TWYCROSS, R.
Sir Michael Sobell House
Churchill Hospital
Headington
Oxford OX3 7LJ, UK

UDÉN, P.
Malmö General Hospital
Department of Surgery
University of Lund
21401 Malmö, Sweden

VAHLENSIECK, W.
University Urological Clinic
Sigmund-Freud-Strasse 25
5300 Bonn, FRG

VALAGUSSA, P.
Istituto Nazionale per lo
Studio e la Cura dei Tumori
Via Venezian, 1
20133 Milano, Italy

VENTAFRIDDA, V.
Istituto Nazionale per lo
Studio e la Cura dei Tumori
Divisione di Terapia del Dolore e Cure
Palliative
Via Venezian, 1
20133 Milano, Italy

VERONESI, P.
Divisione di Chirurgia II
Ospedale San Raffaele
Via Olgettnia, 60
20090 Segrate (Mi), Italy

VERONESI, U.
Direttore Generale
Istituto Nazionale per lo
Studio e la Cura dei Tumori
Via Venezian, 1
20133 Milano, Italy

WALLIN, G.
Karolinska Hospital
10401 Stockholm 60, Sweden

WHITE, H.
95, Harley Street
London W1N IDF, UK

WILLEMS, G.
Department of Heelkunde
Akademisch Ziekenhuis V. U. S.
Laarbeeklaan 101
1090 Bruxelles, Belgium

WOLFF, J. P.
Service de Gynécologie
Institut Gustave Roussy
Rue Camille Desmoulins
94805 Villejuif Cedex, France

ZEDERFELDT, B.
Malmö General Hospital
Department of Surgery
University of Lund
21401 Malmö, Sweden

ZIRNGIBL, H.
Chirurgische Klinik mit Poliklinik
Universität Erlangen-Nürnberg
Maximiliansplatz
8520 Erlangen, FRG

Introduction: The Role of Surgery in Cancer Treatment

U. VERONESI

Surgical Oncology and the Surgical Oncologist

Oncology is a science which investigates the pathological phenomen of uncontrolled cell proliferation in all its multifarious aspects. The various characteristics connected with this abnormal process and with its clinical consequences can be divided into a number of different disciplines grouped under the main headings of experimental oncology, clinical oncology and social oncology. Such a wide range of scientific and cultural interests and of specific competences requires, by definition, very strict multidisciplinary connections between the persons involved in the various fields. Interdisciplinary collaboration is therefore the essential prerequisite for the development and progress of sound research and for the effective control of the disease. The final objective of all efforts remains the patient, and this is the reason why, among all the various disciplines, it is the clinical problem which deserves our greatest attention.

It is indisputable that, in this context, the primary and central role in the treatment of the majority of neoplasias is taken by surgery. In fact, although at times surgery plays a purely palliative role and at others it is simply diagnostic, it is of prime importance in the therapeutic strategy. If there is something dawning in this frontier area of medicine, it is the development of a new attitude towards this centrality. Paradoxically, it is the surgical oncologists themselves who are at the forefront in questioning the real position of their speciality within the world of cancer therapy. Thus it is that these surgical oncologists, who are most aware of the more advanced developments in research, have recently adopted certain initiatives which represent true tendencies and indications for the future. Studies on the natural history of cancer, which are becoming more and more significant, and the work on the biological variables that control cancer growth have greatly influenced the surgical oncologists, who see new areas of research and planning opening up beyond the restrictive confrontation of diverse techniques.

Much of the research on biological markers, on the application of monoclonal antibodies, on chemopreventive agents, and on cellular kinetic tests is carried out by surgical oncologists, and all this means not only that they feel the need to widen their horizons, but also that the biological behaviour of the neoplasia is, for them, even more acutely an element of continual confrontation with their manual intervention.

Any attempt to define the role of surgery in the treatment of tumours, moreover, cannot ignore a distinction which is only apparently a purely academic one, that is, the definition of the role of surgery and that of the surgeon. Whereas observations on the speciality can be made whereby its confines can be firmly established, it is more difficult with regard to the specialist as other factors come into play which relate not only to medicine as a science, but also to psychology and sociology. If, on the one hand, the central role of the surgeon can and must be subjected to dispute, due to new concepts on the treatment of tumours, on the other hand, this central role is still widely evident. It is a fact that, in cases of a suspected tumour, more than 80 percent of patients go first to a surgeon, and he or she remains the main point of reference throughout treatment and follow-up for most of them. On the other hand, this more or less corresponds with the frequency with which surgery is required in the therapy of the cancer patient. There is, however, most certainly something more, i.e. the kind of charismatic figures which surgeons continue to represent, not only in the eyes of the patient and his or her family, but also with regard to their other colleagues.

This situation has without doubt given rise to the significant changes in mentality which have characterized modern oncological surgery, so much so that it has caused it to become less oncological surgery and more surgical oncology: there is also an acceptance of the multidisciplinary approach as an essential characteristic in the treatment of tumours and, therefore, the abandonment of the subjective isolated decision, as well as the collective outlook. One must recall the impressive cultural revolution inherent in the progressive abandonment of mutilating surgery and the frantic search for safe conservative techniques. This evolution has led the surgeon to collaborate in all the areas of diagnosis and to have closer contacts with the pathologist, the radiologist, the endoscopist and the biology, immunology and nuclear medicine laboratories in order to provide histological evidence of the presence of the disease (staging of lymphomas, mediastinic biopsies, "second look" in pelvic tumours etc.) and to supply the laboratory with material which will be more suitable for the study of the kinetic, antigenic, hormonal and other biological and biomolecular characteristics of the tumour being studied. Finally, the effort to enhance reconstructive techniques is the expression of the wish to contribute as much to the quality of survival as to its duration.

Although the traditional role of surgery is today undergoing an undoubted period of crisis, there are already many signs emerging which indicate the will, on the part of the new surgical oncologists, to renew their contribution to the cancer problem. The main emphasis of such a contribution will surely fall on research on the biological characteristics of tumours, on a re-thinking of the doctor/patient relationship and on the wish to keep alive a tradition of learning.

The Historical Centrality of Surgery in Oncology

Surgical exeresis is the oldest form of treatment of malignant tumours. It has maintained its role of primacy through the centuries and is still the treatment of choice in a high percentage of cases. Nevertheless, surgery is becoming more and more a part of a wider programme of interdisciplinary therapy. The surgeon, in fact, is less often the sole person responsible for the treatment of the cancer patient, and ever more frequently, decisions are being taken together with the radiotherapist and the chemotherapist.

Until 1950, the most important achievements in the treatment of cancer were the results obtained by innovative surgical procedures. Table 1 shows the importance, from the historical point of view, that surgery has had in the control of neoplastic disease. What is often forgotten, however, is the role which has been played by surgeons in extending the knowledge of tumours beyond the confines of surgery (Table 2). A few historical facts will serve to illustrate this observation: for example, the first description of a professional tumour, cancer of the scrotum in chimney sweeps, was made by a surgeon, Sir Percival Pott; the

Table 1. The principle steps in the history of surgical oncology

Surgeon	Date	Procedure
Billroth	1881	Gastrectomy
Halsted	1890	Radical mastectomy
Wertheim	1900	Radical hysterectomy
Miles	1908	Abdominoperineal resection of the rectum
Torek	1913	Oesophagectomy
Graham and Singer	1933	Pneumonectomy

Table 2. Contribution of surgeons in various oncological fields

Surgeon	Date	Contribution
P. Pott	1775	Scrotum cancer among chimney sweeps
J. Rehn	1895	Bladder cancer among laundry workers
D. Rigoni-Stern	1842	Incidence of breast cancer among nuns
V. Mickulitz	1881	Gastric endoscopy
G. T. Beatson	1896	Hormone treatment in breast cancer
Ch. Huggins	1940	Hormone treatment in prostate cancer
S. Cade	1935	Interstitial radioactive implant in breast cancer
P. Denoix	1960	TMN classification of tumours
D. Burkitt	1962	Viral lymphoma in Africa
B. Fisher	1965	Adjuvant treatments in breast cancer

important role of hormonal therapy in cancer was demonstrated by another surgeon, G. W. Beatson, who also introduced the oophorectomy into breast cancer; the first epidemiological evidence of a tumour due to a virus was described by D. Burkitt, a surgeon; interstitial therapy of breast cancer with radium was proposed in 1930 by Sir S. Cade, surgeon; and the TNM classification of tumours was thought up by yet another surgeon, P. Denoix.

Moreover, as regards controlled clinical trials, suffice it to say that the first international randomised clinical trial was organised in 1962 by a group of surgeons in order to study the role of dissection of the internal mammary nodes in breast cancer; that the highest number of patients submitted to adjuvant therapies has been accrued by the National Surgical Adjuvant Breast Project (NSABP) chaired by a surgeon, B. Fisher; and that the most extensive controlled clinical studies on the many treatments of malignant melanoma have been carried out by an international group of surgeons.

The long history of cancer surgery has not come to an end, however, on the contrary, today, in a large number of cases, even if part of a multidisciplinary therapeutic strategy, surgery maintains its primary role as a curative procedure and constitutes an indispensible premise to any further treatment, but it is especially for their commitment to clinical research that the surgeons must hold on to their central role in oncology.

In recent years a new generation of surgeons have dedicated themselves entirely to the treatment of tumours, opening up new lines of clinical research. The creation of scientific realities which constitute the modern "surgical oncology" is slowly being brought about by the development of a new philosophy in primary surgery which has a greater awareness of the quality of life of the patients treated, deriving from new attempts to reduce and minimise mutilation, the introduction of new techniques such as perfusion and infusion of the organs, the use of laser rays associated with injections of hematoporphyrin, microsurgery for reconstruction, transplantation of the organs and the diffusion of ever closer integration between surgery and other therapies.

There are two basic prerequisites to enable surgical oncologists to develop their research. The first is cooperation with laboratory researchers in the study of the biology of human tumours. The surgeon is, in fact, the clinician most suited to the study of the natural history of tumours, with research on their rate of growth by way of multiple successive observations, on the use of monoclonal antibodies, on specific tumour markers and the introduction on a wide scale of chemopreventive therapies (for example, retinoids), etc. The second prerequisite is a closer collaboration with the pathologist. The pathology laboratory is the natural arena for the in-depth study of the problem of tumours in man, carried out by a working group of surgeons and pathologists.

A further means of study for the surgical oncologist in conjunction with specialists in other disciplines is the controlled clinical trial. An encouraging factor is the ever-increasing percentage of clinical trials on surgery (surgery alone or combined with other treatments) out of the total number of randomised clinical trials observed in 1987 (Fig. 1.). This tendency is revealed in the new line of surgical research aimed at an ample revision of the so-called traditional radical procedures for their possible substitution with less mutilating techniques,

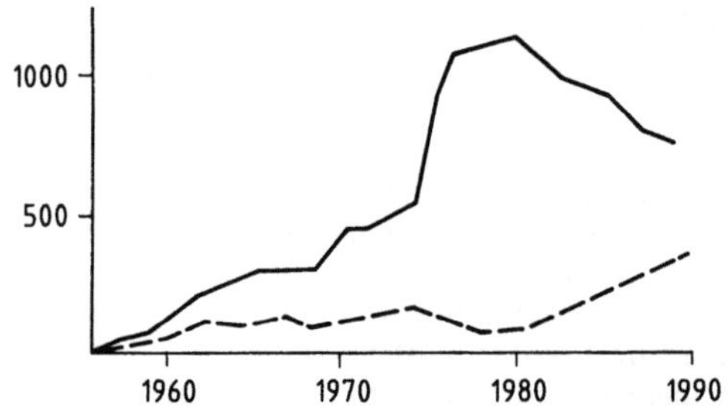

Fig. 1. Number of clinical trials in progress worldwide. **Solid line,** total number of trials; **dotted** line, surgical trials. [From U. Veronesi, A. Costa (1985) The surgical oncologist and clinical research. In: U. Veronesi, G. Bonadonna (eds) Clinical trials in cancer Medicine, part 1. Academic, London, pp 25–34]

especially for tumours of the breast, larynx, rectosigmoid, bone, soft tissue and the thyroid.

It must be recognised that the organisation of a controlled clinical trial for the assessment of the usefulness of a new surgical or radiosurgical treatment for a locoregional tumour will require an immense effort when compared to that needed for preparing and following up a traditional controlled clinical trial.

The Search for Radicality

Malignant tumours develop mostly from one or more sites in an organ and remain confined to that organ for a variable period of time. Although scattered tumour cells can leave the primary foci early, it is unlikely that they will attack distant organs unless they are grouped together in embolisms of a certain size. The probability of successful surgical treatment will therefore depend on: (a) the technical possibility of removing the primary tumour together with a reasonable margin of the surrounding healthy tissue; (b) the absence of metastastic foci. In the presence of these two conditions there is a case for radical surgery.

Surgery would be ill-advised when one of the following conditions exists: (a) when perioperative mortality is too elevated in relation to the probability of cure; (b) when mutilation would be too extensive; (c) when there is a risk of causing the disease to worsen; (d) when the same results can be obtained by conservative or medical treatment.

As far as perioperative mortality is concerned, the present-day techniques of anaesthesia, reanimation and post-operative care have, in all branches of surgery, reduced it to a level where it no longer constitutes an important problem. There are, nevertheless, some radical procedures (for example, on the oesophagus and on the pancreas) where an elevated mortality still exists, especially in the elderly or debilitated patient. The decision to operate must be taken for each individual case, bearing in mind that, should even a slight probability of cure be offered by surgery, it should be proposed even where there is a high operative risk. It is a situation similar to that which presents itself in the case of an emergency, when we are fully aware that the risk is high, but we have no alternative.

With regard to the second limitation, excessive mutilation, there can be no hard and fast rules. Surgeons must evaluate what "excessive" may mean to that particular patient when compared to the physical relief and the probability of cure presented by the operation. They must examine the psychological reactions of the patient, the social and familial environment, his or her needs and the suitability of proceeding in relation to his or her profession. Any decision must depend on a careful analysis of the patient's condition, both with regard to the quality of life following intervention and the duration of that life.

Surgeons must force themselves to be objective and free themselves of their own actual and environmental psychological pressures. They must not allow themselves to be influenced by the fear of criticism on the part of colleagues, or the public. In deciding against a radical intervention they must be sure they are not being unjust to the patient by denying him or her even the slightest probability of cure; they must put aside all pride and, if unable to carry out a particular procedure, they must turn to colleagues who are more expert in the field; they must not find refuge, or an easy way out, in other forms of therapy (radiotherapy, chemotherapy) where these are not equally efficacious. When surgeons are obliged to close an abdomen or a chest without having been able to remove the tumour, they suffer an intense and sad feeling of frustration, but they cannot undertake risky or unreasonable procedures in advanced cases which are biologically incurable just for the sake of "doing something". In the same way, they must not withdraw too early and declare a case inoperable without having considered every possible means of radical removal. These decisions are often arduous, and surgeons will find themselves under pressure to make a quick decision.

Surgeons must be mentally prepared to withstand any influence other than the possibility of curing the patient. A difficult case should never be placed at the end of a day's list when physical fatigue, both that of the surgeon and of the team, could easily influence the decision to undertake a long and complicated operation.

It has long been a point of discussion that surgery can be the cause of accelerating the tumour growth: as far as the dissemination of tumour cells as a result of the manipulation of the tumour is concerned, no clear evidence of this event influencing prognosis has emerged. It should be remembered, however, that incorrect manipulation of the tumour tissue carries a potential risk of dissemination of the tumour cells within the operative field, thus causing local relapse.

Finally, it is logically ill-advised to perform surgery when, in a specific case, the same results can be obtained with conservative procedures. The success of radiotherapy, for instance, obliges us always to consider entrusting the patient to the radiotherapist in cases of radiosensitive tumours. Only when the possibility of a cure tends, objectively, towards surgical treatment can radical surgery be justified. Should the results be the same, the most reasonable choice will be in favour of a non-surgical and less mutilating therapy.

One of the rules expressed during the first half of this century can be summarised in the saying "small tumour, big operation", meaning that surgery had to be wide for the small tumours which had a greater probability of cure and the larger tumours were left to other treatment forms. This rule has been severely criticised in recent years, and the resulting approach has been subjected to considerable revision. It has been observed, in fact, that:

- In the case of a small tumour, serious mutilation and the extensive sacrifice of tissue are often useless.
- It is often the intrinsic biology of the tumour and the host/tumour relationship which condition the result, independently of the type of intervention.
- In the great majority of the cases, with the exception of oropharyngeal and laryngeal tumours, the failure of the treatment is most probably due to the development of distant metastases rather than to local relapse due to incomplete removal of the tissue.

As a result of this new tendency, cancer surgery is diversifying more and more. The number of traditional standard radical procedures (radical mastectomy for breast cancer, abdomino-perineal amputation for rectal cancer, radical clearance of the neck for metastases of the regional lymph nodes, Wertheim-Meigs hysterectomy for cancer of the uterine cervix, etc.) is being replaced by a wider spectrum of surgical procedures which are adapted to the locoregional extension of the disease. Among these new techniques, conservative procedures are on the increase, especially where removal of the organ would create a serious psychological impact. If we take breast cancer as an example, there have been at least 20 groups around the world who have explored the possibilities of reducing the surgical technique with a view to preserving the breast.

Even though combination therapies are dealt with throughout this book, it should be recalled that the possibility of associating surgery with radiotherapy and with chemotherapy can have a notable influence on surgical procedures. It is sufficient to cite the future prospects of more conservative surgery for osteosarcoma when preceded by chemotherapy, the increased indications for removal by radiotherapy and preoperative chemotherapy and the already mentioned conservative surgery for breast cancer when associated with radiotherapy.

An improvement in the 5-year survival rates and reductions in lymph-nodal invasion, local relapses and distant metastases have been obtained by several authors with controlled and large-scale randomized protocols and with preoperative radiotherapy adjuvant to surgery in the treatment of rectal and rectosigmoid tumours.

Conclusions

For many years now, there has been a lively debate on the role of surgical oncology which many would see entrusted, at least partially, to the surgical oncologist. This preference is borne of that very indispensable cultural and interdisciplinary approach of which we have spoken and which is a requirement for the correct treatment of cancer.

The need for a solid surgical formation is indisputable, but over and above the purely technical problems, the therapeutic decision must necessarily be more general and, therefore, oncological. The surgical act is becoming more and more only one of the events (even if fundamental) in the more complex therapeutic process which requires specific and specialised people and structures. This does not mean that the role of surgeons in oncology is redimensioned, on the contrary, they will work the better when they are able to benefit from the progress of the biologists, the pathologists, the radiologists and the chemotherapists, and with them they will be better able to define the limits of intervention with a view to an efficacious attack on the disease which at the same time respects the patient.

The risk for surgeons, should they wish to avoid the problem and should they not want to accept the figure of a surgical oncologist, is that of seeing surgery being progressively reduced to a simple executive act within a therapeutic programme drawn up by medical oncologists and radiotherapists and in which the role of a surgeon would be that of a simple "arm" for the minds of others.

Biology of Cancer

The Cancer Cell

N. S. E. SARGENT and M. M. BURGER

Introduction

Because of the breadth of this topic, we have had to be somewhat selective about what to include in this review: parts of it are simply annotated bibliography while the relatively long section on metastasis reflects both the fact that this is both clinically at least as relevant an area as primary carcinogenesis as well as the fact that research in this area is rapidly expanding. Several topics of general interest are discussed in the section on metastasis, like angiogenesis and treatment. Many of the references quoted are reviews; an additional three are of general interest: Alberts et al. (1983); Anderson (1985) and Cairns (1981).

Cytogenetics

For a long time now the association of chronic myelogenous leukaemia (CML) with the presence of the Philadelphia chromosome (Ph') in the karyotypes of these cells has been known to occur in 90%–95% of patients with CML. This is caused by the translocation of chromosomal material between the long arms of chromosomes 9 and 11 (Rowley 1973). Other translocations specific for Burkitt's lymphoma, t(8;14) (Croce and Klein 1985), and acute monocytic leukaemia, t(9;11) (Diaz et al. 1986), have also been identified and more are reported each week. What is the common mechanism which may explain these and other chromosomal abnormalities in malignant cells? It seems that, in some translocations studied so far, a cellular proto-oncogene on one chromosome is transferred to some regulatory gene element on another, such that the expression of the oncogene is enhanced or that the structure and, therefore, function of the protein product may be modified (Adams 1985).

Such translocations, deletions and inversions are increasingly detected in tumour cells as chromosomal banding techniques become refined. At present up to 5000 bands can be resolved. It becomes obvious that these chromosomal aberrations which can be seen in the microscope are only the tip of the iceberg, and as soon as molecular techniques become efficient enough, one will be confronted with many alterations, some of which may be correlated with malignancy or certain malignancies, and they may have diagnostic and perhaps even prognostic value, but causality will be difficult to assess.

Viral and Chemical Carcinogenesis

After many years of preponderance of viral transformation research, chemical transformation and carcinogenesis have regained proper emphasis again. DNA repair enzymes seem to contribute to homeostasis of tissues since defects such as xeroderma pigmentosum, Bloom's and Fanconi's syndromes lead to an increased incidence of neoplasias. Although the enzymes involved were thought to be known, the repair process seems to be more complicated than originally assumed, and causal correlations for pinpointing the increased tumour incidence have not yet been established.

While it was thought that initiators have to be applied once only and promoters frequently thereafter, it could be shown that under certain circumstances promoters can also be applied once only, and their molecular role may turn out to be similar to that of initiators. Clarification may come with the isolation of a tumour promoter-sensitive gene which codes for a 7100-dalton protein whose function can now be analysed (Lerman et al. 1986). To what degree carcinogens may not act as alkylating agents or otherwise directly upon the DNA, but indirectly via activating proteins or other clastogenic factors which break the DNA or lead to translocations is an avenue of research initiated in several laboratories.

Human viral oncogenesis came onto more solid ground with the evidence that Epstein-Barr virus was found in Burkitt's lymphoma and in the Asian nasopharyngeal carcinoma. Epidemic hepatitis was then added to the list as a precondition for hepatoma. In both cases the evidence is not yet complete that these viruses are sufficient and directly causal for their respective tumours. Human T cell leukaemia virus I is currently the best-accepted culprit for a human neoplasia in only very few instances.

Recently, however, a group of much more common malignancies has become associated with a virus: the DNA of specific human papilloma virus types (HPV 16, 18 and 33) is regularly found in cervical, penile, vulval and perianal cancers. In precursor lesions, viruses of only these three strains are found in a not yet integrated state, while in the carcinoma, in over 90% of cases, viral DNA sequences are now integrated into the human DNA and are actively producing RNA. The fact that male sexual partners have urethral minipapillomas and, in several cases, seem to have the same viral strains promotes the attention given to the human papilloma virus. The available data do not prove but support the concept of a causal relationship of human papilloma virus with these types of human cancer (Hansen 1986).

Oncogenes

There exist in normal eukaryotic cells proto-oncogenes with direct structural counterparts in certain retroviruses which are capable of inducing tumours (carcinomas, sarcomas, leukaemias and neuroblastomas) in certain species of animals (Land et al. 1983; Cooper and Lane 1984: Hunter 1984).

In many human cancer cells activated proto-oncogenes (c-onc) have been found which, when transfected into normal cells, cause tumourigenesis. The fascination of these observations is two-fold: the proto-oncogenes have been found in organisms as diverse as yeast, insects and humans, which means these structures have been highly conserved for perhaps 1000 million years, implying a very fundamental role for the proteins they encode. The other remarkable thing is that cancer-causing retroviruses have genes (v-onc) homologous to the proto-oncogenes. During evolution, these originally non-carcinogenic viruses have incorporated into their genomes the RNA coded for by the proto-oncogenes and are now able themselves to induce cancers. As stated above, eukaryotic proto-oncogenes have to undergo some form of mutation, rearrangement, promotion, or enhancement before they become oncogenic: in their normal form they probably regulate the most basic functions of metabolism, growth control and differentiation of the cell (Müller 1986; Goustin et al. 1986).

Many oncogenes code for growth factors or their receptors, and by this means cancer cells may become independent of local growth control by stimulating their own division (Sporn and Roberts 1985; Klein and Klein 1985; Bishop 1986).

Some scepticism has been displayed as to the role of oncogenes in tumours, i.e. is their expression in cancer cells cause or effect? This question seems to have been answered directly for one oncogene, c-Ha-ras-1, in that it is causative for the initiation of mammary cancer in rats exposed to a chemical mutagen (Zarbl et al. 1985), and more correlative evidence is accumulating (Yokota et al. 1986).

Another key issue which ties in with the concept that tumour progression may be a multi-step process is the question of whether one oncogene can explain the entire process of malignant aberration. In some instances it could be shown that at least two oncogenes are necessary for two defined stages: the first to render the cells immortal, as evidenced by their ability to divide in culture for ever; the second for the fully transformed stage leading to tumourigenic cells in vivo.

Somatic Cell Fusion

An established method for investigating the genetic basis of tumourigenesis is the fusion of cancer cells with normal somatic cells followed by correlating the karyotype of the hybrids with their tumourigenesis or lack of it (Evans et al. 1982; Croce 1980; Harris 1979; Stanbridge et al. 1982; Craig and Sager 1985; Sager 1985). Thus Evans et al. (1982) have assigned to chromosome 4 of normal cells the ability to suppress malignancy in hybrids in a dose-dependent way. Harris (1985) proposes that tumourigenesis of hybrids emerges when they are unable to differentiate to the stage of producing an extracellular matrix (if one parent is of fibroblastic origin).

An important distinction between transformation and tumourigenesis is made in the work of Stanbridge et al. (1982) using HeLa × normal human fibroblast hybrids: they differ in that although both types are immortal, the transformed, but not tumourigenic cells do not grow when transplanted in vivo – their growth is regulated by their host whereas, by definition, that of the tumourigenic (and transformed) cells is not. This is discussed further by Sabin (1981). However, transformed cells can evolve (in the case of hybrids this occurs by chromosomal segregation) to become tumourigenic and this illustrates an extremely important idea in tumour biology: tumour progression.

Tumour Progression, Heterogeneity and Subpopulation Interactions

Nowell (1976) proposed that most tumours are of clonal origin; that is, a single cell undergoes some change which gives it a selective advantage for growth over its neighbouring cells. As clonal expansion occurs, genetic instability of the cells (the mechanism of which is not yet defined) leads to chromosome changes which confer on subgroups within the young tumour various properties, some of which are advantageous to further growth and will cause malignant progression, and some of which are not, and these groups will die out or at least become quiescent or dormant. In this paper Nowell predicted much of what is now known from experimentation in tumour evolution and heterogeneity (Kerbel 1982; Poste and Greig 1982; Rubin 1984). Ling et al. (1985) have developed a slightly different interpretation of heterogeneity (at least as it applies to metastasis and to the development of resistance to cancer chemotherapy) based on the Luria-Delbrück analysis of mutation in bacteria, which they term "dynamic heterogeneity". This makes use of Nowell's idea of the constant generation of variants as a result of genetic instability and regards, say, cells capable of metastasis as occurring only transiently within a tumour because of this instability. Therefore the malignancy of a tumour (defined as its ability to produce metastases: Poste and Fidler 1980) is seen as a balance between the rate of generation of metastatic variants and their rate of loss. This theory has had much success in explaining observations in tumour biology quite apart from metastasis.

Cell-cell and cell-substratum interactions have long been known to play a controlling part in, for instance, embryonic development, adhesion and movement and the activation of immune system cells. More recently such interactions have been shown to occur between populations of tumour cells both in vivo and in vitro (Gorelik et al. 1982; Heppner et al. 1983).

In vivo, this phenomenon is thought to owe much to host-mediated immunity, but in vitro the mechanism is quite unknown. Again taking metastasis as an example, Poste et al. (1981) describe a system for the experimental study of metastasis in which they cloned cells from a mouse melanoma and showed that each clonal population had a metastatic colonisation potential (MCP) which was stably different from that of the parental tumour. Subcloning of these cell lines produced sublines, each of which had stable MCPs different again from *their* parental clone (so far this result is well explained by the theory of Ling et al. (1985) – see above). However, if the clones are now mixed to form a single population, and this is tested for its MCP this property was found to have reverted to that of the parent. Thus in polyclonal populations, interactions are occurring which stabilize and control the behaviour of the complete tumour.

A clinically relevant consequence of these findings is the fact that any therapeutic regimen which kills the majority of tumour cells will leave some single clones which, by definition, have a greater tendency to vary and will thereby develop more variants which carry resistant properties against therapy (chemostatica or others).

Metastasis

This is the ultimate and, for the patient, most devastating manifestation of tumour evolution. It is the process whereby tumour cells escape from the primary and spread to distant sites via the blood and/or lymphatic circulation, or by movement through coelomic spaces, evading or withstanding adverse conditions such as haemodynamic forces (Weiss et al. 1985) and immune attack and then colonise and grow in specific secondary organs (Poste and Fidler 1980; Nicolson and Custead 1982; Schirrmacher 1985). To be able to complete this course, metastatic cells must have many special properties which are discussed below, but bear in mind the discussion of the theories of Nowell (1976) and of Ling et al. (1985) with respect to the generation of tumour cell variants having metastatic ability (see Tumour Progression, Heterogeneity and Subpopulation Interactions).

Somatic Cell Fusion

It has recently been realized that experimental as well as spontaneous fusion of somatic cells with benign cancer cells can lead to the emergence of malignant hybrids (Ramshaw et al. 1983; Larizza et al. 1984 a, b, c; de Baetselier et al. 1981, 1984 a; Kerbel et al. 1983; Roos et al. 1985; reviews: Larizza and Schirrmacher 1984; de Baetselier et al. 1984 b; Lagarde and Kerbel 1985).

It should be noted that in every experiment of this type the tumour cell partner in the hybridization has been derived from a lymphoma or myeloma, and the somatic cell is invariably a T or B lymphocyte or macrophage – i. e. this phenomenon is so far restricted exclusively to the reticuloendothelial system. In the light of this, the site specificity of metastasis of the hybrids (commonly the spleen and liver) is hardly surprising. The usual explanation for the emergence of malignancy in these hybrids is that the somatic cell contributes to the tumour cell the ability to intra- and extravasate, to move in the circulation and to recognise specific tissues (e. g. cytoskeletal and cell surface structures are important for these properties).

Somatic cell fusion has yet to be shown to play a part in the evolution of malignancy in solid tumours, at least in experimental systems. Two recent papers have suggested that cell fusion occurs in human tumours: Kovacs (1985) found evidence of in vivo hybridisation in six malignant tumours of various origins from a sample of 166 and, remarkably, Ruff and Pert (1984) have implicated the fusion of *normal* somatic cells in the *initiation* of a small cell carcinoma of the lung.

Gene Expression

Following the discovery of the role of oncogenes in tumourigenesis, it was natural to consider whether they might be involved in generating metastatic variants within a tumour. Because of the early stage of these investigations the position is currently rather confusing. In one study, mouse NIH/3T3 fibroblasts were made tumourigenic (but not metastatic) by transfection with the c-Ha-ras-activated oncogene. Further transfection with DNA from a hepatic metastasis of a human colonic tumour rendered these cells metastatic in syngeneic mice (Bernstein and Weinberg 1985). The commonly known oncogenes myc and ras could not be found in the human DNA. Similarly Greig et al. (1985) used the same type of cells transfected with DNA from a human primary urinary bladder carcinoma and obtained transfectants having an accelerated ability to metastasise when injected into nude (athymic, immunodeficient) mice. (They found that parental untransfected NIH/3T3 cells *are* tumourigenic and can be metastatic depending upon the site of inoculation – see also Auerbach and Auerbach 1982.) The DNA transfected into these cells contained the activated c-Ha-ras-1 oncogene plus other pieces of the human genome.

Thorgeirsson et al. (1985) undertook much the same study as Greig et al. (1985), coming to similar conclusions with respect to the metastatic ability of NIH/3T3 cells transfected with bladder carcinoma DNA. Their results differed in that they found the activated N-ras oncogene in their transfectants and could not demonstrate that parental NIH/3T3 cells are tumourigenic in nude mice. However, Pozzatti et al. (1986) recently reported that transfection of *primary* rat embryo cells with a cloned activated c-Haras oncogene is sufficient to induce tumourigenesis at low frequency, and that these tumourigenic cells are highly metastatic in nude mice. To complicate matters further, if these cells were additionally transfected with the viral oncogene Ela, then the frequency of tumourigenesis increased ten times, but their metastatic potential was almost abolished. The authors' explanation is that either the Ela gene is coding for an antigen which makes the ras-Ela cells susceptible to immune attack, or that the cells receiving ras alone were a small subset of the total population which already had some of the properties required of metastatic cells, but without the potential for growth conferred by ras.

Gene function can also be altered epigenetically, as with the agent 5-azacytidine which causes hypomethylation of DNA which in turn results in changes of gene expression (Jones 1985; Bird 1986). Trainer et al. (1985), Ormerod et al. (1986) and Olsson and Forchhammer (1984) have all shown that treatment of lowly or non-metastatic tumour cells with 5-azacytidine profoundly increases their metastatic ability.

The Immune System

As with the influence of oncogenes in metastasis, there is also some confusion about the role of the immune status of both the host and the tumour cells within it. Much of this could well be due to the various animal models which are used to study metastasis.

Using a mouse fibrosarcoma system from which a metastatic clone was isolated lacking expression of the H-2K part of the histocompatibility complex, Wallich et al. (1985) have shown that transfection of H-2K genes into these cells led to expression of the H-2K antigens which in turn abolished their capacity to metastasise in immunocompetent mice but had no effect on metastasis in immune-depleted mice. For immune recognition, foreign antigens must be associated with one of the major histocompatibility complex class I antigens and this is thought to be the explanation for these results: that some unknown tumour-associated antigen became recognizable in the presence of the H-2K MHC antigens leading to cytotoxic T cell killing.

However, Taniguchi et al. (1985) demonstrated that the presence of MHC H-2 antigens is necessary for the metastasis of the B_{16} mouse melanoma in immunocompetent syngeneic mice. They proposed two independent mechanisms of immune surveillance of circulating tumour cells, namely that T cells look for the presence of new antigens while natural killer cells become activated when the MHC of the tumour cells does not match that of the host, i.e. loss of H-2 antigens leads to NK cell recognition and killing. A further way in which these two reports may be reconciled is that Taniguchi et al. (1985) were concerned only with total expression of H-2 antigens whereas Wallich et al. (1985) were much more specific – recent evidence indicates that H-2D antigens may suppress the immune response.

One thing that does seem to be clear now is the role of NK cells in host defence against tumour cells (Warner and Dennert 1982): adoptive transfer of NK cells into NK-deficient mice markedly reduced the degree of lung colonisation by melanoma cells injected subsequently.

Angiogenesis

It is well known that both primary and metastatic tumours acquire their own blood circulation as they grow in size – when seen during surgery the major blood vessels supplying some tumours are enormous. Folkman (1986) described an assay in which melanoma cells seeded into a perfused organ grow to a diameter of 1–2 mm and are then forced to stop growing because under these conditions they cannot become vascularized. Now, a number of tumour-derived growth factors have been discovered which stimulate new capillary formation, apparently via an interaction with heparin on the surfaces of endothelial cells. Concurrently, a means of preventing neoangiogenesis (and therefore tumour grwoth) was developed in which penta- or hexa-saccharide fragments of heparin are given to tumour-bearing mice in combination with one of a group of steroids. Interestingly, the heparin fragments do not require anticoagulant activity, and the steroids can be inert with respect to their commonly accepted actions (i.e. as mineralo- and glucocorticoids and as sex hormones). These results have obvious and exciting prospects for clinical application.

Cell Dissociation

This is essential for the initial departure of cells from the primary tumour and involves at least two events:

Decrease in Homotypic Adhesion Between Tumour Cells. This is discussed by Brackenbury (1985) with particular reference to specific cell adhesion molecules, and experiments are described in which the progressive appearance of tumourigenesis in some Rous sarcoma virus-transformed cells is matched by a decrease in the expression of such molecules at the surface of these cells.

Digestion of Connective Tissue to Escape from the Tumour. Collagenase IV and cathepsin B (Sloane et al. 1986) are two proteases which have been strongly implicated in this process. It should be noted that this ability is required at both ends during the course of metastasis, i. e. for escape from the primary and invasion into the stroma of the secondary tissue.

Two recent papers have emphasised the importance of this invasive step in metastasis (Tullberg and Burger 1985; Terranova et al. 1986). Tumour cells were selected for rapid passage through pores in a polycarbonate filter or for invasion through an artificial basement membrane composed of collagens I and IV and laminin. The tumour cells which successfully traversed these barriers when tested for their metastatic ability were found to colonise secondary organs to a much higher extent than their parental (unselected) populations.

Liotta (1986) has reviewed this process and proposes a three-strep sequence for the passage of a tumour cell through the extracellular matrix which is, first, attachment of cell surface laminin receptors to laminin in the matrix followed by release of proteases and then cell movement.

The Cell Surface

The relation between cell surface structure and the ability to metastasise has been approached in a number of ways, initially by treatment of tumour cell surfaces with enzymes, such as neuraminidase, hyaluronidase and trypsin, followed by inoculation into host animals to observe changes in extent or sites of metastatic growth. Where such treatments had any effect, it tended to produce a decrease in the number of lung colonies formed. Humphries et al. (1986 a) used an oligosaccharide-processing inhibitor, swainsonine, to produce just such an effect as that described above. One, more convincing, demonstration of the role of cell surface structure in metastasis was done by Poste and Nicolson (1980). They obtained isolated plasma membranes (without any nuclear material) from a melanoma line having a high lung colonisation potential and fused these into the plasma membranes of another line having a low potential. These cells, when injected into recipient mice, now had a colonisation potential intermediate between that of the two parent lines, showing that there are structures and/or factors on the cell surface which are necessary for such colonisation.

A major problem with such experiments is that one is only altering the membrane phenotype by these experiments, yet cell membranes are turned over (i. e. back to their original form) rapidly. Any effects which are seen must therefore have occurred early (probably within hours) in the comparatively long process of metastasis, making detailed molecular biochemical analysis difficult.

To avoid this, some stable genetic change has to be introduced: one such change is somatic cell fusion (described earlier), and another, aimed specifically at the cell membrane, is the isolation of lectin-resistant mutants.

In particular, the lectin wheat germ agglutinin has been used (Tao et al. 1983; Dennis 1985; and references within both) to produce resistant mutants – WGA^r. These WGA^r cells have a very much lower incidence of metastasis than the parental line, and when the wild-type character (i. e. WGA sensitive phenotype) is restored, either by back selection with a different lectin or somatic cell fusion, the metastatic potential reverts to normal thereby providing more firm evidence (but not proof) for a role for the membrane structure in causing metastasis.

A popular hypothesis as to why membrane structural changes may reduce metastatic potential is that these same changes expose new antigens which render the tumour cells more immunogenic and therefore more readily killed. This idea has been disputed in the form of a report by Mercurio (1986) in which it was shown that expression of novel glycoproteins on tumour cell surfaces decreased their macrophage-mediated lysis (but NK cell and T cell killing were not tested and neither was antibody complement-mediated killing).

Organ Site Specificity

It is common clinical experience that metastasis from a primary neoplasm takes place to certain specific secondary organs, and Paget (1889) described his "seed and soil" hypothesis in which the "soil" (i. e. the secondary organ) provides a congenial environment for the growth of the cancer cells ("seeds"). If the soil environment is hostile, then growth of the seeds is suppressed or inhibited. As examples of this Paget used the bone colonisation typical of breast and thyroid cancers, but virtually unknown in malignant melanoma.

This phenomenon has been reviewed more recently by Hart (1982) and by Kieran and Longenecker (1983), and Paget's hypothesis has received much experimental support from autopsy studies of patients suffering from malignant ascites in whom a peritoneovenous shunt was inserted (Tarin et al. 1984a, b, c; Tarin 1985). In several such patients metastases could not be found even after several months of shunting viable and clonogenic tumour cells directly into their blood.

In experimental metastasis systems (i.e. work done using animal models) where metastasis does occur successfully to specific organs, attention has been largely paid to mechanisms of tumour cell-host cell adhesion to explain this site specificity. Thus Alby and Auerbach (1984) demonstrated specific adherence of glioma cells to brain endothelium and of ovary-derived teratoma cells to ovary endothelium; Netland and Zetter (1984) showed that lung-colonising melanoma cells bound preferentially to lung cryostat sections, while liver-metastatic reticulum cell sarcoma cells do so to liver sections; specific cell surface molecules have been implicated in the adhesion of liver-metastatic lymphoma cells to hepatocytes (Springer et al. 1983; Cheingsong-Popov et al. 1983), and, lastly, Vollmers et al. (1984) described a monoclonal antibody capable of inhibiting lung colonisation of melanoma cells in vivo which also inhibits its adhesion of these tumour cells to laminin in vitro. Much of this work has been prompted by what is, superficially anyway, an analogous system – the homing of lymphocytes to the specialised endothelium of lymph nodes (McConnell 1983; Gallatin et al. 1986). However, lymphocytes are not required to grow at the sites to which they attach, whereas tumour cells must do if they are to form metastases. It is difficult to see how specific adhesion alone can account for site-specific metastasis — it must in some way trigger the growth of tumour cells, or else hold them in a growth-stimulatory environment.

Other mechanisms, which are by no means mutually exclusive, have been suggested as important for site specificity: Hujanen and Terranova (1985) were able partially to purify factors from certain tissues which specifically attracted tumour cells able to metastasise to those tissues, and Szaniawska et al. (1985) showed that substances which are able to stimulate or suppress the growth of human tumour cells are released from cultured lung fragments. Work in this laboratory using a subline of a mouse melanoma which metastasises to the liver (Tao et al. 1979) failed to show any preferential liver colonisation by these cells or rosette formation (indicating adhesion) between them and Kupffer cells or hepatocytes (Madnick and Burger, unpublished). It seems that the reason for their liver tropism lies in the ability of syngeneic hepatocytes to stimulate their growth (Sargent et al. 1988). This is not a chemotactic effect, nor is a diffusible factor responsible, and we have shown that direct contact between hepatocytes and tumour cells is essential for this effect to be seen. Further experiments will concentrate on the role of the cell's membranes and junctional communication.

An additional idea which may be useful in understanding site-specific metastasis lies in the comparative embryological origins of tumour cells and the tissues to which they metastasise.

Treatment

We will not cover classical chemotherapy of cancer here, which in any case has had very disappointing results, but rather concentrate on certain cellular factors which have been largely developed with the help of recombinant DNA techniques. Obviously these factors will be of use in the treatment of primary cancers as well as their metastases. The reasons for the failure of classical chemotherapy are now being understood and these lie in the emergence of resistant mutant cells within tumours. The mechanism seems to be a common one of gene amplification, but two different genes are amplified depending on the drugs administered:

1. Antifolates such as methotrexate are a special case, and here the gene encoding their target enzyme is amplified resulting in overproduction of dihydrofolate reductase which swamps the ability of these drugs to inactivate it (Schimke 1982).
2. A more general mechanism is the amplification of a gene coding for permeability (P)-glycoprotein (Ling et al. 1984; Riordan et al. 1985; Kartner et al. 1985). Treatment of cancer cells with a single drug will give rise to mutants having resistance to this drug and also a wide range of other structurally unrelated drugs. The reason appears to be the overexpression of P-glycoprotein on the cell membrane which somehow protects the resistant cells. This also explains why even combination chemotherapy fails. Unless the P-glycoprotein can be incapacitated, it is difficult to see how chemotherapy can ever be effective except perhaps as an adjunct. It is as such that chemotherapy as well as radiotherapy, hyperthermia treatment and surgery may find a use in a promising treatment using activated macrophages to kill tumour cells.

Macrophages activated in vitro or in vivo with muramyl dipeptide (incorporated into liposomes if in vivo) or macrophage-activating factor (a protein) will non-specifically recognise and kill tumour cells (for instance, horseshoe crab macrophages will kill human tumour cells in vitro – an evolutionary functional conservation of several hundred million years), but they only have a certain capacity to do so. It is proposed that the normal methods mentioned above can be used to knock down the tumour load as much as possible until resistant mutants emerge that start to increase the tumour mass again, at which time activated syngeneic macrophages are infused, ideally to eradicate remaining tumour tissue (see Talmadge et al. 1986; and references therein).

Cachectin is a small protein hormone identical to "tumour necrosis factor" which is produced by macrophages and circulates in the blood (Beutler and Cerami 1986). It is synthesised in response to endotoxin, released after infection with bacteria and also when macrophages recognise tumour cells, and has dual effects when present in large amounts. One is a profound disturbance of normal respiration giving rise to the cachexia typical of advanced cancer, and the other is haemorrhagic necrosis of tumour cells. Very limited clinical trials have begun using the complete structure, but it is hoped that it will be possible to modify it so as to exclude its deleterious effect on metabolism.

Interleukin-2 is a growth factor released from helper T cells which has been found to activate "null" lymphocytes (i.e. non-NK lymphocytes lacking markers for B and T cells, known as LAK cells) to a tumouricidal state. In a group of 25 patients with advanced metastatic cancer of diverse histological origin, combined treatment with autologous LAK cells and interleukin-2 brought about a regression of over 50% of tumour volume in 11 patients and complete remission in one (Rosenberg et al. 1985). Administration of either LAK cells or interleukin-2 alone was ineffectual, so it is probable that the LAK cells, having been activated in vitro and infused back into the patient, require constant stimulation with interleukin-2 in vivo. As with activated macrophages, the best chance for elimination of cancer tissue using this treatment is when the initial tumour burden is as low as possible.

Monoclonal antibodies have great potential in the diagnosis, imaging and treatment of cancer, provided that suitable specific antigen markers can be found on the tumour cell surfaces. One example of this is given in a review by Waldmann (1986). Mature normal resting state T cells do not express the interleukin-2 receptor whereas activated and HTLV-1 infected T cells do. One out of three patients with HTLV-1-induced adult T cell leukaemia showed a marked improvement in health when treated with a monoclonal antibody against the interleukin-2 receptor, although a relapse occurred several months later. Theoretically, monoclonal antibodies can be used in several ways: alone, when they may lyse target cells by a complement-mediated reaction; coupled to a toxin such as ricin A or diphtheria toxin; coupled to a short-range (i.e. α-emitting) radioactive isotope (for treatment) or a γ-emitting (long-range) isotope for imaging disseminated metastases. The power of these techniques will become apparent as new specific tumour markers are discovered.

Recent Developments

Some factors of importance in the control of cell growth have recently been reviewed (Rozengurt 1986), and a report has appeared describing the suppression of mouse malignant melanoma growth by a low molecular weight substance released from cultures of embryonic mouse skin of a certain gestational age and anatomical location (Gerschenson et al. 1986). The morphology of these malignant cells after treatment suggested that they had been induced to differentiate by the embryonic field, and, indeed, it has long been hoped that induction of differentiation would turn out to be a very effective way of treating cancer.

The importance of interactions between extracellular matrix and tumour cells during metastasis has been stressed by the finding that, by specifically blocking the recognition of fibronectin, secondary melanoma growth can be inhibited (Humphries et al. 1986b).

The molecular analysis of the basis for multi-drug resistance (mdr) of cells exposed to cytotoxic cancer chemotherapeutic drugs is receiving much attention, and the genes responsible for this have now been unequivocally identified with the finding that a drug-sensitive cell line can be rendered resistant by transfection into it of specific mdr DNA (Gros et al. 1986).

A characteristic feature of Wilms' tumour is the loss of a large part of chromosome 11 from the malignant cells. Weissman et al. (1987) have now shown that introduction of, specifically, human chromosome 11 into Wilms' tumour cells completely abrogates their malignant phenotype, thereby demonstrating that there exist tumour-suppressing genes and that, in this form of cancer at least, the expression of malignancy is a recessive trait. This has been followed up by the discovery of a piece of normal human DNA, 18 kilobases in size, that can partially suppress the tumourigenicity of a rat tumour cell line (Schaefer et al. 1988). It may not be long before the structure of the specific gene responsible and its protein product is known.

References

Adams JM (1985) Oncogene activation by fusion of chromosomes in leukaemia. Nature 315: 542–543

Alberts B, Bray D, Lewis J, Raff M, Roberts K, Watson JD (1983) Molecular biology of the cell. Garland, New York

Alby L, Auerbach R (1984) Differential adhesion of tumour cells to capillary endothelial cells in vitro. Proc Natl Acad Sci USA 81: 5739–5743

Anderson JR (1985) Muir's textbook of pathology, 12th edn. Arnold, London

Auerbach R, Auerbach W (1982) Regional differences in the growth of normal and neoplastic cells. Science 215: 127–134

Bernstein SC, Weinberg RA (1985) Expression of the metastatic phenotype in cells transfected with human metastatic tumour DNA. Proc Natl Acad Sci USA 82: 1726–1730

Beutler B, Cerami A (1986) Cachectin and tumour necrosis factor as two sides of the same biological coin. Nature 320: 584–588

Bird AP (1986) CpG-rich islands and the function of DNA methylation. Nature 321: 209–213

Bishop JM (1986) Oncogenes as hormone receptors. Nature 321: 112–113

Brackenbury R (1985) Molecular mechanisms of cell adhesion in normal and transformed cells. Cancer Metastasis Rev 4: 41–58

Cairns J (1981) The origin of human cancers. Nature 289: 353–357

Cheingsong-Popov R, Robinson P, Altevogt P, Schirrmacher V (1983) A mouse hepatocyte carbohydrate-specific receptor and its interaction with liver-metastasizing tumour cells. Int J Cancer 32: 359–366

Cooper GM, Lane MA (1984) Cellular transforming genes and oncogenes. Biochim Biophys Acta 738: 9–20

Craig RW, Sager R (1985) Suppression of tumourgenicity in hybrids of normal and oncogene transformed CHEF cells. Proc Natl Acad Sci USA 82: 2062–3063

Croce CM (1980) Cancer genes in cell hybrids. Biochim Biophys Acta 605: 411–430

Croce CM, Klein G (1985) Chromosome translocations and human cancer. Sci Am 252: 44–50

De Baetselier P, Gorelik E, Eshhar Z, Ron Y, Katzav S, Feldman M, Segal S (1981) Metastatic properties conferred on non-metastatic tumours by hybridization of spleen B-lymphocytes with plasmacytoma cells. JNCI 67: 1079–1087

De Baetselier P, Roos E, Brys L, Remels L, Feldman M (1984 a) Generation of invasive and metastatic variants of a non-metastatic T-cell-lymphoma by in vivo fusion with normal host cells. Int J Cancer 34: 731–738

De Baetselier P, Roos E, Brys L, Remels L, Gobert M, de Kegel D, Segal S, Feldman M (1984 b) Non-metastatic tumour cells acquire metastatic properties following somatic hybridization with normal cells. Cancer Metastasis Rev 3: 5–24

Dennis JW (1985) Partial reversion of the metastatic phenotype in a wheat germ agglutinin-resistant mutant of the murine tumour cell line MDAY-D2 selected with Bandeiraea simplicifolia seed lectin. JNCI 74: 1111–1120

Diaz MO, Le Beau MM, Pitha P, Rowley JD (1986) Interferon and c-ets-1 genes in the translocation (9;11) (p22; q23) in human acute monocytic leukaemia. Science 231: 265–267

Evans EP, Burtenshaw MD, Brown BB, Hennion R, Harris H (1982) The analysis of malignancy by cell fusion. IX. Reexamination and clarification of the cytogenetic problem. J Cell Sci 56: 113–120

Folkman J (1986) How is blood vessel growth regulated in normal and neoplastic tissue? G.H.A. Clowes memorial award lecture. Cancer Res 46: 467–473

Gallatin M, St John TP, Siegelaman M, Reichert R, Butcher EC, Weissman IL (1986) Lymphocyte homing receptors. Cell 44: 673–680

Gerschenson M, Graves K, Carson SD, Wells RS, Pierce GB (1986) Regulation of melanoma by the embryonic skin. Proc Natl Acad Sci USA 83: 7307–7310

Gorelik E, Segal S, Shapiro J, Katzav S, Ron Y, Feldman M (1982) Interactions between the local tumour and its metastasis. Cancer Metastasis Rev 1: 83–94

Goustin AS, Loef EB, Shipley GD, Moses HL (1986) Growth factors and cancer. Cancer Res 46: 1015–1029

Greig RG, Koestler TP, Trainer DL, Corwin SP, Miles L, Kline T, Sweet R, et al. (1985) Tumourigenic and metastatic properties of "normal" and ras-transfected NIH/3T3 cells. Proc Natl Acad Sci USA 82: 3698–3701

Gros P, Neriah YP, Croop JM, Houseman DE (1986) Isolation and expression of a complementary DNA that confers multidrug resistance. Nature 323: 728–731

Hansen HZ (1986) Evidence for association between human papilloma virus and neoplasia. Intern Med 7: 66–79

Harris H (1979) Some thoughts about genetics, differentiation and malignancy. Somatic Cell Genet 5: 923–930

Harris H (1985) Suppression of malignancy in hybrid cells: the mechanism. J Cell Sci 79: 83–94

Hart IR (1982) Seed and soil revisted: mechanisms of site-specific metastasis. Cancer Res Rev 1: 5–17

Heppner GH, Miller BE, Miller FR (1983) Tumour subpopulation interactions in neoplasms. Biochim Biophys Acta 695: 215–226

Hujanen ES, Terranova VP (1985) Migration of tumour cells to organ-derived chemoattractants. Cancer Res 45: 3517–3521

Humphries MJ, Matsumoto K, White SL, Olden K (1986 a) Oligosaccharide modification by swainsonine treatment inhibits pulmonary colonization by B16-F10 murine melanoma cells. Proc Natl Acad Sci USA 83: 1752-1756

Humphries MJ, Olden K, Yamada KM (1986 b) A synthetic peptide from fibronectin inhibits experimental metastasis of murine melanoma cells. Science 233: 467–470

Hunter T (1984) Oncogenes and proto-oncogenes: How do they differ? JNCI 73: 773–786

Jones PA (1985) Altering gene expression with 5-aza-cytidine. Cell 40: 485–486

Kartner N, Evernden-Porelle D, Bradley G, Ling V (1985) Detection of P-glycoprotein in multidrug-resistant cell lines by monoclonal antibodies. Nature 316: 820–823

Kerbel RS (1982) Tumour heterogeneity, invasion and metastasis. Invasion Metastasis 2: 61–75

Kerbel RS, Lagarde AE, Dennis JW, Donaghue TP (1983) Spontaneous fusion in vivo between normal host and tumour cells: possible contribution to tumour progression and metastasis studied with a lectin resistant mutant tumour. Mol Cell Biol 3: 523–538

Kieran MW, Longenecker BM (1983) Organ-specific metastasis with special reference to avian systems. Cancer Metastasis Rev 2: 165–183

Klein G, Klein E (1985) Evolution of tumours and the impact of molecular oncology. Nature 315: 190–195

Kovacs G (1985) Premature chromosome condensation: evidence for in vivo cell fusion in human malignant tumours. Int J Cancer 36: 637–641

Lagarde AE, Kerbel RS (1985) Somatic cell hybridization in vivo and in vitro in relation to the metastatic phenotype. Biochim Biophys Acta 823: 81–110

Land H, Parada LF, Weinberg RA (1983) Cellular oncogenes and multistep carcinogenesis. Science 222: 771–778

Larizza L, Schirrmacher V (1984) Somatic cell fusion as a source of genetic rearrangement leading to metastatic variants. Cancer Metastasis Rev 3: 193–222

Larizza L, Schirrmacher V, Graf L, Pflüger E, Peres-Martinez M, Stöhr M (1984a) Suggestive evidence that the highly metastatic variant ESb of the T-cell lymphoma Eb is derived from spontaneous fusion with a host macrophage. Int J Cancer 34: 699–708

Larizza L, Schirrmacher V, Pflüger E (1984b) Acquisition of high metastatic capacity after in vitro fusion of a nonmetastatic tumour line with a bone marrow-derived macrophage. J Exp Med 160: 1579–1584

Larizza L, Schirrmacher V, Stöhr M, Pflüger E, Dzarlieva R (1984c) Inheritance of immunogenicity and metastatic potential in murine cell hybrids from the T-lymphoma ESb08 and normal spleen lymphocytes. JNCI 72: 1371–1381

Lerman MI, Glenn A, Hegameyer B, Colburn NH (1986) Cloning and characterization of putative genes that specify sensitivity to neoplastic transformation by tumour promotors. Int J Cancer 37: 293–302

Ling V, Gerlach J, Kartner N (1984) Multidrug resistance. Breast Cancer Res Treat 4: 89–94

Ling V, Chambers AF, Harris JF, Hill RP (1985) Quantitative genetic analysis of tumour progression. Cancer Metastasis Rev 4: 173–194

Liotta LA (1986) Tumour invasion and metastasis – role of the extracellular matrix: Rhoads memorial award lecture. Cancer Res 46: 1–7

McConnell I (1983) Roving lymphocytes. Nature 304: 17

Mercurio AM (1986) Disruption of oligosaccharide processing in murine tumour cells inhibits their susceptibility to lysis by activated mouse macrophages. Proc Natl Acad Sci USA 83: 2609–2613

Müller R (1986) Proto-oncogenes and differentiation. Trends Biochem Sci 11: 129–132

Netland PA, Zetter BR (1984) Organ-specific adhesion of metastatic tumour cells in vitro. Science 224: 1113–1115

Nicolson GL, Custead SE (1982) Tumour metastasis is not due to adaptation of cells to a new organ environment. Science 215: 176–178

Nowell PC (1976) The clonal evolution of tumour cell populations. Acquired genetic lability permits stepwise selection of variant sublines and underlies tumour progression. Science 194: 23–28

Olsson L, Forchhammer J (1984) Induction of the metastatic phenotype in a mouse tumour model by 5-azacytidine, and characterization of an antigen associated with metastatic activity. Proc Natl Acad Sci USA 81: 3389–3393

Ormerod EJ, Everett CA, Hart IR (1986) Enhanced experimental metastatic capacity of a human tumour line following treatment with 5-azacytidine. Cancer Res 46: 884–890

Paget S (1889) The distribution of secondary growths in cancer of the breast. Lancet 1: 571–573

Poste G, Fidler IJ (1980) The pathogenesis of cancer metastasis. Nature 283: 139–146

Poste G, Greig R (1982) On the genesis of cellular heterogeneity in malignant tumours. Invasion Metastasis 2: 137–176

Poste G, Nicolson GL (1980) Arrest and metastasis of blood-borne tumour cells are modified by fusion of plasma membrane vesicles from highly metastatic cells. Proc Natl Acad Sci USA 77: 399–403

Poste G, Doll J, Fidler IJ (1981) Interactions between clonal subpopulations affect stability of the metastatic phenotype in polyclonal populations of B16 melanoma cells. Proc Natl Acad Sci USA 78: 6226–6230

Pozzatti R, Muschel R, Williams J, Padmanabhan R, Howard B, Liotta L, Khoury G (1986) Primary rat embryo cells transformed by one or two oncogenes show different metastatic potentials. Science 232: 223–227

Ramshaw IA, Carlson S, Wang HC, Badenoch-Jones P (1983) The use of cell fusion to analyse factors involved in tumour cell metastasis. Int J Cancer 32: 471–478

Riordan JR, Deuchars K, Kartner N, Alon N, Trent J, Ling V (1985) Amplification of P-glycoprotein genes in multidrug-resistant mammalian cell lines. Nature 316: 817–819

Roos E, La Rivière G, Collard JG, Stukart MJ, de Baetselier P (1985) Invasiveness of T-cell hybridomas in vitro and their metastatic potential in vivo. Cancer Res 45: 6238–6243

Rosenberg SA, Lotze MT, Muul LM, Leitman S, Chang AE, Ettinghausen SE, Matroy YL, et al. (1985) Observations on the systemic administration of autologous lymphokine-activated killer cells and recombinant interleukin-2 to patients with metastatic cancer. N Engl J Med 313: 1485–1492

Rowley JD (1973) A new consistent chromosomal abnormality in chronic myelogenous leukaemia identified by quinacrine fluorescence and Giemsa staining. Nature 243: 290–293

Rozengurt E (1986) Early signals in the mitogenic response. Science 234: 161–166

Rubin H (1984) Early origin and pervasiveness of cellular heterogeneity in some malignant transformations. Proc Natl Acad Sci USA 81: 5121–5125

Ruff HR, Pert CB (1984) Small cell carcinoma of the lung: macrophage-specific antigens suggest haemopoetic stem cell origin. Science 225: 1034–1036

Sabin AG (1981) Suppression of malignancy in human cancer cells: Issues and challenges. Proc Natl Acad Sci USA 78: 7129–7133

Sager R (1985) Genetic suppression of tumour formation. Adv Cancer Res 44: 43–68

Sargent NSE, Oestreicher M, Haidvogl H, Madnick HM, Burger MM (1988) Growth regulation of cancer metastases by their host organ. Proc Natl Acad Sci USA 85: 7251–7255

Schaefer R, Iyer J, Iten E, Ninkko AC (1988) Partial reversion of the transformed phenotype in HRAS-transfected tumourigenic cells by transfer of a human gene. Proc Natl Acad Sci USA 85: 1590–1594

Schimke RT (ed) (1982) Gene amplification. Cold Spring Harbour Laboratory, New York

Schirrmacher V (1985) Cancer metastasis: experimental approaches, theoretical concepts, and impacts for treatment strategies. Adv Cancer Res 43: 1–73

Sloane BF, Roshin J, Johnson K, Taylor H, Crissman JD, Honn KV (1986) Cathepsin B: Association with plasma membrane in metastatic tumours. Proc Natl Acad Sci USA 83: 2483–2487

Sporn MB, Roberts AB (1985) Autocrine growth factors and cancer. Nature 313: 745–747

Springer GF, Cheingsong-Popov R, Schirrmacher V, Desai PR,

Tegtmeyer H (1983) Proposed molecular basis of tumour cell-hepatocyte interaction. J Biol Chem 258: 5702–5706
Stanbridge EJ, Wilkinson J (1980) Dissociation of anchorage independence from tumourigenicity in human cell hybrids. Int J Cancer 26: 1–8
Stanbridge EJ, Der CJ, Doersen C-J, Nishimi RY, Peehl DM, Weissman BE, Wilkinson JE (1982) Human cell hybrids: Analysis of transformation and tumourigenicity. Science 215: 252–259
Szaniawska B, Majewski S, Kaminski MJ, Noremberg K, Swierz M, Janik P (1985) Stimulatory and inhibitory activities of lung-conditioned medium on the growth of normal and neoplastic cells in vitro. JNCI 75: 303–306
Talmadge JE, Lenz BF, Klabansky R, Simon R, Riggs C, Guo S, Oldham RK, Fidler IJ (1986) Therapy of autochthonous skin cancers in mice with intravenously injected liposomes containing muramyltripeptide. Cancer Res 46: 1160–1163
Taniguchi K, Karre K, Klein G (1985) Lung colonization and metastasis by disseminated B16 melanoma cells: H-2 associated control at the level of the host and the tumour cell. Int J Cancer 36: 503–510
Tao T-W, Matter A, Vogel K, Burger MM (1979) Liver-colonizing melanoma cells selected from B16 melanoma. Int J Cancer 23: 854–857
Tao T-W, Jenkins JM, Vosbeck K, Matter A, Miller M, Jockusch BM, Shen Z-H, Burger MM (1983) Lectin-resistant variants of mouse melanoma cells. II. *In vitro* characteristics. Int J Cancer 31: 239–247
Tarin D (1985) Clinical and experimental studies on the biology of metastasis. Biochim Biophys Acta 780: 227–235
Tarin D, Price JE, Kettlewall MGW, Souter RG, Vass ACR, Crossley B (1984 a) Clinicopathological observations on metastasis in man studied in patients treated with peritoneovenous shunts. Br Med J 288: 749–751
Tarin D, Price JE, Kettlewell MGW, Souter RG, Vass ACR, Crossley B (1984 b) Mechanisms of human tumour metastasis studied in patients with peritoneovenous shunts. Cancer Res 44: 3584–3592
Tarin D, Vass ACR, Kettlewell MGW, Price JE (1984 c) Absence of metastatic sequelae during long-term treatment of malignant ascites by peritoneovenous shunting. Invasion Metastasis 4: 1–12
Terranova VP, Hujanen ES, Loeb DM, Martin GR, Thornburg L, Glushko V (1986) Use of a reconstituted basement membrane to measure cell invasiveness and select for highly invasive tumour cells. Proc Natl Acad Sci USA 83: 465–469
Thorgeirsson VP, Turpeenniemi-Hujanen T, Williams JE, Westin EH, Heilman CA, Talmadge JE, Liotta LA (1985) NIH/3T3 cells transfected with human tumour DNA containing activated ras oncogenes express the metastatic phenotype in nude mice. Mol Cell Biol 5: 259–262
Trainer DL, Kline T, Mallon F, Greig R, Poste G (1985) Effect of 5-azacytidine on DNA methylation and the malignant properties of B16 melanoma cells. Cancer Res 45: 6124–6130
Tullberg KF, Burger MM (1985) Selection of B16 melanoma cells with increased metastatic potential and low intercellular cohesion using nucleopore filters. Invasion Metastasis 5: 1–15
Vollmers HP, Imhof BA, Braun S, Waller CA, Schirrmacher V, Birchmeier W (1984) Monoclonal antibodies which prevent experimental lung metastases. Interference with the adhesion of tumour cells to laminin. FEBS Lett 172: 17–20
Waldmann TA (1986) The structure, function and expression of interleukin-2 receptors on normal and malignant lymphocytes. Science 232: 727–732
Wallich R, Bulbuc N, Hämmerling GJ, Katzav S, Segal S, Feldman M (1985) Abrogation of metastatic properties of tumour cells by de novo expression of H-2K antigens following H-2 gene transfection. Nature 315: 301–305
Warner JF, Dennert G (1982) Effects of a cloned cell line with NK activity on bone marrow transplants, tumour development and metastasis in vivo. Nature 300: 31–34
Weiss L, Dimitrov DS, Angelova B (1985) The haemodynamic destruction of intravascular cancer cells in relation to myocardial metastasis. Proc Natl Acad Sci USA 82: 5737–5741
Weissman BE, Saxon PJ, Pasquale SR, Jones GR, Geiser AG, Stanbridge EJ (1987) Introduction of a normal human chromosome 11 into a Wilms' tumour cell line controls its tumourigenic expression. Science 236: 175–180
Yokota J, Tsunetsugu-Yokota Y, Battifora H, LeFevre C, Cline MJ (1986) Alterations of myc, myb and ras^{Ha} proto-oncogenes in cancers are frequent and show clinical correlation. Science 231: 261–265
Zarbl H, Sukumar S, Arthur AV, Martin-Zanca D, Barbacid M (1985) Direct mutagenesis of Ha-ras-1 oncogenes by N-nitroso-N-methylurea during initiation of mammary carcinogenesis in rats. Nature 315: 382–385

Biology of Cancer Invasion and Metastasis

P. Sträuli

Spread of Cancer: Elementary Considerations

"Spread" is the overall term for one of the chief characteristics of cancer: its capacity to extend in the organism. A crucial feature of spread consists in the fact that host territory is occupied through destruction, not just by displacement, of indigenous tissue constituents.

In its full expression, spread of cancer is a long-range operation both with respect to space and to time. Mainly for didactic reasons, various subdivisions of the whole process have been suggested of which I prefer the following one: preinvasive extension, invasion, dissemination, metastasis formation. One merit of this scheme is that it draws our attention to an important aspect: during each of these phases spread can spontaneously come to a temporary or permanent standstill. The four phases will now be characterized very shortly; more extensive comments will follow in later sections.

Preinvasive extension is spread exclusively in the tissue of origin. It is best known in epithelial malignancies, the carcinomas, in which it takes place during the stages commonly designated as "carcinoma in situ" or "intraepithelial neoplasia."

Invasion begins with transgression of the first tissue border. In most instances, this step coincides with passage of the tumor across the first basement membrane. Continuing invasion often requires the crossing of more tissue borders and, possibly, of more basement membranes. This is an absolute condition for invasion of even the smallest blood vessels, whereas in the lymph system the basement membrane barrier does not exist at the capillary level.

Dissemination consists in the transportation of intravasated cancer elements (single cells, cell groups, tissue fragments) by lymph and blood. With increasing size of cancer elements in transit, traffic is governed more and more by the rules of embolization (see below).

Metastasis formation requires arrest of cancer cells equipped with the capacities of survival and proliferation. Apparently this functional outfit is frequently confined to subsets of the original tumor cell population. This is one of the reasons why metastases are new biological entities and not simply amplifications of the primary tumor.

Concerning spread of cancer as a whole, the question must be asked whether it is *an orderly or disorderly process.* The "classical" concept of metastasis presumed the existence of a regular sequence comprising a first round of spread to lymph nodes and, after exhaustion of the purported barrier function of the latter, a second round to distant organs. This interpretation played a decisive role in the development of surgical oncology, particularly of breast cancer surgery; it has therefore been opposed as "Halstedian" to our current, more biological concept of spread (Fisher et al. 1980). We now consider dissemination in lymph and blood as a predominantly parallel process initiated by an indiscriminate access of cancer to lymph and blood. Exceptions to this rule are well known, e.g., the highly discriminate invasion of lymph and blood vessels by subclasses of thyroid carcinomas. It is also quite clear that an orderly sequence of spread first in lymph and then in blood channels in accordance with the anatomical connection of the two systems can occur. But this is rather an exception, and we must assume that at the time at which lymph node metastases are clinically detected, distant metastatic seeds or micrometastases, if not overt metastases, are already present. Moreover, they can have developed in the absence of any lymph node secondaries. As concerns the localization (organ distribution) of hematogenous metastases, it is influenced by topographical constants depending on the starting point of spread. These constants are the basis for rules that have emerged from the statistical analysis of cancer autopsies (Walther 1948; Viadana et al. 1978). But again, these rules do not justify the conclusion that overall spread follows an orderly pattern. There are too many inconstant factors that modify the basic anatomical scheme, most notably among them the ever-changing and immensely complex interactions of tumor and host. Taken all together, we must, therefore, be aware that for our limited understanding, spread of cancer is characterized by a dominant disorderliness. It is largely this insight that has caused the introduction of new strategies of patient management, especially of adjuvant therapy (Nagel et al. 1985).

Preinvasive Cancer

Confinement of cancer to its tissue of origin can be best assessed in epithelia with their clear-cut basement membrane enclosure. Since, moreover, epithelial cancer is by far the most frequent type of human malignancy, our understanding of preinvasive cancer is largely restricted to carcinomas. Although preinvasive carcinomas occur in all epithelia, the largest number of observations concerns the easily accessible protective epithelia of skin, oral cavity, and uterine cervix.

Owing to such efficient diagnostic tools as colposcopy and exfoliative cytology, *cervical preinvasive carcinoma* has become the most studied pertinent tumor. It has also caused the most extensive debate on terminology (Buckley et al. 1982). Cervical preinvasive carcinoma is preceded by epithelial alterations whose cancerous – or even neoplastic – nature is not always apparent, and many efforts have been made by gynecopathologists to distinguish histologically a possible precancerous stage, dysplasia, from the clear-cut cancerous stage, carcinoma in situ. In many instances, this distinction remains a subjective and arbitrary endeavor. Moreover, progression from dysplasia to carcinoma in situ is not an unequivocal event. In one investigation based entirely on colposcopy and cytology (Richart and Barron 1969), approximately 6% of cases of dysplasia regressed, 22% remained stationary, 28% advanced to a higher degree of dysplasia, and about half of the cases eventually became carcinoma in situ. In view of this situation, it is a reasonable and widely accepted suggestion to consider cervical dysplasia and carcinoma in situ together as an entity of at least diagnostic, but possibly also biological significance, and to call it cervical intraepithelial neoplasia (CIN) (Richart 1967, 1973).

In CIN, proliferation of atypical cells starts in the basal and parabasal layers of the original or of metaplastic squamous epithelium. The neoplastic cells gradually spread through the whole tissue thickness in a manner comparable to the dislocation of differentiating cells during normal epithelial turnover. While vertical extension is uncontested, horizontal spread is a matter of controversy. If one assumes that CIN begins as a single cell or a clone of cells, then intraepithelial extension along the cervical surface is an inescapable conclusion; it has even been termed "intraepithelial invasion" (Richart 1967). There is, however, the opposite concept which presumes development of CIN from a whole, simultaneously transformed segment or field of preexisting epithelium (Burghardt 1984). According to this theory, a neoplastic field remains within its original boundaries, and extension of CIN is only possible by apposition of new fields. The kinetic and morphological data used as pros and cons in this debate cannot be discussed here. But it may be useful to ask whether a preinvasive stage of CIN is a regular feature at all, or whether, as an alternative, the neoplastic cells can fan out immediately or shortly after their coming into being. A few ill-confirmed observations seem to support the latter possibility. At a stage when neoplastic transformation of the cervical epithelium was still confined to the basal zone, newly formed cancer cells were found to have already infiltrated the stroma in a brush- or spray-like configuration (Schiller et al. 1953). An identical observation of the same authors related to the mamilla. The term "carcinoma in situ" would not be applicable to such a behavior. As a more adequate designation "carcinoma invasivo d'emblé" has been suggested (Sirtori 1954), i.e., carcinoma supplied with invasive potential from its very beginning. We are faced here with a problem which has hardly been explored, namely, the cell sociology of invasion: to what extent is invasion a collective cellular endeavor, and how many cells are required for its successful initiation?

CIN can be easily surveyed and therefore causes no major problems of patient management. The contrary in both points is *preinvasiuve carcinoma of the breast.* Its representatives are found in the ducts and in the lobules and are best designated as "intraductal carcinoma" and as "lobular neoplasia" including lobular carcinoma in situ. With this the difference is indicated between the unequivocal cancerous nature of the former and the much less definite character of the latter with its wide spectrum of evolution, the extremes being regression and transition to highly invasive small cell carcinoma. In both tumor types, intraepithelial spread can be very impressive, extending toward the nipple as well as toward the innermost region of the lobules. In encounters with an extending solid tumor, the contiguous normal epithelium vanishes completely, whereas spread of noncohesive carcinoma cells often causes amazingly little damage. A complete myoepithelial layer interposed between tumor and basement membrane can be preserved (Bussolati et al. 1981). And yet, maintenance of the tissue border is only a relative criterion of the preinvasive state, as thoroughly demonstrated by Ozzello (1983). In intraductal carcinoma and, to a lesser degree, also in lobular neoplasia, basement membrane alterations are frequently revealed by the electron microscope: irregular thickness, multilayering, attenuation, and focal or diffuse disruptions. The latter need not be associated with transgression of the basement membrane level by tumor elements. But sometimes, protrusions of cell parts, whole single cells or several cells, through such gaps are recognizable – the very first foci of invasion, practically undetectable by light microscopy. Ozzello (1983) concludes that most, perhaps all, intraductal carcinomas have invasive foci when the first biopsy is examined. The limitations of sampling and microscopic survey explain the occasional occurrence of lymph node metastases in purportedly preinvasive mammary cancers including lobular neoplasia (Rosen 1980).

As concerns nonepithelial preinvasive cancer, we are best informed on an epithelium-associated neoplasia, *malignant melanoma.* It must be emphasized, however, that a genuine preinvasive stage can only be recognized in melanomas arising de novo from epidermal melanocytes. The neoplastic melanocytes spread in the epidermis in a vertical and horizontal direction, but much less regularly than cells of intraepithelial carcinoma. Full epidermal thickness neoplasia is infrequently formed and is by no means a prerequisite of horizontal (so-called radial) spread. The term "melanoma in situ" often applied to this stage has caused and still maintains a similar debate among dermatopathologists as the corresponding cervical affection among gynecopathologists. I share Ackerman's straightforward statement (1984) that the diagnosis of melanoma in situ is a matter of simple morphological observation. The duration of the in situ stage, however, varies enormously in the different types of malignant melanoma: it is very long in lentigo maligna, shorter in superficial spreading melanoma, and practically nonexistent in nodular melanoma.

Invasion and Its Infrastructure

As indicated in the preceding section, spread of preinvasive cancer occurs in two major configurations, solid and dispersed. Combinations of the two patterns are possible either as an original feature or as expression of a transition from a more cohesive to a less cohesive structure. Intraepithelial mammary carcinoma provides many examples for the latter process.

The onset of invasion reflects the tumor structure attained during the preinvasive stage. Squamous cell carcinomas of the uterine cervix begin invading in solid configuration: wedge- and tongue-like tumor projections are extended which, by becoming more numerous and interconnected, build up a complex but completely cohesive structure. In contrast, intraepithelial mammary carcinomas that have spread in dispersed manner during their preinvasive stage infiltrate the periductal stroma in dissociated configuration, the loose cancer cells often forming the characteristic targetoid pattern. Malignant melanoma, for obvious reasons, spreads mainly by means of single cells and small cell groups; but it is noteworthy that it occasionally forms invasive foci consisting of tightly packed – albeit not genuinely cohesive – tumor cells (nodular melanoma).

Invasion of solid carcinomas (squamous cell types as well as adenocarcinomas) can proceed in the original configuration for a considerable time. Indeed, the whole sequence of spread, including intravasation, dissemination, and extravasation, is occasionally accomplished by solid tumor parts and fragments (emboli). In the long run, however, an at least focal (mainly peripheral) dissolution occurs quite often, possibly as a manifestation of tumor progression. Initiation of the single cell state allows the operation of mechanisms such as *tumor cell locomotion* that play a minor or no role during spread in solid form (Sträuli and Haemmerli 1984; Sträuli 1985). Recently, a kind of cyclic transition from solid to dispersed and back, coupled with fluctuations of cell differentiation, has been claimed as key mechanism of invasion in human and rodent carcinomas (Gabbert 1984, 1985). This suggestion must be weighed against the multifactorial nature of the invasion process with the many influences exerted by cancer and host as expression of the ambiguous situation of the tumor within the homeostatic set-up of the organism.

Besides growth pressure and cell motility, *atypical synthetic activity* of cancer cells, both in quantitative and qualitative terms, is an important aspect of the invasion complex. Some facets of this activity are:

- Impaired production of basement membrane constituents
- Synthesis of hydrolases and/or of factors stimulating enzyme synthesis in host cells
- Synthesis of thrombogenic factors and of agents stimulating proliferation and metabolic reactivity of host fibroblasts, osteoblasts/osteoclasts, and capillary endothelial cells
- Release of chemoattractants for host leukocytes

It is instructive to have a look at the operation of some of these factors at the basement membrane level (Porter and Whelan 1984). Normal epithelial cells produce intrinsic basement membrane constituents such as type IV collagen and laminin. With transition to carcinoma this synthetic activity can – but must not – cease; if it does, membrane turnover gradually comes to an end, and membrane attenuation and focal dissolution is the result. On the other hand, cancer cells secrete various proteinases, including a type IV collagenase, with destructive effects on basement membrane architecture. Moreover, chemical messengers, already released by cancer cells in the preinvasive stage and diffusing through the basement membrane, attract leukocytes and capillary loops which, possibly, commit their lytic potential against the peritumoral extracellular matrix.

Such an interaction of tumor and host factors appears fairly realistic in the light of recent (mainly experimental) research (Liotta 1986). And yet, there remains the perplexing question whether this whole machinery is necessary at all. Undoubtedly, it can facilitate basement membrane transgression by solid cancer under the influence of push or pull. But where single cells are concerned, the decisive factor might be a change in the sensory world of these cells, manifesting itself as a loss of basement membrane perception and resulting in simple membrane transmigration in leukocyte fashion (a regular physiological event that has so far remained unexplained).

A special situation exists in *encounters of invading cancer with bone and cartilage.* Certain cancers, particularly squamous cell carcinomas of the oral cavity, nasopharynx, and paranasal sinuses, are prone to invade adjacent bone directly. How this occurs has been partly elucidated by Carter and associates (Carter and Shaw 1980; Carter et al. 1980; Tsao et al. 1981). While the advancing carcinoma is still separated from the bone surface by a zone consisting of granulation tissue and fibrosis, osteoblasts and osteoclasts are already aggregating in the bone periphery. Since the latter outnumber the former, osteoblastic and osteoclastic activity are unbalanced in favor of bone destruction. This allows the tumor to penetrate into and impinge directly on bone substance. As in most aspects of invasion, activation of cells must be considered to derive from both carcinoma and host cells. There appear to be diverse osteoclast stimulants; some are indomethacin sensitive and presumed to be prostaglandins. The same type of invasion is displayed by larynx carcinoma encountering an ossified laryngeal framework. The susceptibility to invasion exhibited by metaplastic cartilage is very different from the resistance of normal cartilage, e.g., of the epiphyseal growth plate contiguous to osteosarcoma. Part of the explanation consists in the presence of osteoclasts in ossified cartilage, whereas normal cartilage does not contain any cell type comparable to the osteoclast. Another reason appears to be the presence of a chondrocyte-derived factor functionally defined as "anti-invasion factor" (AIF). This factor displays several activities which inhibit different aspects of invasion, notably multiplication of cancer cells, collagenase action, and neovascularization (Pauli and Kuettner 1982, 1984).

Spread in the Lymphatic System

In most instances, spread in lymphatics corresponds to the mode of spread before intravasation: it is solid, dispersed, or mixed. In lymph capillaries and small lymphatics, solid spread often occurs in the form of continuous extension, i. e., without interruption between extra- and intralymphatic growth. Extensive networks consisting of fine strands of cancer tissue are thus formed (lymphangiosis carcinomatosa). Embolization of cohesive tumor fragments is only possible in larger lymphatics with a relatively brisk lymph flow.

In spite of almost unlimited possibilities of deviation, lymph flow is essentially unidirectional. It begins in lymph capillaries and ends where the large collecting lymph vessels join the blood vasculature, i. e., at the venular angles. *Lymph nodes* are integrated into this flow system at various levels, of which two are particularly important for the spread of cancer:

1. The *regional level* as center of lymph drainage for a distinct region or organ
2. The *terminal level*, consisting of lymph nodes localized near the venular angles (supraclavicular lymph nodes), as center of lymph drainage for the whole body (*"zentraler Lymphraum des Körpers;"* von Lanz and Wachsmuth 1955)

Statistical analysis shows that cancer of a distinct region most frequently spreads to regional lymph nodes, whereas cancers of all possible sites, taken together, most frequently affect the supraclavicular lymph nodes (Sträuli 1960). If we disregard retrograde extension, cancer elements gain access, via afferent lymphatics, to the subcapsular sinus of lymph nodes. Their further fate depends on various factors. One of them is the functional anatomy of the lymph node which is organized for converting flow into percolation. While lymph is conducted from the subcapsular sinus through the labyrinth of intermediary and medullary sinuses toward the hilus and the efferent lymphatics, transported cells are subject to a kind of filtration process. Transnodal passage is, however, not excluded. Studies in animals have provided evidence for both possibilities: trapping as well as through-passage; they have also shown that cell transit volume and cell transit time are of crucial importance for the results of such experiments. Beginning with a seminal paper subtitled "Effectiveness of the Lymph Node as a Barrier to the Passage of Embolic Tumor Cells" (Zeidman and Buss 1954), extensive experimental work has been devoted to circumstances and extent of cancer cell trapping in lymph nodes. Widely scattered as the results are, they allow the statement that in most instances initial cell retention remains below 100%, in other words: a certain number of cancer cells is regularly capable of traversing lymph nodes (Sträuli 1970). In my opinion, a key observation has been made in recent studies with a transplantable rat mammary carcinoma (Grundmann 1984): in the first few hours after transplantation carcinoma cells rapidly traversed the regional lymph nodes, whereas retention with consecutive metastasis formation only occurred after initiation of tumor growth at the implantation site 4 to 5 weeks later.

Two factors are mainly responsible for departure from a purely filtration-based interaction of lymph nodes and cancer elements (Wallace et al. 1980):

1. The presence of cancer in the drainage area frequently induces reactive lymph node alterations: proliferation of sinus littoral cells (sinus histiocytosis), follicular hyperplasia, and multiplication of interfollicular cells. Thus, lymph-borne cancer is not faced with the text book architecture of lymph nodes, but with structures in dynamic adaptation.
2. Cancer cells carried by percolating lymph need not remain passive. By display of multiplication and translocation, small numbers of cancer cells can escape the regular anatomical pathways of transnodal passage and, for instance, invade blood vessels without ever forming intranodal metastases.

Hyperplastic changes in lymph nodes, particularly the proliferation of lymphocytes and plasma cells, are usually considered as an expression of immune reactivity. It is on this basis that some time ago the preservation of regional lymph nodes, whenever justifiable, was recommended. Various objections to this attitude can be raised. Evidence of cancer cell destruction within lymph nodes under the influence of immune mechanisms is very scarce. Moreover, such mechanisms may entail tumor enhancement instead of inhibition. Besides, induction of immunological host reactivity by a given tumor will be a matter of regional lymph nodes for a limited period only and it will then become systemic by extending to transregional nodes and the spleen. In principle, this development must be expected to have taken its course at the time of clinical diagnosis.

Finally, a strong argument against preservation of inconspicuous regional lymph nodes is the possible presence of micrometastases. Does this threat, in diametrical contrast to attempts at lymph node preservation, justify the general elective dissection of clinically negative regionals? Surgeons have long been and are still looking for a more selective approach.

One exploitable principle is the dependence of metastasis probability upon size of the primary tumor. The example most studied is maximal tumor thickness as decisive prognostic criterion of stage I malignant melanoma (Breslow 1978). Although tumor thickness does not discriminate between the probability of metastasis to regional lymph nodes and to distant sites (WHO 1983), it can be used for handling the former in the following way (Fortner et al. 1985): extirpation is recommended for patients with primary melanomas of a thickness between 1.2 and 4.00 mm, whereas it is not deemed necessary in melanomas below this range (metastases too infrequent) and not considered beneficial in those above it (transregional and hematogenous metastases too frequent).

The terminal pathway of lymphogenous spread is the system of the *thoracic duct*, consisting of the duct itself, the contralateral truncus lymphaceus dexter, and interconnecting channels. In the thoracic duct, cancer elements in transit have repeatedly been demonstrated histologically and cytologically, and good evidence has been presented that such elements can be arrested at hydrodynamically critical sites, the valve pockets, and there give rise to intraductal metastases (Brunner 1960). As long as a lymph flow is not completely obstructed, these foci are insidious sources of cancer cell spilling. Although many of the floating cells may be trapped in supraclavicular lymph nodes, others are directly carried to the venular angles as potential seeds of blood-borne metastases.

Blood-Borne Cancer

In small blood vessels, continuous solid extension of cancer is less frequent than in lymphatics. There are, however, amazing examples of uninterrupted nonoccluding tumor cords in larger veins. It is a characteristic feature of such structures that their distal end is formed by a lymph node metastasis grown into the vascular lumen; the proximal end may project freely into the atrium of the right heart (Walther 1948). But these are exceptional findings. In most instances intravasation of solid cancer results in fragmentation of the invasion edge. Tumor emboli are carried off, and/or detached cancer cells – singly, in small groups, or in whole showers – are transported away. Whereas, in the course of a century, blood-borne cancer fragments have frequently been found in sections from surgical and autopsy material, the identification of *cancer cells in the blood of living subjects* is a relatively recent achievement. Although partly successful attempts were made half a century ago (Pool and Dunlog 1934), a broadly based approach began only in the mid-1950s under the influence of surgeons who tried to analyze the relationship between intraoperative tumor handling, cancer cell dissemination, and prognosis. As a technical corollary of this endeavor, a multitude of methods for concentrating the cancer cells in blood samples were developed (Nadel 1965).

A pioneering and far-sighted study was performed by Engell (1955, 1959) in 125 cancer patients (mostly with intestinal carcinomas). Blood samples were collected from veins draining the tumor site before and after dissection of the carcinoma; in addition, blood was also gained from antecubital veins during the terminal phase of surgery. In local veins cancer cells were found in 42% of the patients before and in 55% after tumor manipulation; 10% of the patients had cancer cells in the peripheral circulation. Important are the follow-up results: 44% of all patients were alive after 5–9 years, although in 51% of them cancer cells had been demonstrated in the blood at the time of operation. With regard to these survivors, Engell (1955) made the statement that "all tumor cells disseminated into the blood must have perished." This led him to conclusions which, although not fully justified by his technically imperfect analysis of a small and heterogenous patient collective, anticipated all-important topics of later discussion in this field: (a) the occurrence of cancer cells in the peripheral blood is so rare as to be of no diagnostic value; (b) the appearance of cancer cells in venous blood from the tumor area is of no prognostic significance; (c) the surgical trauma plays only a minor role with respect to an increased escape of cancer cells into the blood stream. Whereas the first statement has never been seriously jeopardized, Engell's other conclusions have since been relativized. The prognostic significance of blood-borne cancer cells is largely a quantitative problem. Small numbers, as usually identified in occasional samples from the local or peripheral circulation, appear to be innocuous in most instances. On the other hand, prolonged dissemination of large numbers is clearly an ominous sign. In one patient, blood-borne cancer cells comprised 80% of the leukocyte count and justified the term "carcinocythemia" proposed for these exceptional observations (Carey et al. 1976; Gallivan and Lokich 1984).

Regarding the *surgical trauma*, intravasation of cancer elements and mobilization of previously intravasated elements is, in principle, a serious risk. However, massive intraoperative dissemination is largely eliminated by techniques of surgical oncology explicitly developed for preventing recurrence and metastasis (Cole et al. 1954). Nonetheless, small-scale release of cancer cells during surgery is always possible and may be unavoidable, e. g., during mobilization and rotation of a hepatic lobe containing liver carcinoma (Koo et al. 1983), or during thoracotomy initiating surgery of bronchial carcinoma (Pfitzer et al. 1984). Since the quantitative aspect of possible cancer cell spilling can hardly be judged during a surgical intervention, it remains a valid instruction that "every effort should be made to prevent dissemination of cancer cells during operation" (Roberts 1961).

The most striking form of iatrogenic dissemination is the intraoperative embolization or large fragments of lung carcinomas that have invaded the pulmonary vein. The dramatic nature of such an occurrence is well illustrated by a report on the successful removal of a saddle embolus, consisting of squamous cell carcinoma, from the bifurcation of the aorta during lobectomy (Shankar 1981). Less massive arterial embolization from the lungs, eventually resulting in metastases at unusual sites, occurs spontaneously, but is an infrequent event: a review (Vo et al. 1981) lists 25 cases, of which one-half were caused by primary lung cancers and the other half by lung metastases.

Why are circulating cancer cells, unless disseminated in large numbers over prolonged periods, only an insignificant prognostic factor? Engell's assumption that they perish in the blood stream was basically correct; it should be noted, however, that patient survival does not exclude tumor survival, i. e., the dormancy of disseminated and extravasated cancer elements (see The Life History of Metastases). Anyhow, it is now well established that blood-borne cancer cells are in a predominantly hostile environment, and that their best chance of survival lies in a early escape into the perivascular tissue. Our knowledge about this constellation is mainly derived from experimental investigations. The complexity of factors affecting the *fate of blood-borne cancer cells* in animal systems has been thoroughly discussed by Nicolson and Poste (1983). Of the various influences operating in experimental models at least some can be expected to be also active in man. Prominent among them are: (a) forces of shear and distortion to which cancer cells are exposed during transcapillary passage; (b) unspecific cytostatic and cytolytic host reactions mediated by natural antibodies and natural killer cells. In contrast, effects of specific host reactions have hardly been documented so far.

A decisive but incompletely understood facet in the biology of blood-borne cancer is the role of cell surface-controlled interactions during transit and immediately before lodgement. Such interactions can result in homo- and heterotypic adhesion, i. e., in the formation of pluricellular aggregates of cancer cells and of cancer and host cells (platelets and leukocytes), respectively. It appears that, on the whole, aggregates of any kind formed during the transport phase have a better chance of survival and, therefore, a higher metastatic potential. One reason, among other and more complicated causes, is the occurrence of mechanical trapping prior to the dangerous transcapillary passage and, thus, the creation of an earlier chance of extravasation. In the arrest phase, the decisive heterotypic partner of blood-borne cancer cells is the *endothelium* (Warren 1981; Weiss and Glaves 1983). Once contact between cancer cells and endothelium is established, the machinery responsible for maintaining the integrity of the blood vessel luminal surface is challenged, and a complex interaction of plasma constituents, platelets, cancer cells, and endothelial cells takes its course (Gasic 1984).

Although these interactions are important and possibly decisive for the transition of cancer elements from transport to lodgement, it must be emphasized that arrest can be accomplished on a purely mechanical basis by the squeezing of cancer cells into arterioles and capillaries. This mechanism also circumvents the relatively poor adhesion of cancer cells to the endothelium [poor in comparison to their strong attachment to the subendothelial matrix surface, as demonstrated for human and rodent melanoma cells by Kramer et al. (1980)]. If jammed cancer cells are able to display osmotic or mitotic pressure, they destroy the endothelium and eventually the whole vessel wall by a kind of attrition (Chew et al. 1976). This, by the way, is a mode of extravasation that requires no particular mechanisms of "secondary invasion."

Irrespective of the occurrence of mechanical trapping, there is substantial evidence for nonmechanical arrest in relatively large vessels. In these instances association of cancer cells with thrombotic material, established before or during contact with endothelium, must play a role – perhaps a crucial one. Mainly due to the possibility of therapeutic exploitation, this aspect of spread has caused many experimental and clinical investigations. The pertinent ideas and results have been collected in several books (Donati at al. 1981; Jamieson 1982; Honn and Sloane 1984). These monographs show that the relationship between studies in animals and in man is rather loose. This is mainly due to the fact that far-reaching conclusions have been (and occasionally still are) drawn from animal models not concerned with genuine spread, but with the behavior of blood-borne cancer cells introduced into tumor-free animals. Another reason is the complexity of factors interacting in the functional compartment composed of blood plasma, platelets, cancer cells, and endothelium.

For a considerable time, the "coagulation hypothesis of cancer dissemination" (Zacharski 1985) has mainly been concerned with modifications of the classical clotting cascade during cancer dissemination. All available *anticoagulants* have been experimentally tested on this basis, and those with the most consistent antimetastatic (i.e., metastasis-preventing) properties, the hydroxycumarins, have been introduced into clinical trials (Zacharski 1982; Hilgard 1984). In the meantime, a new concept, based on alterations of arachidonic acid metabolism in the critical compartment, has emerged: cancer cells are thought to disturb the balance normally existing between vascular prostacyclin, a potent inhibitor of platelet aggregation, and platelet thromboxane, an equally potent stimulator of platelet aggregation (Honn et al. 1984; Honn and Sloane 1985). Maybe a new clinical approach to metastasis prevention will consist in stimulation of endogenous prostacyclin synthesis.

Even in the absence of any therapeutic intervention, cancer cells in the dissemination phase are in a precarious situation. Their chances of survival, largely coinciding with their chances of escape from the circulation, can only be estimated as a matter of collectives; and these collectives, as a rule, must be large. On a single cell basis and judged by its clinical end effect, metastasis formation, spread of cancer via the blood is an unproductive process ("metastatic inefficiency"; Weiss 1982).

The Life History of Metastases

In the main, hematogenous metastases will be considered in this section. At the end of the dissemination phase, the potential seeds of such metastases range from a single tumor cell to a tumor embolus visible with the naked eye. As mentioned earlier, the size of these seeds is one of the factors responsible for the localization of metastases. All cancer elements transported in the back-to-heart branch of the circulation are ultimately carried to one of the large capillary nets of lung, liver, and vertebral bone marrow. The latter must be included in this general evaluation, since in the vessels connecting central veins and the vertebral venous plexus blood can flow in both directions (Batson 1967). The large capillary nets are critical areas for cancer dissemination: arrest is frequent, but transit is possible. The decision depends not only on size, but also on deformability of the transported material, moreover on anatomical properties of the vasculature (e.g., on the availability of arteriovenous shunts) and on insufficiently understood chemical affinities and interactions between "seed and soil" (Hart 1982).

Due to the potential trapping function of their capillary nets, lung, liver, and bone marrow operate as filter organs (Walther 1948) and key disseminating sites (Viadana et al. 1978; Bross 1980) of hematogenous spread. Use of the term "key" expresses the view that, in accordance with the *cascade or multistep theory of spread*, metastases in lung, liver, and bone marrow are generated first and subsequently constitute the starting points for further dissemination. Indeed, this is a frequent mode of tumor amplification. Nevertheless, the cascade is not a universally valid principle of metastasis (Colombano and Reese 1980). This can be well documented by the mode of spread of gastric carcinoma. As for all other cancers disseminating via the portal vein, the liver is usually considered to act as a generalizing site for the spread of gastric malignancies. However, a new approach to autopsy data analysis (Eder 1984) shows that this is only correct for circumscript (solid) tumors. Diffuse gastric carcinomas do not spread to the liver but to peritoneum, pleura, and spinal column, and even in patients with metastases at several sites, the liver is rarely affected; thus, it cannot be considered as first metastatic target or as filter or key organ for spread of this type of gastric carcinoma (nor can any other organ!).

It is almost a truism that primary cancers and their metastases are different tumors, but the theories behind this statement are controversial. A few simple inferences can provide guidelines across this controversy. The development of any primary cancer is the result of a distinct constellation in which properties of tumor cells and of local host elements are jointly expressed. Tumor transfer to a distant site almost inevitably creates a new and different constellation: although the tumor may be the same, the local anatomical and physiological conditions are not and will, therefore, hardly allow the tumor to repeat the behavior displayed at its original site. Since growth and invasion are the crucial components of this behavior, the conclusion is justified that disseminated and arrested cancer elements are not necessarily able to grow and to invade. Let us, in a first step, simplify the matter by assuming release of cancer cells from a homogenous primary population. At a metastatic site these cells can be expected to display one of the following modes of behavior: (a) they die; (b) they survive without further activity; (c) they multiply; (d) they multiply and invade. The result of b is a dormant metastatic seed, of c a noninvasive, and of d an invasive metastasis. This first level of metastatic diversity is complicated by changes in environmental conditions at the metastatic site with possible induction of transitions between a and d in both directions. Examples are onset of growth in a hitherto dormant cancer focus, or loss of invasiveness of a metastasis (which, in this case, can no longer operate as generalizing site).

We should now approach a further level of metastatic complexity by making the more realistic assumption of heterogeneity (instead of homogeneity) of primary cancer cell populations. Cellular heterogeneity as such is an uncontested property of animal and human cancer (Heppner and Miller 1983) and includes differences between cells of primary and metastatic tumors (Weiss 1980). But does this heterogeneity also comprise the capacity to spread, particularly the potential to survive and multiply at a prospective metastatic site? Should this be the case, then only cells belonging to *subpopulations* (maybe clones) with "metastatic potential" would be able to produce metastases, and metastasic formation would be a kind of selection process for these preexisting cells. Indeed, Fidler and his associates have provided compelling evidence for the occurrence of this whole constellation in mouse tumor systems exposed to distinct experimental conditions (Fidler 1973, 1978; Fidler and Kripke 1977; Fidler and Hart 1982). Directly comparable human data are, of course, not available, and clinical experience regarding the metastatic potential of metastases compared to that of the primary tumor is equivocal. Moreover, other investigations in animals have led to different interpretations (Giavazzi et al. 1980; Mantovani et al. 1981; Weiss et al. 1983). Thus, it appears safe to say that the origin of metastases from preexisting cell subpopulations that have successfully passed through the selective process of premetastatic spread is a possible, but not an exclusive, mechanism. At any rate, dissemination and arrest of cancer cells with diverging functional capacities is a factor that should be integrated into the general and simplistic outline of metastasic formation discussed above. Finally, and as indication of a last level of metastatic complexity, it must be mentioned that cancer cell subpopulations are not autonomously operating units, but prone to interaction with other subpopulations and subject to considerable phenotypic instability (Fidler 1984).

Growth of metastatic seeds requires some comment. Its lack is usually accepted as explanation of dormancy, a condition inferred from experimental studies and from the registration of long latent intervals between elimination of primary cancers and appearance of metastases. Experimental arguments in favor of *dormant metastatic seeds* have been procured in various ways, of which one may be mentioned here: after removal of immunogenic primary tumors in rodents, initiation of growth of hitherto dormant secondary foci in lungs and lymph nodes was achieved by immunosuppression of the host animals (Eccles et al. 1980; Alexander 1983). The dependence of tumor dormancy on host control is convincingly demonstrated in these studies; their relevance for clinical oncology is, however, made doubtful by the lack of human tumors with comparable immunogenicity. This, of course, does not exclude the occasional occurrence of a prolonged nonproliferative state of human cancer cells, originally thought to represent G_0 (Quastler 1963) and now considered possible in other cell cycle phases as well, including G_2 (Post and Sklarew 1985).

On the other hand, latency of metastatic foci might represent pseudodormancy and be due to simple kinetic properties. Unless growth capacity is completely lacking or completely suppressed, all metastatic foci must pass through the *micrometastatic* stage. Whereas the lower size limit of micrometastases is undefined, the upper size limit coincides with clinical visibility which, of course, depends on the diagnostic techniques used. In the skeleton, micrometastases with at least 2 mm diameter are detectable by scintiscans (provided there is an osteoblastic reaction), those with at least 4 mm by radiography (Stoll 1983). If we start from a more generous clinical detection range of micrometastases, 1 mm–1 cm, then we are dealing with hypothetical cancer cell numbers in orders of magnitude of 10^6–10^9. These numbers can be attained in the course of 20–30 rounds of cell division (Collins et al. 1956). The time required for this multiplication is determined by the classical parameters of proliferation kinetics and many additional factors; it can, at any rate, amount to several years. Escape of cancer elements shortly before removal of a primary tumor and more or less constant growth of these elements after dissemination and extravasation should therefore be an acceptable explanation of at least some of the long latent intervals between surgery and appearance of the first metastasis (Allan 1977; Rabes 1984).

Next to growth, invasiveness is the most critical feature of metastases in terms of patient handling. Invasiveness, however, can be lacking, although it is difficult to estimate the frequency of "nonmalignant" metastases. They have the properties of benign tumors growing by expansion and compressing their surroundings. If there are many of these globular foci, severe clinical problems are created. Surgical removal of metastases has become a worthwhile means of diminishing tumor burden, and excision of multiple lung metastases (Weiss and Gilbert 1978) owes its feasibility, at least to a large extent, to the noninvasive nature of many of these tumors.

References

Ackerman AB (1984) Histopathologists can diagnose malignant melanoma in situ correctly and consistently. Am J Dermatopathol [Suppl 1] 6: 103–107

Alexander P (1983) Dormant metastases – studies in experimental animals. J Pathol 141: 379–383

Allan E (1977) Breast cancer: the long latent interval. Eur J Cancer 13: 839–845

Batson OV (1967) The vertebral system of veins as a means for cancer dissemination. In: Ariel IM (ed) Progress in clinical cancer, vol 3. Grune and Stratton, New York, pp 1–18

Breslow A (1978) Evaluation of prognosis in stage I cutaneous melanoma. Plast Reconstr Surg 61: 342–346

Bross IDJ (1980) The biostatistical and biological basis for a cascade theory of human metastasis. In: Grundmann E (ed) Metastatic tumor growth. Fischer, Sutttgart, pp 207–221

Brunner U (1960) Die Entstehung lymphogener Metastasen im Ductus thoracicus. Virchows Arch [Pathol Anat] 333: 241–254

Buckley CH, Butler EB, Fox H (1982) Cervical intraepithelial neoplasia. J Clin Pathol 35: 1–13

Burghardt E (1984) Colposcopy. Cervical pathology. Textbook and atlas. Thieme, Stuttgart

Bussolati G, Botto Micca F, Eusebi V, Betts CM (1981) Myoepithelial cells in lobular carcinoma in situ of the breast: a parallel immunocytochemical and ultrastructural study. Ultrastruct Pathol 2: 219–230

Carey RW, Taft PD, Bennett JM, Kaufman S (1976) Carcinocythemia (carcinoma cell leukemia) due to metastatic carcinoma of the breast. Am J Med 60: 273–278

Carter RL, Shaw HJ (1980) Direct invasion of bone and ossified cartilage by squamous carcinomas of the head and neck: patterns and mechanisms. In: Grundmann E (ed) Metastatic tumor growth. Fischer, Stuttgart, pp 193–205

Carter RL, Tanner NSB, Clifford P, Shaw HJ (1980) Direct bone invasion in squamous carcinomas of the head and neck: pathological and clinical implications. Clin Otolaryngol 5: 107–116

Chew EC, Josephson RL, Wallace AC (1976) Morphologic aspects of the arrest of circulating cancer cells. In: Weiss L (ed) Fundamental aspects of metastasis. North-Holland, Amsterdam, pp 121–150

Cole WH, Packard D, Southwick HW (1954) Carcinoma of the colon with special reference to prevention of recurrence. JAMA 155: 1549–1553

Collins VP, Loeffler RK, Tivey H (1956) Observations on growth rates of human tumors. AJR 76: 988–1000

Colombano SP, Reese PA (1980) The cascade theory of metastatic spread: are there generalizing sites? Cancer 46: 2312–2314

Donati MB, Davidson JF, Garattini S (eds) (1981) Malignancy and the hemostatic system. Raven, New York

Eccles SA, Heckford SE, Alexander P (1980) Effect of cyclosporin A on the growth and spontaneous metastatis of syngeneic animal tumours. Br J Cancer 42: 252–259

Eder M (1984) Die Metastasierung: Fakten und Probleme aus humanpathologischer Sicht. Verh Dtsch Ges Pathol 68: 1–11

Engell HC (1955) Cancer cells in the circulating blood. Acta Chir Scand [Suppl] 201: 1–70

Engell HC (1959) Cancer cells in the blood. A five to nine year follow up study. Ann Surg 149: 457–461

Fidler IJ (1973) Selection of successive tumour lines for metastasis. Nature [New Biol] 242: 148–149

Fidler IJ (1978) Tumor heterogeneity and the biology of cancer invasion and metastasis. Cancer Res 38: 2651–2660

Fidler IJ (1984) Recent concepts of cancer metastasis and their implications for therapy. Cancer Treat Rep 68: 193–198

Fidler IJ, Hart IR (1982) Biological diversity in metastatic neoplasms: origins and implications. Science 217: 998–1003

Fidler IJ, Kripke ML (1977) Metastasis results from preexisting variant cells within a malignant tumor. Science 197: 893–895

Fisher B, Redmond C, Fisher ER, et al. (1980) The contribution of recent NSABP clinical trials of primary breast cancer therapy to an understanding of tumor biology. An overview of findings. Cancer 46: 1009–1025

Fortner JG, Rosen PP, Maclean BJ (1985) Selective use of wide excision with elective lymph node dissection for malignant melanoma. In: Sommers SC, Rosen PP, Fechner RE (eds) Pathology annual, part 1, vol 20. Appleton-Century-Crofts, Norwalk, pp 239–246

Gabbert H (1984) Invasionsmechanismen maligner Tumoren. Verh Dtsch Ges Pathol 68: 18–32

Gabbert H (1985) Mechanisms of invasion: evidence from in vivo observations. Cancer Metastasis Rev 4: 293–309

Gallivan MVE, Lokich JJ (1984) Carcinocythemia (carcinoma cell leukemia). Cancer 53: 1100–1102

Gasic GJ (1984) Role of plasma, platelets, and endothelial cells in tumor metastasis. Cancer Metastasis Rev 3: 99–116

Giavazzi R, Alessandri G, Spreafico F, Garattini S, Mantovani A (1980) Metastasizing capacity of tumour cells from spontaneous metastases of transplanted murine tumours. Br J Cancer 42: 462–472

Grundmann E (1984) Die lymphogene Metastasierung. Verh Dtsch Ges Pathol 63: 33–46

Hart IR (1982) "Seed and soil" revisited: mechanisms of site-specific metastasis. Cancer Metastasis Rev 1: 5–16

Heppner G, Miller BE (1983) Tumor heterogeneity: biological implications and therapeutic consequences. Cancer Metastasis Rev 2: 5–23

Hilgard P (1984) Anticoagulants and tumor growth: Pharmacological considerations. In: Nicolson GL, Milas L (eds) Cancer invasion and metastasis: Biologic and therapeutic aspects. Raven, New York, pp 353–360

Honn KV, Sloane BF (eds) (1984) Hemostatic mechanisms and metastasis. Nijhoff, Boston

Honn KV, Sloane BF (1985) Prostaglandins in tumor cell metastasis. In: Torisu M, Yoshida T (eds) Basic mechanisms and clinical treatment of tumor metastasis. Academic, Orlando, pp 311–333

Honn KV, Menter DG, Onoda JM, Taylor JD, Sloane BF (1984) Role of prostacyclin as a natural deterrent to hematogenous tumor metastasis. In: Nicolson GL, Milas L (eds) Cancer invasion and metastasis: Biologic and therapeutic aspects. Raven, New York, pp 361–388

Jamieson GA (ed) (1982) Interaction of platelets and tumor cells. Liss, New York

Koo J, Fung K, Siu KF, Lee NW, Lett Z, Ho J, Wong J, Ong GB (1983) Recovery of malignant tumor cells from the right atrium during hepatic resection for hepatocellular carcinoma. Cancer 52: 1952–1956

Kramer RH, Gonzalez R, Nicolson GL (1980) Metastatic tumor cells adhere preferentially to the extracellular matrix underlying vascular endothelial cells. Int J Cancer 26: 639–645

Liotta LA (1986) Tumor invasion and metastases – role of the extracellular matrix: Rhoads Memorial Award Lecture. Cancer Res 46: 1–7

Mantovani A, Giavazzi R, Alessandri G, Spreafico F, Garattini S (1981) Characterization of tumor lines derived from spontaneous metastases of a transplanted murine sarcoma. Eur J Cancer 17: 71–76

Nadel EM (ed) (1965) Symposium on tumor cells in the peripheral blood. Acta Cytol 9: 1–93, 95–188

Nagel GA, Wander H-E, Holtkamp W (1985) Prognosefaktoren beim Mammakarzinom. Beitr Onkol 22: 19–43

Nicolson GL, Poste G (1983) Tumor implantation and invasion of metastatic sites. Int Rev Exp Pathol 25: 77–181

Ozzello H (1983) Intraepithelial carcinomas of the breast. In: Hollmann KH, Verley JM (eds) New frontiers in mammary pathology, vol 2. Plenum, New York, pp 147–164

Pauli BV, Kuettner KE (1982) The regulation of invasion by a cartilage-derived anti-invasion factor. In: Liotta LA, Hart IR (eds) Tumor invasion and metastasis. Nijhoff, The Hague, pp 267–290

Pauli BV, Kuettner KE (1984) Host tissue resistance to tumour invasion. In: Mareel MM, Calman KC (eds) Invasion, experimental and clinical implications. Oxford University Press, Oxford, pp 205–227

Pfitzer P, Kamino K, Irlich G (1984) Nachweis zirkulierender Tumorzellen mittels DNA-Cytometrie. Verh Dtsch Ges Pathol 68: 188–193

Pool EH, Dunlop GR (1934) Cancer cells in the blood stream. Am J Cancer 21: 99–102

Porter R, Whelan J (eds) (1984) Basement membranes and cell movement. Ciba Found Symp 108

Post J, Sklarew RJ (1985) The heterogenous proliferation of human cancer cells in vivo. In: Sommers SC, Rosen PP, Fechner RE (eds) Pathology annual, part 1. Appleton-Century-Crofts, Norwalk, pp 359–381

Quastler H (1963) The analysis of cell population kinetics. In: Lamerton LF, Fry RJM (eds) Cell proliferation. Davis, Philadelphia, pp 18–34

Rabes HM (1984) Die Zellkinetik in Metastasen. Verh Dtsch Ges Pathol 68: 147–163

Richart RM (1967) Natural history of cervical intraepithelial neoplasia. Clin Obstet Gynecol 10: 748–784

Richart RM (1973) Cervical intraepithelial neoplasia: a review. Pathol Annu 8: 301–328

Richart RM, Barron BA (1969) A follow-up study of patients with cervical dysplasia. Am J Obstet Gynecol 105: 386–393

Roberts SS (1961) Spread by the vascular system. In: Cole WH, McDonald GO, Roberts SS, Southwick HW (eds) Dissemination of cancer. Prevention and therapy. Appleton-Century-Crofts, New York, pp 61–222

Rosen PP (1980) Axillary lymph node metastasis in patients with occult noninvasive breast carcinoma. Cancer 46: 1298–1306

Schiller W, Daro AF, Gollin HA, Primiano NP (1953) Small preulcerative invasive carcinoma of the cervix: The spray carcinoma. Am J Obstet Gynecol 65: 1088–1098

Shankar PS (1981) Intraoperative systemic tumor embolism. CA 31: 111–113

Sirtori C (1954) Il cancro in situ nella patologia umana e sperimentale, con particolare riguardo al significato della membrana basale. Tumori 40: 42–53

Stoll BA (1983) Natural history, prognosis, and staging of bone metastases. In: Stoll BA, Parbhoo S (eds) Bone metastasis: Monitoring and treatment. Raven, New York, pp 1–20

Sträuli P (1960) Die supraclaviculären Lymphknoten als Zentrum der lymphogenen Krebsmetastasierung. Schweiz Med Wochenschr 90: 529–534

Sträuli P (1970) The barrier function of lymph nodes. A review of experimental studies and their implications for cancer surgery. In: Saegesser F, Pettavel J (eds) Surgical oncology. Huber, Bern, pp 161–176

Sträuli P (1985) The contribution of cancer cell translocation to spread of cancer. Exp Biol Med 10: 249–259

Sträuli P, Haemmerli G (1984) Cancer cell locomotion: its occurrence during invasion. In: Mareel MM, Calman KC (eds) Invasion, experimental and clinical implications. Oxford University Press, Oxford, pp 252–274

Tsao SW, Burman JF, Easty DM, Easty GC, Carter RL (1981) Some mechanisms of local bone destruction by squamous carcinomas of the head and neck. Br J Cancer 43: 392–401

Viadana E, Bross IDJ, Pickren JW (1978) Cascade spread of blood-borne metastases in solid and nonsolid cancers of humans. In: Weiss L, Gilbert HA (eds) Pulmonary metastasis. Nijhoff, The Hague, pp 143–167

Vo NM, Sakurai H, Gambarini AJ (1981) Malignant tumor emboli to the peripheral vessels. J Surg Oncol 17: 151–157

Von Lanz T, Wachsmuth W (1955) Hals. Springer, Berlin Göttingen Heidelberg (Praktische Anatomie, Bd 1/2)

Wallace AC, Josephson RL, Hollenberg NK (1980) Observations on lymph node metastases. In: Grundmann E (ed) Metastatic tumor growth. Fischer, Stuttgart, pp 83–99

Walther HE (1948) Krebsmetastasen. Schwabe, Basel

Warren BA (1981) Cancer cell-endothelial reactions: The microinjury hypothesis and localized thrombosis in the formation of micrometastases. In: Donati MB, Davidson JF, Garattini S (eds) Malignancy and the hemostatic system. Raven, New York, pp 5–25

Weiss L (1980) Metastases: differences between cancer cells in primary and secondary tumors. In: Ioachim HL (ed) Pathobiology annual, vol 10. Raven, New York, pp 51–81

Weiss L (1982) Metastatic inefficiency. In: Weiss L, Gilbert HA (eds) Liver metastasis. Prentice Hall, Boston, pp 126–157

Weiss L, Gilbert HA (eds) (1978) Pulmonary metastasis. Nijhoff, The Hague

Weiss L, Glaves D (1983) Cancer cell damage at the vascular endothelium. Ann NY Acad Sci 416: 681–692

Weiss L, Holmes JC, Ward PM (1983) Do metastases arise from pre-existing subpopulations of cancer cells? Br J Cancer 47: 81–89

WHO (1983) Collaborating Centres of Evaluation of Methods of Diagnosis and Treatment of Melanoma. Tumori 69: 449–454

Zacharski LR (1982) The biologic basis for anticoagulant treatment of cancer. In: Jamieson GA (ed) Interaction of platelets and tumor cells. Liss, New York, pp 113–129

Zacharski LR (1985) The coagulation hypothesis of cancer dissemination. In: Hellmann K, Eccles SA (eds) Treatment of metastasis: Problems and prospects. Taylor and Francis, London, pp 77–80

Zeidman I, Buss JA (1954) Experimental studies on the spread of cancer in the lymphatic system. Cancer Res 14: 403–405

Cancer Epidemiology

C. S. Muir and M.-C. Gran

Introduction

"Epidemiology" has been defined as the use of knowledge on the frequency and distribution of disease to search for determinants, the removal of which would result in a diminution in the frequency of the disease in question. It is customary to consider cancer epidemiology as comprising three major but closely linked areas: descriptive epidemiology, analytical epidemiology and operational epidemiology.

The descriptive epidemiologist measures the occurrence of cancer, preferably in well-defined populations. As will become evident, there are signal differences in the occurrence of cancer, both between and within countries, as there are changes in the occurrence over time. The task of the analytical epidemiologist is to uncover the underlying determinants; once these have been reasonably well established, an intervention study may be mounted to see whether their removal results in a diminution in the frequency of the disease, in other words, operational epidemiology.

Epidemiological methods are mainly observational. While the experimentalist sets the conditions for his experiments and then observes the results, the epidemiologist usually has to observe the results and then determine what the experimental conditions had been. The peculiarity of cancer epidemiology lies in the long (usually decades) interval between the action of the determinant(s) and the occurrence of cancer, and in the multiplicity of determinants which are often dissimilar for different cancers. Further, the same determinant may give rise to cancer in several organs.

The historical background to modern cancer epidemiology has been reviewed by Clemmesen (1965). Although it is quite clear that the epidemiological way of thinking was known to Hippocrates, Ramazzini, in 1700, pointed out that nuns have a different incidence of cancer of the uterus when compared with other females, a finding confirmed in 1844 when Rigoni Stern published a report on cancer of the breast and uterus for the city of Verona, comparing the incidence in unmarried and married females and showing the relationship of marital status to these cancers. Pott, in 1775, suggested the occupational link between scrotal cancer and exposure to soot in English chimney sweeps.

Descriptive Epidemiology

Cancer in a Defined Population

Measures

The impact of cancer on a defined population can be measured in several ways: incidence, mortality and prevalence. Cancer incidence (or morbidity) is the annual number of newly diagnosed cases of cancer occurring in a defined population. Cancer mortality is the annual number of cancer deaths in the population. As measures of cancer risk they are usually expressed as incidence or mortality rates per 100 000 population per annum. The point prevalence is the number of persons with cancer existing in a defined population at a given point of time. This measure (little used) is also usually expressed as so many cases of cancer per 100 000 population. In contrast to these so-called crude rates, age-specific rates are based on the number of cancers occurring in a particular age group. These again are expressed as so many cancers per 100 000 persons in a given age group per annum: age-specific rates are the best measure of cancer risk in a population. They are also used in the calculation of an age-standardised rate (see below). The World Health Organization recommends that age-specific rates be calculated as follows: under one year, 1–4 years, 5–9 years, 10–14 and similar 5-year age groups from 15 to 84 years, ending with 85 years and over. If numbers of cases are rather small, the use of the 10-year age groups is permissible.

To calculate rates, a census population is the most reliable denominator. Although most vital statistics offices issue mid-year and end of year population estimates taking into account births and deaths, such estimates may be distorted by the effect of migration in and out of the area in question. Further, migration is not likely to be uniform for all age groups.

As cancer increases in incidence with age, population age structure can have quite a profound effect on the crude rates (but not on age-specific rates). To remove this effect and thus permit a more valid comparison between populations, it is usual to calculate age-standardised rates. Age-specific rates, calculated by 5-year age groups, are applied to a standard population, and the number of cases of cancer to be expected if the standard population had the same age-specific cancer rates as the population in question is determined. The standard population used for this purpose is usually denoted the "world-standard population". This was based on the age structure of 46 countries in 1950. Examples of age standardisation may be found in Cancer Incidence in Five Continents (Waterhouse et al. 1982). The necessity for age standardisation may be shown by the following example. The crude cancer mortality rate for Polish-born American males in 1959–1961 was over eight times higher than in Poland (754.0 vs. 91.4). Age standardisation corrects for the large differences in the age structure of these populations (only 5% of the migrants were aged below 35 years, compared with 60% of the population of Poland) resulting in age-standardised rates of 176.9 for Polish-born Americans compared to 108.9 for the population of Poland (i. e. 176.9 vs. 108.9).

Doll and Cook (1967) devised a truncated standard rate which examines only the 35–64 age group, a period of life when it is considered cancer diagnosis is most likely to be accurate and complete. Use of this age interval obviates the effect of underregistration in older age groups. Day (1982) has popularised the cumulative rate. This can be regarded as a measure of the probability of dying from or contracting cancer up to a certain age in the absence of other causes of death. A commonly used age interval is 0–74, the result being expressed as a percentage. Thus, in Birmingham, in the United Kingdom, the cumulative incidence rate for lung cancers in males in 1973–1976 was 10.6%: put in another way, about one chance in ten. It must be stressed that while age-standardised rates are required if it is wished to compare the overall cancer risk in populations, such rates are synoptic and conceal the information which can be derived from looking at the age-specific rates. To compare the magnitude of the burden, crude rates are to be preferred.

Cancer Incidence Data

Incidence data are collected by cancer registries which may be national, e.g. Finland, or local, e.g. Varese (Italy). By counting all newly diagnosed cases, an incidence register should provide the most accurate picture of the burden of cancer in a population. Registries expend considerable effort to ensure complete coverage and to avoid duplicate registrations of the same case reported from various institutions or at different times. However, there must be few cancer registries that are sure that *all* cancer cases are recorded. The mechanisms of cancer registration are diverse, being well discussed in the monograph Cancer Registration and its Techniques (MacLennan et al. 1978). While most registries publish an annual report, this is often focused on local interests. For international comparison, the most useful compilations are those of the Cancer Incidence in Five Continents series. The fifth volume (Muir et al. 1987) gives data for 137 populations in 36 countries, presented in a standard form throughout, giving not only age-specific incidence rates by 5-year age groups for various sites of cancer, but also age-standardised and cumulative rates. The range of data collected by registries varies considerably, some record a bare core, others have a very large amount of clinical and treatment detail. While there is always the temptation to collect a large amount of information, there is frequently an inverse ratio between quality and quantity. Table 1 gives the minimal data set recommended in MacLennan et al. (1978).

Several indices can be used to assess the completeness of registration. These are:

1. The ratio of mortality to morbidity which, of course, varies with site.
2. The proportion of persons of unknown age which should not rise above 5% for any site; however, owing to incomplete information often accompanying notification of skin cancer, the proportion may be higher for this site.

Table 1. Minimal data for any cancer registry

Item	Comments
The person	
Personal identification[a]	
Name	According to local usage
Sex	
Date of birth	
Age	Estimate if not known
Demographic	
Address	Usual residence
Ethnic group	When population consists of two or more groups
The tumour	
Topography (site)	Primary if possible
Morphology (histology)	Whenever possible
Incidence date	Month and year
Most valid basis of diagnosis	
Source of information (e.g. hospital record no., name of physician, etc.)	To facilitate subsequent search for additional information

[a] The minimum collected is that which ensures that if the same individual is reported again to the registry, he will be recognised as being the same person.

3. The proportion of individuals for whom registration was based on the mention of cancer on a death certificate only, a figure which should not exceed 10% (a lower figure speaks for completeness only when all deaths in the population are medically certified).
4. The proportion of cases with histological confirmation of diagnosis. A high proportion does not necessarily mean complete registration. It may be that the majority of cases are reported by pathologists with few coming from other sources. With increasing utilisation of biochemical methods of diagnosis of high reliability, these are likely to increase in importance.

Incidence data cannot be better than the hospital case histories and other records on which they are based. Cases of cancer not recognised as such are obviously not registered, and completeness of registration of all the recognised cases and pruning of duplicate registrations varies between registries and over time. There are also considerable differences and changes in registration practice for borderline lesions (e.g. mixed tumours of salivary gland, papillomas of the urinary bladder and benign brain tumours, occult cancers found at autopsy, multiple and multifocal cancers). Diagnostic methods, criteria and terminology as well as coding practices are also not uniform. All this bears on comparability of cancer incidence data.

Cancer Mortality Data

Mortality from cancer is derived from death certificates on which cancer is stated to be either the "disease or condition directly leading to death" or the "underlying antecedent cause".

Mortality data are as good as the death certificates on which they are based. In many countries, not all deaths are certified by physicians, and the quality of those certificates signed by physicians may vary considerably. Mortality data are, by definition, weighted by the lethal cancers. Skin cancer, although frequently diagnosed, is an infrequent cause of death; for lung, oesophagus and pancreas cancers, incidence and mortality are usually very close. While studies of death certificates have shown that some persons were erroneously considered to have cancer, and that for others with the disease the cancer was not stated as the cause of death, such errors have, on the whole, tended to balance out. Cancer diagnosis and death certification in the elderly is often much less accurate than for the younger age groups, and part of the fall in the mortality rates observed in the elderly may be due to this. It has been shown that for patients known to have cancer during their life, malignant disease may not appear on the death certificate, death being due to some other cause. If cancer is mentioned, then the site is frequently less precisely stated than in incidence records, e.g. large bowel rather than rectum.

Several studies have shown that there is considerable international variation in the coding of death certificates; thus in a series of over 1000 death certificates mentioning cancer, 84 were coded to breast cancer in the United States; 95, 89, 87, 65, 93 and 86, respectively, in France, Canada, England and Wales, Federal Republic of Germany, Norway and the Soviet Union (Percy and Dolman 1978). This study does not imply that any one country was "right", only that national coding practices differ.

Mortality data are available from national statistics offices. The most useful compilations are those of the late Professor Segi (Segi and Kurihara 1972) and WHO. Recently, WHO has preferred to make the data available to interested research workers on magnetic tape from the Cancer Mortality Data Bank, rather than by publishing.

The quality of mortality data is indicated to some extent by the percentage of deaths ascribed to "senility, symptoms and other ill-defined conditions", which should not exceed 10%, and by the percentage of deaths certified by physicians (this should be close to 100%).

Cancer in the Absence of a Defined Population

Should the population at risk from which cases come not be definable, rates cannot be calculated. However, some idea of the distribution of cancer can be obtained from examining the relative proportions of the various forms of cancer compared to the total number of cancers (taken as 100%) in a particular series; such series are usually histologically diagnosed cancers or patients treated by radiotherapy or other methods.

Biopsy series have precision of the diagnosis as a chief advantage but are open to serious bias being weighted by the more accessible neoplasms. Further, unless all histological material in an area is pooled and is available for study, an important group may be absent, e.g. gynaecological biopsies. The admission policies of a hospital, the facilities available for diagnosis and treatment, and the interest of the staff may give rise to considerable distortion. Thus, the raised incidence of stomach cancer in Madras in southern India was obscured by the large influx of patients seeking treatment for cancers of the head and neck from a much wider region.

Autopsy series are selected samples of hospital admissions who are themselves selected. Dead males are more likely to be autopsied than dead females, and there is a tendency for the number of necropsies to decline in those dying after the age of 40, the age at which cancer could be expected to be more frequent. In a few regions it may be possible to refer the autopsies to well-defined populations at risk, e.g. Malmö in Sweden. If it is possible to pool biopsy and autopsy results from a region, it may be possible to relate these to a defined population and calculate a minimum incidence rate, as was done for the cities of Algiers, Constantine and Oran in Algeria. Whatever the true rates are, they cannot be less than those obtained by this method. The most useful source of information of this type of material is Cancer Occurrence in Developing Countries (Parkin 1986).

The relative frequency series are more difficult to compare than incidence or mortality data. A commonly used adjustment is to use Tuyns' (1968) method for age correction. This procedure cannot, and does not claim to, correct for the other sources of bias. Experience with relative frequency data has shown that a consistently high frequency for a given site, such as nasopharynx in Singapore or primary liver cancer in southern Africa, with no obvious source of bias points to a common type of cancer. A low relative frequency should be approached with much more caution as the influence of underdiagnosis is usually more difficult to assess.

One of the disadvantages of relative frequency data is that an increased (or decreased) frequency of one cancer decreases (or increases) the relative frequency (percentage) of all the others.

Cancer Variation by Sex

The risk of most cancers is higher among males than among females, particularly for respiratory and upper alimentary tract cancers. More frequent among females are cancers of the breast, of the genital organs, of the gallbladder and of the thyroid.

Cancer Variation by Age

Considering all cancers combined, malignant neoplasms are rare in childhood and adolescence, but after the age of about 25 their risk increases exponentially. With cancer of most sites, as with carcinomas of the alimentary tract, skin and prostate, the relation between risk and age can be approximated by the exponential or power function and is thus approximately linear when plotted on the semi-log or log-log scale (logarithm of risk against either age or logarithm of age) (Fig. 1). Several shapes for the risk-by-age curves have been described: (1) A continuing increase in risk with advancing age, exemplified by lung cancer in males, suggesting the effects of continued exposure to a carcinogen; such curves may turn over in the oldest age groups reflecting either underdiagnosis or the existence of a birth cohort effect, the oldest age groups being less exposed than those born later, as in (2); (3) an age-risk curve consisting of two linear segments, the first having a steeper slope than the second, exemplified by breast or cervix uteri cancers; for breast cancer this has been interpreted as reflecting the existence of two different types of cancer – premenopausal and postmenopausal; (4) a peak of risk in childhood (due to Wilms' tumour), followed by a decline and then a gradient rise representing other kidney cancers.

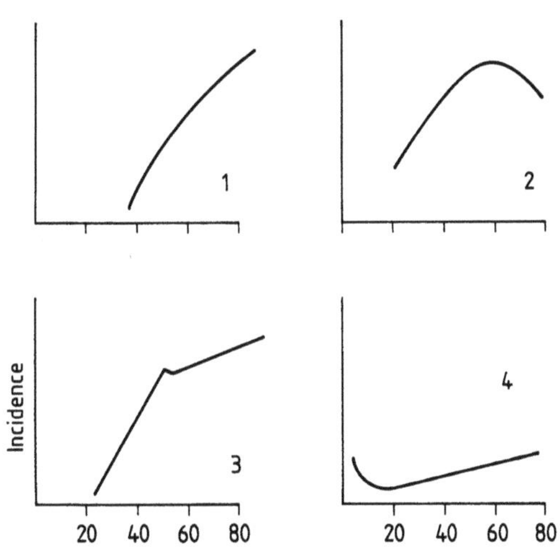

Fig. 1. Cancer age curves indicating differing aetiologies (see text)

Cancer Variation over Space

The geographical distribution of cancer varies greatly with cancer site. For instance, cancer of the mouth is very frequent in India, cancer of the nasopharynx in southern China, cancers of the colon and breast (rather rare in India and China) in occidental countries in which both oral and nasopharynx cancers tend to be rare. Because of these differences, the geography of cancer will be discussed for a few cancer sites of surgical importance separately, and here only a few general remarks are given. Areas of relatively high and low risk can be found also within countries. Cancer mortality and incidence atlases have been published recently for several countries (Mason et al. 1975; Kemp et al. 1985; Cislaghi et al. 1986).

Cancer Variation by Special Population Characteristics: Migrant Studies

Differences in cancer risk between population subgroups have been observed. Examples, to mention only a few, are: ethnicity (low skin cancer risk and high prostate cancer risk for US Blacks as compared with US Whites); religion (low lung, larynx and colon cancer risk among Mormons as compared with total US population) or both (low risk of mouth cancer and high risk of breast cancer among Parsis compared with other Indian religious groups in Bombay); occupation (increased lung cancer risk in asbestos workers and uranium miners); marital status (increased risk of cervix uteri cancer in women who are or have been married); socioeconomic status (decreased stomach cancer risk in high-income groups); residence (the higher risk for most cancers in urban than in rural areas, notable exceptions being lip and skin cancers). It is likely that the demographic characteristic associated with a peculiarity of cancer risk reflects the level of some cancer determinant(s), e.g. low tobacco consumption by Mormons. Hence, population subgroups identifiable by some demographic characteristics may provide special opportunities for studies of cancer causation. Migrant studies take advantage of the great natural experiments that result when populations of a given genetic composition change environments. The ensuing changes in site-specific cancer risk and comparison with the risk in the population of the host country and in those remaining in the country of origin often permit easier identification of the agents responsible and of the mode and time of action of these agents, including the influence of the age when exposures changed. For example, studies on cancer in migrants from such diverse countries as Japan and Poland to the United States have indicated that events early in life, in childhood, determine the risk of stomach cancer, whereas the risk of colon cancer depends on factors acting in adulthood (Haenszel and Kurihara 1968).

Cancer Variation over Time

Overall cancer incidence and mortality are increasing in most male populations while tending to be stable or decreasing slightly in females. Much more meaningful is analysis of time trends for specific cancers. Among the most outstanding features are the increase in the incidence of lung cancer and of cutaneous melanoma and the virtually universal decrease in the incidence of cancers of the stomach and of the cervix uteri.

Time trends are often difficult to evaluate because of chance variation (particularly for rare cancers and in small populations), the lack of data for sufficiently long periods (this pertains more often to incidence than to mortality), changes in cancer classification (decennial changes of the International Classification of Diseases), alternations in diagnostic methods and precision, changes in the completeness and quality of data (here again, incidence data are affected more often) and, for mortality, changes in survival.

The Magnitude of the Cancer Burden

Parkin et al. (1988) have recently attempted to assess the world burden of cancer. Their results appear in Table 2 from which it can be seen that, in 1980, the most common cancer site in the world was stomach, for both sexes combined. However, when males and females are considered separately, lung cancer is first in rank in males and breast cancer in females. The five cancer sites in this table account for over 60% of all malignancies. There are, however, major differences in the patterns when various parts of the world are compared. These are shown for Western and Eastern Europe, North America, Southern Asia and China in the same table.

Interpretation of Descriptive Epidemiology Data

Interpretation of differences in cancer occurrence requires caution. Observed geographical, demographic

Table 2. Most frequent cancers in selected regions of the world around 1980. (Data from Parkin et al. 1988)

Rank	World		Western Europe		Eastern Europe		North America		Southern Asia		China	
	Males	Females	Males	Females	Males	Females	Males	Females	Males	Females	Males	Females
1 Site ’000s	Lung 514	Breast 572	Lung 65	Breast 68	Lung 33	Breast 23	Lung 92	Breast 118	Mouth/pharynx 87	Cervix 91	Stomach 126	Cervix 132
2 Site ’000s	Stomach 409	Cervix 466	Colon/rectum 37	Colon/rectum 39	Stomach 19	Colon/rectum 13	Prostate 82	Colon/rectum 67	Lung 36	Breast 67	Oesophagus 108	Stomach 75
3 Site ’000s	Colon/rectum 286	Colon/rectum 286	Prostate 32	Stomach 17	Colon/rectum 13	Stomach 12	Colon/rectum 64	Lung 39	Oesophagus 30	Mouth/pharynx 45	Liver 78	Oesophagus 59
4 Site ’000s	Mouth/pharynx 257	Stomach 261	Stomach 21	Corpus uteri 16	Prostate 9	Cervix 12	Bladder 31	Corpus uteri 33	Larynx 28	Oesophagus 23	Lung 44	Colon/rectum 37
5 Site ’000s	Prostate 236	Corpus uteri 149	Bladder 18	Cervix 15	Mouth/pharynx 6	Corpus uteri 8	Lymphatic 23	Lymphatic 21	Stomach 21	Ovary 16	Colon/rectum 43	Liver 34
All sites, ’000s	3247	3103	278	262	129	119	441	434	363	367	647	526

or temporal variation may reflect the differences and changes in the completeness of reporting, in the accuracy of diagnosis, in the accessibility of medical facilities or even in medical terminology rather than true differences in cancer frequency due to variation in exposure to cancer determinants. Despite these caveats, the most rational interpretation of the differences described above is that they are largely due to differences in the environment, using that word in its broad sense to include not only air, water and occupational exposures, but also diet, cultural habits (such as age at marriage) and personal habits such as tobacco use.

Analytical Epidemiology

Elucidation of the reasons for the difference in cancer occurrence is the domain of the analytical epidemiologist. The techniques most commonly used are those of the correlation or so-called ecological study as well as case-control and cohort studies.

Cancer Determinants (Risk Factors)

"Cancer determinants" (or "cancer risk factors") is a broad term encompassing not only ionising radiation and chemically discrete carcinogens, co-carcinogens and promoters, but also the characteristics, situations and cultural and personal habits increasing cancer risk.

There is a multitude and diversity of cancer risk factors. For example, among determinants for skin cancer are a genetically based lack of skin pigmentation, solar and ionising radiation, carcinogenic hydrocarbons, arsenic; among lung cancer risk factors are tobacco smoke, uranium mining, ionising radiation, asbestos; among bladder cancer determinants are tobacco smoke, aniline dyes, schistosomiasis; cancer of the cervix uteri is more frequent and cancer of the corpus uteri less frequent in married and parous women. The joint effects of cancer determinants may be multiplicative rather than additive, e.g. tobacco and alcohol in cancer of the oesophagus (Tuyns et al. 1977) and larynx (Tuyns et al. 1988). Furthermore, the end effect of a variety of low-level exposures and the existence of a threshold ("safe") exposure are very difficult to ascertain. There is increasing realisation that promoters are likely to be as important as initiators in the development of cancer.

Correlation Studies

In some studies, the correlation between the occurrence of different cancers is examined. Their geographical distribution or time trends may be compared; for example, a positive correlation between colon and breast cancer suggests some common risk factors (perhaps fat consumption). A correlation between the occurrence of different cancers in individuals rather than in populations may be looked for by investigating the occurrence of multiple cancers. An increased risk of a second primary cancer in the lung or in the urinary bladder observed in patients with laryngeal cancer points to a common determinant (most probably tobacco smoking).

More common are the correlation (ecological) studies which compare the occurrence of a cancer with the occurrence of an exposure or of a variety of exposures, such as national consumption of dairy products or number of cigarettes smoked, to the occurrence of a cancer in a variety of regions. Thus, large bowel cancer mortality correlates well with the total proportion of caloric intake due to fat, and cancer of the rectum with beer. However, there is no guarantee that it is those individuals in the populations compared who consume the larger amounts of fat or of beer who develop the cancers in question. Such items are also interlinked with many other exposures, the heavy alcohol consumer being also frequently a heavy smoker. Historical information on exposure is frequently not available or of poor quality, and many correlations of the type described compare current cancer levels and current consumption, thus ignoring the induction period.

Such studies can be strengthened by taking a probability sample of the populations being compared to give a much better estimate of the spectrum of consumption in the populations, as was done in the international comparison of large bowel cancer in Denmark and Finland which sought to uncover dietary causes (Jensen et al. 1982). Much more confidence can be placed in analytical epidemiological investigations, looking at risk in individuals. Such studies fall into two main groups – case-control and cohort – described below.

Identification of cancer determinants may be sometimes easier for rare cancers, even when the population at risk is not well known. A sudden increase in the incidence of a very rare form of liver cancer, angiosarcoma, was quickly linked with occupational exposure to vinyl chloride, as was the increase in vaginal clear cell adenocarcinoma with maternal exposure to stilboestrol. These examples show the important contribution that the astute clinician can make when he notices the unusual case or recognises the importance of a cluster of a few cases. The much quoted demonstration in 1775 by the surgeon Perceval Pott of the increased risks of scrotal cancer in chimney sweeps falls into this category.

Case-Control (Retrospective) Studies

In the case-control approach, patients (cases) with a given form of cancer are asked a series of questions which the investigator thinks may throw light on past exposure to the determinants of the disease. The same questions are posed to a series of controls without the disease who are generally matched individually to one of the cancer patients by sex and 5-year age group. The answers obtained from cases and controls are then compared to see whether there are any differences. Thus, Wynder and Graham (1950) and Doll and Hill (1952) found that lung cancer cases were more likely to have smoked cigarettes than controls. While case-control studies can be undertaken fairly quickly (2–3 years) and cheaply (US $ 100 000–US $ 250 000), they are not without problems. Such problems are extensively discussed in texts such as that by Schlesselman (1982). The main sources of difficulty lie in: (a) possibility of bias in the selection of the cases and of the controls, e.g. rich patients only taken as cases or as controls; (b) differential recall, i.e. those who have cancer may be more likely to make an effort to try and remember some exposure in the past than those without cancer; (c) memory bias – people genuinely forget what they did in the past particularly in relation to diet; (d) misclassification – if patients without the cancer under study are erroneously considered to have cancer, and vice versa, it is less likely that determinants will be uncovered, and differences in recall by the two groups will again have the same result, misclassification in general tending to diminish the chance of finding a difference between cases and controls.

In the analysis of case-control studies, it is usual to compute the odds ratio, as shown in Table 3, for each of the items considered singly. The differences observed are then tested to see whether those observed are likely to be statistically significant. While the *P* value is of interest, a much more informative measure is the confidence interval which indicates how precise the estimate of risk is likely to be. In general, the smaller the study, the more likely is the confidence interval to be wide. It must always be remembered that for every 100 questions asked, it is likely that five will show a statistically significant difference between cases and controls *by chance alone*, using the conventional 5% level. For this reason, more confidence can be attached to a result which supports a hypothesis written down before the study began. It must also be remembered that probability operates in both directions and a truly "positive" finding may not be uncovered, again by chance.

Table 3. Computation of odds ratio

	With lung cancer	Control	Total
Ever-smoked	80	50	130
Non-smoker	20	50	70
	100	100	200

The odds ratio is $\frac{80 \times 50}{20 \times 50} = 4$ and expresses the likelihood that a lung cancer patient will have smoked compared to persons of the same age and sex without lung cancer.

As many risk factors are interconnected, it is usual to undertake a multivariate analysis to see which of the factors seem to be the most pertinent. Thus, an increased consumption of alcohol by those with lung cancer may only reflect the consumption of cigarettes by heavy drinkers. A well-conducted case-control study can give an indication for the population studied of the proportion of a given cancer due to a given risk factor. Thus in many publications the percentage of lung cancer attributable to tobacco smoking is around 80%–90%. The surgeon can play a major role in this area by encouraging epidemiologists and giving access to his cancer patients and suitable controls.

Cohort (Prospective) Studies

The major advantages of cohort studies lie in the fact that exposure data are recorded before the disease occurs and should therefore be unbiased. Participants are questioned on their current habits and such responses tend to be more accurate than for past exposure. Prospective studies of mortality allow study of a wide spectrum of end-points. It is usual to compare the cancer risk in the cohort with that of the general population of the same age and sex composition.

However, there are disadvantages: a large population sample is needed and the study group needs to be followed for many years as the induction period has to elapse before cancer can arise in cohort members. For this reason, a cohort may be characterised some time in the past, e.g. all working in a factory in

1960, and cancer risk between then and the end of the study determined. However, this approach also has its inconvenience in that it is rarely possible to enquire about the personal habits of cohort members. To get round this difficulty, epidemiologists may try to mount a case-control study within the cohort interviewing cases as they arise and choosing controls from other cohort members. The following studies, that by Dorn and that of man-made mineral fibres followed groups which could be considered to be "preassembled", i.e. insured veterans and employees of an industry, respectively. The Hirayama study comprised a probability sample of an entire population.

The Dorn Study

The Dorn study (Kahn 1966), extending over 8½ years of observation, involved 293,000 holders of life insurance policies, most of them United States Army veterans. Questionnaires on smoking habits were sent to veterans, mainly white males from the middle and upper socioeconomic classes. A total of 46,270 deaths was recorded from 12,265,674 person-years, between the ages of 35 and 84 (July 1954–December 1962). Figure 2 shows mortality ratios for all causes of death, by smoking category. Figure 3 shows mortality ratios among cigarette smokers for lung cancer.

The Hirayama Study

The Hirayama study (1982) was a cohort study of a probability sample of 265,118 adults aged at least 40 in the whole of Japan and was begun in autumn 1965. Cohort members filled in a rather simple questionnaire on personal habits and on the consumption of common dietary items and were followed till death. Among the many interesting findings was the demonstration that daily consumption of yellow-green vegetables (containing more than 1000 IU beta-carotene per 100 g) significantly reduced the risk of cancer of stomach and lung and the possible role of passive smoking in lung cancer. Data are given in Fig. 4.

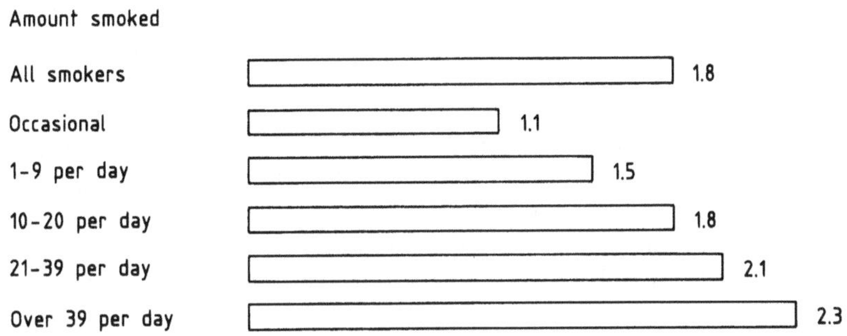

Fig. 2. Overall mortality ratios for deaths from all causes by number of cigarettes smoked daily: comparison with non-smokers. (Data from Kahn 1966)

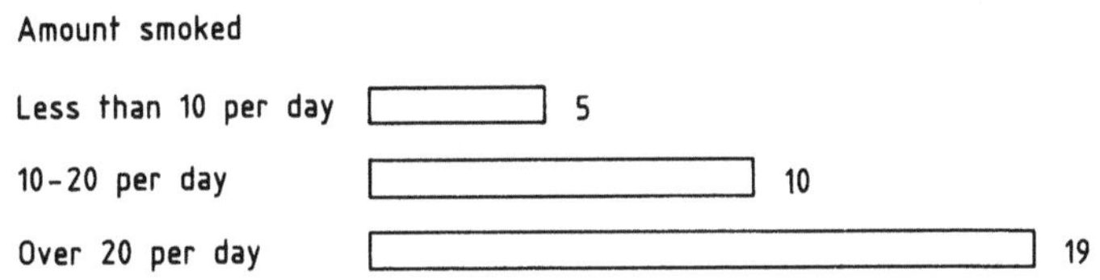

Fig. 3. Lung cancer mortality ratios by number of cigarettes smoked daily: comparison with non-smokers. (Data from Kahn 1966)

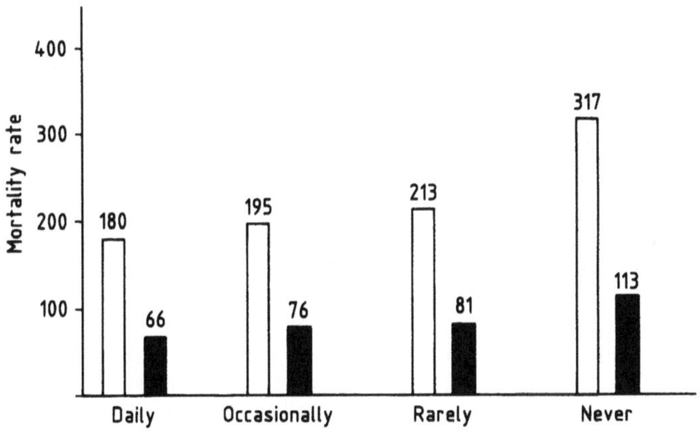

Fig. 4. Stomach *(open bars)* and lung *(solid bars)* cancer mortality rates by consumption of green and yellow vegetables, Japan 1970–1982. (Data from Hirayama 1982)

The Man-Made Mineral Fibres Exposure Study in Seven European Countries

This retrospective study (Saracci 1986) was conducted on a cohort of 25,146 workers in 13 man-made mineral fibre factories (rockwool, slagwool, glasswool and continuous filament). Information was gathered on the past exposure of production workers. Association of chronic respiratory disease or respiratory cancer was evaluated with respect to occupation within the industry. During 309,353 person-years of observation, 1659 deaths were recorded. Exposure to glasswool was not associated with increased risk of lung cancer whereas production of rockwool – using a process now discontinued – gave rise to a modest increase, an increase not observed with the new production method.

Operational Epidemiology

There are many examples of operational epidemiology in the field of infectious disease, vaccination having, for example, eliminated smallpox. Reduction in smoking by British physicians was eventually accompanied by a fall in lung cancer incidence (Doll and Peto 1976) (Fig. 5): appropriate protective measures eliminated skin cancer as an occupational risk for radiologists. Given that most cancers probably have several causes, elimination or reduction in the exposure to one of them is unlikely to result in the disappearance of the disease in question. Nonetheless, for those cancers in which determinants act synergistically, such as alcohol and tobacco in the genesis of oesophageal cancer in western France, reduction in one of the exposures can have a very considerable effect on risk as Tuyns et al. (1977) have shown.

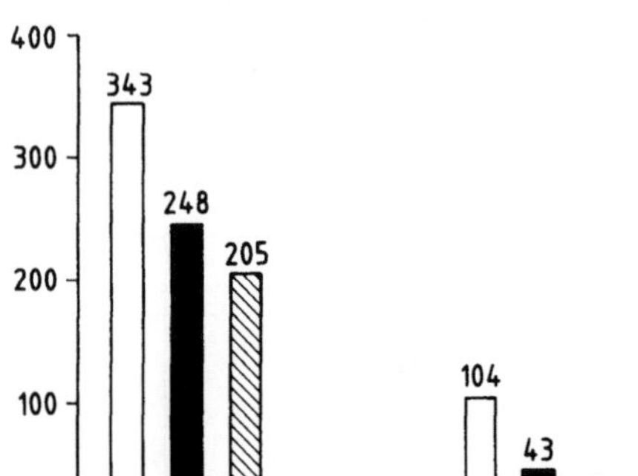

Fig. 5. Annual age-standardised death rate per 100 000. *Open bars,* current smokers of any tobacco; *solid bars,* ex-smokers; *hatched bars,* non-smokers. (Data from Doll and Peto 1976)

Common Cancers of Surgical Importance

In this section, a brief description is given of the geographical distribution of a few cancers of surgical importance selected on the grounds of their high frequency in global terms (Figs. 6 and 7).

Oesophagus

The distribution of oesophageal cancer varies enormously throughout the world. In the Caspian littoral of Iran, age-standardised incidence rates of over 100 in males and nearly 200 in females have been recorded, levels of incidence vastly greater than those observed elsewhere, rates in males being around 25, 29 and 15 in Shanghai, Hong Kong and Bombay, respectively. In parts of France, rates in males are around 30, the disease being however very uncommon in females, in contrast to most of the United Kingdom where, although rates in males are modest, around 6, they are comparatively high, around 3, in females. Within the United States, the Black population of both sexes has rates which are generally four times greater than in Whites.

There appear to be at least two types of oesophageal cancer, that observed in Europe and the Americas where generally there is a very high male/female ratio and the determinants are the consumption of alcoholic beverages (frequently strong) and tobacco, and that occurring in what has been described as the "oesophageal cancer belt" which stretches from eastern Turkey to the north of China via Iran and the southern Soviet Union. The risk factors appear to be different, being possibly strongly influenced by diets low in fresh fruit and vegetables.

Stomach

As noted above, although declining nearly everywhere, stomach cancer is still globally the most frequent of all forms of malignancy. There is a very wide range of incidence, with age-standardised rates varying from 75 per 100 000 in males in Osaka, Japan, to 11 in Connecticut, USA, but even lower rates are seen in India and West Africa. Within Europe there is considerable variation, ranging from 39 in Varese, Italy (with comparable rates in much of eastern Europe) to 18 in Sweden. Within many countries, the disease is much more common in the lower socioeconomic groups (OPCS 1978; Logan 1982).

It has been suggested that a high intake of smoked, salted and pickled foods is related to a high

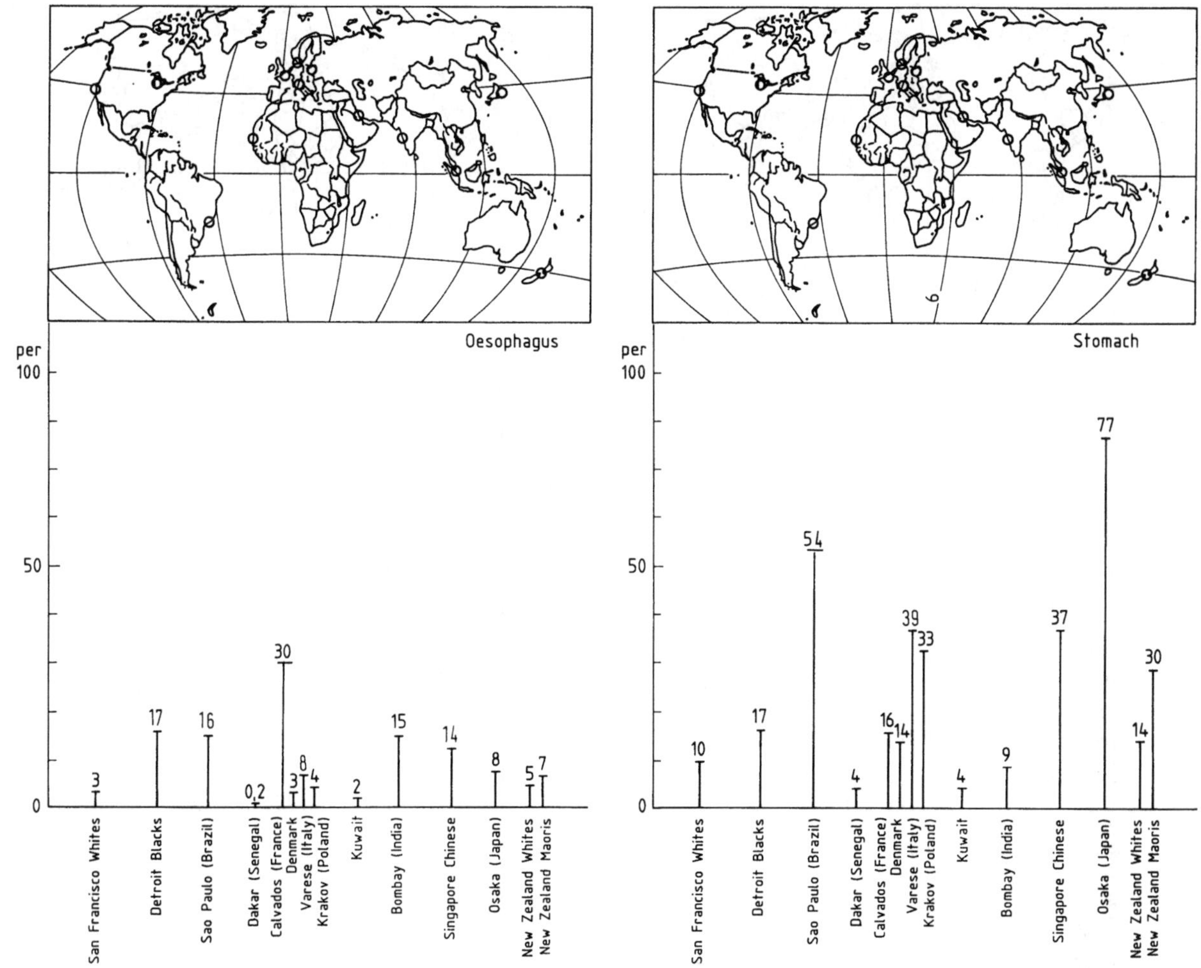

Fig. 6. Incidence of common cancers of surgical importance (oesophagus and stomach) in selected regions of the world (males, 1978–1982)

stomach cancer level. In recent years it has been shown that risk is reduced in those who frequently consume green and yellow vegetables, fresh fruit and milk. These observations have been made in several countries and may thus explain the falling risk as there is a greater availability of dairy products, fresh fruit and vegetables throughout the year in much of the world, with consequent diminution in the consumption of smoked, salted and pickled foods.

Large Bowel

Generally speaking, the rates for large bowel cancer tend to be highest in the more prosperous portions of the world, North America, western Europe and Australasia, with rates of 30–40 per 100 000 in males and 30–35 per 100 000 in females (there is usually a two-fold male excess for rectal cancer, whereas cancer of the colon is frequently slightly commoner in women). These high levels contrast with rates of under 10 in Latin America and of around 17 in much of Japan. In eastern Europe, notably Poland, rates tend to be half of those in western Europe. Rates are under 10 in India and appear to be very low, around 2, in Dakar, Senegal.

A series of epidemiological studies, including the evidence from changes in risk in persons migrating from areas low of incidence, e.g. Japan, to areas of high incidence, e.g. the United States, suggest that environmental factors are of particular importance for these cancers. In brief, diets associated with a large component of meat and fat have been associated with high risk and those with high levels of dietary fibre and cruciferous vegetables (such as cabbage) with a lower risk. Although there is evidence suggesting an association between colonic cancer risk and a high-fat diet, several equally reputable investigators have not been able to confirm this.

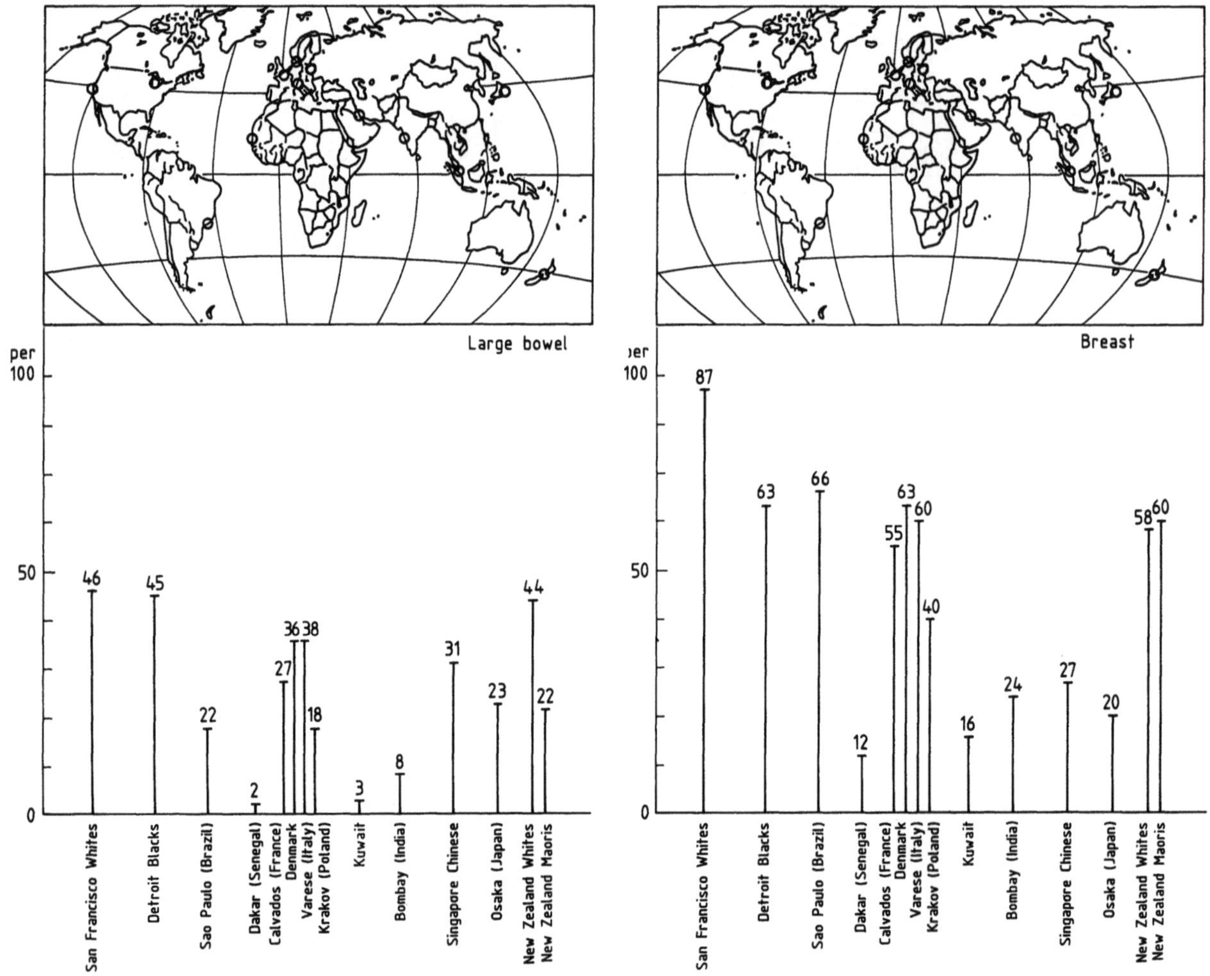

Fig. 7. Incidence of common cancers of surgical importance in selected regions of the world (large bowel – males, 1978–1982; breast – females, 1978–1982)

Breast

Globally the commonest cancer in women, the incidence of breast cancer nonetheless shows very large variations, ranging from nearly 90 per 100 000 in white populations in California to about 20 in Japanese women in Osaka and 12 in Dakar, Senegal. Levels of risk tend to be intermediate in much of Europe, higher in the West, around 60 in much of the United Kingdom, falling to around 20 in rural parts of Poland. In Japan, Singapore and Hong Kong Chinese and in India, the rates are around or over 20. Of great interest are the levels of this cancer seen in Chinese and Japanese living in California and Hawaii which are well over double those seen in the countries of origin, suggesting once again the influence of the new environment as the migrants have not changed their genetic composition.

The risk of breast cancer is influenced by age at first full-term pregnancy, a reduction which is substantial as women who bear a child before the age of 18 have one-third the risk of women whose first child was born after the age of 30. While there seems to be general agreement that pregnancy influences breast cancer through hormonal patterns which may themselves be governed to some degree by diet, notably fat, the fat/breast cancer association has, however, been described as weak in individuals when tested by case-control studies as opposed to correlations examining populations.

Conclusions

The science of epidemiology helps place the work of the surgeon, rightly concerned with diagnosis and treatment of the individual patient, in a larger perspective. As noted above, the surgeon can assist the epidemiologist by encouraging access to his patients for the conduct of case-control studies. As these frequently require large numbers, the collaboration of several surgeons is often needed. The Cancer Registry constitutes a vital element in evaluation of the results of treatment. While the individual clinician will follow his patients closely and thus monitor the results of treatment, the Cancer Registry, which obtains information on all persons with a given cancer diagnosed in a defined population and which matches these cases with death certificates, is in a much better position to evaluate the results of treatment for an entire population. The Cancer Registry is able to take into account patients who were, for various reasons, never treated, as well as those treated without curative intent. Such data permit comparison of "state of the art" therapy by highly skilled teams for selected patients and the survival for the population as a whole. Such information is of the greatest value for those planning the provision of health services. When survival statistics are looked at on a national level, there has unfortunately been little improvement in survival for patients with cancers of lung, stomach, oesophagus and large bowel. While survival for women with breast cancer has improved, mortality in many countries has remained almost constant, which could be interpreted as implying that the definition of breast cancer has changed over the years.

References

Cislaghi C, Decarli A, La Vecchia C, Laverda N, Mezzanotte G, Smans M (1986) Data, statistics and maps on cancer mortality, Italy 1975–1977. Pitagora, Bologna

Clemmesen J (1965) Statistical studies in malignant neoplasms. I. Review and results. Munksgaard, Copenhagen

Day NE (1982) A new measure of age-standardized incidence, the cumulative rate. IARC Sci Publ 15: 443–452

Doll R, Cook P (1967) Summarizing indices for comparison of cancer incidence data. Int J Cancer 2: 269–279

Doll R, Hill AB (1952) A study of the aetiology of carcinoma of the lung. Br Med J 2: 1271–1286

Doll R, Peto R (1976) Mortality in relation to smoking: 20 years' observations in male British doctors. Br Med J 2: 1525–1536

Haenszel W, Kurihara M (1968) Studies of Japanese migrants. I. Mortality from cancer and other diseases among Japanese in the United States. JNCI 40: 43–68

Hirayama M (1982) Does daily intake of green and yellow vegetables induce the risk of cancer in man? An example of the application of epidemiological methods to the identification of individuals at risk. IARC Sci Publ 39: 531–540

Jensen OM, MacLennan R, Wahrendorf J (1982) Diet, bowel function, fecal characteristics and large bowel cancer in Denmark and Finland. Nutr Cancer 4: 5–19

Kahn HA (1966) The Dorn study of smoking and mortality among US veterans: report on eight and one-half years of observation. NCI Monogr 19: 1–126

Kemp I, Boyle P, Smans M, Muir C (eds) (1985) Atlas of cancer in Scotland, 1975–1980. Incidence and epidemiological perspective. IARC Sci Publ 72

Logan WPD (ed) (1982) Cancer mortality by occupational and social class, 1851–1971. IARC. Sci Publ 36

MacLennan R, Muir CS, Steintitz R, Winkler A (eds) (1978) Cancer registration and its techniques. IARC Sci Publ 21

Mason TJ, McKay FW, Hoover R, Fraumeni JF (1975) Atlas of cancer mortality for US countries: 1950–1969, US Government Printing Office, Washington (DHEW publication no 75–780)

Muir C, Waterhouse J, Mack T, Powell J, Whelan S (eds) (1987) Cancer incidence in five continents, vol 5. IARC Sci Publ 88

OPCS (Office of Population Censuses and Surveys) (1978) Occupational mortality. HMSO, London (The Registrar General's decennial supplement for England and Wales, 1970–1972, series DS no 1)

Parkin DM (ed) (1986) Cancer occurrence in developing countries. IARC Sci Publ 75

Parkin DM, Laara E, Muir CS (1988) Estimates of the worldwide frequency of 16 major cancers in 1980. Int J Cancer 41: 184–197

Percy C, Dolman R (1978) Comparison of the coding of death certificates related to cancer in seven countries. Public Health Rep 93 (4): 335–350

Pott P (1775) Chirurgical observations relative to the cataract, the polyps of the nose, cancer of the scrotum, the different kinds of ruptures and the mortification of the toes and feet. Hawes, Clarke and Collins, London

Ramazzini B (1940) De morbis artificum diatriba (1700). University of Chicago Press, Chicago

Sarraci R (1986) Ten years of epidemiologic investigations in man-made mineral fibres and health. Scand J Work Environ Health [Suppl 1] 12: 5–11

Schlesselman JJ (1982) Case-control studies – design, conduct, analysis. Oxford University Press, New York, pp 7–354

Segi M, Kurihara M (1972) Cancer mortality for selected sites in 24 countries, no 6. Japan Cancer Society, Tokyo

Stern Rigoni (1842) I giornale per servire al progressi della pathologia e della terepeutica 2: 507

Stern Rigoni (1844) Annali Universali di Medicina 110: 484

Tuyns AJ (1968) Studies on cancer relative frequencies (ratio studies). A method for computing an age-standardized cancer ratio. Int J Cancer 3: 397–403

Tuyns AJ, Pequignot G, Jensen OM (1977) Le cancer de l'oesophage en Ille-et-Vilaine en fonction des niveaux de consommation d'alcool et de tabac: des risques qui se multiplient. Bull Cancer 64: 45–60

Tuyns AJ, Estève J, Raymond L, Berrino F, Benhamou E, Blanchet F, Boffetta P et al. (1988) Cancer of the larynx-hypopharynx, tobacco and alcohol: the IARC international case-control study in Torino and Varese, Saragossa and Navarra, Geneva and Calvados. Int J Cancer 41: 483–491

Waterhouse JAH, Muir CS, Powell J, Shanmugaratnam K (eds) (1982) Cancer incidence in five continents, vol 4. IARC Sci Publ 42

Wynder EL, Graham EA (1950) Tobacco smoking as a possible etiologic factor in bronchiogenic carcinoma. A study of 684 proved cases. JAMA 143: 329–336

Detection and Diagnosis

Cancer Staging

I. BESZNYÁK

The two most engaging powers of an author are to make new things familiar, familiar things new.

W. M. Thackeray

Introduction

Nowadays the aetiology and mechanism of development of malignant tumours are not clearly understood, there is no exact knowledge on their dissemination, their course is affected by numerous factors, and their incidence shows a rapid growth all over the world. Diagnostics and the successful management of cancer patients require a multidisciplinary team approach. The efforts of medicine are therefore fully justified, that is to say that uniform diagnostic and therapeutic principles should take shape, the data should be presented and evaluated on a common basis and the results obtained should be comparable.

As defined by Mountain et al. (1974) "staging of neoplastic disease is the procedure of assigning a simple coded designator to a patient in accordance with an established set of rules". The staging of cancer represents an attempt to group patients according to the extent of the neoplastic process. The subdivision of all possible presentations of a given malignancy into a limited number of meaningful specific categories or stages is crucial to advancing knowledge about the disease. The widespread use of a single staging system permits investigators to define homogeneous groups for evaluation of natural history and response to therapy.

The TNM System and Its History

Pioneer work on the clinical classification of malignant tumours was done by the League of Nations Health Organization in 1929 (Beahrs and Myers 1983). Between 1942 and 1952 Denoix (1946) developed a classification that can be regarded as the ancestor of the TNM system. In 1950 the International Union Against Cancer (*Union Internationale Contre le Cancer*, UICC) appointed a Committee on Tumour Nomenclature and Statistics and adopted the general definitions of local extension of malignant tumours as a basis for its work on clinical stage classification, which was suggested by the WHO Subcommittee on the Registration of Cases of Cancer as well as their Statistical Presentation (1952). The activity of the International Commission on Stage Grouping and Presentation of Results (ICPR) of the International Congress of Radiology is also noteworthy. The latter and the UICC Committee on Tumour Nomenclature and Statistics held a joint meeting in 1953. The general standpoints on which the tumour classification by anatomical extent can be performed, using the TNM system, were agreed upon (Beahrs and Myers 1983).

In 1954 the UICC Research Commission set up a special Committee on Clinical Stage Classification and Applied Statistics "to pursue studies in this field and to extend the general technique of classification to cancer at all sites". This committee, in 1958 (Paris), selected the breast and larynx as first localisations to discuss and prepared recommendations for the clinical stage classification and for the presentation of results (Spiessl et al. 1982). One year later, also in Paris, they presented their revised proposals for breast tumours for clinical use and evaluation over a 5-year period.

The American Joint Committee on Cancer (AJCC) was first organised on January 9, 1959, as the American Joint Committee for Cancer Staging and End-Results Reporting (AJC) for the purpose of developing a system of clinical staging of cancer by site acceptable to the American medical profession. Each of the six sponsoring organisations designated three members to the committee, under the guidance of the American College of Surgeons which served as administrative sponsor. Subcommittees, called "task forces", were appointed in order to develop classifications of tumours of different anatomical sites.

Between 1960 and 1967 the UICC Committee on Clinical Stage Classification and Applied Statistics published nine brochures describing proposals for the classification of 23 tumour sites. It was recommended that the classification proposals be subjected to prospective and retrospective trial for a 5-year period. These brochures were issued in 1968 in the Livre de Poche series, then in 1969 a complementary booklet was published detailing recommendations for the determination and expression of cancer survival rates and for the setting-up of field trials. This work was subsequently translated into eleven languages.

In the United States the AJC decided to use the TNM system to describe the anatomical extent of the tumour prior to treatment and from this to develop the classification into stages. Task forces (19 up to 1981) were appointed to focus on cancers of particular sites. Results of retrospective studies have been published in separate fascicles and articles recommending stage classifications for cancer at various sites.

The TNM Committee of the UICC and the AJC had been working with similar objectives and along similar lines, although points of view and methods have sometimes differed. To seek closer cooperation and mutual understanding, the representatives of the UICC and AJC gathered on 21–22 November, 1969, in Toronto. Agreement was reached to have previous consultation prior to presenting any of the two groups' classifications. At the International Cancer Congress (1970, Houston) a joint exhibit was presented. Since then numerous joint meetings in Geneva and Houston have been devoted to the classification of the specific cancer sites.

In 1974, a second edition of the Livre de Poche was published by the UICC containing some new site classifications and amendments of previously published classifications, and this was followed by the third edition in 1978. An enlarged and revised edition appeared in 1982 (Spiessl et al. 1982).

The AJC sponsored a National Cancer Conference on Classification and Staging in Atlanta on 27–28 March, 1976. This conference delineated what had been achieved up to that time and brought into focus future activities and needs. The various data in previously published individual-site fascicles with the addition of other material were brought together to form a Manual for Staging of Cancer in 1977. A second edition appeared in 1983 (Beahrs and Myers). The expanding role of the AJC suggested that the original name of the committee no longer portrayed the broader scope of its activities and interests, therefore the name was changed to American Joint Committee on Cancer (AJCC) in 1980.

In developing its classifications, the AJCC has employed the principles of the TNM system as described by the UICC where appropriate but not if other staging recommendations are already accepted and widely used (Beahrs and Myers 1983). The TNM Committee and the AJCC have attempted to come to an agreement on staging of cancer at many anatomical sites. The differences in the recommendations of the two committees are gradually decreasing. In 1985 a UICC classification on eye tumours (UICC 1985a), in 1982 and 1985 a TNM Atlas were published (UICC 1982, 1985b). The fourth edition of the UICC classification was issued in 1987 (Hermanek and Sobin 1987).

National committees and international organisations have taken an increasing interest in the TNM system. They are referred to by initials, as follows:

AJCC,	American Joint Committee on Cancer
BIJC,	British Isles Joint TNM Classification Committee
CNC,	Canadian National TNM Committee
CNU-TNM,	Comité National Uruguayo TNM
DSK,	Deutschsprachiger TNM-Ausschuß (Komitee)
EORTC,	European Organization for Research on Treatment of Cancer
FIGO,	Fédération Internationale de Gynécologie et d'Obstétrique
FTNM,	French TNM Group
ICC,	Italian Committee for TNM cancer classification
ICPR,	International Commission on Stage Grouping in Cancer and the Presentation of Results of the International Society of Radiology
JJC,	Japanese Joint Committee
SIOP,	Société Internationale d'Oncologie Pédiatrique

Cancer staging is not an exact science. As new information becomes available on aetiology, various methods of diagnosis and treatment, the classification and staging of tumours changes. Reflecting the change in our knowledge and the state of the art, the system ought to be revised; this may, however, occur only at reasonable periods. In agreement with the opinion expressed by clinicians of many countries, the UICC has decided that the site classifications should not be changed unless this appears to be unavoidable. It is the intention that the classification published in the 4th edition of the UICC TNM classification (Hermanek and Sobin 1987), should remain unchanged until some major advances in diagnosis and treatment, relevant to a particular site, require reconsideration of the current classification.

Principles and Purposes of Staging

"Staging" comprises all the physical, radiological, surgical and pathological procedures that are supposed to clarify the extent of the tumorous process in order to identify subgroups of patients at a similar stage of development of the disease, supposing that a similar extent would mean a similar prognosis. For most cancer sites the staging recommendations are concerned only with the *anatomical extent* of the disease. At present, staging classifications are based on the determination of the extent of the tumorous process. Their design requires a thorough knowledge, primarily from morphological examinations. An accurate histological diagnosis is, therefore, an essential element in the correct evaluation of the cancer patient. The involvement of WHO in developing internationally acceptable criteria for the histological diagnosis of tumours resulted in the International Histological Classification of Tumours which contains, in a 25-volume series with illustrations, the definitions of tumour types and a nomenclature proposal. A complete and well-known compendium of illustrations and definitions of tumours is the Atlas of Tumour Pathology. Its volumes are also used as basic reference by pathologists throughout the world.

Staging based on the anatomic extent of the disease mostly corresponds to reality. In several instances, however, age of the patient (thyroid) and grade (soft-tissue sarcoma) are also important factors to consider. As the prognosis depends not only on the anatomical extent of the tumorous process, but also on the biological properties of the tumour, more and more research is being devoted to the "biological determinants" of cancer. The evaluation of cell kinetics, pathological characteristics and endocrine receptors, parameters of the immune surveillance system, are becoming more common. Cancer is a biological rather than an anatomical problem. Therefore "it appears likely that the present staging system based on the anatomic extent of cancer will be integrated and perhaps substituted by a more functional, biological staging system" (Veronesi 1984).

Classification and staging based on the TNM system rely on the assumption that cancers of a similar site of origin or histology share similar patterns of extension and growth. The size of the untreated primary cancer (T) is an important characteristic of the stage of the malignant process. As the primary tumour increases in size, at some point (and this event may happen at a very early period of its lifespan) local invasion occurs, followed by involvement of the regional lymph nodes (N) draining the area of the tumour, or by spread to the juxtaregional nodes. The period when this spread is manifest or discernible by currently available clinical examinations is another important marker in the progression of the tumorous process. It is usually later, mainly in the later period of tumour lifespan, that distant metastasis (M) becomes evident with the aid of clinical examinations. Therefore, metastasis is the latest time marker. These three important events (TNM) in the life history of cancer are used to indicate the degree of extension before definitive therapy begins (clinical staging, cTNM). Examination at the time of surgery and histological examination of the tissues removed may also identify the significant markers of the life history of cancer (TNM) as being different from what could be detected clinically prior to therapy. This may also serve as the basis for a stage classification (surgical-evaluative or pathological staging, pTNM). It may be a more accurate piece of information about the period of life history of the tumour and may be valuable for prognostic purposes; however, it cannot be confused with clinical diagnostic staging for evaluative and reporting purposes.

Proper classification and staging of malignant tumours may serve a number of related objectives, namely to:

1. Help the clinician plan treatment for the patient more appropriately. If the prognosis is good, radical treatment can be a major contribution to patient care. On the other hand, if the forecast is hopeless, the physician must refrain from inflicting unnecessary morbidity.
2. Assist in determining prognosis. The need for accurate prognosis is of greater importance when projected new therapies hold promise for only a minor incremental improvement over the existing therapy.
3. Evaluate results of management more reliably.
4. Compare statistics from various institutions more confidently and facilitate the exchange of information between centres. Clinical trials of new treatment modalities require that homogeneous groups of patients be available for comparison.
5. Contribute to the continuing investigation of human cancer and to help evaluate cancer control measures.

The principal purpose is to provide a method of conveying clinical experience to others without ambiguity (Sugarbaker et al. 1982).

General Rules of the TNM System

To standardise its application and to facilitate the use of the TNM system, international organisations have adopted some general rules. The TNM system is based on the assessment of three main components:

1. *T* represents the extent of the primary tumour with appropriate suffixes to describe the size of the tumour or involvement by direct extension.
2. *N* represents the condition of the regional lymph nodes (in certain regions of the juxtaregional lymph nodes), with appropriate suffixes to describe the absence or increasing degrees of the tumorous involvement.
3. *M* represents the absence or presence of distant metastases with appropriate suffixes to describe the degree of dissemination of the tumour.

The general rules according to the UICC principles applicable to all sites are as follows:

1. All cases should be confirmed histologically to classify and establish the extent of the tumour stage. Any other cases must be reported separately.

2.The UICC adopts two classifications:
Pretreatment Clinical Classification, Designated TNM. This is based on evidence acquired prior to the decision as to definitive treatment. Such evidence arises from clinical, radiological, endoscopic and other relevant findings. In some instances, it may be based additionally on the evidence derived from surgical exploration prior to the decision as to definitive treatment. [Note: until 1986 the AJCC distinguished *cTNM* (clinical diagnostic staging) using all information available prior to first definitive treatment, including pathological confirmation of the extent of disease by biopsy or invasive techniques and *sTNM* (surgical-evaluative staging) using all clinical information available plus that obtained on surgical exploration, usually done for a few inaccessible tumours that are not amenable to definitive resection. Furthermore, the AJCC distinguished between *rTNM* (retreatment staging), a classification when restaging was necessary for additional or secondary definitive treatment after an interval following first treatment, and *aTNM* (autopsy staging), used only when the cancer was first diagnosed at autopsy. Since 1987 the AJCC has only used cTNM and pTNM for those patients who have had complete surgical resection of their tumours.]
Postsurgical-Histopathological Classification, Designated pTNM. This is based on the evidence acquired prior to the decision as to definitive treatment, supplemented or modified by the additional evidence acquired from definitive surgery and from the examination of the therapeutically resected specimen.

3. The TNM categories, once established, must remain unchanged. The stage classification should not be modified as a result of information obtained from more definitive observations, for example, pretreatment clinical classification should not be influenced either by the fact that a patient experienced early recurrence or by information from a surgical or pathological report. When restaging is necessary for additional or secondary definitive treatment after a disease-free interval following first treatment, the tu-

mour may be described by TNM but must be identified by the symbol "r" (rTNM or rpTNM). Such cases should not be combined with a primary treatment series but should be grouped together, evaluated and reported separately.

4. In the clinical assessment of a patient, varying amounts of information may be used in determining each stage classification for each primary site. For all sites the minimal requirement for assessing the primary tumour, the regional and, if appropriate, the juxtaregional nodes and distant metastases are listed insofar as these apply to the TNM pretreatment clinical classification.

5. After assigning T, N and M categories, with degrees of extension, these may be grouped into clinical stages.

6. In spite of the fact that originally the TNM system was developed as a dual classification system (TNM and pTNM), it is the clinical TNM classification which is of paramount importance for purposes of reporting and evaluation. It is clear, since a considerable number of cancer patients never undergo surgery and they would thus be excluded from TNM classification if only pTNM were used.

7. If there is doubt concerning the correct T, N or M category to which a particular case should be allotted, then the lower (i.e. less advanced) category should be chosen. This will also be reflected in stage grouping.

8. The use of the certainty factor (C factor) is optional. It reflects the validity of classification according to the diagnostic methods employed.

C1 Evidence from standard diagnostic means
C2 Evidence by special diagnostic means
C3 Evidence from cytology, biopsy of explorative surgery
C4 Evidence following definitive surgery and pathological examination of the resected specimen
C5 Evidence obtained by autopsy

In addition to the above, the AJCC recommends some further considerations. First, at the time of surgical resection of a cancer, gross residual tumour must be identified under *R* to facilitate and aid in additional or further treatment of the patient. *R* does not enter the staging of the tumour.

Secondly, the degree of anaplasia should be recorded as determined on histological study under the letter *G*. If grading is well accepted at an anatomical site by the number 1 to 4, then four groups may be used.

Thirdly, the performance index of the host, considering all co-factors, should be recorded at the time of each stage classification and at follow-up examinations. This should be done under the letter designation *H*.

The Anatomical Regions and Sites

Staging systems have now been developed for nearly all sites. The second edition of the Manual for Staging of Cancer published by the AJCC (Beahrs and Myers 1983) enumerated 41 sites for staging. The fourth edition of UICC TNM classification booklet (Hermanek and Sobin 1987) classified 43 "sites" covering the greater part of malignant tumours.

None of the classifications include tumours of the adrenal, small intestine, parathyroid and pituitary glands. No staging is available for the haemoblastoses and leukaemias. The UICC introduced the staging of the eye and adnexa tumours on 1 January 1985, then that of the tumours of the paranasal sinuses, salivary glands, liver and biliary tract, pancreas and bone. The AJCC introduced staging of cancers of the penis and anal canal from January 1987 on. The latter has been discussed by the UICC since 1 January 1987 together with skin carcinomas. Both organisations introduced staging of tumours of the ampulla Vateri in January 1987. At the present time it is not considered practical to propose a TNM classification for either Hodgkin's disease or for non-Hodgkin's lymphoma (Hermanek and Sobin 1987).

The staging systems of the individual sites are discussed in detail in the relevant chapters.

Definitions of Symbols

In stage classification of tumours at various anatomical sites, an attempt is made to have definitions of the various symbols as similar as possible from one site to another and to simplify the staging as much as possible. Three capital letters are to describe the extent of cancer:

T Primary tumour
N Regional nodes
M Distant metastasis

Chronology of Classification

c Clinical-diagnostic
p Postsurgical treatment-pathological
s Surgical-evaluative
r Retreatment
a Autopsy

TNM Pretreatment Clinical Classification (TNM or cTNM)

T – Primary Tumour

TX The minimum requirements to assess the primary tumour cannot be met
TO No evidence of primary tumour
Tis Preinvasive carcinoma (carcinoma is situ)
T1–T4 Evidence of increasing degrees of size and/or local extent of primary tumour

N – Regional Lymph Nodes

NX The minimum requirements to assess the regional lymph nodes cannot be met
NO No evidence of regional lymph node involvement
N1–N4 Increasing degrees of demonstrable involvement of regional lymph nodes

M – Distant Metastases

MX The minimum requirements to assess the presence of distant metastasis cannot be met
MO No evidence of distant metastases
M1 Evidence of distant metastases

The category of M1 may be subdivided according to the following notations:

Pulmonary	:PUL
Osseus	:OSS
Hepatic	:HEP
Brain	:BRA
Lymph nodes	:LYM
Bone marrow	:MAR
Pleura	:PLE
Peritoneum	:PER
Skin	:SKI
Eye	:EYE
Other	:OTH

pTNM – Postsurgical Histopathological Classification

pT – Primary Tumour

pTX Postsurgical and histopathological extent of invasion cannot be met
pTN No evidence of tumour found on histological examination of specimen
pTis Preinvasive carcinoma (carcinoma in situ)
pT1–pT4 Postsurgical and histopathological evidence of increasing size and/or local extent of primary tumour

Further Information

In certain sites further information regarding the primary tumour may be recorded under the following headings:

G – Histopathological Grading

GX Grade cannot be assessed
G1 Well differentiated
G2 Moderately well differentiated
G3–G4 Poorly to very poorly differentiated; use whichever indicator is most appropriate (term or G plus number).

L – Lymphatic Invasion

LX Lymphatic invasion cannot be assessed
LO No evidence of lymphatic invasion
L1 Evidence of invasion of superficial lymphatics
L2 Evidence of invasion of deep lymphatics

V – Venous Invasion

VX Venous invasion cannot be assessed
VO Veins do not contain tumour
V1 Efferent veins contain tumour
V2 Distant veins contain tumour

pN – Regional Lymph Nodes

pNX The extent of invasion cannot be assessed
pNO No evidence of invasion of regional lymph nodes
pN1–pN3 Evidence of increasing degrees of extent of invasion of regional lymph nodes
pN4 Evidence of invasion of juxtaregional lymph nodes (where applicable)

pM – Distant Metastases

pMX Distant metastases cannot be assessed
pMO No evidence of distant metastases
pM1 Evidence of distant metastases – may be subdivided in the same way as M1

Additional Descriptors

y Symbol

In those cases in which definitive surgery is performed after treatment by other methods, the pTNM categories may be identified by a "y" prefix, e.g. ypT2 pN1 pMO. These cases must be reported separately.

r Symbol

Recurrent tumours may be described by TNM but must be identified by the symbol "r" placed before the appropriate TNM or pTNM category.

C Factor

A flexible system for indicating the information on which the TNM categories are based is recommended for optional use. Named the "level of certainty" or "C factor", it reflects the information available at a point in time and according to the diagnostic methods used (Arnal et al. 1967; Karrer 1983).

The C factor category definitions are as follows:
C1 Evidence from clinical examination only
C2 Evidence obtained by special diagnostic means
C3 Evidence from surgical exploration only
C4 Evidence of the extent of disease following definitive surgery and including the complete examination of the therapeutically resected specimen
C5 Evidence from autopsy

The TNM pretreatment clinical classification is therefore equivalent to C1, C2 and C3 in varying degrees of certainty while the pTNM postsurgical histopathological classification relies on the fact that a particular case may be recategorised from time to time as new evidence comes to light. The whole course of a patient's malignancy through time can therefore be expressed in a chronological manner suitable for computerisation.

R – Residual Tumour

This information does not enter into the establishing stage of tumour but should be recorded on the data form for use in considering additive therapy. When the cancer is treated by definitive surgical procedures, residual cancer, if any, is recorded:
RO No residual tumour
R1 Microscopic residual tumour
R2 Macroscopic residual tumour

Stage Grouping

Classification by the TNM achieves reasonably precise description and recording of the apparent anatomical extent of disease. A tumour with four degrees of T, four degrees of N and two degrees of M will have 32 TNM categories. For purposes of tabulation and analysis, except in very large series, it is necessary to condense these categories into a convenient number of TNM stage groups, usually four in number.

Future Prospects

The staging of malignant diseases is insufficient to help with an accurate prognosis for the individual patient with a given malignant process. A statistical probability for eventual metastasis or death is the best this system can offer. However, the TNM system has provided a major contribution to standardising the morphological classification of neoplastic disease.

It is not too difficult a task to predict some changes in the future of cancer staging. Diagnostic developments, e.g. MRI, may lead to changes because of the ability of these modalities to determine more accurately and noninvasively the anatomical extent of some tumours (Borg and Rosenthal 1984). Moreover, biological markers that reflect tumour distribution and the propensity for tumour invasion will certainly be found. By means of histological markers, it may become possible to improve our diagnostic possibilities, with the aid of histological markers to quantitate differentiation and perhaps even biological behaviour. These new, biological staging variables will be assimilated into new staging systems and even replace the current staging variables that are based on anatomical extent (Henson 1985).

The deficiencies of the TNM system are well known, it should be subject to several corrections and improvements. Its disadvantages are, however, far outweighed by the advantages its application can offer. Therefore, it is beyond doubt that cancer staging and the TNM system have proved their viability and are fully recommended for use in clinical oncology.

References

Arnal ML, Dold U, Ehlers CT, Gögler E, Hamperl H, Karrer K, Oberhoffer G et al. (1967) Zur Klassifizierung der Geschwulstkrankheiten. Der "gesicherte" TNM-Schlüssel. Erweiterungsvorschlag zu den "General Rules" der UICC. Methods Inf Med 6: 70–72

Beahrs OH, Myers MH (eds) (1983) Manual for staging of cancer. Lippincott, Philadelphia

Borg SA, Rosenthal S (1984) Handbook of cancer diagnosis and staging. A clinical atlas. Wiley and Sons, New York

Denoix P (1946) Enquête permanente dans les centres anticancereux. Bull Inst Natl Santé (Paris) 1: 70–75

Henson DE (1985) Staging for cancer. Arch Pathol Lab Med 109: 13–16

Hermanek P (1986) Staging (TNM, pTNM). In: Gall F, Hermanek P, Tonak J (eds) Chirurgische Onkologie. Springer, Berlin Heidelberg New York, pp 121–126

Hermanek P, Sobin LH (eds) (1987) TNM classification of malignant tumours, 4th edn. Springer, Berlin Heidelberg New York

Karrer K (1983) Prognose, Klassifikation. In: Denck H, Karrer K (eds) Chirurgische Onkologie. Edition medizin, Weinheim, pp 27–43

Mountain CF, Carr DT, Anderson WAD (1974) A system for the clinical staging of lung cancer. AJR 120: 130–138

Spiessl B, Dold U, Ott G (1971) Proposal to add a factor of evidence to the TNM System. Int J Cancer 7: 372

Spiessl B, Scheibe O, Wagner O (eds) (1982) TNM-atlas. Illustrated guide to the classification of malignant tumours. Springer, Berlin Heidelberg New York

Sugarbaker PH, Dunnick NR, Sugarbaker EV (1982) Diagnosis and staging. In: De Vita VT Jr, Hellman S, Rosenberg SA (eds) Cancer. Principles and practice of oncology. Lippincott, Philadelphia

UICC (1982) TNM classification of malignant tumours, 3rd edn. UICC, Geneva

UICC (1985a) Classification of opthalmic tumours. UICC, Geneva

UICC (1985b) TNM-atlas. Illustrated guide to the TNM, pTNM classification of malignant tumours, 2nd edn. Springer, Berlin Heidelberg New York

Veronesi U (1984) Staging surgery (Abstr). 2nd Congress of the European Society of Surgical Oncology, Oct 17–19, Geneva

Cancer Detection and Screening: High-Risk Groups

D. M. Parkin

Introduction

Because cancer treatment is most successful, measured as survival, when begun at an early stage, there has been a search for methods capable of identifying early cancers or even premalignant disease. "Screening" as defined as the application of simple tests to a population so as to separate individuals who probably have the disease in question from those who probably do not; positive cases can then be subjected to conventional (more intensive) diagnostic procedures. A distinction is sometimes made from "early diagnosis", where the individuals tested have symptomatic, although unrecognised disease. Since screening programmes are usually applied to subjects who have not specifically sought medical advice, there is a special obligation to ensure that they are effective in reducing morbidity and mortality.

Not all cancers are suitable for screening programmes. The prevalence of preclinical detectable disease in the population may be too low to justify the costs involved both because the duration of this phase of the natural history of the disease may be rather short and because most cancers are relatively rare anyway.

Screening tests, which are applied to large numbers of individuals, should be simple, inexpensive, safe or free from side effects and acceptable to the target population. The validity of a test is expressed in terms of its sensitivity (the proportion of cases which are detected), its specificity (the proportion of non-diseased persons classified as negative) and the predictive value of a positive result (the probability of a positive result being a true positive). In general, the sensitivity of a particular test can only be increased at the expense of a loss of specificity, and vice versa. Occasionally a "positive" test can be defined as a value on a ratio scale (e.g. the level of serum alpha-foetoprotein in liver cancer screening); but usually it is a subjective judgement of clinical findings, X-ray appearance or cytological patterns.

Sensitivity and specificity can also be altered by applying more than one test at a time (e.g. mammography plus palpation for breast cancer) or applying the same test sequentially on several occasions (e.g. tests for faecal occult blood).

Evaluation of Screening

The evaluation of a screening *programme* – whether it is worth introduction – depends upon consideration of the ratio of benefit expected to the costs involved in a specific population. Thus, for rare cancers the yield of cases may be too small to justify the costs of screening the community despite the availability of a valid test, or for common cancers it may be that there is no real advantage to the cancer patient in being diagnosed early. Many important elements contribute to overall effectiveness of a screening programme, other than the biology of the disease concerned, or the characteristics of the screening test. Thus, there should be an agreed policy which includes the identification of the target population and individuals in it; measures to ensure high coverage and attendance; facilities for carrying out, interpreting and ensuring quality control of screening tests; facilities for diagnosis and treatment and a referral system between the individual, laboratory and clinician (Hakama et al. 1985). Variations in these organisational factors can result in different programmes, which use the same screening methods, having quite disparate results.

Benefits of Screening

What to Measure

Since screening aims to detect early disease and improve prognosis, it seems evident that success should be measured in terms of improved survival rates or stage of disease at diagnosis. Whilst absence of change in these parameters may mean that screening has been unsuccessful, they do not provide an adequate measure of effectiveness. There are several biases inherent in such observations (Cole and Morrison 1978). First, if the people undergoing screening are not chosen randomly, there is likely to be some selection bias, which means that those screened are likely to be health-conscious individuals who, even in the absence of screening, may have had a better prognosis than a group that did not accept such tests. Even if allocation were random, however, further bias results from lead time and length bias. "Lead time" is the interval between the time of detection by screening and time at which the disease would otherwise have been diagnosed, so that the gain in apparent survival is due simply to advancing the time of diagnosis. "Length bias" arises because screening tests that are applied to a population at intervals are more likely to detect cancer cases with a long preclinical phase than faster-growing tumours. Cases detected by screening are thus likely to be a biased sample of all cases, with a relatively favourable prognosis. In addition to this, when the condition sought by screening is a precursor of invasive cancer (as in cervical cancer screening), many of the lesions discovered may never have led to cancer, so that their discovery and treatment is of much less benefit to the population than might be supposed.

For these reasons, an appraisal of the effectiveness of screening can be made only by measuring to what degree the objectives of screening are achieved. When screening is for early cancer, these objectives are reductions in mortality (and, perhaps, late complications of disease); when it is aimed at a precancerous condition, reduction in the incidence of invasive disease is a suitable measure. Finally, considerations of the quality of life might be important if early diagnosis leads to a more simple or less traumatic methods of treatment, even though overall mortality is unchanged.

How to Measure

Intervention Studies. The ideal evaluative method is the randomised controlled trial. A less satisfactory alternative is to compare mortality in geographical areas where screening has been introduced with control areas, but this requires high compliance (with screening or non-screening, depending on area) and control of geographical differences.

Observational Studies. Trials of screening are difficult to organise, expensive and time consuming; furthermore, because the benefits of early diagnosis appear obvious there may seem to be no need for a controlled trial in which a proportion of the population is not offered the screening programme, and they may be judged unethical, or the control group may receive screening outside the trial. As a result, the effectiveness of screening must often be assessed from the results of programmes introduced directly as a service. This is still possible, but the interpretation requires consideration of the effect of extraneous variables.

Descriptive studies investigate time trends or geographical variation in disease mortality (or incidence) in relation to the level of screening activity. Although it is almost impossible to exclude multiple alternative explanations for the (expected) inverse association, the sheer volume and coherence of multiple studies may, as in the case of cervical cancer screening (see below), prove persuasive.

Analytical studies compare the risk of mortality (or incidence) of cancer in relation to screening history at the individual level. Cohort studies require the long-term follow-up of individuals, and comparison of disease rates in relation to screening histories. A major problem is selection bias, which is difficult to allow for in the analysis of results. Case-control studies offer an alternative method of obtaining similar results and involve a comparison of screening histories in individuals who do or do not exhibit the outcome which screening aims to prevent (usually this would be death from cancer).

Cost of Screening

The net cost of a screening programme is the difference between the cost of screening activities (considered in this section) and the savings which result from the detection and treatment of disease at an early stage, rather than by conventional methods. The cost of a programme is not simply the financial cost of all the tests which are delivered. Some of these will be false negatives, which give rise to misplaced reassurance and may result in delay in presentation when symptoms do appear. False positive tests result in unnecessary time-consuming and possibly hazardous investigations. Some screening tests may even detect lesions which would never have become clinical cancer. These might be considered as false positives, since as far as the individual is concerned, they result in useless interventions. There may even be a small risk from the test itself, even for the great majority of individuals who are true negatives – in the early years of mammographic screening, when radiation doses were relatively high, it was at least arguable that the risks of radiation-induced cancer outweighed any possible benefit from screening under the age of 50.

High-Risk Groups

Costs of screening can be reduced if examinations are confined to subgroups of the population who are at increased risk, that is with a prevalence of disease considerably greater than in persons at low risk – a difference expressed in terms of relative risk. Selective screening is only useful if a substantial fraction of cases can be found in a high-risk group that is sufficiently small to give rise to worthwhile savings in costs.

In practice, all cancer screening programmes are selective, since they include only certain age groups and may be confined to one sex. Even if screening for breast cancer were equally effective (as measured by sensitivity/specificity) at all ages, there is obviously a lower age limit at which screening is not worthwhile; for example the 57% of the Danish population under age 40 yields only 5.6% of the new cases, and the 51% under 35 only 2.2% (Jensen 1982). The rational choice of a cut-off point would depend primarily on considerations of costs and benefits.

The use of other "risk factors" such as exposures to carcinogens or family or personal history, to define high-risk groups for screening is less satisfactory. This is because in order to identify most potential cases (i.e. achieve high programme sensitivity) the relative risk of the factor concerned has to be large, which is almost never the case, or the risk group must comprise such a large percentage of the population that the advantages of selection are lost (Hakama 1984). Because of this, several attempts have been made to increase programme sensitivity by combining risk factors, and to use such combinations to define a high-risk group. A theoretical example is shown in Table 1 which considers three independent factors combined in various ways to define

Table 1. Combined risk factors in the identification of high-risk groups. (After Hakama 1984)

	A	B	C	A+B	B+C	A+B+C	A or B or C
Size of risk group (% total population)	50	20	10	10	2	1	64
Relative risk	2	5	10	10	50	100	7.6
Proportion of total cases in risk group	67	56	53	53	51	50	93

a high-risk group. This example illustrates that if a high-risk group is sufficiently small to result in a reasonable saving in cost, then the cases deriving from the unscreened population become too numerous (i. e. the sensitivity of the programme is low). In certain industrial settings, potential exposure to carcinogens seems to merit regular examinations – however, the considerations are the same as for other screening programmes – they must be of proven effectiveness and produce an overall benefit commensurate with their cost. Industrial screening is not a substitute for industrial hygiene.

Screening for Cancers at Specific Sites

Cervical Cancer

The first major screening programmes for cancer were those for carcinoma of the cervix by means of exfoliative cytology. Little need was seen in the 1950s for randomised trials since the benefits to be expected seemed obvious; this has led to continuing debate over the value of screening. However, there is a great deal of non-experimental data confirming its overall effectiveness.

Evaluation

Several descriptive studies have shown that the intensity of screening in different areas correlates closely with reductions in incidence or mortality rates from cervical cancer. The most complete analysis is that of incidence in the Nordic countries (Hakama 1982) in each of which the screening experience has been rather different. The fall in incidence was closely related to the coverage offered by the organised mass screening programmes, and time trends in age-specific rates showed that the falls were confined almost entirely to the age groups which had been subjected to screening, with little change or even an increase in incidence in older women.

Several cohort studies, comparing risk of invasive cancer in screened and unscreened women, have been published. Although the effects of selection bias (see What to Measure) cannot be eliminated, the large diminution in risk in screened women (seven- to ten-fold) cannot reasonably be ascribed to such factors. Case-control studies compare screening histories of women with invasive cancer with control subjects. The first such study investigated the screening histories of 212 hospital cases of cancer and of age-matched residential controls (Clarke and Anderson 1979). A relative risk of 2.7 was observed in the unscreened women compared with those who had had at least one test in the preceding 5 years. Subsequent studies all confirmed a protective effect of screening and provided information on the relative protection in relationship to the time elapsed since the last test (see below).

Organisation

The evidence that screening for cervical cancer is an effective procedure is overwhelming, and the fact that some programmes achieve sub-optimal results, for example in the United Kingdom, is a result of defects in the organisational aspects referred to above (see Evaluation of Screening). Analytical studies (case-control and cohort) can be used to estimate the duration of the protection provided by a negative screening test. The pooled data from ten screening programmes in eight countries (IARC Working Group 1986) are shown in Table 2.

These results can be used to estimate the lifetime protection that a woman could acquire provided that she attended regularly for screening and that treatment of detected lesions was completely successful. Three-yearly screening between 25 and 64 (13 tests) would give about 90% protection, 5-yearly screening between 35 and 64 (six tests) would give 70%–75% protection, and even screening every 10 years at these ages should provide 50% protection.

None of the known risk factors appears suitable for identifying a high-risk group for selective screening. However, women who have had a dysplasia or carcinoma in situ treated remain a high risk of developing invasive cervical cancer (Hakama and Pukkala 1977) so that such women may be offered screening tests at shorter than average intervals.

Table 2. Relative protection against cervical cancer in women with two or more negative smears

Time since last negative smear (months)	0–11	12–23	24–35	36–47	48–59	60–71	72–119	120+	Never screened
Relative protection	15.3	11.9	8.0	5.3	2.8	3.6	1.6	0.8	1.0

Breast Cancer

Two methods exist for presymptomatic detection of breast cancer, mammography with or without physical examination of the breasts, and breast self-examination (BSE) performed by the individual herself. Whichever is used, there must be sufficient medical facilities to ensure the rapid diagnostic follow-up of the abnormalities detected and appropriate therapy for any cancers which are found. In contrast to cervical cancer, results from randomised trials evaluating early detection of breast cancer were available before screening had become widespread (Day et al. 1986). The first such study (the Health Insurance Plan of New York) was started in the early 1960s and involved random allocation of 62000 women aged 40–64 to a group offered screening by physical examination and mammography in 4 successive years or to a control group. The reduction in mortality in the screened group was about 30%, principally in women aged over 50 at the time of entry to the trial.

Following this study, screening clinics were introduced in many locations in the United States, and although the results of these so-called breast cancer demonstration and detection projects are difficult to evaluate, they did suggest that mammography was a more sensitive screening method than palpation and they also showed that thermography was of little value because of poor sensitivity and specificity.

Results of improvements in the efficiency of mammography which gives lower radiation exposure and the value of screening in women under 50 are now undergoing evaluation in studies in Sweden, Scotland, Canada and the Netherlands. Preliminary results suggest that mammography alone or combined with palpation can reduce mortality in women over 50 by about one-third. Poor results in younger women seem to be due to a shorter preclinical detectable interval, so that screening in women under 50 may have to be done annually. Although this reduction in risk is not large, because breast cancer is the commonest cancer of women in the world, the potential public benefit is important, and, in western countries at least, breast cancer screening offers the greatest potential impact to the efforts made in the field of preventive medicine.

Because of the high cost of screening by mammography (with or without physical examination), there is a great appeal in BSE programmes, where the subject herself performs the test and can do so as frequently as necessary to detect changes. There are many published reports of BSE projects, often describing reduced size and/or favourable stage distribution of lesions and improved survival in subjects who report practising BSE. However, the contributions of selection, lead time and length bias cannot be assessed, and to date there is no study which evaluates mortality reduction in a population practising BSE versus a suitable control group (Miller et al. 1985). A study in the United Kingdom will compare mortality rates in six districts, in two of which all women aged 45–65 have been invited to BSE classes, and a randomised study using factories as sampling units has been started in the Soviet Union, but it is unlikely that clear-cut results will emerge, at least for many years.

Whatever method of screening is adopted, no high-risk groups suitable for policies of selective screening can be identified (except in terms of age).

Colorectal Cancer

Colorectal cancer appears to be an excellent candidate for screening programmes since it is very common in both sexes in western countries, and survival rates are strongly related to the stage at diagnoses. Furthermore, some cancers arise in adenomatous polyps, which may therefore be a suitable target for early intervention.

Two diagnostic methods have been tried – regular sigmoidoscopic examination and testing for faecal occult blood with guaiac-impregnated paper slides. Sigmoidoscopy ought to be reasonably effective in detecting adenomatous polyps as well as early cancers, at least in the lower part of the colon and the rectum where most tumours arise. Several uncontrolled studies have suggested that regular sigmoidoscopy and removal of adenomas has reduced incidence and improved survival, but they are difficult to interpret. One trial of mulitphasic screening (including sigmoidoscopy) showed a reduction in colorectal cancer deaths in the group receiving regular examinations compared to controls [who were examined only on request (Dales et al. 1979)]; however, the two groups may not have been truly comparable, and the benefits of regular sigmoidoscopy remain questionable. There are considerable reservations, too, concerning acceptability to the general public of regular screening in this way.

The search for a simpler, cheaper, alternative has lead to introduction of tests for occult blood as a means of detecting early cancer (adenomas rarely bleed). Regular testing has become a routine part of the health check-up in several countries, but so far there are no results from controlled trials to indicate its value, although several are underway in the United States, England, Sweden and Denmark.

However, it is clear that the sensitivity of the usual screening test (Haemoccult II) in detecting cancer is relatively low – 40%–80% depending on the method used, and probably below this for adenomatous polyps. Attemps to improve sensitivity generally result in a large number of false positive tests, resulting in a heavy load of costly investigations. Pending the outcome of these studies, screening for colorectal cancer cannot be recommended as a general public health measure (Chamberlain et al. 1986).

The special circumstance of regular surveillance of known high-risk groups, such as the relatives of subjects with familial polyposis syndromes and individuals who have had adenomas or carcinomas resected in the past, is excluded from this conclusion. This is generally done by colonoscopy, although it has been proposed that faecal occult blood testing may have a role in surveillance of these groups, as well as for individuals with a family history suggesting one of the inherited colon cancer syndromes (Winawer et al. 1985). There appears to be no evidence as to whether this would be beneficial.

Stomach Cancer

Stomach cancer is an important cancer worldwide, with a poor prognosis when diagnosed. Experience in screening using photofluorography has been extensive only in Japan, where there are particularly high incidence rates. There were no controlled trials performed before introduction of mass screening, so inferences about effectiveness are based on indirect evidence. Although the declines in mortality rates observed in Japan have largely paralleled declines in incidence, suggesting that screening has played little part, it has been observed that declines are more marked in age groups subjected to screening and in areas where it has been most intense. The many studies which describe favourable stage distribution, survival and mortality in screened versus unscreened groups are of little help in evaluation because of the usual biases (see what to Measure). One case-control study (Oshima et al. 1986) suggests that a reduction of risk of death of up to 50% might be attributable to a past history of screening, and that the reduced risk persists for at least 2 years after the test.

A major drawback of gastric cancer screening is cost. Although double-contrast X-ray examination under image intensifier is relatively sensitive (about 85%), it certainly lacks specificity – a typical value of 86.5% means that the predictive value of a positive test is only 0.7% – so that as many as 14% of those undergoing screening will have to be referred for costly and uncomfortable diagnostic procedures such as gastroscopy. Screening for gastric cancer is not recommended outside Japan (Chamberlain et al. 1986).

Selective screening for groups at higher than average risk for gastric cancer – for example individuals with pernicious anaemia or previous gastric surgery – is likely to be of little value. The relative risk compared to the general population is modest, and such groups account for a very small fraction of gastric cancer cases; furthermore, the benefit of finding early cancers in such subjects is quite unknown (Logan and Langman 1983).

Liver Cancer

Liver cancer provides the (rare) opportunity for selective screening of a high-risk group. The relative risk associated with chronic carriage of hepatitis B surface antigen is high, so that in areas of high incidence, up to 80% of cases occur in a small subgroup (10%–15%) of the population. In China, it appears that follow-up of carriers with regular alpha-foetoprotein examination permits the identification of small, localised tumours amenable to resection. However, the validity of the test and its success in reducing mortality remain to be evaluated.

Oral Cancer

Oral cancer is a major public health problem in certain developing countries, and although primary prevention (avoidance of betel/tobacco chewing) is a more realistic approach, early detection has been considered as an ancilliary method of control. Primary health care workers are capable of successfully identifying oral cancer and pre-cancer, but whether doing so in a mass programme would reduce mortality rates is unknown.

Lung Cancer

Because of its high incidence and poor survival rate, lung cancer screening has been frequently advocated, and the annual chest X-ray forms a common component of many health check-ups. Sputum cytology can also detect early cases. Three randomised trials have been conducted in the United States on middle-aged smokers (Berlin et al. 1984). In two, the value of the addition of sputum cytology to annual X-ray was evaluated, whilst the other compared

4-monthly X-rays plus cytology, with advice for annual radiology. In none of these trials did the more intensively investigated group achieve better mortality than the "controls".

A randomised study in Czechoslovakia compared 6-monthly radiographic and cytologic examinations with a single examination after 3 years (Kubik and Polak 1986). Although cases in the screened group had a better overall stage distribution, mortality rates were similar to the controls (at least during the study period). There is thus no cause for optimism in relation to lung cancer screening, although the value of regular chest X-ray examination versus nothing remains to be assessed.

Conclusions

Screening and early detection are often referred to as "secondary prevention". Although this is clearly a misnomer (disease is not actually prevented), it serves to emphasise the anticipatory nature of such-programmes and the fact that they are generally deployed in the domaine of public health (applied to apparently well persons, rather than those seeking medical help). Screening procedures act as an adjunct to therapy in that they aim to make it more effective - but it is easy to be deluded that *any* early diagnosis is beneficial. At present it appears that only in the case of cervical and breast cancer is this really the case, although it remains possible that screening for stomach and colorectal cancer will prove to be worthwhile, at least in certain areas of the world.

References

Berlin NI, Buncher CR, Fontana RS, Frost JK, Melamed MR (1984) The National Cancer Institute Cooperative Early Lung Cancer Detection Program. Am Rev Respir Dis 130: 545-549

Chamberlain J, Day NE, Hakama M, Miller AB, Prorok P (1986) UICC Workshop of the project on evaluation of screening programmes for gastrointestinal cancer. Int J Cancer 37: 329-334

Clarke EA, Anderson TW (1979) Does screening by ‚Pap' smears help to prevent cervical cancer? A case control study. Lancet 2: 1-4

Cole P, Morrison AS (1978) Basic issues in cancer screening. UICC Tech Rep Ser 40: 7-39

Dales LG, Friedman GD, Collen MF (1979) Evaluating periodic multiphasic health checkups - a controlled trial. J Chronic Dis 32: 385-404

Day NE, Brines CJ, Chamberlain J, Hakama M, Miller AB, Prorok P (1986) UICC project on screening for cancer: report on the workshop on screening for breast cancer. Int J Cancer 38: 303-308

Hakama M (1982) Trends in the incidence of cervical cancer in the Nordic countries. In: Magnus K (ed) Trends in cancer incidence. Hemisphere, New York, pp 279-292

Hakama M (1984) Selective screening by risk groups. UICC Tech Rep Ser 78: 71-80

Hakama M, Pukkala E (1977) Selective screening for cervical cancer: experience of the Finnish mass screening system. Br J Prev Soc Med 31: 238-244

Hakama M, Chamberlain J, Day NE, Miller AB, Prorok PC (1985) Evaluation of screening programmes for gynaecological cancer. Br J Cancer 52: 669-673

IARC Working Group on Evaluation of Cervical Cancer Screening Programmes (1986) Screening for squamous cervical cancer: duration of low risk after negative results of cervical cytology and its implication for screening policies. Br Med J 293: 659-664

Jensen OM (1982) High risk groups and screening for cancer. Cancer Detect Prev 5: 343-348

Kubik A, Polak J (1986) Lung cancer detection. Results of a randomized prospective study in Czechoslovakia. Cancer 57: 2427-2437

Logan RFL, Langman MJS (1983) Screening for gastric cancer after gastric surgery. Lancet 2: 667-670

Miller AB, Chamberlain J, Tsechkovski M (1985) Self examination in the early detection of breast cancer. A review of the evidence with recommendations for further research. J Chronic Dis 38: 527-540

Oshima A, Hirata N, Ubukata TK, Umeda K, Fujimoto I (1986) Evaluation of a mass screening program for stomach cancer with a case-control study design. Int J Cancer 38: 829-833

Winawer SJ, Fath RB, Schottenfeld D, Herbert E (1985) Screening for colorectal cancer. In: Miller AB (ed) Screening for cancer. Academic, Orlando

A Modern View of Histopathological Diagnosis and Classification of Cancer[1]

F. Rilke

Introduction and General Principles

The typing of malignant tumors relies on histopathological diagnoses which are made after the gross and microscopic examination of tissues removed from living patients. This definition usually applies to surgical pathology, the oncological subspeciality of which is certainly a major one, and sets surgical pathology apart from postmortem anatomical pathology. The increasing use of diagnostic cytopathology, particularly of fine needle aspiration, has led many to include this branch of morphology with surgical pathology.

The practice of cooperation between pathologists and surgeons leading to preoperative biopsy diagnosis had its origin in Germany at the end of the last century. From there it spread to other European countries, notably France and the United Kingdom, and then the United States. In the early decades of this century surgical pathologists often began their training as surgeons and later switched to pathology. It is still common that some specialized physicians (gynecologists, dermatologists, gastroenterologists) act as their own pathologists because of the rarity of highly specialized pathologists, such as dermatopathologists, who are available only in large institutions.

It is the responsibility of the surgical pathologist to diagnose, as accurately as possible using all the appropriate technical tools available, abnormalities present in tissue specimens and cell samples. This includes proper cooperation with the clinician, both as to the site selection of the biopsy and the subsequent handling of the samples, in order to achieve maximal diagnostic utility of the biopsy material.

Since the pathologist is a physician, he must have access to all available clinical data. Some types of information should always be written in the request for pathological examination. These include: age,

[1] Unless otherwise specified, all figures show immunohistochemical reactions visualized by the ABC technique.

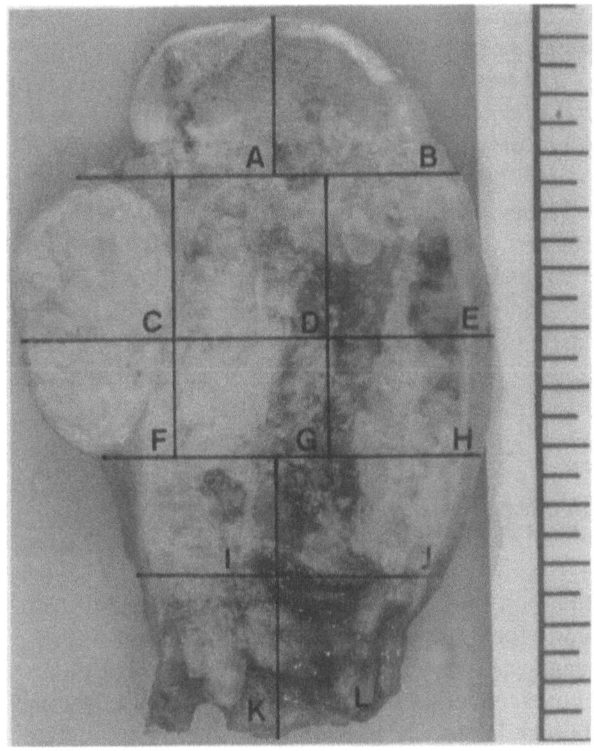

Fig. 1. Osteogenic sarcoma of the distal portion of the right femur of an 8-year-old girl after three cycles (in 2 months) of preoperative chemotherapy, which included vincristine, methotrexate, and cisplatin. The photograph of the cut surface of the bisected surgical specimen of a segmental ablation shows the map of the sampling for histological examination in order to evaluate the degree of necrosis (0%–100%) throughout the tumor in response to treatment. In this case overall response was almost 100%

sex, anatomical site, clinical diagnosis, current surgical procedure, operative findings, previous histological and/or cytological examinations, and previous or present chemo- and/or radiotherapy. There are a few other data which are a sine qua non for histological diagnosis, such as the radiological findings that must accompany the biopsy of a bone lesion and the blood counts when a bone marrow biopsy is submitted for hematopathological diagnosis.

Adequate sampling of the surgical resection specimen is crucial in forming a prognostic opinion and in writing the surgical pathology report. Even though it has to be stressed that unlimited examination is not cost effective, accurate selection of relevant fragments of the surgical specimen contribute significant pieces of information to the final diagnosis. This is best exemplified by the proper examination of breast cancer specimens in order to estimate potential recurrences in relationship to multicentricity (Fisher et al. 1986a) and to assess accurately the resection margins of tumorectomy specimens with special reference to the presence of surrounding intraductal carcinoma (Carter 1986). Another example of practical importance in this respect is in the adenoma-carcinoma continuum of the colon and rectum (Fenoglio and Pascal 1982), where the finding of an area of carcinoma in a large tubular or villous adenoma has to be elaborated upon with reference to the histological grade, depth of invasion, presence or absence of lymphatic involvement, quantification of the malignant component, and freedom of, or involvement by, disease at the resection margin. Finally, the rule that the number of samples should equate the number of centimeters of the largest diameter of an ovarian or testicular tumor should always be observed.

After a complex processing procedure (see Rodriguez, Martinez and Rosai 1981), that shall not be discussed here, the pathologist issues a final report which will become part of the hospital chart because it is a legal document. The report must contain identification of the patient, a gross description, and the final histopathological diagnosis.

The gross description of the specimens must be accurate and complete because no other record will remain in this respect. Photographs (transparencies and instant prints) or even high-quality photocopies may be taken and are often useful for making special sites of sampling or mapping complex lesions such as osteosarcoma (Fig. 1), tumors of the urinary bladder (Koss 1979b), cutaneous melanoma, etc. Simple diagrams may also adequately supplement gross descriptions. Size, shape, color, consistency, and weight are important and well-established descriptive parameters. The various samples of the specimen should be marked with letters or numbers that correlate with the histological slides on a given lesion. The microscopic description can be omitted unless very important points have to be mentioned. We usually produce a brief comment when relevant (rare lesions, special prognostic features, references) after the final diagnosis. For the latter we use the Systematized Nomenclature of Medicine (SNOMED, issued by the College of American Pathologists) with special reference to the incorporated International Classification of Diseases for Oncology (ICD-O; WHO 1976) both for topography (T code) and morphology (M code) of pathological lesions. When all the diagnostic procedures of this department were computerized, these codes were fed into a dedicated computer-assisted reporting system developed in this institution. Anagraphic and diagnostic data are treated by a chain of virtual machines under the VM-CMS system of an IBM 4361 computer. An abstract of diagnostic data is stored in an IBM relational database (SQL).

The reports also routinely include the diagnosis of the previous frozen section examination and all the other procedures which may have been, or will be, performed on the same material (e.g., electron microscopy, receptor studies, biological and kinetic cell markers, etc.). Copies of the report must be kept indefinitely in the department and the same applies to paraffin blocks and histological slides. In recent years, snap-frozen samples of pathological and adjacent normal tissues of selected cases have been kept in deep freezers (−80 °C) for future studies.

Frozen Section Examination

This is a well-established, almost 60-year-old, technique for rapid histopathological diagnosis of tissue samples. The material to be submitted for frozen section examination has to be taken quickly to the pathology laboratory together with the hospital chart. Special requests should be clearly stated by the surgeons since the purpose of a frozen section is to make a therapeutic decision and not to satisfy someone's curiosity or simply to anticipate the final report. The specimens are frozen rapidly, usually in a cryostat at the temperature of about −20 °C, or snap-frozen in cooled 2-methylbutane to reduce artifacts and sectioned with a microtome. The sections are stained with hematoxylin and eosin or other available rapid stains. The written report specifies the type of tissue, the type of lesion and, if appropriate, the extent of resection, i.e., whether the surgical margins are free from tumor involvement. The residual portion of the frozen tissue should then be fixed separately from the other specimens subsequently submitted. The whole procedure can be carried out in 10–15 min.

To make a proper therapeutic decision, the diagnosis of either non-neoplastic lesion, benignancy, or malignancy is sufficient; however, in most cases correct histological typing is feasible. In our experience, deferred diagnoses are in the minority (2%–3%), and their sources are mostly enlarged lymph nodes, soft-tissue and bone lesions, some tumors of the central nervous tissue, and rarely others, such as papillary breast lesions. Except for metastatic carcinoma, all other lesions of lymph nodes are basically unsuitable for frozen section diagnosis.

False positive diagnoses are usually related to the lack of experience on the part of the pathologist, while false negative diagnoses are more often related to the inadequacy of the specimen. The rate of accuracy, i.e., when deferred diagnoses and those at variance are excluded, ranges in most of the reported series between 90% and 95%, whereas the true error rate is less than 3%, with some variation according to the site and type of lesion (Nakazawa et al. 1968).

Breast lesions are among the most common targets for frozen section examination and are rarely wrongly diagnosed; the same applies to tumors of the head and neck region including those of the salivary glands. Follicular proliferations of the thyroid gland and enlargements of the parathyroids may pose diagnostic problems as to their benign or malignant nature. Malignant lesions of the digestive system and of the respiratory tract are often diagnosed on the basis of the regional lymph nodes which, at surgery, appear suggestive of metastatic spread. The same applies to gynecological pathology, except for the not uncommon examination of solid or cystic ovarian tumors, primary or metastatic. Cutaneous tumors are rarely examined as frozen sections since excisional biopsy is usually the rule.

Quick diagnostic decisions may also be made by examining imprint preparations, especially of soft specimens such as lymph nodes and crumbly tumor tissues. In these cases cytological diagnostic criteria prevail over structural histological ones.

Aspiration Biopsy Cytology

This technique is now over 60 years old. It was introduced for the first time in the late 1920s in the United States and extensively developed in Europe after World War II. It is still assuming increasing importance in clinical practice because of the very close cooperation between pathologist, clinician, and/or radiologist.

Crucial points of the procedure are: (a) the use of a thin needle which should measure *less* than 1 mm (gauge 21) in outer diameter; (b) the correct technique of aspiration, which may vary slightly according to the target organ or mass; and (c) the knowledgeable interpretation of the findings. Solid fragments obtained with needles wider than 1 mm are usually not suitable for cytological investigation. The aspirated samples may be processed either as cytological smears or as histological minibiopsies, and small fragments thereof can be stored snap-frozen and/or specifically fixed for electron microscopy. The material obtained can only be fully understood and integrated for the benefit of the patient by pathologists who have wide experience in normal histology and surgical pathology. In this respect, aspiration biopsy cytology represents an ideal integration of the cytopathological and the histopathological approach to tissue diagnosis. Needless to say, cytopathological diagnoses are always expressed with the same terminology as that used for histopathology. Aspiration biopsy cytology has a precise diagnostic purpose and is not used for screening. In fact, cytopathological diagnosis on aspirated material is often the final diagnostic procedure and therefore represents a major responsibility for the cytopathologist (Hajdu and Melamed 1984).

The most common sites of aspiration biopsies are the breasts, prostate, thyroid gland, salivary glands, enlarged superficial lymph nodes, intrathoracic masses, intrahepatic and pancreatic tumors. Since the main purpose of aspiration biopsy cytology of breast lesions is the preoperative diagnosis of carcinoma, to avoid frozen section on a larger biopsy it follows that false positive diagnosis should never occur. False negative diagnoses due to inadequate sampling and/or limited experience are in the range of 5%–25% (Eisenberg et al. 1986).

The same considerations also apply to tumors of the salivary glands except that a number of low-grade carcinomas, such as acinic cell carcinoma and well-differentiated mucoepidermoid carcinoma, may be difficult to recognize cytologically.

Aspiration of non-neoplastic cold thyroid nodules saves quite a large number of unnecessary surgical procedures. Papillary, anaplastic, and medullary carcinomas of the thyroid gland are correctly recognized in most instances, whereas the same cannot be said of well-differentiated follicular carcinomas which may be cytologically undistinguishable from benign follicular hyperplasia and adenomas.

Prostatic tumors are also a frequent target of fine needle aspiration and often yield adequate material for a conclusive diagnosis of carcinoma and even for its grading. Carcinomatous metastatic seeding to lymph nodes is readily identified, and in some instances histological typing is also feasible (e.g., metastatic lymphoepithelial carcinoma of the nasopharynx, papillary carcinoma of the thyroid, small cell carcinoma of the lung, etc.). The same applies to metastatic malignant melanomas, even when unpigmented, since the cells may be identified by proper immunophenotyping. Even though malignant lymphomas may be recognizable in smears, particularly when of the large cell type or when Reed-Sternberg cells are present, as a rule the clinical diagnosis should be followed by an excisional biopsy of a representative lymph node.

Intrathoracic mediastinal and pulmonary masses are currently routinely aspirated percutaneously (Pilotti et al. 1984) when nonivasive procedures such as sputum examination and bronchoscopic brushing are negative. While liver cell carcinomas may be so well differentiated as to mimic benign lesions, ductal carcinomas of the pancreas are almost always easily identified even though metastatic adenocarcinomas to the peripancreatic and retroperitoneal lymph nodes may produce similar findings.

Consultation and Review of Slides

When a patient has undergone a surgical procedure for a neoplasm and further therapy has to be given at a different institution, the original section should always be reviewed for ethical, legal, and technical reasons. From an ethical point of view the patient has to be protected from unnecessary therapeutic procedures, while, legally, the physician should be protected from a malpractice suit if a potentially dangerous therapy is to be administered; and, from a technical point of view, there is always the chance that the previous histopathological diagnosis has to be downgraded, upgraded, slightly modified, or occasionally changed altogether.

In our experience, the most common additions to, or modifications of, previous diagnoses regarding cancer patients to be staged and/or treated at our institution relate to:

1. The adoption of an internationally recognized nomenclature, such as that embodied by ICD-O, to ensure uniformity of diagnosis.
2. The *grading* of malignancy such as for ovarian, endometrial, renal cell and transitional cell carcinomas, and some sarcomas of soft tissues; and the prognostically relevant *subtyping*, such as for squamous cell carcinoma (large cell, small cell, or keratinizing) of the cervix or for carcinoma of the stomach (intestinal, undifferentiated or mixed type).
3. The measurement of the thickness of tumors, such as cutaneous malignant melanoma, or of invasion expressed in millimeters, such as squamous cell carcinoma of the cervix and vulva.
4. The evaluation of the resection margins such as of cutaneous basal cell carcinoma, dermatofibrosarcoma protuberans, etc.
5. The complete listing and the quantification of the various components of testicular germ cell tumors (seminomas vs. nonseminomas) and of dysplasia of the breast (WHO 1981).

6. The correct identification, with the aid of special stains if necessary, of the histological type; examples are: papillary pseudofollicular vs. follicular carcinomas of the thyroid; neuroendocrine tumors of the skin (so-called Merkel's cell carcinoma) and thyroid (medullary carcinoma) vs. not otherwise specified primary or metastatic undifferentiated carcinomas; small blue cell tumors of children and adolescents which include neuroblastoma, embryonal rhabdomyosarcoma, skeletal and extraskeletal Ewing's sarcoma, Askin's tumor of the chest wall (Askin et al. 1979).
7. Plain mistakes, such as spindle cell nevus of the skin vs. malignant melanoma; sclerosing atrophy vs. carcinoma of the prostate in small biopsies; adenoma of the nipple and mammary stellate scars vs. infiltrating duct or tubular carcinomas of the breast; fasciitis and various pseudosarcomatous proliferations including inflammatory pseudotumors of various sites vs. sarcomas of soft parts; infectious mononucleosis and histiocytic necrotizing lymphadenitis (Kikuchi 1972) vs. non-Hodgkin's malignant lymphomas; granular cell tumor with pseudo-epitheliomatous hyperplasia (e.g., of the tongue) vs. squamous cell carcinoma; benign glandular inclusions or nests of benign melanocytes in lymph nodes vs. metastatic disease, etc.
8. In very rare instances, new well-defined and distinct clinicopathological entities with special therapeutic and/or prognostic relevance which may appear in the literature and whose recognition remains restricted to experts for a while. This applies to special types of malignant non-Hodgkin's lymphomas (e.g., the rare peripheral T cell types and the large cell sclerosing type of the mediastinum), the Merkel's cell carcinoma of the skin, the androgen-independent duct carcinomas of the prostate (reviewed by Miller 1988) and perhaps the so-called dysplastic nevus of the skin. This was originally described by Clark et al. in 1978 as a heritable melanocytic lesion in family members of patients with cutaneous malignant melanoma and later (Greene et al. 1985) as an acquired precursor of the latter. The histopathological features of the dysplastic nevus have been fairly well established (Elder 1985) and are reproducible to a major extent.

Special stains should always be performed when they are expected to yield essential information of diagnostic and prognostic value; in such cases, unstained sections should be required from the submitting pathologist. Controversial and difficult cases may still remain unsolved even after multiple consultations, but even in this instance the practice of slide review is of advantage both to the referring and the receiving party and to the patient.

In this context it is only fair to add that nowadays it is not uncommon that wrong histopathological diagnoses, or even not sufficiently precise and detailed ones, are questioned on a short-term basis by alert clinical oncologists, whereas, not too many decades ago, it was the pathologist who had the role of controller, often in the autopsy room.

Classification of Tumors

The classification of tumors is still basically morphological, even though the morphological approach is progressively being supplemented by data regarding the functional activity of the tumor (Williams et al. 1980). Adenomas of the pituitary gland, tumors of the adrenal cortex and medulla and of the parathyroid glands, entopic and ectopic tumors of the endocrine pancreas, functioning benign and malignant tumors of the diffuse endocrine system at various sites are already classified according to the substance(s) synthetized or the functional disturbance produced. One example in this respect is the recently identified, mostly malignant vasoactive intestinal peptide (VIP)-producing tumor (Capella et al. 1983) predominantly of the pancreas.

As a rule, however, classifications of tumors are based on histogenesis and differentiation (Gould 1986). Histogenesis refers to the putative cell of origin of a type of neoplasm, whereas differentiation reflects the degree of similarity to, or dissimilarity from, that putative cell. The concept, however, that is gaining more and more weight is that contrary to this rather static way of thinking, a more dynamic approach should take into consideration the heterogeneity of the tumor cell population, the selection of neoplastic clones, and multidirectional differentiation. Histologically, tumor heterogeneity may be appreciated when making a diagnosis such as mixed germ cell tumors or other mixed tumors (of salivary glands, carcinosarcomas).

Heterogeneity may also become evident following therapeutic interventions such as in neuroblastomas which may differentiate and mature completely, malignant lymphomas which may transform into other morphological subtypes, and small cell lung carcinoma. The latter is presently undergoing a thorough investigation which shows that heterogeneous prognostically significant subtypes exist (Matthews and Gazdar 1985).

In general, the main reference books for an internationally acceptable classification system and terminology are the series of the WHO blue books on histological tumor typing and the United States Armed Forces Institute of Pathology collection of fascicles on tumor pathology, in spite of some exceptions related to rapidly expanding areas, such as the tumors deriving from the lymphatic cells. Monographs on organ-oriented tumor pathology by prominent specialized pathologists are also available and may be of help. It seems, however, that by now tumor histopathology has been fairly well assessed after about three decades (1950–1980) of thorough investigation throughout the world, particularly in the United States and the United Kingdom. Nonetheless, a point that deserves special mention is the change over the years of diagnostic histopathological criteria and standards which may account, at least in part, for some modifications in incidence trends of some types of tumors. The most significant example is adenocarcinoma of the lung, which has increased in incidence since 1974 (Vincent at al. 1974; Dodds et al. 1986) at the expense of squamous cell carcinoma. Similarly, an increase of adenocarcinomas of the proximal stomach including the cardia and the gastroesophageal junction, different from the tumors of the distal stomach, (Wang et al. 1986) has been established.

New entites or prognostically relevant subentities are still being identified or rediscovered and renamed, and the pathologist should constantly be aware of all new information that is being made available. This may involve a steady and substantial effort of the broad area encompassed by oncological pathology, particularly if the new input deriving from other fields such as immunopathology, biochemistry, and cell and molecular biology is also taken into consideration.

Tumors, Uncertain whether Benign or Malignant

The assessment of malignancy, in traditional terms of capability of local invasion and distant metastatic spread, is not always possible on purely morphological grounds. The neoplastic proliferation of certain cell types, such as the cells of the ovarian granulosa, Sertoli's cells, Leydig's cells, paraganglial cells, including those of the adrenal medulla, and the cells of the parathyroid glands, cannot be qualified morphologically. Even though most of these tumors are benign, they may prove to be clinically malignant without an obvious increase in the mitotic index and cellular atypias. These features may still be compatible with a benign nature, whereas massive blood vessel invasion may point toward invasiveness, but not necessarily so. Thymomas are another example of usually benign tumors which are occasionally aggressive. Among tumors of the soft parts, hemangiopericytomas are the most unpredictable: tumors larger than 6 cm in diameter may metastatize and recur more often than smaller tumors with the same type of cellularity. Hence, the terms of "tumor uncertain whether benign or malignant" or "tumor of borderline malignancy" are accepted by ICD-O. In fact, some tumors, such as pulmonary tumorlets, transitional cell papillomas, villous adenomas of the gastrointestinal tract, sex cord stromal gonadal tumors, granulosa cell tumors, paragangliomas (including extra-adrenal paragangliomas), giant pigmented nevi, desmoids, epithelioid leiomyomas, endolymphatic stromal myosis, hemangioendotheliomas, giant cell tumors of bone, etc., should be coded as borderline when the pathological report leaves them not otherwise specified. The term "of borderline malignancy" which identifies a very special subset of epithelial (common), mostly serous and mucinous tumors of the ovary has been replaced, by international agreement, by the one "of low malignant potential," which defines better the low-grade malignant clinical course of only a fraction (5%–15%) of these tumors, while the remaining behave in a benign fashion (Colgan and Norris 1983).

Premalignancy, Atypia, Dysplasia, Borderline Lesions

This area of diagnostic histopathology has been, and in part still is, a long-standing source of uncertainty for the practicing surgical pathologist. Three main points should be mentioned briefly. First, when in a given biopsy a noninvasive atypical lesion is detected, one should ask oneself whether the tissue sample is representative or not. In fact, non uncommonly foci of atypia may be located next to unequivocal overt invasive carcinomas missed by the biopsy. Hence, the adequacy of the biopsy should be discussed with, and ascertained by, the submitting endoscopist, gynecologist, radiologist, etc. Secondly, so-called premalignant lesions are not irreversible, even though the degree of probability not to procede to a carcinoma can never be quantitated in a given case. Thirdly, one should keep in mind that the biology of potentially dangerous atypical lesions and the following clinical and therapeutic attitude are very much dependent upon the anatomic site of the lesion.

For a number of premalignant lesions the pathological diagnostic criteria are well established, and acceptable guidelines for the clinical treatment are also available. This is the case of the dysplasia-carcinoma in situ sequence of the *uterine cervix* (reviewed by Koss 1979 a) – also named cervical intraepithelial neoplasia (CIN) (Richart 1967) – which has unexpectedly become a very important subject in recent years after the discovery of the etiological role of some types of papillomavirus (zur Hausen et al. 1984). This event may, in the near future, change the whole approach towards prevention, early diagnosis, and therapy of preinvasive squamous epithelial lesions not only of the transformation zone of the uterine cervix but also of the vagina, vulva, penis, and extragenital sites such as larynx, esophagus, anus, oral mucosa, and various cutaneous sites. In this respect, of special interest is the detection of viral DNA integrated into cellular DNA of invasive cervical carcinomas as opposed to the episomal viral DNA in the cells of CIN (Shirasawa et al. 1986).

Even though the term "mammary dysplasia," which replaced "fibrocystic disease" (WHO 1981) may not be ideal, it has the advantage of covering a wide spectrum of lesions which range from very bland alterations to epithelial, ductal and lobular, hyperplasia with, or without, cellular atypia. Recent data from a prospective study (Dupont and Page 1985) allows one to identify within the spectrum three groups of lesions (Page 1986) which show a very different prevalence: nonproliferative dysplasia (70%), proliferative lesions without atypia (26%), and atypical hyperplasia (4%). We apply this subgrouping of breast dysplasia as suggested by the authors, and our reports now also include a percentage quantification of the various components. We tend to include lobular carcinoma in situ, also named "lobular neoplasia" (Haagensen et al. 1978), among proliferative lesions with atypia, whereas intraductal carcinoma is kept as a separate entity because of its higher malignant potential (Fisher et al. 1986 b).

Reporting squamous metaplasia with varying degrees (mild, moderate, severe) of atypia of the bronchial mucosa is more commonly a cytological task, however, the same terminology also applies to the corresponding tissue findings in bronchial biopsies. In contrast to most other sites, a carcinoma in situ of the bronchial mucosa is rarely found as a discrete lesion and almost always accompanies an already invasive lesion. The problem with carcinoma in situ of the bronchial mucosa is particularly complex, also in view of its multicentricity and difficult therapeutic approach (Carter 1978). On the contrary, intraepithelial atypias including carcinoma in situ are often found and successfully removed from other sites such as the oral mucosa, the vocal cords, and the esophagus.

In the stomach, dysplastic lesions of the mucosa (excluding adenomas) are not frequently found and recently precise diagnostic criteria have been elaborated (Ming et al. 1984) even though it remains to be shown how and where gastric dysplasia fits into the conventional scheme of progression to invasive carcinoma.

Different yet again is the situation in the large bowel where the most common precursors of carcinoma are villous and tubular adenomas. The latter quite often show a variably sized villous component which can and should be quantified as a percentage of the section. Although the epithelial lining of these adenomas is dysplastic by definition, it has been agreed (Muto et al. 1975) that the presence of areas of dysplasia in adenomas, usually larger than 1 cm in diameter, be mentioned in the report only when an area of adenocarcinoma is recognized which does not trespass on the muscularis mucosae. The absence of any potential spread of these otherwise cytologically malignant lesions either directly or via the lymphatic vessels is the justification for the avoidance of the term "carcinoma" in the report and prevents overzealous surgeons performing unnecessary and dangerous mutilations.

In the urinary tract, and particularly in the bladder, the finding of foci of "atypical hyperplasia" of the transitional epithelium, unless temporarily induced by some drugs, is a serious problem since this alteration falls somewhat short of urothelial carcinoma in situ. The latter is not only an almost invariably irreversible lesion but it progresses quite rapidly to invasion, in contrast to low-grade papillary urothelial tumors (Koss 1975).

There are other sites in which lesions with more or less pronounced malignant potential may occur, such as in the endometrium in which adenomatous hyperplasia with or without atypia may be detected (Kurman and Norris 1982), the prostate in which the criteria for the diagnosis of atypical hyperplasia and carcinoma in situ have still to be defined (Miller 1988), the liver for which the difference between small and large cell type dysplasia has been stressed (Watanabe et al. 1983).

In summary, the term "atypia" is preferable when the cellular changes fall somewhat short of clear-cut malignancy and the pathologist wants to stress the possibly premalignant pathological situation. Atypias may be graded into mild, moderate, and severe. The same applies to dysplasia, even though the latter term is less acceptable since it may also convey a different message that is unrelated to oncology. However, some dysplasias, such as those of the stomach, large bowel, cervix, etc., have found their way into the every day diagnostic language and are probably here to stay. The term "borderline lesion" has already been discussed.

It appears that the concept of morphological atypia as a possibly premalignant state is applicable only to epithelial cells and perhaps melanocytes, but not to connective tissue cells, nerve cells, and lymphoid cells, with the notable exception of hematopoietic cells. In fact, myeloid dysplastic syndromes with varying degrees of severity (Bennett et al. 1982) may precede acute myeloid leukemia.

Special Stains

A number of special stains are of great help, for example, the Alcian blue cationic dye at pH 2.5 for poorly differentiated adenocarcinomas and, in general, for the identification of even minimal amounts of cytoplasmic epithelial acid mucins. This is useful partly for therapeutic reasons, when a squamous cell carcinoma should be ruled out, and partly in order to locate the primary tumor when the biopsy has been taken from a metastatic deposit. A special use of the Alcian blue technique is the separation of various acid mucins with different critical electrolyte concentration points using various concentrations of, for example, magnesium chloride.

Kreyberg's method (WHO 1967) operates in the same direction as Alcian blue, except for the simultaneous visualization of cytoplasmic keratinization by means of safranin O. This is especially useful for the identification of poorly differentiated squamous cell carcinomas and mucoepidermoid carcinomas. It has turned out that the latter are fairly common, not only in the usual sites such as the major and minor salivary glands, but also in the lungs and the upper respiratory tract (Carter and Eggleston 1980) where they may reveal variable degrees of aggressiveness.

The periodic acid-Schiff (PAS) reaction (oxidation to aldehydes and subsequent reaction with fuchsin-sulphurous acid) preceded by an enzyme-linked digestion (amylases or diastase) visualizes the presence of glycogen and can be applied to identify Ewing's sarcoma, renal cell carcinomas, and clear cell carcinomas (for example, of the female genital tract), clear cell sarcoma of tendons and aponeuroses (also called "malignant melanoma of soft parts"), etc. Without prior enzymic digestion, the PAS reaction stains many substances, some of which are diagnostically useful. This applies to cytoplasmic Russell and nuclear Dutcher bodies in lymphoplasmacytoid cells producing oligosaccharide units containing polymeric IgM in benign inflammatory and neoplastic conditions.

Neutral mucins (glycoconjugates) and sialidase-labile sialomucin are also PAS positive, as is the sulfated group of epithelial mucins (some intestinal goblet cells, serous bronchial glands), even though to a variable extent, whereas connective tissue mucins are PAS negative. The basement membrane always appears strongly PAS positive. The PAS reaction (second step) is often combined with the Alcian blue technique at pH 2.5 (first step) to demonstrate the presence of both acid and neutral mucins. This combined method is routinely applied to endoscopic biopsies of the stomach for the demonstration of complete and incomplete intestinal metaplasia and foci of mucin-secreting undifferentiated carcinoma and to lobular invasive carcinoma of the breast, in which mucin droplets may be found as opposed to invasive duct carcinoma.

The Romanowsky-Giemsa staining method (containing azure B and anionic eosin Y) should always be employed when a lymphoproliferative lesion is being investigated since, on a thin section, it allows nuclear details and other features (metachromasia of various substrates) to stand out better than with any other method.

The reticulin fiber silver impregnation methods (Gordon and Sweet; Gomori) are very useful in some circumstances, such as for the demonstration of the reticulin scaffold of soft-tissue tumors, some malignant lymphomas, a few undifferentiated carcinomas, and in some problem cases of cutaneous malignant melanoma.

Many other special stains are available for selected purposes, for example:

- Stein's method for bile, based on the oxidation of bilirubin by a iodine solution
- Masson-Fontana's silver method for melanin
- The bleaching method of melanin by strong oxidizing agents for the visualization of the melanocytes
- Von Kossa silver method and the Alizarin red S stain for calcium
- Weigert's resorcin-fuchsin stain for elastic fibers (or the Orhoeff technique)
- Masson trichrome technique for the demonstration of collagen (blue/green) and muscle (red)
- Hale's dialysed iron technique for acid mucin, es-

pecially weakly reactive hyaluronic acid deposits in mesotheliomas
- Perls Prussian blue reaction for ferric iron (hemosiderin)
- Mallory's phosphotungstic acid-hematoxylin (PTAH) stain for fibrin and CNS
- Congo red staining accompanied by polarized light examination (green birefringence of dichroism) for amyloid
- Bromine or standard Sudan black and oil red O for lipids on cryostat sections postfixed in calcium-formol.

Electron Microscopy

In surgical pathology conventional transmission electron microscopy (EM) is useful for diagnostic purposes in only a minority of cases, especially since the development of immunohistochemical procedures. In our laboratories, from 1975 onward, we have embedded about 7%–8% of all surgical specimens in Epon and examined between 30% and 50% of these. These percentages have decreased considerably during the last 2 years. This leaves untouched all the potential of this powerful investigative tool, which may also be coupled with immunological techniques for the ultrastructural localization of various substances (peptides, immunoglobulins, etc.). In addition, EM technology is expensive, slow, sample dependent, and needs specially trained personnel. Nonetheless, the saving of samples of tumor tissue(s) embedded in Epon costs little, and it occupies very little space. The availability of fragments for EM is of great value for retrospective studies of both single cases and extensive series. In our experience protracted storage in a phosphate buffer after glutaraldeyde prefixation of tissue samples allows good preservation of ultrastructural details for routine and cytochemical studies (Sabatini et al. 1963). Also fixation and storage in buffered formalin is frequently useful, while reprocessed tissue fragments from paraffin blocks are rarely profitable.

In our laboratories we have found that EM is a useful complement in fine needle aspiration cytopathology. When a thin cylinder of compact tissue is aspirated, a fragment thereof should be processed for EM, particularly if the remaining tissue is insufficient for all desirable immunohistochemical procedures. In general, for the understanding of findings obtained by high-sensitivity immunohistochemical procedures, integration with the ultrastructural morphology is illuminating.

At a routine level we have found EM helpful in identifying some tumors of soft parts (e.g., S-100 protein-negative epithelioid schwannomas, factor VIII-related antigen-negative vascular tumors displaying Weibel-Palade bodies; clear cell sarcomas containing a few melanosomes); some neuroendocrine tumors, whose cytoplasmic content in dense core granules can then be compared with the degree of argyrophilia/argentaffinity and the results of the immunohistochemical search for several neuropeptides; some cases of neuroblastomas vs. Ewing's sarcoma or primitive neuroectodermal tumors; some cases of mesothelioma. Occasionally, we have obtained some valuable information from the identification of papillomavirus virions in biopsies of the uterine cervix and vulva showing dysplasia of the epithelium (Della Torre et al. 1978) and of various kinds of bacteria such as in Whipple's disease and mycobacteria in opportunistic infections.

As a corollary it should be noted that technical developments in EM have led to the use of resins as embedding media. High-resolution light microscopy can be performed on sections of suitable resin-embedded tissue(s) less than 1 μm thick, such as bone marrow and lymph nodes. Epoxy and acrylic resins are widely used to embed glutaraldehyde-, formalin-, or Bouin-fixed material. With some modifications, many special stains can be applied to resin-embedded sections, including some enzyme-histochemical and immunohistochemical techniques.

Enzyme Histochemistry

Among enzymes a few have diagnostic significance if present in large quantities in certain cell types. Enzyme histochemistry has considerable importance and a large number of methods are available to demonstrate in situ hydrolytic (hydrolases) and oxidative (oxidases and dehydrogenases) enzymes. It should, however, be pointed out that a number of enzymes can also be visualized by immunohistochemistry inasmuch as the antigenic properties of the proteins are exploited in order to generate antibodies which are usually polyclonal. Nonetheless, the lability of many enzymes often requires special treatment of the tissue.

Among hydrolytic enzymes, the phosphatases (acid, alkaline, and specific) hydrolize phosphate esters at various pH levels. The demonstration of high acid phosphatase activity in metastatic carcinoma strongly indicates that the primary site is in the prostate even though other neoplasms, such as carcinoids and insulinomas, may react, whereas, on the contrary, a poorly differentiated prostatic primary may be negative. Nowadays this marker is more often visualized immunohistochemically using polyclonal sera, sometimes together with the prostate-specific antigen.

Dipeptidylaminopeptidase IV activity, which cleaves glycylproline-ß-naphtylamide in the human hematopoietic system, is almost entirely restricted to the cell surface of normal helper/inducer T lymphocytes and is a reliable marker for most lympho-proliferative diseases derived from them, such as T4+/T8-T(CD4+/CD8-)-CLL. Also, this enzyme is recognized by a monoclonal antibody (Feller et al. 1986). β-Naphtyl acetate esterase (NAE) can be visualized in imprints of lymph nodes with histiocytic proliferative disorders since it is extensively present in normal and neoplastic cells derived from the macrophage-phagocytic system (MPS) (van Furth et al. 1972). NAE is also present in globular form in T lymphocytes. Naphtol AS-D chloroacetate esterase (CAE), muramidase and myeloperoxidase activities are present in mature, and even in immature, myeloid cells (e.g., of granulocytic sarcoma), and the first two can be detected in fixed paraffin-embedded material. A strong CAE activity is shown by neutrophils and mast cells, but not by eosinophilic granulocytes, whose granules are PAS negative, contrary to those of neutrophils. A strong cytoplasmic lysozyme activity is shown by mature histiocytes, but its intensity decreases rapidly in immature cells and cannot, therefore, be used as a marker for neoplasms of histiocytic lineage (e.g., malignant histiocytosis).

Immunohistochemistry

This technique is based on the localization of tissue constituents with antigenic properties by means of labeled antibodies as specific reagents. The first labels used were fluorescent and even now indirect immunofluorescent techniques are still widely used. However, peroxidase later replaced fluorescein as the antibody label until the high-sensitivity peroxidase-antiperoxidase (PAP) complex method was developed (Sternberger 1979). Further advances were represented by the use of the alkaline phosphatase-antialkaline phosphatase method (APAAP) (Cordell et al. 1984), the double or multiple staining of antigens (Sternberger and Joseph 1979), the colloidal gold-labeling method (with silver enhancement) (Danscher and Norgaard 1983) and the now widely accepted avidin-biotin complex (ABC) technique (Hsu et al. 1981).

After the first phase of the immunohistochemical revolution in surgical pathology, which was characterized by the dichotomy between the high expectations of specific results and the availability of insufficiently well-characterized antibodies, the current second phase allows pathologists to rely on those findings which can be technically controlled and critically evaluated before acceptance and integrated into the rational elaboration of the final diagnosis (Erlandson 1984). Both monoclonal (Köhler and Milstein 1975) and polyclonal antibodies are available in very large numbers nowadays - several thousands are listed in various specialized directories - and can be obtained either commercially or from scientific institutions and investigators.

For medium-sized pathology laboratories it is advisable to select only a small number of reliable reagents that can be used before the expiration date in view of their high cost. Since no one fixative is ideal for the preservation of all antigens, it would be also advisable to store at −80 °C small snap-frozen fragments of representative tissue of the tumor (and of the surrounding uninvolved tissue, if possible) for immunohistochemical analysis on frozen sections. In general, 10% formalin (4% formaldehyde plain or buffered), Bouin's fluid (picric acid, formaldehyde, acetic acid) and B5 solution (mercuric chloride, sodium acetate, formaldehyde) are the most popular fixatives, even though each has its own limitations. Hence, there is no reason to change the fixation method one is accustomed to, as long as one is aware of its pros and cons.

The main targets for immunohistochemistry in surgical pathology may be grouped as follows:

1. Intermediate filaments and other constituents of the cytoskeleton, such as actin
2. Special cell products, including hormone receptors and oncogene-encoded proteins
3. Oncodevelopmental tumor markers
4. Hormone-containing cells
5. Surface antigens, particularly of T and B lymphocytes, myeloid cells, and MPS-derived cells
6. Immunoglobulins and their light and heavy chains
7. Enzymes
8. Cell cycle-linked antigens (e.g., Ki 67; transferrin receptor)
9. Any simple or conjugated structural or transport protein against which an antibody has been generated, including extracellular substances such as collagen types II and IV, laminin (Ekblom et al. 1982), fibronectin (Stenman and Vaheri 1981), and so-called tumor-associated antigens (Fig. 2)
10. Bacterial and viral organisms or components thereof

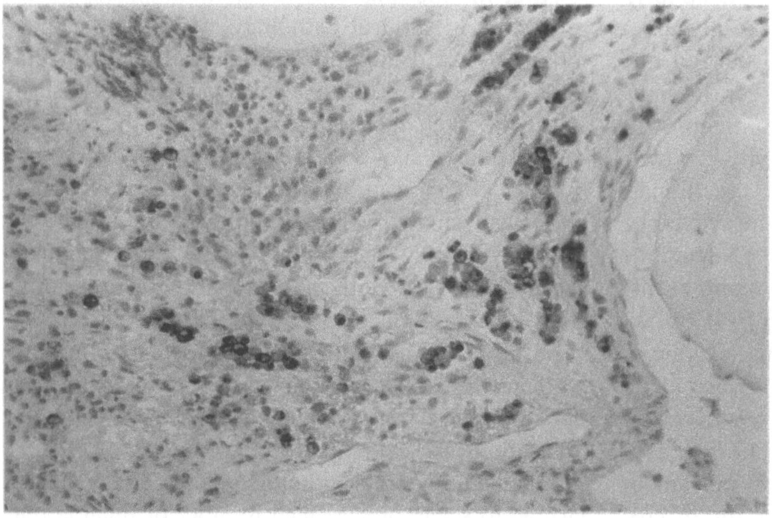

Fig. 2. Metastatic lobular carcinoma of the breast. Scattered malignant cells are visualized by the monoclonal antibody MBr1 (Mariani-Costantini et al. 1984). ×70

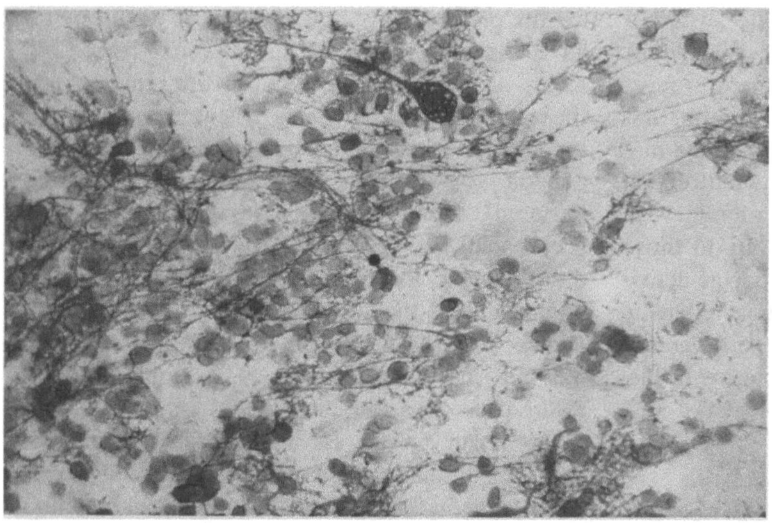

Fig. 3. Smear of fine needle aspirate of neuroblastoma. The cytoplasms and the neurites are stained by an antineurofilament (68 kd) antiserum. ×105

Intermediate filaments are a major target for polyclonal and the more recent monoclonal antibodies. Intermediate filaments are proteins which show a nonspecific fibrous structure at EM, except when cytokeratins form tonofilaments which are easily identified. Intermediate filaments measure between 8 and 11 nm and are hence wider than microfilaments (6 nm) and thinner than microtubules (25 nm); all these structures are part of the cytoskeleton (Osborn and Weber 1983). The five recognized classes of intermediate filaments differ in the peptidic structure, which is encoded by different gene families, and are classified as follows:

1. Cytokeratins, 19 of which are known and are contained in epithelial cells and epithelioid mesothelial cells. Individual proteins are designated by molecular mass expressed in kilodaltons (kd) and by the number of the numerical classification (Moll et al. 1982). Various types of epithelium, such as simple and multistratified epithelia, cutaneous and corneal epithelia, contain specific couples ("keratin pairs") made up of an acid and a basic protein of various molecular weights, ranging from 40 to 68 kd (Cooper et al. 1985).
2. Vimentin (57 kd) which is present in connective tissue cells and commonly coexpressed in variable amounts by tumors, including carcinomas, in addition to desmin or other intermediate filaments.
3. Desmin (53 kd), which is essentially restricted to muscle cells.
4. Neurofilaments, a triplet of 68, 160, and 200 kd expressed by neurons (Fig. 3).
5. Glial fibrillary acidic protein (55 kd) contained by glial cells.

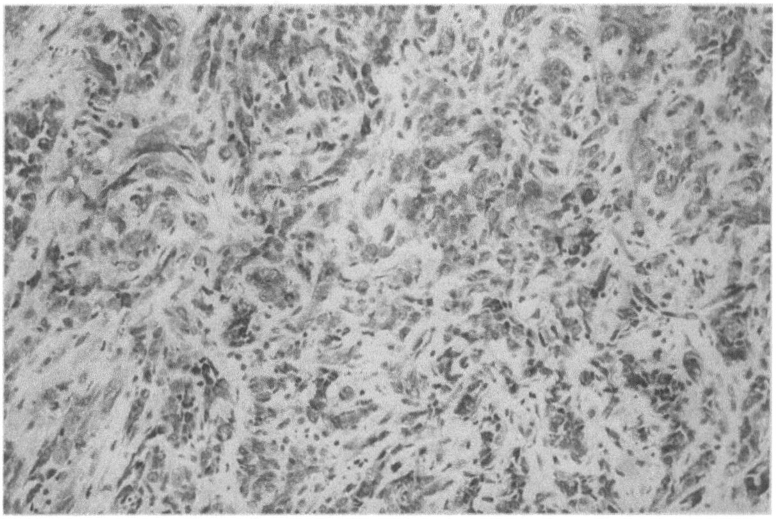

Fig. 4. Bronchiolo-alveolar carcinoma of the lung metastatic to the bone marrow. The tumor shows an equivocal structure which simulates a vascular malignancy; the cells are, however, positive for cytokeratin. ×60

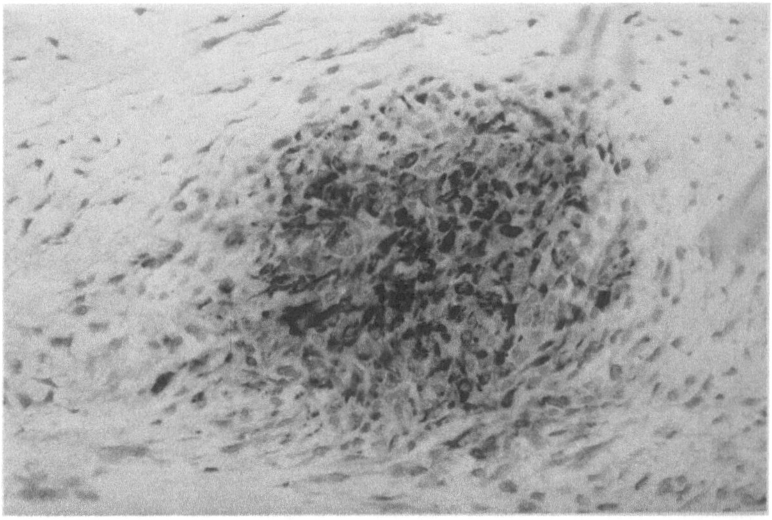

Fig. 5. Epithelioid sarcoma. A large number of neoplastic cells are positive for cytokeratin. ×80

In general, tumors preserve the intermediate filament characteristic of the corresponding normal tissue, and metastases reproduce the cytoskeletal pattern of the primary. All carcinomas, no matter how poorly differentiated (Fig. 4), including nasopharyngeal carcinoma, are usually the target of a full spectrum specificity panel of monoclonal antibodies against cytokeratins (Corson 1986). Some notable exceptions, such as renal cell carcinoma, liver cell carcinoma, and adrenal cortical carcinoma, may remain unstained if an antibody against low molecular weight cytokeratin is not included in the panel. Also among germ cell tumors, seminomas are not stained, even though they contain vimentin, whereas embryonal carcinomas and yolk sac tumors are (Miettinen et al. 1985). Carcinoids and, in general, neuroendocrine carcinomas of varying degrees of differentiation do contain cytokeratins, often in a dot-like fashion, whereas less commonly they show the diffuse type of cytoplasmic stain. These tumors, however, express neuroendocrine markers in addition to epithelial cytoskeletal proteins (Blobel et al. 1985).

Sarcomas of soft parts do not contain cytokeratins, except the epithelial-like pseudoglandular component of synovial sarcomas, most cells of epithelioid sarcomas (Fig. 5), and glandular formations (Fig. 6) in malignant schwannomas. Among bone tumors, adamantinoma and chordoma are understandably keratin positive, as are a number of mesothelial-derived adenomatoid tumors and all malignant epithelioid mesotheliomas (Fig. 7) (Battifora and Kopinski 1985). The not uncommon pseudosarcomatous squamous cell carcinoma (Fig. 8) of the skin and mucous membranes consists predominantly of kera-

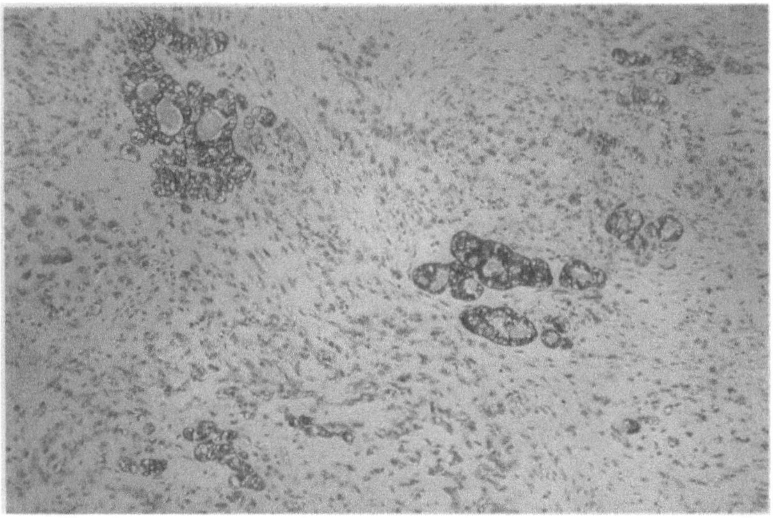

Fig. 6. Same case as in Fig. 9. The glandular component is decorated by a panel of anticytokeratin antibodies. × 30

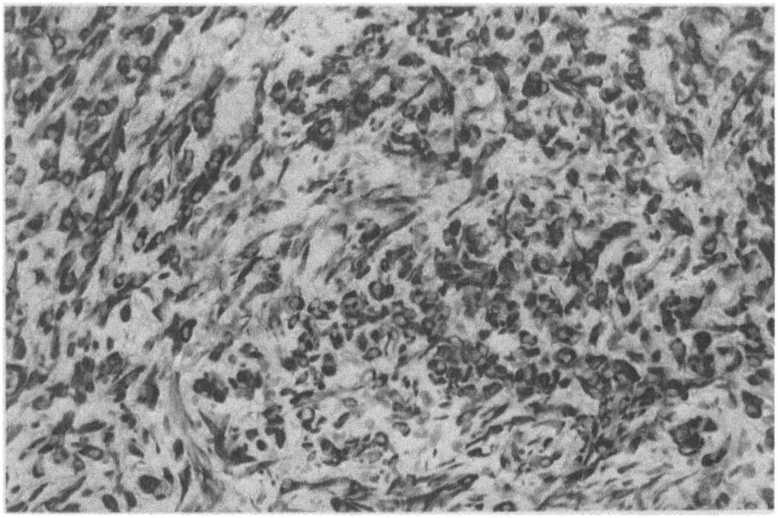

Fig. 7. Malignant biphasic peritoneal mesothelioma. Positivity for cytokeratin of both epithelioid and sarcomataous cell types. × 70

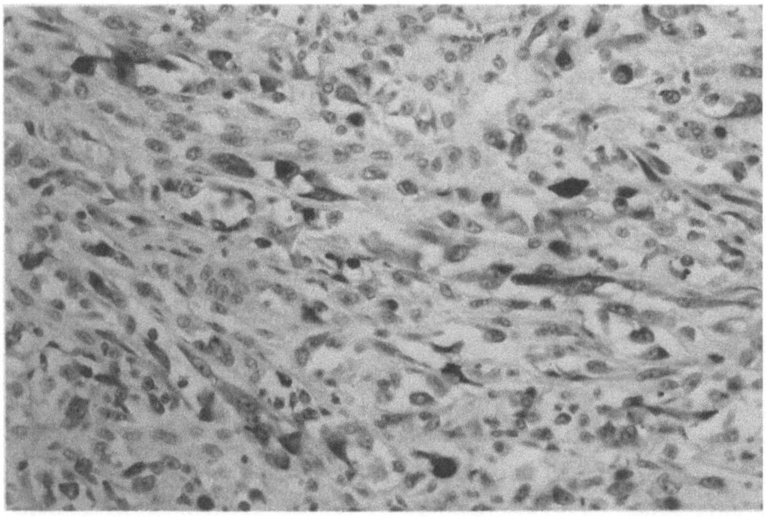

Fig. 8. Pseudosarcomatous squamous cell carcinoma of the vulva. A large number of spindle-shaped cells are positive for cytokeratin. × 80

tin-containing cells, and the same applies to the carcinomatous component of carcinosarcomas.

The frequent coexpression of vimentin in addition to cytokeratin by many nonmesenchymal tumors is a significant exception to the rule of the monotypic expression of intermediate filaments and limits the usefulness of its visualization. Vimentin immunoreactivity is shown by some carcinoma cells of kidney, thyroid gland, ovary, and salivary glands; sarcomatous mesothelioma; rhabdo- and leiomyosarcomas; and several tumors of the CNS. Coexpression of one of the other intermediate filaments is rare; notable examples are the cutaneous neuroendocrine carcinoma (Toker 1972) and some small cell carcinomas of the lung, in whose cells neurofilaments and cytokeratin may be detected simultaneously.

Desmin can be visualized on paraffin-embedded material and is a more reliable marker for rhabdo- and leiomyosarcomas than myoglobin (Figs. 9 and 10). One major component of the cytoskeleton which does not belong to intermediate filaments and can be easily visualized is actin, which is particularly abundant in myoepithelial cells, pericytes, and smooth muscle fibers (Mukai et al. 1981). It is a general indicator of "myoid" or cytoplasmic contractile differentiation.

Because of its great usefulness in clinical practice, in spite of the relatively high percentage of nonresponders to endocrine therapy, the determination of estrogen and progesterone receptor content in breast cancer patients has become a common tool in the last two decades. Steroid receptors are deter-

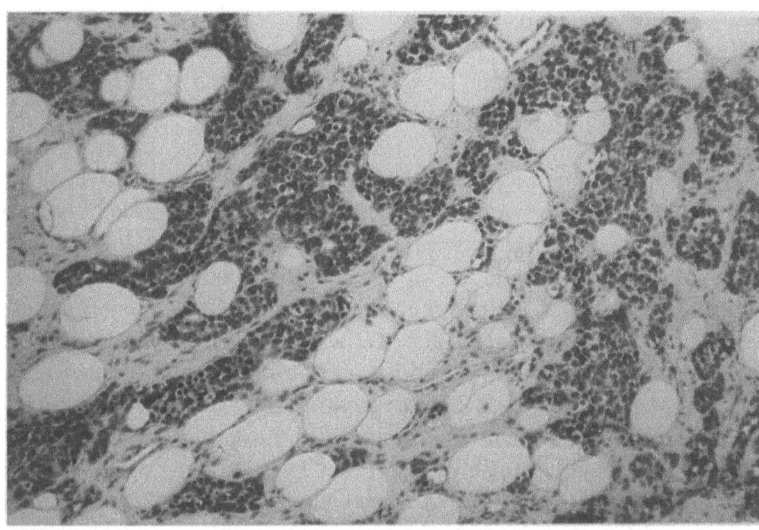

Fig. 9. Alveolar rhabdomyosarcoma of the perineum with unusual structure. The cells are positive for desmin. × 35

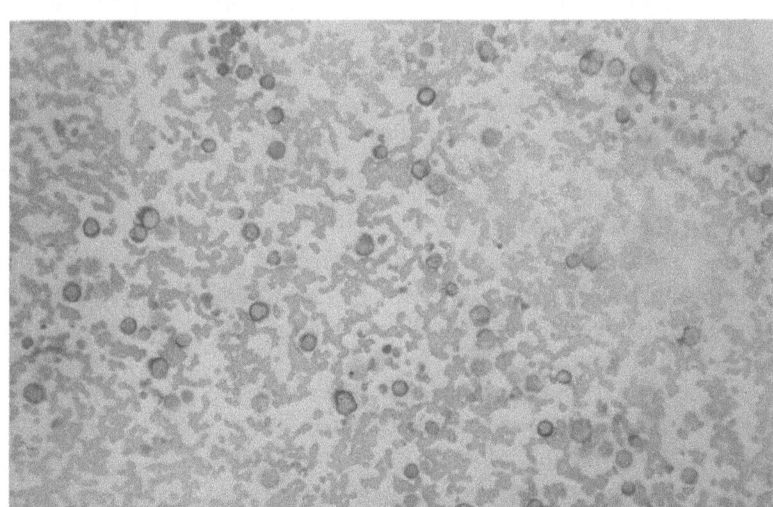

Fig. 10. Bone marrow smear containing numerous cells of a metastatic rhabdomyosarcoma. Desmin, × 40

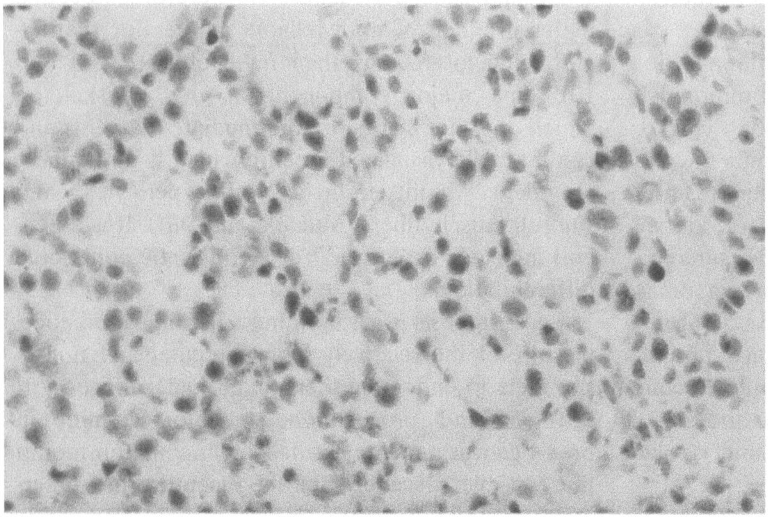

Fig. 11. Carcinoma of the breast. Immunostain of estrogen receptor (ER) – containing nuclei visualized by the H222 monoclonal antibody ER assay kit (Abbott). Note the presence of a few negative nuclei. ×130

mined almost exclusively by radioligand binding methods; immunological methods (enzyme immunoassay) have recently been added by virtue of the development of monoclonal antibodies as probes for receptor detection (Greene et al. 1980). Histochemical fluorescence methods and later immunohistochemical methods (reviewed by Chamness et al. 1980) challenged all previous techniques (King et al. 1985). Monoclonal antibodies which identify both the progesterone and the estrogen receptor proteins in the nuclei of the target cells (King and Greene 1984; Press et al. 1986) were used for immunoperoxidase staining, preferably of frozen sections (Fig. 11), and the results correlated favorably with those of traditional methods (Poulsen et al. 1985; Di Fronzo et al. 1986). However, in spite of the feasibility of the method and the soundness of the underlying principle, some caution is warranted and the time has not yet come to switch from the latter to the former approach. Immunocytochemical methods allow one to find an intriguing inverse relation between the presence of estrogen receptors and that of epidermal growth factor receptor in carcinomas of the breast (Sainsbury et al. 1985). This cell marker may become prognostically even more significant in the near future, particularly in combination with other new parameters. For example, the cell surface receptor for the iron-transport protein transferrin has also been investigated immunohistochemically in breast cancer with uncertain results.

Antigens other than intermediate filaments are commonly looked for during the attempt to characterize malignant tumors. Most of them are proteins produced by one or a few cell types. Factor VIII-related antigen is produced by differentiated endothelial cells, including those of the recently identified epithelioid hemangioendothelioma (Weiss and Enzinger 1982) of soft parts, bone, and viscera (e.g., intravascular bronchioloalveolar tumor of the lung) but not sufficiently by poorly differentiated angiosarcoma cells. The latter cells are, however, often provided with a receptor for Ulex Europeaus agglutinin 1 (Fig. 12), which is a lectin[1] obtained from a spring shrub. The decoration is helpful, but not specific, as some epithelial cells exhibit the same receptor.

Thyroglobulin and calcitonin are products of specific cell types of the thyroid gland in normal conditions, as well as of tumors of the thyroid (Fig. 13) and of other sites (e.g., ovarian thyroglobulin-producing struma, calcitonin-producing neuroendocrine carcinomas). Neuron-specific enolase (NSE), an isomer of the glycolytic enzyme enolase, is thought to be fairly specific for neuronal and neuroendocrine tumors (Fig. 14) but with notable exceptions (Pahlman et al. 1986). S-100 protein, originally believed to be specific for neural tissue-derived tumors because of its presence in bovine brain extracts, in addition to its presence in a large number of neurogenic tumors, is also found in some non-neurogenic tumors, including malignant melanomas, chondrosarcomas, schwannomas (Fig. 15) and some liposarcomas.

In difficult cases, however, for a broad preliminary distinction between a carcinoma, a melanoma, and a malignant lymphoma, the simultaneous use of antisera, respectively, against cytokeratins of low and

[1] Lectins are proteins or glycoproteins, exctracted from plants, invertebrates, and lower vertebrates, that have the capacity to bind sugars specifically.

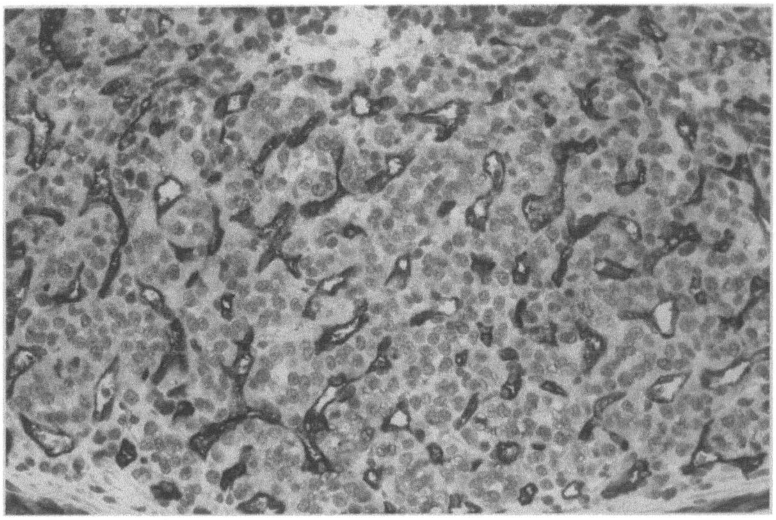

Fig. 12. Malignant hemangiopericytoma. The endothelial cells are decorated by *Ulex europeaus* lectin I, while the surrounding malignant pericytes are negative. × 80

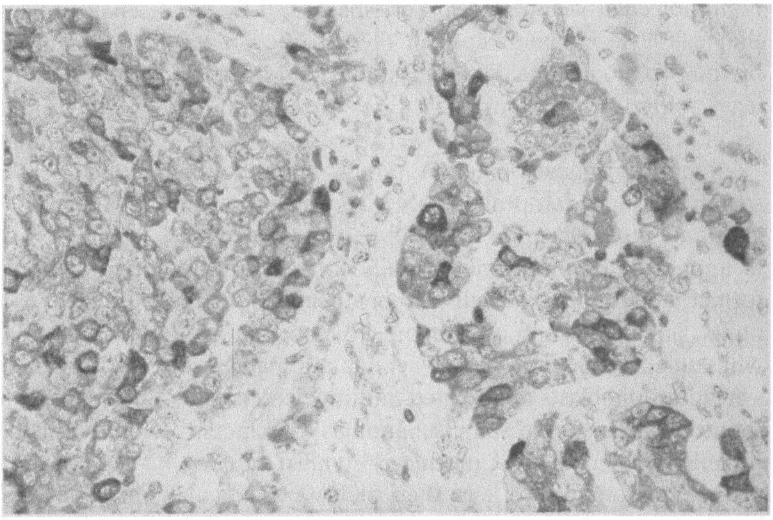

Fig. 13. Medullary carcinoma of the thyroid gland. Variable intensity of the decoration of tumor cells by an anticalcitonin antiserum. × 130

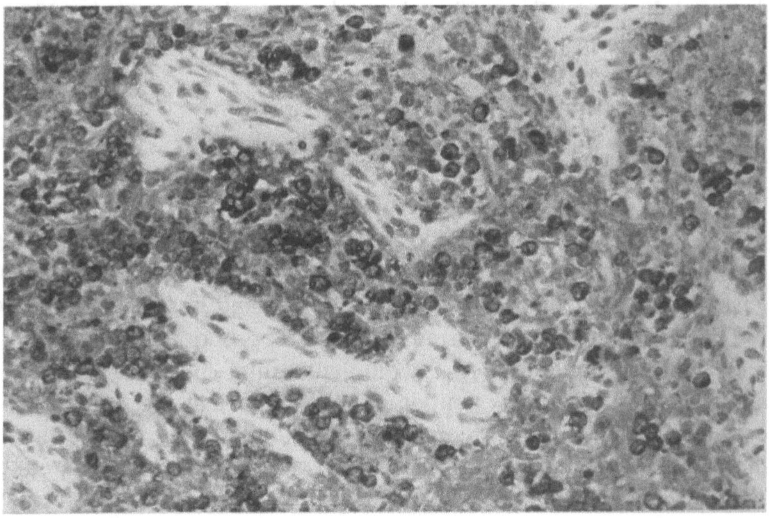

Fig. 14. Small cell carcinoma of the lung. A substantial number of tumor cells are positive for neuron-specific enolase. × 80

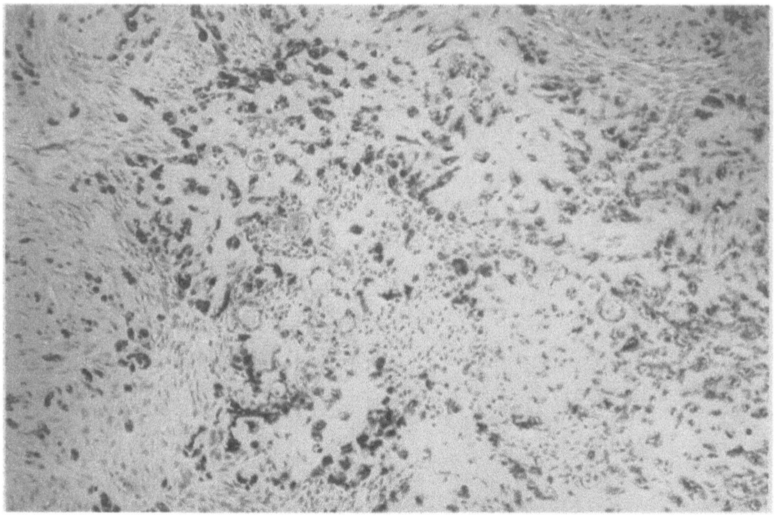

Fig. 15. Schwannoma with glandular differentiation. Most of the Schwann's cells are positive for S-100 protein. × 30

high molecular weight, S-100 proteins A and B, and the leukocyte common antigen (T200) (recognized by the two monoclonal antibodies 2B11 and PD7/26) leaves only 10% of the problem cases unsolved (Gatter et al. 1985).

Among oncodevelopmental tumor markers the search for alpha-fetoprotein (aFP) and beta human chorionic gonadotrophin (β-HCG) has a narrow area of application, but may yield significant results. The former is present in the cells of hepatocellular carcinomas and some germ cell tumors (yolk sac tumors), while the latter is produced by benign and malignant syncytiotrophoblasts and related multinucleated cells found, for example, in some seminomas. Carcinoembryonic antigen (CEA) is produced by most carcinomas of the large bowel and their metastases. Its alleged absence from malignant mesotheliomas and presence in pulmonary adenocarcinomas appears to be helpful only in a limited number of cases for differential diagnosis. The epithelial membrane antigen (EMA) (Heyderman et al. 1979) and the human milk fat globule membrane antigens (Ceriani et al. 1977) as markers for epithelial cells have lost part of their interest since the availability of the anticytokeratin antibodies. A large number of hormonal peptides synthetized by functioning cells of several amphicrine (Chejfec et al. 1985), endocrine, and neuroendocrine cell-derived neoplasms, most notably of the gastro-entero-pancreatic system, of the lungs, and of the pituitary, can be visualized with the appropriately labeled antibodies. An incomplete listing includes gastrin-releasing peptide (the mammalian counterpart of amphibian bombesin), calcitonin, somatotropin, somatostatin, insulin, glucagon, gastrin, ACTH, leu-enkephalin, VIP, and HCG (α and β chain). Peptide hormone-producing endocrine tumors and multiple endocrine neoplasias also synthetize and release chromogranine A, which is a 68-kd acidic monomeric protein that can be visualized immunohistochemically (O'Connor and Deftos 1986).

Polyclonal and monoclonal antisera for the immunocytochemical identification of cytoplasmic immunoglobulins have been used for the last decade in order to establish the monoclonality of B-lymphoproliferative disease, with special reference to anti-light chains (κ and λ) antisera. For the detection of the fixation-labile surface immunoglobulins the method is not completely reliable, and immunofluorescence on frozen sections (or live cell suspensions) may be preferable. More stable are other antigens which enable the identification, respectively, of B and T cells, even in paraffin sections, by means of anti-pan B (Salter et al. 1985) and anti-pan T (Norton et al. 1986) antibodies, even though freshly frozen tissue is still preferable for immunophenotyping lymphoid tissue. A variety of recently clustered monoclonal antibodies is now available against lymphocytes and their various subsets, myeloid cells, MPS-derived cells, other reticulum cells, platelets, etc. It should be pointed out that malignant lymphomas, when investigated by large panels of immunophenotyping reagents may show aberrant patterns of antigen expression, not only by the presence of unexpected positive findings, but also by the loss of markers and abnormal coexpression.

A large number of recently recognized proteins have been described and generally they have been designated only by their molecular mass (in kd). Some of them, such als p21 (Tanaka et al. 1986), re-

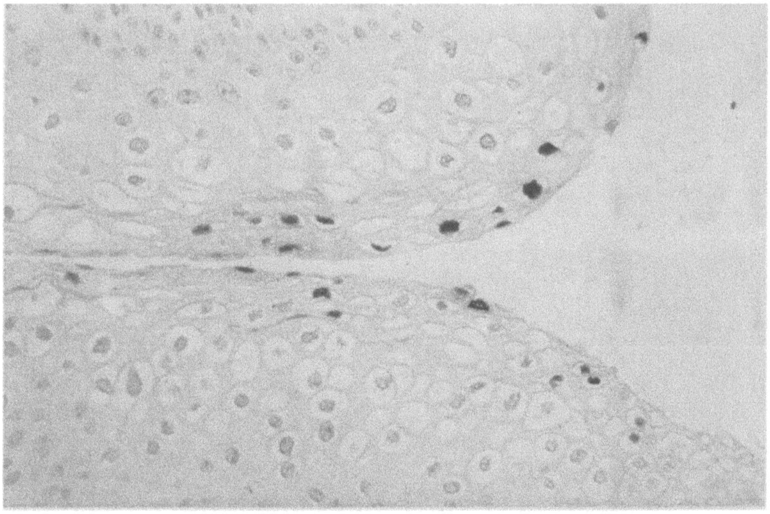

Fig. 16. Papillomavirus infection of the squamous cell epithelium of the uterine cervix. The nuclei stained within the superficial cell layers contain assembled virions and are visualized by a species-nonspecific antibody against the internal capsid antigen. × 80

present products encoded by oncogenes (Weinberg 1985) whose enhanced activity or amplification can be so established (Yokota et al. 1986), such as c-*myc*-encoded p62 in some malignant lymphomas (Jack et al. 1986).

Of special interest for the evaluation of cellular growth fractions in various malignancies, such as breast cancer (Gerdes et al. 1986) and malignant lymphomas, is a recently generated antibody Ki 67 (Gerdes et al. 1983), which reacts with a nuclear antigen present in proliferating cells and expressed throughout the cell cycle. Among components of viruses, a special mention should be made regarding (a) the internal capsid antigen of the genus papillomavirus, which can be easily detected by means of a polyclonal antibody in the infected nuclei of permissive squamous cells of the vulva, vagina, cervix (Fig. 16), larynx, skin etc.; (b) the proteins encoded by the core and surface genes of HBV (HEPADNA); and (c) several antigens of herpesvirus simplex types I and II and cytomegalovirus.

Finally, it should be stressed that histochemical and immunohistochemical investigations are of no value unless adequate positive and negative controls are carried out. Both false positive and negative results may occur for a variety of technical reasons (errors in fixation and processing, weak antisera, etc.). As a positive control, appropriate known positive paraffin blocks or frozen material can easily be retrieved from one's own files. As negative controls, the reaction should be performed (a) with the replacement of the specific primary antibody with an immunoglobulin from the same source and species, but directed against an unrelated antigen; and (b) after preadsorption of the primary antiserum with the purified antigen to be detected. Control slides should always be filed together with the diagnostic ones and shown together with them.

In Situ Hybridization

This is a new histochemical tool (Gall and Pardue 1969) which identifies specific DNA or RNA sequences in individual cells in smears or histological sections (reviewed by Sklar 1985). The method is highly sensitive, chemically precise, and has a high spatial resolution. In situ hybridization involves a specific reaction between a defined labeled nucleotide sequence (the probe) and a complementary target sequence under appropriate conditions. The probes are generated with the recombinant DNA technique and may be labeled with radionuclides such as ^{3}H, ^{32}P, ^{35}S, and ^{125}J. However, there is a current tendency to use nonradioactive markers, such as fluorochromes, enzymes, various haptens, and biotin, which is particularly promising (Leary et al. 1983). Nonautoradiographic hybridization by hybridocytochemical means has a number of advantages (low cost, absence of radiation hazard, disposal, etc.) and the major disadvantage of a lesser sensitivity, which may be overcome in due course. Biotinylated deoxynucleotides can be incorporated into DNA fragments by nick translation (Maniatis et al. 1976) and detected either with avidin-linked enzymes (ABC) or antibiotin antibodies.

At the present time in situ hybridization is used for the detection of viral mRNA and DNA in infected cells, the identification of specific sequences of

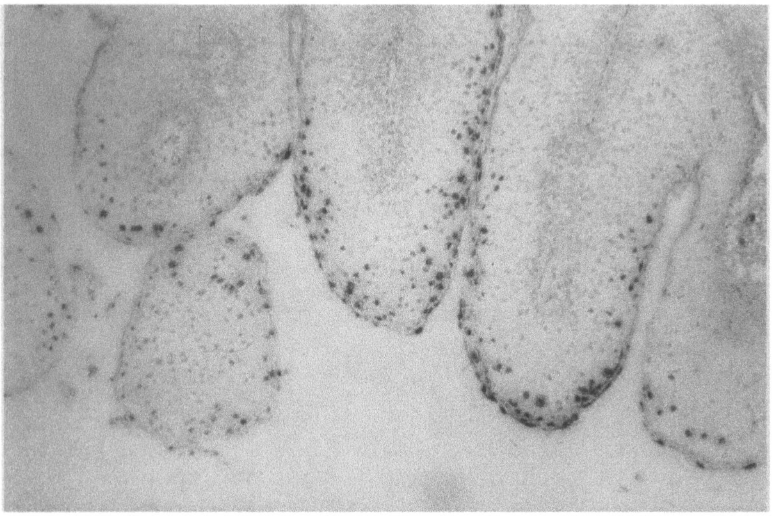

Fig. 17. Juvenile papillomatosis of the larynx. In situ hybridization of viral episomal DNA with a 35S-labeled probe for HPV types 6 and 11 (kindly supplied by Prof. H zur Hausen). Hematoxylin nuclear counterstain. × 25

mRNA in discrete cell populations which synthetize special products (e.g., hormones by restricted cell groups) at a low level, and for the chromosomal localization of genes, including oncogenes (Le Beau et al. 1985). For example, in situ hybridization has allowed investigators to (a) identify the distribution of HBV DNA within individual liver cells and make semiquantitative estimates of numbers of infected cells (Blum et al. 1984); (b) visualize type-specific HPV DNA in vulvar, cervical, penile, and laryngeal (Fig. 17) lesions and identify potentially dangerous HPV-16 and HPV-18 infections (Gupta et al. 1985); (c) detect HIV in glial cells in patients with AIDS encephalopathy (Shaw et al. 1985), etc.

The advances in cloning nucleotide sequences and producing monoclonal antibodies to specific antigens permitted the simultaneous detection by in situ hybridization and immunocytochemistry in the same cells of specific nucleic acid fragments and proteins. Discordant results of the two methods may indicate uptake or storage without synthesis or, vice versa, active secretion.

Appropriate controls should prevent false positive results, which may be produced by nonspecific hybridizations (plasmid DNA), endogenous peroxidase and biotin, pigmented material, etc.

Genotyping

The diagnosis of non-Hodgkin's malignant lymphomas has acquired a totally new dimension in recent years as the techniques of molecular biology for the detection of immunoglobulin and T cell receptor gene rearrangements have become available. The DNA hybridization principle allows the identification of even a small number of cells in which the same configuration of rearranged genes is present. This objective and highly sensitive method is unique in detecting clonal populations of cells which have a very high probability of being malignant. Polyclonal populations of lymphocytes will not show non-germ line extrabands of rearranged DNA fragments. Small numbers of lymphomatous cells (<5%) may be detected in cell suspensions of lymph nodes, extranodal sites, bone marrow, blood, etc., allowing not only primary diagnoses, but also the early identification of relapses of the disease.

References

Askin FB, Rosai J, Sibley RK, Dehner LP, McAlister WH (1979) Malignant small cell tumor of the thoracopulmonary region in childhood: A distinctive clinicopathologic entity of uncertain histogenesis. Cancer 43: 2438–2451

Battifora H, Kopinski MI (1985) Distinction of mesothelioma from adenocarcinoma. An immunohistochemical approach. Cancer 55: 1679–1685

Bennett JM, Catovsky D, Daniel MT, Flandrin G, Galton DAG, Gralnick HR, Sultan C (1982) Proposal for the classification of the myelodysplastic syndromes. Br J Haematol 51: 189–199

Blobel GA, Gould VE, Moll R, Lee I, Huszar M, Geiger B, Franke WW (1985) Coexpression of neuroendocrine markers and epithelial cytoskeletal proteins in bronchopulmonary neuroendocrine neoplasms. Lab Invest 52: 39–51

Blum HE, Haase AT, Vyas GN (1984) Molecular pathogenesis of hepatitis B virus infection simultaneous detection of viral DNA and antigens in paraffin-embedded liver sections. Lancet 2: 771–775

Capella C, Polak JM, Buffa R, Tapia FJ, Heitz U, Usellini L,

Bloom SR, Solcia E (1983) Morphologic patterns and diagnostic criteria or VIP-producing endocrine tumors. A histologic, histochemical, ultrastructural, and biochemical study of 32 cases. Cancer 52: 1860–1874

Carter D (1978) Pathology of early squamous cell carcinoma of the lung. Pathol Annu 13: 131–147

Carter D (1986) Margins of "lumpectomy" for breast cancer. Hum Pathol 17: 330–332

Carter D, Eggleston JC (1980) Tumors of the lower respiratory tract. AFIP, Washington, pp 193–199

Ceriani AL, Thompson K, Petersson JA, Abraham S (1977) Surface differentiation antigens of human mammary epithelial cells carried on the human milk fat globule. Proc Natl Acad Sci USA 74: 582–586

Chamness GC, Mercer WD, McGuire WL (1980) Are histochemical methods for estrogen receptor valid? J Histochem Cytochem 28: 792–798

Chejfec G, Capella C, Solcia E, Jao W, Gould VE (1985) Amphicrine cells, dysplasias, and neoplasias. Cancer 56: 2683–2690

Clark WH Jr, Reimer RR, Greene M, Ainsworth AM, Mastrangelo MJ (1978) Origin of familial malignant melanomas from heritable melanocytic lesions: "the B-K mole syndrome". Arch Dermatol 114: 732–738

Colgan TJ, Norris HJ (1983) Ovarian epithelial tumors of low malignant potentials: a review. Int J Gynecol Pathol 1: 367–382

Cooper D, Schermer A, Sun TT (1985) Biology of disease. Classification of human epithelial and their neoplasms using monoclonal antibodies to keratins: strategies, applications and limitations. Lab Invest 52: 243–256

Cordell JL, Falini B, Erber WN, Ghosh AK, Abdulaziz Z, MacDonald S, Pulford KAF, et al. (1984) Immunoenzymatic labeling of monoclonal antibodies using immune complexes of alkaline phosphatase and monoclonal anti-alkaline phosphatase (APAAP complexes). J Histochem Cytochem 32: 219–229

Corson JM (1986) Keratin protein immunohistochemistry in surgical pathology practice. Pathol Annu 21: 47–81

Danscher G, Norgaard JO (1983) Light microscopic visualization of colloidal gold on resinembedded tissue. J Histochem Cytochem 31: 1394–1398

Della Torre G, Pilotti S, de Palo G, Rilke F (1978) Viral particles in cervical condylomatous lesions. Tumori 64: 594–553

Di Fronzo G, Clemente C, Cappelletti V, Miodini P, Coradini D, Ronchi E, Andreola S, Rilke F (1986) Relationship between ER-ICA and conventional steroid receptor assays in human breast cancer. Breast Cancer Res Treat 8: 35–43

Dodds L, Davis S, Polissar L (1986) A population-based study of lung cancer incidence trends by histologic type, 1974-81. JNCI 76: 21–29

Dupont WD, Page DL (1985) Risk factors for breast cancer in women with proliferative breast disease. N Engl J Med 312: 146–151

Eisenberg AJ, Hajdu SI, Wilhelmus J, Melamed MR, Kinne D (1986) Preoperative aspiration cytology of breast tumors. Acta Cytol (Baltimore) 30: 135–146

Ekblom P, Miettinen M, Rapola J, Foidart JM (1982) Demonstration of laminin, a basement membrane glycoprotein, in routinely processed formalin fixed human tissues. Histochemistry 75: 301–307

Elder DE (1985) The dysplastic nevus. Pathology 17: 291–297

Erlandson RA (1984) Diagnostic immunohistochemistry of human tumors. An interim evaluation. Am J Surg Pathol 8: 615–624

Feller AC, Radzun HJ, Heymann E, Haas H, Scholz W, Parwaresch MR (1986) A monoclonal antibody detecting dipeptidylpeptidase IV in human tissue. Virchows Arch [A] 409: 263–273

Fenoglio CM, Pascal RR (1982) Colorectal adenomas and cancer. Pathologic relationship. Cancer 50: 2601–2608

Fisher ER, Sass R, Fisher B, Gregorio R, Brown R, Wickerham L (1986a) Pathologic findings from the National Surgical Adjuvant Breast Project (Protocol 6). II. Relation of local breast recurrence to multicentricity. Cancer 57: 1717–1724

Fisher ER, Sass R, Fisher B, Wickerham L, Paik SM (1986b) Pathologic findings from the National Surgical Adjuvant Breast Project (Protocol 6). I. Intraductal carcinoma (DCIS). Cancer 57: 197–208

Gall JB, Pardue ML (1969) Formation and detection of RNA-DNA hybrid molecules in cytological preparations. Proc Natl Acad Sci USA 63: 378–383

Gatter KC, Alcock C, Heryet A, Mason DY (1985) Clinical importance of analysing malignant tumours of uncertain origin with immunohistological techniques. Lancet 1: 1302–1305

Gerdes J, Lelle RJ, Pickartz H, Heidenreich W, Schwarting R, Kurtsiefer L, Stauch G, Stein H (1986) Growth fractions in breast cancers determined in situ with monoclonal antibody Ki-67. J Clin Pathol 39: 977–980

Gerdes J, Schwab U, Lemke H, Stein H (1983) Production of a mouse monoclonal antibody reactive with a human nuclear antigen associated with cell proliferation. Int J Cancer 31: 13–20

Gould VE (1986) Histogenesis and differentiation: a re-evaluation of these concepts as criteria for the classification of tumors. Hum Pathol 17: 212–215

Greene MH, Clark WH, Tucker MA, Elder DE, Kraemer KH, DuPont G, Witmer WK et al. (1985) Acquired precursors of cutaneous malignant melanoma. The familial dysplastic nevus syndrome. N Engl J Med 312: 91–97

Greene GL, Nolan C, Engler JP, Jensen EV (1980) Monoclonal antibodies to human estrogen receptor. Proc Natl acad Sci USA 77: 5115–5119

Gupta J, Gendelman HE, Naghashfar Z, Gupta P, Rosenshein N, Sawada E, Woodruff JD, Shah KV (1985) Specific identification of human papillomavirus type in cervical smears and paraffin sections by in situ hybridization with radioactive probes: a preliminary communication. Int J Gynecol Pathol 4: 211–218

Haagensen CD, Lane N, Lattes R, Bodian C (1978) Lobular neoplasia (so-called lobular carcinoma in situ) of the breast. Cancer 42: 737–769

Hajdu SI, Melamed MR (1984) Limitations of aspiration cytology in the diagnosis of primary neoplasms. Acta Cytol (Baltimore) 28: 337–345

Heyderman E, Steele K, Ormerod MG (1979) A new antigen on the epithelial membrane: its immunoperoxidase localisation in normal and neoplastic tissue. J Clin Pathol 32: 35–39

Hsu SU, Raine L, Fanger H (1981) Use of avidin-biotin-peroxidase complex (ABC) in immunoperoxidase techniques: a comparison between ABC and unlabeled antibody (PAP) procedures. J Histochem Cytochem 29: 577–580

Jack AS, Kerr IB, Evan G, Lee FD (1986) The distribution of the c-myc oncogene product in malignant lymphomas and various normal tissues as demonstrated by immunocytochemistry. Br J Cancer 53: 713–719

Kikuchi M (1972) Lymphadenitis showing focal reticulum cell hyperplasia with nuclear debris and phagocytes: a clinicopathological study (in Japanese). Nippon Ketsueki Gakkai Zasshi 35: 379–380

King JW, DeSombre ER, Jensen EV, Greene GL (1985) Comparison of immunocytochemical and steroid-binding assays for estrogen receptor in human breast tumors. Cancer Res 45: 293–304

King JW, Greene GL (1984) Monoclonal antibodies localize oestrogen receptor in the nuclei of target cells. Nature 307: 745–747

Köhler G, Milstein C (1975) Continuous cultures of fused cells secreting antibody of predefined specificity. Nature 256: 495–497

Koss LG (1975) Tumors of the urinary bladder. AFIP, Washington (Atlas of tumor pathology, 2nd ser, fasc 11)

Koss LG (1979 a) Diagnostic cytology and its histopathologic bases, 3rd edn. Lippincott, Philadelphia

Koss LG (1979 b) Mapping of the urinary bladder: its impact on the concepts of bladder cancer. Hum Pathol 10: 533–548

Kurman RJ, Norris HJ (1982) Endometrial neoplasia: hyperplasia and carcinoma. In: Blaustein A (ed) Pathology of the female genital tract, 3rd edn. Springer, Berlin Heidelberg New York, pp 311–351

Leary JJ, Brigati DJ, Ward DC (1983) Rapid and sensitive colorimetric method for visualizing biotinlabeled DNA probes hybridized to DNA or RNA immobilized on nitrocellulose: bioblots. Proc Natl Acad Sci USA 80: 4045–4049

Le Beau MM, Westbrook CA, Diaz MO, Rowley JD, Oren M (1985) Translocation of the p53 gene in t(15;17) in acute promyelocytic leukaemia. Nature 316: 826–828

Maniatis T, Kee SG, Efstratiadis A, Kafatos FC (1976) Amplification and characterization of a globin gene synthetized in vitro. Cell 8: 163–182

Mariani-Costantini R, Barbanti P, Colnaghi MI, Menard S, Clemente C, Rilke F (1984) Reactivity of a monoclonal antibody with tissues and tumors from the human breast. Am J Pathol 115: 47–56

Matthews MJ, Gazdar AF (1985) Changing histology in malignant tumors: diagnostic and therapeutic significance. Eur J Cancer Clin Oncol 21: 549–552

Miettinen M, Virtanen I, Talerman A (1985) Intermediate filament proteins in human testis and testicular germ-cell tumors. Am J Pathol 120: 402–410

Miller GJ (1988) An atlas of prostatic biopsies: dilemmas of morphologic variance. Prog Surg Pathol VIII: 81–110

Ming SC, Bajta A, Correa P, Elster K, Jarvi OH, Munoz N, Nagayo T, Stemmerman GN (1984) Gastric dysplasia. Significance and pathologic criteria. Cancer 54: 1794–1801

Moll R, Franke WW, Schiller DL (1982) The catalog of human cytokeratins: patterns of expression in normal epithelia, tumors and cultured cells. Cell 31: 11–24

Mukai K, Schollmeyer JV, Rosai J (1981) Immunohistochemical localization of actin: its application in surgical pathology. Am J Surg Pathol 5: 91–97

Muto T, HJR Bussey, Morson BC (1975) The evolution of cancer of the colon and rectum. Cancer 36: 2251–2270

Nakazawa H, Rosen P, Lane N, Lattes R (1968) Frozen section experience in 3000 cases. Accuracy, limitations and value in residency training. Am J Clin Pathol 49: 41–51

Norton AJ, Ramsay AD, Smith SH, Beverley PCL, Isaacson PG (1986) Monoclonal antibody (UCHL1) that recognises normal and neoplastic T cells in routinely fixed tissues. J Clin Pathol 39: 399–405

O'Connor DT, Deftos LJ (1986) Secretion of chromogranin A by peptide-producing endocrine neoplasms. N Engl J Med 314: 1145–51

Osborn M, Weber K (1983) Tumor diagnosis by intermediate filament typing. A novel tool for surgical pathology. Lab Invest 48: 372–394

Page DL (1986) Cancer risk assessment in benign breast biopsies. Hum Pathol 17: 871–874

Pahlman S, Esscher T, Nilsson K (1986) Expression of γ-subunit of enolase, neuron-specific enolase, in human non-endocrine tumors and derived cell lines. Lab Invest 54: 554–560

Pilotti S, Rilke F, Gribaudi G, Damascelli B, Ravasi G (1984) Transthoracic fine needle aspiration biopsy in pulmonary lesions: updated results. Acta Cytol (Baltimore) 28: 225–232

Poulsen HS, Ozzello L, King WJ, Greene GL (1985) The use of monoclonal antibodies to estrogen receptors (ER) for immunoperoxidase detection of ER in paraffin sections of human breast cancer tissue. J Histochem Cytochem 33: 87–92

Press MF, King WJ, Greene GL (1986) Immunocytochemical localization of progesterone receptor in breast carcinoma. Lab Invest 54: 51A

Richart RM (1967) The natural history of cervical intraepithelial neoplasia. Clin Obstet Gynecol 10: 748–784

Rodriguez Martinez HA, Rosai J (1981) Gross techniques in surgical pathology. In: Rosai J (ed) Ackerman's surgical pathology, 6th edn. Mosby, St Louis, pp 19–38

Sabatini DD, Bensch K, Barrnett RJ (1963) Cytochemistry and electron microscopy. The preservation of cellular structures and enzymatic activity by aldehyde fixation. J Cell Biol 17: 19–58

Sainsbury JRC, Farndon JR, Sherbet GV, Harris AL (1985) Epidermal-growth-factor receptors and oestrogen receptors in human breast cancer. Lancet 8425: 364–366

Salter DM, Krajewski AS, Dewar AE (1985) Immunohistochemical staining of non-Hodgkin's lymphoma with monoclonal antibodies specific for the leucocyte common antigen. J Pathol 146: 345–353

Shaw GM, Harper ME, Hahn BH, Epstein LG, Gajdusek DC, Price WR, Navia BA, et al. (1985) HTVLV-III infection in brains of children and adults with AIDS encephalopathy. Science 227: 177–182

Shirasawa H, Tomita Y, Kubota K, Kasai T, Sekiya S, Takamizawa H, Simizu B (1986) Detection of human papillomavirus type 16 DNA and evidence for integration into the cell DNA in cervical dysplasia. J Gen Virol 67: 2011–2015

Sklar J (1985) DNA hybridization in diagnostic pathology. Hum Pathol 16: 654–658

Stenman S, Vaheri A (1981) Fibronectin in human solid tumors. Int J Cancer 27: 427–435

Sternberger LA (1979) Immunocytochemistry, 2nd edn. Wiley and Sons, New York, pp 1–354

Sternberger LA, Joseph SA (1979) The unlabeled antibody method. Contrasting colour staining of paired pituitary hormones without antibody removal. J Histochem Cytochem 27: 1424–1429

Tanaka T, Slamon DJ, Battifora H, Cline MJ (1986) Expression of p21 ras oncoproteins in human cancers. Cancer Res 46: 1465–1470

Toker C (1972) Trabecular carcinoma of the skin. Arch Dermatol 105: 2308–2311

Van Furth R, Cohn ZA, Hirsch JG, Humphrey JH, Spector WG, Langevoort HL (1972) The mononuclear phagocyte system: A new classification of macrophages, monocytes and their precursor cells. Bull WHO 46: 845–852

Vincent RG, Pickren JW, Lane WW, Bross I, Takita H, Houten L, Gutierrez AC, Rzepka T (1977) The changing histopathology of lung cancer. A review of 1682 cases. Cancer 39: 1647–1655

Wang HH, Antonioli DA, Goldman H (1986) Comparative features of esophageal and gastric adenocarcinomas. Hum Pathol 17: 482–487

Watanabe S, Okita K, Harada T, Kodama T, Numa Y, Takemoto T, Takahashi T (1983) Morphologic studies of the liver cell dysplasia. Cancer 51: 2197–2205

Weinberg RA (1985) The action of oncogenes in the cytoplasm and nucleus. Science 230: 770–776

Weiss SW, Enzinger FM (1982) Epithelioid hemangioendothelioma. A vascular tumor often mistaken for a carcinoma. Cancer 50: 970–981

WHO (1967) Histological typing of lung tumours. WHO, Geneva, pp 27–28

WHO (1976) International classification of diseases for oncology, 1st edn. WHO, Geneva

WHO (1981) Histological typing of breast tumours, 2nd edn. WHO, Geneva, pp 23–25

Williams ED, Siebenmann RE, Sobin LH (1980) Histological typing of endocrine tumours. WHO, Geneva

Yokota J, Tsunetsugu-Yokota Y, Battifora H, Le Fevre C, Cline MJ (1986) Alterations of myc, myb, and ras^{Ha} proto-oncogenes in cancers are frequent and show clinical correlation. Science 231: 261–265

Zur Hausen H, Gissmann L, Schlehofer JR (1984) Viruses in the etiology of human genital cancer. Prog Med Virol 30: 170–186

Modern Imaging Techniques in Diagnosis Staging and Follow-up of Cancer

P. HAEHNEL, M. DREYFUS, and D. JAECK

Introduction

The recent introduction of new techniques in medical imagery should lead to a comparison of their respective merits. As is often the case in medicine, the latest discovery tends to supplant the previous techniques, and it is only after some years that the advantages of the various methods may be weighed up. Unfortunately, the appearance of a new technique often leads doctors to confuse modernism with truth. This is why it would now seem interesting to take stock of the results obtained by new techniques in the diagnosis of most cancers, notably by magnetic resonance imaging (MRI), computed tomography (CT), and ultrasonography (US).

Schematically, the field of application of MRI would be in the diagnosis of CNS, abdominal, and pelvic cancers. CT diagnosis is more efficient in retroperitoneal diseases (lymph nodes and adrenal glands) as well as in bile duct and pelvic cancer extension diagnosis.

Interventional radiology is becoming more and more important, especially in therapeutic methods (which do not figure in this paper), such as arterial embolization of hepatic metastasis of carcinoid tumors of the bowel. Conventional radiology has lost none of its significance, especially in breast cancer, where it is the only technique revealing signs of occult breast carcinoma.

Digestive Tract

Esophagus

MRI has already shown considerable potential in the study of the thorax and especially in the evaluation of the heart, the great vessels, the mediastinum, and the pulmonary hila (Webb et al. 1984a; Cohen et al. 1983). Application to esophageal carcinoma has also received attention (Ross et al. 1984; Smith et al. 1981). However, the results of a recent study (Quint et al. 1985a, b) strongly suggest that the current technique of nonrespiratory gated spin echo magnetic resonance is inaccurate in staging esophageal carcinoma. MRI, like CT, also appears inaccurate in assessing local features (aortic and tracheobronchial invasion) that are important in determining resectability. In the series of Quint et al. (1985b), the MR images of 25% of patients with esophageal carcinoma were indeterminate for aortic invasion because of the absence of a fat plane over 45°–90° of the aortic circumference at the plane of the esophageal tumor. Previous investigation done by the same authors showed relatively low CT staging accuracy (Quint et al. 1985a). The inaccuracy in tumor staging by both CT and MRI was mainly due to difficulty in detecting tumor spread through the muscular wall of the esophagus into adjacent mediastinal soft tissue (Quint et al. 1985b).

Stomach

CT is a proven imaging modality for the evaluation of primary gastric tumors (Kressel et al. 1979; Lee et al. 1979). In a recent series of 38 patients (Mullin and Shirkhoda 1985) CT was helpful in the diagnosis of local recurrence and distant metastasis, in guiding the biopsy of the suspected abnormalities, and in the evaluation of the results of the treatment. In this study, recurrent carcinoma was seen as a soft tissue mass averaging 3 cm in size. Secondary signs, such as obliterations of the fascial plane between the area of anastomosis and pancreatic bed, were helpful in confirming the diagnosis (Moss et al. 1980). CT seemed to be better than conventional barium studies in demonstrating recurrent local disease. Of course, CT yields more information about distant metastasis and adenopathy and can be used for percutaneous guided biopsy.

Small Bowel

US may be helpful in both detection and staging of malignancies of the small bowel (Fakhri and Berk 1981). These malignancies may produce rounded masses involving the small bowel and mesentery. The "target" or "bull's-eye" appearance, sometimes simulating a transverse section of a kidney, and the additional presence of focal bowel wall thickening are helpful signs. Extensive mesenteric or hepatic metastases may also be detected.

Abdominal Carcinoid Tumor

CT evaluation of carcinoid tumor has received scant attention in the literature, consisting of only a few case reports (Bernardino et al. 1979; Damgaard-Petersen and Stage 1979; Siegel et al. 1980). A recent report of ten patients (Cockey et al. 1985) showed in four cases a pattern that has been considered as strongly suggestive of carcinoid tumor: many small punctate or linear mesenteric densities due to reactive desmoplasia and adenopathy, with either rounded mesenteric masses or hepatic masses. Focal thickening of small bowel was a helpful additional sign. Of course, clinical history and biological findings are also necessary.

Kaposi's Sarcoma

The CT characteristics in Kaposi's sarcoma and lymphadenopathy syndrome have been studied (Moon et al. 1984). Mesenteric lymphadenopathy was seen, but there was no associated fibrosis or mesenteric retraction. The clinical history was usually helpful in making diagnosis.

Rectal Tumors

Conventional radiography and US have been inadequate for preoperative staging of these neoplasms (Nicholls et al. 1982). CT has permitted more definitive assessment of perirectal involvement (Meyer et al. 1983; Thoenl et al. 1981; Dixon et al. 1981; Grabbe et al. 1983; Sperber et al. 1983); however, the accuracy in evaluating perirectal fat and lymph node invasion is variable. The efficacy of transrectal sonography (endosonography) has been evaluated (Rifkin and Marks 1985) in 31 patients. Transrectal US was able to image all masses situated within 12 cm of the anus. Malignant infiltration of perirectal fat and perirectal node involvement were detected at least as accurately with US as with CT, suggesting that this technique is a cost-effective and reliable adjunct for staging rectal cancers, at least in the hands of well-trained sonographers.

However, the efficiency of CT in the staging and follow-up study of carcinoma of the rectum has been reinforced (Clark et al. 1984; Butch et al. 1986); it has virtually replaced the excretory urogram in the preoperative assessment of patients with this carcinoma. It has also been shown to be very helpful in the demonstration of tumor extension, especially in the presacral area and the pelvic side walls.

In early preoperative detection of local or regional recurrences, CT is very accurate. In a prospective evaluation (McCarthy et al. 1985) of CT and clinical factors in detection of recurrent rectosigmoid carcinoma [including carcinoembryonic antigen (CEA)], CT appeared to be the most sensitive test. The best screening period for recurrence is between 6 months and 2 years after surgery (Grabbe et al. 1983). CT provides both a nonoperative survey of the pelvis and a method of directing fine needle biopsy. Therefore, the use of CT at specific time intervals (6 months) is particularly important for detection of recurrence (Kelvin et al. 1983).

Anal Canal Tumors

Anal canal tumors constitute only a small percentage of colorectal malignancies. However, preoperative evaluation of patients with these tumors is helpful in planning appropriate therapy and determining an accurate prognosis. CT evaluation has been shown to be beneficial both before and after therapy (Cohan et al. 1985).

Pancreas

CT has replaced arteriography as the primary imaging method of choice in the diagnosis of carcinoma of the pancreas (Breatnach et al. 1985; Whalen 1979). The value of CT in endocrine tumors has been emphasized in recent studies (Breatnach et al. 1985; Rossi et al. 1985). Previous reports had shown low accuracy with US and even CT (Rossi et al. 1985). However, considerable advances have recently been made with CT in the detection of pancreatic lesions as well as local and hepatic metastases. In particular, Rossi et al. (1985) have stressed the importance of a proper CT technique using fast scanners (five to ten scans per minute) and repeated bolus injections of contrast medium. CT should, therefore, be the initial step in examining patients with suspected endocrine tumors of the pancreas. If necessary, arteriography and, in a few cases, transhepatic selective venous sampling may be used. Breatnach et al. came to the same conclusions in CT evaluation of glucagonomas (Breatnach et al. 1985).

MRI of the pancreas using conventional techniques has been limited by low signal to noise ratio and respiratory or peristaltic artifacts (Simeone et al. 1985). High-resolution surface coil imaging offers more diagnostic information than comparable T2-weighted images. Simeone et al. (1985) concluded that normal pancreatic anatomy and pancreatic abnormalities can be demonstrated with prototype MR surface coil technology. In some cases, this method can demonstrate normal structures and pathological features better than conventional body coil MRI or X-ray CT. In contrast to previous pessimism about the prospect of MRI of the pancreas, surface coil MRI may become a valuable clinical technique for examination of the pancreas.

In postoperative evaluation after pancreatectomy, CT appears to be extremely useful during the postoperative period as well as during the follow-up. Heiken et al. (1984) evaluated a group of patients, who had undergone radical pancreatic section, for

1 week in 11 years after surgery. CT demonstrated postoperative complications or tumor recurrence and was 100% accurate in patients who were followed up. Heiken et al. (1984) used a CT protocol including intravenous administration of glucagon immediately before scanning; this drug helps fill the afferent loop and prevents misinterpretation of this loop as a soft tissue mass. Administration of intravenous contrast material helped to delineate anatomy and to differentiate para-aortic lymph nodes.

Liver

Malignant involvement of the liver, both primary and metastatic, is more frequent than benign hepatic tumors. The radiographic diagnosis of primary hepatocellular carcinoma is usually difficult. To determine the true extent of the tumor is even more difficult since these tumors often occur in cirrhotic livers. CT, particularly with dynamic bolus contrast medium enhancement, has brought about a significant advance in the diagnosis of hepatomas. However, early diagnosis is of prime importance in the treatment of hepatocellular carcinoma.

Matsui et al. (1985) introduced infusion hepatic angiography and reported its effectiveness in early detection of small liver cancers. However, in the case of hypovascular hepatic tumors, they developed dynamic sequential CT with table incrementation during arterial portography. They compared this method with other imaging methods including radionuclide liver scans, US, CT, selective celiac angiography, and infusion hepatic angiography in the detection of hepatocellular carcinomas of less than 3 cm in diameter. Dynamic sequential CT with table incrementation during arterial portography appeared to be the most sensitive method.

Vermess et al. (1985) compared the definition of liver tumors at MRI with the definition of liver tumors at CT. MRI was particularly useful in differentiating the tumor from otherwise abnormal areas of the liver, mostly focal cirrhosis. MRI has the advantage of demonstrating major vessels in relation to the hepatoma without injection of any contrast agent.

La Berge et al. (1984) published a series with surgical correlation: CT correctly predicted the extent of the tumor in 13 out of 16 cases. However, in 20% of the patients the true extent of the tumor was not determined preoperatively. MRI seems to be more capable than CT of determining the extent of hepatic involvement (Moss et al. 1984) and of differentiating hemangioma and hepatic malignancies (Ohtomo et al. 1985). Disadvantages of MRI are that calcifications within the tumor are not demonstrated and that venous invasion and extrahepatic spread are not well shown. The greatest obstacle to MRI of the liver is respiratory and transmitted cardiac motion. Finally, the capability of MRI to demonstrate small hepatomas or metastatic lesions has not yet been convincingly demonstrated. Development of combined cardiac/respiratory gating will probably improve liver images.

In children, hepatic tumor diagnosis may be improved using a protocol involving a combination of US, CT, and scintigraphy (Miller and Greenspan 1985).

In patients with primary carcinomas of the gallbladder or with biliary ductal carcinoma, CT accurately identifies the site of obstruction in the major bile ducts and is able to evaluate extraductal extension (Thorsen et al. 1984).

The ability of MRI and CT in helping to detect hepatic metastases has been shown to be comparable (Heiken et al. 1985). The MRI technique that is most reliable in detecting metastases is inversion recovery and a relatively T2-weighted spinecho technique (TR = 1500 ms, TE = 60 ms). Heiken et al. (1985) after performing MRI and CT studies in 50 patients with hepatic metastases, concluded that CT, because of its shorter imaging time, greater spatial resolution, and lower cost, should remain the preferred screening test for hepatic metastases. MRI should be reserved for patients with equivocal CT findings and for patients in whom there is persistent clinical suspicion of hepatic metastases despite a negative CT examination. However, in a randomized controlled comparison of detection of hepatic metastases, the accuracy of a single T1-weighted (10-min) pulse sequence was superior to that of contrast-enhanced CT (Stark et al. 1987).

Abdominal and Pelvic Lymphadenopathies

Several studies have recently been reported comparing the ability of MRI and CT to demonstrate normal and abnormal lymph nodes, especially in the abdomen (Lee et al. 1984; Dooms et al. 1984, 1985a). MRI detected all lymphadenopathy originally documented by CT and easily distinguished blood vessels from lymph nodes; on the other hand, CT offered better spatial resolution and could be completed in a shorter time (Lee et al. 1984). Even though MRI displayed the nodes better because of its excellent soft-tissue contrast resolution, differentiation between benign and malignant lymph nodes could not be achieved using current MRI parameters (Dooms et al. 1985 a).

Soft-Tissue Neoplasms

CT is useful for demonstrating the location, size, and extent of the tumor and its effect on adjacent organs and neurovascular structures. CT is also useful for the detection of tumor recurrence and for following tumor response to radiation or chemotherapy (Weekes et al. 1985). Differentiation between lipomas and liposarcomas is achieved by both MRI and CT (Dooms et al. 1985 b).

Thyroid

CT has proven valuable in the evaluation of cervical masses of various etiologies (Kier et al. 1985; Silverman et al. 1983). CT has recently been utilized for the evaluation of thyroid masses as a complementary technique to radionuclide and US imaging (Silverman et al. 1983; Reede et al. 1982). No specific criteria are available for determining the benign or malignant nature of a thyroid lesion by CT; however, the findings of a poorly marginated mass, central necrosis, and associated lymphadenopathy are consistent with a malignant tumor (Kier et al. 1985).

Radecki et al. (1984) compared US and CT in 48 patients with a clinical diagnosis of thyroid abnormality and also correlated these data with biopsy or surgery. Both techniques lacked histopathological specificity. CT appeared to be advantageous in detecting external thyroid extension, while US was better in detecting small nodules and evaluating intrinsic thyroid abnormalities.

In medullar carcinoma of the thyroid, CT is probably helpful in detecting abnormal lymph nodes in the neck but more so in detecting them in the mediastinum (Reiners et al. 1983) in the case of a recurrent high CEA level after thyroidectomy.

Bone

Recently, some studies have attempted to use MRI in bone tumor evaluation and to compare this method with CT (Shirkhoda et al. 1985). MRI is not able to differentiate benign from malignant tumors. Some signs could only give a suspicion of a benign (well-defined low signal rim between lesion and adjacent marrow) or malignant nature (poorly defined inhomogeneities within tumors). Further studies will be necessary to see if each type of tumor has specific T1 and T2 relaxation times. However, at present plain films still remain the best technique for diagnosing bone tumors.

On the other hand, MRI is the best technique for evaluating bone marrow extension. In this case, sagittal sections are extremely useful; longitudinal involvement of the marrow can be predicted, and thus, the level of resection or amputation can be determined. MRI is also better in the depiction of soft tissue extension as contrasts are better. CT remains superior to MRI in describing normal cortex, pathological fractures, and mineralization.

In describing neurovascular structures and joints, MRI seems to be better than CT. In the follow-up of the patients already treated, CT is able to determine whether the mass has decreased or remained the same. This technique is a good predictor of healing processes. But in some patients with nonferromagnetic metallic protheses, MRI is better than CT in the diagnosis of recurrent tumors.

Evaluation of bone tumors by P31 MR spectroscopy tries to determine specific tumor spectra by examination of local metabolism. This work is still in progress, and so far few teams have reported their results (Nidecker et al. 1985).

Thorax

Many studies have compared MRI with CT in diagnosis and staging of hilar and mediastinal masses (Webb et al. 1984 a; Gamsu et al. 1983). Most authors think that CT still remains the best method, but that MRI could provide a lot of information. In fact, both have similar accuracy in describing lymph nodes. CT, with better spatial resolution, is superior in showing lesions, while MRI, which provides excellent contrast, allows differentiation between nodules and vascular structures.

CT is more reliable in defining bronchial involvement and depicting masses located close to the diaphragm or pleura. In detecting mediastinal nodes MRI seems to have slightly higher sensitivity but lower specificity than CT. MRI also seems to have better accuracy in the evaluation of soft-tissue tumors.

MRI has some drawbacks: artifact formation during respiratory motion, a long examination time, and it is unsuitable for patients with ferromagnetic material. It is particularly indicated for patients who are allergic to CT contrast injection.

During staging, both techniques present diverse advantages. One study (Webb et al. 1984 b) reports on the usefulness of combining transaxial and coronal sections for MRI; these combined images provide better preoperative anatomic relationships and improve the diagnostic results. The increase in evaluation accuracy allows a better selection of patients who have to undergo mediastinoscopy (only with mediastinal lymph nodes).

Heart

Until recently the only technique for diagnosing cardiac tumors was echocardiography. Now gated cardiac MRI is a new noninvasive process for displaying cardiac neoplasms. MRI could be superior in imaging and be complementary to two-dimensional echocardiography (Go et al. 1985). It seems to be more precise regarding the size, shape, and surface characteristics of the tumor. Its wider viewing field provides better data on eventual valvular obstruction and cardiac chamber size. Both techniques provide high accuracy on tumor localization.

MRI is also able to diagnose pericardial disease (Stark et al. 1984) and especially masses. The sensitivity of this method allows differentiation of pericardial masses from fat pad and diaphragmatic eventration.

In fact, two-dimensional echocardiography does have some limitation: obesity; chest wall thickness and configuration, and degree of pulmonary hyperinflation are all difficulties which do not affect MRI. On the other hand, two-dimensional echocardiography is cheaper, easier, and can be used in patients with severe *rythmical* disturbances. Thus MRI could provide results where two-dimensional echocardiography is not successful and will very soon become a complementary technique to those commonly in use.

Kidneys

MRI could be a helpful method in preoperative evaluation and staging of retroperitoneal neoplasms. The usefulness of MRI in kidney cancer has already been emphasized (Hricak et al. 1985; Parienty et al. 1985). A very high degree of accuracy was obtained in the diagnosis and the extent of perirenal involvement. The MRI features were compared with surgical data: 100% of MRI diagnoses were reliable, and of 27 cases 26 stagings were correct. This technique seems to be highly effective in describing thrombosis or venous involvement. Extension to adjacent organs is well defined. Advantages of MRI versus CT could be in preoperative localization of perirenal neoplasms.

Another author has reported that CT is a good method for preoperative distinction between renal cysts and cystic cancers (Parienty et al. 1985). Some signs could help diagnoses: Cysts larger than 10 cm, localized thickening of cyst walls seen with contrast enhancement, implantation of an irregular and poorly defined cyst. In fact, MRI could be better in classifying the few cases where CT is not able to differentiate benign from malignant tumors.

Bladder

Fisher et al. (1985 b) compared MRI and CT for the evaluation and staging of bladder neoplasms. MRI is highly accurate in detecting the site, size, and pattern of growth of a tumor. When tumor size is more than 1.5 cm, diagnosis is easy using transversal and sagittal sections, but carcinoma in situ cannot be detected. MRI has some advantages over CT; first, diagnosis is possible whether the bladder is distended or not; but most important is the better possibility provided for staging cancer. Variation of intensity between the different pelvic organs and inside the bladder wall permits identification of involvement and TNM staging. Thus T2 (TNM) is distinguishable from T3a, and the latter is different on MR images from T3b. The lack of fat pads around the bladder explains the difficulties experienced with CT staging as contrast differences are too weak. However, although MRI is a good method for evaluation, histological proof by means of a biopsy is still required for diagnosis.

Uterus

Some reports have studied the use of MRI in detecting, uterine lesions, (Lee et al. 1985; Hamlin et al. 1985 a). This method allows different tissues to be identified in relation to intensity signals, so correlation between MRI data and histological findings has been established (Lee et al. 1985). The endometrium forms a central high-intensity zone, whereas the myometrium is an area with a medium-intensity signal. Most abnormalities can be seen with MRI, especially endometrial and cervical carcinoma. Endometrial cancer is represented by a small zone of slightly higher intensity than the myometrium but lower than the endometrium.

MRI could be interesting in the staging of endometrial carcinoma. The method is able to define the depth of myometrial invasion (Hricak et al. 1987; Powell et al. 1986 a). However, some papers give the limits of this procedure (Hricak et al. 1987; Michel et al. 1987). Firstly, MRI was not able to differentiate endometrial carcinoma from adenomatous hyperplasia or blood clots. Secondly, the method failed to diagnose carcinomas limited to the endometrium, particularly in postmenopausal women in whom the junctional zone is frequently missing (Hricak et al. 1987; Michel et al. 1986).

Transvaginal ultrasound scanning could be a new way of investigating the depth of myometrial invasion (Fleischer et al. 1987). The cervix has an MRI signal with a lower intensity than the myometrium due to the high proportion of connective tissue. Cases of cervical carcinoma are indicated by areas of high intensity as compared with the normal structures. In fact, abnormalities are recognized more by the changes in intensity than by morphological variations. The interest of MRI in cervical carcinoma is to provide multiplanar facilities allowing the study of the volume and extension of the tumor (Powell et al. 1986 b). It could also determine the response to preoperative radiotherapy by showing any residual tumor (Michel et al. 1987). Finally, one of the most important contributions of MRI is its ability to distinguish radiation fibrosis and recurrent tumor (Glazer et al. 1985).

Trophoblast

Up until now, evaluation of trophoblastic disease has depended on HCG tests. Ultrasound findings are not specific enough, and angiography is quite an invasive method. Recently, dynamic CT has seemed more reliable (Miyasaka et al. 1985). Images are specific from invasive mole and choriocarcinoma. After bolus injection, Miyasaka et al. (1985) found contrast-enhanced areas in the myometrium with low-density areas in or around lesions. These features could be representative of hydatid moles penetrating uterine muscle.

For choriocarcinoma Miyasaka et al. (1985) described a large hypodense zone *surrounded* by a contrast area. This image is related to the angiographical results, i.e., central avascularity and peripheral pooling. These authors therefore consider dynamic CT to be the most reliable technique for evaluation of trophoblastic disease.

Ovaries

It is now well known that MRI findings are wholly reliable in pelvic diseases (Hamlin et al. 1985 b). Thus, ovarian masses can be depicted quite easily. Some reports (Dooms et al. 1986; Hricak et al. 1983 a) tend to classify ovarian lesions using T1 and T2 relaxation times values. They believe that each type of histological mass provides a specific value. Thus, hemorrhagic cysts have shortest T1 and T2 relaxation times, while cystic ovarian tumors, like mucinous cystadenoma, have the longest. MRI is also able to evaluate the stage of the hematoma, the intensity of which depends on iron concentration (Bradley and Schmidt 1984; Nishimura et al. 1987). Difficulties, however, exist in distinguishing the complex benign cysts from ovarian stromal carcinoma and inflammatory masses; MRI appearances are quite similar with each of these abnormalities presenting a structural heterogeneity.

Another author writes about the effectiveness of CT in diagnosing Krukenberg's tumors (Cho and Gold 1985). No specific signs can be described, but CT seems to be superior to sonography for the evaluation of recurrent ovarian carcinoma and depiction of the extent of the disease. CT is also to be preferred in the evaluation of response to treatment. MRI is useful in identifying recurrent pelvic neoplasm and distinguishing it from post-treatment fibrosis (Ebner et al. 1988).

Testicles

As the treatment of a nonseminomatous testicular tumor depends on staging, some authors (Poskitt et al. 1985) have tried to determine what the most cost-efficient protocol is. They have compared sonography, CT, lymphangiograms, tumor marker determination, and excretory urograms. The last three techniques had a high false negative rate (35%, 61%, 78%, respectively). Sonography and CT had no significant differences in accuracy (90%) and false negative rate (13% and 18%, respectively). Neither sonography nor CT was able to differentiate stages A1, B1, and B2 on the one hand, and B3 and C on the other, but these results do not affect therapy. Indeed, because there is no close relation between CT features and histology, the first three stages need retroperitoneal lymph node dissection, whereas the last two stages require preoperative chemotherapy. So, the authors proposed the use of sonography as a screening method and performed CT only when sonographic examination was inadequate (because of obesity or bowel gas), or negative.

Recently, Stomper et al. (1985) examined correlation between CT findings after chemotherapy and histology. They recommended continuing surgery in order to have histological evidence on which further treatment could be based. Node size and density cannot be used as indications of remaining malignancy. Even changes during chemotherapy are not related to histological types.

Prostate

CT staging for prostate cancer must be very logical. One begins to expose the pelvic section and then continues up to the aortic bifurcation. If no lymphadenopathy is revealed, investigation may be stopped. The examination should be extended to the distal para-aortic area (renal arteries level) if large iliac nodes are found (Styles and Seltzer 1985). Rifkin and Marks (1985) proposed transrectal sonourethrography to examine the prostatic urethra. In this way it is possible to diagnose intrinsic pathology. Recently, Fleischer (1987) proposed prostatic endosonography as a potential screening test. This method could diagnose preclinical prostatic carcinoma. It could also improve the results of needle biopsy. One of the important aspects is its ability to determine the precise location of a nonpalpable nodule, as it is well known that peripheral tumors are more likely to be cancerous.

There are many reports on the use of MRI in examining the prostate where carcinoma gives high-intensity signals (Steyn and Smith 1982; Hricak et al. 1983b). In a recent report, a normal prostate was compared with benign hypertrophic disease and carcinoma (Poon et al. 1985). Normal anatomy showed a bright rim around the gland corresponding to periprostatic venous plexus. Preservation of this rim would show absence of extraglandular extension. On the other hand, however, Poon et al. (1985) were not able to differentiate either benign from malignant tumors, or normal from pathological tissue. So MRI seems to be better for staging prostate carcinoma than for diagnosing very precise disease.

CNS

MRI has been found to be capable of obtaining excellent results in the exploration of certain anatomical regions, in particular the CNS, the osteoarticular and muscular body, and the pelvic cavity (Bilanik et al. 1984a, b). MRI appears to be superior to CT in that it permits a more precise differentiation of the tumor itself and of the surrounding *edema*, as well as the peritumoral tissue. However, when CT is combined with iodinated contrast substances, it can obtain better results. This is why new contrast materials specific for MRI are being developed in addition to those, such as gadolinium-DTPA, already in use (Felix et al. 1985; Bydder et al. 1985). The examination of a subject before and after using gadolinium – DTPA is undoubtedly more informative in that the real extent of the tumor can be better observed, thus allowing for its complete excision. These results are similar for both cerebral and for spinal cord tumors. In the latter localization, contrast enhancement permits the differentiation of intermedullary and extramedullary tumors. The use of gadolinium-DTPA should, however, be reserved for specific cases, especially as it makes examination more expensive and time-consuming.

These characteristics are true for all intracranial tumors, especially *sellar and extrasellar* tumors (Enzmann et al. 1985; Lee and Deck 1985). No other technique can give such precise information distinguishing between a pituitary mass and the adjacent structures, in particular the optic *channels* and the vessels. At the other end of the vertebral column, the sacrococcygeal chordoma can be detected more easily using MRI. When the *craniocaudial* extension of the lesion becomes primordial, only MRI permits real evaluation because of the *possibility of using coronal and sagittal* sections. Similarly, the differentiation between peritumorous tissues and tumors is facilitated, which can help in diagnosing a recurring tumor.

Ocular Tumors

The advantage of MRI in the diagnosis of pituitary lesions has already been established, essentially through the visualization of the relation between the tumor and optic tracts. The diagnosis and staging of choroidal melanoma has been greatly facilitated by CT and also by ultrasound, the results of which were practically identical in the measuring of the thickness of the lesion. The advantage, particularly of CT, is considerable in the follow-up of patients treated conservatively as well as in the search of further lesions in the vicinity (Peyster et al. 1985).

Nasopharynx

As in all exploration of soft tissue, MRI has undeniable advantages over other techniques. It permits a better characterization of pathological tissue because of the quality of the image and the excellent contrast. Not only does MRI show the exact extent of the tumor, but it also reveals the extension toward the ganglions without the aid of any contrast material. At the same time, it permits the differentiation between recurrent malignant disease and fibrous postradiation tissue (Dillon et al. 1984).

In conclusion, in all tumoral pathology of the CNS and the head and neck, MRI shows advantages over CT. Soft-tissue contrast and the clear separation of normal and pathological tissue are determining elements for the therapeutic procedure, whether surgical or radiotherapeutical. The advantages of MRI will increase with the inclusion of special contrast materials, but these, in our opinion, should be reserved for specific pathological research because of the high cost and, particularly, the harmful side effects.

Breast

Breast cancer remains the highest cause of mortality in a certain group of women. Approximately one in thirteen females will have breast cancer. The mortality rate for this disease has remained nearly unchanged for the past 40 years, and the incidence rate is rising in females under 40 years of age. The only way of reducing the mortality rate lies in early detection – that is, detecting breast cancer in women in apparently good health. Breast cancer still remains, from a pathological point of view, a grave problem. Despite greatly improved diagnostic techniques, the chances of survival have not increased significantly. Early diagnosis of breast cancer encounters two problems: (a) the difficulty of characterizing, by medical imagery, the nature of tissue classified as "precancerous"; (b) the difficulty of diagnosing cancer at the start of its development.

It would appear desirable to take stock of the different methods of evaluating breast cancer, as this would lead to a better understanding and deeper knowledge of mammary pathology. Investigation combining clinical examination, radiography, and cytological biopsy has always been the basis of early detection of breast cancer and currently permits diagnosis in 95% of cases.

The techniques which were introduced in the late 1960s, such as thermography and echography, have met with varying degrees of success. Thermography, apart from its diagnostic properties, had the added advantage that it used no ionizing radiation. This was one of the reasons why this method was put forward as a screening technique. Unfortunately, credibility was lost due to the exaggerated arguments of the advocates of thermography. At present, because of the methodology used, thermography can make no diagnosis as to the benign or the malignant nature of a lesion. Nevertheless, thermography still occupies an important place in breast cancer prognosis in determining the choice of *treatment*, and in the follow-up of high-risk diseases such as fibrocystic mastopathy.

Echography has been highly successful in differentiating between solid and cystic tumors. It has made significant progress in cancer imagery with the appearance of certain specific signs of malignancy. Unfortunately, the correlation between x-ray and echographical examination has not always been easy. Echography can claim to be part of the battery of diagnostic tests, but it is not sufficiently reliable in comparison to radiology.

Radiology remains at present by far the most informative, reliable, and easily reproduced method. It should not be necessary to stress the importance of a strict technique in its use. Radiography permits diagnosis of infraclinical cancers; when too small, however, a complete picture of the tumor is not shown as radiological opacity. In this case, the only early signs of breast cancer are indirect ones: (a) microcalcification; (b) structural rupture linked to epithelium proliferation and, elsewhere, to changes in the conjunctival matrix around the growing tumor. These indirect signs show up very well in breast radiography, but not in other screening methods.

New methods must at present be assessed by comparison with radiography. It appears from work by authors with experience of MRI and CT (Lindfors et al. 1985; El Yousef et al. 1985; J. L. Lamarque et al. 1988, unpublished) that MRI does not improve diagnosis of breast cancer. MRI would seem to be in the early stages of its technological development and could have interesting applications in the study of tumor extension. On the other hand, no case has yet been published concerning an infraclinical breast cancer that has not been shown up by radiography.

Some authors consider that MRI might reveal certain indications in cases where mammography is not conclusive (El Yousef et al. 1985; J. L. Lamarque et al. 1988, unpublished, R. Amalric 1988, unpublished). However, this gain in information may be offset by the high cost and difficulty of MRI examination, especially as surgery would, in any case, be necessary.

MRI would thus appear to be a method for the future, confined, at present, to research and evaluation. Research should be aimed at obtaining a better characterization of breast tissue. Analysis of fibrosis, fibrocystic disease, and adenosis should eventually allow definition of tissular risk. This is where the real interest of MRI lies in diagnostic evaluation.

Stereotactic breast puncture allows great precision in bringing the tip of the biopsy needle in contact with the radiological abnormality. This is achieved with safety and comfort for the patient. The stereotactic method allows insertion of a hooked wire in the breast during the same operation (Denarnaud et al. 1987).

Conclusion

The ability of MRI and CT to visualize soft-tissue tumors has revolutionized diagnostic medical imagery. Their properties have been investigated in several studies. However, the cost of these methods, especially in relation to general screening, has necessitated a limitation of their use to those areas where they will show real benefits. While in diagnostics complementarity of methods is the ideal, financial restraints make this line of research uncertain.

References

Alfidi RJ, Haaga JR, El Yousef SJ, et al (1982) Preliminary experimental results in humans and animals with a superconducting whole-body nuclear magnetic resonance scanner. Radiology 143: 175–181

Amalric R (1988) Fiabilité de la tomographie par résonance magnétique dans les carcinomes

Axel L, Kressel HY, Thickman D, et al (1983) NMR imaging of the chest at 0.12 T: clinical experience with a resistive magnet. AJR 141: 1157–1162

Balfe DM, Koehler RE, Karstaedt N, Stanley RJ, Sagel SS (1981) CT of gastric neoplasms. Radiology 140: 431–436

Balthazar EJ, Subramanyam BR, Lefleur RS, Barone CM (1984) Solid and papillary epithelial neoplasm of the pancreas. Radiology 150: 39–40

Bernardino ME, Jing BS, Wallace S (1979) Computed tomography diagnosis of mesenteric masses. AJR 132: 33–36

Bilaniuk LT, Zimmerman RA, Wehrli FW, Goldberg HI, Grossman RI, Bottomley PA, Edelstein WA, et al (1984a) Cerebral magnetic resonance: comparison of high and low field strength imaging. Radiology 153: 409–414

Bilaniuk LT, Zimmerman RA, Wehrli FW, Snyder PJ, Goldberg HI, Grossman RI, Bottomley PA, et al (1984b) Magnetic resonance imaging of pituitary lesions using 1.0 to 1.5 T field strength. Radiology 153: 415–418

Bradley W, Schmidt P (1984) Effect of methemoglobin formation on the MR appearance of subarachnoid hemorrhage (Abstr). Radiology 153 (P): 166

Breatnach ES, Han SY, Rahatzad MT, Stanley RJ (1985) CT evaluation of glucagonomas. J Comput Assist Tomogr 9 (1): 25–29

Butch RJ, Stark DD, Wittenberg J, Tepper JE, Saini S, Simeone JF, Mueller PR, Ferrucci JT Jr (1986) Staging rectal cancer by MR and CT. AJR 146: 1155–1160

Bydder GM, Brown J, Niendorf HP, Young IR (1985) Enhancement of cervical intraspinal tumors in MR imaging with intravenous gadolinium-DTPA. J Comput Assist Tomogr 9 (5): 847–851

Cho KC, Gold BM (1985) Computed tomography of Krukenberg tumors. AJR 145: 285–288

Clark J, Bankoff M, Carter B, Smith TJ (1984) The use of computerized tomography scan in the staging and follow-up study of carcinoma of the rectum. Surg Gynecol Obstet 159: 335–342

Cockey BM, Fishman EK, Jones B, Siegelman SS (1985) Computed tomography of abdominal carcinoid tumor. J Comput Assist Tomogr 9 (1): 38–42

Cohan RH, Silverman PM, Thompson WM, Halvorsen RA, Baker ME (1985) Computed tomography of epithelial neoplasms of the anal canal. AJR 145: 569–573

Cohen AM, Creviston S, Lipuma JP, Bryan PJ, Haaga JR, Alfidi RJ (1983) NMR evaluation of hilar and mediastinal lymphadenopathy. Radiology 148: 739–742

Damgaard-Petersen K, Stage JG (1979) CT scanning in patients with Zollinger-Ellison syndrome and carcinoid syndrome. Scand J Gastroenterol [Suppl] 1453: 117–122

Dedrick CG, McLoud TC, Shepard J-AO, Shipley RT (1985) Computed tomography of localized pleural mesothelioma. AJR 144: 275–280

Denarnaud Y, Haehnel P, Isnard A, Chaintreuil J (1987) Stereotactic breast puncture: new step in breast screening. Diagn Imag 3: 189–192

Dillon WP, Mills CM, Kjos B, Degroot J, Brant-Zawadzki M (1984) Magnetic resonance imaging of the nasopharynx. Radiology 152: 731–738

Dixon AK, Kelsey Fry I, Morson BC, Nichols RJ, Mason AY (1981) Pre-operative computed tomography of carcinoma of the rectum. Br J Radiol 54: 655–659

Dooms GC, Hricak H, Crooks LE, Higgins CB (1984) Magnetic resonance imaging of the lymh nodes: comparison with CT Radiology 153: 719–728

Dooms GC, Hricak H, Moseley ME, Bottles K, Fischer M, Higgins CB (1985a) Characterization of lymphadenopathy by magnetic resonance relaxation times: preliminary results. Radiology 155: 691–697

Dooms GC, Hricak H, Sollitto RA, Higgins CB (1985b) Lipomatous tumors and tumors with fatty component: MR imaging potential and comparison of MR and CT results. Radiology 157: 479–483

Dooms G, Hricak H, Tscholakoff D (1986) Adnexal structures: MR imaging. Radiology 158: 639–646

Ebner F, Kressel HY, Mintz MC, Carlson JA, Cohen EK, Schiebler M, Gefter W, Axel L (1988) Tumor recurrence versus fibrosis in the female pelvis – differentiation with MR imaging at 1,5 T. Radiology 166: 333–340

El Yousef SJ, O'Connell DM, Duchesneau RH, Smith MJ, Hubay CA, Guyton SP (1985) Benign and malignant breast disease: magnetic resonance and radiofrequency pulse sequences. AJR 145: 1–8
Enzmann DR, Wheat R, Marshall WH, Bird R, Murphy-Irwing K, Karbon K, Hanbery J, et al (1985) Tumors of the central nervous system studied by computed tomography and ultrasound. Radiology 154: 393–399
Fakhry JR, Berk RN (1981) The target pattern. AJR 137: 969–972
Felix R, Schorner W, Laniado M, Niendorf H-P, Claussen C, Fiegler W, Speck U (1985) Brain tumors: MR imaging with gadolinium-DTPA. Radiology 156: 681–688
Fisher MR, Hricak H, Reinhold C, Proctor E, Williams R (1985a) Female urethral carcinoma: MRI staging. AJR 144: 603–604
Fisher MR, Hricak H, Tanagho EA (1985b) Urinary bladder MR imaging. II. Neoplasm. Radiology 157: 471–477
Fleischer A (1987) Prostatic endosonography – a potential screening test. Diagnostic Imaging International 3: 68–72
Fleischer A, Dudley S, Entman S, Baxter J, Kalemeris G, James E (1987) Myometrial invasion by endometrial carcinoma: sonographic assessment. Radiology 162: 307–310
Gale ME, Robbins AH (1985) Computed tomography of the gallbladder: unusual diseases. J Comput Assist Tomogr 9 (3): 439–443
Gamsu G, Webb WR, Sheldon P, et al (1983) Nuclear magnetic resonance imaging of the thorax. Radiology 147: 473–480
Glazer GM, Aisen AM, Francis IR, Gyves JW, Lande I, Adler DD (1985a) Hepatic cavernous hemangioma: magnetic resonance imaging. Radiology 155: 417–420
Glazer H, Lee J, Levitt R, Heiken J, Ling D, Totty W, Balge D, Emani B, Wasserman T, Murphy W (1985b) Radiation fibrosis: differentiation from recurrent tumor by MR imaging. Radiology 156: 721–726
Go RT, O'Donnell JK, Underwood DA, Feiglin DDH, Salcedo EE, Pantoja M, McIntyre WJ, Meaney TF (1985) Comparison of gated cardiac MRI and 2D echocardiography of intracardiac neoplasms. AJR 145: 21–25
Grabbe E, Lierse W, Winkler R (1983) The perirectal fascia: morphology and use in staging of rectal carcinoma. Radiology 149: 241–246
Haehnel P (1983) Les pièges de la radiographie mammaire. In: Renaud R, Gairard B (eds) Contraception et sein. Masson, Paris pp 196–210 (Formation médicale continue en sénologie)
Haehnel P, Kleitz C (1984) Sémiologie radiologique des cancers du sein. Radiologie 4: 263–275
Haehnel P, Kleitz C (1985) Apport de la radiologie dans le diagnostic des cancers du sein infra-cliniques. In. Demaille A, Delecour M, Adenis L, Crepin G, Cappelaere C (eds) Les maladies du sein en 1985. Masson, Paris, pp 46–56 (Formation médicale continue en sénologie)
Hamlin DJ, Pettersson H, Fitzsimmons J, Morgan LS (1985a) MR imaging of uterine leiomyomas and their complications. J Comput Assist Tomogr 9 (5): 902–907
Hamlin DJ, Fitzsimmons JR, Pettersson H, Riggall FC, Morgan L, Wilkinson EJ (1985b) Magnetic resonance imaging of the pelvis. AJR 145: 585–590
Heiken JP, Balfe DM, Picus D, Scharp DW (1984) Radical pancreatectomy: postoperative evaluation by CT. Radiology 153: 211–215
Heiken JP, Lee JK, Glazer HS, Ling D (1985) Hepatic metastases studied with MR and CT. Radiology 156: 423–427
Hricak H, Alpers C, Crooks L, Sheldon P (1983a) Magnetic resonance imaging of the female pelvis; initial experience. AJR 145: 1119–1128
Hricak H, Williams R, Spring D (1983b) Anatomy and pathology of the male pelvis by magnetic resonance imaging. AJR 141: 1101–1110
Hricak H, Demas BE, Williams RD, McNamara MT, Hedgcock MW, Amparo EG, Tanagho EA (1985) Magnetic resonance imaging in the diagnosis and staging of renal and perirenal neoplasms. Radiology 154: 709–715
Hricak H, Stern J, Fisher M, Shapeero L, Winkler M, Lacey C (1987) Endometrial carcinoma by MR imaging. Radiology 162: 297–305
Kelvin F, Korobkin M, Heaston D, Grant J, Akwari O (1983) The pelvis after surgery for rectal carcinoma: serial CT observations with emphasis on nonneoplastic feature. AJR 141: 959–964
Kier R, Silverman PM, Korobkin M, Wain S, Leight G, Burch W Jr (1985) Malignant teratoma of the thyroid in an adult: CT appearance. J Comput Assist Tomogr 9 (1): 174–176
Kim SY, Kim JH, Lee JD (1985) Papillary carcinoma of the pancreas: findings of US and CT. Radiology 154: 338
Kressel HY, Callen PW, Montage JP, et al (1978) Computed tomographic evaluation of disorders affecting the alimentary tract. Radiology 129: 451–455
La Berge JM, Laing FC, Federle MP, Jeffrey RB Jr, Lim RC Jr (1984) Hepatocellular carcinoma: assessment of resectability by computed tomography and ultrasound. Radiology 152: 485–490
Lamarque JL, Rodiere MJ, Pujol J, Prat X, Martin JM, Barneon G, Rouanet JP (1988) IRM et sein – Mythe ou réalité. Aujourd' hui ou demain peut-être? (in press)
Lee BCP, Deck MDF (1985) Sellar and juxtasellar lesion detection with MR. Radiology 157: 143–147
Lee JKT, Heiken JP, Ling D, Glazer HS, Balfe DM, Levitt RG, Dixon WT, Murphy WA (1984) Magnetic resonance imaging of abdominal and pelvic lymphadenopathy. Radiology 153: 181–188
Lee JKT, Gersell DJ, Balfe DM, Worthington JL, Picus D, Gapp G (1985) The uterus: in vitro MR-anatomic correlation of normal and abnormal specimens. Radiology 157: 175–179
Lee KR, Levine E, Moffit RE, Bigongiari LR, Hemreck AS (1979) Computed tomographic staging of malignant gastric neoplasms. Radiology 133: 151–155
Lindfors KK, Meyer JE, Bussee PM, Kopans DB, Munzenrider JE, Sawicka JM (1985) CT evaluation of local and regional breast cancer recurrence. AJR 145: 833–837
Matsui O, Takashima T, Kadoya M, Ida M, Suzuki M, Kitagawa K, Kamimura R et al (1985) Dynamic computed tomography during arterial portography: the most sensitive examination for small hepatocellular carcinomas. J Comput Assist Tomogr 9 (1): 19–24
Meyer JE, Dosoretz DE, Gunderson LL, Stark P, Kopans DB (1983) CT evaluation of locally advanced carcinoma of the distal colon and rectum. J Comput Assist Tomogr 7 (2): 265–267
McCarthy SM, Barnes D, Deveney K, Moss AA, Goldberg HI (1985) Detection of recurrent rectosigmoid carcinoma: prospective evaluation of CT and clinical factors. AJR 144: 577–579
McMillin KI, Gross BH (1985) CT demonstration of peripelvic and periureteral non-Hodgkin lymphoma. AJR 144: 945–946
Michel G, Galakhoff C, Masselot J, Vanel D, Heran F, Charpentier P, Castaigne D, Gerbaulet A, George M (1987) Interêt de l'imagerie par resonance magnétique des cancers du col et du corps de l'uterus. Etude préliminaire à propos de

9 cas de cancer du corps et de 20 cas de cancer du col. J Radiol 68: 167–175

Miller JH, Greenspan BS (1985) Integrated imaging of hepatic tumors in childhood. Radiology 154: 83–90

Miyasaka Y, Hachiya J, Furuya Y, Seki T, Watanabe H (1985) CT evaluation of invasive trophoblastic disease. J Comput Assist Tomogr 9 (3): 459–462

Moldofsky PJ, Sears HF, Mulhern CB Jr, Hammond ND, Powe J, Gatenby RA, Steplewski Z, Koprowski H (1984) Detection of metastatic tumor in normal-size retroperitoneal lymph nodes by monoclonal antibody imaging. Engl J Med 311: 106–107

Moon KL Jr, Federle MP, Abrams DI, Volberding P, Lewis BJ (1984) Kaposi sarcoma and lymphadenopathy syndrome: limitations of abnormal CT in acquired immunodeficiency syndrome. Radiology 150: 479–483

Moss AA, Schnyder P, Candardjis G, Margulis AR (1980) Computed tomography of benign and malignant gastric abnormalities. J Clin Gastroenterol 2: 401–409

Moss AA, Schnyder P, Marx W, Margulis AR (1981) Gastric adenocarcinoma: a comparison of the accuracy and economics of staging by computed tomography and surgery. Gastroenterology 80: 45–50

Moss AA, Goldberg HI, Stark DB, et al (1984) Hepatic tumors: magnetic resonance and CT appearance. Radiology 150: 141–147

Mullin D, Shirkhoda A (1985) Computed tomography after gastrectomy in primary gastric carcinoma. J Comput Assist Tomogr 9 (1): 30–33

Nicholls RJ, Mason AY, Morson BC, Dixon AK, Kelsey Fry I (1982) The clinical staging of rectal cancer. Br J Surg 69: 404–409

Nidecker AC, Muller S, Aue WP, Seelig J, Fridrich R, Remagen W, Hartweg H, Benz UF (1985) Extremity bone tumors: evaluation by P-31 MR spectroscopy. Radiology 157: 167–174

Nishimura K, Togashi K, Itoh K, Fujisawa I, Noma S, Kawamura Y, Nakano Y, Itoh H, Torizuka K, Osaza H (1987) Endometrial cysts of the ovary: MR imaging. Radiology 162: 315–318

Ohtomo K, Itai Y, Furui S, Yashiro N, Yoshikawa K, Iio M (1985) Hepatic tumors: differentiation by transverse relaxation time (T2) of magnetic resonance imaging. Radiology 155: 421–423

Parienty RA, Pradel J, Parienty I (1985) Cystic renal cancers: CT characteristics. Radiology 157: 741–744

Pearlberg JL, Sandler MA, Kvale P, Beute GH, Madrazo BL (1985) Computed-tomographic and conventional linear-tomographic evaluation of tracheobronchial lesions for laser photoresection. Radiology 154: 759–762

Peyster RG, Augsburger JJ, Shields JA, Satchell TV, Markoe AM, Clarke K, Haskin ME (1985) Choroidal melanoma: comparison of CT, fundoscopy, and US. Radiology 156: 675–680

Pillari G, Weinrel J, Jernace F, et al (1983) CT of gastric masses: image patterns and a note on potential pitfalls. Gastrointest. Radiol 8: 11–17

Poon P, McCallum R, Henkelman M, Bronskill M, Sutcliffe S, Jewett M, Rider W, Bruce A (1985) Magnetic resonance imaging of the prostate. Radiology 154: 143–149

Poskitt KJ, Cooperberg PL, Sullivan LD (1985) Sonography and CT in staging nonseminomatous testicular tumors. AJR 144: 939–944

Powell M, Womack C, Buckley J, Worthington B, Symonds E (1986a) Pre-operative magnetic resonance imaging of stage 1 endometrial adenocarcinoma. Br J Obstet Gynaecol 93: 353–360

Powell M, Worthington B, Sokal M, Wastie M, Buckley J, Symonds E (1986b) Magnetic resonance imaging – its application to cervical carcinoma. Br J Obstet Gynaecol 93: 1276–1285

Quint LE, Glazer GM, Orringer MB, Gross BH (1985a) Esophageal carcinoma: CT findings. Radiology 155: 171–175

Quint LE, Glazer GM, Orringer MB (1985b) Esophageal imaging by MR and CT: study of normal anatomy and neoplasms. Radiology 156: 727–731

Radecki PD, Arger PH, Arenson RL, Jennings AS, Coleman BG, Mintz MC, Kressel HY (1984) Thyroid imaging: comparison of high-resolution real-time ultrasound and computed tomography. Radiology 153: 145–147

Reede DL, Bergeron RT, McCauley DI (1982) CT of the thyroid and of other thoracic inlet disorders. J Otolaryngol 11: 349–357

Reiners C, Baum K, Wiedemann W, Schick F, Spiegel W (1983) Special diagnostics in follow-up C Cell (medullary) carcinoma of the thyroid. Acta Endocrinol (Copenh) 252: 61–62

Rifkin MD, Marks GJ (1985) Transrectal US as an adjunct in the diagnosis of rectal and extrarectal tumors. Radiology 157: 499–502

Rosenthal DI, Scott JA, Mankin HJ, Wismer GL, Brady TJ (1985) Sacrococcygeal chordoma: magnetic resonance imaging and computed tomography. AJR 145: 143–147

Ross JS, O'Donovan PB, Novoa R, et al (1984) Magnetic resonance of the chest: initial experience with imaging and in vivo T1 and T2 calculations. Radiology 152: 95–101

Rossi P, Baert A, Passariello R, Simonetti G, Pavone P, Tempesta P (1985) CT of functioning tumors of the pancreas. AJR 144: 57–60

Shirkhoda A, Jaffe N, Wallace S, Ayala A, Lindell MM, Zornoza J (1985) Computed tomography of osteosarcoma after intraarterial chemotherapy. AJR 144: 95–99

Siegel RS, Kuhns LR, Borlaza GS, McCormick TL, Simmons JL (1980) Computed tomography and angiography in ileal carcinoid tumor and retractile mesenteritis. Radiology 134: 437–440

Silverman PM, Korobkin M, Moore AV (1983) Computed tomography of cystic neck masses. J Comput Assist Tomogr 7: 488–502

Silverman PM, Newman GE, Korobkin M, Workman JB, Moore AV, Coleman RE (1984) Computed tomography in the evaluation of thyroid disease. AJR 142: 897–902

Simeone JF, Daniels GH, Mueller PR, et al (1982) High-resolution real-time sonography of the thyroid. Radiology 145: 431–435

Simeone JF, Edelman RR, Stark DD, Wittenberg J, White EM, Butch RJ, Mueller PR, et al (1985) Surface coil MR imaging of abdominal viscera. Radiology 157: 437–441

Smith FW, Hutchison JMS, Mallard JR, et al (1981) Oesophageal carcinoma demonstrated by whole-body nuclear magnetic resonance imaging. Br Med J 282: 510–512

Sperber M, Marks GJ, Mohiuddin M, Mapp E (1983) Rectal cancer: extent of disease and radiotherapeutic effects by computed tomography. Comput Radiol 7 (4): 209–214

Stanley RJ, Sagel SS, Evens RG (1980) The impact of new imaging methods on pancreatic arteriography. Radiology 136: 251–253

Stark DD, Moss AA, Goldberg HI, Davis PL, Federle MP (1984a) Magnetic resonance and CT of the normal and diseased pancreas: a comparative study. Radiology 150: 153–162

Stark DD, Higgins CB, Lanzer P, Lipton MJ, Schiller N, Crooks LE, Botvinick EB, Kaufman L (1984b) Magnetic resonance imaging of the pericardium: normal and pathologic findings. Radiology 150: 469–474

Stark D, Wittenberg J, Butch RJ, Ferrucci JF Jr (1987) Hepatic metastases: randomized, controlled comparison of detection with MR imaging and CT. Radiology 165: 399–406

Steyr J, Smith F (1982) Nuclear magnetic resonance imaging of the prostate. Br J Urol 54: 726–728

Stomper PC, Jochelson MS, Garnick MB, Richie JP (1985) Residual abdominal masses after chemotherapy for nonseminomatous testicular cancer: correlation of CT and histology. AJR 145: 743–746

Styles RA, Seltzer SE (1985) CT staging of prostate cancer. Radiology 157 (3): 838

Takashima T, Matsui O (1980) Infusion hepatic angiography in the detection of small hepatocellular carcinomas. Radiology 136: 321–325

Thoenl RF, Moss AA, Schnyder P, Margulis AR (1981) Detection and staging of primary rectal and rectosigmoid cancer by computed tomography. Radiology 141: 135–138

Thorsen MK, Quiroz F, Lawson TL, Smith DF, Foley WD, Stewart ET (1984) Primary biliary carcinoma: CT evaluation. Radiology 152: 479–483

Vermess M, Leung AW-L, Bydder GM, Steiner RE, Blumgart LH, Young IR (1985) MR imaging of the liver in primary hepatocellular carcinoma. J Comput Assist Tomogr 9 (4): 749–754

Webb WR, Gamsu G, Stark DD, Moore EH (1984a) Magnetic resonance imaging of the normal and abnormal pulmonary hila. Radiology 152: 89–94

Webb R, Jensen B, Gamsu G, Sollitto R, Moore E (1984b) Coronal magnetic resonance imaging of the chest: normal and abnormal. Radiology 153: 729–735

Weekes RG, McLeod RA, Reiman HM, Pritchard DJ (1985) CT of soft-tissue neoplasms. AJR 144: 355–360

Whalen JP (1979) Caldwell lecture. Radiology fo the abdomen: impact of new imaging methods. AJR 133: 586–618

Zimmer WD, Berquist TH, McLeod RA, Sim FH, Pritchard DJ, Shives TC, Wold LE, May GR (1985) Bone tumors: magnetic resonance imaging versus computed tomography. Radiology 155: 709–718

Zirinsky K, Auh YH, Rubenstein WA, Kneeland JB, Whalen JP, Kazam E (1985) The portacaval space. CT with MR correlation. Radiology 156: 453–460

Endoscopy in the Diagnosis and Treatment of Cancer

P. Spinelli

Introduction

Endoscopy represents the desire in Man to continue learning more and more from the medical and scientific point of view. The first attempts at endoscopy date back to ancient times, but it was only in the last century that methods approached a true and diagnostic procedure capable of viewing the internal cavities of the body in line with its external contours. The very first endoscopes were rigid tubes, ingeniously lit and totally compatible with the existing, restricted technological know-how of the last century. The original attempts at lighting were made by reflecting sunlight or candlelight through the tube into the cavity to be examined. Great progress was made, however, with the miniaturisation of incandescent lamps. Artificial light had partially resolved the problem of cavity illumination, but these small lamps tended to overheat and burn the inner wall of the cavity being studied, or even break during examination. The use of rigid tubes meant very few cavities could be explored, and exploration was further limited, in the case of cranial districts, by the deviation of the spine or by impediments in the mouth opening. In the 1930s, the creation of the first semi-flexible endoscopes seemed to have opened up new horizons, but, unfortunately, due to their high cost, fragility and difficult handling, they were very scarce. The real progress of endoscopy began in the late 1950s with the creation of Hirschowitz's flexible endoscope which was based on fibre optic technology (Hopkins and Kapany 1954; Hirschowitz et al. 1958).

These new instruments facilitate endoscopic examination by making insertion easier and less traumatic and they make endoscopy an objective, diagnostic tool as they allow intracavitary pictures to be taken by connecting a camera to the ocular. It may seem trivial, but the possibility of showing images of the body's most profound cavities in their original colour and of taking specimens from these same places has truly conquered novel scientific frontiers in the field of medicine.

In recent years, the endoscopic science of light has stimulated the improvement of the radiological science of shadows. With the first gastroscopes came the gastrocameras, miniaturised cameras mounted on the tip of the fibrescope, with which photographs could be taken of all the stomach walls, even by a technician, and the images could be interpreted later by a physician. In the late 1970s, following a period of general use of endoscopic cinematography, the telecamera became the most widely used form of documentation and teaching. Besides the application of a camera to the endoscope eyepiece, miniaturisation has also allowed for the introduction of the telecamera onto the tip of the endoscope. The images of the internal organs are no longer transmitted on optic fibres, but electronically via this video-endoscopy. The method is very precise, can be computerised and has proved to be very useful for teaching (Classen et al. 1987; Schapiro et al. 1987).

Indications for endoscopy have also changed, particularly, in the study of tumours: from the diagnosis of advanced tumours, which was the first objective, we have passed on to the detection of early and minute forms of cancer. Endoscopy has thus made it possible to separate advanced and early stages of tumours. Recently, moreover, the therapeutic area has broadened, methods have become more numerous, less traumatic, shorter and with fewer risks of complications.

Endoscopy is now running the same course that made radiology a highly individual science, with diagnostic and therapeutic units and with its own administration. The fundamental "endoscopy unit" is an organised group, consisting of a physician and an assistant working with a source of light, an endoscope, the necessary accessories for histological and cytological specimens and complete photographic equipment. A series of diagnostic, operative and teaching procedures can also be added.

The diagnostic procedures benefit from the still image, the spontaneous and caused mobility (cough due to intrathoracic endoscopy), the direct and transmitted pulsations, the sampling of tissue specimens and the recording of the images. The endoscopic image is first evaluated by an overall glance into the cavity being investigated. One must consider the integrity of the morphology and the surface of the walls, the presence and the quality of any secretion, any lesions present, their shape, size, colour, consistency, mobility and relation to the surrounding organs when assessable. When organs with peristalsis are examined, this should be checked as functioning and regular. If alterations of the cavity are noted, a decision should be reached whether or not to take samples. Histological and cytological specimens can be taken from the cavities, either by visual control or by transparietal sampling. It is interesting to note the application of staining methods in endoscopy, different colours being given to healthy tissue and pathological tissues as a guide to correct sampling. An evaluation of the dimensions, as with an X-ray, cannot be obtained easily with endoscopy mainly because of the distortion of the images: on occasion, a centrimetrical, folding probe may be used.

Alongside the staining procedures, the study of fluorescence is becoming more and more important for the diagnosis of cancer. Every tissue gives off a natural characteristic fluorescence, but it can also be increased by injecting photosensitising drugs. They can be selectively concentrated in malignant and premalignant tissues, allowing the identification of tumours even when they are not microscopically visible (Profio et al. 1983).

Recognition of fluorescent signals is difficult because of their faintness; possible fluorescent elaboration by procedures of image withdrawal might be obtained in the near future by the use of video-endoscopes. Radiological control is widely used in endoscopy to identify the positioning of the endoscopes and sampling accessories (colonoscopy, peripheric bronchoscopy), or to obtain images from cavities which have been endoscopically injected with a radiopaque medium. In this way radiologists and endoscopists work together and form the basis of a correct exploitation of their respective tasks.

Therapeutic methods are developing daily, both in number and in variety. Various forms of energy are used, from mechanical to thermal (in the form of electric waves, electromagnetic radiation by laser or microwaves) and to photodynamic. Generally, it can be said that mechanical energy helps the dilation of the lumen in the internal organ, while thermal energy is adopted in the destruction of tumoral lesions and haemostasis. Today the practice of endoscopy is most widely used in the digestive, respiratory and urinary tracts, where necrosing substances can be injected, and cryotherapy can be adopted to remove obstruction of the gut.

Oesophagus

Endoscopy has helped greatly in the diagnosis of oesophageal carcinomas due to the fact that each time an examination of the gastric and duodenal mucosa is necessary, the oesophagus comes under examination, and it is possible to identify asymptomatic oesophageal cancers quite casually. These are generally early stage lesions with a good prognosis.

Endoscopic Anatomy

The oesophagus has a tubular shape and has a calibre which varies depending on the segment under examination. It is about 25–27 cm long and is related to the height of the individual, the distance from the cardia to the upper dental arch is 38–42 cm. Because of the intrinsic shape of the organ, or because of its connections with the surrounding anatomical parts, the oesophagus has three strictures:

1. The so-called cricopharyngeal stricture which corresponds to the upper oesophageal sphincter, or Killian's ostium, and consists of cricopharyngeal muscle and cricoid cartilage.
2. The bronchoaortic stricture, situated about 9–11 cm below the previous tract, is related to the aortic arch and the main left bronchus.
3. The cardial stricture is formed by the oesophago-diaphragmatic structures.

The calibre of the oesophagus varies depending on the peristalsis, the mediastinal tension and insufflation by the endoscope. The inner oesophageal layer is made of flat, pluristratified epithelium which is characteristically slightly transparent.

Instruments Used

The oesophagus is examined using rigid or flexible instruments, the latter being the most commonly used. A typical oesophagoscope has axial vision and is about 50 cm long. Today, however, most oesophagoscopies are carried out with gastroscopes, which are about 110–120 cm long and enable the examination to be made distally up to the duodenum. Instruments with frontolateral fields of vision are very useful for gathering samples from the oesophageal walls.

Diagnosis

The endoscopic diagnosis of advanced oesophageal carcinoma is easily accomplished and is coupled with histological and cytological sampling. On the whole, this procedure is diagnostic in more than 90% of cases (Bruni and Nelson 1975; Prolla et al. 1977).

The diagnosis of early oesophageal carcinoma and the endoscopic follow-up of precancerous lesions has proved to be very interesting. Certain conditions, such as tilosis which is associated with papillomatosis of the oesophagus and hypercheratosis of the sole of the foot and the plam of the hand, are associated with oesophageal epidermoid carcinoma in 70% of cases. Long-lasting achalasia, stenoses and Plummer-Vinson syndrome are conditions related to a higher incidence of carcinoma.

The diagnosis of carcinoma at an early stage is of extreme importance given the high percentage of survival in these patients. These forms are identified by the alterations in the mucosa which can be of minimal size; the colouration of the mucosa is sometimes useful for this, but the possibilities of investigation offered by modern endoscopes limit the indications.

Therapy

Endoscopic therapy of oesophageal carcinoma is used in both early and advanced stages. Endoscopic therapy is needed in the early stages when there are contraindications to traditional therapy, particularly in high-risk patients. On the other hand, in cases of advanced carcinomas, circumstances change considerably. The oesophagus is immersed in mediastinum, which is a space rich in lymphatic vessels allowing oesophageal carcinoma to spread easily: on the whole, fewer than 10% of patients operated on for this type of cancer survive 5 years. The majority of operations performed therapeutically are not really radical and prove to be palliative, having a high risk of morbidity and mortality, either from surgery or from its consequences. Surgery should be reserved for those patients who will really benefit from this form of treatment, and whenever the aim of therapy is palliation, the method of choice is endoscopy.

Endoscopic methods differ according to the stage of the disease – early or advanced. In the case of early disease, treatment aims to be complete. If the lesion presents as a polypoid or elevated lesion, it can be removed by using an electrocoagulating snare, whereas if it is flat or excavated, an electro- or laser photocoagulation is used. Photodynamic therapy has only recently been introduced, but it has given very satisfactory results (Gluckman and Weissler 1986), especially in cases where the tumoral tissue is reduced in thickness (superficial forms).

In advanced stages the aim of endoscopic therapy is purely palliation of the symptoms, in particular those symptoms closely linked to the organ, such as obstruction of the secretion passage, dysphagia, malnutrition and pain. The methods at our disposal are: dilation, electrocoagulation, laser photocoagulation and photodynamic therapy.

The dilation of a stenotic lumen can be obtained by introducing dilators which slide on a guide wire previously inserted through the restricted tract. These dilators can be cylindro-conic or olive shaped: in these cases the dilation is obtained by manual pulsion; there are also pneumatic dilators with cylindrical balloons at the distal end; they are inflated under controlled pressure. In some cases the guide wire cannot be inserted into the restricted tract, and then it can be helpful to place some small fragments of highly hydrophilous seaweed into the stenosis so that, after a couple of hours, the algae will reinflate. Whereas the dilated tracts will generally tend to close in about 2–8 weeks, the methods which destroy the tissues and clear the tract by means of laser or electrocoagulation normally take longer. The application of a prosthesis ensures less risk of a rapid recurrence of stenosis. Polypoid lesions (which may be sessile or pedunculated papillomas) in the oesophagus, as well as in the rest of the digestive tract, can also be removed by electroresection.

Stomach

Endoscopic Anatomy

The stomach is examined with the patient in left lateral decubitus. Having passed the cardia, one looks for two points of reference. The first is the "mucus lake", i.e. the area where the gastric contents accumulate marking the side of the big curve towards the fundus and the gastric angle which is on the small curve where the horizontal and vertical portions meet. The pyloris is the second point of reference. During inflation the mucosa loses its characteristic plicae in the antral region, but retains them in the fundus and in the body. Lesions of the surface are described referring to the points mentioned above.

Instruments Used

The stomach can be examined using frontal, oblique or lateral vision instruments. Oblique vision instruments are better for bioptic sampling and for a more detailed study of the small curve in the vertical portion.

Diagnosis

Endoscopy has allowed for the individualisation of smaller and smaller malignant neoplasms. For this reason, in 1962, the Japanese Society of Gastrointestinal Endoscopy drew up a classification, based on the endoscopic report, of gastric carcinomas with limited growth and, therefore, a better prognosis. Diagnosis of gastric epithelial tumours will also serve to identify early and advanced forms. The first type, typically, does not extend below the submucosal layer (Spinelli 1981).

In general, the macroscopical classification can also be applied to endoscopy: Borrmann's classification, which has always been referred to in the past, indicates three forms of cancer, i.e. vegetating, infiltrating and ulcerated, and from this one tries to derive a prognostic evaluation based on form and size. It is quite easy to individualise a gastric carcinoma which corresponds to traditional Borrmann typing and to take samples which confirm the presence of lesions and allow the classification on a histological basis. On the other hand, it is much harder to individualise a gastric carcinoma in its early form when it has very limited growth and its morphology can easily be mistaken for gastritic lesion. In the case of these lesions, histological and cytological sampling becomes absolutely necessary for diagnosis to be made.

Once a lesion with the endoscopic features of an early carcinoma is detected, it is of the utmost importance to check whether the deep layers of the walls are involved and to what extent. At this point it is useful to observe the lesion during the peristaltic movements of the organ and its passive mobility, i.e. under pressure/traction with the endoscopic forceps. Even though these actions have no definite significance, they contribute to the formation of a diagnostic impression which will be communicated to the surgeon. The surgeon will also be informed of the precise location of the lesion (distance from the main points of reference) bearing in mind that early lesions are not often palpable and, therefore, can only be partially included in the resected piece.

Local recurrence, due to unsuccessful radical surgery of early carcinomas, is one of the most frustrating events in our field. The ecographic endoscope has been introduced only very recently. It is an ultrasound probe situated at the tip of a special endoscope which is capable of identifying the depth of infiltration of a cancerous growth (Di Magno et al. 1982; Tio et al. 1986). Apart from carcinomas, malignant lymphomas represent about 5% of malignant stomach tumours. They are usually non-Hodgkin's lymphomas; the gastric location can be secondary to a lymph-nodal location: in these cases it is possible to locate a parietal compression that is projected inside the gastric cavity. On the other hand, primary tumours are responsible for complete involvement of the gastric walls which have infiltrative and ulcerative aspects producing a reduction in the volume of the stomach.

One of the most important aspects of endoscopic diagnosis is the possibility it offers in monitoring precancerous lesions such as atrophic gastritis, intestinal metaplasia and adenomas, which are all conditions which appear by themselves and can be associated with pernicious anaemia, the lesions, in this disease, being located on the gastric fundus. Follow-up and attentive observation of the gastric mucosa during routine examination will permit the identification of a high percentage of early carcinomas relative to the diagnosis of advanced forms. Since early carcinomas are known to heal in over 90% of cases, their detection creates an important therapeutic implication in diagnostic endoscopy.

Therapy

Gastric polypectomy permits the removal of lesions protruding into the lumen. These are mainly hyperplastic polyps and, noticeably less frequently, adenomas. It is only the latter which can become malignant. The safest method is the complete removal and histological testing of these polyps. Adenomas can contain malignant tissue foci, which occur more frequently in the larger adenomas. The method used in these cases is practically the same as that normally adopted when the same situation occurs in the large intestine, to which we shall refer later.

Hemostasis and destruction of malignant tumoral lesions can be achieved by means of localised variations of rapidly increasing or decreasing temperature, the latter as in the case of cryotherapy in which flexible cryoprobes introduced through the endoscope are used. Hyperthermal methods consist of laser technology, endoscopic electrosurgery and microwaves (Spinelli 1984; Tabuse et al. 1985). Laser technique has already been mentioned. Electrosurgery, when laser sources are not available, tends to be extremely useful, enabling us to obtain unipolar, bipolar or multipolar coagulation. Microwave apparatus is composed of a source, placed outside the patient, and an antenna, the tip of which can be introduced through the endoscope and made to contact the tissue. Endoscopy offers a reliable and safe therapeutic method for bleeding tumours; coagulated tissue will necrose, so multiple coagulations are able to destroy tumoral masses and allow the recanalisation of the obstructed tracts.

Duodenum

Primary neoplasms of the duodenum are infrequent, except for those of Vater's papilla originating from the duodenal, choledochal or pancreatic mucosa.

Endoscopic Anatomy

Once the pyloric sphincter has been passed, the lumen of the digestive tract widens again in the duodenal bulb, where the mucosal wall appears smooth after insufflation. At the upper bend, the transverse Kerckring's plicae begin to emanate from the mucosal and submucosal layers. When the upper two-thirds pass into the lower third, there is a longitudinal plica on the posteromedial wall with Vater's papilla situated at its superior extremity. The papilla, in its turn, can be found at the inferior end of a longitudinal prominence caused by the intramural presence of the distal choledochus and is more evident when the choledochus is dilated. In the intermediate tract of the third portion of the duodenum, the aortic pulsation is observed on the posterior wall, whereas that of the superior mesenteric artery can occasionally be recognised on the anterior wall. The duodenojejunal angle is peculiar because the lumen is markedly bent making it extremely difficult for the scope to pass beyond it.

Instruments Used

On the whole, the duodenum can be studied endoscopically by fibrescopes with axial and with wide fields of vision, or others with frontolateral vision. Instruments with lateral vision are used to operate endoscopically on the papilla and the above-mentioned fibrescopes can only be a substitute for them in cases where patients have undergone a Billroth II resection of the stomach.

Diagnosis and Therapy

Duodenoscopy permits us to examine Vater's papilla by direct vision, and the biliary or pancreatic ducts by injection of radiopaque medium and radiological visualisation (Cotton, 1972). Adenomas and carcinomas can originate from papillary or ampullar epithelium: endoscopic resection can be performed with radical therapeutic aims in the first case and with palliation in mind in the second case. In a patient with vegetating papillary carcinoma we removed the papilla, and surgery proved itself to be radical because during the cephalopancreasectomy performed afterwards, no more malignant tissue was found. Most frequently, endoscopic surgery is indicated in patients with jaundice deriving from biliary or pancreatic neoplasms, or even from lymphnodes compressing the biliary tree. In these cases, the papillary orifice must be opened by papillotomy, and then stents can be inserted to restore the biliary flow and achieve a palliative therapy of jaundice (Huibregtse and Tytgat, 1984).

Perendoscopic biliary drainage is, on the one hand, part of preoperative preparation, so that the patient can undergo surgery without the aggravation of biliary retention, and on the other hand, it is a form of definitive palliation, as happens with those patients who cannot undergo surgery.

In respect of transcutaneous biliary drainage, the perduodenoscopic method has the advantage of being complication-free, of giving information about the stomach and the duodenum, and of providing the possibility of follow-up and pancreatography. Furthermore, in those cases where the biliary tract is big enough (from 8 mm upwards), an endoscope can be inserted after having performed a sphincterectomy. This permits detailed observation of the biliary and pancreatic tracts, even when they are dilated. Today, with biliary stenoses, it is possible to obtain dilation mechanically or pneumatically, before or as an alternative to stenting.

Jejunum

The jejunum is generally investigated in cases of stomach resection with gastrojejunal anastomosis, and its neoplastic pathology is limited to lymphomas and carcinomas of the duodenojejunal angle. The former appear in the form of stenotic muffs, the latter with ulcerations. Carcinomatous infiltrations which occur on anastomosis following resection for gastric carcinoma are treated by dilation or thermal electrocoagulation.

Ileum

As well as lymphomas, carcinomas may also be localised in the ileum, generally in the last loop, with similar aspects to the jejunal carcinoma. The last loop can usually be examined during coloscopy. Recanalisation can be carried out.

Large Intestine

Neoplasms of the large bowel are becoming more and more frequent in Western countries. Coloscopy is most important for early diagnosis, prevention, therapy and palliation of obstructing lesions.

Endoscopic Anatomy

The anal verge, situated at the caudal end of the large intestine, can be seen by opening the buttocks wide apart. It corresponds to the beginning of the anal canal, which is 4–5 cm long, and terminates where the lining changes from mucosal epithelium to squamous epithelium. There is a clear line, called the line of Hilton, 1 cm above the anal verge; it can be seen and palpated better by traction of the perineal skin towards the ischiatic bones. The pectinate line is situated 2 cm proximally; it is formed by the outline of the semilumar valves, protecting crypts and the bases of Morgagni's columns which separate the crypts. These crypts are the site where the anal glands empty. The anal canal terminates at the top of Morgagni's columns where the dilation of the rectal ampulla begins. In the erect position it is directed downwards and backwards. If prolonged upwards, its axis would meet the umbilicus.

The rectum, in its initial tract, has three curves bordered by plicae, or valves; the superior and the inferior plicae are situated on the left side and the middle one on the right side. The ampullar mucosa is smooth, but the sigmoid mucosa becomes smooth after inflation. The endoscopic limits of the sigmoid colon are identified by the changes of intestinal direction at the rectosigmoid and the colosigmoid junctions. With experience, one learns to recognise the position of the endoscope by abdominal palpation and identification of the light transmitted through the abdominal wall. It is also useful to identify a first straight tract with a circular lumen, which is the left colon, a second straight tract with a triangular lumen, which is the transverse and, eventually, a third straight tract which is the right colon ending at the cecum where the valve and, sometimes, the appendix lumen can be seen.

Examination of the large intestine can be carried out by rigid tubes for the 30 cm caudally and flexible instruments for the remaining parts. The latter can be long (up to 180 cm), short (up to 60 cm) or medium. They have wide channels which allow clearing when faeces are found.

Diagnosis

Early diagnosis and prevention of carcinoma of the large bowel are possible mainly because polyps with malignant evolution, the adenomas, can be identified and resected. As is well known, most cancers of the large intestine develop from adenomas. When they are removed, their malignant transformation is prevented. In fact, the premalignant lesion of the large bowel is dysplasia, without any peculiar macroscopic findings. It can be observed in long-lasting aspecific chronic inflammatory diseases (ulcerative colitis or Crohn's disease). The problem concerning the endoscopic identification of dysplastic areas, by methods employing staining or fluorescence, is an important field of research at the moment (Bottiroli et al., 1987). Diagnosis of carcinoma of the large intestine is not usually difficult; the earliest forms are, generally, those which modify the normal aspect in a few details, such as the regularity of the surface, the integrity of the mucosal lining, easy bleeding and fragility. Polyps, especially when sessile with a villous aspect and large in size (more than 2 cm), most frequently show cancerous areas. For the large bowel, too, the term "early carcinoma" is adopted to indicate a form of which the depth is confined to the submucosal layer. Advanced carcinoma can be seen as a polypoid lesion, or an ulcerated plaque, or even a stenotic muff, when the infiltration reaches most of the parietal circumference. Endoscopic diagnosis must be confirmed by histological diagnosis.

In some cases, diagnosis of a carcinoma is difficult because the tumour is inside a stenotic tract as a result of diverticolitis or an inflammatory disease. Such stenoses can only be passed when examination is carried out under general anaesthesia.

Therapy

The most important application of endoscopy is polypectomy: first, it allows the removal of penduncultated polyps, but also large sessile polyps can be removed (polyps obstructing the intestinal lumen can be resected) (Christie and Shina, 1982). When histological examination reveals the presence of carcinomatous tissue in the adenoma, endoscopic removal will be followed by surgical resection of the bowel, if the carcinomatous tissue is poorly differentiated, or polypectomy has been performed fragmentarily, or the malignant tissue reaches the resection line (in pedunculated adenomas). Apart from patients at high surgical risk, these are the principles on which the radicality of endoscopic therapy for colorectal carcinoma is based. However, a wide therapeutic field concerns the endoscopic palliation of carcinoma. It is indicated for patients at high surgical risk, or those not responding to traditional forms, or who refuse derivative surgery. Palliation aims at restoring the natural passage of faeces and at stopping haemorrhage from bleeding lesions. Neodimium - YAG or argon laser, or electrocoagulation can be used (Mathus-Vliegen and Tytgat, 1986). Stenoses can also be treated by mechanical or pneumatic dilation.

Respiratory Apparatus

The tracheobronchoscope (TBS) is indicated in the diagnosis and staging of tracheobroncho-oesophageal and mediastinic neoplasms. It is a method which has gained much from the introduction of fibre-optic instruments which are thin (4–6 mm), simple to use and can be introduced even in cases of lockjaw and significant deviations of the thoracic skeleton.

The explorable areas of mucosa have been greatly enlarged thanks to their use and the IV-V-VI orders of bronchi can now be visualised, and histological and cytological specimens can be taken even below the pleura by guiding the endoscopic probe with a radioscope. The fibrobronchoscope can be introduced by the nose or the mouth, and, by giving a local anaesthetic in the larynx, the epiglottis, the vocal chords, the trachea, the carina and the bronchial tree can be examined, starting from the supposedly healthy side.

Indications for a TBS may be a suspected neoplasm, based on results of an objective radiological or cytological examination, or on the presence of recurring haemoptysis or a persistant cough which is not responsive to treatment. Wherever a lesion has been ascertained, the bronchoscope will determine the extension of resection, of a pneumonectomy, of any other surgical intervention, or it will establish the impossibility of, or contraindications to surgery (Robbins et al., 1981). The endoscopic specimens of carcinoma can be classified according to the different aspects, in relation to the depth of invasion and the histotypes. In the case of squamous cell carcinoma, the presence of intraepithelial lesions is difficult to show. There can be thickening of the mucosa, with alterations in the shine of the surface. If the lesion, even though invasive, remains above the cartilaginous level, the thickening of the mucosa will take the form of granulous stain with neoformations of vessels. The lesion which invades the whole of the bronchial wall presents like a clear swelling growing upwards on the inside of the bronchus, with a roughly irregular surface and disappearance of the cartilaginous pattern, and bleeding when touched, due to intense vascularization.

The appearance of adenocarcinomas and small cell anaplastic carcinomas is, generally, different. They have prevalently infiltrating aspects with submucosal growth which can cause the blockage of a bronchus with a mucosa-covered funnel-like stricture which, at biopsy, may prove normal.

In these cases microscopic diagnosis will be obtained from deep histology and transtenotic brushing cytology. When malignant tumour cells (MTC) in the sputum are not supported by radiographic evidence of pulmonary carcinoma, one speaks of "occult lung cancer". This term was coined by Papanicolau and Koprowska in 1951. The presence of MTC in the sputum can be due to the desquamation of a microinvasive intraepithelial carcinoma, invasive either in early or advanced stage. Whereas it is rare that a carcinoma in the advanced stage should not be visible, it is more frequent in the early stage. "Early lung cancer" defines the central carcinoma which has not invaded the bronchial wall and the peripheral lesion in which the maximal diameter has not exceeded 20 mm. These tumours rarely have bronchial metastases. In the early stage they are, generally, curable by surgery, even with conservative operations. Intraepithelial or microinvasive carcinomas can be treated with conservative methods, such as endoscopy, as has been shown in the most recent literature from Japan, and this leads to an added interest in detecting these form (Hayata and Dougherty, 1983). When tumoral cells have been found in the sputum of a patient, but the traditional radiological investigation has given a negative result, we carry out bronchial washing, washing the right side and then the left separately and then each bronchus alone.

Today new methods consisting of fluorescent imaging are being introduced alongside these procedures. There are two ways of revealing the fluorescence of the tissues: looking for the fluorescence of the tissue itself (autofluorescence) and the search for fluorescence due to the absorption of a substance by a particular tissue (drug-induced fluorescence of a selective type). This is the procedure with substances which are retained in a higher concentration and are eliminated more slowly by the tumoral tissue in comparison to the surrounding normal tissue. The most commonly used of these substances is a haematoporphyrin derivate, which is fixed in the malignant tissue at concentrations of four to ten times more than in normal tissue.

By illuminating the bronchial tree with light radiation at low wave lengths, an emission of fluorescence is produced from which the site of the tumour can be detected (Spinelli, 1983).

Therapy

The traditional therapies open to bronchoscopy (instillation of drugs, aspiration of the abscess cavity, electrocoagulation) have now been joined by several laser therapies. The first experience was with CO_2 laser guided along rigid bronchoscopes, but with the advent of optic fibres, which can be used with the flexible bronchoscope (Neodimium-YAG and Argon laser), haemostatic and, particularly, obstruction-freeing applications have increased both at the level of the trachea and the main bronchi and lobes (the freeing of an obstruction of a bronchial segment or subsegment has no clinical relevance). This obstruction-freeing therapy can be associated with any other type of treatment. Just recently a photodynamic therapy has acquired great interest, and it can be used both therapeutically and palliatively. The Japanese (Hayata et al., 1982) have reported, in fact, the complete disappearance of small cancers with little damage to the surrounding healthy tissue.

Pleural Cavity

Already used for the treatment of some complications, in particular adherences, in tuberculosis, the pleuroscope is used today for the examination of pleural fluids. Although several other uses have been proposed for the pleuroscope, such as, for example, the staging of lung cancer, it is still indicated for fluids which do not respond to therapy and for which no cause has been found, as well as in those cases where pleural biopsy is required without the need to open the thorax. There are several occasions when a pleuroscope is necessary, for example, when fluid is present. If the fluid appears in patients who have undergone irradiation of the mediastinum, it is necessary to establish whether this formation of fluid is due to a recurrence of the disease or whether it is of postactinic origin. It is the same in the case of patients irradiated in the region of the breast; the fact that there are no tumoral cells in the fluid does not imply that it is not of neoplastic origin, but that there is no desquamation of the cells in the pleural cavity. This can occur because the infiltrating cells which are responsible for the lymphatic blockage, causing the formation of pleural fluid, may come from the subpleural spaces and may not have come to the surface yet. In these cases, both a transpleuroscopic histological examination and an endoscopic investigation will help to clarify the situation.

Mediastinoscopy

Mediastinoscopy was designed by Carlens and published in 1959. It allows the exploration of the upper mediastinum up to the main bronchi. We can divide the mediastinum into three areas: the anterosuperior area limited by the sternum, the anterior heart border and ascending aorta; the posterior area lying dorsal to the anterior margin of the dorsal spine; and the middle between these two spaces. Generally, masses located in the anterior mediastinum belong to the thyroid or thymus, or else they are lymphomas, teratomas, lipomas or cystic and vascular enlargements. In the posterior mediastinum one finds neurogenic, vascular, infectious or, rarely, other masses; in the middle there are vascular, lymphomas, metastatic, oesophageal and tracheal tumours. All the lesions located in the anterior mediastinum and in the middle mediastinum, in front of the trachea, can be considered as indications for mediastinoscopy. It can be used to biopsy accessible lymph nodes in the paratracheal and hilar locations.

Mediastinoscopy is performed through a 4-cm cervical incision 2 cm above the sternal manubrim. A rigid tubular endoscope is introduced through this incision and progresses by blunt dissection under general anaethesia. Mediastinoscopy is a widespread diagnostic technique and, in the last 10 years, it has been suggested that it should be included in the staging of lung cancer. Recently, alternative and less invasive procedures, such as computed tomography and nuclear magnetic resonance imaging, transparietal aspiration through the skin, or through bronchoscopic or oesophagoscopic procedures, have enormously reduced the need for mediastinoscopy. Classical indications for this technique are an assessment of resectability of lung cancer and diagnosis of lymphoma. The complication rate is less than 1%, and the mortality rate is also less than 1%. The use of computed tomography gives good resolution among the structures of the thoracic inlet and allows the density and, consequently, the nature of the mediastinal lesions to be evaluated. Recently, endoscopic ultrasonography has provided further possibilities of studying the mediastinum and, in particular, a clearer definition of lesions adjacent to the oesophagus (Tio et al., 1986). Nuclear magnetic resonance imaging differentiates vascular from nonvascular structures, makes it unnecessary to adopt contrast media and, consequently, impedes the reaction associated with their use. This is a method which is ideal for children since they do not have to be irradiated.

References

Bottiroli G, dal Fante M, Spinelli P (1987) HpD fluorescence emission in samples of human pre-malignant and malignant lesions of the bowel. In: Sottini S, Trigari S (eds) Proceeding of ECOOSA. Spie, Bellingham, Washington, p 320

Bruni HC, Nelson RS (1985) Carcinoma of the esophagus and cardia. Diagnostic evaluation in 113 cases. J Thorac Cardiovasc Surg 70: 367

Carlens E (1959) Mediastinoscopy: a method for inspection and tissue biopsy in the superior mediastinum. Dis chest 36: 343–352

Christie JP, Shina H (1982) Technique of colonoscopic polypectomy. Surg Clin North am 62: 877

Classen M, Knyrim K, Seidlitz HK, Hagenmuller F (1987) Electronic endoscopy: the latest technology. Endoscopy 19: 118

Cotton PB (1972) Cannulation of the papilla of Vater by endoscopy and retrograde cholangiopancreatography (ERCP). Gut 13: 1014

Di Magno E, Regan PT, Clain J, et al. (1982) Human endoscopic ultrasonography. Gastroenterology 83: 824

Gluckman JL, Weissler MC (1986) Role of photodynamic therapy in the management of early cancers of the upper aerodigestive tract. Lasers Med Sci 1: 217

Hayata Y, Dougherty TJ (eds) (1983) Lasers and hematoporphyrin derivative in cancer. Igaku-Shoin, Tokyo

Hayata Y, Kato H, Konaka C, et al. (1982) Hematopophyrin derivative and laser photoradiation in the treatment of lung cancer. Chest 81: 269

Hirschowitz BI, Curtis LE, Peters CW, et al. (1958) The fiberscope. Gastroenterology 35: 50

Hopkins HH, Kapany NS (1954) A flexible fiberscope. Nature 173: 39

Huibregtse K, Tytgat GNJ (1984) Endoscopic placement of biliary prostheses. Gastrointest Endosc 1: 219–231

Mathus-Vliegen EMH, Tytgat GNJ (1986) Laser photocoagulation in the palliation of colorectal malignancies. Cancer 57: 2212

Papanicolau GN, Koprowska I (1951) Carcinoma in situ of right lower bronchus; case report. Cancer 4: 141–146

Profio AE, Doiron DR, Balchum OJ, Huth GC (1983) Fluorescence bronchoscopy for localization of carcinoma in situ. Med Phys 10: 35

Prolla JC, Reilley RW, Kirsner JB (1977) Direct vision endoscopic cytology and biopsy in the diagnosis of esophageal and gastric tumours: current experience. Acta Cytol (Baltimore) 21: 399

Robbins HM, Sweet ME, Jefferson SE, et al. (1981) The determination of resectability of lung cancer by fiberoptic bronchoscopy. Arch Intern Med 141: 649

Schapiro M, Auslander MO, Schapiro MB (1987) The electronic video endoscope: clinical experience with 1200 diagnostic and therapeutic cases in the community hospital. Gastrointest Endosc 33: 63

Spinelli P (1981) Early gastric cancer. Arch Atti Soc Ital Chir 37

Spinelli P (1983) Endoscopie au laser avec fluorescence et photochimio therapie du cancer. Acta Endosc 13: 201

Spinelli P (1984) Laser in endoscopy. In: Angelini L, Fegiz G, Wells PNT (eds) Emerging technologies in surgery. Masson, Paris, p 187

Tabuse K, Katsumi M, Nagai Y, et al. (1985) Microwave tissue coagulation applied clinically in endoscopic surgery. Endoscopy 17: 139

Tio TL, den Hartog JF, Tytgat GNJ (1986) The role of endoscopic ultrasonography in assessing local resectability of oesophagogastric malignancies. Accuracy, pitfalls, and predictability. Scand J Gastroenterol [Suppl 123] 21: 78

Monoclonal Antibodies in the Diagnosis and Management of Colorectal Carcinomas

J. P. Mach, F. Buchegger, J. Pettavel, A. Bischof-Delaloye, and B. Delaloye

Introduction

In this chapter, we shall review the usefulness and limitations of monoclonal antibodies (MAbs) directed against markers associated with colorectal carcinomas in the diagnosis, the follow-up, and, potentially, the therapy of colorectal carcinomas. The chapter will be divided into two major parts: first, the in vitro use of MAbs for the measurement of circulating markers in colorectal carcinoma patients; secondly, the application of MAbs in vivo, where the tumor markers are considered as a target for the localization of injected MAbs into the tumor. Since carcinoembryonic antigen (CEA) (Gold and Freedman 1965) appears to remain the best marker of colorectal carcinomas for both types of applications, we shall illustrate this chapter with personal results obtained with MAbs directed against this antigen and only mention, by way of comparison, the progress made by the use of MAbs against different colorectal carcinoma markers.

MAbs for In Vitro Assay of Colorectal Carcinoma Markers

Carcinoembryonic Antigen

There is something particular about the CEA assay, which is one of the most utilized blood tests for the follow-up of cancer patients. Since the discovery of CEA, the different assays described to measure this antigen in patients' serum or plasma have been the subject of controversy concerning the cancer specificity of this test. The first assay developed by the group of Gold was an inhibition radioimmunoassay (RIA) performed on perchloric acid extracts of serum. It was initially reported to detect elevated circulating CEA levels exclusively in the blood from patients with carcinomas derived from digestive organs (Thomson et al. 1969).

The perfect tumor and organ specificity of CEA suggested by these early results was not, however, confirmed in the abundant literature on this subject (Mach et al. 1973; Hansen et al. 1974). It is now evident that elevated levels of ciculating CEA (up to 2000 μg per liter of serum) can be observed in some cases of different types of carcinomas derived from secretory epithelial cells, including, in order of frequency: carcinomas of the large bowel, pancreas, stomach, lung, breast, prostate, uterus, liver, ovary, and esophagus. A particular case is represented by medullary thyroid carcinomas where almost every patient displays elevated circulating CEA level. In addition, moderate elevations of serum CEA levels up to 30 μg per liter, as compared to less than 5 μg per liter in normal individuals, can be observed in 5%–40% of patients with nonmalignant inflammatory diseases such as ulcerative colitis, Crohn's disease, liver cirrhosis, and chronic bronchitis, as well as in normal individuals with heavy smoking habits (Mach et al. 1973, 1974a; Hansen et al. 1974; Zamchek 1974).

In view of these results, obtained mostly with RIA using polyclonal antibodies (on serum samples extracted by perchlorid acid treatment or by heating at 70 °C), it was logical to evaluate whether or not the use of highly selected anti-CEA MAbs could improve the cancer specificity of the CEA test.

MAbs for the Enzyme Immunoassay of CEA

MAbs represent the optimal reagents for solid phase enzyme immunoassay (EIA) because of their homogeneity, their exquisite specificity for individual epitopes of the measured antigen, and their availability in unlimited amounts. Thus, as soon as we obtained the first MAb directed against CEA, MAb 23 (Accolla et al. 1980), we used this antibody in the immunoadsorbent solid phase of an EIA in conjunction with purified polyclonal goat anti-CEA antibodies coupled to alkaline phosphatase (Buchegger et al. 1982a). The results were almost identical to those obtained in the conventional inhibition RIA, using radiolabeled CEA and polyclonal anti-CEA antibodies, as determined on the same blood samples of 125 patients with colorectal carcinomas, 15 patients

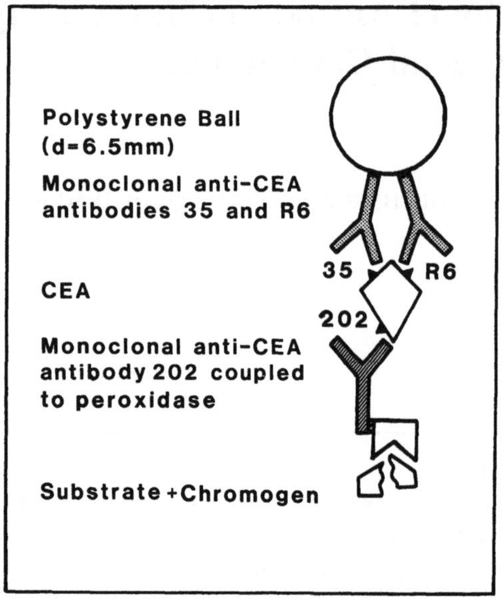

Fig. 1. Schematic description of a solid phase noncompetitive EIA using three monoclonal antibodies for the direct measurement of CEA in patients' serum

with liver cirrhosis, and 59 normal individual with heavy smoking habits (Buchegger et al. 1982a).

Furthermore, the selection of new anti-CEA antibodies with higher affinity and no reactivity with normal granulocyte cross-reacting antigens (NCA) (Buchegger et al. 1984) allowed the development of several forms of EIA with two anti-CEA MAbs on the solid phase and a third anti-CEA MAb coupled to peroxidase as described in Fig. 1 (Buchegger and Mach 1986).

Despite these optimal reagents and very good sensitivity as demonstrated in the standard curve in Figs. 2 and 3, it was not possible to eliminate some results of elevated CEA values in nonmalignant diseases. Figure 4 compares the results obtained with the old RIA with those obtained with the most modern direct EIA using three anti-CEA MAbs in serum samples from 25 colon carcinoma patients and from a selected group of 21 patients with liver cirrhosis (Buchegger and Mach 1986). No major qualitative difference between the two assays is demonstrated.

Thus, the results suggest that the CEA detected in the blood of some patients with nonmalignant inflammatory diseases is immunogenically undistinguishable from colon carcinoma CEA. These results have now been confirmed by several groups using commercially available solid phase CEA assays with excellent anti-CEA MAbs. There was, however, an occasional provocative report suggesting that the use of a new anti-CEA MAb with a unique specificity, could drastically reduce the percentage of posi-

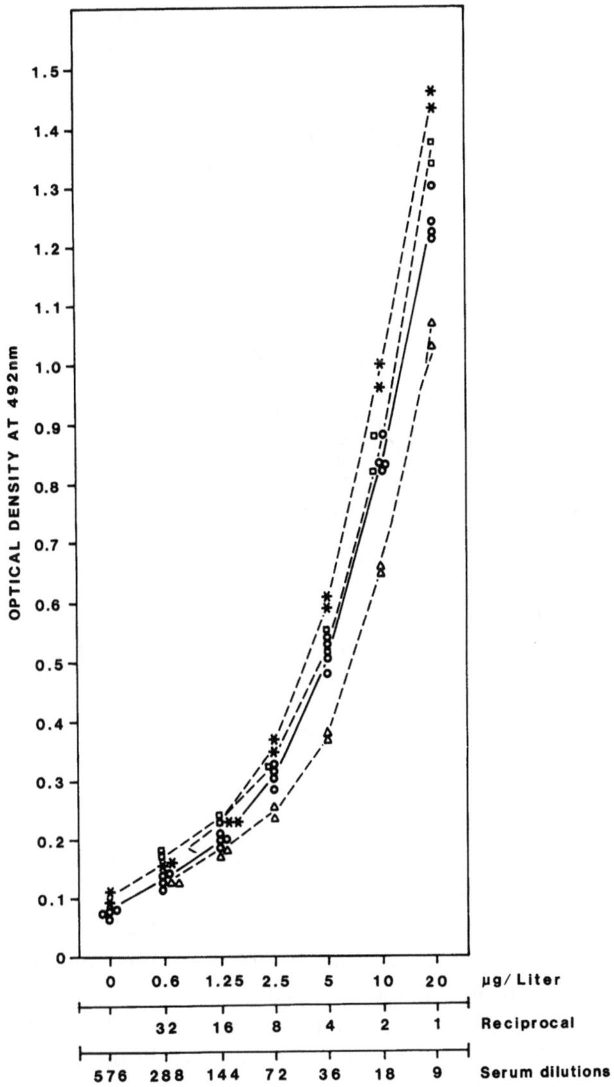

Fig. 2. Standard curves comparing normal bovine serum enriched with various amounts of CEA purified from metastases of colon carcinoma *(circles)* (two duplicate values obtained on 2 separate days) with serial dilutions from the sera of three patients with moderately elevated CEA levels *(triangles* and *squares)* or highly elevated CEA level *(asterisk). Ordinate* shows the optical density at 492 nm on an arithmetic scale, the *abscissa* shows CEA values and reciprocal serum dilutions on a log scale (Buchegger and Mach 1986)

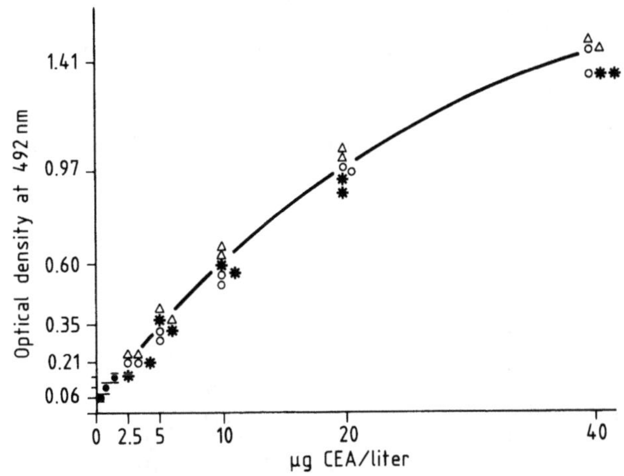

Fig. 3. Standard curve drawn by computer according to the results obtained with standard amounts of CEA measured in duplicate by direct m-EIA on three different days *(circles, triangles,* and *asterisks). Ordinate* and *abscissa* are on arithmetic scales (Buchegger and Mach 1986)

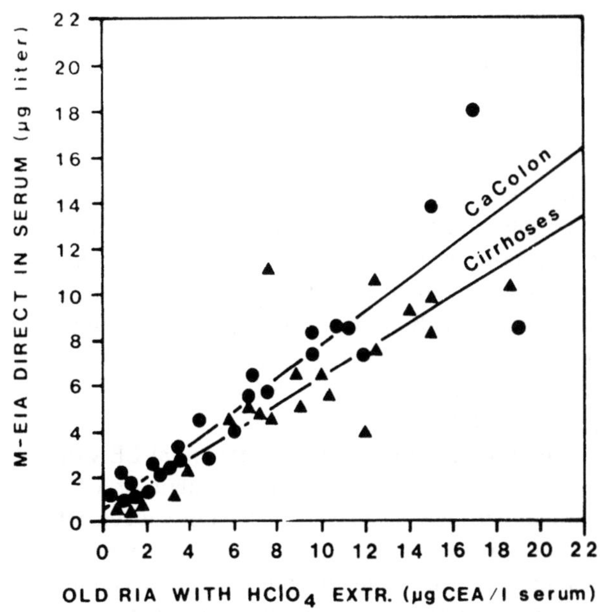

Fig. 4. Comparison of results obtained for 25 colorectal carcinoma patients *(circles)* and 21 patients with liver cirrhosis *(triangles)* measured either by the old inhibition RIA after perchloric acid extraction of the sample *(abscissa)* or by the direct enzyme immunoassay described in Fig. 1 *(ordinate).* The correlation between the two assays for the colorectal carcinoma patients was 0.90, whereas for the liver cirrhosis patients it was 0.84 (Buchegger an Mach 1986)

tive CEA results in nonmalignant digestive diseases (Hedin et al. 1983). But these results, published in 1983, have not yet been confirmed on large series of patients with carcinomas or nonmalignant diseases.

Practical Recommendations for the Clinical Use of the CEA Assay

Because of the moderately elevated CEA values observed in numerous types of nonmalignant diseases, the CEA assay is not recommended as a cancer-screening test. The most rational application of the CEA test consists in the follow-up of colorectal carcinoma patients, to detect early recurrences or dissemination (Mach et al. 1974 a, 1978; Martin et al. 1976) (as illustrated in Fig. 5), as well as for the evaluation of the efficacy of surgical resection or of

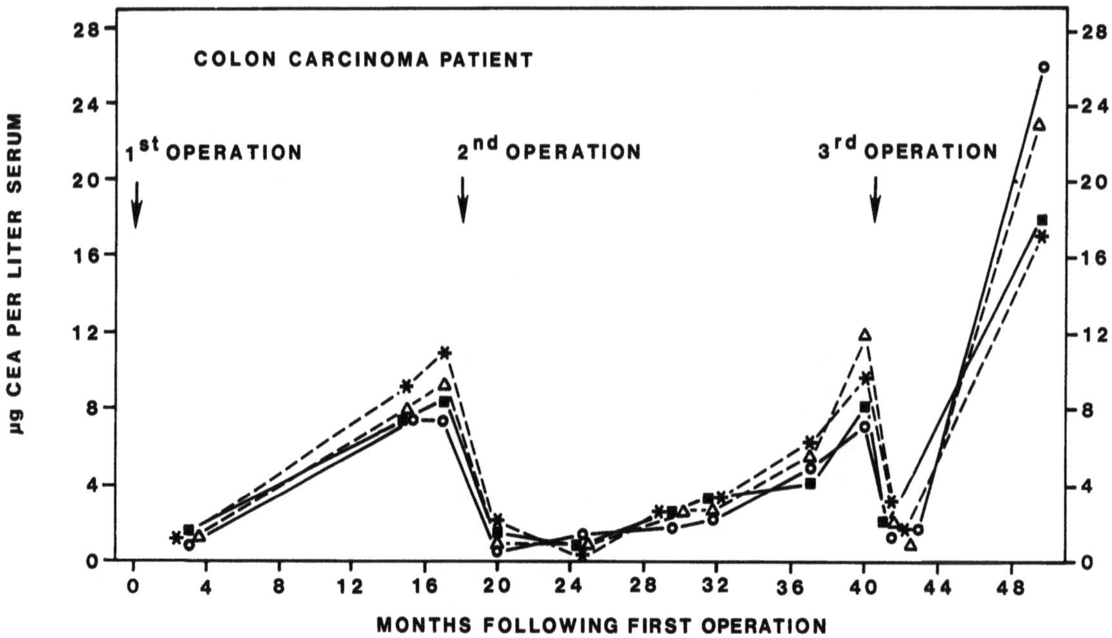

Fig. 5. Comparison of CEA measurements performed by four methods on the same sequential serum samples from a patient who had three recurrences after removal of a primary colon carcinoma and was twice reoperated on the basis of CEA results. The four methods were: RIA using goat antiserum *(asterisks)*, two EIA involving heat extraction of serum samples *(triangles)* and *(open circles)*, the direct m-EIA without heat extraction described here *(squares)* (Buchegger and Mach 1986)

chemotherapy. In all these situations, sequential CEA determinations before and after treatment are much more meaningful than isolated results. In this context, one should recommend the use of the same CEA assay for the follow-up of the same patients in order to avoid some changes in numerical values which may exist between different methods using different CEA standard curves.

An exception to the rule of sequential CEA determinations consists in the measurement of CEA in patients strongly suspected of having cancer, where a single markedly elevated CEA value (>30–50 µg per liter) will indicate the presence of a carcinoma derived from secretory epithelium and justify further investigations, including the use of immunoscintigraphy which will be described in the second part of this chapter.

In general, the most modern CEA assays are performed directly on 0.025–0.2 ml serum or plasma without prior extraction by perchloric acid (Thomson et al. 1969; Zamchek 1974; Mach et al. 1974a) or by heating in acetic acid (Buchegger et al. 1982b) methods which were recommended in the early CEA assays. These extraction procedures do not appear to be necessary any more, particularly in the assays where the MAbs linked to a solid phase are absorbing CEA during a first incubation followed by the elimination of unreactive serum proteins by washing before adding the tracer antibody for a second incubation (Fig. 1).

It should be mentioned, however, that even in such two-step assays and, a fortiori, in the single incubation assays, the presence of antimouse antibodies in the serum sample to be analyzed can give false positive results in direct assays by bridging the mouse antibodies linked to the solid phase and the second mouse antibody used as tracer. This type of artifact can be markedly inhibited by adding 5–10 µg normal mouse IgG and 10 µl heat aggregated normal human serum in each tube with the serum sample and with the tracer antibody (Buchegger and Mach 1986). In addition to the problem of antimouse antibodies, we have recently observed a few (very rare) cases, where patients with no evidence of cancer had moderate elevations of CEA levels (10–13 µg per liter) in the direct assay, which decresed to undetectable values after heat extraction. The patients had no detectable antimouse Ig antibodies, and the addition of an excess of normal mouse Ig did not decrease the elevated values observed in the direct assay. Thus, in addition to antimouse Ig antibodies, there may be some heat-labile products which can provoke nonspecific binding of the tracer antibody to the solid phase. These very rare cases are presently under investigation in our and other laboratories.

New Colon Carcinoma Markers Detectable in the Circulation

Several new markers, which are released into the blood of patients with various types of carcinomas, have been identified by MAbs. None of these new secreted markers are, however, restricted to colorectal carcinoma, and their assays have not detected a higher percentage of positivity in colorectal carcinoma than the CEA assay. The marker which comes the closest to CEA in terms of percentage detection rates in colorectal carcinoma patients is the 19-9 antigen. According to Ritts et al. (1984) it is above the normal limit of 40 units per ml in 18% of colorectal carcinomas at different stages, as compared to 38% of positivity for the CEA assay. Importantly, the 19-9 antigen can detect a higher percentage of pancreatic and hepatobiliary carcinomas than the CEA assay.

Another antigen defined by a MAb which is more often present in pancreatic carcinoma (68%) than colorectal carcinomas (10%) is the DU-PAN-2 antigen (Metzgar et al. 1984).

One should also mention an antigen which has been identified by the MAb B-72.3 raised against membrane-enriched fractions of a mammary carcinoma. This "pancarcinoma"-associated antigen, called TAG-72 (Paterson et al. 1986), has been detected by competition RIA in the sera of seven out of 20 (35%) patients with advanced colon carcinomas and in a similar percentage of cases with other types of carcinomas.

Finally, the ovarian carcinoma marker Ca-125 (Bast et al. 1983) has also been found positive in a small percentage of cases with advanced colorectal carcinomas.

Several authors have proposed adding one or all of these four assays for new carcinoma markers to the CEA assay in order to increase the percentage of detection of colorectal carcinomas. Indeed, it is true that some cases of colorectal carcinoma can have a normal CEA level and an elevated 19-9 or DU-PAN-2 antigen value. However, one should be aware that by increasing the number of tests one might also increase the number of false positive results. It is important to note in this context that several authors (Mezger et al. 1988; A. Ruibal, Barcelona, and M. Gerard, Brussels, personal communications) have found elevated values of 19-9 or Ca-125 antigen in nonmalignant liver diseases and in cases of ascites with no tumor.

Thus, while the concept of using a cocktail of carcinoma tests to detect a large variety of epithelial malignancies remains attractive, the real clinical usefulness of such an approach has not yet been convincingly demonstrated.

Radiolabeled MAbs for In Vivo Diagnosis and Therapy of Colorectal Carcinomas

First Experimental Models for Studying the In Vivo Tumor Localization of Radiolabeled Antibodies

More than 30 years ago, Pressman and Korngold (1953) and Bale and Spar (1957) reported the first experiments indicating that radiolabeled antibodies injected into a tumor-bearing animal could localize preferentially into the tumor, which could be detected by external scanning. These early studies were, however, performed with poorly characterized antibodies obtained by absorption and elution from tumor cells or crude tumor fractions. Thus, these types of antibodies could not be used for clinical applications.

It took 30 years until our group (Mach et al. 1974b), in parallel with Goldenberg's group (Goldenberg et al. 1974), proposed using antibodies against a well-defined human tumor-associated antigen, CEA, to localize colon carcinomas. We introduced into this field the model of nude mice bearing well-differentiated xenografts of human colon carcinoma and demonstrated that ^{131}I-labeled, affinity purified, goat anti-CEA antibodies localized specifically into the colon carcinoma, as compared to ^{125}I-labeled purified normal goat IgG, injected simultaneously as an internal control (Mach et al. 1974b).

First Generation of Immunoscintigraphy

Goldenberg et al. (1978) reported the first successful detection of carcinomas by external photoscanning in patients injected with ^{131}I-labeled purified goat anti-CEA antibodies. From their initial series of 18 patients up to the numerous more recent publications, however, this group has always claimed the detection of almost all tumors with no false positive results. In contrast, we have reported a critical appraisal of this method of tumor detection and a more complete analysis of the clinical results (Mach et al. 1980a). In our first series of 27 patients, we reported only 41% of tumor detection despite the use of the same methodology as Goldenberg's group, i.e., highly purified ^{131}I-labeled goat anti-CEA antibodies, external photoscanning and the Tc-99m subtraction technology (DeLand et al. 1980). In addition to our critical evaluation of the clinical usefulness of immunoscintigraphy, confirmed by an enlarged series of 53 patients from our group (Mach et al. 1980b) and

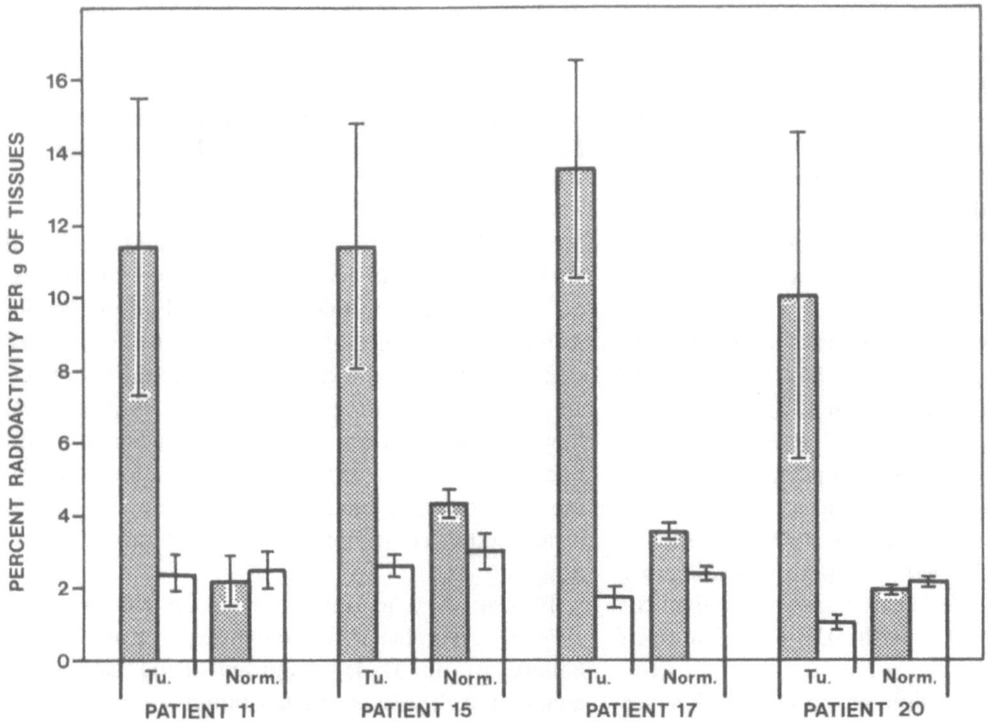

Fig. 6. Demonstration of the specific tumor localization of goat anti-CEA antibodies *(shaded bars)* as compared to normal goat IgG *(open bars)* injected into patients with colorectal carcinomas. *Tu.* resected tumor fragments; *Norm.*, adjacent normal mucosa; *vertical lines*, standard deviation. (From Mach et al. 1980 a)

by others (Sullivan et al. 1982), our positive observation was that direct measurement of radioactivity in tumor and adjacent normal tissues (surgically resected after injection of ^{131}I-labeled anti-CEA antibodies and ^{125}I normal IgG) showed a definitely higher tumor uptake of antibody as compared to control IgG (Fig. 6) (Mach et al. 1980 a, b). Thus, despite a marked background of radioactivity in the liver and spleen observed after injection of ^{131}I-labeled polyclonal intact antibodies, we provided evidence of the specific tumor localization of the antibodies.

Second Generation of Immunoscintigraphy

The improvements introduced in the second generation of immunoscintigraphy were due to the use of MAbs instead of polyclonal antibodies and single photon emission computerized tomography (SPECT or ECT) instead of planar scintigraphy.

The obvious advantage of MAbs for immunoscintigraphy is not their monoclonality per se, but the fact that a single population of antibodies with a particular specificity and affinity for one antigenic determinant of a tumor marker can be selected and produced in unlimited amounts. In the field of radiolabeled antibodies, it is of utmost importance to eliminate any antibody directed against a cross-reacting antigen (Buchegger et al. 1984). The second advantage of the MAb technology is that it permits the production of large amounts of antibodies against cell surface markers which are not yet purified or not even precisely identified.

Soon after the production of the first MAb against CEA (Accolla et al. 1980), we reported on a series of patients injected with this antibody labeled with ^{131}I and tested either by planar scintigraphy (Mach et al. 1981) or by ECT, in collaboration with Tubiana's group Berche et al. (1982). The use of MAbs markedly decreased the background of radioactivity present in the reticuloendothelial system (RES), and the use of ECT allowed a better three-dimensional spatial resolution. The signal to noise ratio was not, however, very high due in part to the poor detection efficiency of ^{131}I by the camera and in part to the relatively low affinity of the first anti-CEA MAb used in this study.

MAbs against other tumor markers associated with colon carcinoma discovered by the MAb technology, such as MAb 17-1A produced by Koprowski's group Herlyn et al. (1979), were also tested because it was important to determine which type of

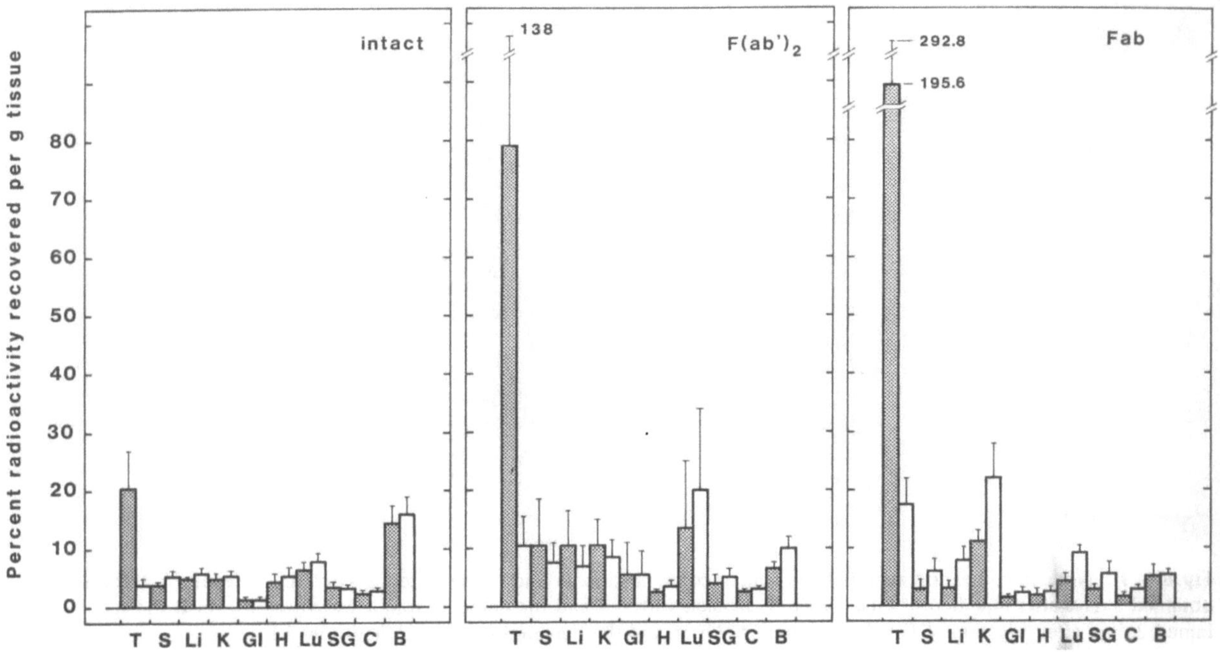

Fig. 7. Biodistribution of MAb 35 or its fragments *(shaded bars)* and control mouse IgG or fragments *(open bars)* injected simultaneously into nude mice bearing xenografts of human colon carcinoma. The *vertical line* represents standard deviations calculated from groups of four to seven mice per MAb or fragment. *T*, tumor; *S*, spleen; *Li*, liver; *K*, kidney; *GI*, gastrointestinal tract; *H*, heart; *Lu*, lung; *SG*, salivary gland; *C*, carcass and head; *B*, blood. (From Buchegger et al. 1983)

target antigen was the best for immunoscintigraphy. We analyzed a series of 53 colorectal carcinoma patients, injected with ^{131}I-labeled MAb 17-1A (Mach et al. 1983), by planar scintigraphy and ECT, but did not find the results superior to those obtained with anti-CEA MAbs. Namely, the tumor to normal tissue ratios determined in resected tumors were not very high with the MAb 17-1A.

Fragments of MAbs

Preliminary results of immunoscintigraphy obtained in patients injected with F(ab')$_2$ fragments of goat anti-CEA antibodies showed a decrease of background radioactivity in the RES (Mach et al. 1980a, b). Clinical results are, however, always difficult to interpret objectively. Thus, an experimental study was necessary to determine the advantages and limitations of fragments as compared to intact antibodies. F(ab')$_2$ and Fab fragments from two newly selected anti-CEA MAbs of high affinity (Haskell et al. 1983) were prepared and tested for their capacity to localize, in the human colon carcinoma, Co-112 grafted in nude mice (Buchegger et al. 1983). Groups of mice were injected simultaneously with intact antibodies or fragments labeled with ^{131}I and with normal IgG or their corresponding fragments labeled with ^{125}I. The mice were dissected 2–5 days later. The results obtained with MAb 35 or its fragments, expressed as a percentage of the total radioactivity recovered for each isotope per gram tumor and normal tissue, are shown in Fig. 7 (Buchegger et al. 1983).

It is evident that the ratios of tumor to normal organ antibody concentration increase dramatically with the use of fragments. These ratios were 7 for intact antibody, 24 for F(ab')$_2$, and 82 for Fab. The specificity indices calculated by dividing the tumor to normal organ ratios obtained for antibody by the corresponding ratio obtained for control IgG were 3.4 for intact antibody, 8.2 for F(ab')$_2$, and 19 for Fab (Buchegger et al. 1983).

The scanning results obtained with intact antibodies and fragments were in agreement with those obtained by direct measurements of radioactivity. With intact antibodies, tumor grafts of 0.5–1 g gave contrasted positive scans only 3 days after injection (Fig. 8 A), whereas fragments of antibodies allowed the detection of smaller tumors earlier (1–2 days). The best results were obtained with Fab fragments of MAb 35, which allowed the clear detection of a tumor graft of 0.1 g 2 days after injection (Fig. 8 B).

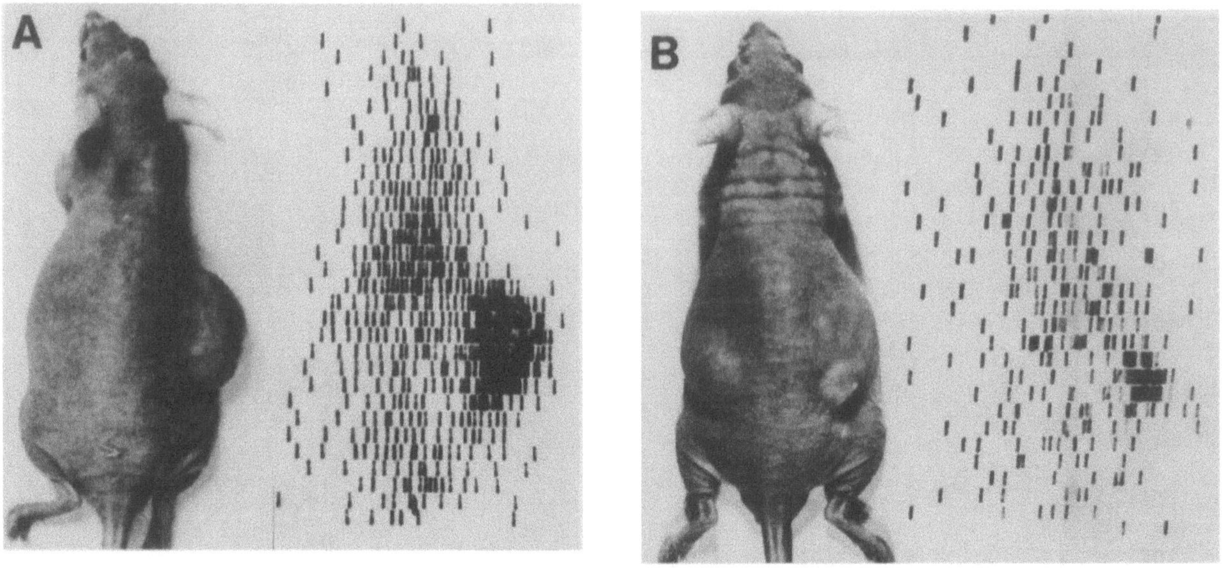

Fig. 8 A, B. Nude mice bearing xenograft of human colon carcinoma and corresponding whole body scans. In **A** the scan was obtained 3 days after injection of intact MAb 35 labeled with ^{131}I and the detected tumor weighed 1.2 g. In **B** the scan was obtained 2 days after injection of Fab fragments of MAb 35 and the detected tumor weighed only 0.1 g

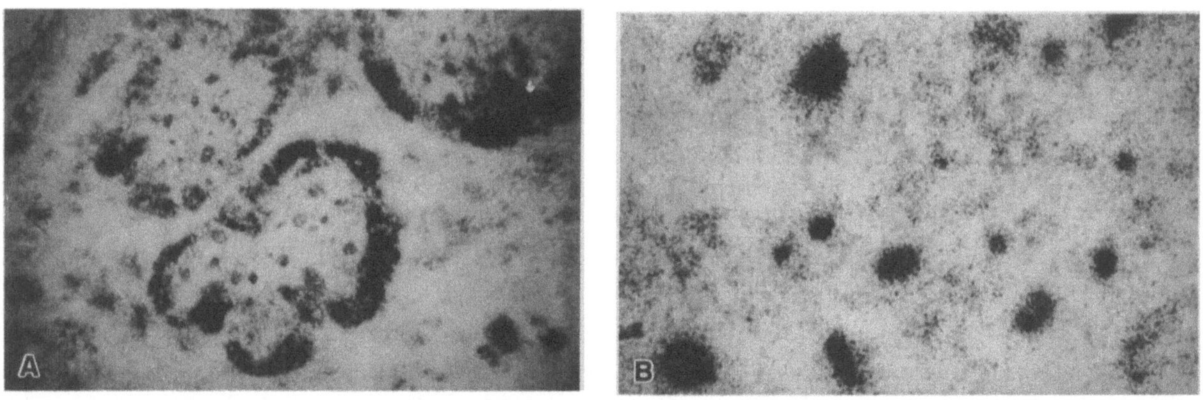

Fig. 9 A, B. Autoradiographs of 8-μm frozen sections from the human colon carcinoma Co-112 grafted in nude mice, obtained 3 days after injection of either intact MAb 35 (**A**) or its Fab fragments (**B**) both labeled with ^{125}I. The *small dots* and *dark areas* correspond to the silver grains due to the radioactivity localized in vivo, whereas the light staining corresponds to the immunoperoxidase reaction obtained by incubating the tissue sections with anti-CEA MAb. A × 200, B × 400

Autoradiographs of tumor sections from mice injected with intact antibodies labeled with ^{125}I and fragments showed first, that they both localized in the tumor nodules and not in the stromal connective tissue of mouse origin. However, the intact MAbs were localized mostly at the periphery of tumor nodules (Fig. 9 A), whereas the $F(ab')_2$ and Fab fragments penetrated deeper into the tumor nodules, often localizing within the pseudolumen of the malignant glands where the concentration of CEA is the highest (Fig. 9 B).

In addition to the better penetration of Fab fragments, Fig. 9 also shows that both the intact antibodies and Fab fragments gave a patchy distribution of radioactivity in malignant tissues, with some areas of intense radioactivity and others with almost no radioactivity. These results indicate that if these types of antibody were to be used for radioimmunotherapy, it would be necessary to select an isotope capable of destroying tumor cells within a radius of 100–500 μm.

From the presentation of these results, one could conclude that fragments of antibodies have only advantages over intact MAbs. This impression is in part due to the fact that in Fig. 7, the results are expressed as a percentage of the total radioactivity recovered at the day of dissection. If we now consider the percentage of the injected dose of radioactivity, we see that the amount of radioactivity delivered to the tumor is higher with intact antibodies than with fragments. We reported 9.1% of the injected dose per gram of tumor at days 4–5 for intact MAbs, as compared to 2.5% per gram of tumor at days 2–3 for the Fab fragments (Buchegger et al. 1983).

Third Generation of Immunoscintigraphy

Antibody fragments, which have been shown experimentally to penetrate better and more rapidly into the tumor (Buchegger et al. 1983; Halpern et al. 1984), but which have a short biological half-life, needed to be labeled with an isotope such as ^{123}I which can be detected by the gamma cameras with much better efficiency than ^{131}I and is optimal for imaging by ECT. We performed a clinical study including 31 patients with known colorectal carcinomas who were injected with $F(ab')_2$ and Fab fragments from MAb 35 (1–1.5 mg labeled with 2–8 mCi ^{123}I) (Delaloye et al. 1986 a). Representative examples of detections from small tumors (3 and 5 g), as well as the demonstration of the slow penetration of fragments in a large liver metastasis, are shown in Fig. 10 A–C. Another advantage of ECT is that it does not require the use of subtraction techniques which are susceptible to the formation of artifacts (Ott et al. 1983). The tumor detection rate of this retrospective study was high: 89% for the 27 patients

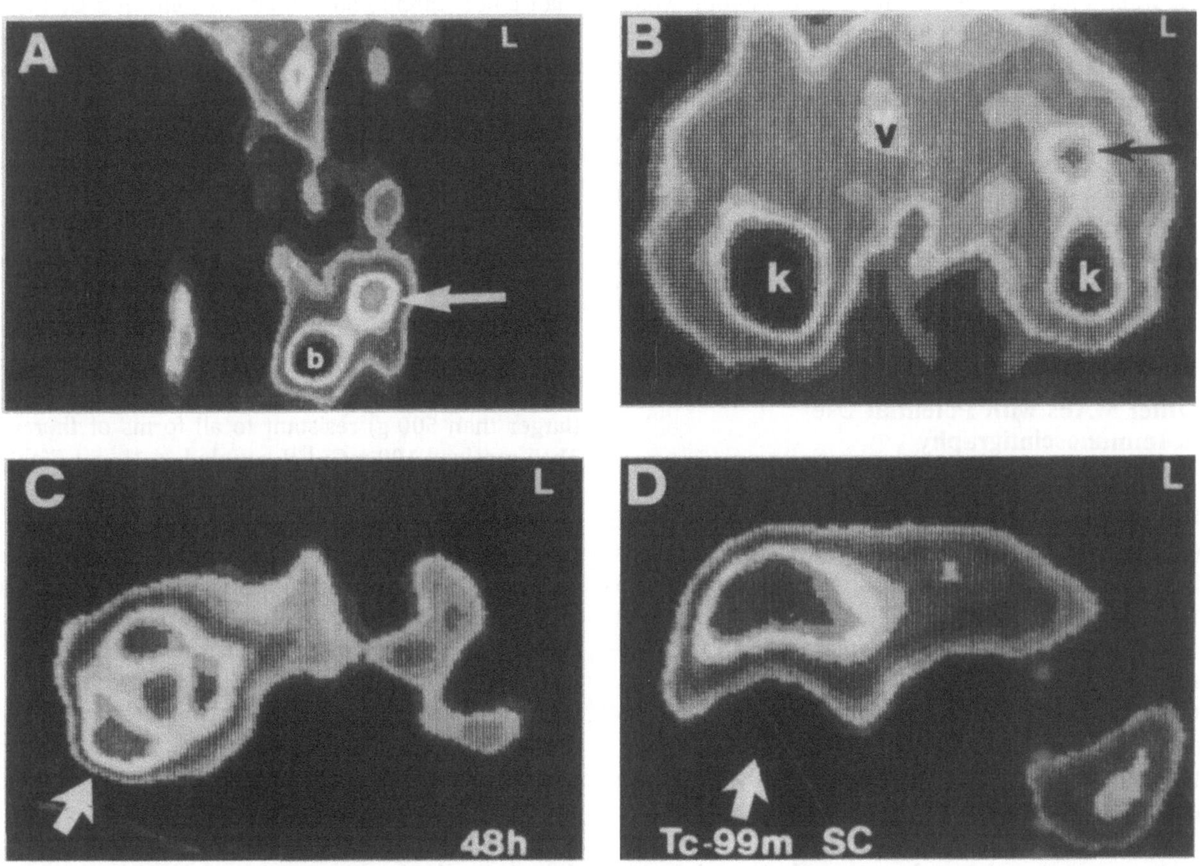

Fig. 10 A–D. Detection of colon carcinoma in patients by ECT after injection of fragments from anti-CEA MAb 35 labeled with I-123. **A** Visualization of a 5-g sigmoid tumor on a coronal section of the pelvis obtained 24 h after injection of Fab fragments. Tumor *(arrow)* and bladder *(b)* are well defined. The relatively high tumor uptake of Fab fragments was confirmed by direct counting of the resected tumor and adjacent normal tissues. The tumor to normal mucosa ratio was 5.0. **B** illustrates the detection of a relatively small carcinoma (3 g) located in the splenic angle of the large bowel. The transverse ECT section taken 6 h after injection of Fab fragments shows an uptake of radioactivity (colored red in the original scintigraph, *arrow*) corresponding to the tumor, just anterior to the left kidney. The tumor activity exceeds the vascular activity *(v)* but is lower than the kidney activity *(k)*. **C** demonstrates in a transverse ECT section the penetration of $F(ab')_2$ mostly at the periphery of a large liver metastasis, located in the posterior part of the right liver lobe. **D** confirms the presence of the metastasis detected by a photon-deficient area in the corresponding section of a sulfur colloid ECT, left. (From Delaloye et al. 1986)

injected with Fab and $F(ab')_2$ fragments. More important than the detection rate (which can depend on patient selection) was the quality of the tumor images, mostly those obtained with Fab fragments, which gave much better tumor contrast than in the previous generation of immunoscintigraphy. Interestingly, nine of the 23 cases of primary carcinomas and local recurrences (all but one of which were detected) had almost normal CEA values at the time of positive immunoscintigraphy. A prospective clinical study is ongoing to determine the potential clinical usefulness of this form of third generation immunoscintigraphy.

We agree with Larson et al. (1983), who also showed, using antimelanoma MAbs, that Fab fragments from high-affinity antibodies (10^9 M^{-1}) represent the best tracer for diagnostic immunoscintigraphy. Fab fragments are optimal reagents, in particular when they are labeled with ^{123}I, an isotope which has already been recommended for use in immunoscintigraphy by Epenetos et al. (1982). We are not convinced, however, that Fab can be used for radioimmunotherapy as proposed by Larson et al. (1983), because of their too short circulating half-life resulting in a relatively low percentage of injected dose delivered into the tumor. For therapy, our experimental results suggest that $F(ab')_2$ represents the best fragments (Buchegger et al. 1988).

Other MAbs with Potential Use in Immunoscintigraphy

In addition to the MAb 17-1A already mentioned (Herlyn et al. 1979; Mach et al. 1983), another antibody from Koprowski's group which detects the 19-9 antigen (Ritts et al. 1984), has been successfully used in the form of $F(ab')_2$ fragments mixed with the same fragment of an anti-CEA antibody for the detection of colon carcinoma by Chatal et al. (1984) and several European groups. Of great potential interest is also the MAb B-72,3 directed against the pancarcinoma antigen TAG-72 (Paterson et al. 1986). This antibody was recently shown to give relatively high uptakes in colorectal carcinomas by Colcher et al. (1987).

Outside the field of digestive carcinomas, one should also mention the large clinical experience obtained by Buraggi's group and several other Italian groups in the detection of melanoma after injection of the MAb 225.289 (Buraggi et al. 1985).

In the field of ovarian carcinomas, the intraperitoneal injection of the MAbs developed by the groups of Bast et al. (1983), Epenetos et al. (1982), or Miotti et al. (1987) may be of great interest, either for tumor detection or for radioimmunotherapy.

First Approach to Radioimmunotherapy

Large doses of ^{131}I-labeled antibodies have been injected intravenously into patients for the treatment of primary hepatic carcinoma (Order et al. 1980), of melanoma (Larson et al. 1983), and lymphoma (De Nardo et al. 1987). Intracavitary injection has been proposed by Epenetos et al. (1984) as an alternative route of administration of ^{131}I-labeled antibodies in order to increase the amounts of radioactivity delivered in metastases localized in these cavities.

After extensive experimentations in nude mice showing that doses of 150 μCi of ^{131}I per gram of human colon carcinoma xenografts delivered by intravenous injection of anti-CEA MAbs and $F(ab')_2$ fragments could provoke tumor regressions and remissions (Buchegger et al. 1988), we started a pilot radioimmunotherapy trial in patients with liver metastases from colon carcinoma in collaboration with the group of Delaloye et al. (1986 b; Mach et al. 1988). Anti-CEA MAbs labeled with therapeutic doses of ^{131}I were injected into the hepatic artery through the side port of an infusion pump, already placed to deliver chemotherapy, or through a catheter placed for the duration of the antibody perfusion (3 h). The first four patients had extensive metastases (larger than 500 g) resistant to all forms of therapy. They received 100 mCi ^{131}I coupled to 10 mg $F(ab')_2$ fragments (three patients) or 10 mg intact anti-CEA MAbs. The radiation doses delivered to these large tumor masses never reached values higher than 2000 rad. No tumor regression was observed but the patients tolerated the treatment very well with no side effects. Thus, we recently treated three patients with smaller liver metastases (50–150 g) and low serum CEA levels (12–35 ng per milliliter) with the same amount of ^{131}I coupled to 40 mg of a mixture of two intact MAbs directed against two different epitopes of the CEA molecules.

As a representative example, we will describe here the results obtained in the first of the three patients. This patient had two liver metastases of 3 and 5 cm diameter (from a resected sigmoid carcinoma) detectable on two distinct transverse CT sections (Fig. 11 A and D). The patient received a single injection into the hepatic artery of 100 mCi ^{131}I coupled to 40 mg of two intact MAbs. Four days later the ECT transverse section taken at the same level as the previously described CT sections showed a selective

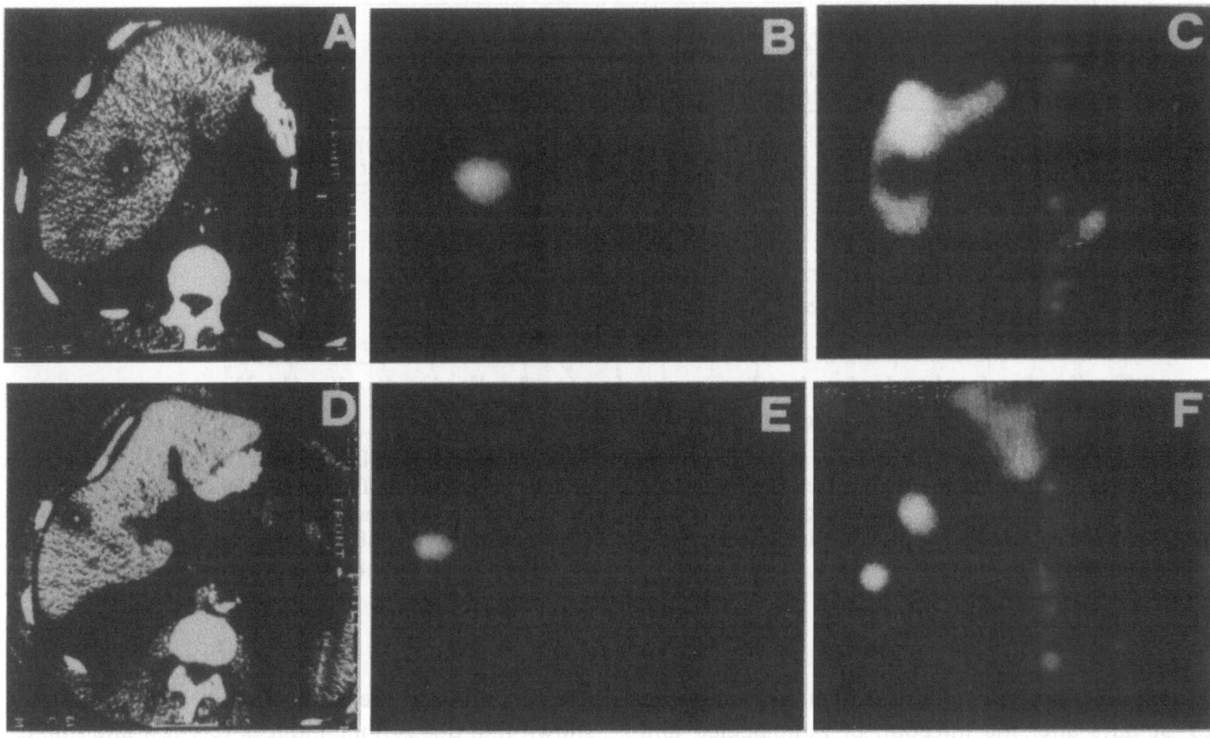

Fig. 11. A–F. Localization of therapeutic doses of ^{131}I-labeled intact anti-CEA MAbs in liver metastases from colon carcinoma after injection into the hepatic artery. **A** CT transverse section demonstrates 5-cm diameter liver metastasis. **B** Corresponding ECT transverse section shows that most of the detected radioactivity is localized in the metastasis. **C** Tc99m sulfur colloid ECT shows a photon-deficient area corresponding to the metastasis. **D** Lower CT transverse section demonstrates a 3-cm diameter liver metastasis on the right edge of the liver. **E** Corresponding ECT transverse section shows that most of the radioactivity detected is localized into the metastasis. **F** ECT coronal section across both metastases confirms the radioactivity uptake in the two metastases plus some radioactivity at the base of the heart. (Results obtained in collaboration with Delaloye et al. 1986 and reproduced from Mach et al. 1988)

uptake of radioactivity in both metastases (Fig. 11 B and E). The larger, more central metastasis was also detectable by a photon-deficient area in the sulfur colloid ECT (Fig. 11 C) corresponding exactly to the well-defined spot of antibody uptake (Fig. 11 B). In the coronal section (Fig. 11 F) the two spots of radioactivity uptake corresponding to the two liver metastases are clearly visible, as well as some radioactivity corresponding to the base of the heart. The tumor to normal liver ratios calculated from the ECT sections were 3-4. Dosimetric estimation (MIRD) gave values of 4300 rad in the metastases, 1075 rad in normal liver and 88 rad in the bone marrow.

The estimated radioactivity in the tumor was calculated from the following parameters: (a) the whole body half-life (56 h, determined by urinary elimination); (b) the percentage of radioactivity localized in the liver (31%, determined by a modified dual probe whole body counter during the first 3 days after injection); and (c) the tumor to normal liver ratios determined by ECT at day 4. The calculated values were of 50–80 μCi per gram of tumor representing 0.05%–0.08% of the injected dose per gram of tumor. We believe that the higher percentages of injected dose in tumor, as compared to values observed in diagnostic immunoscintigraphy, are due in part to the intra-arterial route of injection and in part to the larger amounts of antibody used. Our percentages of injected dose in tumor are definitely higher than the values of 0.005% per gram of tumor which lead Vaughan et al. (1986) to conclude that radioimmunotherapy of cancer with ^{131}I was completely unrealistic.

We do not claim to have reached our goal yet, since we did not obtain evidence of tumor regression by the criteria of repeated CT or by CEA monitoring (Fig. 12), but we have demonstrated by ECT the specific uptake of radioactivity in liver metastases from colon carcinoma (Fig. 11 B, E, F) after intra-arterial injection of therapeutic doses of ^{131}I-labeled anti-CEA MAbs.

An essential factor was that our patient did not suffer from any major side effects except for a moderate drop in peripheral blood leukocytes and plate-

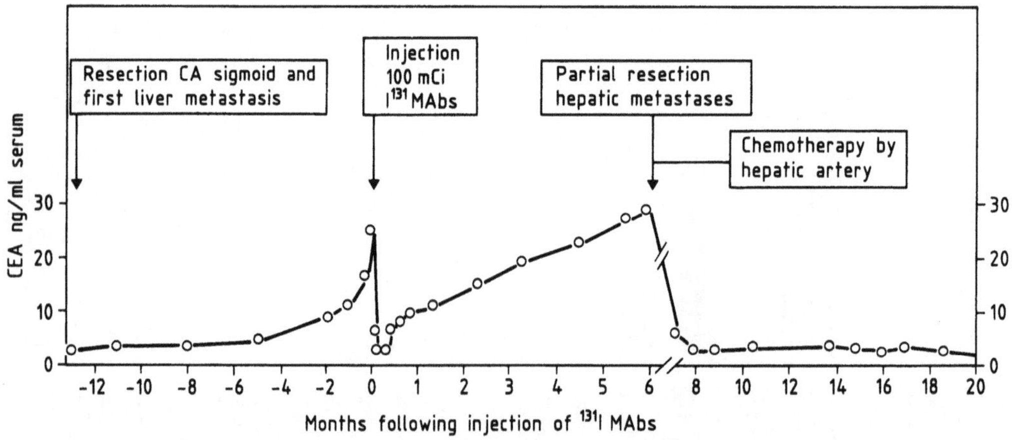

Fig. 12. Evolution of serum CEA level in patient after injection of 40 mg anti-CEA MAb labeled with 100 mCi ^{131}I, followed by partial resection of hepatic metastasis and chemotherapy delivered via the hepatic artery. The elevation of circulating CEA levels occurring 12–48 h after injection may be due to a direct effect of the MAbs on the tumor, whereas the following decrease of CEA levels lasting 7–10 days is probably due to complexing of CEA by the injected MAb. The CEA was measured by a sandwich solid phase EIA after heat extraction of CEA samples (Buchegger et al. 1982b) to avoid interference by circulating antibodies (Mach et al. 1988)

let counts to about one-third of their normal values 25–30 days after the injection of radiolabeled antibodies. Six months after the radioimmunotherapy, the liver metastases were partially resected surgically and the patient was treated with 5-fluorouracil injected into the hepatic artery. Following this, the serum CEA levels decreased to normal (Fig. 12). Nineteen months after initiation of chemotherapy the patient is well with no evidence of disease on liver CT, and serum CEA levels are still normal.

Conclusions from the In Vivo Use of Radiolabeled MAbs

For diagnostic immunoscintigraphy, we consider that I-123, in particular when it is coupled to fragments of MAbs which penetrate relatively rapidly into the tumor and are also rapidly eliminated in the urine, represents an optimal tracer. Alternatively, In-111 is a good, promising isotope despite the fact that the In-111-labeled antibodies presently available (by DTPA chelation) have a tendency to accumulate in the liver.

For radioimmunotherapy, we consider that ^{131}I is still one of the best radionuclides presently available to label antibodies for the following reasons: (a) as already seen, injection of antibodies labeled with iodine isotopes does not provoke accumulation of radioactivity in the RES; since we are mostly limited by the toxicity of radioactivity in bone marrow and liver, this low deposition in RES represents an essential factor; (b) as reported by Tubiana (1982) and others, long-term experience in the use of large doses of ^{131}I for the treatment of thyroid carcinomas has shown that this isotope induces very few late side effects.

We realize that we have not yet reached the appropriate dose of radioactivity in the tumor to be curative or even palliative in the cases reported here. We think, however, that the ECT images presented in Fig. 11, which will be soon completed with two additional case reports with similar or higher radioactivity uptakes in metastases (Delaloye et al., in preparation) represent very encouraging evidence of specific accumulation of radioactivity in liver metastases from colon carcinoma after injection of therapeutic doses of radiolabeled MAbs. We definitely need to multiply by a factor of 3 or 4 the doses of radioactivity that we have already delivered to the liver metastases in order to obtain a useful therapeutic effect. This increase of radiation to the tumor could be achieved by several approaches: (a) by repeated injections of the same dose of antibody and ^{131}I followed by autologous bone marrow rescue; (b) by provoking a vasodilatation and increasing the perfusion of the tumor metastases before injection of radiolabeled MAbs; (c) by the addition of conventional radiation doses on the larger tumor masses by selective transcutaneous radiotherapy, as recommended by Order et al. (1980).

With cautious optimism, we believe that by using these approaches and by constantly improving the quality of the radiolabeled MAbs, we will be able to offer, in the not too distant future, a more rational treatment for liver metastases from colorectal carcinoma.

References

Accolla RS, Carrel S, Mach J-P (1980) Monoclonal antibodies specific for carcinoembryonic antigen and produced by two hybrid cell lines. Proc Natl Acad Sci USA 77: 563–566

Bale WF, Spar IL (1957) Studies directed toward the use of antibodies as carriers of radioactivity for therapy. Adv Biol Med Phys 5: 285–356

Bast RC Jr, Klug TL, St John E, Jenison E, Niloff JM, Lazarus H, Berkowitz RS, et al. (1983) A radioimmunoassay using a monoclonal antibody to monitor the course of epithelial ovarian cancer. N Engl J Med 309: 883–887

Berche C, Mach J-P, Lumbroso JD, Langlais C, Aubry F, Buchegger F, Carrel S, et al. (1982) Tomoscintigraphy for detecting gastrointestinal and medullary thyroid cancers: first clinical results using radiolabelled monoclonal antibodies against carcinoembryonic antigen. Br Med J 285: 1447–1451

Buchegger F, Mach J-P (1986) Carcinoembryonic antigen. Enzyme-immunoassay of CEA in unextracted patients' serum, using three different monoclonal antibodies. In: Bergmeyer HU (ed) Methods of enzymatic analysis vol 9. VCH, Weinheim, pp 143–160

Buchegger F, Phan M, Revier D, Carrel S, Accolla RS, Mach J-P (1982a) Monoclonal antibodies against carcinoembryonic antigen (CEA) used in a solid-phase enzyme immunoassay. First clinical results. J Immunol Methods 49: 129–139

Buchegger F, Mettraux C, Accolla RS, Carrel S, Mach J-P (1982b) Sandwich enzyme-immunoassay using three monoclonal antibodies against different epitopes of carcinoembryonic antigen "CEA". Immunol Lett 5: 85–91

Buchegger F, Haskell CM, Schreyer M, Scazziga BR, Randin S, Carrel S, Mach J-P (1983) Radiolabeled fragments of monoclonal anti-CEA antibodies for localization of human colon carcinoma grafted into nude mice. J Exp Med 158: 413–427

Buchegger F, Schreyer M, Carrel S, Mach J-P (1984) Monoclonal antibodies identify a CEA crossreacting antigen of 95 kD (NCA-95) distinct in antigenicity and tissue distribution from the previously described NCA of 55 kD. Int J Cancer 33: 643–649

Buchegger F, Vacca A, Carrel S, Schreyer M, Mach J-P (1988) Radioimmunotherapy of human colon carcinoma by ^{131}I labeled monoclonal anti-CEA antibodies in the nude mouse model. Int J Cancer 41: 127–134

Buraggi GL, Callegaro L, Mariani G, Turrin A, Cascinelli N, Attili A, Bombardieri E, et al. (1985) Imaging with ^{131}I-labeled monoclonal antibodies to a high-molecular-weight melanoma-associated antigen in patients with melanoma: Efficacy of whole immunoglobulin and its F(ab')$_2$ fragments. Cancer Res 45: 3378–3387

Chatal J-F, Saccavini J-C, Fumoleau P, Douillard J-Y, Curtet C, Kremer M, Le Mevel B, Koprowski H (1984) Immunoscintigraphy of colon carcinoma. J Nucl Med 25: 307–314

Colcher D, Esteban JM, Carrasquillo JA, Sugarbaker P, Reynolds JC, Bryant G, Larson SM, Schlom J (1987) Quantitative analyses of selective radiolabeled monoclonal antibody localization in metastatic lesions of colorectal cancer patients. Cancer Res 47: 1185–1189

Delaloye B, Bischof-Delaloye A, Buchegger F, von Fliedner V, Grob JP, Volant JC, Pettavel J, Mach J-P (1986a) Detection of colorectal carcinoma by emission-computerized tomography after injection of I-123-labeled Fab or F(ab')$_2$ fragments from monoclonal anti-carcinoembryonic antigen antibodies. J Clin Invest 77: 301–311

Delaloye B, Bischof-Delaloye A, Buchegger F, Mach J-P (1986b) Fundamental biokinetic measurements with respect to radioimmunotherapy. In: Schubiger PA, Hasler PA (eds) Radionuclides for therapy. Roches, Basel, pp 149–159

DeLand FH, Kim EE, Simmons G, Goldenberg DM (1980) Imaging approach to radioimmunodetection. Cancer Res 40: 3046–3049

DeNardo SJ, DeNardo GL, O'Grady LF, Macey DJ, Mills SL, Epstein AL, Peng J-S, McGahan JP (1987) Treatment of a patient with B cell lymphoma by 1-131 LYM-1 monoclonal antibodies. Int J Biol Markers 2: 49–53

Epenetos AA, Mather S, Granowska M, Nimmon CC, Hawkins LR, Britton KE, Shepherd J, et al. (1982) Targeting of I-123-labelled tumourassociated monoclonal antibodies to ovarian, breast and gastrointestinal tumours. Lancet 2: 999–1005

Epenetos AA, and Hammersmith Oncology Group (1984) Antibody-guided irradiation of malignant lesions: three cases illustrating a new method of treatment. Lancet 1: 1441–1443

Gold P, Freedman SO (1965) Demonstration of tumor-specific antigens in human colonic carcinomata by immunological tolerance and absorption techniques. J Exp Med 121: 439–462

Goldenberg DM, Preston DF, Primus FJ, Hansen HJ (1974) Photoscan localization of GW-39 tumors in hamsters using radiolabeled anticarcinoembryonic antigen immunoglobulin G. Cancer Res 34: 1–9

Goldenberg DM, Deland F, Kim E, Bennett S, Primus FJ, van Nagell JR, Estes N, et al. (1978) Use of radiolabeled antibodies to carcinoembryonic antigen for the detection and localization of diverse cancers by external photoscanning. N Engl J Med 298: 1384–1388

Halpern SE, Buchegger F, Schreyer M, Mach J-P (1984) Effect of size of radiolabeled antibody and fragments on tumor uptake and distribution in nephrectomized mice. J Nucl Med 25: 112

Hansen HJ, Snyder JJ, Miller E, Vandervoorde JP, Miller ON, Hines LR, Burns JJ (1974) Carcinoembryonic antigen (CEA) assay: a laboratory adjunct in the diagnosis and management of cancer. Hum Pathol 5: 139–147

Haskell CM, Buchegger F, Schreyer M, Carrel S, Mach J-P (1983) Monoclonal antibodies to carcinoembryonic antigen: ionic strength as a factor in the selection of antibodies for immunoscintigraphy. Cancer Res 43: 3857–3864

Hedin A, Carlsson L, Berglund A, Hammarstrom S (1983) A monoclonal antibody-enzmye immunoassay for serum carcinoembryonic antigen with increased specificity for carcinomas. Proc Natl Acad Sci USA 80: 3470–3474

Herlyn M, Steplewski Z, Herlyn D, Koprowski H (1979) Colorectal carcinoma-specific antigen: detection by means of monoclonal antibodies. Proc Natl Acad Sci USA 76: 1438–1442

Larson SM, Carrasquillo JA, Krohn KA, Brown JP, McCuffin RW, Ferens JM, Graham MM, et al. (1983) Localization of I-131-labeled P97-specific Fab fragments in human melanoma as a basis for radiotherapy. J Clin Invest 72: 2101–2114

Mach J-P, Puszaszeri G, Dysli M, Kapp F, Bierens de Haan B, Loosli RM, Grob P, Isliker H (1973) Dosage radioimmunologique de l'antigène carcino-embryonnaire (CEA) dans le plasma de malades atteints de carcinomes. Conclusion des premiers résultats d'une étude collaborative en Suisse. Schweiz Med Wochenschr 103: 365–371

Mach J-P, Jaeger PH, Bertholet MM, Ruegsegger CH, Loosli RM, Pettavel J (1974a) Detection of recurrence of large bowel carcinoma by radioimmunoassay of circulating carcinoembryonic antigen (CEA). Lancet 2: 535–540

Mach J-P, Carrel S, Merenda C, Sordat B, Cerottini J-C (1974 b) In vivo localization of radiolabeled antibodies to carcinoembryonic antigen in human colon carcinoma grafted into nude mice. Nature 248: 704–706

Mach J-P, Vienny H, Jaeger P, Haldemann B, Egely R, Pettavel J (1978) Long-term follow-up of colorectal carcinoma patients by repeated CEA radioimmunoassay. Cancer 42: 1439–1447

Mach J-P, Carrell S, Forni M, Ritschard J, Donath A, Alberto P (1980 a) Tumor localization of radiolabeled antibodies against carcinoembryonic antigen in patients with carcinoma. A critical evaluation. N Engl J Med 303: 5–10

Mach J-P, Forni M, Ritschard J, Buchegger F, Carrel S, Widgren S, Donath A, Alberto P (1980 b) Use and limitations of radiolabeled anti-CEA antibodies and their fragments for photoscanning detection of human colorectal carcinomas. Oncodev Biol Med 1: 49–69

Mach J-P, Buchegger F, Forni M, Ritschard J, Berche C, Lumbroso JD, Schreyer M, et al. (1981) Use of radiolabelled monoclonal anti-CEA antibodies for the detection of human carcinomas by external photoscanning and tomoscintigraphy. Immunol Today 2: 239–249

Mach J-P, Chatal J-F, Lumbroso J-D, Buchegger F, Forni M, Ritschard J, Berche C, et al. (1983) Tumor localization in patients by radiolabeled monoclonal antibodies against colon carcinoma. Cancer Res 43: 5593–5600

Mach J-P, Buchegger F, Bischof-Delaloye A, Curchod S, Studer A, Douglas P, Leyvraz S, Grob J-P, et al. (1988) Progess in diagnostic immunoscintigraphy and first approach to radioimmunotherapy of colon carcinoma. In: Srivastava S (ed) NATO Advanced Study Institute of Radiolabeled Monoclonal Antibodies for Imaging and Therapy. Plenum, New York, pp. 95–110

Martin EW Jr, Kibbey WE, di Vecchia L, Anderson G, Catalano P, Minton JP (1976) Carcinoembryonic antigen, clinical and histological aspects. Cancer 37: 62–81

Metzgar RS, Rodriguez N, Finn OJ, Lan MS, Daasch VN, Fernstein PD, Meyers WC, et al. (1984) Detection of a pancreatic cancer-associated antigen (DU-PAN-2 antigen) in serum and ascites of patients with adenocarcinoma. Proc Natl Acad Sci USA 81: 5242–5246

Mezger F, Witmanns W, Lamerz R (1988) Elevated serum CA 125 levels in patients with benign ascitic or pleural effusions. Tumor Biol 9: 47–52

Miotti S, Canevari S, Ménard S, Mezzanzanica D, Porro G, Pupa SM, Regazzoni M (1987) Characterization of human ovarian carcinoma-associated antigens defined by novel monoclonal antibodies with tumor-restricted specificity. Int J Cancer 39: 297–303

Order SE, Klein JL, Ettinger D, Alderson P, Siegelman S, Leichner P (1980) Phase I–II study of radiolabeled antibody integrated in the treatment of primary hepatic malignancies. Int J Radiat Oncol Biol Phys 6: 703–710

Ott RJ, Grey LJ, Zivanovic MA, Flower MA, Trott NG (1983) The limitations of the dual radionuclide subtraction technique for the external detection of tumours by radioiodine-labelled antibodies. Br J Radiol 56: 101–108

Paterson AJ, Schlom J, Sears HF, Bennett J, Colcher D (1986) A radioimmunoassay for the detection of a human tumor-associated glycoprotein (TAG-72) using monoclonal antibody B72.3. Int J Cancer 37: 659–666

Pressman D, Korngold I (1953) The in vivo localization of anti-Wagner-osteogenic-sarcoma antibodies. Cancer 6: 619–623

Ritts RE Jr, del Villano BC, Go VLW, Herberman RB, Klug TL, Zurawski VR Jr (1984) Initial clinical evaluation of an immunoradiometric assay for CA19.9 using the NCI serum bank. Int J Cancer 33: 339–345

Sullivan DC, Silva JS, Cox CE, Haagensen DE, Harris CC, Briner WH, Wells SA (1982) Localization of I-131-labeled goat and primate anti-carcinoembryonic antigen (CEA) antibodies in patients with cancer. Invest Radiol 17: 350–355

Thomson DMP, Krupey J, Freedman SO, Gold P (1969) The radioimmunoassay of circulating carcinoembryonic antigen of the human digestive system. Proc Natl Acad Sci USA 64: 161–167

Tubiana M (1982) Risk associated with the use of radiopharmaceuticals. Proc World Congr Nucl Med Biol 3: 2603–2629

Vaughan ATM, Bradwell AR, Dykes PW, Anderson P (1986) Illusions of tumour killing using radiolabelled antibodies. Lancet 1: 1492–1493

Zamchek N (1974) Carcinoembryonic antigen. Quantitative variations in circulating levels in benign and malignant digestive tract diseases. Adv Intern Med 19: 413–418

General Concepts in Cancer Treatment

Principles of Surgery in the Primary Treatment of Cancer

I. BURN

The extraordinary developments in the management of malignant disease during the last 30 years have caused considerable problems for surgeons. Older surgeons remember the dominant role of surgery during the middle years of the century, when surgical technique perhaps was the most important consideration. Despite its shortcomings, surgery consistently provided cure for tens of thousands of sufferers from cancer throughout the world each year. However, there is no doubt that during the period of surgical dominance, much surgery for malignant disease was overambitious and not infrequently aggravated the condition. This often was the fault of case selection rather than of the procedure concerned.

There are three reasons for carrying out surgery in primary cancer treatment. First, whenever the situation permits, determined surgery is used with the object of eradicating the disease totally. Second, surgery is used as part of a combined therapeutic programme, aimed hopefully at curing the disease in situations where surgery alone is not sufficient to achieve this. Third, surgery is used for obviously incurable cancer, for a variety of reasons. In this last category, surgery may play a part in attempted prolonged control of the disease, it may be used to reduce the bulk of a cancer preparatory to other palliative treatment and it may be used simply to alleviate temporarily an otherwise intolerable situation.

As well as the above roles of surgery in the primary treatment of malignant disease, some form of surgical biopsy frequently is necessary as a preliminary to treatment. There are some cancers where primary treatment is carried out without biopsy, such as cancer of the kidney and some cancers of the gastrointestinal tract, but these are exceptions to the general rule.

Biopsy

Although biopsy primarily is associated with the diagnosis of neoplasms, increased use is now being made in the diagnosis of non-neoplastic conditions, such as those of the kidney, liver and reticuloendothelial system. The development of new methods of obtaining samples for analysis, and in particular the advances in endoscopic techniques, have increased the range of biopsy considerably during the past two decades.

As well as its use in establishing the diagnosis of the primary lesion, biopsy is assuming an ever-increasing role in providing early information about the biological nature of various tumours. The histological type and the grade of malignancy may be assessed from biopsy tissue and may have a profound influence on subsequent treatment as, for example, in cancers of the urinary bladder. The determination of receptor activity and ploidy studies are other sources of information which may be influential in planning treatment for various cancers.

Another developing role of biopsy is in the staging of malignant disease. The precise definition of the extent of a cancer is becoming accepted as a necessary preliminary to planning primary therapy. This practice undoubtedly will increase with the general acceptance of the international TNM system of classification and increasing availability of equipment for identifying occult metastatic disease.

Biopsy may have an important function as part of the staging process and there are a number of currently practised examples. In breast cancer, it is customary in some units to carry out deliberate biopsy of axillary and internal mammary lymph nodes as part of the staging process. In some cases, a more determined dissection of the axillary nodes is regarded more as a means of obtaining information on staging rather than as definitive therapy.

Another example of the use of biopsy for the purpose of staging is in Hodgkin's disease and other lymphomas. Although there is some evidence that the practice of staging laparotomy is on the wane, it is still customary in many centres to regard biopsy of the liver and para-aortic lymph nodes as an integral part of planning primary treatment.

Methods

There are many ways in which tissue may be obtained for histological examination, employing either the surgeon's knife, a curette, or some form of needle, cannula or trephine. A small section of tissue may be removed from the main bulk of the tumour by incision with a small blade, as in biopsy of certain lesions of the skin, buccal cavity and liver. In many instances of biopsy, excision of the whole lesion may be more appropriate, for example when dealing with small tumours of the breast and skin and with suspicious lymph nodes. General anaesthesia is usually recommended for most forms of incision and excision biopsy. Local anaesthesia may be feasible for the biopsy of certain non-pigmented tumours of the skin.

Biopsy material may be obtained by curettage of certain soft tumour masses, examples of which occur within bone, the brain and the uterus. Many organs are now accessible to the passage of some form of endoscope, with biopsy material being obtained by the removal of small fragments of tissue with cutting forceps or punch. Tumours of the bronchus, colon, common bile duct, duodenum, larynx, mediastinum, oesophagus, peritoneal cavity, rectum, stomach, urethra and urinary bladder are examples of lesions which can be biopsied in this way.

Finally, increasing use is now made of needles and cannulae for obtaining cores of tissue for the purpose of a biopsy. In the strictest sense, simple syringe and needle aspiration techniques should *not* be included within this definition, the material obtained being more suitable for cytological examination. Needle biopsy, although usually done under local anaesthetic, must provide a core of tissue adequate for full histological examination and possibly other tests, such as the assessment of receptor activity.

A variety of needles and cannulae, such as the Vim-Silverman, the Tru-Cut and the high-speed drill, are now available. Needle biopsy has a real place in the diagnosis of suspected neoplasms of the breast, prostate, thyroid, uterus, lungs, liver, bone and connective tissue.

Rules

Whatever the method used, it should never be forgotten that surgeons have a major responsibility in safeguarding the proprieties of biopsy. It should always be regarded as a serious commitment in a patient who at the time of biopsy may have a curable cancer. Nothing should be done which might jeopardize the chance of cure, bearing in mind that any method of biopsy may release cells from a malignant tumour into tissue which previously was uncontaminated. Also, great care should be taken to ensure that adequate material is obtained on the first occasion.

In respect of the responsibility of biopsy, the World Health Organization (WHO) in 1966, in its Technical Reports series, recommended that a number of general rules should apply:

1. The tissue removed should be representative of the whole lesion. In certain circumstances, multi-

ple specimens might be advantageous, as, for example, in taking small punch biopsies through an endoscope or when sampling from a region of suspected lymphadenopathy.

2. Zones of haemorrhage, necrosis and obvious infection should be avoided when selecting the site for biopsy.
3. Crushing and charring of removed tissue should be avoided.
4. When taking biopsies from lesions of the skin and mucosal surfaces, healthy marginal tissue should be included in the specimen. Biopsies of polypoid and other proliferative lesions should include tissue from the base of the lesion.
5. During biopsy, the tumour and the surrounding tissues always should be handled with extreme care, to avoid massaging cancer cells into the circulation.
6. When a deep lesion is being biopsied, extreme care should be taken to avoid direct implantation of released malignant cells into adjacent healthy tissue. This is especially important when closing a wound over the site of a biopsy. Drainage tubes preferably should be avoided and separate stab drainage *never* used.
7. Repeated biopsies of the same lesion should be avoided, every effort being made to obtain adequate material at the first occasion.

The WHO also stressed that the closest cooperation should exist between surgeon and pathologist. The pathologist always should be provided with all the relevant clinical information to assist in making the diagnosis. These recommendations from the WHO are as pertinent today as they were 20 years ago.

In the context of biopsy the continuing role of frozen-section histology is currently under scrutiny. Immediate frozen-section histology of fresh specimens always has involved a slight but definite risk of misdiagnosis. Apart from this, the technique also has other disadvantages.

It is becoming accepted that, for many cancers, primary treatment is only decided after staging the disease. This requirement usually nullifies the concept of immediate frozen-section histology as a preliminary to definitive surgery under the same anaesthetic. Possibly of even greater importance nowadays is the increasing commitment to adequate and complete discussion with the patient before operation.

Staging

As stated, accurate definition of the extent of a cancer is an important prerequisite to treatment. This means full assessment of the primary tumour complex and a search for metastases, including those which are symptomless. One of the most impressive contributions of the UICC has been the introduction of the international TNM system of classification, the use of which is now widespread.

The planning of modern primary therapy requires full information about the extent of the disease. The recognition of clearly incurable states will avoid the use of inappropriate local therapy. This is as important as providing determined local therapy for those patients with genuine early cancers who have every chance of complete cure.

Such techniques as lymphography, hepatic ultrasonography, bone scans, lung tomography, brain scans and mediastinoscopy during the past 20 years, have immeasurably improved the accuracy of staging. Surgeons have been heavily involved in the development of such techniques and they are becoming increasingly familiar with the requirements of staging. The era of rushing into the treatment of cancer without careful preliminary staging should now be behind us.

Primary Cancer Surgery

Real progress has been made in the management of the more common "solid" cancers. It is now possible to diagnose the disease in many organs at a very early stage and to be reasonably confident that no occult distant metastases are present. The careful surveillance of recognizable premalignant states and of patients at high risk for a variety of malignancies, the growing impact of cancer screening programmes and the increasing awareness among the general population of the early symptoms of cancer means the stage is set for an era of truly early diagnosis of malignant disease. Many cancers are now being diagnosed at such an early stage of their existence that the likelihood of even minimal involvement of the regional lymph nodes is very low indeed. Such patients have curable disease and must be treated accordingly.

Even with advanced disease, it is often possible to control the process much longer than hitherto and certainly way beyond the natural history of the untreated disease.

Despite the enormous volume of research in oncology, a truly fundamental understanding of the cancerous process still eludes us. Until the process is unravelled, we must persevere with two major objectives, namely early diagnosis and adequate treatment. The surgeon's involvement in both of these is paramount.

As a result of modern methods of early, even presymptomatic, diagnosis, an increasing number of patients with minimal disease are revealed. The introduction of cervical screening in the Western World, the Japanese experience with stomach cancer, and the emerging programmes of screening for breast, buccal cavity, colon, lung and other cancers, are all examples of current determined attempts to diagnose very early asymptomatic cancer.

Another developing area is the increasing recognition of premalignant states, both by the clinician and by the pathologist. Surgeons increasingly will be responsible for dealing with ever-increasing numbers of patients with premalignant histology and in situ cancer.

For practical purposes, five stages of malignant disease may be considered when planning treatment. These are in situ cancers, minimal cancers, early disease, middle-stage disease and advanced disease. The surgical approach needs to be defined according to these five stages. It will vary from site to site, but some basic points are common to all.

In Situ Cancer

The importance of in situ cancer is that a boundary has been crossed. The label "cancer" is full of implications. The term "in situ" has been used most commonly in connection with the uterine cervix, but it is now being applied in a variety of organs and tissues. Sometimes areas of in situ cancer occur in association with an established invasive lesion nearby.

The initial treatment of in situ cancer has to take into consideration the future vulnerability of the remainder of the organ concerned. In situ cancer alone is never associated with metastatic disease. Eradication of the diseased tissue is guaranteed by its surgical excision or by some other form of ablation, such as cryosurgery. How to deal with the apparently healthy remainder of the affected organ is a difficult decision. For example, a good case can be made for advising the immediate removal of a breast containing in situ cancer because of the high risk of further disease. The alternative is very careful surveillance and the introduction of such preventive measures as are relevant to the organ concerned.

There is no easy answer, and often the decision has to be made on an individual basis for the patient concerned.

Minimal Cancer

The term "minimal cancer" is now being used with increasing frequency and has much to commend it. It implies a very small volume of established malignant disease, which historically has been found rarely to be associated with spread beyond the site of origin, even to the nearest lymph nodes. In TNM terms, the tumour stage is T_0 or sometimes T_1, T_0 implying no obvious clinical abnormality and T_1 referring to the very smallest clinically evident tumours. Minimal cancers may be diagnosed as a result of early detection through screening programmes, the cervix, breast and stomach providing examples. They may be diagnosed as a result of the thorough examination of tissue removed for some unrelated reason, as in the prostate, thyroid or breast. Or they may be identified with certainty after prompt action in patients with minimal symptoms, for example the removal of a very early malignant melanoma.

Minimal cancer is very different from in situ cancer. In situ cancer contains no invasive features and has a total freedom from the risk of dissemination. Minimal cancer, despite a very low probability of dissemination, nevertheless does show invasive features. For this reason, the treatment of minimal cancer poses a particular dilemma.

The limited nature of the lesion makes it tempting to consider limited surgery as the primary treatment of choice. Against this is the real concern that the chance of total cure may be missed if primary therapy is not adequate. Current practice reflects different needs at different sites. The most early forms of malignant melanoma may be treated perfectly safely by excision with a relatively small margin, considerably less than that advocated for more established lesions. Minimal superficial cancers of the stomach are still considered best treated by gastrectomy, although extensive lymph node removal is not necessary. Minimal cancers of the prostate or thyroid not infrequently are diagnosed in tissue removed for some other pathology, such as benign prostatic hypertrophy or multinodular goitre. Whether further surgery is considered depends very much upon the extent of the original procedure. Minimal cancer of the breast rarely justifies immediate treatment of the regional lymph nodes, but debate continues whether or not the whole breast should be removed.

The breast exemplifies the problem of treating minimal cancer. For the majority of organs, surgery is the most appropriate therapy, with little justification for adjuvant radiotherapy or systemic drug therapy. As stated, there would seem to be little justification for routine dissection of the regional lymph nodes, and the main concern is deciding the extent of surgery in the organ concerned. It is doubtful whether any form of clinical trial will ever help to solve the problem. The best approach would seem to be to weigh up all the prevailing circumstances and make an individual decision for each patient affected.

There is some enthusiasm for the use of surgical methods other than scalpel excision in the treatment of certain minimal cancers, for example the use of cryosurgery on the tongue and buccal cavity. Such methods should continue to be investigated, but it is not yet appropriate to regard any of them as standard therapy.

Early Cancer

It is not particularly satisfying to use the terms "early" and "advanced" in the context of malignant disease, but the terms have become customary. The implication of "early" is a stage of disease where there is a good chance of total eradication of the cancer by local treatment alone. Usually this means a small tumour with at most minimal evidence of involvement of the nearest regional lymph nodes. There are situations, however, where relatively large lesions may still be regarded as early. Examples are certain superficial varieties of malignant melanoma, low-grade epitheliomas of the skin and well-differentiated cancers of the thyroid gland. Also, not all small cancers can be regarded as early simply because of their size. Poorly differentiated anaplastic cancers of the lung, breast and ovary may metastasize widely whilst still very small.

The attitude to the staging of cancer probably is as good an indication of the true surgical oncologist as any other factor. The surgeon who is prepared to stage a cancer well is a surgical oncologist.

The conclusion that a patient has an early cancer, with all its implications, must be preceded by careful attention to the staging process. Different criteria will be used for tumours arising at different sites, and these criteria undoubtedly change according to increasing experience of treating the disease. As data accumulate and genuine long-term survival figures emerge, we can better predict the future for new patients. The response to modern methods of treatment will certainly influence the definition of "early" as the years go on.

The role of surgery in early cancer continues to be pre-eminent for the majority of the common solid tumours. These generally are the cancers for which radical surgery was most successful in the past. Early cancers of the breast, testis, skin, uterus, colon, rectum, tongue, lip, buccal cavity, larynx, thyroid, urinary bladder and prostate, and even such high-mortality cancers as those of stomach and lung, all showed high cure rates after radical surgery for those patients who survived the procedures. The disease was curable by such surgery if treated early. Unfortunately, for some of these cancers, e.g. those of the stomach and urinary bladder, there was initial high operative mortality. Also, such radical procedures often necessitated permanent disfigurement and morbidity.

It is in the realm of the initial treatment of early cancer that radical surgery has been called into question. Although understandable, this perhaps is ironic in a situation where such surgery has proved to be the most effective at curing cancer.

By definition, traditional radical cancer surgery has implied the complete or nearly complete removal of the organ or tissue bearing the primary tumour, together with the regional lymph nodes draining the tumour-bearing site and such intervening tissue as is necessary to achieve this as a monobloc procedure. The lymph node dissection was included because it was recognized long ago that this represented the first site of spread and that early involvement of the regional nodes was still compatible with cure so long as treatment was adequate.

The introduction of such operations about a century ago coincided with, and indeed was responsible for, the first recorded genuine cures of malignant disease. Nowadays, because of the failure of such methods to control the more advanced stages of cancer and because of the often considerable morbidity caused, radical cancer surgery has come under critical scrutiny. The role of radical surgery for cancers of the buccal cavity, thyroid, urinary bladder, breast, rectum, and skin has been questioned. In some sites, such as breast and rectum, there has been widespread abandonment of the procedure. These are the very organs where such procedures had proved their ability to cure early malignant disease.

The proposed alternatives to traditional radical surgery for early cancers have been many. Modified radical procedures (so-called), simple removal of tissue and organs without nodal dissection, and very limited surgery have all been advocated. Adjuvant radiotherapy, endocrine therapy and systemic chemotherapy have been used variously.

In breast cancer, for example, the past two decades have seen a gradual decline in the surgical role in line with these trends. Modified radical mastectomy with preservation of the pectoralis major muscle, simple total mastectomy with or without postoperative radiotherapy, and, more recently, limited surgery of numerous designs, have all been fashionable. Often the declared justification for such procedures has been the evidence of clinical trials, the validity of which has been at best questionable.

The rectum is another prominent site where there has been a reduction in radical surgery for early cancer. The move has been away from the traditional abdominoperineal resection of the rectum towards lesser techniques which preserve the anal sphincter but sacrifice the principle of monobloc dissection.

Surgeons of the present generation are privileged to work in an era when general anaesthesia has never been more capable, and when technical advances and supportive measures have made major surgery as safe as it has ever been. The high mortality seen with radical cancer surgery in the past should not occur in the modern age. I am firmly of the opinion, therefore, that for early cancers previously shown to be curable by radical surgery, alternative limited methods must be shown definitively to be every bit as effective before they are transferred from the area of research to general use.

The role of limited surgery for early cancers needs to be investigated fully by those capable of being totally objective about its use. To date, the case for limited surgery certainly has not been proved.

Those surgeons who treat early curable cancer, whatever the site, and who themselves are not involved in the investigation of limited techniques, should continue to consider traditional radical surgery for their patients. If they do not, we may well find ourselves faced with an unprecedented incidence of recurrent local disease in years to come.

Middle-Stage Cancer

In may seem artificial to introduce "middle-stage" cancer as a separate category but it is necessary if "early" curable disease is defined strictly, as has been done above.

Middle-stage disease represents real uncertainty. These are patients with larger primary lesions but no recognizable evidence of late-stage lymph node disease or distant metastases. The category also includes patients with smaller primary lesions but a worrying amount of regional lymph node involvement. It must also include those patients with such adverse biological features within the tumour that although metastatic disease appears to be absent, the probability of its presence is actually very high. Poorly differentiated tumours are obvious examples.

In the past such cancers have often erroneously been labelled 'early'. Clinical trials reported as studying early cancer are full of such cases. These tumours should, however, be regarded in an entirely different way.

Whereas the role of radical surgery in early cancer is under scrutiny for the reasons given earlier, its record of achieving cure in genuine early disease is undisputed. Its record in middle-stage disease is not nearly as impressive, nor indeed is that of any other form of primary therapy.

In middle-stage disease, the role of surgery as primary therapy varies according to the circumstances. Included in the category of middle-stage disease are various connective tissue sarcomas, bone tumours, pelvic malignancies, retroperitoneal and mediastinal tumours and large cancers of the head and neck region. For these tumours massive extirpation procedures often are indicated and are fully justified. Surgeons must continue to be bold in such circumstances, for massive surgery, however mutilating, provides the only chance of continued survival. There certainly remains a place for such procedures as hindquarter amputation, pelvic exenteration and the facial commando operations, practised on a highly selective basis by surgeons skilled in the techniques. Modern methods of reconstruction and rehabilitation have gone a long way towards softening the blow of such procedures.

In the case of the more common solid cancers, allocation to the category "middle-stage disease" is not necessarily an indication for massive surgery. The use of conventional radical monobloc surgery may be justified, but the real need is to consider the early use of additional treatments because of the increased risk of local recurrent and metastatic disease. These are patients for whom the use of preoperative or postoperative local radiotherapy often is necessary and where the surgical procedure may well be modified because of this. In some circumstances, apart from the initial biopsy, surgery may give way entirely to radiotherapy as the preferred method of primary treatment. Middle-stage cancers of the middle third of the oesophagus and certain cancers of the buccal cavity come into this category, for example. What must be avoided is making matters worse by inappropriate surgery.

As well as the variations in local therapy to suit the particular circumstances, the early use of additional systemic therapy has to be considered. If the risk of occult metastatic disease is high, as for example in patients with multiple involved regional nodes, then the early use of appropriate systemic chemotherapy, or endocrine therapy, may well delay the onset of overt metastases and will probably prolong life. In some instances of middle-stage disease, such as Wilm's tumour, certain tumours of the testis and osteogenic sarcomas, determined multimodal therapy from the outset may even effect cure.

The primary treatment of middle-stage cancer perhaps is the most demanding of all stages of the disease. If the right decisions are made, cure may even be achieved in unfavourable situations or life prolonged in tolerable circumstances for long periods. If the wrong decisions are made, the situation may be worsened to a point that the disease is aggravated and the patient's life perhaps shortened.

Advanced Cancer

The connotation of the term "advanced cancer" is a gloomy one. It implies the inevitability of death from the disease, yet any prognostication may be confounded by the idiosyncracies of the cancer. Even this late in the twentieth century, it is a regrettable fact that many cancers are recognizably advanced when first diagnosed. The first therapy the patient receives is given knowing that the disease is at an advanced stage.

The features of advanced disease will vary according to the site of origin of the cancer. Generally, cancer has to be regarded as advanced when there is extensive local invasion by the tumour, especially if this includes widespread involvement of the lymphatics of the organ. Advanced disease also includes local invasion of surrounding structures and adjacent viscera, marked involvement of the regional lymph nodes, especially if many nodes are affected, and obvious involvement of veins in the vicinity of the primary tumour. Any evidence of distant metastases, even if occult, must also be included within the category of advanced disease.

The methods of assessment needed to arrive at the decision that a cancer is advanced vary from site to site, but must be thorough. The implications of labelling the disease "advanced", especially in a previously untreated patient, are considerable.

The role of the surgeon in the primary treatment of patients with advanced disease has changed considerably during the past two decades. This represents a major development in surgical oncological responsibility.

Realistically, the objective in patients with advanced cancer being treated for the first time has to be control of the disease for as long as possible, with amelioration of unpleasant symptoms. Generally, this will require the proper application of multiple therapies. In some instances, primary major surgery will still be justified, for example the removal of an advanced offensive obstructing cancer of the gastrointestinal tract. Often surgery must be of a temperate nature or may well best be avoided altogether. Examples of this are many advanced cancers of the breast, which are more suitably treated by combinations of endocrine therapy and radiotherapy.

Often the requirements are very individual, such as careful removal of solitary hepatic, pulmonary or cerebral metastases, debulking procedures preparatory to determined chemotherapy or radiotherapy, limb or hepatic perfusion with cytotoxics, endocrine ablation surgery for selected cases of advanced breast cancer, and the internal fixation of certain pathological fractures. All these may be required as primary therapy.

In the case of advanced cancer, surgery has to be even more circumspect than for middle-stage disease, because of the risk of aggravating the situation. Great experience is needed for dealing effectively with advanced cancer, and surgeons often have to resist the temptation to use the knife.

Concluding Remarks

In this chapter, no attempt has been made to define operative procedures for the many sites of malignant disease. Simple guidelines and principles are suggested, based predominantly upon the stage of the disease when first diagnosed. There are many different requirements regionally, but the objectives of primary treatment have a fundamental similarity.

Oncological surgery now is a very complex subject, requiring deep knowledge of the cancer process as well as expertise in surgical technique.

The surgeon's responsibility in the primary treatment of cancer continues to be all-important. The atmosphere surrounding cancer has changed. Patients are now more willing to discuss their condition frankly and accept that malignant disease can be cured if treated early and effectively. It is mandatory that surgeons continue to provide the means of cure whenever appropriate. There must be no lessening of surgical intent in the primary treatment of cancer.

Selected Further Reading

Butcher HR (1970) Surgery of cancer. In: Ackerman LV, del Regato JA (eds) Cancer: diagnosis, treatment and prognosis. Mosby, St. Louis, pp 69–73

Forrest APM, Cant ELM (1976) Surgery and malignant disease: a re-appraisal. In: Symington T, Carter RL (eds) Scientific foundation of oncology. Heinemann, London, pp 605–611

Forrest APM, Carter DC, MacLeod IB (1985) Surgery of cancer. In: Forrest APM, Carter DC, Machead IB (eds) Principles and practice of surgery. Churchill Livingstone, Edinburgh, pp 156–167

International Union Against Cancer (1982) Principles of treatment. In: Sherman CD (ed) Manual of clinical oncology, 3rd edn. Springer, Berlin, Heidelberg, New York, pp 77–89

McKenna RJ, Murphy GP (1986) Fundamentals of surgical oncology, MacMillan, New York, pp 379–850

Najarian JS, Delaney JP (1976) Advances in cancer surgery. Stratton, New York

Nealon TF Jr (1976) Management of the patient with cancer. Saunders, Philadelphia

Surgery in the Treatment of Recurrent and Metastatic Cancer

J. Pettavel, J. Costa, P. Douglas, A. Besson, M. Savary, and N. de Tribolet

"Palliation is not simply the duration of life, but rather, the measure of comfortable living the individual enjoys in the remainder of his life".

George T. Pack

"Cancer surgery rather than being maximal should be optimized and adjusted to a cancer situation".

Felix Harder

Recurrent carcinoma is the name given to cancer in part of an organ, or adjacent tissue, left intact at the time of initial, supposedly curative surgery. An interval between primary resection and secondary exploration is important. Late recurrence must be distinguished from a second independent primary tumour and from the late development of multifocal cancer. Correct staging of recurrent cancer must be carried out in order to ascertain whether curative treatment is still possible or whether only palliation can be considered. The surgical oncologist must be familiar with the more common sites of dissemination, routes of invasion and failure patterns, so as to know where to look and for what. A good knowledge of high-risk categories facilitates the choice of optimal therapy for a given patient. The development of cancer markers (including the most recent monoclonal antibodies) should be kept in mind. Our goal is not to discover all imaginable recurrences with the risk of spoiling what is left of the patient's life, but to give him the best chance of a good (and if possible long) life. With the progress of chemotherapy, despite the still frequent occurrence of local recurrences, major surgery for recurrent cancer is not so frequently relied upon as it used to be in the past. Surgical skill deserves some emphasis.

Considerations on the Pathology of Recurrent Cancer

The diagnosis of local recurrence and that of distant metastases often needs to be confirmed by examination of a tissue sample or an effusion. In the identification of recurrences, fine-needle aspiration cytology has become a reliable tool, especially when coupled with the use of immunological markers (Martin et al. 1984). The recurrence of a lymphoma can be proven by the immunological study of cells obtained by fine-needle aspiration, avoiding an open biopsy.

When evaluating cells or tissues in a patient with a possible recurrence, the pathologist must bear in mind a set of "rules" that apply specifically to this situation. Some of these principles are as follows:

1. *Tumours are heterogeneous.* Perhaps the most dramatic example of this heterogeneity and cell selection in the metastatic process is provided by embryonal carcinoma of the testis, where metastatic deposits "mature" or differentiate with marked changes in their histology (Willis and Hajdu 1973). Heavily pigmented metastases can be observed secondary to an amelanotic clear cell sarcoma of the soft tissues. Progression of tumours can also manifest itself by the selection, at the metastatic site, of cells that lack histotype differentiation: it is not uncommon for lung metastases of sarcomas to be so undifferentiated as to be unclassifiable from the histological point of view.

2. *The tumour and the tumour bed are modified by therapy.* It is of the utmost importance to avoid interpreting tissue and cell changes induced by irradiation as a recurrence. High doses of radiation therapy applied to a tumour bed in order to treat soft tissue sarcoma can make identification of a late recurrence difficult. Postsurgical fibrosis in the perineum can be difficult to distinguish from recurrence of a well-differentiated neurofibrosarcoma. At the time when histological evaluation of a metastasis is performed, tumour cells may be absent. When clinical and radiological examinations show a persistent mass, with a good tumour response at other sites, the clinician and pathologist need to decide whether the mass could represent residual active tumour. Walled off, focally calcified, necrotic material or dense sclerotic fibrous tissue can simulate persistent or recurrent disease. Careful pathological study will often solve the problem. Although immunochemical techniques are useful in identifying isolated tumour cells (Ghosh et al. 1985), adequate gross and microscopic sampling of the tissues should not be neglected.

Tumour tissues are also modified by the therapeutic measures, and treated persistent disease can offer a picture very different to that when it was first studied. Exemplary of this situation are the changes in carcinoma of the prostate after estrogen therapy (Wattenberg 1947).

3. *When evaluating a late local recurrence* or a single distant metastasis, the pathologist must consider the possibility of a second primary tumour. The second tumour may reflect a familial predisposition to second primaries (Mulvihill 1977), or may be related to therapy (induced second primary). Most of the therapeutically induced malignancies are leukaemias, followed by lymphomas and sarcomas. The latter tumours types are perhaps more frequent in patients who have received aggressive multimodality therapy.

4. *Before an interpretation and diagnosis* is rendered the pathologist must review all the previous material.

5. *Tissues from metastatic lesions* should be handled with the same care as that from primary lesions. Evaluation of margins should be detailed and accurate, the lesions adequately sampled and material set aside for special studies (e.g. electron microscopy, histochemistry). One situation in the management of metastatic disease taxes the diagnostic resources of the pathologist and deserves special comment. This is the patient presenting with an "occult primary": An initial biopsy shows a malignant tumour unlikely to be a primary of the biopsied site. Often the first step for the oncologist evaluating such a patient is the review of the biopsy. The pathologist must then decide whether he has adequate tissue to do all the required studies, or whether he has to press his clinical colleagues for a second tissue sample. Immunochemistry has proven of great value in the evaluation of undifferentiated tumours. Often differentiation among lymphoma, carcinoma, melanoma, sarcoma,

can be achieved by using antibodies directed against intermediate filaments and other antigenic determinants. The question in the case of carcinoma concerns its origin. The presence in the tumour cells of immunoreactivity for certain products can occasionally pinpoint the primary (e.g. thyroglobulin for thyroid carcinoma), or orientate the search (neuropeptides for neuroendocrine tumours). Because few proteins, or surface binding sites (e.g. lectins), are restricted to one tissue cell type, it is good policy to use extended batteries of markers. These batteries should be used systematically in all cases, so that experience is gained in the antigenic profiles of primary tumours and their metastases.

Surgery After Radiotherapy

Surgeons need no longer be apprehensive when it comes to performing selective surgery for relapse after curative radiotherapy. Gone are the days when the only devices used to administer high doses were conventional therapy machines. Such doses from these machines provoked cutaneous changes such as teleaniectasia, ischaemia and fibrosis, all of which caused innumerable problems for the surgeon. The use of orthovoltage treatment equipment in the curative treatment of cancer must today be avoided at all cost, except when one is dealing with superficial skin neoplasms, as it is fraught with surgical problems, such as excessive bleeding and poor post-operative healing. High-energy devices, with their tissue-sparing effect, provide far better results. When local relapse occurs after definitive irradiation it is important to consider the possibility of performing salvage surgery. However, certain important clinical factors must be borne in mind before the decision to perform salvage surgery is made, namely, the patient's general condition, the extent of the disease and the quality of life after surgery.

But are there any radiotherapeutic factors which may influence the decision to carry out salvage surgery, such as dosage, fractionation and interval from conclusion of definitive irradiation to time of relapse? A useful clinical model to illustrate the use of salvage surgery after definitive irradiation and which casts some light on the questions above, is cancer of the head and neck. It is generally accepted that if one pools all the stages in head and neck cancer, relapse occurs on average 2 years following irradiation. This interval affords ample time for tissue healing, and therefore when salvage surgery is carried out, surgical morbidity stays at a respectable level.

In curative irradiation doses range from 5000 cGy to 7000 cGy, given in fractions varying from 20 Gy to about 35 Gy over a period of about 4–7.5 weeks. When treatment regimens are contained within these schedules (time, dose, fractionation), salvage, when necessary, can be carried out without any increase in surgical morbidity.

Goodman et al. (1981), in their series of bladder cancer patients treated by definitive irradiation followed by selective cystectomy for relapse, recorded operative mortality of 11%. His patients received a tumour dose of 5000 cGy in 15 fractions over a period of 3 weeks.

Moderate but curative radiation doses given over relatively short periods and high radiation doses given over moderately long fractionation periods do not impede salvage surgery when high-energy beams are used. There is adequate tissue recovery when relapse occurs on a time scale of months: surgeons need no longer worry about treading on previously irradiated ground.

Recurrent Head and Neck Cancer

Tumours of the Parotid Gland

So-called benign tumours of the parotid gland may behave (i.e. recur), or later develop, as if potentially malignant from the beginning. Recurrent mixed tumours should be treated radically (in our opinion without preliminary histological examination). The standard operation is then total parotidectomy with preservation of the facial nerve. Adenoid cystic carcinoma is an aggressive, extremely neurotropic tumour which shows a marked tendency to spread along the lymphatic sheaths of the nerves. Facial nerve resection is mandatory but does not always succeed in preventing deeper recurrences. Pulmonary and bony metastases appear late in the course of the disease. Lymph nodes are rarely invaded.

Mucoepidermoid tumours of the parotid gland should be considered malignant. Metastases, when present, are located in lymph nodes, bones and skin. Carcinomas of this site are usually highly infiltrating and necessitate extended resections, especially in the case of recurrence, however small. Severance of the facial nerve should be completed with immediate grafting.

Tumours of the Thyroid

Each type of recurrent tumour of the thyroid should be treated differently according to histology and to the extensiveness of the primary treatment. One should keep in mind that the age of the patient is almost more important a factor than a microscopic appearance of the tumour, even in the case of a recurrent cancer. A decrease of TSH secretion is mandatory for all organoid (differentiated) carcinomas.

Papillary Carcinoma. Treatment of the recurrence differs according to whether the primary was treated by subtotal lobectomy or total thyroidectomy. The initial treatment of choice is, for us, total lobectomy on the affected side, completed by subtotal lobectomy on the other side. Totalization of the resection remains possible in case of recurrence. Radical node dissection is questionable, since lymph node involvement does not seem to alter the prognosis, at least in young patients.

Follicular Carcinoma. One-third of recurrences are exclusively local, one-third are distant metastases and one-third a combination of both. If the disease was initially treated by total lobectomy and isthmectomy, treatment of all types of recurrences necessitate total thyroidectomy. Follicular carcinomas "function" and take up significant amounts of radioiodine. Total thyroidectomy eliminates competition for the isotope and renders nuclear treatment more effective.

Anaplastic Carcinomas. "Very little remains for the boldest to devise, or the most dexterous to perform", as Sir John Erichsen said in the Lancet (1873) in another context. Decompression of the trachea and some kind of neck dissection may alleviate the course of recurrent medullary carcinomas.

Other Head and Neck Cancer

Salvage surgery for relapse of cancer of the mouth, the pharynx and the larynx, when possible, is justified oncologically by the low incidence of distant metastases. On a functional basis salvage surgery is recommended because the quality of life is improved and the operation has the advantage that subsequent nursing care is relatively easy for the family. In the pre-treatment work-up, upper aerodigestive panendoscopy must be carried out because of the high incidence (20%) of simultaneous multiple sites of ENT, oesophageal and bronchial tumours, as demonstrated by Savary and co-workers (1984). The recent progress in reconstructive surgery, in particular the introduction of myocutaneous flaps, as described by Ariyan (1979), has made excision of a malignant relapse and buccopharyngolaryngeal reconstruction possible in a single session. For lesions of the floor of the mouth, and also for lesions involving the tongue, the glossoamygdaline region and the oropharynx, excision is usually carried out across the mandible and reconstruction is generally accomplished using myocutaneous flaps from the large pectoral and trapezius muscles. With this procedure Brupbacher et al. (1983) have shown a failure rate of 10%. For the hypopharynx, the same workers have documented a failure rate of 20% after myocutaneous flap reconstruction using the large pectoral muscle following circular pharyngolaryngectomy as selective surgery. In view of this high failure rate, Davidge-Pitts and Mannel (1983) have advocated using a colonic or gastric tube after oesophageal stripping associated with pharyngolaryngectomy. When local relapse occurs following radiotherapy to the larynx for cancer, the surgery of choice is total laryngectomy. However, when the relapse is supraglottic or glottic, supraglottic horizontal partial laryngectomy or reconstructive subtotal laryngectomy (cricohyoidopexy) are of value according to Wigand et al. (1984).

Recurrent Breast Cancer

Thorough cancer evaluation is necessary before planning treatment of a relapse. Mammography of the other breast, skeletal scintigraphy and possibly radiographic bone scan, thoracic radiography and computer-assisted tomography of the liver (or, if this is not available, ultrasonography or isotopic scintigraphy) complete the physical examination. In rare cases aspiration cytology or preliminary biopsy might help identify an unexpected radio-induced sarcoma mimicking a late locoregional recurrence of the primary cancer. Modalities of treatment of locoregional recurrence depend on the type of initial surgery, use or otherwise of initial radiotherapy, duration of free interval, concomitant distant recurrence, level of hormone receptors (in the primary, but also in the secondary tumour). Lastly, treatment of a lymph-borne metastasis is not the same as treatment of a haematogenous deposit in skin traumatized by surgery or radiotherapy.

After conservative surgical treatment of the primary cancer, secondary amputation is followed by a

5-year survival rate of more than 50%. Such secondary amputation may be necessitated by local failure. After conventional amputation of the breast, Donegan and Skibba (1983) describe only 15% of purely local relapses versus 75% of distant recurrence with or without local relapse. Gilliland et al. (1983) cite 60%–80% of local recurrence within 2 years after treatment of a primary and almost 90% within the first 5 years. No patient survived more than 23 years after the first manifestation of relapse. Local surgery for local relapse makes sense, at least for the first and possibly the second local relapse. Ablative endocrine surgery or hormonal manipulation, if advisable in light of the level of hormone receptors, should not be postponed too long. Surgical treatment of pleuropulmonary or hepatic secondaries is rarely indicated. Relapse occuring in axillary vessels or nerves and/or the thoracic wall can be managed by compound operations such as interscapulo(mammo)thoracic amputation including the relevant part of the thoracic wall. Use of flaps from the amputated extremity, possibly together with omental transposition flaps and synthetic mesh for stabilization of the thoracic wall, causes no problems.

Recurrent Limb and Girdle Cancer

Forequarter Amputation

Crosby of Dartmouth Medical College (1836) is credited with the first successful treatment of cancer by forequarter amputation. This operation, otherwise known as interscapulothoracic amputation, is described in Moseley's (1957) classic monograph. The indications are bulky sarcomas of the soft parts, or bony sarcomas of the upper limb, especially in the shoulder region, and skin carcinoma, or melanoma, with massive axillary involvement. The operation is technically simple, the only critical factor being, sometimes, the control of the subclavian vessels behind the clavicle if this is already surrounded by actinic fibrosis and a possible tumour. Resection of the second rib and intrathoracic ligation of the subclavian artery and vein should be considered. Proceeding from the anterior aspect is easier, in our opinion, than from the posterior aspect of the shoulder. A good knowledge of the regional anatomy is mandatory. Five-year cure rates vary between 35% and 45%, depending on the nature of the primary. Operation for recurrent cancer does not alter the end results [34% vs 37% in Pack's (1956) series]. Forequarter amputation can be extended to the breast and thoracic wall. These exarticulations are routine surgical oncology procedures and should not need the assistance of an orthopaedic surgeon.

Hindquarter Amputation

The first successful attempt is attributed to Girard of Bern in 1895. Hindquarter amputation, also known as interilioabdominal amputation or hemipelvectomy, is considered when simple exarticulation of the hip joint does not seem to suffice. This amputation includes part or all of the pelvic girdle. Sparing of the pubic symphysis or part of the iliac bone, in order to facilitate rehabilitation, should be contemplated. On the other hand, resection of the pubic symphysis or partial resection of the sacrum may in itself be curative. The more complete (in the anatomical sense) the amputation, the easier it is to perform. Hindquarter amputation can be extended to any part of the pelvic viscera, combining exenterative resection with exarticulation in the hope of achieving cure.

Indications for hindquarter amputation are sarcomas of the innominate bone or proximal femur invading the hip joint. The possibility of using flaps from the amputated extremity should be kept in mind. These operations are easy to perform and the operative mortality is minimal. Five-year end results vary according to the histology of the primary tumour (20%–40%). Recurrent cancer only moderately alters end results (29% vs 42%) in Pack's data (1956).

Translumbar Amputation

Translumbar amputation, or hemicorporectomy, may occasionally achieve cure in patients with otherwise incurable disease. The operation is once again technically simple, but a highly specialized rehabilitation centre must be available and the patient *and* his family must be willing, conditions which are rarely met.

Regional Hyperthermic Chemotherapy Perfusion

Creech et al. (1958) had the idea of potentiating regional chemotherapy by means of isolated extracorporeal circulation, permitting the use of normally lethal dosages of oncolytic drugs. This opened a new era in the treatment of recurrent tumours of the extremities, decreasing the incidence of exarticulations.

Temperatures of 37 °C and hyperoxygenation were used. Cavaliere et al. (1967) demonstrated the sensitivity of cancer cells to hyperthermia reaching tissue temperatures of 42°–43 °C. Problems are local toxicity (combination of high temperatures and specific agents) and general toxicity (overcome by leakage monitoring). The 10-year survival rate for recurrent melanoma of the lower limb with satellite or in-transit metastases is 23% (Krementz 1986).

Recurrent Gastrointestinal Cancer

Bowden (1967) demonstrated that 60% of gastric or duodenal stump relapses are resectable. He noted that the duration of the relapse-free interval is important: it was 50 months on average in 24 operable patients and only 17 months in 33 inoperable cases. Very late local recurrences, although exceptional, may be found after 10–15 years. The degree of anaplasia of the primary tumour does not seem to influence the operability of the secondary. Survival rate in Bowden's experience was 5 months for 33 palliative operations, but 15 months for "curative" procedures (with four postoperative deaths and four long-term survivals: 3.5, 4.5, 7 and 11 years). The standard operation for recurrence is total gastrectomy with pancreatosplenectomy. When the upper suture line seems invaded after primary surgery, our policy is to wait for 3 months before performing endoscopic examination, repeat endoscopy after 6 months and possibly carry out a second-look operation following this delay.

Recurrent Colon Carcinoma

The results of surgery for symptomatic recurrence after extended resection of colon cancer are disappointing. Of 34 patients operated on by Eldar et al. (1985), only eight had curative intent procedures, with a 5-year survival rate of 50% (compared to 7% for the remaining 26 patients). At 10 years, all the patients had died of recurrent disease.

Second-look Surgery

Most of the time-recurrent abdominal cancers are only reoperated on when symptomatic, which is often too late for a possible cure. Wangensteen (1954) started reoperating on all those patients who previously (4–9 months earlier) benefitted from the resection of a cancer of the stomach, colon, rectum, ovaries, or retroperitoneal sarcoma. When second-look surgery yielded evidence of operable relapse of the primary, the patient was urged to accept a third-look operation and so on, until there was either no more evidence of disease, or the patient died. The end results were disappointing, except for cancer of the colon, where a salvage rate of 14% was demonstrated. With the routine measurement of tumour markers (especially CEA), new hopes were raised. Some surgeons, e.g. Minton et al. (1985) and Staab et al. (1985), claim good results and even cancer cures with CEA-monitored second-look operations. From our series of 1,367 patients, we have selected 25 patients who underwent surgery for cure of their primary tumour and who were reoperated on a total of 38 times because of an elevation of the previously normal CEA. At the time of the CEA-suspected relapse, 20 patients were asymptomatic, although more detailed evaluation, including CT scan, ultrasonography, angiography and colonoscopy, demonstrated some evidence of cancer; 13 asymptomatic patients patients underwent second-look surgery in the absence of any preoperative evidence of cancer.

Recurrence involved the liver in 14 patients, in 13 of whom metastasectomy and/or long-term arterial chemotherapy was feasible. Two new primaries were discovered in the colon and resected with curative intent, as were four metastatic involvements of the small bowel, five of the colon and six pelvic recurrences. CEA values returned to normal 13 times after second-look surgery. Many patients were thought to have benefitted, but in fact we did not observe one single long-term cure of cancer. This does not mean that we should discontinue measuring CEA or other markers in the course of follow-up and forego second-look surgery in selected cases of colon cancer.

Minton et al. (1985) are probably right when they suggests measuring CEA levels at 6-week intervals and reoperating immediately when CEA elevation is confirmed.

Recurrent Pelvic Cancer

Pelvic Exenteration

Pelvic exenteration was well described by Brunschwig as early as 1948 and was reviewed by the same author in 1964. The long-term results of 756 cases were then analyzed in detail and critical comment given.

Anterior pelvic exenteration is restricted to total cystectomy including the distal part of the ureter and total hysterosalpingo-oophorectomy. Posterior pelvic exenteration adds hysterosalpingo-oophorectomy to rectum amputation. These resections are en-bloc procedures which must include pelvic lymph node dissection (see below for discussion of urinary diversion procedures). The usual indications for pelvic exenteration are advanced cancer of the cervix uteri after failure of initial actinic treatment, sarcoma of the urinary bladder and some locally advanced cancers of the prostate, vulva, vagina or rectum without evidence of distant recurrence. Extended pelvic exenteration is a combination of the above-mentioned procedure with some form of hindquarter amputation or conservative excision of the pelvic girdle. All aspects of these operations should be familiar to surgical oncologists; they are well described in Brunschwig's papers and books. Brunschwig's overall mortality (1964) was 15.8% (756 patients) and more than 20% of these patients were alive and well after 5 years. In today's medical context, with the improvement of anaesthetic techniques and the wide array of better antibiotics, the results would surely be better.

Urinary and Fecal Stream Diversion

Urinary obstruction is a complication frequently met with in oncology. Urinary diversion is technically simple but carries an important responsibility for the surgeon and should not be advised if the only result is to prolong the patient's suffering from severe pain due to the progress of intractable disease. However, it may alleviate unpleasant problems due to urinary fistula or painful tenesmus after urinary bladder irradiation. Unilateral or bilateral nephrostomy may be considered in emergency situations, but this procedure is increasingly being replaced by the endoscopic insertion of pigtail catheters. Ureterostomies and ureteral implantations in the colon should be avoided, except for short-term survivors. An ileal conduit, as described by Bricker (1950) and McAfee and Bricker (1967), undoubtedly yields the best possible quality of life after pelvic exenteration. Procedures for fecal stream diversion, including small bowel short-circuit and ileotransversostomy, are too well known to need description here. Continent ileostomies are helpful after total proctocolectomy for familial polyposis and cancer if ileo-anal anastomosis is impossible. Continent colostomies are not yet advisable.

Metastases of Occult Primary Tumours

Patients with metastases of unknown primaries should be treated like other cancer patients. Of all cancers, 0.5%–7% are initially presented as metastatic disease. Long survival, although rare, is not exceptional. The median survival time is 3–4 months, but one may find 25% survival at 1 year and 10% survival at 5 years. Holmes and Fouts (1970) report 2-year survival of 10%, 5-year survival of 5% and 10-year survival of 3% among 686 patients. The most common sites, in decreasing order of frequency, were bones, lungs, liver, generalized CNS and cervical lymph nodes. The most frequent sites of the primary are pancreas and lung (Nyström et al. 1977), while breast and prostate primaries are rare.

Cancerous Cervical Nodes. Metastases in the upper and lower levels of the cervical lymph node chains have different origins and prognoses. Metastases of the upper nodes originate in the nose and throat territories and are epidermoid carcinomas with a better prognosis than low cervical metastases, which originate from digestive adenocarcinomas, or epidermoid tumours appearing in older patients, often alcoholics or heavy smokers. MacComb (1972) insists that a thorough check-up and aspiration biopsy should be considered before any node excision, radical neck dissection being ultimately performed if possible.

Axillary Metastases. Axillary metastases most often originate in the homolateral breast and necessitate some form of radical breast amputation, with the exception of a very small and easy to investigate breast, where a wait-and-see policy is advisable. In the case of melanoma, radical axillary dissection should always be undertaken to avoid ulceration and inextirpability of the lesion later on.

Inguinal Metastases. Melanoma is the most frequent primary. Krementz (1986) reports a 47% 10-year survival rate after inguinal dissection and isolated extracorporeal chemotherapy perfusions.

Brain Metastases

Approximately 20% of cancer patients have intracranial metastases at autopsy. The most frequent sites of origin are lung, breast, kidney and skin (melanoma). The clinical presentation consists of focal neurological deficit, seizures or increased intracranial pressure. Patients with multiple brain metastases are treated by steroids and whole-brain radiotherapy. Patients with a solitary metastasis undergo evaluation of the extent of the disease and, if the systemic disease seems to be under control, the brain lesion should be resected where surgically accessible. Classically, postoperative radiotherapy is considered, since small, undetected metastases may be present in other regions of the brain. It is doubtful whether surgical treatment of a single brain metastasis increases survival in comparison with radiotherapy alone. On the other hand, the immediate improvement in the quality of life which may be brought about by surgical extirpation may be compromised by the disabling side effects of radiotherapy. Thus the best treatment of a solitary brain metastasis remains an open question (Cairncross and Posner 1983). Chemotherapy for brain metastases has, up to now, yielded poor results.

Pulmonary Metastases

Presentation

Precocious metastases are those recognized prior to the diagnosis of the primary tumour. Synchronous metastases are discovered at the same time as the primary. Both these situations are much less frequent than metachronous metastases. Twenty years ago this last group of metastases used to be found in 50% of patients with symptoms. Today, however, almost all are detected by systematic screening examination (Saegesser 1970). This screening generally consists of a periodic plain chest X-ray. Nowadays, the most accurate (but still quite expensive) method is the computerized thoracic scan, which can detect smaller metastatic foci ($\geqslant$7 mm) with 90% sensibility (Roth 1985).

Indication for Surgery

All surgeons recommend excision of pulmonary metastases (a) in low-risk patients, (b) in the case of controlled primary tumour that has been treated or excised for cure, (c) when there is no evidence of extrapulmonary metastases and (d) when the number of pulmonary deposits is relatively small (bilateral localization is not always a contraindication) (Roth 1985; Saegesser et al. 1970).

The nature and histology of the primary, the disease interval (which is still somewhat controversial and should be related to the histology of the primary) and the doubling time, number and dimensions of the metastases basically do not represent contraindications but rather prognostic factors that should be kept in mind.

Doubling time is a useful criterion only for small metastases, because larger ones may grow more slowly, for vascular reasons. Generally speaking, possible metastases should not be left to grow for too long.

Surgical Treatment

As pulmonary metastases are usually located just underneath the pleura and "daughter metastases" in the lymph nodes are rarely present (~30% of cases), the technique of excision should be as conservative as possible. The use of automatic stapling devices to remove the metastases with a small margin of 1 cm of healthy lung tissue has improved functional results and has allowed resection of more numerous deposits. In the case of bilateral lung metastases, the trans-sternal route allows simultaneous bilateral excisions (Johnston 1983). Tumours with lung metastases that are often amenable to surgery are, in decreasing order of operability and also from good to poor prognosis: osteogenic sarcoma, soft tissue sarcoma, renal carcinoma, testicular carcinoma, ENT tumours, colorectal cancer, uterus carcinoma, breast carcinoma, endocrine tumours, melanomas. In the case of primary tumours of other locations, the appearance of pulmonary coin lesions most probably represents a new primary lung cancer (Saegesser et al. 1970).

Prognosis

After excision of a documented metastasis the prognosis is quite good, with 5-year survival rates often superior to those of primary lung cancer. Twenty-five to thirty per cent of patients will still be alive after this time (Beattie 1984; Saegesser et al. 1970), the actual figures varying from 15% to 50% depending on the histological type of the primary tumour. Long or even very long survival is by no means rare (Saegesser et al. 1970; Roth 1985).

Hepatic Metastases

Between 1970 and 1977 we operated on 451 patients with colorectal cancer and discovered evidence of hepatic metastases in 110 cases (24.4%). The presen-

Table 1. Presentation of hepatic metastases ($n = 110$)

Metastases	Bilateral	Right-side only	Left-side only
Multiple	58%	13%	3%
Solitary	7%	16%	3%

tation of these metastases at laparotomy is shown in Table 1.

Liver scanning reveals that some "solitary" metastases are actually multiple. Radical excision is the only potentially curative treatment for hepatic metastases, but no more than 1%–3% of patients will in fact be cured. Metastasectomy with a 1-cm margin is sufficient for a solitary deposit. A margin of 3–4 cm normal tissue is safer for excision of a confluent group of metastases. Lobectomy should be considered if it is feasible. Peroperative ultrasonography is helpful. Excision of more than three independent foci is thought excessive by most surgeons. The results of excision of hepatic metastases of colorectal origin are shown in Table 2. When surgical treatment is not advisable, long-term arterial chemotherapy should be considered at least for metastases of colorectal origin. An objective response rate of 40%–80% and about 20% complete disappearance of scanned lesions may be expected. Prolongation of survival is not yet established.

The therapeutic role of liver ischaemia (induced by arterial ligation, embolization or microspheres) is being studied, and this technique may prove curative in some metastases of endocrine tumours like insulinoma. The only way to compare the results of different therapeutic procedures is to classify and to stage hepatic metastases. Van de Velde and Sugarbaker (1984) proposed an international staging system which should replace all previous classifications (Table 3).

Table 3. International staging system for hepatic metastases

Stage 0	: Curatively resected metastases
Stage I	: P_1 (PHR 25%), no E, no S
Stage II	: P_2 (PHR 25–75%), no E, no S
Stage III	: P_3 (PHR 75%), no S or any P with E and/or S
PHR:	percent of hepatic replacement by tumor;
E:	concurrent extrahepatic disease;
S:	symptoms attributable to liver metastases

From Van de Velde and Sugarbaker (1984)
P and PHR, partial hepatic replacement.

Table 2. Results of resection of hepatic metastases of colorectal origin

Reference	City/clinic	Year of publication	No. of patients	Major hepatic resections/ wedge resections	Postoperative mortality (%)	Survival (%) 1 year	3 years	5 years	10 years	Medians survival (months)
Flanagan and Foster (1967)	Collective review	1967	45					23		18
Foster and Berman (1977)	Collective review	1974	88					18		
Wilson and Adson (1976)	Mayo Clinic	1976	60	21/39	1.6			28	19	
				solitaries				42	28	
Morrow et al. (1982)	Minneapolis	1982	29					27		
Mühe et al. (1982)	Erlangen	1982	21					20	15	
Balser and Rohner (1982)	Geneva	1982	21	21/0	14					
Thompson et al. (1983)	Los Angeles	1983	22		0	80	38	31		27
Iwatsuki et al. (1983)	Pittsburgh	1983	24	24/0	0	91	73	52		
Fortner et al. (1984)	Memorial, New York	1984	65	65/0	9	89	57	40		
Steele et al. (1984)	Boston	1984	43		5	90	65			
Adson and Van Heerden (1984)	Mayo Clinic	1984	141	67/74	4/0	88	44	25		
Petrelli et al. (1985)	Buffalo	1985	36	19/17	14	45	30			22
August et al. (1984)	NCI, Bethesda	1985	33	13/20	0	72	53			38
Huguet et al. (1985)	Paris, Monaco	1985	49		6	58	28			
			Total: 667					Average: 29.5%		

References

Adson MA, van Heerden JA, Adson MH, Wagner JS, Ilstrup DM (1984) Resection of hepatic metastases from colorectal cancer. Arch Surg 119: 647–651

Ariyan S (1979) The pectoralis major myocutaneous flap – a versatile flap for reconstruction on the head and neck. Plast Reconstr Surg 63: 73

August DA, Ottow RT, Sugarbaker PA (1984) Clinical perspective of human colorectal cancer metastasis. Cancer Metastasis Rev 3: 303–324

Balser S, Rohner A (1982) 21 Résections hépatiques partielles pour métastases colo-rectaux. Elvetica chirurgica Acta 49: 179–181

Beattie EJ (1984) Surgical treatment of pulmonary metastases. Cancer 54: 2729–2731

Bowden L (1967) Surgery of locally recurrent gastric cancer. In: McNeer G, Pack G (eds) Neoplasms of the stomach. Lippincott, Philadelphia, pp 332–339

Bricker EM (1950) Bladder substitution after pelvic exenteration. Surg Clin North Am 30: 1511

Brunschwig A (1948) Complete excision of pelvic viscera for advanced cancer. Cancer 1: 177–183

Brunschwig A (1964) L'exentération pelvienne. Masson, Paris

Brupbacher JP, Klaus E, Savary M, Meyer R (1983) Les lambeaux myocutanés du grand pectoral, du sterno-cléïdo-mastoïdien et du trapèze transverse dans la reconstruction maxillo-faciale après chirurgie d'exérèse de cancers de la bouche et de l'oropharynx: à propos de 65 cas. Aktuel Probl Otolaryngol 6: 132–139

Cairncross JG, Posner JB (1983) The management of brain metastases. In: Oncology of the nervous system. Martinus Nijoff, The Hague

Cavaliere R, Ciogatto EC, Giovanella BC et al. (1967) Selective heat sensitivity of cancer cells: biochemical and clinical studies. Cancer 20: 1351–1381

Creech O Jr, Krementz ET, Ryan RF et al. (1958) Chemotherapy of cancer. Regional perfusion utilizing an extracorporeal circuit. Ann Surg 148: 616–632

Davidge-Pitts KJ, Mannel A (1983) Pharyngo-laryngectomy with extra thoracic esophagectomy. Head Neck Surg 6: 571

Donegan WL, Skibba JL (1983) Patterns of survival and disease recurrence after mastectomy for cancer of the breast. Cancer Treat Symp 2: 107–116

Eldar S, Kemeny MM, Terz JJ (1985) Extended resections for carcinoma of the colon and rectum. Surg Gynecol Obstet 161: 319–322

Flanagan LJ, Foster JH (1967) Hepatic resection for metastatic cancer. Am J Surg 113: 551–557

Fortner JG, Silva JS, Golbey RB, Cox EB, Maclean BJ (1984) Multivariate analysis of a personal series of 247 consecutive patients with liver metastases from colorectal cancer. I. Treatment by hepatic resection. Ann Surg 199: 306–316

Foster JH, Berman MM (1977) Solid liver tumors. Saunders, Philadelphia

Ghosh AK, Erber WN, Haffon CSR et al. (1985) Detection of metastatic tumor cells in routine bone marrow smears by immuno-alkaline phosphatase labelling with monoclonal antibodies. Br J Haematol 61: 31

Gilliland MD, Barton RM, Copeland EM III (1983) The implication of local recurrence of breast cancer as the first site of therapeutic failure. Ann Surg 197: 284–287

Goodman G, Hislop T, Elwood MJ, Balfour J (1981) Conservation of bladder function in patients with invasive bladder cancer treated by definitive irradiation and selective cystectomy. Int J Radiat Oncol Biol Phys 7: 569–573

Griffen WD, Wangensteen OW (1965) The second-look operation in the management of abdominal cancers. In: Ariel IM (ed) Progress in clinical cancer, vol 1. Grune and Stratton, New York, pp 154–159

Holmes FF, Fouts TI (1970) Metastatic cancer of unknown primary site. Cancer 26: 816–820

Huguet C, Nordlinger B, Curci O (1985) Résection chirurgicale des métastases hépatiques des cancers du côlon et du rectum. A propos de 49 cas. In: Lemerte J (ed) Actualités carcinologiques. Masson, Paris

Iwatsuki S, Shaw BW, Starzl TE (1983) Experience with 150 liver resections. Ann Surg 197: 247–253

Johnston MR (1983) Median sternotomy for resection of pulmonary metastases. J Thorac Cardiovasc Surg 85: 516–522

Krementz ET (1986) Regional perfusion. Cancer 57: 416–432

MacComb WS (1972) Diagnosis and treatment of metastatic cervical cancerous nodes from unknown primary site. Am J Surg 124: 441–449

Martin SE, Zhang HZ, Magyarosy E et al. (1984) Immunological methods in cytology: Definitive diagnosis of non-Hodgkin's lymphomas using immunological markers for T and B cells. Am J Clin Pathol 82: 32–39

McAfee CA, Bricker EM (1967) Palliation by diversion of the urinary and fecal stream. In: Hickey RC (ed) Palliative care of the cancer patient. Churchill, London

Minton JP, Hoehn JL, Gerber DM et al. (1985) Results of a 400-patient carcinoembryonic antigen second-look colorectal cancer study. Cancer 55: 1284–1290

Morrow CE, Grage TB, Sutherland DER, Najarian JS (1982) Hepatic resection for secondary neoplasms. Surgery 92: 610–614

Moseley HF (1957) The forequarter amputation. Livingstone, Edinburgh

Mühe E, Gall FP, Angermann B (1982) Resection of liver metastases. World J Surg 6: 210–215

Mulvihill JJ (1977) Genetic repertory of human neuroplasia. In: Mulvihill JJ, Milten RW, Fraumeni JF Jr (eds) Genetics of human cancer. Raven, New York

Nyström JC, Weiner Heffelfinger-Juttner J et al. (1977) Metastatic and histologic presentations in unknown primary cancer. Semin Oncol 4: 53–58

Pack GT (1956) Major exarticulations for malignant neoplasms of the extremities. J Bone Joint Surg [Am] 38: 249–262

Petrelli NJ, Nambisan RN, Herrera L, Mittelman A (1985) Hepatic resection for isolated metastasis from colorectal carcinoma. Am J Surg 149: 205–209

Roth AJ (1985) Treatment of metastatic cancer to lung. In: De Vita VT, Helmann S, Rosenberg SA (eds) Principles and practice of oncology, 2nd ed. Lippincott, Philadelphia, pp 2104–2117

Saegesser F, Besson A, Kafai F (1970) Pulmonary coin lesions and metastases. In: Saegesser F, Pettavel J (eds) Surgical oncology. Huber, Berne, pp 539–610

Savary M, Pasche R, Monnier PH (1984) Endoscopic screening for multiple squamous cell carcinoma of the upper digestive and respiratory tracts (oncologically oriented upper aero-digestive pan-endoscopy). In: Wigand ME, Steiner W, Stell PM (eds) Functional partial laryngectomy. Conservation surgery for carcinoma of the larynx. Springer, Berlin Heidelberg New York, pp 51–58

Staab HJ, Anderer FA, Stumpf E et al. (1985) Eighty-four potential second-look operations based on sequential carcinoembryonic antigen determination. Am J Surg 149: 198–204

Steele G, Osteen RT, Wilson RE, Brooks DC, Mayer RJ, Zamcheck N, Ravikumar TS (1984) Patterns of failure after surgical care of large liver tumors. Am J Surg 147: 554–559

Thompson HH, Tompkins RK, Longmire WP Jr (1983) Major hepatic resection. A 25-year experience. Ann Surg 197: 375–388

Van de Velde CJH, Sugarbaker PH (eds) (1984) Liver metastasis. Basic aspects, detection and management. Nijhoff, Boston, pp 292–312

Wangensteen OH, Lewis JF, Arhelger SW, Muller JJ, Machean LD (1954) An interim report upon the "second-look" procedure for cancer of the stomach, colon and rectum for "limited intraperitoneal carcinosis." Surg Gynecol Obstet 99: 257–267

Wattenberg CA (1947) Bone changes and variations in skeletal metastases due to diethylstilbestrol and orchiectomy during treatment of cancer of the prostate. J Virol 58: 378–383

Wigand ME, Steiner W, Stell PM (1984) Functional partial laryngectomy. Conservation surgery for carcinoma of the larynx. Springer, Berlin Heidelberg New York

Willis GW, Hajdu SI (1973) Histologically benign teratoid metastasis of testicular embryonal carcinoma: report of five cases. Am J Clin Pathol 59: 338–343

Wilson SM, Adson MA (1976) Surgical treatment of hepatic metastases from colorectal cancers. Arch Surg III: 330–334

Irradiation in Cancer Treatment

M. Tubiana

Radiotherapy (RT) is, with surgery, one of the two main methods for the locoregional treatment of cancer. Its modern era started in 1920, when Regaud showed that with proper fractionation it was possible to reduce the toxic effects of radiation on normal tissue without a correspondingly large loss of therapeutic effect on the tumor. This differential effect takes advantage of the strong regulatory mechanisms that exist in normal tissues. The roles of the dose per fraction (fractionation) and of the overall duration of the radiotherapy course (protraction) have recently been further elucidated (Tubiana et al. 1986b; Fowler 1984).

A second important advance was the measurement of dose distribution within the patient. The study of the dose-effect relationship for tumor control and injury to the normal surrounding tissues underlined the paramount importance of precise delivery of a cancericidal dose to the whole of the tumor, while sparing as much of the surrounding normal tissues as possible. A tumor was regarded as radioresistant if it could not be locally controlled by the maximum doses which provoked a small incidence of complications in the surrounding tissues. Hence, tumors were classified into three categories: the radiosensitive, including lymphomas and seminomas; those of limited sensitivity, such as squamous carcinomas and adenocarcinomas; and the radioresistant, in particular sarcomas, melanomas and tumors of the gastrointestinal tract. The philosophy of accepted risks led to the concept of the optimum dose, which is that giving the highest incidence of tumor control with the lowest rate of severe complications. The numerical value of the optimum dose varies with the histologic type of the tumor and with its size, the fractionation regimen and the technique of radiotherapy.

The current renewed interest in radiotherapy is explained by three considerations: (1) combination of surgery and RT have made conservative treatment possible; (2) chemotherapy has a relatively limited effectiveness on most solid tumors; (3) improved local control of the primary tumor does not suffice to cure the patient, but is in some patients translated into improved long-term survival.

Relationship Between Local Control and Survival

The reality of the improvement has been a subject of debate. If all patients with bulky tumors which are difficult to control already have occult metastases at the time of treatment, a gain in the frequency of local control would only result in an increased incidence of death due to distant metastases. However, a sizeable proportion of relatively large tumors have not yet metastasized. For several sites, salvage treatment for local failures results in long-term survival (Suit 1982). Moreover, metastatic spread is more frequent in those patients with uncontrolled or recurrent local tumors.

There is often a discrepancy between the reduction in the incidence of local recurrences obtained with preoperative or postoperative RT and the relatively small impact on survival. This is not surprising, since local recurrence has an impact on survival only under two conditions: (1) if the patient had no distant metastases at the time of initial treatment; (2) if the recurrence initiated a metastasis before being detected and treated (Tubiana et al. 1986a). Let us take, for example, breast cancer. Postoperative RT is able to reduce the incidence of locoregional recurrence; however, an increase in survival is observed in only a small subset of patients, namely those with a tumor located in the inner quadrants and with positive axillary nodes. For tumors of the outer quadrants, the lymphatic drainage leads to an involvement of the axillary nodes and the internal mammary chain is seldom involved. For tumors of the inner quadrants, involvement of the internal mammary chain is observed in approximately one-third of the patients with metastasis-bearing axillary nodes. It is only in this last group of patients that postoperative radiotherapy improves survival. This result is easy to interpret. A breast cancer usually initiates a metastatic spread only when it has exceeded a threshold volume of a few cubic centimeters (Koscielny et al. 1984). Thus, locoregional recurrences will initiate distant metastases only when they reach this size. Axillary recurrences are easy to detect and are likely to be treated before they can initiate metastases. Conversely, internal mammary chain recurrences are not detected early and, thus, are a likely nidus for further dissemination (Tubiana et al. 1986a).

Biological Bases of Radiotherapy

The aim of curative radiotherapy is to control the tumor. A small proportion of tumor cells (ca. 0.1%) have the capacity for unlimited division; these are called stem cells. The other tumor cells are more differentiated and can undergo only a few divisions or cannot divide at all. Tumor control can be achieved only if all the stem cells have lost their proliferating ability. Cell death after irradiation is defined by the inability to proliferate. Morphologically intact cells may not be able to proliferate. The proportion of cells surviving is related to the dose delivered. Lethal radiobiological damage is inflicted at random. Moreover, the repair of non-lethal damage is terminated in less than 1 day. Therefore, during a fractionated course of irradiation the dose-response relationship for cell killing is exponential (Fletcher 1980). Consequently, a given dose per fraction kills a fixed proportion of cells, and it takes the same number of fractions to reduce a cell population from one billion (10^9) cells to one million (10^6) as it does to reduce that population from one thousand (10^3) to one (10^0).

A partial regression is generally defined as 50% reduction in tumor size. At a first approximation this corresponds to the death of 50% of the cells. If this is obtained with a dose D_{50}, total clinical disappearance (complete regression) of a tumor of 100 g (10^{11} cells) requires that at least 999 cells out of 1000 are killed, as a lump of 100 mg is no longer detectable. This is obtained with a dose 10 times larger: 10 D_{50}. If all the tumor cells are stem cells, to obtain an average of less than one surviving stem cell per tumor would, for a tumor of 100 g, require a dose equal to 36 D_{50}. If only 0.1% of the tumor cells are clonogenic, which appears more likely, then a dose equal to 26 D_{50} would suffice. Whatever the proportion of stem cells, the tumor control dose is approximately 30 times larger than that which achieves a significant partial regression and at least 3 times larger than that which achieves complete clinical remission. In these calculations no allowance is made for tumor repopulation during the course of RT; this would correspond to 4–5 D_{50}. For most human tumor cell lineages the D_{50} varies between 2 and 2.5 Gy (Fertil and Malaise 1985).

On the basis of this dose-effect relationship it is possible to generate a theoretical curve of radiation dose against likelihood of tumor cure. At a low dose there is insufficient cell kill to cause tumor control, since only tumors with zero stem cells are cured. As the dose is raised (close to about one lethal event per cell) the probability of control increases from 25% to 75% with a relatively small dose increment (approximately 5 Gy). To increase the probability of control from 85% to 95% requires a disproportionately large increase in dose because the curve flattens. The calculation shows that a small underdosage in part of the tumor (a dose inferior by 20% to the tumor control dose in one-tenth of the tumor mass) would practically annihilate the likelihood of tumor control.

A similar sigmoid relationship exists between the likelihood of complications and the dose, but for radioresponsive tumors the dose which bears a 50% likelihood of complications is on average 5–15 Gy higher than the dose which controls 50% of the tumor. This small margin explains both the potential and the difficulties of radiotherapy. For example, for bladder tumors the doses which control 25% and 50% of the tumors induce complication rates of 10% and 30% respectively. The dose response curve for complications in a given tissue or organ applies to all patients because the radiosensitivity of normal tissue is approximately identical in all normal individuals. Conversely, there are occasional large variations in tumor response which is affected by at least four factors: (1) the intrinsic radiosensitivity of the tumor cells; (2) the presence of hypoxic cells; (3) the kinetics of tumor cell proliferation; (4) the volume of the tumor.

Intrinsic Radiosensitivity of Tumor Cells

In tissue cultures, after a dose of 2 Gy (the average dose per fraction in RT) the survival of the different types of tumor cells varies widely. There is a significant correlation between histologic type and cell survival, although there is relatively large variability among the cell lines of a histologic type. In vitro cell survival is higher in tumors of radioresistant histologic types (Fertil et al.).

The Presence of Hypoxic Cells

Damage produced by ionizing radiation is decreased by the absence of oxygen; the radiation dose necessary to sterilize hypoxic cells is approximately 3 times greater than that necessary for cells exhibiting normal oxygen tension. There are anoxic cells in all animal tumors with a diameter larger than a few millimeters, because as tumors grow they outstrip their blood supply. It is probable that there are also hypoxic components in human tumors. In most cases the proportion of hypoxic cells decreases during a fractionated course of irradiation due to reoxygenation caused by various factors, in particular the shrinkage of the tumor. However, in some human tumors reoxygenation is less effective, as evidenced by the beneficial effect of radiosensitizers and hyperbaric oxygen and the adverse effect of uncorrected anemia.

Kinetics of Tumor Cell Proliferation

Cell kinetics can exert an influence on the radiosensitivity of tumors and normal tissues in several ways.

Variations in Cell Radiosensitivity Throughout the Intermitotic Cycle. The overall cell survival in a tissue depends upon the radiosensitivity of cells in each phase and the number of cells in that phase. There is little variation in the duration of the cell cycle for the various types of human tumors, but the proliferative fraction ranges from less than 1% to nearly 100%. The proliferative fraction varies with the histologic type of the tumor; however, there is a wide distribution of individual values within each histologic type (Malaise et al. 1973). Among tumors of the same histologic type, the less differentiated tumors are those with the highest proliferative fraction.

Repopulation. In normal tissues with a rapid cell turnover, after an injury the excessive loss of differentiated cells triggers the recruitment of quiescent cells into the proliferative pool; it also causes a shortening of the cell cycle. Repopulation also occurs in some tumors following irradiation and may explain radioresistance during fractionated radiotherapy; in human tumors a shortening of doubling time has been observed after irradiation, and some data suggest the existence of a significant repopulation during a course of radiotherapy. Split-course radiotherapy of head and neck tumors has given a smaller percentage of local control than that obtained with continuous courses. In a few types of tumors, repopulation is sufficiently rapid to cause radioresistance; a notable example is Burkitt's lymphoma. However, in most human tumors the influence of repopulation appears to be smaller although not negligible (Tubiana 1988).

Volume of Tumor

Bulky tumors require higher radiation doses for control than do smaller ones and there is a relationship between tumor volume and the tumor control dose. In the case of tumors of the upper respiratory and digestive tract, for example, the dose for control increases from 60 Gy for tumors of less than 2 cm in diameter, to 75 Gy for tumors of 4–6 cm in diameter and 80 Gy for tumors of more than 6 cm in diameter

(Fletcher 1980). The number of cells in a tumor of diameter 6 cm is approximately 30 times greater than in a tumor of diameter 2 cm. Thus, the tumor control dose should theoretically be increased by 5 D_{50}, that is by about 10–12 Gy. However, this increase in dose is not sufficient to maintain at the same level the proportion of tumor control. This is probably due to the influence of other factors such as hypoxia, because the hypoxic compartment is greater in large tumors; a larger proportion of quiescent or slowly dividing cells which are more radioresistant; and possibly the presence of radioresistant subclones.

Let us now consider the largest occult metastatic foci (diameter 4 mm). Since their volume is 1000-fold smaller than that of a tumor of 4 cm, the tumor control dose should be 10 D_{50} less than the dose which controls a tumor of 4 cm. In effect, in clinical practice, a dose of 50 Gy appears to be sufficient. This dose is well tolerated by normal tissues, whereas the high doses required for the control of gross tumors may induce sequelae (Dutreix et al. 1988).

Size of Irradiated Volume and Normal Tissue Tolerance. For a given dose the tissue reactions are more severe when the field size is larger. For example, in patients with cervix carcinoma an increase in major complications (from 5% to 22%) is observed in patients treated with an extended field to include para-aortic nodes instead of the standard pelvic field (Fletcher 1980).

Hence, the tolerance dose is less for large fields than for small, while large lesions require higher doses than small ones. Two techniques are usually employed to solve this dilemma. The shrinking field technique takes advantage of the regression of the tumor; the field size is progressively reduced, and a higher dose is delivered to the center of the tumor where irradiation is likely to fail. In the booster technique the residual tumor receives a dose supplement of about 20 Gy at the end of the radiotherapy course.

Volume Change Following Irradiation

The tumor volume regression following irradiation in a tumor is the result of three mechanisms: cell killing, rate of dead cell removal, and repopulation. The delay after which nonviable cells will actually die is correlated with the cell turnover rate of the tumor. Thus, there is no direct proportionality between the rate of response and the proportion of cells that have become unable to proliferate and are doomed to die.

It is not advisable to adjust the total dose delivered to the tumor on the basis of the initial response; indeed, rapid tumor regression should not lead to a reduction of the planned dose, since the radiation dose which induces complete clinical remission is equal to only one-third of the tumor control dose.

Early and Late Complications

The doses are limited by the risk of radiation injury to normal tissues, which is related to the dose delivered and the size of the volume irradiated. *Early complications* are mainly observed in tissue with a rapid cell turnover (bone marrow, skin, mucosa, etc.). They are due to an imbalance between cell killing and compensatory cellular proliferation. After completion of irradiation they are reversible.

Late complications of RT manifest themselves months or years after completion of irradiation. They are not reversible. Their incidence does have some relation to the total dose, but the dose per fraction is critical. Late complications are mainly observed in tissues with a slow cell turnover: subcutaneous tissue, liver, lung, etc. When severe they may be incompatible with a normal life.

Role of Immunocompetence. The theory of immunosurveillance attributes to the immune system a major role in the reaction of the host against tumor cells. This gave rise to the fear of a detrimental effect of irradiation on the immune system regarding tumor growth. In fact, despite claims to the contrary, no clinical study demonstrates that irradiation enhances the onset of metastatic disease in man.

Technique of Radiotherapy

The high-energy beams generated by telecobalt units and linear accelerators liberated RT from the constraints of skin and superficial tissue reactions. Their high penetration made it possible to deliver sufficient doses to deep-seated tumors anywhere in the body.

The sharply defined edges of these beams allow for treatment of lesions located near critical tissues, such as the eye. It is also possible to shape the beam with lead shields, filter wedges and compensators, and thus to use large, complex fields tailored to the needs of the individual patient.

Computer dosimetry enables mapping of the dose distribution in the plane through the center of the tumor and in any other parallel or perpendicular plane. Three-dimensional display of the dose is becoming possible, a technique which will further ensure the precision and adequacy of dose distribution within the target.

Tumor localization is a prerequisite for precise RT. New imaging techniques, in particular computed tomography, have improved the quality of tumor delineation, which in turn has resulted in much better treatment protocols. Since a slight geographic error or an underdosage to a small part of the tumor, will greatly increase the probability of local failure, it can be hoped that these new techniques will result in an increased incidence of tumor control and a decreased incidence of injury to critical normal tissues.

The replacement of radium by radioactive isotopes such as iridium wires and cesium seeds has, in conjunction with afterloading techniques and computer dosimetry, greatly improved the efficacy of interstitial and intracavitary therapy. These localized irradiations of tumors are particularly useful in the treatment of carcinoma of the cervix, the bladder and the oral cavity. At Villejuif, for example, when radium was replaced by iridium wires the 5-year survival rate of patients with cancer of the anterior portion of the tongue increased from 18% for those treated between 1960 and 1965 to 50% for those treated between 1971 and 1973.

Quality Control. The sophistication of the RT being delivered in the specialized centers should not disguise the fact that the quality of RT is not the same in all centers. Several studies performed in the USA and in Europe have revealed that in many institutions the value of the treatment delivered is questionable. This may be due to a lack of training of personnel (radiotherapist and physicist), or to inadequate instrumentation (obsolete radiotherapy equipment, absence of computer facilities and simulators, etc.). Faulty radiotherapy techniques result in lower rates of tumor control (Kramer 1984).

Clinical Practice of Radiotherapy

Radiotherapy can be used alone or in combination with other treatment modalities: surgery and chemotherapy (CT).

Radiotherapy Alone

The advantage of treatment by RT alone is the preservation of the organ and/or the function, for example the preservation of the voice after treatment of cancer of the larynx. The target volume should encompass the tumor plus a safety margin around it and the regional lymph node areas which are likely to be involved, unless they are treated by surgery. The choice of tumor dose should take into account the characteristics of the tumor, the size of the target volume and the radiosensitivity of the critical normal tissues located near the tumor.

Some tumors, such as seminomas or lymphomas, can be controlled by doses of 40–45 Gy. Others are more radioresistant and the tumor control dose averages around 60–75 Gy, among them are, for example, cancers of the URDT or the uterus. The tumor control dose for breast tumors is even larger, from 70 to 80 Gy. In some subtypes of tumors (for example infiltrating or ulcerating tumors of the URDT), or when the tumor is very large, RT is less effective. In these patients the dose giving a high probability of tumor control entails an unacceptable risk of complications, and treatment by RT alone is inadvisable. However, RT still can play a role in conjunction with other treatment modalities, in particular surgery; if there is a medical contraindication to surgery, RT may be considered alone with a curative or palliative aim, or in combination with CT. Only in a few highly radioresistant tumors, such as those of the stomach or the colon, does RT have no role to play.

Combination of Radiotherapy and Surgery

Radiotherapy and surgery are associated in various circumstances. RT can control local recurrence after surgical excision of the tumor (e.g., breast and bladder tumors), and a local failure following treatment by radiotherapy alone can be salvaged by extended surgery. For example, transmaxillary buccopharyngectomy yields a 30% local control rate in cases of residue or relapse of a tumor of the oropharynx treated by RT.

The rationale for planned combined of irradiation and surgery is that the mechanism of failure for the two techniques is different. Irradiation failure occurs with bulky masses and not at the periphery of tumors where cells are small in number, unless it is performed without a safety margin around the tumor. Conversely, surgical resection is limited by the preservation of critical normal tissues adjacent to the tumor; microscopic disease extending beyond the macroscopic border of the tumor may be left behind.

Thus the two modalities are complementary: surgery can excise the gross masses, irradiation can eradicate microscopic disease.

A few decades ago postoperative RT was used infrequently because the prevailing concept held that one should wait for recurrence in order to have something tangible to irradiate. When it was recognized that higher doses are required to eradicate gross masses than subclinical disease, prophylactic irradiation of clinically uninvolved areas at risk of containing occult deposits was enhanced. This method is now widely used with excellent clinical results.

Preoperative Irradiation

Preoperative irradiation has a few theoretical advantages. (1) The blood supply has not been disturbed and microscopic disease is euoxic. (2) The incidence of distant metastases may be decreased because fewer viable malignant clonogenic cells may be dislodged by surgical manipulation. Theoretically, a relatively small dose (20 Gy) is sufficient for achieve this, and irradiation can be immediately followed by the surgical procedure; however, the few controlled clinical trials which have been performed have shown no significant decrease in the frequency of distant metastases. (3) The size of the tumor is reduced and unresectable tumors may become operable. However, it is not clear how often this actually results in local control, since the gross tumor may only be changed to a microscopic tumor and tumor recurrence will still result. Nevertheless, some data suggest that it may be of benefit in certain cases.

The main limitation of preoperative irradiation is the risk of significant increase in the incidence of complications associated with subsequent extensive surgical procedures. Thus 50 Gy is the maximum dose, and when this dose is given, it is then necessary to allow the tissues to recover from the irradiation (3–5 weeks). Low-dose preoperative irradiation (20 Gy) does not cause a delay in healing, so surgery can be performed immediately after irradiation, but the locoregional control rate is low.

Preoperative irradiation has another disadvantage: if a few weeks' interval was allowed between RT and surgery, irradiation prevents ascertainment of the initial anatomic extent, in particular of lymph node involvement. Likewise the assessment of histologic grade can be difficult.

Postoperative Irradiation

The main advantage of postoperative irradiation is that a higher dose may be given without significant risk. Furthermore, the subgroup of patients who might benefit from irradiation can be defined accurately as a consequence of surgical exploration and pathologic review. Unnecessary irradiation can be avoided, and if complete excision of the tumor is impossible a boost can be given to the appropriate area.

Another advantage is that time can be allowed for wound healing so that the radiation will not interfere with this process; however, it has been shown that the incidence of recurrence is higher when the irradiation has been delayed for over 6 weeks (Vikram et al. 1984).

In the peritoneal cavity surgery may cause loops of bowel to be fixed and this will increase the likelihood of small intestine damage by irradiation.

Both schedules require close cooperation between the surgeon and the radiotherapist. When postoperative RT is planned the surgeon must adapt his technique and the surgical excision may be less radical. Likewise, the radiotherapist must take into account in preoperative RT the type of surgical procedure which is planned, and in postoperative RT the extent of residual disease. For example, if there is a microscopically uninvolved surgical margin of more than 5 mm the radiation dose may be lower than when there is disease near the cut surface.

Conservative Treatment

Full advantage of the combination of RT and surgery is taken in conservative treatment. The surgical excision is limited to the removal of the gross mass, for example lumpectomy in the treatment of breast cancer. Subsequent irradiation, with relatively modest doses, eradicates the surrounding subclinical disease. This method has been recently proven effective for breast cancer and soft tissue sarcoma.

Spatial Cooperation

For several types of cancer RT and surgery are directed against different target volumes. For example, in laryngeal carcinoma RT is used for the treatment of the primary tumor so as to preserve normal phonation while surgery is used for the treatment of cervical lymph nodes; and in testicular seminoma orchidectomy is combined with irradiation of the abdominal lymph nodes.

Intraoperative Radiotherapy

In intraoperative RT, direct-view irradiation with high-energy electrons of surgically exposed tumor allows a good protection of uninvolved tissue. Thereafter, conventional fractionated external beam RT is administered. The preliminary results are promising; however, the technique is time-consuming and requires sophisticated equipment.

Combination of Radiotherapy and Chemotherapy

The association of RT and CT has two main purposes. The first is the addition of the effects of the two modalities on the primary tumor. The second is a spatial cooperation, RT being directed against the primary tumor and CT being used to control disseminated disease (Tubiana et al. 1985).

Tumor mass reduction by means of cytotoxic drugs prior to irradiation of the residual tumor may increase the effectiveness of RT in a less bulky tumor. Promising results have been reported in the treatment of breast tumors, soft tissue sarcoma, oropharynx and hypopharynx, rectum and anal canal. However, the future will show whether the shrinkage of the tumor obtained by CT actually results in therapeutic gain. One point is already clear: the radiation dose should not be significantly lowered because of the reduction in tumor size, since a decrease in local control rate was observed when lower tumor doses were used. This is in accordance with theoretical considerations. If a radiation dose of approximately 30 D_{50} is required to control a tumor treated by RT alone, it follows that when CT is used first and has been able to decrease the tumor volume by half, the necessary RT dose is 29 D_{50}. If CT has reduced the tumor diameter by half, the necessary RT dose is 26 D_{50}. It is only when CT has produced complete regression of the tumor that RT can be reduced to 20 D_{50}. Even when this is the case, a combination of RT and CT is useful only if the sum of the effects of the two modalities is less for the normal tissues than for the tumor. The additive effect of RT and CT on the local disease is shown by the lower incidence of local recurrences of breast tumors in patients who had received CT and RT than in those treated by RT only; the incidence of local recurrence is high in patients treated only by surgery and CT (Fisher et al. 1985).

A *sequential regimen* avoids interaction between the two modalities and reduces the cumulative effect on normal tissue. However, the therapeutic gain is often relatively small because (a) the efficacy of cytotoxic drugs on bulky tumors is often limited, and (b) under CT the clones of cells resistant to the cytotoxic drugs administered will expand. *Concomitant administration* of drugs and ionizing radiation delivers the two modalities without undue delay, but the risk is that the effect on normal tissues is often as great as that on the tumor, and the decrease in the tolerated radiation dose may outweigh the increase in the effect on neoplastic tissues.

Two methods have been used to obtain a therapeutic gain: (1) administration of drugs which do not provoke serious toxic effects on the critical tissues included in the irradiated volume, and (2) introduction of a sufficiently long interval between the completion of one modality and the initiation of the other. However, a delay of CT until after the completion of RT, or an interruption of CT during the course of RT, allows the occult metastases located outside the radiation field to increase in size.

Undue delays are avoided in *integrated regimens* in which CT is started with the usual scheduling of one cycle every month and RT courses are interdigitated between CT cycles. The results obtained with this alternating regimen are excellent in small cell lung carcinoma and in non-Hodgkin's lymphoma; the early and late tolerances are satisfactory (Tubiana et al. 1985).

However, such regimens, like other types of combination of RT and CT, are effective only on tumors which are both radiosensitive and chemosensitive. Otherwise, the toxic effects of both modalities are accumulated without much of an increase of the effect on neoplastic tissues.

References

Dutreix J., Tubiana M., Dutreix A. (1988) An approach to the interpretation of clinical data on the tumour control probability dose relationship. Radiotherapy Oncology 11: 239–248

Fertil B, Malaise EP (1985) Intrinsic radiosensitivity of human cell lines is correlated with radioresponsiveness of human tumors. Int J Radiat Oncol Biol Phys 11: 1699–1707

Fisher B, Bauer M, Margolese R et al. (1985) Five-year results of a randomized clinical trial comparing total mastectomy and segmental mastectomy with or without radiation in the treatment of breast cancer. N Engl J Med 312: 665–673

Fletcher GH (1980) Textbook of radiotherapy, 3rd edn. Lea and Febiger, Philadelphia

Fowler JF (1984) What next in fractionated radiotherapy? The first James Kirk memorial lecture. Br J Cancer 49 [Suppl VI]: 285–300

Koscielny S, Tubiana M, Le MG et al. (1984) Breast cancer: relationship between the size of the primary tumour and the probability of metastatic dissemination. Br J Cancer 49: 709–715

Kramer S (1984) The patterns of clinical cure in radiation therapy in the United States. Int J Radiat Oncol Biol Phys 10: 49–53

Malaise EP, Chavaudra N, Tubiana M (1973) The relationship

between growth rate, labelling index and histological type of human solid tumours. Eur J Cancer 9: 305–312

Suit H (1982) Potential for improving survival rates for the cancer patient by incrasing the efficacy of treatment of the primary lesion. Cancer 50: 1227–1234

Tubiana M. (1988) Repopulation in human tumors – A biological background for fractionation in radiotherapy. Acta Oncologica 27: 83–88

Tubiana M, Arriagada R, Cosset JM (1985) Sequencing of drugs and radiation. Cancer 55: 2131–2139

Tubiana M, Arriagada R, Sarrazin D (1986 a) Human cancer: natural history, radiation induced immunodepression and post-operative radiation therapy. Int J Radiat Oncol Biol Phys 12: 477–485

Tubiana M, Dutreix J, Wambersie A (1986 b) Radiobiologie humaine, vol 1. Hermann, Paris

Vikram B, Strong EW, Shah JP, Spiro R (1984) Failure in the neck following multimodality treatment for advanced head and neck cancer. Head Neck Surg 6: 724–729

Intraoperative Radiotherapy

H. J. Hoekstra and F. A. Calvo

Introduction

Today combined modality therapies comprising surgery, chemotherapy, and radiation procedures are used in the treatment of a variety of malignancies and have shown an improvement in the 5-year survival rates. New surgical techniques have been developed, and new and effective chemotherapeutics have become available. Progress is still being made in the development of new chemotherapeutic agents and less toxic drug dose schedules. Progress in radiation therapy has been achieved by the improvements in technical equipment and technical advances in methods of radiation therapy, including the use of computerized planning of radiation therapy and multiple fields. The aim has been to increase the dose to the tumor and minimize the dose to the adjacent normal tissues, thereby increasing the local control rate without increasing the complication rate. The delivery of tumoricidal doses of radiation with external beam techniques, especially the treatment of intra-abdominal, retroperitoneal, or pelvic malignancies, can be accompagnied by a short- or long-term toxicity to normal tissues.

Intraoperative radiotherapy (IORT) is a technique in which a single high dose of electron beam irradiation is delivered during a surgical procedure to a tumor or tumor bed and/or areas of possible local regional spread, with the ability to shield or physically move normal tissues and organs out of the treatment field. Interest has grown in this experimental treatment modality as a method of potentially overcoming the limitations of conventional fractionated external beam radiotherapy (EBRT) by limiting the radiation exposure of normal tissues and, therefore, limiting the radiation toxicity.

History

At the beginning of this century, only low-energy X-rays (50–100 kV) were available in the treatment of cancer. It was impossible to treat intra-abdominal malignancies by irradiation because of the poor penetration and dose distribution of the radiation equipment. To overcome these limitations Beck (1909) decided to perform a laparotomy in which the gastric or colon tumor was surgically exposed and submitted to dermopexy. Now it was possible to irradiate the tumor with low-voltage contact roentgen. The so-called eventration treatment earned limited popularity for the treatment of intra-abdominal malignancies, and the technique was modified by Eloesser (1937) in the early 1930s. A laparotomy was performed, followed by an excision or dissection of the tumor, and a large cylinder was placed over the area to be irradiated. The small bowel was packed off with gauze, the skin protected with lead, and the tumor or tumor bed irradiated with 2500–4500 roentgen using 200–250-kV X-rays. No short- or long-term complications were described (Eloesser 1937; Schumann 1933; Pack and Livingston 1940). Several years later the technique of IORT was combined with pre- or postoperative EBRT (Fairchild and Shorter 1947; Barth and Meinel 1959). However, the poor penetration of the low-energy radiation prevented its extensive use.

The introduction of megavoltage irradiation in the 1960s hampered the further use of orthovoltage. Now it seemed to be possible to treat intra-abdominal malignancies with a sufficient dose of irradiation, but the results were not satisfactory. Interest in IORT was awakened in the mid-1970s mainly through the efforts of Abe et al. (1974), who demonstrated that megavoltage IORT could safely and effectively be used in areas within the abdomen. Today this experimental treatment modality of electron beam IORT is being utilized and investigated in several institutions in Japan, the United States, and Europe (Abe and Takahashi 1981; Gunderson et al. 1983; Hoekstra et al. 1987).

Tissue Tolerance

Until recently, the radiobiological effects of varying doses of IORT were unknown. Although the biological efficacy of a single fraction is unknown, it is probably equivalent biologically to a dose of a factor 2–2.5 greater than that given by conventional fractionated EBRT (Suit 1973).

Abe and Arakawa (1967) investigated the effect of a single massive dose ranging from 25 Gy to 30 Gy from a cobalt - 60 unit to the stomach and intestine with various field sizes in a canine model. There was severe morbidity and mortality. Only two out of 11 dogs survived more than 1 month. However, radiation damage to tissue and organs outside the treatment volume was minimized. Subsequently, IORT tissue tolerance studies were initiated at the National Cancer Institute (NCI) at Bethesda to study the tissue tolerance of normal and surgically manipulated tissues to IORT before clinical treatment was started. A canine model was used to provide guidelines for the clinical IORT doses. Because the theoretical biological advantage of IORT seemed to be most compelling in the treatment of abdominal malignancies, initial experimental IORT tissue tolerance of retroperitoneal and intra-abdominal tissues were investigated by Sindelar et al. (1983b) and later also for mediastinal and thoracic organs and tissues.

Intraoperative irradiation of the retroperitoneum, including aorta, vena cava, inferior portion of the left kidney, and distal portion of the left ureter, was investigated at five dose levels: 0, 20, 30, 40, and 50 Gy. The kidney and ureter appear to be highly sensitive to IORT. The kidney showed parenchymal atrophy and hyalinization necrosis at 20 Gy. The radiosensitive ureter showed dose-related ureteral fibrosis, which regularly led to ureteral stricture and therefore hydronephrosis and secondary kidney damage. In contrast to this, the aorta and vena cava tolerated a single dose of up to 50 Gy well. Subintimal and medial fibrosis of the aorta and vena cava may occur at doses of over 30 Gy (Sindelar et al. 1982a). The tolerance of aortic anastomosis up to 20, 30, and 40 Gy IORT was studied. An adequate healing of the anastomosis at all dose levels with no suture failure was found. Stenosis may occur at any dose level (Tepper et al. 1983). The radiation-induced decrease in cell turnover appears to abate with time (Sindelar et al. 1983a).

Although the small and large bowel are, in general, excluded from the IORT field, because of their relatively high radiation sensitivity, the small bowel tolerance to IORT was investigated at three dose levels: 20, 30, and 45 Gy. Mucosal ulceration and muscular fibrosis developed at a dose of 20 Gy, while at doses of 30 and 45 Gy obstruction through fibrosis or perforation of the bowel were found, especially in normal functional bowel. Defunctionalized small bowel tolerates doses at these levels slightly better (Tepper et al. 1983; Sindelar et al. 1983b). Intestinal anastomosis demonstrated an adequate healing up to 45 Gy and the radiation-induced decrease in cell turnover appears to normalize after a certain time period (Sindelar et al. 1983a).

IORT is frequently used in pancreatic and gastric malignancies. Intraoperative irradiation of these tumors, or resected tumor beds, and areas of loco regional spread will include the porto hepatic area. Therefore, the tolerance of the liver hilum of rabbits to IORT was investigated by Todoroki (1978). Slight fibrosis, atrophy, and degeneration was detected in the bile duct, portal vein, hepatic artery, and surrounding liver tissues after 30 Gy. The effect of IORT to the bile duct and surrounding tissues was also investigated in a canine model at 20, 30, and 45 Gy. Dose-related fibrosis and partial obstruction with secondary hepatic changes of the liver-parenchyma were found, and no changes were observed in the irradiated portions of the portal vein and hepatic artery (Sindelar et al. 1982b). Biliary enteric anastomosis fail to heal at 20 Gy, suggesting that the bile duct does not tolerate any therapeutic irradiation after surgical manipulation (Sindelar et al. 1982b, 1983b).

IORT may have a role in the treatment of superficial bladder tumors. Therefore, the tolerance of the bladder to IORT was investigated at six dose levels: 0, 20, 25, 30, 35, and 40 Gy. The bladder trigone and one of the ureteral orifices were irradiated. Above 25 Gy, fibrosis of the ureteral orifice induced hydronephrosis. The bladder epithelium did not show any macroscopic erosion or ulceration. Microscopically the mucosa remained intact up to 45 Gy, but dose-related submucosal fibrosis and inflammation was found (Kinsella et al. 1988).

Peripheral nerve radiation damage is an uncommon complication after conventional fractionated EBRT, but clinical evidence of peripheral nerve injury was found after clinical IORT (Kinsella et al. 1985). Therefore, the tolerance of peripheral nerves to IORT was investigated at dose levels ranging from 20 to 75 Gy. A linear relation between radiation dose versus hind limb paresis was found. The nerve loss and fibrosis, which appeared was dose-time related, and no vascular injury such as occlusion or thrombosis was found. Therefore, in IORT the peripheral nerve is one of the other dose-limiting normal tissues (Kinsella et al. 1985).

The tolerance of mediastinal structures to IORT was investigated at four dose levels: 0, 20, 30, and 40 Gy. Intact mediastinal structures tolerate IORT up to doses of 30 Gy, although 30- or 40-Gy IORT may induce cardiac and lung damage without clinical significance (Barnes et al. 1987). An intact canine esophagus tolerated 20-Gy IORT without significant toxicity, but higher doses of 20–30 Gy may induce esophagitis with ulceration and stricture (Sindelar et al. 1988a). IORT to the bronchial stump after left pneumectomy was investigated at 0, 20, 30, and 40 Gy. Esophagitis occurred in the majority of the animals, but no stump dehiscence occurred (Pass et al. 1987).

A summary of the results of the IORT tissue tolerance studies in a canine model is shown in Table 1.

Radiation Physics and Surgical Aspects

IORT can be performed with both orthovoltage or megavoltage equipment. Although orthovoltage is less expensive, it is not recommended for IORT because of its poor depth-dose characteristics, wide-angled setting, absorbed dose enhancement in bone, and the low exposure rate requiring long treatment time. There is also interest in the use of orthovoltage IORT (Rich et al. 1984). An electron beam is preferred because of the "flat" dose distribution (penetration quality) and the sharp fall-off of the beam. With proper energy selection of the accelerator, a tumor or tumor bed can be effectively treated while sparing the adjacent normal tissues (Fig. 1).

There are two opinions concerning the use of IORT. In the beginning IORT was utilized at Kyoto University, Howard University, and the NCI as an adjunct to gross surgical resection of various intra-abdominal, retroperitoneal, or pelvic malignancies. In contrast to this, the Massachusetts General Hospital (MGH) and Mayo Clinic combined ± 50 Gy EBRT with an intraoperative "boost" of 15–20 Gy (Abe and Takahasi 1981; Gunderson et al. 1983). Although the optimal use of IORT is still unknown, it is believed that IORT has its greatest value in combination with maximal surgical resection of the tumor, with or without EBRT. Initial clinical experience with IORT involved the use of single fields of EBRT. In modern IORT treatment, extensive surgical resections have necessitated the use of extensive IORT fields which are constructed utilizing field-matching techniques (Sindelar et al. 1988b).

The IORT applicator has three functions: (a) collimation of the electron beam; (b) delineation of the

Table 1. Tolerance of normal and surgically manipulated tissues to single-dose intraoperative electron beam irradiation based on a canine model

Organ or tissue	Maximal dose without severe complications (Gy)	Comments and findings
Normal tissues		
Aorta	50	Patency to 50 Gy; fibrosis over 30 Gy
Vena cava	50	Patency to 50 Gy; fibrosis over 30 Gy
Intestine (functional)	20	Ulceration, fibrosis, stenosis over 20 Gy
Intestine (defunctionalized)	45	Intact to 45 Gy; fibrosis over 20 Gy
Bile duct	20	Fibrosis, stenosis over 20 Gy
Kidney	20	Parenchymal atrophy and hyalinization necrosis over 20 Gy
Ureter	30	Fibrosis, stenosis over 30 Gy
Nerve	25	Fibrosis, fiber loss over 25 Gy; paralysis over 40 Gy
Bladder	30	Stenosis of the ureteral-vesical junction over 25 Gy; bladder mocosa intact up to 45 Gy, dose-related fibrosis
Esophagus	20	Esophagitis and ulceration over 30 Gy
Bronchial stump	40	No stump dehiscence to 40 Gy
Mediastinal structures	20	Cardiac and lung fibrosis over 30 Gy
Surgically manipulated tissues		
Aortic suture line	45	Intact to 45 Gy; fibrosis, stenosis over 20 Gy, sometimes producing late occlusion
Intestinal suture line	45	Intact to 45 Gy; fibrosis, stenosis over 20 Gy
Biliary suture line	20	Suture line disruption at 20 Gy
Bladder suture line	30	Dose-related contraction over 30 Gy, no suture line disruption

treatment volume; and (c) retraction of tissue and organs outside the electron beam.

The lucite, acrylic electron beam applicators are not available commercially. Different applicator systems, circular, rectangular, pentagonal and horseshoe-shaped applicators, different sizes and bevels have been described (McCullough and Anderson 1982; Biggs et al. 1983; Fraass et al. 1985; McCullough and Gunderson 1988). Isodose curves for each applicator are crucial for IORT delivery and need to be individually measured for all various electron energies and applicators for single and multiple field matching (Shaw et al. 1987). The applicators are gas-sterilized at 50 °C with an outgas time of 24 h. The rectangular and square applicators are difficult to use intra-abdominally, and circular applicators do not allow multiple field matching. The horse-shoe-shaped or "squircle" (one square and one circular end) slightly bevelled applicator, can easily be used intra-abdominally and facilitates multiple field matching (Sindelar et al. 1988b). A stainless steel shield placed around the applicator, decreases the peripheral dose to normal structures to approximately 2% of the total delivered dose, sparing the adjacent structures, and also acts as a tissue retractor for intestinal viscera (Fraass et al. 1985). When the treatment field is identified, the appropriate applicators are selected. When necessary, immobile tissues or viscera may be shielded with customized, sterilized

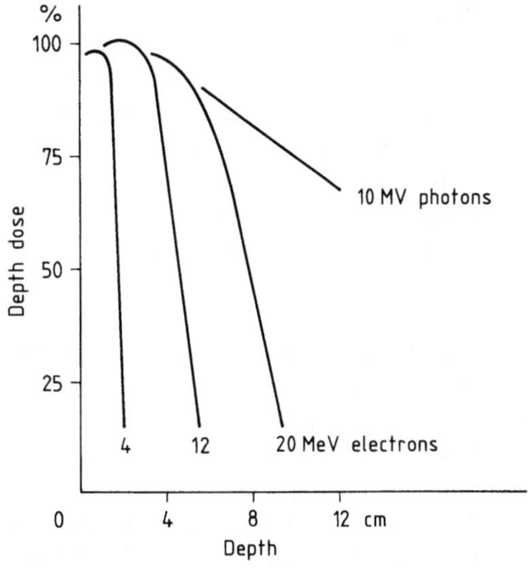

Fig. 1. Depth dose curves for 4-, 12-, and 20-MeV electron beams and 10-MV photons

lead wafers. The stainless steel shield is placed, and the acrylic applicator placed within the shield and docked to the linear accelerator head. A modified surgical table allowing fine lateral, longitudinal, and vertical motions, while preserving the pitch and roll motions of a standard surgical operating table, can reduce the difficulty of docking the electron applicators to the head of the linear accelerator during IORT procedures (Fraass et al. 1985).

Visualization and documentation of treatment fields during IORT is crucial to ensure adequate field coverage as well as exclusion of normal tissue from the electron beam. Various systems, such as periscopes, mirrors, and television verification systems, have been described for use in IORT (Fraass et al. 1983). Treatment field verification and documentation are both essential for IORT treatment, especially when multiple fields are used.

Optimal surgical exposure is needed for IORT treatment. Typically, IORT procedures may require more extensive incisions than routinely performed for comparable tumors in order to achieve adequate mobilization and exposure to IORT. In general, first the resection is performed, followed by IORT to the resected tumor bed and/or areas of loco regional spread. Surgical reconstructions are performed after the irradiation procedure (Sindelar et al. 1988b). When necessary, immobile tissue or viscera may be shielded with customized, sterilized lead sheets. All IORT electron doses are quoted at the 90% isodose line and at D max, and it has also been established that the 90% dose be the minimal dose to the tumor. The applicator needs to be larger than the treatment field by at least 1 cm. If possible, one field is used, otherwise multiple fields are necessary (Shaw et al. 1987). When multiple fields are used, considerable care must be exercised in the positioning of fields after the first to ensure accurate and adequate abutment of fields. For homogeneity of field dose, the inside edge of the applicator is overlapped for a distance of 3 mm. A smaller overlap would lead to areas of underdosing, and a greater overlap would lead to areas of excessive dose (Fraass et al. 1985; Shaw et al. 1987).

During the IORT procedure, the patient and the anesthesia equipment are monitored by closed circuit television from outside the treatment room. With integrated devices, close continuous monitoring of ECG, arterial blood pressure, central venous pressure, and temperature are possible. In case of emergency, access to the patient is available within seconds if malfunction of anesthesia equipment or other difficulties occur (Ashayeri et al. 1986).

Clinical Results

Almost 2500 patients have been treated with IORT in Japan, the United States, and Europe, with or without EBRT, the majority with resectable or unresectable abdominal and pelvic malignancies. The largest experience in IORT has been published by Kyoto University in Japan, followed by the MGH, Mayo Clinic, Howard University, National Cancer Institute (NCI), New England Deaconess Hospital and Joint Center for Radiation Therapy (NED-JCRT), and Navarra University. Only the NCI is performing prospective randomized clinical trials with IORT in gastric, pancreatic, retroperitoneal malignancies, and pelvic tumors (NIH 1984). Therefore, it is difficult to draw any conclusions from the literature. The Radiation Therapy Oncology Group (RTOG) has developed the first cooperative multi-institutional effort to explore IORT in prospective, multicentric trials.

Gastric Cancer

At Kyoto University Hospital, Abe et al. (1974) have performed a prospective nonrandomized study in patients with stage I–IV gastric cancer in which surgical resection was combined with or without a single fraction of IORT (28–35 Gy), 28 Gy to microscopic residuals, and 30–35 Gy to gross or macroscopic residual disease. The results show an improvement over surgery alone – IORT for stage II (84% versus 62%), stage III (62% versus 37%), and stage IV (15% versus 0%). No benefit in survival was found for stage I disease patients (87% versus 93%) (Abe et al. 1987).

The NCI is performing a randomized prospective clinical trial in gastric cancer which extends through the serosa, positive locoregional nodes, or gross residual disease: surgical resection with 20 Gy IORT versus surgical resection and postoperative EBRT, 45–50 Gy over 5–6 weeks (Sindelar et al. 1983b; Kinsella and Sindelar 1985). Until now no difference in local control or survival has been demonstrated. The MGH is trying to accrue patients into a study of preoperative 45 Gy EBRT, followed by gastrectomy and IORT to the tumor bed. At the Mayo Clinic patients receive low-dose preoperative EBRT and surgery. If there is any residual disease after surgery, they receive an intraoperative boost within 10 days postoperatively, followed by EBRT with or without chemotherapy (Tepper et al. 1984).

IORT has a possible therapeutic utility in controlling locally advanced gastric cancer, without increasing the treatment morbidity and with no long-term complications.

Pancreatic Cancer

The effect of IORT has been mainly studied as a single treatment modality with locally advanced pancreatic cancer. In general, 15–30 Gy IORT was delivered, sometimes in combination with 50 Gy pre- or postoperative EBRT and/or chemotherapy (Goldson et al. 1981; Sindelar et al. 1983b; Abe 1984; Shipley et al. 1984; Tepper et al. 1984; Gunderson et al. 1985; Kinsella and Sindelar 1985; Tepper 1985; Sindelar and Kinsella 1986a, b). There was an improvement in local control, but no improvement in survival (Goldson et al. 1981; Abe 1984; Shipley et al. 1984; Gunderson et al. 1985; Tepper 1985; Sindelar and Kinsella 1986a, b). Improvement in local control may be possibly enhanced with the use of intravenous misonidazole (3.5 mg/m^2), a radiosensitizer, given 20 min prior to IORT in order to decrease the radioresistance of hypoxic cells to IORT (Shipley et al. 1984). Pain relief was found within 1 week in 70% of the patients receiving more than 20 Gy IORT (Abe and Takahashi 1981; Tepper 1985). Severe upper gastrointestinal bleeding from duodenal ulceration, and endocrine and exocrine pancreatic insufficiency are the major long-term complications (Sindelar et al. 1983b; Hoekstra et al. 1985). Intraoperative mobilization of the stomach, exclusion of at least a part of the duodenum and gastric and biliary bypasses are recommended in the IORT treatment of unresectable pancreatic cancer.

Prospective randomized clinical trials for unresectable and resectable pancreatic cancer are performed at the NCI. Patients with unresectable pancreatic cancer receive either 25 Gy IORT, 50 Gy EBRT and 5-fluorouracil (5FU), or 50 Gy EBRT and 5FU (Sindelar and Kinsella 1986b). Patients with resectable pancreatic cancer who have positive resection margins, positive regional lymph nodes, or gross residual disease receive either 20 Gy IORT or 50 Gy EBRT (Sindelar and Kinsella 1986a). No preliminary conclusions can be drawn. IORT in combination with EBRT has demonstrated an improvement in the local control rate for unresectable pancreatic cancer without an improvement in survival. Detailed autopsy analyses of radiation effects on the pancreas and adjacent tissues showed that IORT can induce a progressive retroperitoneal fibrosis and fibrosis of the porta hepatis in patients with resectable pancreatic carcinoma. In unresectable pancreatic carcinoma the major expression of IORT with EBRT is a progressive fibrosis of the pancreas with vascular sclerosis, nerve degeneration, atrophy of acinar cells, and atypical changes in the ducts of the pancreas, as well as degenerative changes of the pancreatic tumor (Hoekstra et al. 1988b). The value of IORT in resectable pancreatic cancer is still unknown.

Colorectal Cancer

Unresectability and local failure after surgical resection are the two major problems in the treatment of rectal cancer. To improve local control, investigators at the MGH and Mayo Clinic have treated patients with locally advanced rectal cancer with 50 Gy preoperative EBRT, followed by low anterior resection or abdominoperineal resection and 15–20 Gy IORT to the resected tumor bed. A dose of 15 Gy is used in patients with only microscopic residual disease, whereas a dose of 20 Gy is delivered to patients with gross residual disease. These studies show a strong survival advantage and local control compared with patients treated with 50 Gy EBRT and surgery alone (Tepper et al. 1984; Gunderson et al. 1985, 1988). IORT used in combination with EBRT and surgery did not significantly increase severe complications (Tepper et al. 1984). IORT may significantly improve the local control of patients with locally advanced rectal cancer treated with high-dose preoperative EBRT, surgery, and IORT, without increasing the complication rate. There is an increased risk of peripheral neuropathy and ureteral obstruction (Shaw et al. 1988).

Biliary Tract Cancer

Cancer of the biliary tract is frequently unresectable and the anatomical area prohibits sufficient doses of EBRT. In a multicenter study 25–30 Gy IORT was delivered to unresectable biliary tract cancer. Approximately 90% of the patients had recanalization of the obstruction portion of the bile duct. A single dose of 35 Gy IORT is safe and can be a potentially curative dose, as long as the lesion is smaller than 3 cm in diameter (Todoroki et al. 1980; Abe and Takahashi 1981). At the Mayo Clinic patients with unresectable biliary tract cancer are preoperatively treated with 45–50 Gy EBRT, followed by 15–20 Gy IORT as a booster dose and 20–30 Gy with transcatheter sources. The early results are encouraging but the numbers of patients are too small (Buskirk et al. 1984; Gunderson et al. 1985). IORT may enhance local control especially for extrahepatic biliary tract cancer without increasing morbidity.

Retroperitoneal Sarcomas

Adequate surgical resection of retroperitoneal sarcomas is in general difficult, retroperitoneal sarcomas, therefore, have a tendency to recur locally. High-dose postoperative radiotherapy (50 Gy) may improve local control but also induce severe intestinal morbidity (Glenn et al. 1985). The NCI is performing a prospective clinical trial in patients with retroperitoneal sarcomas. All the patients are treated with surgery and randomized to receive 20 Gy IORT to the resected tumor bed and 35–40 Gy postoperative EBRT or standard therapy consisting of high-dose, 50–55 Gy postoperative EBRT (Kinsella et al. 1988). At the MGH in contrast to the NCI, patients with a retroperitoneal sarcoma receive 45–50 Gy EBRT preoperatively, followed by surgery and an intraoperative boost of 15–20 Gy IORT (Tepper et al. 1984). At Kyoto University patients receive only surgery and 30–45 Gy IORT to the tumor bed and no EBRT (Abe and Takahashi 1981).

All three institutions achieved satisfactory local control rate with low treatment morbidity. The NCI retroperitoneal soft tissue sarcoma study demonstrated no improvement in survival but a lower treatment morbidity and better local control (Kinsella et al. 1988). Therefore, in the treatment of retroperitoneal sarcomas, IORT is promising.

Cervical Cancer

In patients with an advanced stage of cervical cancer, there is a high incidence of involvement of the para-aortic and pelvic lymph nodes. The treatment of these metastases with high-dose EBRT induces severe intestinal morbidity. Consequently, Delgado et al. (1984), at Howard University, are investigating the role of surgery, IORT, and postoperative EBRT. After laparotomy the intestine and ureters are mobilized and the para-aortic lymph node area is treated from the renal vessels to the aortic bifurcation; the pelvic nodal region is also treated while avoiding field overlap. Patients with pathologically negative nodes were treated with 10 Gy IORT, and patients with grossly involved lymph nodes received 25 Gy IORT. Some patients received intracavitary radiation, as well as 25–45 Gy EBRT. The combination therapy was well tolerated, but no further conclusion can be drawn (Delgado et al. 1984). IORT for advanced cervical cancer seems attractive and reasonable in comparison to conventional radiotherapy techniques.

Bladder and Prostate Cancer

The IORT experience in bladder and prostate malignancies is limited to the Japanese experience. Matsumoto et al. (1981) initiated a multi-institutional study in which superficial bladder tumors were treated through an open cystostomy and 25–30 Gy IORT, without any other surgical or nonsurgical treatment, followed by 30–40 Gy EBRT. Good bladder function was preserved with a local (5-year) recurrence rate of only 19%. The uretheral orifice and bladder trigone were included in the IORT portal if necessary, without serious short- or long-term complications.

At Kyoto University, localized prostate cancer was treated with 20–35 Gy IORT to the prostate tumor by a perineal or transpubic approach. A single IORT dose of 35 Gy or a lower booster dose of 25 Gy and EBRT can be curative in localized prostate cancer. Acute complications such as dysuria and hematuria were encountered in all patients (Takahashi et al. 1985). The IORT treatment for superficial bladder tumors and localized prostate cancer is feasible, but further studies are necessary (Shipley et al. 1987).

Brain Tumors

Kyoto and Howard Universities have treated a small number of patients with brain tumors, primary glial and meningeal tumors with IORT and EBRT. At Kyoto University patients were first treated with 30–40 Gy EBRT, followed 4 weeks later by craniotomy, removal of necrotic tissue, and 10–20 Gy IORT to the residual tumor or tumor bed. Patients treated with EBRT and IORT react significantly better than those receiving EBRT only (Terao 1981 quoted by Abe and Takahashi 1981). In contrast to this, patients at Howard University first underwent surgical resection and decompression, followed by 15 Gy IORT to the tumor bed. After surgical recovery the patients received 55 Gy EBRT. The combined treatment modality was well tolerated when the cranial vault was decompressed (Goldson et al. 1984).

Preliminary results show promise for surgical debulking and an IORT boost to the tumor bed for meningeal tumors. Large animal studies are necessary for tissue toxicity and morbidity studies, prior to the further clinical use of IORT for brain malignancies.

Pediatric Tumors

One of the more challenging problems in pediatric oncology is the management of children with extensive intra-abdominal, retroperitoneal, or pelvic malignancies. Small children tolerate EBRT well, but the extreme sensitivity of their normal tissue to radiation may cause severe morbidity. The experience with IORT for pediatric malignancies is very limited.

A few institutions have treated experimentally several patients with unresectable or marginally resectable retroperitoneal tumors, such as neuroblastoma, rhabdomyosarcoma, Wilms' tumors, and Ewing's sarcomas, in combination with EBRT and chemotherapy. The limited experience has show the feasibility of IORT for pediatric malignancies (Kaufman et al. 1984; Hoekstra et al. 1986). The future of IORT in pediatric oncology remains to be explored. Particularly, areas of residual disease may benefit from a boost of IORT. As survival rates with some tumors improve, the side effects of conventional EBRT become relatively more significant. By allowing a reduction of the dose given with external beams, IORT may reduce the impact without sacrificing results previously achieved.

Lung and Mediastinal Tumors

IORT experience in lung cancer is very limited. Abe and Takahashi (1981) reported on IORT for unresectable lung cancer and concluded that lung cancer is no indication for IORT in contrast to mediastinal tumors. Howard University, the University of Graz and the NCI have also treated some patients with lung cancer (Pass et al. 1987; Gunderson et al. 1983, 1987; Arian-Schad et al. 1988). It is too early to draw any conclusion, but the IORT treatment could induce esophagitis when the esophagus was in the IORT portal. The acute and late normal tissue tolerance of bronchial stump and esophagus as well as mediastinal structures is currently being investigated at the NCI (Barnes et al. 1987; Pass et al. 1987; Sindelar et al. 1988a). Based on these experimental studies, the further clinical use of IORT for lung and mediastinal tumors needs to be planned.

Complications

When a new combined modality therapy is introduced, it is necessary to evaluate carefully treatment-related complications. IORT is used in combination with or without EBRT, with or without surgical resection. Although more than 2000 patients have been treated with IORT, it is very difficult to analyze the IORT data about the specific toxicity and complications related to this new treatment technique (Hoekstra et al. 1985, 1987). Experimental IORT tissue tolerance studies have shown the tissue tolerance in a variety of intact and surgically manipulated tissues (Abe and Arakawa 1967; Todoroki 1978; Sindelar et al. 1982a; Sindelar et al. 1982b, 1983a, b, 1986, 1988a; Tepper et al. 1983; Kinsella et al. 1984; Kinsella et al. 1985; Barnes et al. 1987; Pass et al. 1987). Autopsy studies of patients with IORT has demonstrated the validity of the canine model for IORT tissue tolerance studies (Sindelar et al. 1986).

In the majority of the IORT centers, patients are transported from the operating theater to the radiation department and back to the operating theater. No anesthetic- or transportation-related complications attributable to exposure to nonsterile conditions have been described (Tepper et al. 1984; Hoekstra et al. 1985). Complications in docking procedures can be expected, especially in the upper abdomen and pelvis, where the patient anatomy makes it difficult to irradiate the defined areas. Multiple field matching is especially difficult in these areas.

The dose tolerance of the pancreas to IORT, or in combination with EBRT and/or chemotherapy, is still unknown, as is the secondary induced morbidity when IORT is performed for unresectable pancreatic cancer. About 25% of the patients develop an upper gastrointestinal bleeding from necrotic tumor or "benign ulcer" from an IORT dose of more than 25 Gy (Sindelar et al. 1985). Postirradiation edema of the pancreas, ulcers, and gastritis may be the result of direct irradiation of duodenum or stomach. Irradiation of stomach and duodenum should therefore be avoided when possible, or bypass procedures performed after IORT. Irradiation of pancreas or bile duct will induce stenosis of the bile duct. Biliary bypasses can prevent biliary obstruction due to tumor or irradiation-induced fibrosis. Pancreatic endo- and exocrine insufficiency is common in pancreatic cancer, but can also be the expression of radiation-induced pancreatic fibrosis, requiring supplementation with oral pancreatic enzymes. The pancreas is also at risk for complications when IORT in the upper abdomen is performed after gastrectomy (Sindelar et al. 1983b; Tepper 1985). Pancreatitis, pancreatic fistula, pseudocyst formation, and late endocrine and exocrine pancreatic insufficiency are common complications (Sindelar et al. 1983b; Tepper 1985). In general, careful surgery and positioning of the treatment cone can prevent this kind of complication.

Nerve injuries are uncommon after conventional radiotherapy in contrast to IORT. Kinsella et al. (1985) studied the effect of IORT on peripheral nerves in a canine model and found linear dose-time correlation with hind limb paresis over the dose ranges of 20–27.5 Gy IORT. Histological examinations showed dose-related nerve fiber loss and fibrosis. These kind of peripheral nerve injuries were also documentated in patients treated with IORT and EBRT for pelvic or retroperitoneal malignancies (Kinsella et al. 1985; Shaw et al. 1988). Tepper et al. (1984) found no increase in severe complications with the addition of 10–20 Gy IORT in patients with locally advanced rectal cancer treated with 50 Gy preoperative radiotherapy and surgery.

The IORT working group has developed quality control parameters for the use and evaluation of IORT (Tepper et al. 1986). The areas of expertise necessary for appropriate IORT delivery and accurate data analysis can be divided into five basic areas: physics, surgical procedure, pathological evaluation of the specimens, actual delivery of the IORT, and patient selection and follow-up. Unfortunately, no published data are available in which the scoring system for IORT complications was used. It is clear that IORT has a potential morbidity which must be considered in the treatment planning, relative to its potential advantage in tumor control and dose sparing of normal tissues. The ureter, kidney, and peripheral nerves are the primary IORT dose-limiting structures within the retroperitoneum, and intraoperative irradiation should be avoided.

Project Development

Intraoperative delivery of radiation is not a simple procedure. An IORT program requires cooperation and input from a variety of disciplines such as surgeons, radiation oncologists, anesthesists, physicists, theater nurses, and radiation technologists. For the evaluation of the IORT treatment the support of a radiation biologist and pathologist cannot be missed for clinical pathological correlations of therapeutic efficacy on neoplastic tissue and possible toxic effects on normal tissues (Table 2). One surgeon and one radiation oncologist need to coordinate the IORT group, and they are primarily responsible for the IORT program and general treatment philosophy. Although it is not essential that they perform all the IORT procedures, it is preferable at the beginning of an IORT program.

Table 2. IORT group participants

Surgery	Delivery of IORT	IORT patients' follow-up	Treatment evaluation
Surgeon Anesthesist Theater nurse Radiation therapist	Radiation therapist Surgeon Theater nurse Physicist Radiation technologist	Surgeon Radiation therapist	Surgeon Radiation therapist Pathologist Radiobiologist Physicist

It is important to determine which methods of performing the IORT are the most convenient and cost effective. IORT treatment should not be done on a casual basis. First, the cost of this experimental treatment modality is substantial, and, secondly, there is a need for IORT treatment evaluation of palliative and curative IORT cases requiring a certain input per year. Therefore, it is recommended that potential patients be identified for this new treatment modality and that attempts be made to estimate the overall cost effectiveness.

Where should IORT be carried out? Should we build an operating theater in the radiation department, or a radiation room in the operating theater? A specific IORT suite is justified when an IORT research program exists, and a certain number of patients are treated with IORT. To maximize the efficacy of IORT, the Groningen IORT group decided to construct a specific IORT facility within the general operating theater of their new hospital. This is a unique situation, with the opportunity of treating patients with IORT at any time and, if necessary, more than one IORT procedure can be performed on the same day (Hoekstra et al. 1988a). When such a facility is not available, the patient needs to be transported. Transportation of an IORT patient from the operating theater to the radiation area and back is not hazardous (Hoekstra et al. 1985).

There is no doubt about the advantage of megavoltage intraoperative irradiation over orthovoltage irradiation. A high-energy electron beam linear accelerator provides a range of electron energies which allows a spectrum of tumor volume to be treated. The sharp fall-off dose at specific depths allows accurate treatment of defined volume while limiting irradiation of underlying structures. Although orthovoltage equipment is less expensive, it is not recommended for IORT because of its poor depth-dose characteristics, wide angle setting, absorbed dose enhancement in bone, and the low exposure rate requiring long treatment time. However, a linear acceleator requires more shielding of the treatment room, necessary for safe operation, and can add substantially to the initial cost of an IORT program.

Although the NCI has made a through study of the effect of IORT on a variety of tissues and organs, the radiobiological effects of single high dose electron beam irradiation combined with conventional fractionated external beam irradiation are still unknown. The effect of IORT and EBRT to normal tissue and organs needs to be studied. When an IORT project is developed, an IORT research project should just be initiated.

Future Prospects

The efficacy of IORT depends not only on the dose, but also on the stability of the patient's circulation, which is related to the tissue perfusion, the arterial PO_2, and level of temperature of the various tissues and organs located in the IORT portal. Hypoxic cells are radioresistant. The effect of radiation will be more effective when perfusion is maximal, the saturation optimal, and the tissue temperature as high as possible. Radiosensitizers can increase the radiosensitivity of the hypoxic cells. Local hyperthermia may increase radiation-induced cell death or reduce the cell repair capacity. Hyperthermia and radiosensitizers may possibly enhance the cancericidal effect of IORT (Hahn 1982; Phillips 1985). Further radiobiological and tissue tolerance studies are therefore necessary: the effect of the combination IORT and EBRT, IORT and local hyperthermia, IORT and sensitizers, as well as other combinations of IORT, EBRT, local hyperthermia, and sensitizers needs to be studied.

The technical and physics aspects of IORT are also underdeveloped. Have we already designed the optimal applicators for IORT? Is there a need for a color television verification system, allowing continuous visualization of the treatment field during the docking and irradiation procedure? Dose calculation and verification of IORT treatment is under investigation and seems to be promising (Bakker et al. 1984). Special physics computerized investigation programs are necessary for a scientific documentation of the treatment planning of IORT, as well as the EBRT dose, for detailed treatment failure analysis. Further physics IORT research programs need to be initiated.

Summary

IORT is feasible for various intra-abdominal, retroperitoneal, pelvic, and various other malignancies. IORT can be delivered to a certain tumor volume or resected tumor bed and areas of loco regional spread without producing significant toxicity to normal tissues and organs and without increasing the morbidity. With IORT it is possible to increase the total radiation dose, thereby improving the therapeutic ratio. Optimal IORT-EBRT dosages are under investigation. It is still an experimental treatment modality, combining surgery, radiation therapy, and, if necessary, chemotherapy. It is important to determine which method of treatment is the best and most convenient for the patient and most cost effective. The answer can only be given when prospective randomized clinical IORT trials are initiated. At present IORT is a promising treatment modality, and cooperative efforts among IORT researchers should be stressed.

References

Abe M (1984) Intraoperative radiation therapy for gastrointestinal malignancy. In: DeCosse JJ, Sherlock P (eds) Clinical management of gastrointestinal cancer. Nijhoff, Boston, pp 327–351 (Cancer treatment and research, vol 18)

Abe M, Shibamoto Y, Takahasi M, Manabe T, Tobe T, Inamoto T (1987) Intraoperative radiotherapy in carcinoma of the stomach and pancreas. World J Surg 11: 459–464

Abe M, Arakawa M (1967) Fundamental studies on surgical irradiation. Histological and hematological changes following irradiation during laparotomy of dogs. Jpn Soc Cancer Ther 2: 271–278

Abe M, Takahashi M (1981) Intraoperative radiotherapy: the Japanese experience. Int J Radiat Oncol Biol Phys 7: 863–868

Abe M, Yabumoto E, Takahashi M, Tobe T, Mori K (1974) Intraoperative radiotherapy of gastric cancer. Cancer 34: 2034–2041

Arian-Schad K, Leitner M, Jüttner F, Kohek P, Hackl A, Friehs G, Combined intraoperative (IORT) and external radiation therapy in patients with nonresectable non-small-cell lung cancer (NSCLC). In progress in radio-oncology IV. Kärcher, Kogelnik, Szepesi (eds). Vienna 1989: submitted/in press

Ashayeri E, Dallas T, Goldson AL, Seton M, Conseption DT, Manning JC (1986) Anesthesia in intraoperative radiotherapy patients. J Natl Med Assoc 78: 193–199

Bakker D, Kruize HH, Hoekstra HJ, Mehta DM, Crommelin MA (1984) Electron beam treatment: clinical, technical and dosimetric aspects. Med Phys 11: 410

Barnes M, Pass H, DeLuca A, Tochner Z, Potter O, Terrill R, Sindelar WF, Kinsella TJ (1987) Response of the mediastinal and thoracic viscera of the dog to intraoperative radiation therapy (IORT). Int J Radiat Oncol Biol Phys 13: 371–378

Barth G, Meinel F (1959) Intraoperative Kontakttherapie in den großen Körperhöhlen. Strahlentherapie 109: 386–395

Beck C (1909) An external roentgen treatment of internal structures (eventration treatment). NY Med J 89: 621–622

Biggs PJ, Epp ER, Ling CC, Novack DH, Michaels HB (1983) Dosimetry, field shaping and other considerations for intraoperative electron therapy. Int J Radiat Oncol Biol Phys 7: 875–884

Buskirk SJ, Gunderson LL, Adson MA, et al. (1984) Analysis of failure following curative irradiation of gall bladder and extrahepatic bile duct carcinoma. Int J Radiat Oncol Biol Phys 10: 2013–2023

Delgado G, Goldson AL, Ashayeri E, Hill LT, Petrill ES, Hatch KD (1984) Intraoperative radiation in the treatment of advanced cervical cancer. J Obstet Gynecol 63: 246–252
Eloesser L (1937) The treatment of some abdominal cancers by irradiation through the open abdomen combined with cautery excision. Ann Surg 645–652
Fairchild GC, Shorter A (1947) Irradiation of gastric cancer. Br J Radiol 20: 511–522
Fraass BA, Harrington FS, Kinsella TJ, Sindelar WF (1983) Television system for verification and documentation of treatment fields during intraoperative radiotherapy. Int J Radiol Oncol Biol Phys 9: 1409–1411
Fraass BA, Miller RW, Kinsella TJ et al. (1985) Intraoperative radiation therapy at the National Cancer Institute: technical innovations and dosimetry. Int J Radiat Oncol Biol Phys 11: 1299–1311
Glenn J, Sindelar WF, Kinsella TJ et al. (1985) Results of multimodality therapy of resectable soft tissue sarcomas of the retroperitoneum. Surgery 97: 316–325
Goldson AL, Ashayeri E, Espinoza MC, et al. (1981) Single dose intraoperative electrons for advanced stage pancreatic cancer: phase 1 pilot study. Int J Radiat Oncol Biol Phys 7: 869–874
Goldson AL, Sheeter OE, Ashayeri E, Collier-Manning J, Barber JB, Fan KJ (1984) Intraoperative radiotherapy for intracranial malignancies. Cancer 54: 2807–2813
Gunderson LL, Tepper JE, Biggs PJ, Goldson AL, Martin JK, McCullough EC, Rich TA, et al. (1983) Intraoperative ± external beam irradiation. Curr Probl Cancer 7: 11
Gunderson LL, Martin JK, O'Conell MJ, Beart RW, Kuols LK, Nagorney DM (1985) Residual, recurrent, or unresectable gastrointestinal cancer. Cancer 55: 2250–2258
Gunderson LL, Martin JK, Beart RW, Nagorney DM, Fieck JM, Wiland HS, Martinez A, O'Connell MJ, Martenson IA, McIlrath DC (1988) Intraoperative and external beam irradiation for locally advanced colorectal cancer. Ann Surg 207: 52–60
Hahn GM (1982) Hyperthermia and cancer. Plenum, New York
Hoekstra HJ, Kinsella TJ, Maher M, Smith R, Tochner ZA, Sindelar WF (1985) Treatment complications related to intraoperative radiotherapy (Abstr C-989). Proceedings of the American Society of Clinical Oncology. Waverly Baltimore, p 252
Hoekstra HJ, Mehta DM, Humphrey GB, Vermeij J, Oldhoff J (1986) Intraoperative radiotherapy. A new combined modality therapy in pediatric oncology. Pediatr Res 20: 1045
Hoekstra HJ, Sindelar WF, Kinsella TJ, Oldhoff J (1987) History, preliminary results, complications and future prospects of intraoperative radiotherapy. J Surg Oncol 36: 175–182
Hoekstra HJ, Mehta DM, Oldhoff J, Vermeij J, Crommelin M (1988 a) The development of an intraoperative radiotherapy program – the Groningen IORT project. In: Dobelbower RR, Abe M (eds) Intraoperative radiation therapy. CRC, Boca Raton (in press)
Hoekstra HJ, Restrepo C, Kinsella TJ, Sindelar WF (1988 b) Histopathological effects of intraoperative radiotherapy on pancreas and adjacent tissues: a postmortem analysis. J Surg Oncol 37: 104–108
Kaufman BH, Gunderson LL, Evans RG, Burgert EO, Gilchrist GS, Smithson WA (1984) Intraoperative irradiation: a new technique in pediatric oncology. J Pediatr Surg 19: 861–862
Kinsella TJ, Sindelar WF (1985) Intraoperative radiotherapy. In: DeVita VT, Hellman S, Rosenberg SA (eds) Cancer, principles and practice of oncology. Lippincott, Philadelphia, pp 2293–2304
Kinsella TJ, Sindelar WF, DeLuca A, Barnes M, Tochner Z, Mixon A, Terrill R (1988) Tolerance of the bladder to intraoperative radiotherapy (IORT): an experimental study. Int J Radiat Oncol Biol Phys 14: 939–946
Kinsella TJ, Sindelar WF, DeLuca AM, Pezekkpour G, Smith R, Maher M, Terrill R, et al. (1985) Tolerance of peripheral nerve to intraoperative radiotherapy (IORT): clinical and experimental studies. Int J Radiat Oncol Biol Phys 11: 1579–1585
Kinsella TJ, Sindelar WF, Lack E, Glatstein E, Rosenberg SA (1988) Preliminary results of a randomized study of adjuvant radiation therapy in resectable adult retroperitoneal soft tissue sarcomas. J Clin Oncol 6: 18–25
Matsumoto K, Kakizoe T, Mikuriya S, Tanaka T, Kondo J, Umegaki Y (1981) Clinical evaluation of intraoperative radiotherapy for carcinoma of the urinary bladder. Cancer 47: 509–513
McCullough EC, Anderson JA (1982) Dosimetric properties of an applicator system for intraoperative electron beam therapy utilizing a Clinac-18 accelerator. Med Phys 9: 261–268
McCullough EC, Gunderson LL (1988) Energy as well as applicator size and shape utilized in over 250 intraoperative electron bean procedures. Int J Radiat Oncol Biol Phys 15: 1041–1042
NIH, National Institutes of Health (1984) Intraoperative radiation therapy. JAMA 251: 3086–3087
Pack GT, Livingston EM (1940) Treatment of cancer and allied diseases, 2nd edn. Hoeber, New York, pp 1088–1109
Pass HI, Sindelar WF, Kinsella TJ, DeLuca A, Barnes AM, Kurtzman S, Hoekstra HJ et al. (1987) Delivery of intraoperative radiation therapy after pneumectomy: experimental observations and early clinical results. Ann Thorac Surg 44: 14–20
Phillips TL (1985) Radiation sensitizers and protectors. In: DeVita VT, Hellman S, Rosenberg SA (eds) Cancer, principles and practice of oncology. Lippincott, Philadelphia, pp 2256–2271
Rich TA, Cady B, McDermott WV, Kase KR, Chaffey JT, Hellmann S (1984) Orthovoltage intraoperative radiation therapy: a new look, an old idea. Int J Radiat Oncol Biol Phys 10: 1957–1965
Schumann EA (1933) Direct intraabdominal radiation in advanced pelvic carcinoma. Am J Obstet Gynecol 26: 260–263
Shaw EG, Blackwell CR, McCullough EC, Gunderson LL (1987) Matching intraoperative electron beam fields: dosimetric and clinical considerations. Int J Radiat Oncol Biol Phys 13: 1303–1307
Shaw EG, Gunderson LL, Martin JK, Beart RW, Nagorney AM, Podratz KC (1988) Peripheral nerve and ureteral tolerance to intraoperative radiation therapy: clinical and dose-response analysis. Int J Radiat Oncol Biol Phys (in press)
Shipley WU, Wood WC, Tepper JE et al. (1984) Intraoperative electron beam irradiation for patients with unresectable pancreatic carcinoma. Ann Surg 200: 289–296
Shipley WU, Kaufman DS, Prout GR (1987) Intraoperative radiation therapy in patients with bladder cancer. A review of techniques allowing improved tumor doses and providing high cure rates without loss of bladder function. Cancer 60: 1485–1488
Sindelar WF, Kinsella TJ (1986 a) Randomized trial of intraoperative radiotherapy in resected carcinoma of the pancreas. Int J Radiat Oncol Biol Phys [Suppl 1] 12: 148
Sindelar WF, Kinsella TJ (1986 b) Randomized trial of intraop-

erative radiotherapy in unresectable carcinoma of the pancreas. Int J Radiat Oncol Biol Phys [Suppl 1] 12: 148

Sindelar WF, Tepper J, Travis EL, Terrill R (1982a) Tolerance of retroperitoneal structures to intraoperative radiation. Ann Surg 96: 601–608

Sindelar WF, Tepper J, Travis EL (1982b) Tolerance of bile duct to intraoperative irradiation. Surgery 92: 533–540

Sindelar WF, Morrow BM, Travis EL, Tepper J, Merkel AB, Kranda K, Terrill R (1983a) Effects of intraoperative electron irradiation in the dog on cell turnover in intact and surgically-anastomosed aorta and intestine. J Radiol Oncol Biol Phys 9: 523–532

Sindelar WF, Kinsella TJ, Tepper J, Travis EL, Rosenberg SA, Glatstein E (1983b) Experimental and clinical studies with intraoperative radiotherapy. Surg Gynecol Obstet 157: 205–219

Sindelar WF, Kinsella TJ, Hoekstra HJ, Tochner ZA, Smith R, Maher M (1985) Duodenal hemorrhage as a complication of intraoperative radiotherapy for unresectable carcinomas of the pancreas (Abstr C-1075). Proceedings of the American Society of Clinical Oncology, Waverly, Baltimore, p 277

Sindelar WF, Hoekstra HJ, Restrepo C, Kinsella TJ (1986) Pathological tissue changes following intraoperative radiotherapy. Am J Clin Oncol 9: 504–509

Sindelar WF, Hoekstra HJ, Kinsella TJ, Barnes M, DeLuca AM, Tochner Z, Pass HI, Kranda KC et al. (1988a) Tolerance of canine esophagus to intraoperative electron beam radiotherapy. Int J Radiat Oncol Biol Phys 15: 663–669

Sindelar WF, Hoekstra HJ, Kinsella TJ (1988b) Surgical approaches and techniques in intraoperative radiotherapy for intraabdominal, retroperitoneal and pelvic neoplasms. Surgery 103: 247–256

Suit HD (1973) Radiation biology. In: Fletcher GH (ed) A basis for radiotherapy. Textbook of radiotherapy. Lea and Febiger, Philadelphia, pp 75–121

Takahashi M, Okada K, Shibamoto Y, Abe M, Yoshida O (1985) Intraoperative radiotherapy in the definitive treatment of localized carcinoma of the prostate. Int J Radiat Oncol Biol Phys 11: 147–151

Tepper JE (1985) Intraoperative radiation therapy for pancreatic carcinoma. In: Fortner JG, Roads JE (eds) Accomplishments in cancer research 1984. Lippincott, Philadelphia, pp 249–257

Tepper JE, Sindelar WF, Travis EL, Terrill R, Padikal T (1983) Tolerance of canine anastomosis to intraoperative radiation therapy. Int J Radiol Oncol Biol Phys 9: 987–991

Tepper JE, Gunderson LL, Orlow E, Cohen AL, Hedberg SE, Shipley WU, Blitzer PH, Rich T (1984) Complications of intraoperative radiotherapy. Int J Radiat Oncol Biol Phys 10: 1831–1839

Tepper JE, Wood WC, Cohen AM et al. (1985) Intraoperative radiation therapy. In: DeVita VT, Hellman S, Rosenberg SA (eds) Important advances in oncology 1985. Lippincott, Philadelphia, pp 226–242

Tepper JE, Gunderson LL, Goldson AL, et al. (1986) Quality control parameters of intraoperative radiation therapy. Int J Radiat Oncol Biol Phys 12: 1687–1695

Todoroki T (1978) The late effects of single massive irradiation with electrons of the liver hilum in rabbits. Jpn J Gastroenterol Surg 11: 169–177

Todoroki T, Iwasaki Y, Okamura T, et al. (1980) Intraoperative radiotherapy for advanced carcinoma of the biliary system. Cancer 46: 2179–2184

The Biologic Basis of Cancer Chemotherapy

M. BROWER and D. CARNEY

The treatment of cancer with antineoplastic drugs has improved tremendously since the discovery over 40 years ago that nitrogen mustard can palliate advanced malignancies. Curative therapy is now available for such cancers as acute leukemia, testicular carcinoma, and aggressive non-Hodgkin's lymphoma, while substantial prolongation of life is possible for patients with many other forms of cancer. Although many of the ways in which the anticancer drugs are used have evolved empirically over the last four decades, our understanding of the biologic principles underlying cancer chemotherapy has increased as well, providing the foundation for more effective cancer treatment in the future.

In this chapter, we shall describe the mechanisms of action of the most important anticancer drugs, and we shall discuss the methods now used to screen potential new agents for activity. The principles of the cell cycle and of certain mathematical models relevant to the design of cancer treatment will be described, along with the principles of adjuvant and neo-adjuvant chemotherapy. We will briefly summarize attempts to predict drug sensitivity by in vitro testing. We will then present a summary of our rapidly expanding understanding of the mechanisms of cellular resistance to anticancer drugs and discuss the relationship between dose and response in oncology and the basic principles of combination chemotherapy.

Mechanisms of Action of Anticancer Drugs

Most anticancer drugs damage specific cellular constituents, usually DNA. Detailed monographs describing the anticancer drugs and what is known about their mechanisms of action are available (Chabner 1982; Pratt and Ruddon 1979). The alkylating agents, including nitrogen mustard, were the first class of anticancer drugs to achieve wide use (Table 1). Nitrogen mustard is a bifunctional alkylating agent containing two reactive CH_2CH_2Cl groups which ionize to $CH_2CH_2\cdot$ and react with DNA and other molecules at two sites (Fig. 1) (Brower and Loughner 1985). Although there are several targets for the reactive alkyl groups on the DNA molecule, the primary site of attack is the N-7 position of guanosine, causing cross-linkage between the N-7 guanosines in complementary DNA strands. The in vivo cytotoxicity of alkylating agents such as nitrogen

Table 1. Mechanisms of action of anticancer drugs

Drug	Mechanism
Alkylating agents	
Nitrogen mustard	Alkylates DNA, forming crosslinks
Cyclophosphamide	Alkylates DNA, forming crosslinks
Ifosfamide	Alkylates DNA, forming crosslinks
Busulfan	Alkylates DNA, forming crosslinks
Chlorambucil	Alkylates DNA, forming crosslinks
Melphalan	Alkylates DNA, forming crosslinks
BCNU	Alkylates DNA and carbamoylates proteins
CCNU	Alkylates DNA and carbamoylates proteins
Streptozocin	Alkylates DNA and carbamoylates proteins
Antimetabolites	
Methotrexate	Blocks dihydrofolate reductase
5-Fluorouracil	Inhibits thymidylate synthetase
6-Mercaptopurine	Inhibits purine ring synthesis
6-Thioguanine	Inhibits purine ring synthesis
Cytosine arabinoside	Competitive inhibitor of incorporation of dCTP into DNA
Plant alkaloids	
Vincristine	Spindle poison, disrupts microtubules
Vinblastine	Spindle poison, disrupts microtubules
Vindesine	Spindle poison, disrupts microtubules
Etoposide	Inhibits DNA topoisomerase II
Antibiotics and analogs	
Doxorubicin	Intercalates between DNA base pairs
Daunorubicin	Intercalates between DNA base pairs
Epirubicin	Intercalates between DNA base pairs
Mitoxantrone	Intercalates between DNA base pairs
Bleomycin	Causes DNA strand breaks
Actinomycin D	Intercalates between DNA base pairs
Mitomycin C	Probably alkylates DNA
Miscellaneous	
Cisplatin	Attacks DNA, forms intrastrand crosslinks
Carboplatin	Attacks DNA, forms intrastrand crosslinks
Procarbazine	Nonclassical alkylator of DNA
Dacarbazine	Nonclassical alkylator of DNA
Hydroxyurea	Inhibits ribonucleotide reductase
L-Asparaginase	Depletes cells of L-asparagine
Hormones	
Tamoxifen	Antiestrogen
Medroxyprogesterone acetate	Progestational agent
Megestrol acetate	Progestational agent
Fluoxymesterone	Androgenic agent
Diethylstilbestrol	Estrogenic agent
Prednisone	Glucocorticoid
Aminoglutethimide	Inhibits adrenal steroid synthesis
Leuprolide	LHRH agonist
Flutamide	Antiandrogen
Cyproterone acetate	Antiandrogen

mustard closely correlates with the amount of DNA cross-linking.

Because nitrogen mustard must be administered intravenously, causes severe nausea, must be solubilized immediately before use, and causes severe tissue damage if extravasated, chemists have developed many other alkylating agents wich are widely used (Table 1). Cyclophosphamide, ifosfamide, melphalan, and chlorambucil are nitrogen mustard derivatives with side chains that increase the stability of the molecule. Busulfan and thiotepa are two other drugs that function as alkylating agents. Cyclophosphamide is the alkylating agent most widely used today to treat lymphomas and breast, ovarian, lung, and other cancers.

Minor changes in chemical structure can result in marked differences in drug activity and toxicity. Ifosfamide is a structural isomer of cyclophosphamide which was first synthesized in 1965 and which is active in cisplatin-resistant testicular cancer, while cyclophosphamide lacks activity. The dose-limiting side effect of cyclophosphamide is hematologic, bladder toxicity only occasionally being seen, while ifosfamide frequently causes severe bladder damage, but is only mildly myelosuppressive.

The nitrosoureas are a group of drugs that function primarily as alkylators and were discovered through systematic in vitro screening sponsored by the drug development program of the National Cancer Institute (NCI) of the USA (Weiss and Issell 1982). Although they function mainly by alkylating DNA, these drugs also have the ability to generate isocyanate moieties that can react with amino groups to carbamoylate proteins. The nitrosoureas are more lipid soluble than the classic alkylating agents and therefore they can cross the blood-brain barrier efficiently, making these drugs clinically useful against central nervous system tumors. Other anticancer drugs, including procarbazine and dacarbazine though not sharing the classic alkylator chemical structure of nitrogen mustard, function as alkylating agents.

Antimetabolites are the second-oldest group of anticancer drugs, first used by Sidney Farber against childhood leukemia in 1948. Reduced folic acid derivatives are required for DNA synthesis, and rapidly proliferating tumor cells synthesize DNA more rapidly than normal cells. The folic acid analogs like methotrexate are taken up by cancer cells and act as metabolic poisons. They bind tightly to and inhibit the key enzyme dihydrofolate reductase (DHFR; Fig. 2), which is needed to supply reduced folates. The effect of methotrexate can be reversed by supplying leucovorin, a reduced folate which bypasses

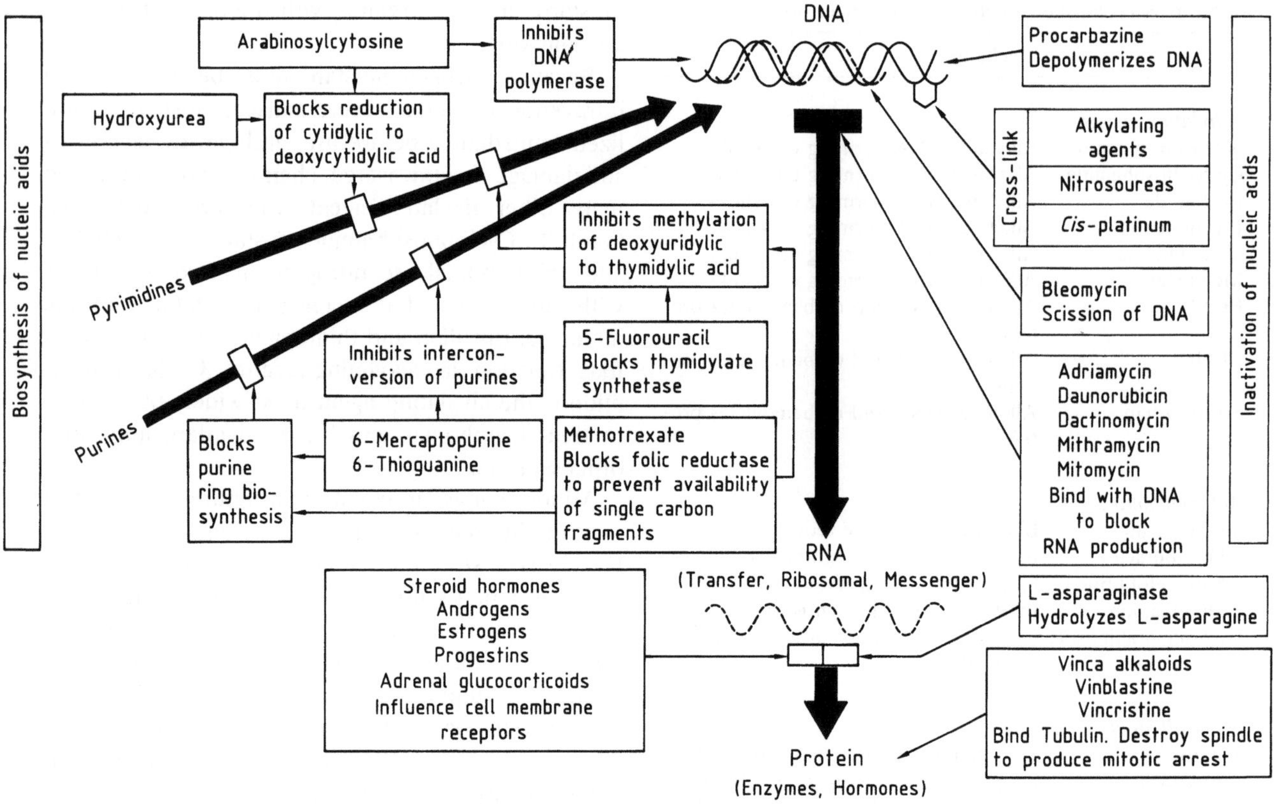

Fig. 1. Sites of action of common antineoplastic drugs. (From Krakoff 1981)

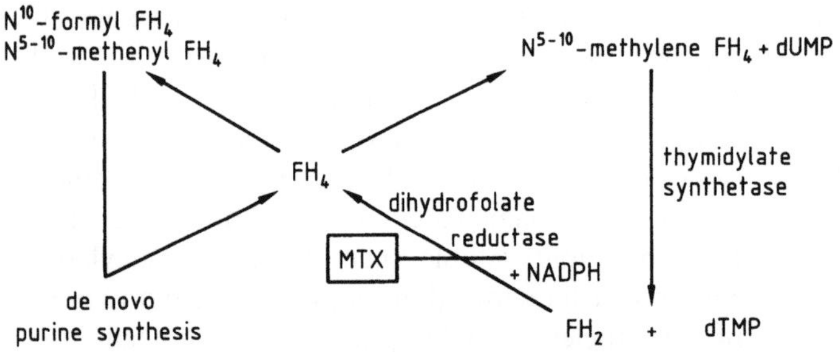

Fig. 2. Central role of dihydrofolate reductase in maintaining intracellular pool of tetrahydrofolic acid **(FH_4)**. FH_4 serves as a source for the active folate cofactors required for synthesis of purines and pyrimidines. Methotrexate **(MTX)** inhibits the reductase reaction, leading to accumulation of intracellular folates as FH_2. (From Chabner 1982)

the block induced by methotrexate in the synthesis of substances needed for the manufacture of purines. Because so much is understood about the biochemistry of methotrexate, attempts to improve its therapeutic ratio biochemically are ongoing (Jolivet et al. 1983).

Other antimetabolites in common use are listed in Table 1. Only 5-fluorouracil (5-FU) is widely used in nonhematologic malignancies. 5-FU is a "false metabolite" differing from the pyrimidine uracil by the substitution of one fluorine for one hydrogen atom. One metabolite of 5-FU, 5-FdUMP, inhibits the key enzyme thymidylate synthetase, which is needed for the manufacture of DNA, while another metabolite is incorporated into the RNA molecule. Methotrexate can increase 5-FU's conversion into its active metabolite, and extensive research has been carried out on how best to sequence these two drugs (Anonymous 1983). The inhibition of thymidylate synthetase by 5-FdUMP increases with high intracellular levels of reduced folates. This laboratory observation led directly to phase II clinical trials suggesting increased activity of the combination of 5-FU and leucovorin (folinic acid) in common gastrointestinal malignancies (Grem et al. 1987).

The antitumor antibiotics, discovered by systematic screening of fungal products, interact with DNA. Extensive research has elucidated their mechanism of action. Doxorubicin (Adriamycin), first used in 1970, has a broad spectrum of antineoplastic activity, and is an integral part of the therapy of lymphomas, small cell lung cancer, breast and ovarian cancer, and sarcomas. Doxorubicin and the closely related antileukemic drug daunorubicin share a characteristic tetracyclic ring structure that binds by intercalation with the DNA molecule, interfering with DNA replication (Fig. 3). Use of these drugs can be limited by cardiotoxicity, which may be due to free radical formation and which may be reduced by prolonged drug infusions, or by using small weekly drug doses rather than large doses every 3 weeks (Young et al. 1983). Understanding of the structure-function relationship of the doxorubicin molecule has led to the synthesis of newer drugs, including epirubicin (an isomer of doxorubicin) and mitoxantrone (an anthraquinone with a tricyclic ring structure), which retain intercalating activity and antitumor activity but which are less toxic than the parent compound (Cersosimo and Hong 1986; Shenkenberg and Van Hoff 1986).

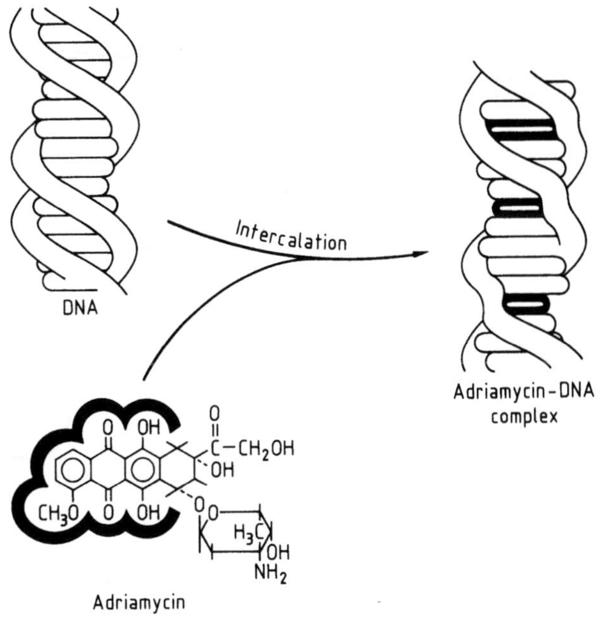

Fig. 3. Diagrammatic model of the intercalation of Adriamycin into DNA showing that local unwinding of the helical structure must occur as the base pairs are moved apart by intercalation. The open, wafer-shaped units represent the base pairs and the coils the deoxyribose phosphate backbone of the DNA double helix. The solid, wafer-shaped units on the right represent Adriamycin (viewed in the plane of the anthracycline portion of the molecule) intercalated between base pairs. In a more detailed model, the amino sugar moiety of the drug would be seen to be located in the major groove of the DNA. (From Pratt and Ruddon 1979)

Bleomycin, discovered in Japan in 1966, is used against lymphoma, testicular cancer, and squamous cell carcinomas. This drug binds to DNA and causes DNA strand scission in a reaction mediated by free oxygen radicals produced by oxidation of a bleomycin-iron complex. The drug causes virtually no myelosuppression (Blum et al. 1973). Its major dose-limiting toxicity is pulmonary fibrosis, and attempts to find useful bleomycin analogs lacking pulmonary toxicity continue.

The plant products used in cancer chemotherapy include the vinca alkaloids derived from the periwinkle and the epidophyllotoxins derived from the mandrake. The epidophyllotoxins are closely related to podophyllin, long used to treat warts. The antitumor activity of the vinca alkaloids was discovered during the screening of thousands of plant products in the late 1950s. They are mitotic inhibitors, acting by binding to tubulin, the major component of the microtubules of the mitotic spindle. Vincristine and vinblastine, the two periwinkle alkaloids in widest use, differ in clinical structure by only a single side chain substitution, yet vincristine is minimally myelotoxic and its dose-limiting toxicity is peripheral neuropathy, while the dose-limiting toxicity of vinblastine is myelosuppression. The epidophyllotoxins interfere with DNA synthesis, apparently by inhibiting the essential DNA repair enzyme topoisomerase II (Ross et al. 1984). The plant products are particularly active in acute leukemia, lymphomas, small cell lung cancer, and testicular cancer.

Cisplatin is a unique drug. In 1965, Rosenberg observed the inhibition of *E. coli* replication by electric current given via platinum electrodes, due to an electrolysis product of the electrode. Rosenberg proceeded to identify cisplatin as the active agent, and determine that it had antitumor activity. Initially deemed too toxic for clinical administration, cisplatin advanced into the clinic after it was found that intense intravenous hydration and diuresis could ameliorate its dose-limiting nephrotoxicity. Cisplatin is vital to the combination chemotherapy regimens that cure testicular cancer, and is also useful in small cell lung, ovarian, bladder, and head and neck cancer. Its major toxicities are severe nausea and vomiting, peripheral neuropathy, ototoxicity, and nephrotoxicity. As with doxorubicin, scientists are synthesizing cisplatin analogs that retain antitumor activity with less toxicity. Carboplatin (CBDCA) and iproplatin (CHIP) are the two new platinum analogs that appear most useful, although they are more myelosuppressive than cisplatin. Cisplatin and its analogs function as alkylating agents, generally after reactions with water replacing the chloride ion with H_2O. As with the alkylating agent, cytotoxicity correlates with DNA cross-linking (Loehrer and Einhorn 1984).

Lastly, we will consider hormonal agents. The use of hormones in cancer therapy dates back to 1941,

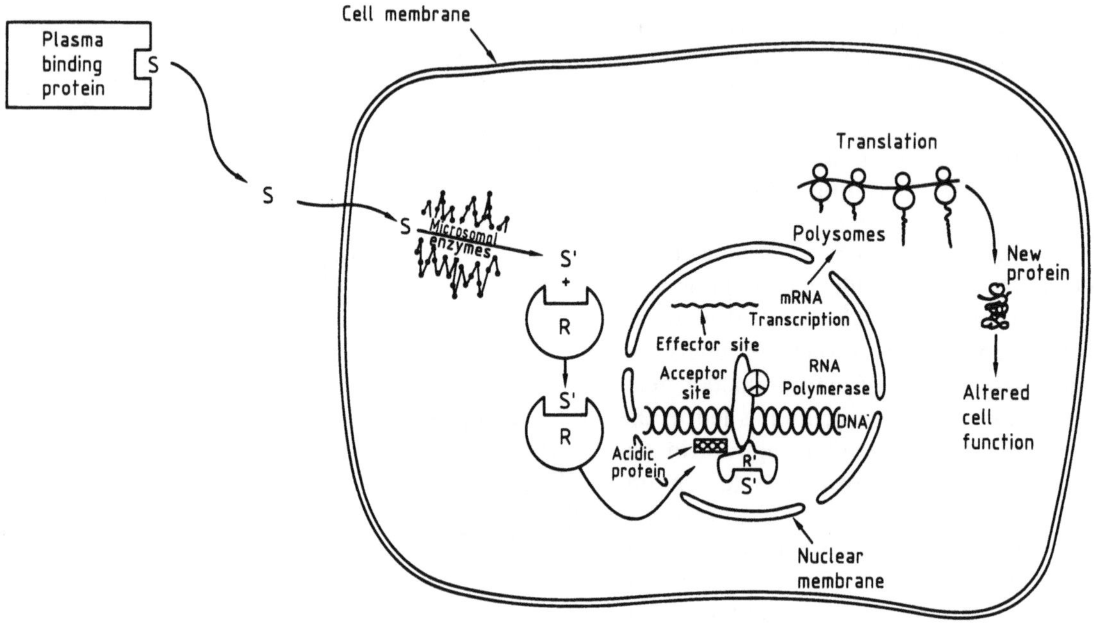

Fig. 4. Schematic representation of the mechanisms of steroid hormone action. (From Chabner 1982)

when Huggins first used estrogens to treat prostate cancer. Today, many hormonal agents are available to oncologists (Table 1). They are invaluable in the treatment of breast, prostate, and endometrial cancer, and, in addition, corticosteroids are a cornerstone in the management of lymphoblastic leukemia, myeloma, and lymphomas. Extensive research has demonstrated that steroid hormones exert their influence via cytoplasmic receptors. The hormone-receptor complex formed after exposure to the hormone translocates to the cell nucleus, where it binds to the chromosome at specific sites and causes synthesis of new messenger RNA (mRNA) signals and eventually of new proteins (Fig. 4). The development of methods to assay for estrogen receptor and other steroid hormone receptors in tumor tissue is a major scientific advance, permitting the selection of patients for hormonal therapy in a rational manner.

Development of New Drugs

Many of the 40 useful anticancer drugs were discovered by chance observation, but most were found during careful, systematic development and screening programs. In the past, rapidly growing murine leukemias were the targets against which as many as 40 000 compounds were tested each year for antiproliferative activity. If anticancer activity was found against L1210 or P388 leukemia, then further animal testing, including testing with xenografts of human tumor cell lines grown in athymic nude mice, would be carried out. After anticancer activity was confirmed, toxicity trials in rodents preceded clinical trials in humans. Extensive research is often required to formulate pharmacologically useful drugs from compounds with promising initial results, with attention to factors such as solubility and stability (Driscoll 1984). Clinical trials of new drugs in humans are classified as phase I–IV trials (Table 2).

Table 2. Phases in clinical testing of new anticancer drugs

Phase I	Determination of maximum tolerated dose, toxicities, schedule, and human pharmacology of new drug; any observation of antitumor responses is incidental
Phase II	Determination of response rate in specific tumors
Phase III	Determination of effectiveness in comparison with existing standard chemotherapy in patients with advanced disease
Phase IV	Determination of effectiveness in comparison with existing standard therapy in early disease (combined modality, adjuvant therapy)

It may be inappropriate to rely entirely on the rapidly growing murine leukemia model to screen anticancer drugs. Most common cancers in adult patients are slow growing and resistant to most common drugs, in contrast to the rapidly growing and drug-sensitive L1210 and P388 tumors. Therefore, the NCI recently developed a panel of human tumor cell lines representative of the broad range of common neoplasms. Initial drug screening can be carried out in these cell lines in vitro in parallel with the standard mouse tests. The hope is that drugs may be discovered with specific activity against the slowly growing, inherently refractory tumors (Shoemaker 1986).

Cell Kinetics, Mathematical Models and Cancer Therapy

Multiple factors are involved in determining resistance and sensitivity to chemotherapy, but in general (with many exceptions), rapidly dividing cells are usually more sensitive to chemotherapy than quiescent or slowly dividing cells. If a single malignant cell is implanted in a mouse (for example an L1210 leukemia cell), the tumor cell population grows exponentially until the mouse is killed. Classic work by Schabel in the 1960s showed that with L1210 leukemia, tumor cell kill follows first-order kinetics; that is, the proportion of tumor cells killed by a given drug is constant regardless of cell number. Thus, if a given drug dose kills 99% of an initial population of 10^{12} L1210 cells, then six doses of the drug will be required to reduce the tumor burden to 10^0 cells and theoretically attain a cure. This is the scientific basis for the standard practice of repeated intermittent drug dosing in cancer chemotherapy.

Tumor cell kill is logarithmic: the same dose of drug is required to reduce 100 cells to 10 cells (a reduction of 90 cells) as to reduce 100 million cells to 10 million (a reduction of 90 million cells). If we assume that a gram of tumor ($\simeq 10^9$ cells) is at or below the limit of detectability at most sites, a patient with this amount of residual tumor would be considered to have had a complete response. If a kilogram of tumor ($\simeq 10^{12}$ cells) is close to a lethal burden, it will take three logs of cell kill to reduce a tumor mass from a lethal cell burden to a state of complete response. However, it will take nine logs of cell kill to go from a state of complete response to a state approaching total cell kill. With chemotherapy alone, the amount of treatment required to bring a patient from a lethal tumor burden to complete response is thus only one-quarter of the total amount of treatment required for cure, in the absence of factors influencing cell kill. Therefore, clinicians usually administer maintenance chemotherapy after achieving an initial remission, although the role for such therapy has not been clearly established in most adult cancers and, in fact, has been shown to be ineffective in testicular cancer.

Most human tumors exhibit Gompertzian rather than exponential growth. A tumor in which all the cells are in continuous cycle would have a growth fraction of 100%. The growth of such a tumor would be logarithmic, or exponential, the number of cells at time T being equal to C_0e^{KT}, where C_0 is the number of cells initially and K is the growth rate constant. It is thought that very small tumor masses, such as micrometastases, may conform to this pattern. As the tumor becomes larger, its growth fraction will fall as an increasing number of cells enter the resting phase G_0 of the cell cycle (Fig. 5), presumably because of the limitation in blood supply to the center of the tumor mass.

This, together with increased cell loss and possibly lengthening of the cell cycle, will cause the kinetics of the increase in tumor volume to become slower than exponential. This is called "Gompertzian kinetics". Tumor cells are usually much less susceptible to anticancer drugs when they are not actively proliferating. This may help to account for the resistance of many human cancers to treatment. However, when tumor cell number is decreased by initial induction and maintenance chemotherapy, the proportion of cells actively growing might increase, rendering the tumor more sensitive to chemotherapy. A mathematical model based on this concept, developed by Norton and Simon, has been used to justify "late intensification" chemotherapy (Norton and Simon 1986).

The cell cycle is illustrated in Fig. 5. The cycle begins with mitosis and proceeds to G_1 (first growth phase), S (DNA synthesis phase), and G_2 (second growth phase). In addition, cells can enter the resting G_0 phase, in which they may be relatively impervious to chemotherapy. Certain chemotherapeutic agents are "cycle specific," killing cells more effectively during certain phases of the cell cycle. Antimetabolites, including methotrexate and cytosine arabinoside, are most effective on cells in S phase. The vinca alkaloids specifically arrest cells in mitosis. Cycle-specific drugs usually demonstrate a plateau in cell kill with increasing dose when administered in large intermittent boluses, because cells not in the sensitive part of the cell cycle at the time of treatment will not be affected by the drug. Therefore, when cytosine arabinoside is used to treat acute leukemia, the drug is usually given by prolonged continuous infusion, so that most of the leukemia cells will pass through S phase during treatment. In contrast to the antimetabolites, the alkylating agents and antitumor antibiotics are cell cycle nonspecific. Genetic damage caused by these agents can be lethal regardless of the time of drug administration. Unfortunately, cell cycle considerations alone are not

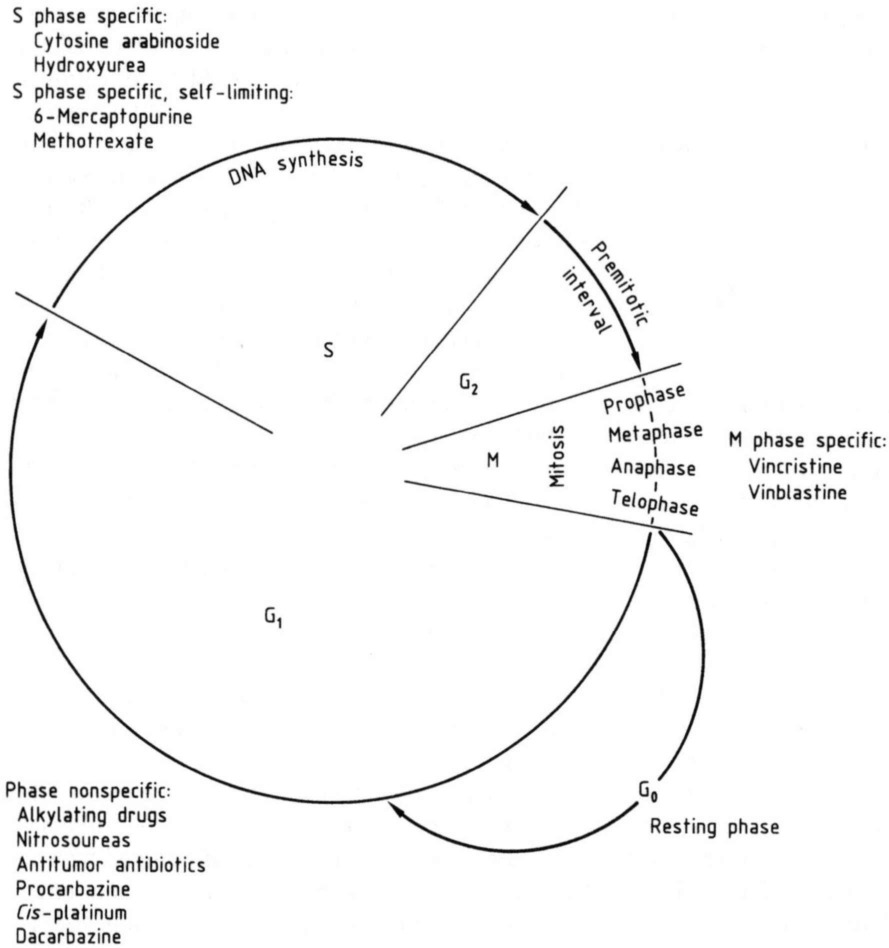

Fig. 5. The cell cycle and the relationship of antitumor drug action to the cycle. G_1 is the period between mitosis and the beginning of DNA synthesis. Resting cells (cells that are not preparing for cell division) are said to be in a subphase of G_1, G_0. S is the period of DNA synthesis, G_2 the premitotic interval, and M the period of mitosis. Examples of cell cycle-dependent anticancer drugs are listed next to the phase at which they act. Drugs that are cytotoxic for cells at any point in the cycle are called cycle phase-nonspecific drugs. (From Pratt and Ruddon 1979)

sufficient to explain all facets of resistance to chemotherapy (Tannock 1978). It is well known that large tumors (or patients with large tumor burdens) are usually refractory to chemotherapy, and cell kinetic theory explains this by stating that a large number of cells in such tumors are not proliferating because they are hypoxic, poorly vascularized, and lacking nutrients.

A mathematical model developed by Goldie and Coldman of Vancouver provides an alternative explanation for the inherent resistance of large tumors to chemotherapy (Goldie and Coldman 1979). In their model, cancer cells have an inherent rate of spontaneous mutation from a drug-sensitive to a drug-resistant phenotype. As a tumor grows from a single cell to a clinically detectable neoplasm, the probability that at least one cancer cell has become drug-resistant, thereby rendering the cancer incurable with chemotherapy, increases very rapidly (Fig. 6). This mathematical model predicts that inherent drug resistance might be overcome by early administration of multiple "non-cross-resistant" chemotherapeutic agents, or regimens, before the tumor has time to evolve cell populations resistant to all of the chemotherapeutic agents used. Thus, alternating the MOPP regimen with the ABVD regimen in the initial management of Hodgkin's disease should give superior results to initial treatment with MOPP alone and reserving ABVD for MOPP failures, and this indeed appears to be the case (Bonadonna et al. 1986). Trials are currently underway in a variety of cancers in an effort to further confirm the validity of the Goldie-Coldman hypothesis. For example, the model predicts that administering the four drugs of MOPP on days 1 and 29 and giving ABVD on days 8 and 36 of a 2-month cycle will be superior to giving MOPP on days 1 and 8 and ABVD on days 29 and 43 as is usually the case, since deferring ABVD until day 29 gives the Hodgkin's cells an extra 3 weeks to mutate to the drug-resistant phenotype.

The Goldie-Coldman model explains why adjuvant chemotherapy can be curative in diseases such as breast cancer and osteogenic and soft tissue sarcomas when curative chemotherapy in patients with clinically detectable metastases is not available. Moreover, the model provides a justification for neo-

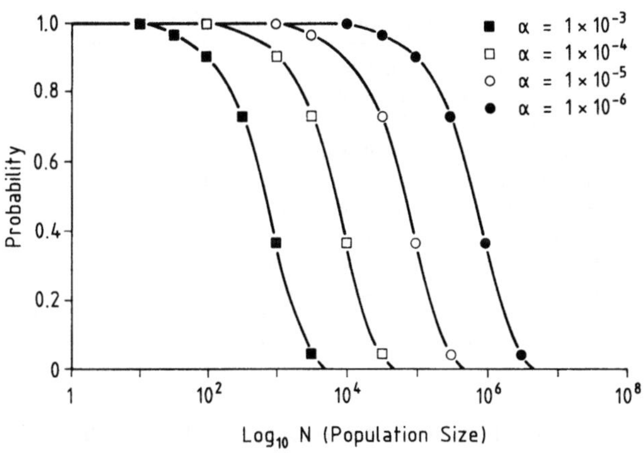

Fig. 6. Probability of the existence of no resistant phenotypes as a function of the mutation rate (α) and tumor size (N). The almost identical profile of each curve reflects the independence of the time required for a class of tumors to proceed from the state when only 5% have resistant phenotypes to that when 95% have such phenotypes. (From Goldie and Coldman 1979)

adjuvant chemotherapy, or the administration of adjuvant chemotherapy prior to definitive local therapy. The hypothesis states that resistance to chemotherapy depends on the duration of the tumor's existence, so that delaying chemotherapy until after surgery may give tumor cells enough time to mutate to the resistant phenotype. In tumors such as squamous carcinomas of the head and neck, the response rate to chemotherapy is much lower in patients who have failed surgery or radiation therapy than in patients not previously treated. Neo-adjuvant chemotherapy attempts to take advantage of such observations. It is most commonly used in head and neck and esophageal cancers and in soft tissue and osteogenic sarcomas, and it is being investigated in breast and bladder cancer. It should be noted that despite the appeal of the concept of neo-adjuvant chemotherapy, no randomized trial of such treatment has yet shown prolonged survival in any cancer.

Goldie and Coldman recently offered an explanation for the observation that slow-growing, well-differentiated tumors tend to be less likely to respond to chemotherapy than rapidly growing undifferentiated tumors. In the slowly growing tumor, many cells terminally differentiate and die during the development of the cancer, so the cells present in the tumor at any given time have been through many more cell divisions. They have therefore had an increased opportunity to undergo spontaneous mutation to the drug-resistant phenotype than cells in the rapidly dividing, undifferentiated tumor. Given a fixed mutation rate, tumors in which loss of stem cell capacity occurs with high frequency will have a higher proportion of resistant stem cells than those in which such loss is infrequent (Goldie and Coldman 1983).

In Vitro Drug Sensitivity Testing

Because most adult cancers are either resistant to most chemotherapy when treatment is started or acquire drug resistance during treatment, scientists have developed in vitro systems that ideally would be able to rapidly and accurately determine the pattern of drug sensitivity of an individual patient's tumor. This would permit rational selection of antineoplastic therapy, analogous to using in vitro antibiotic testing in infectious diseases. In the 1970s, Hamburger and Salmon's development of the "human tumor stem cell assay" and Courtenay's independent development of a similar assay stimulated interest in in vitro drug sensitivity testing. The basis of these "clonogenic" assays is the stem cell model of tumor growth, in which only a small population of tumor cells have an unlimited capacity for self-renewal and are responsible for tumor growth. The survival of these clonogenic stem cells (assayed by determining the percentage of anchorage-independent cell clones surviving in vitro drug exposure) is used to predict drug response in the patient.

Unfortunately, these assays suffer from multiple problems (Selby et al. 1983). Only a small proportion of human tumors grow with a colony-forming efficiency that allows drug testing. Several weeks elapse after biopsy before in vitro drug data can be generated. Most human tumors are resistant to most chemotherapeutic agents, and although the ability of clonogenic assays to predict resistance is good, their utility regarding selection of clinically useful drugs is limited.

Many other in vitro predictive tests are under investigation, including dye exclusion assays, radionuclide precursor incorporation assays, and human tumor xenograft culture (Carney and Winkler 1985). Other groups use cell culture to rapidly expand the number of available tumor cells from a patient's biopsy prior to attempting drug sensitivity testing.

Mechanisms of Drug Resistance

We have already indicated that the phenomenon of drug resistance is perhaps the most vexing problem in clinical oncology. Cancers can be divided into those that are usually inherently resistant to chemotherapy (for example renal cell carcinoma and melanoma) and those that are initially sensitive but rapidly acquire drug resistance (such as small cell lung cancer and breast cancer). Acquisition of drug resistance is, in a sense, a characteristic of malignant cells, related to the genetic instability and mutability of cancer cells and the associated phenomenon of tumor progression (Klein and Klein 1985). Non malignant cells such as normal bone marrow cells never become resistant to cytotoxic drugs.

In experimental models, there is a clear dose-response curve with chemotherapy (Frei and Canellos 1980). "Drug resistance" can be a manifestation of inadequate drug dosing, and even a slight reduction of dose may drastically impair clinical activity. In most adult cancers, for example in the majority of patients with extensive stage small cell lung cancer, the goal of chemotherapy is palliative, so the improved response obtainable with very high dose chemotherapy may be outweighed by the toxicities and impaired quality of life resulting from therapy (Brower et al. 1983). However, when cure is the therapeutic goal, as in Hodgkin's disease or in the adjuvant therapy of breast cancer, results appear better when maximally tolerated doses of chemotherapy are administered (Bonadonna and Valagussa 1981). Further evidence for the relationship between dose and response in cancer medicine is the ability to salvage occasional patients with "incurable" tumors with very high dose treatment regimens, such as high-dose chemotherapy with allogeneic marrow rescue in chronic myelogenous leukemia, and very high dose cisplatin with hypertonic saline in refractory testicular or ovarian tumors (Ozols et al. 1984).

Cancers can be resistant to chemotherapy because of failure of drug to reach tumor in sanctuary sites such as the meninges, brain, or testes, or because of the inability of drug to penetrate into large, poorly vascularized tumor masses. Individual variations in drug metabolism and pharmacology may result in differences in drug levels or in products of drug concentration × time in different patients given identical drug doses (Zimm et al. 1983). However, resistance to chemotherapy at the level of the cell has attracted the most scientific interest in recent years.

Table 3 lists cellular mechanisms of drug resistance that have been found to be relevant to anticancer drugs (Ozols and Cowan 1986). We will comment on some of these mechanisms.

Decreased metabolic activation of drug has been found to be a mechanism of resistance to two drugs studied in small cell lung cancer. Cells resistant to methotrexate may be unable to form an active polyglutamated form of the drug (Curt et al. 1985). Cells resistant to the experimental agent tiazofurin may lack the ability to transform the drug to its analog tiazofurin adenine dinucleotide (Carney et al. 1985).

Table 3. Cellular mechanisms of drug resistance

1. Decreased drug uptake by cell
2. Increased drug elimination by cell
3. Decreased metabolic activation of drug
4. Increased catabolism of drug
5. Alterations in cellular repair mechanisms
6. Alterations in cofactors required for drug effect
7. Alterations in target proteins
8. Increased concentration of target protein
9. Increased concentration of protective protein

Adapted with permission from Ozols and Cowan (1986).

Alterations in cellular repair mechanisms may permit cells to become resistant to alkylating agents. Glutathione is a cellular constituent that protects cells from drug effects by direct detoxification of anticancer drugs or of free radical species induced by the drug. Glutathione may also help repair DNA cross-links induced by alkylating agents. Resistance to alkylating agents in experimental models is often associated with elevation of cellular glutathione content. Based on these observations, it may be worth combining drugs that inhibit glutathione synthesis with alkylating agents (Ozols and Cowan 1986).

The effect of methotrexate on its target enzyme DHFR is the classic example of increased concentration of target protein as a mechanism of drug resistance. Exposure of tumor cells to methotrexate leads to an increase in the amount of DNA and mRNA coding for DHFR, along with an increase in the amount of DHFR protein. This increase in DHFR is associated with the development of drug resistance. The amplified DNA coding for extra copies of the DHFR gene is either found in peculiar elongated chromosomes containing homogeneously staining regions (HSRs), or in small "double-minute" chromosomes that are not present in normal cells. When the amplified DHFR gene copies are in HSRs, they are stably reproduced and the resistance to methotrexate is permanent, but when the amplified gene copies are on double-minute chromosomes, the gene can be lost over time with cell replication and methotrexate sensitivity redevelops. This latter phenomenon has been observed in human small cell lung cancer (Curt et al. 1983). Gene amplification is a common phenomenon in cancer cells, and in particular, amplification of oncogenes such as *c-myc* is seen in many neoplasms. The tendency to gene amplification seen in cancer cells, but not in normal cells, may help explain why cancer cells, but not normal cells, seem to have the inherent ability to develop drug resistance.

Increased concentration of a protective protein is a phenomenon associated with "pleiotropic drug resistance". Clinicians have long known that patients treated with one anticancer drug can become resistant to many other drugs, including ones with completely different mechanisms of action and molecular structures. Thus, doxorubicin is an active drug in untreated patients with ovarian cancer, but in patients previously treated with the alkylating agent melphalan, doxorubicin is devoid of activity.

Victor Ling of the University of Toronto developed the most widely used model for the in vitro study of pleiotropic drug resistance (Ling et al. 1983). Exposure of Chinese hamster ovary cells to colchicine leads to resistance not only to colchicine but also to the vinca alkaloids, etoposide, the anthracycline antibiotics, and melphalan. A high molecular weight basic glycoprotein, gp 170, appears in the cell membrane of these cells, and this glycoprotein may be responsible for drug resistance, probably by facilitating the egress of positively charged anticancer drugs of diverse structure and class from the cell. The gene coding for gp 170 (also known as "P-glycoprotein" or "mdr gene") has been cloned, and transfection of the gene into sensitive cells confers drug resistance (Guild et al. 1988). The amino acid sequence deduced from the nucleotide sequence of the cloned gene indicates strong homology with bacterial transport proteins that mediate energy-dependent drug efflux (Gros et al. 1986). The P-glycoprotein may be present in normal epithelial cells such as those lining the colon to eliminate noxious foreign substances from cells, leading to inherent resistance to chemotherapy of tumors originating from such epithelial cells.

Tsuruo (1983) has demonstrated that in certain cell lines, drug resistance can be overcome by calcium channel-blocking drugs such as verapamil, apparently by reducing P-glycoprotein-mediated drug efflux. Clinical trials testing verapamil in combination with doxorubicin in doxorubicin-refractory patients are ongoing (Ozols and Cowan 1986).

Non-small cell lung cancer is usually inherently resistant to chemotherapy and small cell lung cancer is usually inherently sensitive; it is notable that two-dimensional gel electrophoresis of the cell membranes of human lung cancer cell lines demonstrate high molecular weight glycoproteins in non-small cell cancer lines, while they are not present in small cell cancer lines (Baylin et al. 1982).

Principles of Combination Chemotherapy

The use of drugs in combination largely evolved out of the clinics, because treatment with single agents, unlike the treatment of bacterial infections, was unable either to produce significant remissions or to cure patients with cancer. The era of effective combination chemotherapy began with the treatment of leukemias and lymphomas and has now extended to the treatment of more common malignancies. It now seems likely that drug combinations are effective because they accomplish three important feats which are not possible with single agent treatments:

1. They provide maximal cell kill within the range of toxicity tolerated by the host for each drug.
2. They provide a broader range of coverage of de novo resistant cell lines in the heterogeneous tumor population.
3. They prevent, or slow down, the development of new resistant lines.

Failure of combination chemotherapy to work in marginally sensitive tumors seems related to the absence of a dose-response curve for cytoreduction within the range of doses tolerable to the host. A classic example of such a drug combination is MOPP for Hodgkin's disease, combining nitrogen mustard (dose-limiting toxicity: early myelosuppression), vincristine (dose-limiting toxicity: peripheral neuropathy), procarbazine (dose-limiting toxicity: late myelosuppression), and prednisone. In testicular cancer, vinblastine or etoposide (dose-limiting toxicity: myelosuppression), bleomycin (dose-limiting toxicity: pulmonary), and cisplatin (dose-limiting toxicity: renal) are combined at full single-agent doses.

The Goldie-Coldman hypothesis suggests that better results should be achieved with combination cancer chemotherapy, just as optimal antituberculosis therapy requires combination antibacterial chemotherapy. If a given cancer has 10^{12} cells, and one in 10^{6} cells are resistant to drug A and one in 10^{6} cells to drug B because of different spontaneous mutations, only therapy with drug A and drug B combined can sterilize the tumor.

Optimal scheduling and sequencing of drugs is an active area of clinical investigation. Tumor regrowth between courses of chemotherapy after an initial response is common in rapidly proliferating cancers such as aggressive non-Hodgkin's lymphomas. To prevent this, non myelosuppressive chemotherapy can be added in midcycle between intermittent courses of myelosuppressive therapy, using drugs such as bleomycin, vincristine, prednisone, or high-dose methotrexate with leucovorin rescue. In non-

Hodgkin's lymphoma, a large randomized trial recently demonstrated the superiority of using non myelosuppressive drugs in midcycle rather than at the beginning of each 3-week cycle (Johnson et al. 1983). Weekly non myelosuppressive therapy with weekly bleomycin is used in testicular cancer chemotherapy, and a new Canadian regimen alternating myelosuppressive with non myelosuppressive therapy with weekly dosing has shown exceptional promise in diffuse large cell lymphoma (Klimo and Connors 1985).

Conclusions

Our nascent understanding of the biologic basis of cancer chemotherapy is just beginning to be applied to clinical cancer medicine. New methods are being applied to search for effective drugs, both analogs of existing useful compounds and drugs with novel structure and activity. The optimal timing, sequencing, and dosing of drugs are under intense study, and there is an increasing trend toward integrating chemotherapy into the primary management of cancer (adjuvant and neo-adjuvant chemotherapy). Methods of protecting normal tissues from the toxic effects of chemotherapy or of sensitizing tumor tissue to chemotherapy are under investigation. As we have described, studies of methods to circumvent drug resistance, including calcium-channel blockers and glutathione-depleting drugs, are ongoing.

Direct delivery of drug to tumors by intra-arterial infusion is an old technique that is in widespread use and may prove superior to standard therapy. Drugs that cause differentiation of tumor cells to a nonmalignant phenotype are being tested. Finally, conventional chemotherapy will be used in the future with biologic response modifiers, and exhaustive scientific effort will be required to determine how best to combine these modalities.

References

Anonymous (1983) Sequential methotrexate and 5-fluorouracil in the management of neoplastic disease. Semin Oncol 10 [Suppl 2]: 1-39

Baylin SB, Gazdar AF, Minna JD, Bernal SD, Shaper JH (1982) A unique cell surface protein phenotype distinguishes human small-cell from non-small cell lung cancer. Proc Natl Acad Sci USA 79: 4650-4654

Blum RH, Carter SK, Agre K (1973) A clinical review of bleomycin: a new antineoplastic agent. Cancer 31: 903-913

Bonadonna G, Valagussa P (1981) Dose response effect of adjuvant chemotherapy in breast cancer. N Engl J Med 30: 10-15

Bonadonna G, Valagussa P, Santoro A (1986) Alternating non-cross-resistant combination chemotherapy or MOPP in Stage IV Hodgkin's disease. Ann Intern Med 104: 739-746

Brower M, Loughner J (1985) Cancer chemotherapy, part 1: the alkylating agents. Hosp Formul 20: 1060-1070

Brower M, Ihde DC, Johnston-Early A et al. (1983) Treatment of extensive stage small cell bronchogenic carcinoma: effects of variation in intensity of induction chemotherapy. Am J Med 75: 993-1000

Carney DN, Winkler CF (1985) In vitro assays of chemotherapeutic sensitivity. In: De Vita VT, Hellman S, Rosenberg SA (eds) Important advances in oncology 1985. Lippincott, Philadelphia

Carney DN, Ahluwalia GS, Jayaram HN, Cooney DA, Johns DG (1985) Relationship between the cytotoxicity of tiazofurin and its metabolism by cultured human lung cancer cells. J Clin Invest 75: 175-182

Cersosimo RJ, Hong WK (1986) Epirubicin: a review of the pharmacology, clinical activity, and adverse effects of an adriamycin analog. J Clin Oncol 4: 425-439

Chabner B (1982) Pharmacologic principles of cancer treatment. Saunders, Philadelphia

Curt GA, Carney DN, Cowan KH et al. (1983) Unstable methotrexate resistance in human small cell carcinoma associated with double minute chromosomes. N Engl J Med 308: 199-202

Curt GA, Jolivet J, Carney DN et al. (1985) Determinants of the sensitivity of human small cell lung cancer cell lines to methotrexate. J Clin Invest 76: 1323-1329

Driscoll JS (1984) The preclinical and new drug research program of the National Cancer Institute. Cancer Treat Rep 68: 63-76

Frei E, Canellos GP (1980) Dose: a critical factor in cancer chemotherapy. Am J Med 69: 585-594

Goldie JH, Coldman AJ (1979) A mathematical model relating the drug sensitivity of tumors to their spontaneous mutation rate. Cancer Treat Rep 63: 1727-1733

Goldie JH, Coldman AJ (1983) Quantitative model for multiple levels of drug resistance in clinical tumors. Cancer Treat Rep 67: 923-931

Grem JL, Hoth DF, Hamilton JM, King SA, Leyland-Jones B (1987) Overview of current status and future direction of clinical trials with 5-fluorouracil in combination with folinic acid. Cancer Treat Rep 71: 1249-1264

Gros P, Croop J, Housman D (1986) Mammalian multidrug resistance gene: complete cDNA sequence indicates strong homology to bacterial transport proteins. Cell 47: 371-380

Guild BC, Mulligan RC, Gros P, Housman DE (1988) Retroviral transfer of a murine cDNA for multidrug resistance confers pleiotropic drug resistance to cells without prior drug selection. Proc Natl Acad Sci USA 85: 1595-1599

Johnson GJ, Costello WB, Oken MM et al. (1983) Sequential cyclophosphamide-prednisone and vincristine-bleomycin (CPOB): an effective schedule-dependent treatment for advanced diffuse histiocytic lymphoma. Cancer 52: 1133-1141

Jolivet J, Cowan KH, Curt GA, Clendeninn NJ, Chabner BA (1983) The pharmacology and clinical use of methotrexate. N Engl J Med 309: 1094-1104

Klein G, Klein E (1985) Evolution of tumors and the impact of molecular oncology. Nature 315: 190-195

Klimo P, Connors JM (1985) MACOP-B chemotherapy for the treatment of diffuse large cell lymphoma. Ann Intern Med 102: 596-602

Krakoff IH (1981) Cancer chemotherapeutic agents. CA 31: 130-140

Ling V, Kartner N, Sudo T, Siminovitch L, Riordan JR (1983)

Multidrug resistance phenotype in Chinese hamster ovary cells. Cancer Treat Rep 67: 869–874
Loehrer PJ, Einhorn LH (1984) Cisplatin. Ann Intern Med 100: 704–713
Norton L, Simon R (1986) The Norton-Simon hypothesis revisited. Cancer Treat Rep 70: 163–169
Ozols RF, Cowan K (1986) New aspects of clinical drug resistance: the role of gene amplification and the reversal of resistance in drug refractory cancer. In: De Vita VT, Hellman S, Rosenberg SA (eds) Important advances in oncology 1986. Lippincott, Philadelphia, pp 129–157
Ozols RF, Corden BJ, Jacobs J, Wesley MN, Ostchega Y, Young RC (1984) High-dose cisplatin in hypertonic saline. Ann Intern Med 100: 19–24
Pratt WB, Ruddon RW (1979) The anticancer drugs. Oxford University Press, New York
Ross W, Rowe T, Glisson J, Yalowich J, Liu L (1984) Role of topoisomerase II in mediating epipodophyllotoxin-induced DNA cleavage. Cancer Res 44: 5857–5860
Selby P, Buick RN, Tannock I (1983) A critical appraisal of the "human tumor stem-cell assay". N Engl J Med 308: 129–134
Shenkenberg TD, Van Hoff DD (1986) Mitoxantrone: a new anticancer drug with significant clinical activity. Ann Intern Med 105: 67–81
Shoemaker RH (1986) New approaches to antitumor drug screening: the human tumor colony forming assay. Cancer Treat Rep 70: 9–12
Tannock I (1978) Cell kinetics and chemotherapy: a critical review. Cancer Treat Rep 62: 1117–1133
Tsuruo T (1983) Reversal of acquired resistance to vinca alkaloids and anthracycline antibiotics. Cancer Treat Rep 67: 889–894
Weiss RB, Issell BF (1982) The nitrosoureas: carmustine (BCNU) and lomustine (CCNU). Cancer Treat Rev 9: 313–330
Young RC, Ozols RF, Myers CE (1981) The anthracycline antineoplastic drugs. N Engl J Med 305: 139–153
Zimm S, Collins JM, Riccardi R et al. (1983) Variable bioavailability of oral mercaptopurine. N Engl J Med 308: 1005–1009

Chemotherapy in Cancer Treatment

E. Boven and H. M. Pinedo

In the past decade, chemotherapy has dramatically improved long-term disease-free survival in various advanced malignancies. Progress can be attributed to (1) higher response rates to combination chemotherapy than to single-agent therapy; (2) the possibility of eradicating subclinical disease by means of adjuvant chemotherapy; (3) enhancement of the effectiveness of other modalities, such as surgery and radiotherapy, by pretreating patients with chemotherapy; or (4) regional administration of cytotoxic drugs in the case of localized disease. In advanced hematologic malignancies the benefit of chemotherapy is unquestionable, with long-term disease-free survival (cure) in more than 50% of patients with acute lymphocytic leukemia, Hodgkin's disease or aggressive types of non-Hodgkin's lymphoma and in smaller percentages of patients with acute nonlymphocytic leukemia and indolent types of non-Hodgkin's lymphoma (Chabner et al. 1984). Excellent long-term palliation with chemotherapy can be expected in multiple myeloma and chronic leukemia. In advanced solid tumors improved treatment results are frequently attributable to chemotherapy as part of a multimodality approach. Presently, the majority of patients with advanced testicular cancer, gestational trophoblastic disease and some childhood tumors will be cured. High response rates with increasing numbers of long-term disease-free patients are observed in ovarian cancer and small cell lung cancer. Benefit from chemotherapy, expressed in prolonged survival, can also be expected in breast cancer and gastric cancer.

Major advances in multimodality cancer therapy are achieved exclusively by close collaboration of surgeon, radiotherapist and medical oncologist. Without doubt, aggressive chemotherapy should be handled by an experienced oncologist with knowledge of acute and long-term hazards to the patient. Also, steps forward have to be made by participating in multicenter clinical trials prospectively comparing standard therapy to new approaches (see Staquet, this volume). Those patients with lesions not amenable to conventional treatment are potential candidates for clinical trials studying the interaction of surgery with radiation and/or chemotherapy, innovative chemotherapy, antitumor effects of biologic response modifiers, etc. (Chabner et al. 1984; Wilson 1984; Oldham 1985). In the present chapter we will discuss the state of the art of chemotherapy in solid tumors.

Head and Neck Cancer

Squamous Cell Cancer. Only one-third of patients with squamous cell cancer of the head and neck present with localized disease easily curable by surgery and radiation. These treatment modalities, however, have not provided for adequate tumor control in locally advanced and regional disease. Local recurrences occur in up to 60% of all patients, and distant metastases develop in 20%–30%. Previously, only the latter group of patients would have been considered for chemotherapy. In the past few years considerable efforts have been put into developing protocols to study the role of intra-arterial chemotherapy, chemotherapy combined with radiotherapy or induction chemotherapy.

Three drugs – methotrexate, bleomycin and cisplatin – have consistently shown antitumor activity in head and neck cancer (Mead and Jacobs 1982). Methotrexate has undergone extensive evaluation of its optimal dose, schedule and method of delivery. Weekly administration appears to be more effective than the administration of either monthly high doses or daily small doses. High-dose methotrexate plus leucovorin rescue does not significantly increase the response rate or the duration of survival (Woods et al. 1981). Remissions on single agents have generally been shorter than 6 months. Compared to standard single agents, a combination of active drugs has not made a major impact on the course of this stage of disease (Rozencweig et al. 1984; Williams et al. 1986). However, recent results with the combination of cisplatin plus 5-fluorouracil continuous infusion are encouraging, with response rates from 70% to 90% and an overall median duration of survival of 27 weeks (Kish et al. 1985). The efficacy of the regimen was less if 5-fluorouracil was administered as a bolus injection. Superior results of combination chemotherapy in advanced disease have yet to be confirmed in prospectively randomized trials in which one treatment arm consists of single-agent therapy.

Intra-arterial chemotherapy has usually been studied only in cancers of the oral cavity, oropharynx and maxillary sinus. Despite considerable clinical experience, the advantage of intra-arterial over intravenous treatment has yet to be proven. This modality is unable to control neck disease and other areas of distant metastases. The introduction of implantable infusion pumps has brought about a renewal of interest in this treatment approach (Wheeler et al. 1984).

Previous studies combining methotrexate or bleomycin with radiation in an attempt to achieve better efficacy in locally advanced, inoperable head and neck cancer have failed to demonstrate increased disease-free survival. Preliminary data on simultaneous irradiation and administration of cisplatin (a drug with radiosensitizing properties), either alone or with 5-fluorouracil infusions, suggest a remarkable improvement of locoregional control (Leipzig 1983; Taylor et al. 1985). It is not yet known whether concomitant use of these modalities is superior to sequential treatment in terms of improving long-term disease-free survival.

Recently, emphasis has been put on the use of chemotherapy as inital treatment in locally advanced disease (stages III and IV). The response rate of 50%–80% with chemotherapy in previously untreated patients is clearly superior to the rate in patients who have undergone prior surgery, irradiation or both (Mead and Jacobs 1982). Because of these dramatic regressions, it is reasonable to predict enhanced local control with subsequent surgery or radiotherapy. Results of studies prospectively randomizing patients to conventional local treatment with or without induction chemotherapy have to be awaited. Moreover, it has yet to be shown whether this type of therapy is more beneficial than adjuvant chemotherapy following regional treatment.

Salivary Gland Tumors. Adenoid cystic cancer, mucoepidermoid cancer and acinous cell cancer all respond to a variety of single agents. Most experience has been obtained in adenoid cystic cancer, where the single agents with which the highest activities have been observed are cisplatin, 5-fluorouracil and doxorubicin (Suen and Johns 1982).

Cancer of the Lungs, Mediastinum and Pleural Cavity

Small Cell Lung Cancer (SCLC). SCLC is a common malignancy with a distinct feature of early widespread metastasis. From several randomized trials it became clear that combination chemotherapy can significantly prolong the median duration of survival in patients with SCLC. Prognosis in SCLC strongly depends on disease stage, classified in two categories: patients with limited disease (lesions confined to one hemithorax, including hilar and mediastinal nodes, but excluding malignant pleuritis), and those with extensive disease. Combination chemotherapy is indicated in practically all patients. Objective response rates can be achieved in more than 75% of cases, with approximately 50% of limited-disease patients and 20% of extensive-disease patients achieving complete remission (Greco et al. 1985; Elliot et al. 1984). The best results are obtained with simultaneous administration of at least three cytostatic agents active in SCLC, such as cyclophosphamide, methotrexate and lomustine; cyclophosphamide, doxorubicin and vincristine; or cyclophosphamide, doxorubicin and etoposide. Median survival periods with the various regimens are similar, ranging from 9 to 14 months depending on disease stage. Many centers still irradiate the primary tumor in cases of complete remission documented on bronchoscopy (Bleehen et al. 1983). Also, prophylactic cranial irradiation is advised in such cases. Unfortunately, only 5%–10% of all patients survive free of disease for more than 2 years, the majority of whom initially had limited disease. Attempts to improve therapeutic strategies with existing drugs, new drugs and combinations of drugs include studies of alternating non-cross-resistant chemotherapy and intensive induction chemotherapy, with or without autologous bone marrow transplantation. Reviving interest can be observed in the surgical treatment of patients with operable, limited-disease SCLC (Osterlind et al. 1985). Whether this small subgroup will benefit from surgery in terms of survival has to be determined in a prospectively randomized trial.

Non-Small Cell Lung Cancer (NSCLC). Surgery is the treatment of choice for patients considered potentially curable of NSCLC. In inoperable, locally advanced disease, radiotherapy is primarily chosen, but results have been generally disappointing in prolonging survival. Thus far, chemotherapy in patients with recurring or advanced NSCLC is still associated with a very low response rate without overall benefit. Cisplatin, etoposide and vindesine are presently the three most frequently investigated drugs, but objective response rates are below 20% (Hoffman et al. 1983; Klastersky and Sculier 1985). Cisplatin-containing regimens appear to achieve a response rate of approximately 30%, and responders may benefit from such therapies. The presently available regimens should not be considered as standard treatments. The role of combined modalities, such as concomitant chemotherapy and radiotherapy in patients with locally advanced inoperable NSCLC, is under investigation. In this respect, 5-fluorouracil and cisplatin have been added individually to radiation, but it is too early to draw conclusions with regard to long-term efficacy (Reimer et al. 1981; Byfield et al. 1983).

Thymoma. Invasive thymoma is a rare, malignant tumor leading to death in about 50% of patients within 5 years (Verley and Hollmann 1985). Those 20% of patients not suitable for surgery and/or radiotherapy, or with distant metastases, are potential candidates for chemotherapy. Little information is available regarding the efficacy of cytostatic agents. Cisplatin-containing regimens, such as a combination of the drug with doxorubicin, vincristine and cyclophosphamide, appear to yield the best outcome (Fornasiero et al. 1984).

Mesothelioma. Information on the clinical course and treatment of mesothelioma remains anecdotal. The role of chemotherapy in the management of these tumors is currently unclear. The assessment of response has been facilitated by the use of computerized tomography. The best agent in mesothelioma appears to be doxorubicin, with response rates of 21%–44% (Aisner and Wiernik 1981; Chahinian et al. 1982). Recently, intracavitary cisplatin has shown activity against mesothelioma (Pfeifle et al. 1985).

Gastrointestinal Cancer

Esophageal Cancer. In approximately 50% of patients with squamous-cell cancer of the esophagus, the disease is already incurable at the time of diagnosis. In patients with metastatic lesions, vindesine, bleomycin, and cisplatin have shown moderate activity. Combination regimens including two or three of these drugs will result in a response rate of 26%–33% with a median duration of response of 5–7 months (Kelsen et al. 1983; De Besi et al. 1984), but are not advised on a routine basis. Preoperative chemotherapy is gaining a more important role in the treatment of locoregional esophageal cancer, the aim being to improve cure rate and survival. Two approaches are being studied: (1) preoperative chemotherapy, and (2) the addition of chemotherapy to preoperative radiation. After preoperative treatment with combined cisplatin, vindesine and bleomycin, Kelsen et al. (1983) observed a response rate of 63% and the presence of resectable disease in 50% of all patients. Preliminary results of simultaneous radiation and chemotherapy employing a combination of 5-fluorouracil and cisplatin (Leichman et al. 1984), or 5-fluorouracil and mitomycin C (Keane et al. 1985), not only indicate that this regimen is advantageous in terms of achieving resectability, but also suggest that it is superior to radiation alone in controlling locoregional disease. It is obvious that such treatments should be restricted to highly specialized centers. At present, the role of postsurgical adjuvant chemotherapy has not been established.

Gastric Cancer. Stomach cancer is the gastrointestinal cancer most sensitive to chemotherapy. In 1979, MacDonald et al. reported the first results of a study in patients with advanced disease using the regimen of 5-fluorouracil, doxorubicin and mitomycin C (FAM). Their final results showed a 42% response rate with a median survival time of 14 months for responders (Schein 1985). Since then, many investigators have confirmed the activity of FAM and the combination is generally regarded as the treatment of choice. The best results are observed in patients with a good performance score. Results of current studies comparing FAM with single-agent chemotherapy or with other drug combinations in patients with advanced stomach cancer have to be awaited. Thus far, adjuvant chemotherapy following surgery has failed to be of any benefit.

Cancer of the Pancreas and Biliary Tract. The development of chemotherapy for pancreatic cancer has proceeded slowly due to a variety of factors. In many patients it is difficult to obtain an objective tumor parameter to assess the effect of treatment. In addition, many patients are not eligible for clinical trials, because this tumor characteristically causes marked debility as a result of pain, anorexia and malabsorption. Limited activity in pancreatic cancer has been observed with 5-fluorouracil, mitomycin C and streptozocin (Schein 1985). Some benefit in survival has also been observed in patients responding to combination chemotherapy (FAM), but gains have been generally small. Overall, chemotherapy should not be given on a routine basis in pancreatic cancer. The combination of radiotherapy and chemotherapy is a continuous area of research in patients with locally advanced pancreatic cancer, but no advantage regarding survival has yet been demonstrated.

Cancer of the biliary tract is uncommon and chemotherapy data are scanty. It appears that mitomycin C is the most active single agent. A trial with this drug appears justified in patients with an evaluable lesion. The FAM regimen was reported as having achieved a response rate of 31% in a very small group of patients (Harvey et al. 1984), but should not be considered as standard treatment.

Hepatocellular Cancer. In unresectable primary liver cancer, there is no widely accepted standard chemotherapy. Most patients die rapidly of progressive disease. Doxorubicin appears to be the most active drug (Falkson et al. 1978). Innovative therapy using ^{131}I-labeled antiferritin as part of a multimodality approach (Order et al. 1985) seems to provide better results, but should still be regarded as a highly experimental measure.

Colorectal Cancer. The chemotherapeutic management of advanced colorectal cancer has been disappointing so far. The most commonly used cytostatic agent is 5-fluorouracil, with approximately 20% of patients achieving objective responses. The slightly better results obtained with a combination of methyl-CCNU, vincristine, 5-fluorouracil and streptozocin (MOF-Strep) need confirmation in larger groups of patients (Weltz et al. 1983; Kemeny et al. 1983). At present, interest in 5-fluorouracil has revived, with experimental studies of various doses, routes and schedules of administration, as well as attempts to increase its therapeutic efficacy by biochemical modulation (Sugarbaker et al. 1985; Nadajewicz et al. 1984; Van Groeningen et al. 1986). To date, adjuvant chemotherapy in colorectal cancer must be considered investigational and thus should not be applied on a routine basis. In view of the importance of this malignancy and the potential toxicity of therapeutic regimens, controlled clinical trials employing randomized patient groups should include a control arm (Metzger et al. 1985). The role of intra-arterial chemotherapy in hepatic metastases of colorectal cancer will be discussed in the next chapter (Liver Infusion Chemotherapy).

Anal Cancer. Management of squamous cell cancer of the anus has been primarily surgical in the past. Recent reports indicate that concomitant chemotherapy and radiation may be considered a therapeutic equivalent to radical surgery in anal cancer. Long-term local control can be achieved with the addition of mitomycin C and 5-fluorouracil to radical radiotherapy (Cummings et al. 1982; Flam et al. 1983).

Cancer of the Urogenital Tract

Renal Cell Cancer. At the time of diagnosis, about half the patients with renal cell cancer have advanced metastatic disease. Unfortunately, no clearly effective chemotherapeutic regimen has yet been developed. Future studies with biologicals will hopefully improve the prognosis in these patients.

Bladder Cancer. Transitional cell cancer of the urothelial tract (renal pelvis, ureter, bladder and urethra) is a chemotherapeutically responsive tumor. The most important drugs in advanced disease are cisplatin, methotrexate and doxorubicin, with response rates of 20%–45% and median duration of response of 3–6 months (Yagoda 1980; Stoter 1985). Cisplatin-containing combinations previously showed no therapeutic advantage over single-agent cisplatin. Recently introduced regimens containing cisplatin and methotrexate appear more effective, with response rates of 46%–72% and a definite increase in duration of response and survival, particularly in complete responders (Stoter 1985). However, the high incidence of toxicity (mucositis, myelosuppression, renal insufficiency) warrants the establishment of safer treatment before introducing these drugs for routine application in advanced disease or in an adjuvant setting after local treatment of invasive bladder cancer.

With cisplatin being most active in bladder cancer, studies have been initiated to combine this drug with external beam radiation in the treatment of patients with inoperable clinical stage T2–T4 tumors after transurethral resection. Animal studies have indicated a significant activity of this approach in transitional cell tumors (Soloway et al. 1979). Indeed, approximately 60% of patients experience complete remission on the combined modality regimen, while toxicity is acceptable (Shipley et al. 1984). Longer follow-up is required to determine whether responses are maintained and will result in lasting benefit.

In patients with superficial bladder cancer (stage Tis, T1a, T1) a variety of drugs have been used for intravesical instillation, either as adjuvant therapy after transurethral resection or as treatment for surgically inaccessible disease. Epodyl, thiotepa, doxorubicin and mitomycin C are each active in destroying superficial bladder tumors. Mitomycin C (40 mg in 40 ml water once weekly for 8 weeks) is probably the least toxic agent (Issell et al. 1984). It is unclear whether intravesical chemotherapy will alter the ultimate course of the disease.

Prostate Cancer. Patients with advanced prostatic cancer should first be treated with hormones. Chemotherapy has been poorly evaluated, primarily due to difficulties in staging and uncertainty about the value of indicator lesions. Drugs with activity in endocrine-refractory advanced disease are doxorubicin (Torti et al. 1983) and mitomycin C (Jones et al. 1986). While objective response rates are low, a large but yet to be defined proportion of patients experience relief of pain and improvement of performance status.

Penile Cancer. Advanced epidermoid cancer of the penis is a rare disease. Methotrexate, cisplatin and bleomycin were reported to be active in this tumor, but the majority of responses are only partial and of short duration (Ahmed et al. 1984).

Testicular Tumors. Nonseminomatous testicular cancer is the solid tumor in adults most sensitive to chemotherapy. Combination chemotherapy is the treatment of choice for patients with bulky stage II–IV disease. Also, in limited stage II disease radical lymph node dissection tends to be replaced by chemotherapy. The most commonly used combination has been cisplatin, vinblastine and bleomycin (PVB), which cures approximately 75% of patients (Stoter et al. 1984). A similarly effective but somewhat more toxic regimen is a combination of cisplatin, bleomycin, vinblastine, actinomycin D and cyclophosphamide (VAB-6) (Vugrin et al. 1983). Recently, a less toxic combination consisting of bleomycin, etoposide and cisplatin (BEP) has proved equally effective to PVB (Peckham et al. 1983), and should now be considered first-line chemotherapy for testicular nonseminomas. The most important prognostic factor for response is tumor volume, with only 50% of patients with bulky disease achieving long-term disease-free survival. Studies of the efficacy of etoposide and cisplatin without bleomycin (EP) in reducing toxicity in patients with small-volume metastases have recently been initiated. Preliminary results indicate a high complete response rate (75%) and reduction of toxicity, but a randomized trial is necessary to evaluate the therapeutic outcome of EP vs BEP (Peckham et al. 1985a). Testicular cancer patients not achieving complete remission after four chemotherapy cycles, assessed either by computerized tomography or by the inadequate fall of initially elevated tumor markers (alpha-fetoprotein, human chorionic gonadotropin), should undergo cytoreductive surgery if feasible (Donohue et al. 1980). In the presence of residual vital tumor cells in the pathologic specimen, the patient should continue on chemotherapy for at least two additional cycles. Maintenance chemotherapy does not add to the number of complete responders. In patients not achieving complete remission, and in those presenting with a relapse after initial adequate therapy, salvage treatment including new drugs (Loehrer et al. 1986) or high-dose chemotherapy with autologous bone marrow transplantation can still be effective. Intensified chemotherapy is also being studied as primary treatment in patients with high-volume metastases.

In general, orchidectomy should always be performed before chemotherapy. The testis may behave as a sanctuary and still contain viable tumor at the end of chemotherapy (Greist et al. 1984).

Testicular seminoma is also extremely sensitive to chemotherapy. Cisplatin-containing regimens should be considered as initial treatment in advanced, bulky disease. Schedules such as VAB-6, PVB and BEP, have resulted in 80%–90% patients becoming free of disease (Vugrin and Whitmore 1984; Peckham et al. 1985b). The value of post-treatment irradiation of the sites of the initial lesions has yet to be definitively evaluated, but with our present knowledge it should be given in case of residual disease after four cycles of chemotherapy.

Presently, extragonadal germ cell tumors are essentially just as responsive as testicular cancer to cisplatin-containing chemotherapy (Logothetis et al. 1985). However, patients with these tumors appear to have a less favorable prognosis, which may not only be caused by the extent of the disease at the time of presentation.

Gynecologic Malignancies

Epithelial Ovarian Cancer. In patients with ovarian cancer, the prognostic factors include stage of disease, histologic grade, extent of tumor lesions after surgery and response to chemotherapy. At diagnosis, the majority of patients present with FIGO stage III or IV disease, which cannot be cured by surgery alone. With the introduction of cisplatin-containing combination chemotherapy after cytoreductive surgery, there has been a significant increase in response rate, median duration of survival, 5-year survival rate, and cure rate (Piver 1984; Ozols and Young 1984). The most active drugs in ovarian cancer are the alkylating agents (cyclophosphamide, melphalan), cisplatin, hexamethylmelamine and doxorubicin. Young et al. (1978) were the first to demonstrate that combination chemotherapy yields better results than single-agent melphalan in terms of an increased response rate, more complete responders and longer median overall survival. Various prospectively randomized trials have since confirmed this observation (Ozols and Young 1984). The present regimens containing both cisplatin and cyclophosphamide yield the best results, such as a response rate of approximately 68% and a median duration of overall survival of 18–23 months (Neijt et al. 1984). Patients with minimal residual disease after surgery (largest diameter of tumor deposits less than 1–1.5 cm) fare better on chemotherapy than patients with bulky disease. In the case of initial failure of cytoreductive surgery a second attempt at tumor debulking seems justifiable in patients responding to chemotherapy (Ozols and Young 1984; Berek et al. 1983). Results of salvage chemotherapy for relapsing disease are generally disappointing. Efforts have continued to find new effective combinations.

Former studies in stage I or II ovarian cancer indicated that approximately 50% of patients eventually presented with a relapse after adequate surgery with or without radiotherapy. Most likely, a number of these patients would have been classified as having disease of a higher stage if a more rigorous staging procedure had been employed (Piver 1984). Therefore, both the role of radiotherapy and that of chemotherapy as an adjunct to surgery in stage I and II ovarian cancer need to be reassessed in carefully staged patients.

Some new chemotherapy approaches with relevance to ovarian cancer are of interest. First, carboplatin, a cisplatin analog without evidence of significant renal toxicity or ototoxicity, has shown antitumor activity in ovarian cancer comparable to that of the parent compound (Thigpen et al. 1984). It is not yet known whether clinical efficacy is maintained at the same level with carboplatin-containing regimens as with regimens including cisplatin. Second, the impact on survival of intraperitoneal chemotherapy as a measure to eradicate minimal residual or microscopic disease needs further investigation in various stages of ovarian cancer (Myers 1984) (see Schlag and Herfarth, this volume).

Germ Cell Tumors of the Ovary. Malignant germ cell tumors of the ovary are rare and aggressive neoplasms affecting young women. Localized dysgerminoma is frequently curable with surgery followed by radiotherapy. Prior to the use of combination chemotherapy, the majority of patients with endodermal sinus tumors or immature teratomes died of their disease. The cure rate has increased with the introduction of adjuvant chemotherapy. While the combination of vincristine, actinomycin D and cyclophosphamide (VAC) has been considered the standard treatment for all stages of disease in the past, cisplatin-containing regimens such as VAB-6 or PVB, known for their activity in nonseminomatous testicular cancer, have further improved response rates to over 75% in advanced disease (Bradoff et al. 1982; Carlson et al. 1983). The PVB regimen should also replace VAC in an adjuvant setting following surgery for localized disease.

Endometrial Cancer. Because of the frequency of localized disease in endometrial cancer, the results of surgery, radiotherapy or a combination of the two modalities are rewarding, with approximately 70% of patients surviving for 5 years. Progestins represent the first-line treatment in recurrent or advanced disease, with one-third of patients responding. Nonhormonal chemotherapy as second-line treatment has not been studied extensively. Doxorubicin, cyclophosphamide and cisplatin have the highest activity. In two small studies on the combination of these drugs, response rates of 47% and 81% were observed, with a median duration of overall survival of 10 months in both studies (Turbow et al. 1985; Pasmantier et al. 1985). Presently there is no role for adjuvant chemotherapy in patients with a high risk of recurrence after primary surgery followed by radiation.

Cancer of the Cervix. Until recently, chemotherapy did not play an important role in the treatment of cervical cancer because initial therapy with other modalities was fairly effective. Several factors are responsible for the difficulties in assessing the antitumor activity of cytotoxic agents in advanced or recurrent disease, including inevaluability of pelvic disease in previously operated and/or irradiated areas, limited bone marrow reserve after previous radiation, impaired renal function due to ureteral obstruction and limited chemotherapy access to previously treated pelvic tumor lesions. Several agents have shown activity in cervical cancer, of which cisplatin, vincristine, mitomycin C, methotrexate and bleomycin have been most widely used in combination regimens. Small studies on combination chemotherapy reported response rates of 40%–66% with a median duration of response of generally less than 7 months (Baker et al. 1976; Krebs et al. 1980; Rosenthal et al. 1983). Prospective randomized trials are required to assess the relative contribution of each single agent to the efficacy of combination chemotherapy in this type of disease.

As part of a multimodality approach in the treatment of locally advanced cervical cancer (nodal metastases), combination chemotherapy is gaining interest in an attempt to increase the number of patients with initial control of disease. A higher proportion of patients are likely to respond to cytotoxic agents as first-line treatment, which will facilitate irradiation or even surgical resection of residual tumor lesions (Friedlander et al. 1984).

Gestational Trophoblastic Disease (GTD). Considering the good results that can be achieved with methotrexate or actinomycin D in GTD, current work focusses on efforts to decrease toxicity in low-risk patients and to introduce more aggressive approaches in those with poor-prognosis features. Low-risk disease is characterized by a low circulating level of human chorionic gonadotropin (HCG), no cerebral or hepatic metastases, a short interval between prior gestation and the appearance of GTD and no prior chemotherapy. In nonmetastatic GTD complete sustained responses are obtained with chemotherapy in 90% of cases without hysterectomy (Goldstein and Berkowitz 1982). In order to preserve fertility, methotrexate with leucovorin rescue is the treatment of choice in good-prognosis patients. Patients on treatment should be carefully monitored for normalization of HCG levels. Generally, it is recommended to continue chemotherapy for at least three cycles after normalization of HCG levels. In the case of primary hysterectomy, adjuvant single-agent chemotherapy is indicated. Relapsing patients with GTD can still be cured with actinomycin D or with multiple-drug regimens.

In high-risk GTD, deaths from drug resistance still occur. Initial chemotherapy consists of a multiple-drug regimen, such as the CHAMOCA regimen designed by Bagshawe, rather than single agents (Begent and Bagshawe 1982; Surwit 1982). Attempts are being made to integrate two newer drugs, cisplatin and etoposide, which have substantial activity in GTD, into the initial chemotherapy for patients with a poor prognosis. In the course of the disease, additional surgery of potentially resectable sites of active disease should be considered.

Miscellaneous Tumors. Cancer of the fallopian tube has some parallels with ovarian cancer. Tumors not completely resected, or recurring, may respond to regimens containing cisplatin, cyclophosphamide and doxorubicin (Deppe et al. 1980).

Squamous cell cancer of the vulva occurs rarely and at an advanced age. Bleomycin, methotrexate or doxorubicin may achieve regression of tumor lesions in the case of recurrent or metastatic disease after initial surgery with or without radiation (Deppe et al. 1979).

Breast Cancer

The traditional treatment for patients with primary breast cancer has been radical surgery with or without radiotherapy, while that for patients with advanced disease has been palliative hormonal therapy followed by chemotherapy. These treatments have met with limited effectiveness in terms of eradicating the disease. Studies in the past decade have given cause for optimism. Adjuvant systemic therapy after local treatment appears beneficial to certain subsets of patients with primary breast cancer. Estrogen receptor is an important prognostic factor and can reliably predict which patients will respond to hormonal therapy.

Premenopausal patients with advanced disease with a negative estrogen receptor, patients refractory to hormonal therapy and those with rapidly progressive disease regardless of the receptor status are candidates for chemotherapy. Postmenopausal patients with negative estrogen receptor and slowly progressive disease should be considered for initial hormonal treatment, because of their 10%–20% chance of responding to this treatment. A wide range of cytostatic agents has been shown to induce regression of breast cancer metastases. Cyclophosphamide and doxorubicin are considered the most active agents, with response rates of 35%–40%, followed by methotrexate, 5-fluorouracil, vinca alkaloids and mitomycin C (Lyss and Loeb 1984; Perlow and Holland 1984). Several drug combinations have been studied, of which cyclophosphamide, methotrexate and 5-fluorouracil (CMF) and 5-fluorouracil, doxorubicin and cyclophosphamide (FAC) are most popular. Presently, all forms of first-line combination chemotherapy in advanced disease can be expected to yield comparable results. In women given appropriate dose levels, the response rate may range from 45% to 75%, with a median duration of response of 7–13 months and an overall survival rate of 2–24 months (Bonadonna and Valagussa 1983; Hryniuk and Bush 1984). Patients with progressive disease refractory to first-line combination chemotherapy may still respond to salvage chemotherapy. The combination of hormones and cytostatic agents in the treatment of advanced breast cancer has given controversial results. From recent studies it appears that postmenopausal patients, and especially those with receptor-rich tumors, benefit from this approach in terms of survival (Mouridsen et al. 1985; Kiang et al. 1985). Most likely, survival will be at least as long with the sequential use of both modalities. However, in receptor-positive patients with rapidly progressive disease the addition of hormones to combination chemotherapy should be considered in order to increase the chance of a fast and long-lasting response.

Prospectively randomized trials have investigated the role of adjuvant chemotherapy in patients with primary resected breast cancer with or without local radiotherapy. At the consensus meeting of the National Institutes of Health in 1985, it was recommended that for premenopausal women with axillary node involvement, treatment with established combination chemotherapy (CMF) should become standard care (Glick 1985). This recommendation was based on data suggesting that in these patients adjuvant chemotherapy provided slight but significant improvements in both relapse-free and overall survival. Thus far, it appears that maximum tumor cell kill is achieved within the first few months after mastectomy. Presently, effective adjuvant chemotherapy is considered to consist of intensive chemotherapy using full drug doses for a period of 6 months (Bonadonna and Valagussa 1983). Further studies will have to define subsets of patients deriving most benefit from adjuvant chemotherapy (number of involved nodes, receptor status, etc.), select the best chemotherapeutic regimen (multiple non-cross-resistant combinations, chemohormonotherapy, etc.), and determine the risk of long-term side effects. At the same consensus meeting (Glick 1985) adjuvant hormonal therapy was recommended for postmenopausal women with axillary node involvement.

Male Breast Cancer. Male breast cancer is a rare malignancy with many similarities to female breast cancer. In patients with advanced disease, not responding or refractory to hormones, CMF or doxorubicin-based chemotherapy regimens are moderately effective (Yap et al. 1980 a).

Endocrine Tumors

A variety of endocrine tumors are capable of producing hormones that are either endogenous to the organ of origin or ectopic, such as polypeptides with ACTH action. Systemic therapy for functioning tumors not amenable to surgery can be divided into two distinct forms of management: antihormonal and anticancer. Also, nonfunctioning advanced tumors have incidentally been treated with chemotherapy. The combination of streptozocin plus 5-fluorouracil has shown activity in advanced islet cell cancers and in metastatic carcinoid tumors (Moertel et al. 1980; Engstrom et al. 1984). In advanced adrenal cortical carcinoma, o,p′-DDD (mitotane) is the first treatment (Boven et al. 1984). Refractory patients may benefit from a combination of cyclophosphamide, doxorubicin and cisplatin (Van Slooten and Van Oosterom 1983). The ergot derivative bromocriptine is known to effectively reduce the size of pituitary tumors of varying histology (Wollesen et al. 1982). Doxorubicin may achieve regression of metastatic thyroid cancer (Leeper and Shimaoka 1980).

Malignant Melanoma

Systemic chemotherapy of advanced malignant melanoma is still as unsatisfactory as it was in 1972, when Luce published an analysis of data on the use of single-agent chemotherapy. No single-agent or combination chemotherapy (with or without immunotherapy) appears to yield better results than the 20% partial responses and the less than 5% complete responses being achieved with dacarbazine (DTIC). Although adjuvant chemotherapy after excision of primary tumors or regional metastases is still being studied, so far no benefit has been observed.

For metastases localized in one extremity, (hyperthermic) regional isolation perfusion with melphalan is the treatment of choice (Hafström and Jönsson 1980). There are no hard data to recommend its use as an adjunct to surgical treatment of uncomplicated primaries. Prophylactic (hyperthermic) perfusion with melphalan in poor-prognosis patients (Clark level IV/V, Breslow thickness over 1.5 mm) is now propagated by several groups (Schraffordt Koops et al. 1981; Ghussen et al. 1984), but additional randomized studies are urgently needed to establish whether the procedure is of any benefit and whether hyperthermia is necessary.

Sarcomas

Soft Tissue Sarcoma. Doxorubicin is the most effective single agent in the treatment of advanced soft tissue sarcomas, with a response rate of about 25% in nonpretreated patients. Data on the efficacy of combination chemotherapy are controversial. Any combination to be used should include doxorubicin. With the widely used CYVADIC regimen (cyclophosphamide, vincristine, doxorubicin, dacarbazine) an overall response rate of 38%–50% may be expected with a median survival time of 16–21 months for responders (6–14 months for nonresponders) (Pinedo et al. 1984; Yap et al. 1980b). Complete responders fare significantly better than partial responders, and a small fraction may even be cured with or without additional surgery. Of late, ifosfamide with mesna has proved active in soft tissue sarcoma, with a response rate of 23%–38% (Brade et al. 1985). Results of combination chemotherapy in which ifosfamide and doxorubicin are included have to be awaited.

The growing interest in the role of postsurgical adjuvant chemotherapy in soft tissue sarcomas is clear from various studies dealing with this subject. In a prospective randomized trial by Rosenberg et al. (1983), it was demonstrated that in patients with locally treated high-grade sarcoma of the extremities, a group receiving adjuvant chemotherapy (doxorubicin, cyclophosphamide, and high-dose methotrexate) showed significantly prolonged disease-free survival compared to the control group. Other studies on adjuvant chemotherapy in soft tissue sarcomas of the extremities reported controversial results (Edmonson et al. 1984; Antmann et al. 1984). Also in sarcomas of head and neck, breast, and trunk this approach did not demonstrate any benefit for survival (Glenn et al. 1985). Therefore, postsurgical adjuvant chemotherapy cannot yet be recommended as standard treatment.

Osteosarcoma. Three major changes in chemotherapy for osteosarcomas have taken place since the early 1970s. This treatment modality has been introduced as a postsurgical adjuvant, as a more aggressive management of metastatic disease followed by surgery and as a measure to allow limb preservation. The most active single agents in osteosarcoma are doxorubicin and high-dose methotrexate with leucovorin rescue, with response rates of 30%–40% in advanced disease (Goorin et al. 1985). A recent study has pointed out the possible activity of cisplatin, with a response rate of 19% in pretreated patients (Gaspanni et al. 1985).

The beneficial effect of postsurgical adjuvant chemotherapy, as advocated by Rosen et al. (1984a), has been confirmed by various prospectively randomized trials (Eilber and Eckhardt 1985; Link et al. 1985). The combined modality approach with intensive chemotherapy has increased the relapse-free rates of patients with nonmetastatic osteosarcoma from 20% to 60%–80% at 2 years.

The responsiveness of osteosarcomas to chemotherapy has led to more aggressive therapy for metastatic disease. Removal of solitary lung metastases with or without prior chemotherapy nowadays results in a 5-year survival rate of approximately 40% (Goorin et al. 1985).

The type of chemotherapy employed to facilitate limb-salvage surgery is similar to that in use for postoperative adjuvant therapy. The drugs are given either intravenously or intra-arterially (Eilber et al. 1984). The advantage of the latter route over the former has yet to be proven. Subsequent histologic assessment of tumor destruction may identify the best agent(s), to be used after removal of the primary. Although preliminary reports have indicated that it may be possible to preserve the limb in many patients, further investigation is necessary to ascertain whether this type of therapy might not negatively influence the disease-free survival rate.

Childhood Solid Tumors

Two trends in therapeutic approaches can be observed in the design of clinical trials in childhood tumors. First, there is the attempt to reduce late side effects in diseases which are usually cured by combined modality treatments, such as Wilms' tumor. Second, trials with very intensive treatments are being performed with the aim of improving the prognosis of resistant tumors, such as stage III and IV neuroblastomas. We will briefly discuss the major childhood tumors.

Hepatic Malignancies. The prognosis for children with incompletely resected hepatic malignancies has been very poor. Radiation is usually ineffective in decreasing the size of the tumor prior to surgery, since the required tumor dose is above the hepatic tolerance. A combination of doxorubicin with cyclophosphamide, vincristine and 5-fluorouracil, however, may significantly reduce tumor burden in both hepatoblastomas and hepatocellular carcinomas, enabling successful surgery (Evans et al. 1982; Weinblatt et al. 1982). As an adjunct to primary surgery, the combination also appears to increase the number of cures. Of the newer drugs, cisplatin combined with doxorubicin achieved remarkable responses in each of three hepatoblastoma patients (Quinn et al. 1985).

Wilms' Tumor. After the introduction of combination chemotherapy consisting of actinomycin D, vincristine and doxorubicin (VAC), the 2-year disease-free survival rate of all patients with Wilms' tumor increased to 70% (Clouse et al. 1985). Management may now be refined with regard to extent of disease and histopathologic appearance, the major prognostic factors. For patients with stage I disease this means that chemotherapy seems an adequate substitute for postoperative radiation. The International Society of Paediatric Oncology (Lemerle et al. 1983) has pointed out the importance of preoperative chemotherapy in all disease stages to facilitate surgery. The investigators of the National Wilms' Tumor Study (D'Angio et al. 1981) focussed their treatment approach on operative findings not affected by prior chemotherapy. Both methods of management have their advantages and both can be expected to have very good overall results.

Neuroblastoma. Before the introduction of multimodality approaches including regional radiation and intensive chemotherapy, neuroblastoma had a dismal prognosis, with 70% of children dying of their disease. Survival mainly depends on the stage of the disease and the age at diagnosis, with children under 1 year of age having a better outcome. There is no uniform treatment approach in neuroblastoma. Nowadays, stages I and II usually undergo radiotherapy with or without chemotherapy after surgery, which is reported to result in a survival rate of over 85% (Rosen et al. 1984b). Multimodality approaches in stages III and IV include aggressive chemotherapy such as combinations of vincristine, doxorubicin, cisplatin, an alkylating agent, and dacarbazine. Survival rates are 45%–80% in stage III neuroblastoma and in stage IV patients under 1 year of age, but less than 10% in stage IV patients over 1 year of age. Stage IV neuroblastoma without roentgenographic evidence of bone metastases has been recognized as a separate entity with a more favorable prognosis than stage IV disease with bone metastases (Stokes et al. 1984).

Mesenchymal Tumors. Rhabdomyosarcoma is the most common of the soft tissue malignancies encountered in childhood, accounting for over 50% of all pediatric sarcomas. Prognostic factors for children with soft tissue sarcoma are stage of disease at presentation and site of the primary tumor, with sarcomas arising in the perineum, gastrointestinal tract, retroperitoneum or extremities being at greatest risk of relapse after initially effective therapy (Raney et al. 1983). The present trends in the treatment of rhabdomyosarcomas are to decrease long-term sequelae due to mutilating surgery and radiation and to use chemotherapy as the major treatment modality. The most effective chemotherapy regimen is VAC, with doxorubicin added (VACAd) in poor prognosis patients. For stage I tumors amenable to complete resection, postoperative radiotherapy appears unnecessary if the patient is given adjuvant VAC chemotherapy (Flamant and Hill 1984; Donaldson 1985). Cure rates in localized disease are 65%–75%. Patients with higher stages of disease are treated either by preoperative chemotherapy, limited surgery and/or radiotherapy followed by chemotherapy, or by surgery/biopsy followed by radiotherapy and chemotherapy. Cure rates may be expected from approximately 50% in stage II patients to below 20% in stage IV patients, depending on the primary tumor site.

Few data are available regarding the efficacy of combined modality approaches for childhood soft tissue sarcomas other than rhabdomyosarcomas. Chemotherapy in advanced disease has included VACAd and additional drugs, but responses have often been partial and of limited duration (Donaldson 1985).

Ewing's Sarcoma of Bone. During the past 15 years the multimodality approach with inclusion of combination chemotherapy has dramatically altered survival in Ewing's sarcoma. The value of adjuvant chemotherapy, usually consisting of VACAd with or without additional drugs, in localized disease has resulted in projected 5-year disease-free survival rates of 65%–79% (Rosen et al. 1981; Bacci et al. 1985). Tumors of the extremities have a better prognosis than those of the pelvis, spine, ribs or jaw. Because of the high effectiveness of combination chemotherapy, much interest has been focussed on its use as initial treatment followed by less aggressive surgery or moderate-dose radiation therapy to preserve the patient's functional capabilities.

In advanced Ewing's sarcoma it appears that VACAd combination chemotherapy and radiotherapy to all sites of overt disease can produce prolonged disease-free survival and possible cures in a significant proportion of patients (Pilepich et al. 1981).

Malignant Germ Cell Tumors. Malignant germ cell tumors are rare malignancies in childhood, occurring either in the gonads or in the midline area of the body. Localized testicular seminomas and ovarian dysgerminomas can be cured with surgery and radiotherapy. Nongerminomas are less radiosensitive, and even in localized disease relapses or metastases are frequent. Recent experience gained from chemotherapy in testicular or ovarian germ cell tumors, other than germinomas, in adults has been applied successfully to the treatment of such tumors in children. Cisplatin-containing regimens (PVB) have improved survival rates in advanced disease in children (Brodeur et al. 1981; Flamant et al. 1984). Comparable to studies in adults, new therapeutic approaches in children should include the introduction of effective, less toxic drugs (etoposide) and the design of treatment regimens according to the extent of disease.

References

Ahmed T, Sklaroff R, Yagoda A (1984) Sequential trials of methotrexate, cisplatin, and bleomycin for penile cancer. J Urol 132: 465–468

Aisner J, Wiernik PH (1981) Chemotherapy in the treatment of malignant mesothelioma. Semin Oncol 8: 335–343

Antman K, Smit H, Carson J, Wood W, Proppe K, Harman D, Carey R, Greenberger J, Blum R, Wilson R (1984) Preliminary results of a randomized trial of adjuvant doxorubicin for sarcomas: lack of apparent difference between treatment groups. J Clin Oncol 2: 601–608

Bacci G, Picci P, Gherlinzoni F, Capanna R, Calderoni P, Putti C, Mancini A, Campanacci M (1985) Localized Ewing's sarcoma of bone: ten years' experience at the Istituto Ortopedico Rizzoli in 124 cases treated with multimodal therapy. Eur J Cancer Clin Oncol 21: 163–173

Baker LH, Opipari MI, Izbicki RM (1976) Phase II study of mitomycin-C, vincristine, and bleomycin in advanced squamous cell carcinoma of the uterine cervix. Cancer 38: 2222–2224

Begent RHJ, Bagshawe KD (1982) The management of high-risk choriocarcinoma. Semin Oncol 9: 198–203

Berek JS, Hacker NF, Lagasse LD, Nieberg RK, Elashoff RM (1983) Survival of patients following secondary cytoreductive surgery in ovarian cancer. Obstet Gynecol 61: 189–193

Bleehen NM, Bunn PA, Cox JD, Dombernowsky P, Fox RM, Host H, Joss R, White JE, Wittes RE (1983) Role of radiation therapy in small cell anaplastic carcinoma of the lung. Cancer Treat Rep 67: 11–19

Bonadonna G, Valagussa P (1983) Chemotherapy of breast cancer: current views and results. Int J Radiat Oncol Biol Phys 9: 279–297

Boven E, Vermorken JB, Van Slooten H, Pinedo HM (1984) Complete response of metastasized adrenal cortical carcinoma with o,p′-DDD. Cancer 53: 26–29

Brade WP, Herdrich K, Varini M (1985) Ifosfamide – pharmacology, safety and therapeutic potential. Cancer Treat Rev 12: 1–47

Bradoff JE, Hakes TB, Ochoa M, Golbey R (1982) Germ cell malignancies of the ovary. Cancer 50: 1070–1075

Brodeur GM, Howarth CB, Pratt CB, Caces J, Hustu HO (1981) Malignant germ cell tumors in 57 children and adolescents. Cancer 48: 1890–1898

Byfield JE, Stanton W, Sharp TR, Frankel SS, Koziol J (1983) Phase I–II study of 120-hour infused 5-FU and split-course radiation therapy in localized non-small cell lung cancer. Cancer Treat Rep 67: 933–936

Carlson RW, Sikic BI, Turbow MM, Ballon SC (1983) Combination cisplatin, vinblastine, and bleomycin chemotherapy (PVB) for malignant germ-cell tumors of the ovary. J Clin Oncol 1: 645–651

Chabner BA, Fine RL, Allegra CJ, Yeh GW, Curt GA (1984) Cancer chemotherapy. Cancer 54: 2599–2608

Chahinian AP, Pajak TF, Holland JF, Norton L, Ambinder RM, Mandel EM (1982) Diffuse malignant mesothelioma. Ann Int Med 96 (1): 746–755

Clouse JW, Thomas PRM, Griffiths RC, Perez CA, Vietti TJ, Fineberg B (1985) The changing management of Wilms' tumor over a 30-year period. Cancer 56: 1484–1489

Cummings BJ, Rider WD, Harwood AR, Keane TJ, Thomas GM, Erlichman C, Fine S (1982) Combined radical radiation therapy and chemotherapy for primary squamous cell carcinoma of the anal canal. Cancer Treat Rep 66: 489–492

D'Angio GJ, Evans A, Breslow N, Beckwith B, Bishop H, Farewell V, Goodwin W, Leape L, Palmer N, Sinks L, Sutow W, Tefft M, Wolff J (1981) The treatment of Wilms' tumor. Cancer 47: 2302–2311

De Besi P, Salvagno L, Endrizzi L, Sileni VC, Fosser V, Cartei G, Paccagnella A, Pardo EL, Tremolada C, Peracchia A, Fiorentino MV (1984) Cisplatin, bleomycin and methotrexate in the treatment of advanced oesophageal cancer. Eur J Cancer Clin Oncol 20: 743–747

Deppe G, Cohen CJ, Bruckner HW (1979) Chemotherapy of squamous cell carcinoma of the vulva: a review. Gynecol Oncol 7: 345–348

Deppe G, Bruckner HW, Cohen CJ (1980) Combination chemotherapy for advanced carcinoma of the Fallopian tube. Obstet Gynecol 56: 530–532

Donaldson SS (1985) The value of adjuvant chemotherapy in the management of sarcomas in children. Cancer 55: 2184–2197

Donohue JP, Einhorn LH, Williams SD (1980) Cytoreductive surgery for metastatic testis cancer: considerations of timing and extent. J Urol 123: 876–880

Edmonson JH, Fleming TR, Ivins JC, Burgert EO, Soule EH, O'Connell MJ, Sim FH, Ahmann DL (1984) Randomized study of systemic chemotherapy following complete excision of nonosseous sarcomas. J Clin Oncol 2: 1390–1396

Eilber F, Guiliano A, Eckhardt J, Patterson K, Moseley S, Goodnight J (1987) Adjuvant chemotherapy for osteosarcoma: a randomized prospective trial. J Clin Oncol 5: 21–26

Eilber FR, Eckhardt J, Morton DL (1984) Advances in the treatment of sarcomas of the extremity. Cancer 54: 2695–2701

Elliott JA, Østerlind K, Hansen HH (1984) Cyclic alternating "non-cross resistant" chemotherapy in the management of small cell anaplastic carcinoma of the lung. Cancer Treat Rev 11: 103–113

Engstrom PF, Lavin PT, Moertel CG, Folsch E, Douglass HO (1984) Streptozotocin plus fluorouracil versus doxorubicin therapy for metastatic carcinoid tumor. J Clin Oncol 2: 1255–1259

Evans AE, Land VJ, Newton WA, Randolph JG, Sather HN, Tefft M (1982) Combination chemotherapy (vincristine, adriamycin, cyclophosphamide, and 5-fluorouracil) in the treatment of children with malignant hepatoma. Cancer 50: 821–826

Falkson G, Moertel C, Lavin P, Pretorius FJ, Carbone PP (1978) Chemotherapy studies in primary liver cancer. Cancer 42: 2149–2156

Flam MS, John M, Lovalvo LJ, Mills RJ, Ramalho LD, Prather C, Mowry PA, Morgan DR, Lau BP (1983) Definitive nonsurgical therapy of epithelial malignancies of the anal canal. Cancer 51: 1378–1387

Flamant F, Hill C (1984) The improvement in survival associated with combined chemotherapy in childhood rhabdomyosarcoma. Cancer 53: 2417–2421

Flamant F, Schwartz L, Delons E, Caillaud JM, Hartmann O, Lemerle J (1984) Nonseminomatous malignant germ cell tumors in children. Cancer 54: 1687–1691

Fornasiero A, Daniele O, Sperandio P, Morandi P, Fosser VP, Cartei G, Fiorentino MV (1984) Chemotherapy of invasive or metastatic thymoma: report of 11 cases. Cancer Treat Rep 68: 1205–1210

Friedlander ML, Atkinson K, Coppleson JVM, Elliot P, Green D, Houghton R, Solomon HJ, Russell P, Tattersall MHN (1984) The integration of chemotherapy into the management of locally advanced cervical cancer: a pilot study. Gynecol Oncol 19: 1–17

Gasparini M, Rouesse J, Van Oosterom A, Wagener T, Somers R, Rusel JA, Voute PA, Bramwell V, Thomas D, Sylvester R, Rozencweig M (1985) Phase II study of cisplatin in advanced osteogenic sarcoma. Cancer Treat Rep 69: 211–213

Ghussen F, Nagel K, Groth W, Müller JM, Stützer H (1984) A prospective randomized study of regional extremity perfusion in patients with malignant melanoma. Ann Surg 200: 764–768

Glenn J, Kinsella T, Glatstein E, Tepper J, Baker A, Sugarbaker P, Sindelar W, Roth J, Brennan M, Costa J, Seipp C, Wesley R, Young RC, Rosenberg SA (1985) A randomized, prospective trial of adjuvant chemotherapy in adults with soft tissue sarcomas of the head and neck, breast, and trunk. Cancer 55: 1206–1214

Glick JH (1985) Adjuvant chemotherapy for breast cancer. National Institutes of Health Consensus Development. JAMA 254: 3461–3463

Goldstein DP, Berkowitz RS (1982) Nonmetastatic and low-risk metastatic gestational trophoblastic neoplasms. Semin Oncol 9: 191–197

Goorin AM, Abelson HT, Frei E (1985) Osteosarcoma: fifteen years later. N Engl J Med 313: 1637–1642

Greco FA, Johnson DH, Hainsworth JD, Wolff SN (1985) Chemotherapy of small-cell lung cancer. Semin Oncol 12 [Suppl 6]: 31–37

Greist A, Einhorn LH, Williams SD, Donohue JP, Rowland RG (1984) Pathologic findings at orchiectomy following chemotherapy for disseminated testicular cancer. J Clin Oncol 2: 1025–1027

Hafström L, Jönsson PE (1980) Hyperthermic perfusion of recurrent malignant melanoma on the extremities. Acta Chir Scand 146: 313–318

Harvey JH, Smith FP, Schein PS (1984) 5-Fluorouracil, mitomycin, and doxorubicin (FAM) in carcinoma of the biliary tract. J Clin Oncol 2: 1245–1248

Hoffman PC, Bitran JD, Golomb HM (1983) Chemotherapy of metastatic non-small cell bronchogenic carcinoma. Semin Oncol 10: 111–122

Hryniuk W, Bush H (1984) The importance of dose intensity in chemotherapy of metastatic breast cancer. J Clin Oncol 2: 1281–1288

Issell BF, Prout GR, Soloway MS, Cummings KB, Brannen G, Veenema R, Flanagan M, Block NL, Summers JL, Levin EA, Defuria MD (1984) Mitomycin C intravesical therapy in noninvasive bladder cancer after failure on thiotepa. Cancer 53: 1025–1028

Jones WG, Fosså SD, Bono AV, Croles JJ, Stoter G, de Pauw M, Sylvester R, members of EORTC Genito-Urinary Tract Cancer Co-operative Group (1986) Mitomycin-C in the treatment of metastatic prostate cancer: report on an EORTC phase II study. World J Urol 4: 182–185

Keane TJ, Harwood AR, Elhakim T, Rider WD, Cummings BJ, Ginsberg RJ, Cooper JC (1985) Radical radiation therapy with 5-fluorouracil infusion and mitomycin C for oesophageal squamous carcinoma. Radiother Oncol 4: 205–210

Kelsen D, Hilaris B, Coonley C, Chapman R, Lesser M, Dukeman M, Heelan R, Bains M (1983) Cisplatin, vindesine, and bleomycin chemotherapy of loco-regional and advanced esophageal carcinoma. Am J Med 75: 645–652

Kemeny N, Yagoda A, Braun D (1983) Metastatic colorectal carcinoma. Cancer 51: 20–24

Kiang DT, Gay J, Goldman A, Kennedy BJ (1985) A randomized trial of chemotherapy and hormonal therapy in advanced breast cancer. N Engl J Med 313: 1241–1246

Kish JA, Ensley JF, Jacobs J, Weaver A, Cummings G, Al-Sarraf M (1985) A randomized trial of cisplatin (CACP) + 5-fluorouracil (5-FU) infusion and CACP + 5-FU bolus for recurrent and advanced squamous cell carcinoma of the head and neck. Cancer 56: 2740–2744

Klastersky J, Sculier JP (1985) Chemotherapy of non-small-cell lung cancer. Semin Oncol 12 [Suppl 6]: 38–48

Krebs HB, Girtanner RE, Nordqvist SRB, Mineau I, Helmkamp BF, Averette HE (1980) Treatment of advanced cervical cancer by combination of bleomycin and mitomycin-C. Cancer 46: 2159–2161

Leeper RD, Shimaoka K (1980) Treatment of metastatic thyroid cancer. Clin Endocrinol Metab 9: 383–404

Leichman L, Steiger Z, Seydel HG, Dindogru A, Kinzie J, Toben S, MacKenzie G, Shell J (1984) Preoperative chemotherapy and radiation therapy for patients with cancer of

the esophagus: a potentially curative approach. J Clin Oncol 2: 75–79
Leipzig B (1983) Cisplatin sensitization to radiotherapy of squamous cell carcinomas of the head and neck. Am J Surg 146: 462–465
Lemerle J, Voute PA, Tournade MF, Rodary C, Delemarre JFM, Sarrazin D, Burgers JMV, Sandstedt B, Mildenberger H, Carli M, Jereb B, Moorman-Voestermans CGM (1983) Effectiveness of preoperative chemotherapy in Wilms' tumor: results of an International Society of Paediatric Oncology (SIOP) clinical trial. J Clin Oncol 1: 604–609
Link MP, Goorin AM, Miser AW, Green AA, Pratt CB, Belasco JB, Pritchard J, Malpas JS, Baker AR, Kirkpatrick JA, Ayala AG, Shuster JS, Abelson HT, Simone JV, Vietti TJ (1986) The effect of adjuvant chemotherapy on relapse-free survival in patients with osteosarcoma of the extremity. N Engl J Med 314: 1600–1606
Loehrer PJ, Einhorn LH, Williams SD (1986) VP-16 plus ifosfamide plus cisplatin as salvage therapy in refractory germ cell cancer. J Clin Oncol 4: 523–536
Logothetis CJ, Samuels ML, Selig DE, Dexeus FH, Johnson DE, Swanson DA, von Eschenbach AC (1985) Chemotherapy of extragonadal germ cell tumors. J Clin Oncol 3: 316–325
Luce JK (1972) Chemotherapy of malignant melanoma. Cancer 30: 1604–1615
Lyss AP, Loeb V (1984) Chemotherapy of advanced breast cancer. Cancer 53: 778–782
MacDonald JS, Woolley PV, Smythe T, Ueno W, Hoth D, Schein PS (1979) 5-Fluorouracil, adriamycin, and mitomycin-C (FAM) combination chemotherapy in the treatment of advanced gastric cancer. Cancer 44: 42–47
Madajewicz S, Petrelli N, Rustum YM, Campbell J, Herrera L, Mittelman A, Perry A, Creaven PJ (1984) Phase I–II trial of high-dose calcium leucovorin and 5-fluorouracil in advanced colorectal cancer. Cancer Res 44: 4667–4669
Mead GM, Jacobs C (1982) Changing role of chemotherapy in treatment of head and neck cancer. Am J Med 73: 582–595
Metzger UF, Ghosh BC, Kisner DL (1985) Adjuvant treatment of colorectal cancer. Cancer Chemother Pharmacol 14: 1–8
Moertel CG, Hanley JA, Johnson LA (1980) Streptozotocin alone compared with streptozotocin plus fluorouracil in the treatment of advanced islet-cell carcinoma. N Engl J Med 303: 1189–1194
Mouridsen HT, Rose C, Engelsman E, Sylvester R, Rotmensz N (1985) Combined cytotoxic and endocrine therapy in postmenopausal patients with advanced breast cancer. A randomized study of CMF vs CMF plus tamoxifen. Eur J Cancer Clin Oncol 21: 291–299
Myers C (1984) The use of intraperitoneal chemotherapy in the treatment of ovarian cancer. Semin Oncol 11: 275–284
Neijt JP, Ten Bokkel Huinink WW, Van der Burg MEL, Van Oosterom AT, Vriesendorp R, Pinedo HM (1984) Current status of systemic chemotherapy in the treatment of advanced ovarian cancer with emphasis on CHAP-5. Radiother Oncol 2: 19–29
Oldham RK (1985) Biologicals and biological response modifiers: new approaches to cancer treatment. Cancer Invest 3: 53–70
Order SE, Stillwagon GB, Klein JL, Leichner PK, Siegelmann SS, Fishman EK, Ettinger DS, Haulk T, Kopher K, Finney K, Surdyke M, Self S, Leibel S (1985) Iodine 131 antiferritin, a new treatment modality in hepatoma: a radiation therapy oncology group study. J Clin Oncol 3: 1573–1582
Østerlind K, Hansen M, Hansen HH, Dombernowsky P, Rorth M (1985) Treatment policy of surgery in small cell carcinoma of the lung: retrospective analysis of a series of 874 consecutive patients. Thorax 40: 272–277
Ozols RF, Young RC (1984) Chemotherapy of ovarian cancer. Semin Oncol 11: 251–263
Pasmantier MW, Coleman M, Silver RT, Mamaril AP, Quiguyan CC, Galindo A (1985) Treatment of advanced endometrial carcinoma with doxorubicin and cisplatin: effects on both untreated and previously treated patients. Cancer Treat Rep 69: 539–542
Peckham MJ, Barrett A, Liew KH, Horwich A, Robinson B, Dobbs HJ, McElwain TJ, Hendry WF (1983) The treatment of metastatic germ-cell testicular tumours with bleomycin, etoposide and cis-platin (BEP). Br J Cancer 47: 613–619
Peckham MJ, Horwich A, Blackmore C, Hendry WF (1985a) Etoposide and cisplatin with or without bleomycin as first-line chemotherapy for patients with small volume metastases of testicular nonseminoma. Cancer Treat Rep 69: 483–488
Peckham MJ, Horwich A, Hendry WF (1985b) Advanced seminoma: treatment with cis-platinum-based combination chemotherapy or carboplatin (JM8). Br J Cancer 52: 7–13
Perlow LS, Holland JF (1984) Chemotherapy of breast cancer. Med Oncol Tumor Pharmacother 1: 169–192
Pfeifle CE, Howell SB, Markman M (1985) Intracavitary cisplatin chemotherapy for mesothelioma. Cancer Treat Rep 69: 205–207
Pilepich MV, Vietti TJ, Nesbit ME, Tefft M, Kissane J, Burgert EO, Pritchard D (1981) Radiotherapy and combination chemotherapy in advanced Ewing's sarcoma-intergroup study. Cancer 47: 1930–1936
Pinedo HM, Bramwell VHC, Mouridsen HT, Somers R, Vendrik CPJ, Santoro A, Buesa J, Wagener T, Van Oosterom AT, Van Unnik JAM, Sylvester R, De Pauw M, Thomas D, Bonadonna G (1984) Cyvadic in advanced soft tissue sarcoma: a randomized study comparing two schedules. Cancer 53: 1825–1832
Piver MS (1984) Ovarian carcinoma. Cancer 54: 2706–2715
Quinn JJ, Altman AJ, Robinson HT, Cooke RW, Hight DW, Foster JH (1985) Adriamycin and cisplatin for hepatoblastoma. Cancer 56: 1926–1929
Raney RB, Crist WM, Maurer JM, Foulkes MA for the Intergroup Rhabdomyosarcoma Study Committee (1983) Prognosis of children with soft tissue sarcoma who relapse after achieving a complete response. Cancer 52: 44–50
Reimer RR, Gahbauer R, Bukowski RM, Hewlett JS, Groppe CW, Weick JK, Antunez AR (1981) Simultaneous treatment with cisplatin and radiation therapy for advanced solid tumors: a pilot study. Cancer Treat Rep 65: 219–222
Rosen G, Caparros B, Nirenberg A, Marcove RC, Huvos AG, Kosloff C, Lane J, Murphy ML (1981) Ewing's sarcoma: ten-year experience with adjuvant chemotherapy. Cancer 47: 2204–2213
Rosen G, Caparros B. Groshen S, Nirenberg A, Cacavio A, Marcove RC, Lane JM, Huvos AG (1984a) Primary osteogenic sarcoma of the femur: a model for the use of preoperative chemotherapy in high risk malignant tumors. Cancer Invest 2: 181–192
Rosen EM, Cassady JR, Frantz CN, Kretschmar C, Levey R, Sallan SE (1984b) Neuroblastoma: the Joint Center for Radiation Therapy/Dana-Farber Cancer Institute/Children's Hospital experience. J Clin Oncol 2: 719–732
Rosenberg SA, Tepper J, Glatstein E, Costa J, Young R, Baker A, Brennan MF, De Moss EV, Seipp C, Sindelar WF, Sugarbaker P, Wesley R (1983) Prospective randomized evaluation of adjuvant chemotherapy in adults with soft tissue sarcomas of the extremities. Cancer 52: 424–434

Rosenthal CJ, Khulpateea N, Boyce J, Mehrotra S, Tamarin S (1983) Effective chemotherapy for advanced carcinoma of the cervix with bleomycin, cisplatin, vincristine, and methotrexate. Cancer 52: 2025–2030

Rozencweig M, Dodion P, Bruntsch U, Gallmeier W, Clavel M, Gignoux B, Cortes Funes H, Cavalli F, Kirkpatrick A, Dalesio O, Van Rijmenant M (1984) Combination chemotherapy with cisplatin, methotrexate, bleomycin, and vincristine (CABO) in advanced squamous cell carcinoma of the head and neck. Cancer 54: 1499–1503

Schein PS (1985) The role of chemotherapy in the management of gastric and pancreatic carcinomas. Semin Oncol 12 [Suppl 6]: 49–60

Schraffordt Koops H, Beekhuis H, Oldhoff J, Oosterhuis JW, Van der Ploeg E, Vermey A (1981) Local recurrence and survival in patients with (Clark Level IV/V and over 1.5-mm thickness) Stage I malignant melanoma of the extremities after regional perfusion. Cancer 48: 1952–1957

Shipley WU, Coombs LJ, Einstein AB, Soloway MS, Wajsman Z, Prout GR, National Bladder Cancer Collaborative Group A (1984) Cisplatin and full dose irradiation for patients with invasive bladder carcinoma: a preliminary report of tolerance and local response. J Urol 132: 899–903

Soloway MS, Morris CR, Sudderth B (1979) Radiation therapy and cis-diammine-dichloroplatinum (II) in transplantable and primary murine bladder cancer. Int J Radiat Oncol Biol Phys 5: 1355–1360

Stokes SH, Thomas PRM, Perez CA, Vietti TJ (1984) Stage IV-S neuroblastoma. Cancer 53: 2083–2086

Stoter G (1985) Chemotherapy for metastatic bladder carcinoma. World J Urol 3: 110–114

Stoter G, Vendrik CPJ, Struyvenberg A, Sleyfer DT, Vriesendorp R, Schraffordt Koops H, Van Oosterom AT, Ten Bokkel Huinink WW, Pinedo HM (1984) Five-year survival of patients with disseminated nonseminomatous testicular cancer treated with cisplatin, vinblastine, and bleomycin. Cancer 54: 1521–1524

Suen JY, Johns ME (1982) Chemotherapy for salivary gland cancer. Laryngoscope 92: 235–239

Sugarbaker PH, Gianola FJ, Speyer JL, Wesley R, Barofsky I, Myers CE (1985) Prospective randomized trial of intravenous v intraperitoneal 5-FU in patients with advanced primary colon or rectal cancer. Semin Oncol 12 [Suppl 4]: 101–111

Surwit EA (1982) The management of poor prognosis trophoblastic disease. Semin Oncol 9: 204–207

Taylor SG, Murthy AK, Showel JL, Caldarelli DD, Hutchinson JC, Holinger LD, Kramer T, Kiel K (1985) Improved control in advanced head and neck cancer with simultaneous radiation and cisplatin/5-FU chemotherapy. Cancer Treat Rep 69: 933–939

Thigpen J, Vance RB, Balducci L, Khansur T (1984) New drugs and experimental approaches in ovarian cancer treatment. Semin Oncol 11: 314–326

Torti FM, Aston D, Lum BL, Kohler M, Williams R, Spaulding JT, Shortliffe L, Freiha FS (1983) Weekly doxorubicin in endocrine-refractory carcinoma of the prostate. J Clin Oncol 1: 477–482

Turbow MM, Ballon SC, Sikic BI, Koretz MM (1985) Cisplatin, doxorubicin, and cyclophosphamide chemotherapy for advanced endometrial carcinoma. Cancer Treat Rep 69: 465–467

Van Groeningen CJ, Leyva A, Kraal I, Peters GJ, Pinedo HM (1986) Clinical and pharmacokinetic studies of prolonged administration of high-dose uridine intended for rescue from 5-fluorouracil toxicity. Cancer Treat Rep 70: 745–750

Van Slooten H, Van Oosterom AT (1983) CAP (cyclophosphamide, doxorubicin, and cisplatin) regimen in adrenal cortical carcinoma. Cancer Treat Rep 67: 377–379

Verley JM, Hollmann KH (1985) Thymoma. Cancer 55: 1074–1086

Vugrin D, Whitmore WF (1984) The VAB-6 regimen in the treatment of metastatic seminoma. Cancer 53: 2422–2424

Vugrin D, Whitmore WF, Golbey RB (1983) VAB-6 combination chemotherapy without maintenance in treatment of disseminated cancer of the testis. Cancer 51: 211–215

Weinblatt ME, Siegel SE, Siegel MM, Stanley P, Weitzman JJ (1982) Preoperative chemotherapy for unresectable primary hepatic malignancies in children. Cancer 50: 1061–1064

Weltz MD, Perry DJ, Blom J, Butler WM (1983) Methyl-CCNU, 5-fluorouracil, vincristine, and streptozotocin (MOF-Strep) in metastatic colo-rectal carcinoma. J Clin Oncol 1: 135–137

Wheeler RH, Baker SR, Medvec BR (1984) Single-agent and combination-drug regional chemotherapy for head and neck cancer using an implantable infusion pump. Cancer 54: 1504–1512

Williams SD, Velez-Garcia E, Essessee I, Ratkin G, Birch R, Einhorn LH (1986) Chemotherapy for head and neck cancer. Cancer 57: 18–23

Wilson RE (1984) Surgical oncology. Cancer 54: 2595–2598

Wollesen F, Andersen T, Karle A (1982) Size reduction of extrasellar pituitary tumors during bromocriptine treatment. Ann Intern Med 96: 281–286

Woods RL, Fox RM, Tattersall MHN (1981) Methotrexate treatment of squamous-cell head and neck cancers: dose-response evaluation. Br Med J 282: 600–602

Yagoda A (1980) Chemotherapy of metastatic bladder cancer. Cancer 45: 1879–1888

Yap HY, Tashima CK, Blumenschein GR, Hortobagyi GN, Eckles N (1980 a) Chemotherapy for advanced male breast cancer. JAMA 243: 1739–1741

Yap BS, Baker LH, Sinkovics JG, Rivkin SE, Bottomley R, Thipgen T, Burgess MA, Benjamin RS, Bodey GP (1980 b) Cyclophosphamide, vincristine, adriamycin, and DTIC (CYVADIC) combination chemotherapy for the treatment of advanced sarcomas. Cancer Treat Rep 64: 93–98

Young RC, Chabner BA, Hubbard SP, Fisher RI, Bender RA, Anderson T, Simon RM, Canellos GP, DeVita VT (1978) Advanced ovarian adenocarcinoma. N Engl J Med 299: 1261–1266

Liver Infusion Chemotherapy

P. Schlag and C. Herfarth

Primary liver tumors characteristically remain confined to the liver for a long time, and colorectal carcinoma displays a particularly strong tendency to metastasize to the liver alone (Eder 1984; Pikren et al. 1984; Russel et al. 1984). Nevertheless, tumor size and extension often preclude operative resection despite the regionally limited growth, unless liver transplantation is considered (Hughes et al. 1986; Iwatsuki et al. 1985; Malt 1985; Neuhaus et al. 1986). The results of transplantation, however, remain disappointing in hepatic malignancy. The choice and the potential of the therapies currently available, particularly of systemic cytostatic therapy for primary liver tumors and for most hepatic metastases, is extremely limited. New treatment modalities are thus being sought (Friedmann 1986; Kemeny et al. 1984; Schreml 1986). One approach under investigation is regional cytostatic chemotherapy. The value of such chemotherapy in liver tumors cannot yet be judged definitively, however, and development of the technique cannot be regarded as concluded.

Pharmacokinetics and Pharmacodynamics

The rationale for regional cytostatic chemotherapy is supported by the fact that most cytostatics display high and dose-related toxicity and therapeutic efficacy when given by this means (Frei and Canellos 1980). Even when intravenous administration has no influence on tumor growth, regional administration of the same cytostatic may well achieve improved efficacy (Chen and Gross 1980; Collins 1986). Regional administration can result in maximal exposure of the tumor to the cytostatic while avoiding dose-limiting toxicity to bone marrow and other organ systems. This property of regional chemotherapy is particularly marked in the treatment of liver tumors owing to the high metabolic activity encountered in this organ. Normal liver cells are able to inactivate cytostatic substances before they spread throughout the organism. It follows that the principal dose-limiting factors are the proportion and the functional capacity of normal hepatic tissue, so that the dose is restricted in cases of cirrhosis or advanced tumor (Aguiar 1986).

The efficacy of regional cytostatic therapy is, in addition, determined by drug elimination in the total circulation (Chen and Gross 1980; Ensminger et al. 1982), but the effect depends too on regional blood flow (Chen and Gross 1980; Collins 1986; Ensminger and Gyves 1984). An increase in systemic toxicity through arteriovenous shunt must also be assumed. Regional administration is of little advantage when intravenous administration is very effective in the first place or when the tumor is extremely sensitive to cytostatics (Friedmann 1986; Schreml 1986), and will have no effect on a tumor which has shown itself resistant to high-dose cytostatic therapy (Ensminger and Gyves 1984). Up to the present time, however, few criteria for prediction of resistance to cytostatics have been identified. In particular, it remains unclear to what extent testing of cytostatics on tumor may be helpful (Link et al. 1985). In addition, it remains an open question whether tumor vascularity predicts response to therapy (Daly et al. 1985; Kaplan et al. 1980; Lehner et al. 1988). Especially suitable for regional chemotherapy of the liver are drugs which are not only metabolized primarily in the liver (first-pass effect) but also evince a short plasma half-life and a high total-body clearance (Ensminger et al. 1978; Ensminger and Gyves 1984). These requirements are met most fully by the fluorinated pyrimidines. 5-Fluorouracil, for example, is 100 times more effective regionally than intravenously, FUDR 400 times more effective. Dichloromethotrexate, mitomycin C, and cisplatin are also more beneficial when administered regionally (Ensminger et al. 1981; Kelsen et al. 1980; Tseng et al. 1981). Both the whole-body extraction rate and the first-pass effect of the liver are affected by the size of the dose administered, so that with higher doses the selective advantage of regional administration may be nullified. This may also occur when two substances are administered together, the one affecting the extraction of the other (Ensminger and Gyves 1984; Kirkwood et al. 1980).

Intra-arterial vs Intraportal Infusion

Two routes are possible for the regional administration of cytostatics to liver tumors, the intra-arterial and the intraportal (Chen and Gross 1980; Gerard et al. 1986; Laufmann et al. 1984). By reason of the greater intraportal blood flow and on the basis of the pharmacokinetics (see above), the intra-arterial approach is the procedure of choice. This approach is also indicated by what we know of the vascularization of liver tumors (Ackermann and Heckmer 1980; Ackermann and Hodgson 1986; Lin et al. 1984; Strohmeier et al. 1986). As a rule, the arterial perfusion of a tumor determines the drug concentration achieved. Indeed, the efficacy of regional therapy of liver tumors has been shown to depend on vascularization. Animal experiments investigating various routes of administration of regional cytostatics have also demonstrated the superiority of the intra-arterial over the intraportal approach for liver tumors (Cotino and Zwaveling 1976; Schlag et al. 1988 b). A probable exception is adjuvant cytostatic perfusion of the liver, but this procedure is undertaken for a different purpose, namely to destroy tumor cells in the portal circulation during primary resection, as well as any micrometastases that might be present (Ackermann 1986; Metzger 1986; Taylor 1978).

Prerequisites

General

A general prerequisite for regional chemotherapy is the exclusion of extrahepatic tumor. The main indications are hepatocellular carcinoma and hepatic metastases of colorectal carcinoma. Particularly with hepatic metastases from other forms of carcinoma, regional cytostatic therapy is seldom indicated, as in most cases a generalized systemic disease is present. The sole exception is provided by some cases of endocrine malignant tumors. No definitive statement can yet be made concerning the indication for liver infusion chemotherapy in patients with heavy metastatic invasion of the liver and a correspondingly low life expectancy. Tumor invasion of the liver should not be so far advanced that a priori no adequate detoxification of cytostatics can be expected after direct intrahepatic administration. In this situation regional chemotherapy would no longer be superior to intravenous systemic chemotherapy.

In addition to staging of the tumor, liver infusion chemotherapy must be preceded by demonstration of vascularization of the liver by means of celiac and mesenteric angiography. Variations from the normal arterial vascularization are found in 50% of cases. It should also be ascertained from the angiogram that no occlusion of the portal vein is present. This is necessary because of the risk involved in intra-arterial catheter implantation in the presence of such an occlusion: arterial thrombosis may result in liver failure (Gerard et al. 1986). Angiographic demonstration of massive shunting signifies additional toxicity problems and is a factor to be considered when deciding the indication for regional chemotherapy.

Methodological

Despite the theoretical advantages, the technical difficulties involved in carrying out regional cytostatic therapy meant that this technique took a long time to replace intravenous therapy as the method of choice (Clouse et al. 1977; Petrek and Minton 1979; Reed et al. 1981). In the past, regional treatment was impracticable because of the high risk of infection and thrombosis associated with repeated insertion of intravascular catheters. Not until the introduction of fully implantable catheter systems did this mode of treatment receive fresh impetus (Blackshear et al. 1972; Buchwald et al. 1980). The catheter materials available today go a long way toward satisfying the requirements for safe, secure implantation and unproblematic long-term treatment (Lokich and Ensminger 1983; Schlag 1985). The catheters are placed in position operatively and connected either to an implantable drug pump or to an injection port. The advantages of the implantable pump are better patient comfort and improved practicability. Disadvantages are the considerable costs and the fact that as a rule FUDR is the only cytostatic that can usefully be administered with the pumps currently available. The reasons for this are first, the difference between the size of the pump reservoir and the necessary dose, and second, the nonvariable flow rate. External pumps display much greater variability and can be connected to the injection port via special cannulas with a feed line (Civalleri et al. 1986 a). Reservoir size is greater and there is a choice between pumps with set infusion pattern and rate and those with variable infusion rates or pulsed infusion (Roemeling et al. 1986 a; Wright et al. 1986). Depending on the arterial supply of the liver, the implantation of two catheters may under certain circumstances be necessary in order to achieve complete liver perfusion, and corresponding pump and port models are now commercially available. Dual arteriovenous catheter systems can be implanted in order to combine arterial with central-venous systemic chemotherapy. This dual therapy is being increasingly promulgated because of the frequency of later extrahepatic tumor progression observed in patients treated intra-arterially (Balch et al. 1983; Kemeny et al. 1984; Schwartz et al. 1985).

Operative Catheter Insertion and Checking of Catheter Position

One of two approaches is recommended for catheter implantation: either a right subcostal incision or a transrectal incision in the right epigastrium. Before the final decision to insert the catheter, the abdominal cavity should be carefully explored for extrahepatic metastases, since if any are present intraperitoneal chemotherapy may be more appropriate (Speyer 1984; Sugarbaker et al. 1985). Any enlarged lymph nodes in the hepatoduodenal ligament must be checked for tumor intraoperatively by means of microscopic examinations of frozen sections (August et al. 1985). In the case of normal arterial supply of the liver the catheter is inserted in the gastroduodenal artery, using the method described by Watkins et al. (1970) and schematically shown in Fig. 1. It is essential to ligate all arteries not running to the liver which may arise from the common hepatic artery after the origin of the gastroduodenal artery (e.g., right gastric artery) (Hohn et al. 1985). Careful preparation is necessary in order to prevent later complications (ulceration, gastritis, etc.) (Chuang et al. 1981; Gluck et al. 1985; Narsete et al. 1977; Petras et al. 1985; Shike et al. 1986), and cholecystectomy is also recommended in this regard. One should remember that it is currently unclear to what extent devascularization of the extrahepatic bile ducts favors induction of sclerosing cholangitis on subsequent cytostatic therapy (Bergmann et al. 1986; Doria et al. 1986; Kemeny N et al. 1984; Kemeny MM et al. 1985; Shepard et al. 1985). Dual arterial supply may necessitate the insertion of two catheters, one placed as a rule in the gastroduodenal artery by the usual method and the other in the accessory vessel (Fig. 2). In the case of a narrow lumen, and especially in the absence of lateral branches suitable for catheter implantation according to Watkin, a Holder catheter should be used (Niederhuber and Ensminger 1983). Dual arterial supply of the liver may also be dealt with by ligation of one artery. Obligatory left – right arterial shunts of the liver ensure that collateralization of the area usually supplied by the ligated artery takes place within a very short time (Bengmark and Rosengren 1970). The completeness of liver perfusion can be checked intraoperatively using fluorescein and Wood's lamp. This method can provide no more than a certain degree of orientation, however, as only the superficial areas of the liver are accessible to inspection.

The implanted catheter is connected either to an implantable drug pump or an injection port. It has been found advantageous to place the injection port

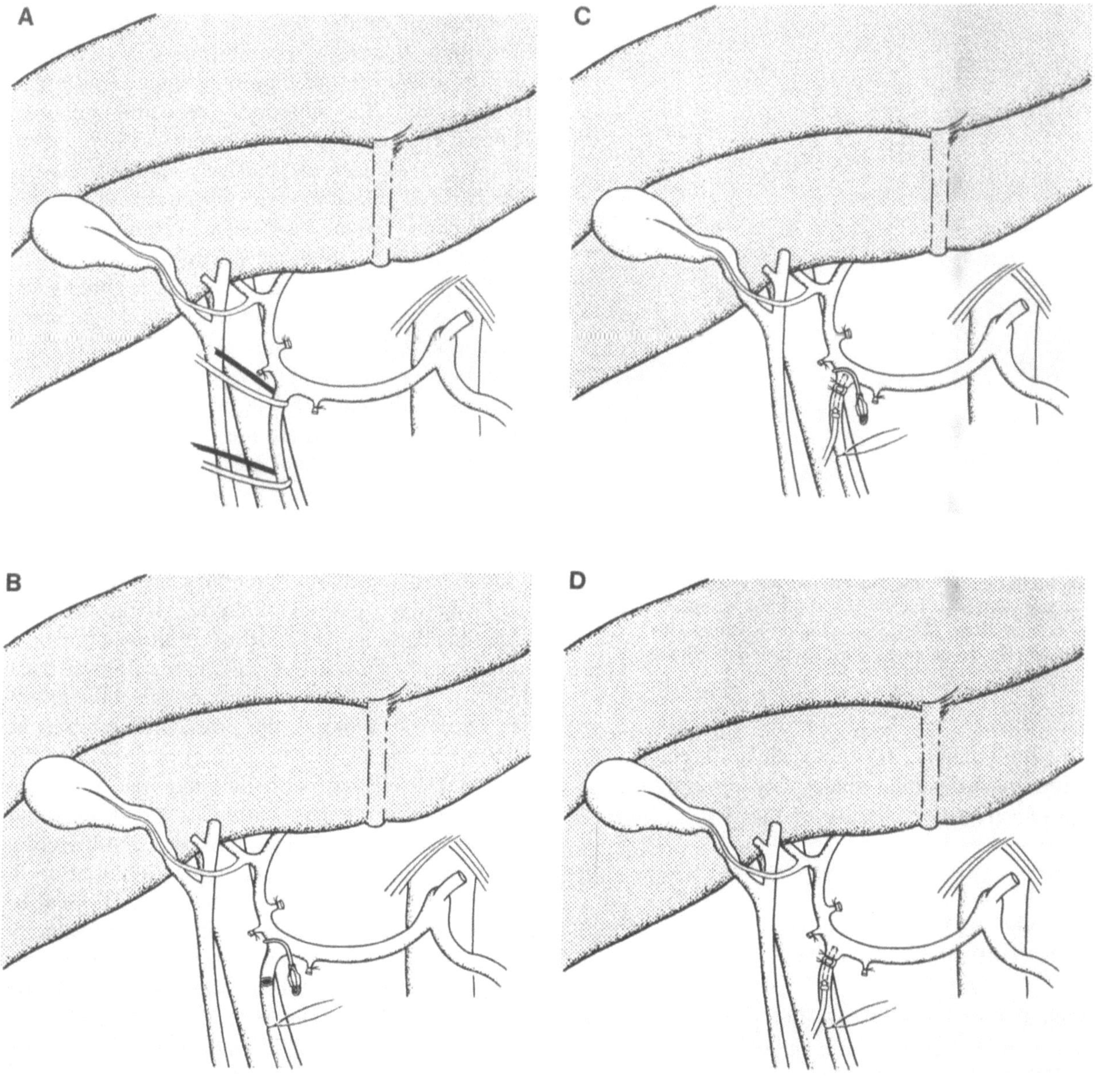

Fig. 1 A–D. Operative procedure of the implantation of an arteria hepatica catheter. **A** The arteria gastroduodenalis is tied and recurrent branch arteries of the arteria hepatica are ligated. **B** After the placement of a Yasergil clamp at the branching off of the arteria gastroduodenalis and its distal ligation, the artery is opened by a cross arteriectomy. **C** The catheter is placed via arteriotomy and fixed by means of vascular ligature. **D** After removal of the Yasergil clamp, the tip of the catheter is in a tangential position to the arteria hepatica

on a firm foundation, for example on the costal arch or subcutaneously over the sternum, whereas the drug pump is better placed in a skin pocket in the hypogastrium. Postoperatively, the completeness of liver perfusion should be demonstrated by means of technetium-MAA scintigraphy before cytostatic therapy is commenced (Daly et al. 1985; Kaplan et al. 1980; Lehner et al. 1988; Yang et al. 1982). Control phytate scintigraphy should be carried out for purposes of adequate comparison to rule out the possibility of incorrect interpretation. If this should reveal additional extrahepatic perfusion (gastroduodenal area), there must be nonligated extrahepatic collateral vessels, which can then be occluded by mean of transfemoral selective catheterization and embolization (Wallace et al. 1984). If some areas of tumorous liver are not covered with the catheter in the chosen position, one can consider combining intra-arterial and systemic therapy from the outset. In the event of large arteriovenous shunts, as encountered particu-

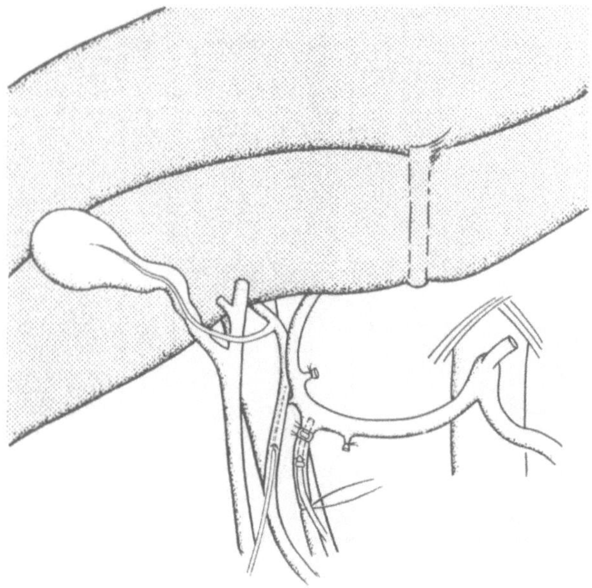

Fig. 2. In the case of a dual arterial vascular supply, a supplementary catheter is introduced into the liver artery which has no branch artery. The catheterization is done with a special catheter (Holder catheter) directly via an arteriotomy

larly, for example, in hepatocellular carcinoma of a cirrhotic liver, caution is necessary in setting the dosage of cytostatics because of the risk of increased systemic toxicity.

Execution of the Therapy

While the implantation of a drug pump usally means that a strict and continuous chemotherapy regimen has been selected, an injection port permits various forms of drug administration (Civalleri et al. 1986 a; Clark 1986; Schlag et al. 1987). The reservoir of the implanted pump can be filled and also emptied via a transcutaneous puncture. As a rule, the treatment regimen comprises alternating 14-day periods of continuous FUDR infusion and administration of heparinized saline. Continuous chemotherapy seems clearly superior to bolus or short-term treatment for FUDR (Lokich 1986; Moertel et al. 1967; Seifert et al. 1975), but the same is not necessarily true for other cytostatics. Thus for alkylating substances, brief, repeated peak concentrations are more beneficial than continuously consistent levels, since the latter permit swifter and simpler DNA repair processes which make lethal cell damage impossible. Antimetabolites, in contrast, are most effective with continuous administration (Ensminger and Gyves 1984). Clinical confirmation of the theoretical considerations behind these treatment recommendations is difficult, and up to the present time only some aspects have been verified. The superiority of continuous locoregional chemotherapy with fluorinated pyrimidines, however, has been conclusively demonstrated in standardized animal models (Bartkowski et al. 1986). In this context, there have been some interesting reports of fluctuations in sensitivity to cytostatics according to the time of day, and these phenomena should be taken into account when planning therapy (Hrushesky 1985; Roemeling et al. 1986 b).

Various external pump systems are available for continuous therapy. The technology has now advanced to the point where the treatment can be carried out on an outpatient basis (Schlag et al. 1987). The catheter occlusion rate with port systems is slightly higher than with implantable pumps because there is no constant irrigation of the catheter. The introduction of a heparin-saline lock into the catheter system between periods of therapy is thus strongly advised. (With implanted drug pumps, of course, continuous heparin irrigation is carried out at these times.) If despite these precautions the catheter system becomes occluded, the problem may often be resolved be means of an injection of streptase (Rubin 1983). Persisting occlusion suggests thrombosis of the common hepatic artery, so that operative catheter revision must always be preceded by repeat celiacography or mesentericography. If the artery is still patent, reimplantation of the catheter may be considered. The most frequent complication of long-term chemotherapy via an injection port is needle dislocation. Provided the problem is noticed soon enough, there are generally no harmful consequences, particularly if fluorinated pyrimidines are being administered. A greater amount of extravasation, especially if other cytostatics (e.g., doxorubicin or mitomycin C) are involved usually leads to necrosis of the skin (Argenta et al. 1983; Johnston-Early and Cohen 1981). Surgical revision with skin grafting is indicated, especially to protect the implant against superinfection

Results

Although regional chemotherapy of liver tumors is theoretically attractive, there is still controversy surrounding its ultimate effectiveness (Clark 1986; Schwartz et al. 1985; Taylor 1985).

In the case of hepatocellular carcinoma other forms of treatment are largely ineffective (Falkson

Table 1. Studies evaluating regional chemotherapy in hepatocellular carcinoma

Reference	Patients (*n*)	Drugs	Response Type	(%)	Median survival (months)	Toxicity		
						Cardio-toxicity (%)	Alopecia (%)	Myelo-toxicity (%)
Reed et al (1981)	13	FUDR	CR+PR	70	8		ND	
Patt et al. (1983 a)	12	FUDRAM	CR PR SD	8 58 25	14	0	100	23
Balch et al. (1983)	13	ADR	PR SD	46 46	20	38	23	8
Hottenrott et al (1987)	9	ADR	CR+PR	78	5	0	ND	33
Own unpublished results (1987)	8	FUDRAM	PR SD	25 25	8	0	80	80

CR, complete remission; PR, partial remission; SD, stable disease; ND, no data.

Table 2. Studies evaluating intra-arterial FUDR chemotherapy using implantable pumps in colorectal liver metastases

Reference	Patients (*n*)	Response		Survival	
		Imaging technique (%)	CEA (%)	From start of therapy (months)	From time of diagnosis (months)
Balch et al. (1983)	110	–	88	–	24
Niederhuber et al. (1984)	93	76	91	18	25
Kemeny et al. (1986)	41	52	69	15	–
Shepard et al. (1985)	62	32	–	17	–
Rothmund et al. (1986)	22	64	77	15	26
Hottenrott and Lorenz (1987)	52	46	75	16	–

and Coetzer 1986) and a trial of regional cytostatic therapy is worth considering. In this context the experience of treatment with an intra-arterially administered combination of FUDR, doxorubicin, and mitomycin C is often of particular interest (Patt et al. 1983 a). The treatment regimen, however, is relatively toxic and difficult to control, especially in the presence of cirrhosis of the liver (Table 1). These problems essentially stem from the reduction in first-pass effect frequently associated with cirrhosis. We have demonstrated this lowered metabolization of intra-arterially administered cytostatics in animal experiments, using the model of glucosamine-induced cirrhosis of rat liver (Aguiar 1986). Long term, the cirrhotic rats displayed higher concentrations of cytostatics in the peripheral venous circulation than did the animals with healthy livers. This resulted in persisting myelosuppression. Our clinical experience also shows the necessity for the utmost caution in intra-arterial chemotherapy of primary liver malignancies, especially with associated cirrhosis of the liver. Timely dose reduction and further optimization of the intra-arterial therapy are essential.

Most experience of intra-arterial chemotherapy has been gained with hepatic metastases of colorectal carcinoma. The majority of trails have involved long-term continuous FUDR therapy using fully implantable drug pumps (Balch et al. 1983; Barone et al. 1982; Ensminger et al. 1982; Hodgson et al. 1986; Johnson et al. 1985; Kemeny and Daly 1986; Shepard et al. 1985; Schwartz et al. 1985). Table 2 shows the results of the largest such studies carried out so far. The apparent discrepancy of the findings is explained above all by lack of consistency of criteria for assessing the results. On applying a comparable standard (Jeppson and Bengmark 1986; Lokich and Ensminger 1983; Van de Velde et al. 1984 b), however, the following picture emerges: the median survival from the time of catheter implantation lies between 14 and 16 months. The rate of tumor regression according to uniformly applied WHO criteria is around 40%, higher than achieved with systemic chemotherapy (Kemeny 1983; Kemeny and Daly 1986; Huberman 1983). The median progression-free survival is 8 months. Up to the present time there has been no unequivocal demonstration, either in

Table 3. Randomized trials evaluating intra-arterial versus intravenous FUDR chemotherapy using implantable pumps in colorectal liver metastases

Reference	Drug administration	Patients (n)	Cross over	Response (%)	Median survival (months)	Extrahepatic tumor progression (%)
Kemeny et al. (1986)	i.a.	45	+	46	15	43
	i.v.	49		22.5	15	15
Hohn et al. (1987)	i.a.	50	+	42	ND	
	i.v.	64		9		
Chang et al. (1987)	i.a.	32	–	62	17	50
	i.v.	29		17	13	20
Hottenrott et al. (1987)	i.a.	26	–	52	16	54
	i.a. + i.v. (5-FU)	20		65	16	40

ND, no data.

Table 4. Side effects of intra-arterial FUDR chemotherapy using implantable pumps

Reference	Patients (n)	FUDR dosage (× 14 days every 28 days)	Chemical hepatitis (%)	Biliary sclerosis (%)	Gastrointestinal toxicity (%)
Balch et al. (1983)	110	0.3 mg/kg per day for 4 months, then 0.2 mg/kg per day	90	K.A.	17
Niederhuber et al. (1984)	93	0,3 mg/kg per day	32	24	56
Hohn et al. (1986)	55	0.1–0.3 mg/kg per day	96	56	K.A.
Kemeny et al. (1986)	73	0.1.–0.3 mg/kg per day	47	19	33
Kemeny et al. (1984)	45	0.3 mg/kg per day	71	5	46
Chang et al. (1987)	32	0.2/kg per day	79	21	51

retrospective or in prospective randomized studies of comparable populations, of longer survival with intra-arterial than with systemic cytostatic chemotherapy among patients with hepatic metastases of colorectal carcinoma (Table 3). The advantage of intraarterial therapy over intravenous treatment therefore consists less in prolongation of survival than in a lower rate of side effects (Hohn et al. 1986; Hubermann 1983; Kemeny 1983; Kemeny and Daly 1986). One reason for this is that in spite of tumor control in the liver, extrahepatic tumor progression occurs in the great majority of patients under regional cytostasis (Balch et al. 1983; Hohn et al. 1986; Kemeny and Daly 1986). Combined simultaneous intra-arterial and intravenous cytostatic therapy, however, has also failed so far to produce improvement of results (Hottenrott et al. 1987). On the other hand, intra-arterial cytostatic chemotherapy can be expected to achieve tumor regression in half the patients who evince progression of hepatic metastases under intravenous therapy (Patt et al. 1983 b). The principal disadvantages of intra-arterial chemotherapy are the hepatobiliary side effects, such as chemical hepatitis and, most important, sclerosing cholangitis (Bergmann et al. 1986; Botet et al. 1985; Hohn et al. 1986; Kemeny et al. 1984, 1985; Shepard et al. 1985). The last-mentioned is dose-dependent and occurs above all during long-term FUDR therapy (Table 4). We have found that long-term intra-arterial 5-fluorouracil therapy is equally effective (Table 5) while causing considerably less severe side effects, and for this reason it is our agent of choice (Schlag et al. 1988 a).

Further Developments

Isolated liver perfusion represents the logical development of an exclusively local cytostatic treatment procedure which attemps to achieve a maximal concentration of cytostatics in the tumor without risking toxicity of the whole organism (Sindelar 1985; Schwemmle and Aigner 1986; Van de Velde et al. 1984 a). Apart from the considerable expense and technical input involved in operation, the major disadvantage of isolated organ perfusion is that expo-

Table 5. Studies evaluating intra-arterial 5-FU long-term chemotherapy in patients with colorectal liver metastases

Reference	Patients (*n*)	Drug administration	Response (%)	Median survival (months)	Side effects			Technical problems (%)
					Hemato-logic (%)	Gastro-intestinal (%)	Hepato-biliary (%)	
Denck (1984)	50	6–7g 5-FU for 3–6 days q 6–8 weeks	58	14		minimal		<5
Rougier et al. (1987)	43	1g/m² body surface for 6 h weekly	56	12 (79%)	18	9	–	65
Own unpublished results (1987)	33	1g/m² body surface for 5 days q 6–8 weeks	27	14	5	30	5	20

sure to the cytostatics is short (1–2 h) and is generally not repeated. On grounds of tumor biology alone such a procedure cannot have the desired therapeutic effect, especially using antimetabolite cytostatics, because sufficient cell damage can be expected only on longer-term administration (Ensminger and Gyves 1984). Thus the clinical results of liver perfusion chemotherapy of primary and secondary liver tumors have also been disappointing. In particular, the results that can be achieved bear no relation to the morbidity and mortality associated with the treatment. More promising, however, are developments of regional chemotherapy based on pharmacodynamic and tumor biological considerations. Since tumor exposure to cytostatics depends, among other factors, on intravasal hepatic blood flow, reduction of flow velocity would be expected to produce an increase in concentration. Attempts are currently being made to influence blood flow in the common hepatic artery by mechanical and pharmacological means in order to obtain greater effectiveness and broaden the therapeutic application (Aronson et al. 1979; Bengmark and Jeppson 1986; Fujimote et al. 1985; Hafström et al. 1980; Iwaki et al. 1978). The most promising developments of liver infusion chemotherapy are chemoembolization, in which cytostatics are administered mixed with degradable microparticles, and techniques involving administration of cytostatics incorporated in microsomes. Finally, investigations are under way with the aim of clarifying to what extent local administration of special tumoraffin and tumoricidal products and cells (monoclonal antibodies, radionuclides, activated killer cells, etc.) might increase therapeutic effectiveness compared with systemic application (Freeman and Mayhew 1986; Order et al. 1986; Steplewski et al. 1986). The experience with intra-arterial infusion chemotherapy of liver tumors and the analysis and discussion of the technique has, particularly in the past few years, contributed to an improved knowledge of tumor biology and to a more differentiated pharmacokinetic understanding of cytostatic therapy. On this basis it is hoped that development of this strategy will eventually yield improvements in the treatment of primary and secondary liver tumors.

References

Ackerman NB (1986) Experimental studies on the role of the portal circulation in hepatic tumor vascularity. Cancer 58: 1653–1657

Ackerman NB, Heckmer PA (1980) The blood supply of experimental liver metastases. V. Increased tumor perfusion with epinephrine. Am J Surg 140: 625–631

Ackerman NB, Hodgson WB (1986) Vascular patterns of liver tumors and their consequences for different therapeutic approaches. In: Herfarth C, Schlag P, Hohenberger P (eds) Therapeutic strategies in primary and metastatic liver cancer. Springer, Berlin Heidelberg New York Tokyo, pp 248–255

Aguiar JLA (1986) Pharmacokinetics and toxicity of 5-fluorouracil in experimental thioacetamide-induced cirrhosis after intra-arterial liver administration to rats. Thesis, University of Heidelberg

Argenta LC, Manders EK (1983) Mitomycin C extravasation injuries. Cancer 51: 1080–1082

Aronsen KF, Hellekant C, Holmberg J, Rothman U, Teder H (1979) Controlled blocking of hepatic artery flow with enzymatically degradable microspheres combined with oncolytic drugs. Eur Surg Res 11: 99–106

August DA, Sugarbaker PH, Schneider PD (1985) Lymphatic dissemination of hepatic metastases: implications for the follow-up and treatment of patients with colorectal cancer. Cancer 55: 1490–1994

Balch CM, Urist MM, McGregor ML (1983) Continuous regional chemotherapy for metastatic colorectal cancer using a totally implantable infusion pump. Am J Surg 145: 285–290

Barone RM, Byfield JE, Goldfarb PB, Frankel S, Ginn C, Greer S (1982) Intraarterial chemotherapy using an implan-

table infusion pump and liver irradiation for the treatment of hepatic metastases. Cancer 50: 850–862
Bartkowski R, Berger MR, Aguiar JLA, Henne TH, Dörsam J, Geelhaar GH, Schlag P, Herfarth C (1986) Experiments of the efficacy and toxicity of locoregional chemotherapy of liver tumors with 5-fluoro-2′-deoxyuridine (FUDR) and 5-fluorouracil (5-FU) in an animal model. J Cancer Res Clin Oncol 111: 42–46
Bengmark S, Jeppson B (1986) Permanent hepatic arterial ligation versus temporary dearterialization in the treatment of hepatic tumors. In: Herfarth C, Schlag P, Hohenberger P (eds) Therapeutic strategies in primary and metastatic liver cancer. Springer, Berlin Heidelberg New York Tokyo, pp 268–275
Bengmark S, Rosengren K (1970) Angiographic study of the collateral circulation to the liver after ligation of the hepatic artery in man. Am J Surg 19: 620–624
Bergmann JF, Rougier P, Liguory C (1986) Sclerosing cholangitis after continuous hepatic artery infusion of FUDR. Gastroenterol Clin Biol 10/2: 177–179
Blackshear PJ, Dorman FD, Blackshear PL et al. (1972) The design and initial testing of an implantable infusion pump. Surg Gynecol Obstet 143: 54–56
Botet JF, Watson RC, Kemeny N, Daly JM, Yeh S (1985) Cholangitis complicating intraarterial chemotherapy in liver metastasis. Radiology 156 (2): 335–337
Buchwald H, Grage TB, Vassilopoulos PP, Rohde TD, Varco RL, Blackshear PJ (1980) Intra-arterial infusion chemotherapy for hepatic carcinoma using a totally implantable infusion pump. Cancer 45: 866–869
Chang AE, Schneider PD, Sugarbaker PH, Simpson C, Culname RNM, Steinberg SM (1987) A prospective randomized trial of regional versus systemic continuous 5-fluorodeoxyuridine chemotherapy in the treatment of colorectal liver metastases. Ann Surg 206: 685–693
Chen HSG, Gross JF (1980) Intra-arterial infusion of anticancer drugs: theoretic aspects of drug delivery and review of responses. Cancer treat Rep 64: 31–40
Chuang VP, Wallace S, Stroehlein J, Yap HY, Patt YZ (1981) Hepatic artery infusion chemotherapy: gastro-duodenal complications. AJR 137: 347–350
Civalleri D, Cafiero F, Cosimelli M, Craus W, Doci R, Repetto M, Simoni G (1986 a) Regional arterial chemotherapy of liver tumours. I. Performance comparison between a totally implantable pump and a conventional access system. Eur J Surg Oncol 12: 277–282
Civalleri D, Scopinaro G, Simoni G, Claudiani F, Repetto M, DeCian F, Bonalumi U (1986 b) Starch microsphere-induced arterial flow redistribution after occlusion of replaced hepatic arteries in patients with liver metastases. Cancer 58: 2151–2155
Clark CG (1986) Implantable vascular access devices in the treatment of colorectal liver metastases. Br J Surg 73: 419–421
Clouse MD, Ahmed R, Ryan RB, Oberfield RA, McCaffrey JA (1977) Complications of long term transbrachial hepatic arterial infusion chemotherapy, AJR 129: 799–803
Clouse ME (1983) Roentgenographic techniques for diagnosis and management of liver tumors. Semin Oncol 2: 159–175
Collins JM (1986) Pharmacologic rationale for hepatic arterial therapy. In: Herfarth C, Schlag P, Hohenberger P (eds) Therapeutic strategies in primary and metastatic liver cancer. Springer, Berlin Heidelberg New York Tokyo, pp 140–147
Collins JM, Dedrick RL, King FG, Speyer JL, Meyers CE (1980) Non-linear pharmacokinetic models for 5-fluorouracil in man: intravenous and intraperitoneal routes. Clin Pharmacol Ther 25: 235–246
Cotino H, Zwaveling A (1976) Treatment of experimental liver tumors by continuous intra-arterial chemotherapy. Eur J Cancer 12: 177–180
Daly JM, Kemeny N, Oderman P, Botet J (1984) Long-term hepatic arterial infusion chemotherapy. Arch Surg 119: 936–941
Daly JM, Butler J, Kemeny N, Yeh SDJ, Ridge JA, Botet J, Bading JR, DeCosse JJ, Benua RS (1985) Predicting tumor response in patients with colorectal hepatic metastases. Ann Surg 202: 384–393
Denck H (1984) Ergebnisse einer intraarteriellen intermittierenden Chemotherapie mit 5-FU bei Metastasenleber sowie inoperablen Tumoren des Gastrointestinal- und Urogenitaltraktes. Onkologie 7: 167–176
Doria MI, Shepard KV, Levin B, Riddell RH (1986) Liver pathology following hepatic arterial infusion chemotherapy: hepatic toxicity with FUDR. Cancer 58: 855–861
Eder M (1984) Die Metastasierung: Fakten und Probleme aus Humanpathologischer Sicht. Verh Dtsch Ges Pathol 68: 1–11
Ensminger WD, Gyves JW (1984) Regional cancer chemotherapy. Cancer Treat Rep 68: 101–115
Ensminger WD, Rosowsky A, Raso V, Levin DC, Glode M, Come S, Steele G, Frei E III (1978) A clinical pharmacologic evaluation of hepatic arterial infusions of 5-fluorouracil-2′-deoxyuridine and 5-fluorouracil. Cancer Res 38: 3784–3792
Ensminger WD, Dakhil S, Doan K, Cho K, Wheeler R, Pollard HM (1981) Clinical pharmacology of dichloromethotrexate in hepatic infusions. Proc Am Assoc Cancer Res and ASCO 22: 271
Ensminger W, Niederhuber J, Gyves J, et al. (1982) Effective control of liver metastases from colon cancer with an implanted system for hepatic arterial chemotherapy. Proc Am Assoc Cancer Res 1: 94
Falkson G, Coetzer BJ (1986) Application and results of different chemotherapy regimens in primary liver malignancies. In: Herfarth C, Schlag P, Hohenberger P (eds) Therapeutic strategies in primary and metastatic liver cancer. Springer, Berlin Heidelberg New York Tokyo, pp 103–111
Freeman AI, Mayhew E (1986) Targeted drug delivery. Cancer 58: 573–583
Frei E III, Canellos GP (1980) Dose: a critical factor in cancer chemotherapy. Am J Med 69: 585–594
Friedman MA (1986) Systemic therapies for patients with liver tumors: prospects for the future. In: Herfarth C, Schlag P, Hohenberger P (eds) Therapeutic strategies in primary and metastatic liver cancer. Springer, Berlin Heidelberg New York Tokyo, pp 112–119
Fujimoto S, Miyazaki M, Endoh F, Takahashi O, Okui M, Morimoto Y (1985) Biodegradable mitomycin C microspheres given intra-arterially for inoperable hepatic cancer. Cancer 56: 2404–2410
Gerard A, Dalesio O, Duez N, Lise M, Pector JC, Bleiberg H, Nitti D, Willems G, Delvaux G (1986) Hepatic arterial ligation and portal vein infusion: a clinical trial by the Gastrointestinal Tract Cancer Group of the European Organization for Research and Treatment of Cancer. In: Herfarth C, Schlag P, Hohenberger P (eds) Therapeutic strategies in primary and metastatic liver cancer. Springer, Berlin Heidelberg New York Tokyo, pp 276–281
Gluck WL, Akwari OE, Kelvin FM, Goodwin BJ (1985) A reversible enteropathy complicating continuous hepatic ar-

tery infusion chemotherapy with 5-fluoro-2′-deoxyuridine. Cancer 56: 2424–2427

Hafstrom L, Nobin A, Persson B, Sundquist K (1980) Effects of catecholamines on cardiovascular response and blood flow distribution to normal tissue and liver tumor in rats. Cancer Res 40: 481–485

Hodgson WJB, Mittelman A, Katz S, Friedland M, Berman H, Morgan J, Ahmed T, Byrne D (1986) Treatment of colorectal hepatic metastases by intrahepatic chemotherapy alone or as an adjuvant to complete or partial removal of metastatic disease. Ann Surg 203: 420–425

Hohn DC, Stagg RJ, Price DC, Lewis BJ (1985) Avoidance of gastroduodenal toxicity in patients receiving hepatic arterial 5-fluoro-2′-deoxyuridine. J Clin Oncol 3: 1257–1260

Hohn DC, Rayner AA, Economou JS, Ignoffo RJ, Lewis BJ, Stagg RJ (1986) Toxicities and complications of implanted pump hepatic arterial and intravenous floxuridine infusion. Cancer 57: 465–470

Hohn D, Stagg R, Rayner A, Lewis B (1987) The NCOG randomized trial of intravenous (IV) vs. hepatic arterial (IA) FUDR for colorectal cancer metastatic to the liver. 3rd International Conference on Advances in Regional Cancer Therapy, Neu Ulm 1987 (Abstr B 6)

Hottenrott C, Lorenz M (1987) Stellenwert der regionalen Chemotherapie der Leber, Z Gastroenterol 25: 364–373

Hottenrott C, Lorenz M, Encke A (1987) Kann der Erfolg einer lokalen Chemotherapie der Leber durch eine zusätzliche systemische Zytostase verbessert werden? Eine randomisierte Multicenterstudie. Langenbecks Arch Chir, Kongressbericht 1987

Hrushesky WJM (1985) Circadian timing of cancer chemotherapy. Science 228: 73–75

Huberman MS (1983) Comparison of systemic chemotherapy with hepatic arterial infusion in metastatic colorectal carcinoma. Semin Oncol 102: 238–248

Hughes KS, Simon R, Songhorabodi S et al. (1986) Resection of the liver for colorectal carcinoma metastases: A multi-institutional study of patterns of recurrence. Surgery 100: 218–284

Iwaki A, Nagasue N, Kobayoshi M, Inokuchi K (1978) Intraarterial chemotherapy with concomitant use of vasoconstrictors for liver cancer. Cancer Treat Rep 62: 145–146

Iwatsuki S, Gordon RD, Shaw BW, Starzl TE (1985) Role of liver transplantation in cancer therapy. Ann Surg 202: 401–407

Jeppsson B, Bengmark S (1986) Determinants of survival after intraarterial infusion of 5-fluorouracil for liver metastases from colorectal cancer: a multivariate analysis. J Surg Oncol 31: 246–254

Johnson LP, Wassermann PB, Rivkin SE (1985) The implanted pump in metastatic colorectal cancer of the liver. Am J Surg 149: 595–598

Johnston-Early A, Cohen MH (1981) Mitomycin C-induced skin ulceration remote from infusion site. Cancer Treat Rep 65: 529

Kaplan WD, Ensminger WD, Come SE, Smith EH, D'Orsi CJ, Levin DC, Takvorian RW, Steele GD Jr (1980) Radionuclide angiography to predict patient response to hepatic artery chemotherapy. Cancer Treat Rep 64: 1217–1222

Kelsen DP, Hoffman J, Alcock N et al. (1980) Pharmacokinetics of regional infusion of cisplatin. Proc Am Assoc Cancer Res 21: 745

Kemeny MM, Battifora H, Blayney DW et al. (1985) Sclerosing cholangitis after continuous hepatic artery infusion of FUDR. Ann Surg 202: 176–181

Kemeny N (1983) The systemic chemotherapy of hepatic metastases. Semin Oncol 2: 148–158

Kemeny N, Daly J (1986) Preliminary results of a randomized study of intrahepatic infusion versus systemic infusion of 5-fluoro-2′-deoxyuridine for metastatic colorectal carcinoma. In: Herfarth C, Schlag P, Hohenberger P (eds) Therapeutic strategies in primary and metastatic liver cancer. Springer, Berlin Heidelberg New York Tokyo, pp 171–178

Kemeny N, Daly J, Oderman P, Shike M, Chun H, Petroni G, Geller N (1984) Hepatic artery pump infusion: toxicity and results in patients with metastatic colorectal carcinoma. J Clin Oncol 2: 595–600

Kemeny N, Reichmann B, Oderman P, Daly J, Geller N (1986) Update of a randomized study of intrahepatic (H) vs. systematic (S) infusion of fluorodeoxyuridine (FUDR) in patients with liver metastases from colorectal carcinoma (CRC). Proc Asco 5: 345

Kirkwood J, Ensminger W, Rosowsky A (1980) 5-fluorouracil and thymidine: pharmacokinetic observations in a phase I trial comparing 5-fluorouracil and 5-fluorouracil with concurrent thymidine infusions. Cancer Res 40: 107–113

Laufman L, Nims T, Guy JT, Guy JF, Courter S (1984) Hepatic arterial ligation and portal vein infusion for liver metastases from colorectal cancer. J Clin Oncol 2: 1382–1389

Lehner B, Kretzschmar U, Bubeck B, Hölting T, Schlag P (1988) Results of liver angiography and perfusion scintigraphy do not correlate with response to hepatic artery infusion chemotherapy. J Surg Oncol 39: 73–78

Lin G, Lunderquist A, Hägerstrand I, Boijsen E (1984) Postmortem examination of the blood supply and vascular pattern of small liver metastases in man. Surgery 96: 517–526

Link KH, Aigner KR, Kühn W, Roetering N, Schwemmle K (1985) Chemosensitivitätsbestimmung in vitro bei regionaler Chemotherapie von Lebertumoren. Tumor Diagn Ther 6: 238–243

Lokich J (1983) Determination of response in treatment of hepatic neoplasia. Semin Oncol 2: 228–237

Lokich J (1986) Systemic, infusional chemotherapy for liver metastases; an improved schedule for 5-fluorouracil. In: Herforth C, Schlag P, Hohenberger P (eds) Therapeutic strategies in primary metastatic cancer. Springer, Berlin Heidelberg New York Tokyo, pp 131–139

Lokich J, Ensminger W (1983) Ambulatory pump infusion devices for hepatic artery infusion. Semin Oncol 2: 183–191

Lokich J, Bothe A, Fine N, Perri J (1982) The delivery of cancer chemotherapy by constant venous infusion. Cancer 50: 2731–2735

Malt RA (1985) Surgery for hepatic neoplasms. N Engl J Med 313: 1591–1596

Metzger U (1986) Prevention of liver metastases of colorectal carcinoma. In: Herfarth C, Schlag P, Hohenberger P (eds) Therapeutic strategies in primary and metastatic liver cancer. Springer, Berlin Heidelberg New York Tokyo, pp 29–34

Moertel CG, Reitemeier RJ, Hahn R (1967) A controlled comparison of 5-fluoro-2′-deoxyuridine therapy administered by rapid intravenous injection and by continuous intravenous infusion. Cancer Res 27: 549–552

Narsete T, Ansfield F, Wirtanen G, Ramirez G, Wolfberg W, Jarrett F (1977) Gastric ulceration in patients receiving intrahepatic infusion of 5-fluorouracil. Ann Surg 186: 734–736

Neuhaus P, Brölsch CE, Ringe B, Pichlmayr R (1986) Liver transplantation for liver tumors. In: Herfarth C, Schlag P, Hohenberger P (eds) Therapeutic strategies in primary and metastatic liver cancer. Springer, Berlin Heidelberg New York Tokyo, pp 221–228

Niederhuber JE, Ensminger WD (1983) Surgical considerations in the management of hepatic neoplasia. Semin Oncol 10: 135–147
Niederhuber E, Ensminger WD, Gyves J, Thrall J, Walker S, Cozzi E (1984) Regional chemotherapy of colorectal cancer metastatic to the liver. Cancer 53: 1336–1343
Order SE, Stillwagon GB, Klein JL, Leichner PK, Siegelman SS, Fishman EK, Ettinger DS, Haulk T, Kopher K, Finney K, Surdyke M, Self S, Leibel S (1985) Iodine 131 antiferritin, a new treatment modality in hepatoma: a Radiation Therapy Oncology Group study. J Clin Oncol 3: 1573–1582
Patt YZ, Chuang VP, Wallace S, Benjamin RS, Fuqua R, Mavligit GM (1983 a) Hepatic arterial chemotherapy and occlusion for palliation of primary hepatocellular and unknown primary neoplasms in the liver. Cancer 51: 1359–1363
Patt YZ, Peters RE, Chuang VP, Wallace S, Mavligit G (1983 b) Effective retreatment of patients with colorectal cancer and liver metastases. Am J Med 75: 237–240
Petras RE, Hart WR, Bukowski RM (1985) Gastric epithelial atypia associated with hepatic arterial infusion chemotherapy. Cancer 56: 745–750
Petrek JA, Minton JP (1979) Treatment of hepatic metastases by percutaneous hepatic arterial infusion. Cancer 43: 2182–2188
Pikren JW, Tsukuda Y, Lane WW (1984) Liver metastases: analysis of autopsy data. In: Weiss L, Gilberg HA (eds) Liver metastases. Hall, Boston
Reed ML, Vaitkevicius VK, Al-Sarraf M, Vaughn CB, Singhakowinta A, Sexon-Porte M, Izbicki R, Baker L, Straatsma GW (1981) The practicality of chronic hepatic artery infusion therapy of primary and metastatic hepatic malignancies: ten-year results of 124 patients in a prospective protocol. Cancer 47: 402–409
Roemeling von R, MacDonald M, Langevin T, Buchwald H, Hrushesky WJM (1986 a) Chemotherapy via implanted infusion pump: new perspectives for delivery of long-term continuous treatment. Oncology Nursing forum 13: 17–24
Roemeling von R, Hrushesky WJM, Kennedy BJ, Buchwald H (1986 b) Programmed automatic FUDR chronotherapy improves therapeutic index. In: Pannell M (ed) Surgical Forum, XXXVII. American College of Surgeons, 55 East Eric Street, Chicago, IL 60611
Rothmund M, Brückner R, Keller E, Quint B, Knutz A, Schicketanz K (1986) Chemotherapie bei Lebermetastasen colorectaler Carcinome mit implantierbaren Gasdruckpumpen – Ergebnisse einer prospektiven Studie. Dtsch Med Wochenschr III: 652
Rougier P, Laser P, Elias D, Ghosn M, Droz JP, Sidibe S, Theodore C, Lumbroso J (1987) Intraarterial hepatic chemotherapy (IAHC) for liver metastasis (LM) from colorectal (CR) origin (Abstr). Proc Am Soc Clin Oncol 6: 369
Rubin RN (1983) Local installation of small doses of streptokinase for treatment of thrombotic occlusions of long-term access catheters. J Clin Oncol 1: 7
Russel AH, Tong DT, Dawson LE, Wisbeck W (1984) Adenocarcinoma of the proximal colon: sites of initial dissemination and patterns of recurrence following surgery alone. Cancer 53: 360–367
Schlag P (1985) Continuous cancer chemotherapy – rationale and prerequisites for treatment at home. Int J Tech Assoc Health Care 1: 18–20
Schlag P, Feil H, Ruoff G, Hohenberger P, Hölting T, Buhl K (1987) Onkologische Behandlung zu Hause: Erfahrungen mit einer ambulanten intraartiellen Chemotherapie von Lebermetastasen. Schweiz Med Wochenschr 117: 1342–1346
Schlag P, Hohenberger P, Hölting T, Buhl K, Herfarth C (1988 a) Intraarterielle 5-Fluorouracil-Chemotherapie bei Lebermetastasen kolorektaler Karzinome. Med Klin 83: 705–709
Schlag P, Dörsam J, Aguiar JLA, Bartkowski R, Berger M (1988 b) Hepatic arterial infusion (HAI) chemotherapy proves to be advantageous in the treatment of experimental liver tumors. Eur J Clin Oncol 24: 1013–1018
Schreml W (1986) Indications for treatment and determination of treatment effects with primary and secondary liver tumors. In: Herfarth C, Schlag P, Hohenberger P (eds) Therapeutic strategies in primary and metastatic liver cancer. Springer, Berlin Heidelberg New York Tokyo, pp 91–102
Schwartz SI, Jones LS, McCune CS (1985) Assessment of treatment of intrahepatic malignancies using chemotherapy via an implantable pump. Ann Surg 201: 560–567
Schwemmle K, Aigner K (1986) Requirements and results of liver perfusion. In: Herfarth C, Schlag P, Hohenberger P (eds) Therapeutic strategies in primary and metastatic liver cancer. Springer, Berlin Heidelberg New York Tokyo, pp 229–233
Seifert P, Baker LH, Reed ML, Vaitkevicius K (1975) Comparison of continuously infused 5-fluorouracil with bolus injection in treatment of patients with colorectal adenocarcinoma. Cancer 36: 123–126
Shepard KV, Levin B, Karl RC, Faintuch J, DuBrow RA, Hagle M, Cooper RM, Beschorner J, Stablein D (1985) Therapy for metastatic colorectal cancer with hepatic artery infusion chemotherapy using a subcutaneous implanted pump. J Clin Oncol 3: 161–169
Shike M, Gillin JC, Kemeny N, Daly JM, Kurtz RC (1986) Severe gastroduodenal ulcerations complicating hepatic artery infusion chemotherapy for metastatic colon cancer. Am J Gastroenterol 81: 176–179
Sindelar WF (1985) Isolation-perfusion of the liver with 5-fluorouracil. Ann Surg 201: 337–343
Speyer JL (1984) Intraperitoneal chemotherapy. A possible role in the treatment of hepatic metastases. In: Van de Velde CJH, Sugarbaker PH (eds) Liver metastatis: basic aspects, detection and management. Martinus Nijhoff, Boston
Steplewski Z, Sears HF, Koprowski H (1986) Monoclonal antibody infusion in gastrointestinal cancer patients. In: Herfarth C, Schlag P, Hohenberger P (eds) Therapeutic strategies in primary and metastatic liver cancer. Springer, Berlin Heidelberg New York Tokyo, pp 321–323
Strohmeier T, Haugeberg G, Lierse W (1986) Vaskularisation von Lebermetastasen: eine korrosionsanatomische Studie. Acta Anat 12: 172–176
Sugarbaker PH, Gianola FJ, Speyer JL, Wesley R, Barofsky I, Myers CE (1985) Prospective randomized trial of intravenous v intraperitoneal 5-FU in patients with advanced primary colon or rectal cancer. Semin Oncol [Suppl 4] 12: 101–111
Taylor I. (1978) Cytotoxic perfusion for colorectal liver metastases. Br J Surg 65: 219–222
Taylor I (1985) Colorectal liver metastases – to treat or not to treat? Br J Surg 72: 511–516
Tseng MH, Luch J, Mittelman A et al. (1981) Chemotherapy of advanced colorectal cancer with regional arterial mitomycin C infusion and concomitant measurement of serum drug level. Proc Am Assoc Cancer Res 22: 359
Van de Velde CJH, Tjaden UR, Kothuis BJL (1984 a) Isolated regional liver perfusion in the treatment of hepatic metastases. In: Van de Velde CJH, Sugarbaker P (eds) Liver metastases. Nijhoff, Amsterdam, pp 292–312
Van de Velde CJH, Veenhof CHN, Sugarbaker PH (1984 b)

Methodology in the clinical study of hepatic metastases. In: Van de Velde CJH, Sugarbaker PH (eds) Liver metastasis: basic aspects, detection and management. Martinus Nijhoff, Boston, pp 358–375

Wallace S, Charnsangavej C, Carrasco CH, Bechtel W, Wright K, Gianturco C (1984) Radiological intervention technique in the percutaneous treatment of liver metastases. In: Van de Velde CJH, Sugarbaker PH (eds) Liver metastasis: basic aspects, detection and management. Martinus Nijhoff, Boston, pp 214–229

Watkins E, Khazei AM, Nahra KS (1970) Surgical basis for arterial infusion chemotherapy of disseminated carcinoma of the liver. Surg Gynecol Obstet 130: 581–605

Wright KC, Wallace S, Kim EE, Haynie T, Charnsangavej C, Carrasco H, Chuang VP, Gianturco C (1986) Pulsed arterial infusions - chemotherapeutic implications. Cancer 57: 1952–1956

Yang PJ, Thrall JH, Ensminger WD, Niederhuber JE, Gyves JW, Tuscan M, Doan K, Cozzi E (1982) Perfusion scintigraphy (Tc-99m MAA) during surgery for placement of chemotherapy in hepatic artery: concise communication. J Nucl Med 23: 1066–1069

Adjuvant Systemic Therapy

G. BONADONNA, F. FOSSATI-BELLANI, and P. VALAGUSSA

Introduction

There is unchallenged evidence that cancer chemotherapy has made progress in many tumors since the mid-1970s. In particular, certain neoplasms can now be cured only after the administration of adequate polydrug regimens. New strategies have been proposed and applied during the past 10 years to improve the clinical results in various tumors. These consist mainly in adjuvant chemotherapy for patients at high risk of recurrence following standard locoregional treatment, and in the delivery of non-cross-resistant regimens to overcome the problem of primary cell resistance.

Principles of Systemic Adjuvant Therapy

Systemic adjuvant therapy was introduced into clinical trials on a full scale in the 1970s and has continued to evolve, as second- and third-generation trials have become based on human cancer models rather than preclinical models. The possibility of complementary therapeutic action of various modalities was recognized when chemotherapy was first introduced. Subsequently, the demonstration of the successful application of various modalities when directed toward the early stages of Wilms' tumor led to the concept of combined modality treatment. After many abortive attempts to utilize chemotherapy in the early stages of adult solid tumors in the late 1950s and the 1960s, the concept of postsurgical treatment of minimal residual disease emerged. Reflecting an additional evolution are terms such as neo-adjuvant or protoadjuvant chemotherapy which refer to the use of primary systemic therapy, before a local intervention. This chapter will review the preclinical foundations of adjuvant systemic therapy and will specifically discuss how concepts have evolved with the application of the strategic principles to the management of various tumors.

Preclinical Basis

The experimental foundations of adjuvant therapy were derived to a great extent from studies performed by Skipper and Schabel (1984) and coworkers at the Southern Research Institute in Birmingham, Alabama, USA. Their observations on the survival of mice with transplantable solid tumors of varying age and size subjected to resection led them to postulate a great variability in metastatic body burden at the time of surgery. Because of this, empirical considerations have to be utilized in the selection of drugs, the treatment schedule and the duration of treatment. Surgical cure rates in solid tumors of mice also show a relationship to tumor size. Interestingly, the "break" point in the survival curves, after which no further recurrences were noted, occurred at similar times after surgery, although the proportion of animals surviving mostly varied. This indicated that the biology of the tumor was similar in the various animals, but the tumor burden accounted for the variability. As a corollary to this, definitive conclusions with regard to therapeutic effectiveness must be withheld until this break point is reached, since it is the patients with large tumor burdens who are less likely to benefit from adjuvant therapy that make up the first portion of the survival curves. As for selection of drugs and treatment schedules, these must be effective in achieving a net reduction in cell burden by the next cycle; it is apparent that the optimal intensity must, generally, be identical to the intensity that yields the optimal results in advanced disease. Martin et al. (1975) demonstrated that both drug combinations and surgery were optimal in making an impact on the survival of mice bearing mammary tumors. However, since the tumor burden is generally lower if treatments are started in adjuvant situations, the duration of treatment necessary for eradication is likely to be less. Emergence of resistance is likely to parallel advanced disease as a major cause of adjuvant therapy failure. However, in accordance with the hypothesis advanced by Goldie and Coldman (1985) and Schilsky (1985), with lower tumor burdens the emergence of resistant cells is less.

Immunotherapeutic agents were attractive drugs for the adjuvant setting in view of the unlikelihood of long-term toxicities and the postulated efficacy of these approaches at low tumor burdens. Experiments in general indicated that agents such as *Corynebacterium parvum* acted in antimetastatic fashion and had an effect only when given a specific time prior to surgery in circumstances when surgery alone was also clearly beneficial.

Hormones are receiving renewed attention as potential adjuvant treatments. In carcinogen-induced mammary tumors of mice, the demonstration that tamoxifen can both delay the appearance of tumors and decrease their overall frequency in a dose-dependent and schedule-dependent manner has been of great interest, not only for adjuvant treatment of breast cancer, but also for possible inhibition of carcinogenic influences. In animal models, interruption of tamoxifen may partially eliminate the benefit, as tumors will begin to recur.

The complexities of human disease may require additional models for proper interpretation. For example, one may be able to explain late recurrence using the concept of "dormant" stem cells which have metastatized and escaped eradication. Early recurrence, on the other hand, indicates a failure to eradicate "committed" stem cells expected to be sensitive to chemotherapy, unless their numbers were such as to allow emergence of drug resistance. Strategies of adjuvant therapy are in fact dependent on the intrinsic efficacy of the chemotherapy as well as on the patterns and site of relapse.

Theoretical Considerations

In the absence of reliable biochemical tumor markers, adjuvant treatment must be chosen empirically, based on the treatment of advanced disease, and used in situations where staging provides some estimate of risk of recurrence (and thus tumor burden). Hence, the effective treatment should be administered to patients at risk at an intensity equal to that employed in advanced disease but for a shorter time. Early treatment at a time of minimum tumor burden is to be preferred (noting that preoperative treatment may mask staging information). Guidance for proper administration of systemic adjuvant therapy must be based on comparative experience with a similarly staged group of patients not receiving treatment. Relapse-free survival and overall survival comparisons will indicate the benefit that might be achieved from adjuvant treatment.

The other side of the coin, however, is the risk of the side effects from adjuvant therapy which are experienced by 100% of the population treated. The relapsing population receives what we term "salvage" therapy. Cost/benefit analyses are central to the decision on whether to use adjuvant strategies or salvage treatments. When the risk has been well delineated, and the relapsing population forms a high proportion of the total and is not likely to be cured (such as in breast cancer), the rationale for adjuvant therapy is powerful, favoring any potential benefit, whatever the cost. On the other hand, in testicular cancer the ability to salvage patients with chemotherapy has been well demonstrated. The fulcrum of the balance in this instance shifts towards the cost side. In all these considerations, however, the overriding factor is efficacy. When the efficacy or contribution of the adjuvant treatment is likely to be modest, then considerations of the cost to the treated population become most important. Such situations often require trials with concomitant untreated controls.

Since the treatment given is empirical, its administration has been designed according to certain guiding principles derived from advanced disease. However, for the specific purpose of adjuvant therapy some drugs may be avoided. In particular, drugs which may have long-term sequelae should be excluded. Drugs which could affect the patient's fertility and gonadal function should not be used when equally effective therapeutic alternatives are available.

Other theoretical rationales for adjuvant therapy are: (a) a lower tumor burden with presumed smaller primary drug-resistant fraction; (b) kinetically more favorable circumstances; (c) a less disturbed microenvironment at commencement of therapy; (d) a less compromised host.

Primary Chemotherapy

Primary, (neo-adjuvant, protoadjuvant) chemotherapy is used in those tumors that have traditionally been treated initially, or entirely, with locoregional ablative surgery or intensive irradiation. As previously mentioned, if chemotherapy is administered in these situations to high-risk patients, it is used as an adjuvant *after* locoregional control procedure. The concept of primary chemotherapy is to deliver drug treatment *before* the locoregional control procedure to further assure local control and, more generally, to kill cancer cells in metastatic regional and systemic distributions. Thus, while in the classical postoperative or postirradiation adjuvant setting complete remission is induced by surgery and/or radiotherapy, in the neo-adjuvant approach the initial tumor response is induced by drug treatment, followed by consolidation with surgery, radiotherapy, different chemotherapy, or a combination of these modalities.

The scientific rationale of primary chemotherapy (Frei 1985; Norton 1985; Schilsky 1985; Ragaz et al. 1986) can be summarized as follows: (a) The analysis of experimental tumors shows that surgical removal of the primary neoplasm results in a temporary enhancement of growth rate in the residual secondary tumors. Appropriately timed chemotherapy can prevent the deleterious consequences of increased tumor growth. (b) The use of primary chemotherapy may result in significant regression of the primary tumor, rendering it possible to carry out less extensive, or intensive, locoregional treatment with the preservation of physiological, cosmetic and psychological functions. There are, at present, important indications from retrospective as well as from prospective clinical trials that neo-adjuvant chemotherapy may be beneficial in specific circumstances. The tumors in which primary chemotherapy has been administered are as follows: head and neck cancer (stage III), bone and soft tissue sarcomas, bladder cancer, breast cancer (stage I–III), anal carcinoma, Hodgkin's disease (intermediate stages), and non-Hodgkin's lymphomas (stages I and II).

Clinical Findings

Wilms' Tumor

The current standard treatment of Wilms' tumor (nephroblastoma) is considered the first classical example of a successful coordinated multidisciplinary approach to a specific neoplasm. The survival rate, originally less than 10%, was raised to 40% in the 1950s with development in surgical techniques and the use of preoperative and postoperative irradiation. The subsequent introduction of chemotherapy, notably the agents dactinomycin and vincristine, as an adjuvant to surgery and radiotherapy completely revolutionized the therapy of this tumor (D'Angio 1985).

The efficacy of multiple courses vs a single paraoperative course of dactinomycin or vincristine alone, and of combination chemotherapy, was tested within cooperative groups, whose studies allowed recognition of factors influencing prognosis. The results of the first, second, and third National Wilms' Tumor Study group trials can be summarized as follows: (a) patients with stage I anaplastic tumors who received treatment identical to that of patients with stage I tumors of favorable histology have the same excellent prognosis; (b) in group II and III patients, the combination of dactinomycin and vincristine is superior to either agent alone; (c) routine, postoperative radiation therapy of the flank is not necessary for children with stage I tumors of favorable histology or stage I anaplastic tumors, nor for those with stage II tumors of favorable histology when post-nephrectomy combination chemotherapy consisting of dactinomycin and vincristine is administered; (d) the prognosis for patients with stage III tumors of favorable histology is best when the treatment program includes either a three-drug combination with dactinomycin, vincristine, and doxorubicin plus 1000 rad radiation therapy to the flank, or dactinomycin and vincristine plus 2000 rad radiation therapy to the flank; (e) the four-drug regimen consisting of cyclophosphamide, vincristine, dactinomycin, and doxorubicin may benefit patients with stages II–IV anaplastic tumors; (f) in general, stages II and III tumors of favorable histology can be successfully treated with less intensive regimens.

Preoperative treatment (radiation with or without chemotherapy) was tested in the European trials of the International Society of Pediatric Oncology (SIOP). The essential results can be summarized as follows: (a) preoperative radiotherapy or chemotherapy reduces intraoperative tumor spillage; (b) preoperative chemotherapy using dactinomycin plus vincristine is preferable to radiation; (c) multiple courses of dactinomycin plus vincristine for 15 months vs 6 months failed to improve survival. In the United Kingdom, the first trial of the Medical Research Council compared intensive vincristine therapy to dactinomycin treatment. The 2-year relapse-free survival was superior in patients receiving vincristine alone (Morris Jones et al. 1978).

Before the introduction of chemotherapy, 60% of children with Wilms' tumor died as a result of metastatic involvement of lungs, liver, and abdomen. Today, the long-term survival rate is in excess of 80%. National and international cooperative groups are now attempting to refine treatments to achieve maximal survival benefit with minimal toxicity.

Bone Sarcomas

In osteosarcoma and Ewing's sarcoma the multimodal treatment approach has resulted in a real improvement in survival and also in cure rate. Although progress in treatment and cure of bone sarcomas is slow, during the past decade a better knowledge of natural history and prognostic factors has been achieved, along with improvement of diagnostic procedures and refinements of surgical and radiotherapeutic methods. Improvement in overall survival reflects aggressiveness in tumor treatment. A new direction in the treatment of both types of bone sarcoma is the use of preoperative or preirradiation chemotherapy. This sequential approach provides a window of time to plan the definitive therapy of primary tumor more adequately by properly selecting individualized treatment modalities.

Ewing's Sarcoma

Ewing's sarcoma is a malignant bone neoplasm of children, adolescents, and young adults the cure rate of which was less than 20% before the introduction of chemotherapy. Radiation may achieve local tumor control, which is related to the total dose delivered, with or without subsequent surgery. Intensive systemic chemotherapy combined with radiation has improved the 2-year survival rates to 50%. A number of chemotherapeutic agents have been tested: vincristine plus dactinomycin plus cyclophosphamide (VAC) and vincristine plus dactinomycin plus cyclophosphamide plus doxorubicin (VACA) represent the two major drug combinations investigated.

In the Intergroup Ewing's Sarcoma Study, differences in the incidence of pulmonary metastases were found when patients were treated with postirradiation adjuvant VAC or VACA and pulmonary radiation (Perez et al. 1981; Donaldson 1985).

In spite of the addition of lung or total-body irradiation to systemic chemotherapy, metastatic spread still represents the major problem. A different sequential approach to Ewing's sarcoma – cytoreduction by intensive chemotherapy before definitive irradiation with or without surgery – is under evaluation in many institutions. In fact, more effective systemic chemotherapy through adjustment of drug schedules is needed to further improve survival in this tumor, whose natural history was changed with modern antitumor treatments.

Osteosarcoma

The concept for multidisciplinary treatment of osteogenic sarcoma has considerably changed during the past decade. Historically, prognosis and cure rates following surgical therapy alone were poor: 80% of patients developed overt metastatic disease by 2 years after diagnosis. An increase in survival rates was observed when high-dose methotrexate (HDMTX) and doxorubicin were used as adjuvant therapy following mutilating surgery (Goorin et al. 1985). After 1977, numerous drug combinations, including HDMTX plus doxorubicin plus cisplatin and cyclophosphamide plus dacarbazine plus bleomycin, have been used in various studies in the USA and Europe. Results were very similar among reported trials, with 2-3 year relapse-free survival ranging from 40% to 58%.

Up to a few years ago, the surgical treatment of choice for primary tumors of the long bones was amputation or limb disarticulation followed by adjuvant chemotherapy. Today, the strategy has changed and includes preoperative chemotherapy to achieve initial tumor control followed by a limb-sparing procedure and further chemotherapy based on the histopathological findings in the surgical specimen. This strategy was first proposed by the Memorial Hospital group in New York (Rosen et al. 1983). The limb preservation program starts with HDMTX, cisplatin, and doxorubicin given in various combinations prior to surgery. The effectiveness of chemotherapy is demonstrated pathologically by evaluating the extent of necrosis in the primary tumor specimen. With tissue destruction in approximately 90% of the tumors the relapse-free survival ranges from 80% to 92%. Present findings, however, need confirmation through more prolonged follow-up. More recently, preoperative chemotherapy was administered intra-arterially by several research centers with the intention of obtaining maximal local tumor necrosis. Doxorubicin, cisplatin and HDMTX were utilized with favorable results. Thus, preoperative systemic chemotherapy may actually have an important impact not only on subsequent adjuvant systemic therapy, but also on local tumor control avoiding amputation. Conversely, intra-arterial chemotherapy may not only result in excellent local control but may also identify important agents to be used systematically. It will be crucial, however, to confirm in appropriately designed clinical trials the value of chemotherapy modification based on gross in vivo tumor destruction.

The efficacy of adjuvant HDMTX following mutilating surgery has been questioned by investigators of the Mayo Clinic, through a prospective randomized trial where no significant total survival improvement in comparison with concomitant untreated control group was detectable (Edmonson et al. 1984). For this reason, two other randomized trials were undertaken, one by a cooperative group and the other by a single institution (Goorin et al. 1985). Both trials were conducted on nonmetastatic extremity osteosarcoma and compared the results of the six-drug adjuvant therapy regimen (T-10 regimen) of the Memorial Hospital with those of surgery alone. The 2-year results from both the above-mentioned controlled studies indicate that the natural history of osteosarcoma was not changed, thereby validating the data from historical controls. In spite of the short follow-up periods, these two important studies have shown that intensive, multidrug adjuvant chemotherapy, as predicted by the sequential trials by G. Rosen at Memorial Hospital (1983), has a significant favorable impact on relapse-free and overall survival among patients with nonmetastatic high-grade osteosarcoma of the extremities.

Soft Tissue Sarcomas

Rhabdomyosarcoma in Children

During the past decade, effective combination chemotherapy used in coordinated programs with radiation and surgery has increased the 2-year survival rate for rhabdomyosarcoma to nearly 60%. Combination regimens including vincristine, dactinomycin, and cyclophosphamide have commonly been utilized (Donaldson 1985). The benefit from adjuvant systemic chemotherapy in the treatment of rhabdomyosarcoma was demonstrated through a prospective randomized trial where patients classified as group I and receiving chemotherapy showed a survival rate of 82% compared to 47% for those not treated with chemotherapy.

In 1972 the Intergroup Rhabdomyosarcoma Study (IRS) initiated the first cooperative trials to test the relative merits of chemotherapy and radiotherapy in the various disease stages. The conclusions were as follows (Table 1): (a) in localized completely resected disease (group I), radiotherapy is unnecessary if patients receive adjuvant VAC chemotherapy (vincristine, dactinomycin, and oral cyclophosphamide); (b) in group II tumors a three-drug regimen (VAC) was as effective as a two-drug regimen (vincristine plus dactinomycin) when postoperative irradiation was given; (c) in group III-IV disease the addition of doxorubicin to "pulse VAC" failed to improve the

Table 1. First trial of the Intergroup Rhabdomyosarcoma Study: 5-year relapse-free and overall survival rates

Group	Treatment	RFS (%)	OS (%)
I	S+VAC	81	93
	S+RT+VAC	79	81
II	S+RT+VAC	72	73
	S+RT+VA	65	70
III	RT+VACA	61	51
	RT+VAC	58	53
IV	RT+VACA	41	26
	RT+VAC	19	14

S, surgery; RT, radiotherapy; RFS, relapse-free survival; OS, overall survival. For chemotherapy acronyms see text.

Table 2. Second trial of Intergroup Rhabdomyosarcoma Study: 3-year relapse-free and 2-year overall survival rates

Group	Treatment	RFS (%)	OS (%)
I	S+VAC	87	100
	S+VA	83	92
II	S+VA+RT	81	94
	S+VAC+RT	70	79
III	VAC+RT		
		80–83	71–79
	Vadr–VAC+RT		
IV	VAC+RT		
		43–62	37–40
	Vadr–CVAC+RT		

S, surgery; RT, radiotherapy; RFS, relapse-free survival; OS, overall survival. For chemotherapy acronyms see text.

outcome of patients who were routinely irradiated. The preliminary data from the second IRS trials, initiated in 1978 (Maurer et al. 1983), are summarized in Table 2. The relapse-free survival in group I and II patients was similar in both trials. However, in the second study the relapse-free survival for groups III and IV appeared significantly superior to that in the first. These findings indicated that an aggressive chemotherapy program produced a superior outcome in patients with more advanced disease.

Future combined treatment strategies for rhabdomyosarcoma should take into consideration variables such as primary tumor location, tumor bulk, and nodal status, which all affect prognosis. Complications from the disease itself, as well as from therapeutic modalities, are also being considered in the design of new treatment approaches or drug regimens in the attempt to decrease treatment-related sequelae.

Soft Tissue Sarcomas in Adults

Soft tissue sarcomas in adults respond differently to treatment than the rhabdomyosarcoma of childhood. Adjuvant therapy in the former is still under development and not totally established, whereas combined modality therapy has been an essential component of the management of childhood sarcomas. Nevertheless, the same strategy is increasingly applicable to all types of adult soft tissue sarcomas. The histological types have varied somewhat in frequency according to pathologist's classifications, with malignant fibrohistiocytoma recently being recorded as the most common, and synovial sarcoma also increasing in incidence. Most important in determining the prognosis and the likelihood of local and hematogenous spread are the grade of the tumor and the size of the initial primary, with documentation of whether the margins of resection were clear of tumor.

The role of more conservative, function-sparing operations followed by radiation has been well established in randomized studies by the National Cancer Institute (1985). In some centers, regional (intra-arterial) chemotherapy, in combination with radiotherapy and surgery, has been used in limb-sparing treatment of soft tissue sarcomas. The results of this approach have not been established as superior to those of other multimodality approaches. Adjuvant systemic chemotherapy with doxorubicin-containing regimens has yielded conflicting results. The National Cancer Institute study has documented the superiority of adjuvant chemotherapy with doxorubicin and cyclophosphamide followed by HDMTX over observation in both relapse-free survival and overall survival. Other studies performed in the USA and in Europe, however, indicate no such advantage with regimens that on the surface appear equivalent (National Cancer Institute 1985). Thus, at present, the role of adjuvant systemic chemotherapy in the treatment of high-grade soft tissue sarcomas of the extremities remains unsettled. Moreover, the use of doxorubicin as an adjuvant has resulted in a documented decline in cardiac ejection fraction in the majority of patients. For this reason, it is imperative that additional prospective randomized studies be performed to establish the efficacy of adjuvant systemic chemotherapy in a reproducible way.

Breast Cancer

There is convincing evidence that the natural history of operable breast cancer can be perturbed by adjuvant medical intervention. During the past 15 years the search for optimal systemic adjuvant therapy in high-risk patients has represented a major research effort in cancer medicine. The initial reports of randomized trials performed by the National Surgical Adjuvant Breast Project (NSABP) in the USA and by the Milan Cancer Institute in Italy have stimulated, all over the world, similar research studies which have contributed a large body of information. Findings from prospective clinical trials were recently discussed during the second NIH Consensus Development Conference. Admittedly, few questions have been answered and many more remain to be solved. Nonetheless, it is undeniable that significant reductions in death rates following systemic adjuvant therapy have been documented. The present findings are summarized below while many details are available in the medical literature (Bonadonna and Valagussa 1985; Bonadonna et al. 1985; Bonadonna 1986).

Adjuvant Chemotherapy

So far, adjuvant chemotherapy has almost always been administered to patients with histologically positive axillary lymph nodes, in whom the 3-year relapse rate following radical or modified radical mastectomy is approximately 50%. The initial studies performed by the NSABP utilizing melphalan and by the Milan Cancer Institute utilizing cyclophosphamide, methotrexate and fluorouracil (CMF) were recognized to yield results of considerable biological and clinical interest requiring additional study evolution. The essential findings obtained by research teams whose case series included a concomitant control arm are reported in Table 3. After more than a decade of trials the following conclusions can be drawn:

a) Adjuvant chemotherapy can exert significantly prolonged therapeutic activity in some patients bearing micrometastases.
b) Both premenopausal and postmenopausal women can benefit from effective adjuvant chemotherapy, albeit with differences in treatment outcome in favor of the former.
c) The degree of nodal involvement affects treatment results. Patients with > 10 involved nodes benefit only minimally from presently utilized regimens.
d) Overall, combination chemotherapy was reported to be superior to single agents.
e) The maximum kill of drug-sensitive tumor cells probably occurs within the first few cycles, thus suggesting that prolonged treatment duration with the same drugs is unnecessary.

Table 3. Adjuvant chemotherapy studies with a concomitant control group with locoregional treatment alone in node-positive patients

First author	Adjuvant treatment	Essential findings in treated groups
Fisher	PAM	Increased RFS and OS in premenopause, one to three nodes
Bonadonna	CMF	Increased RFS and OS in premenopause
Senn	LMF + BCG	Increased RFS in postmenopause, no OS difference
Wheeler	CVFM	Increased RFS (mainly in postmenopause), no OS difference
Rubens	PAM	No significant difference after PAM
Rubens	CMF	CMF superior in premenopause, no OS difference
Morrison	AVCMF	Increased RFS in premenopause, no OS difference
Smith	CMF vs CMF + RT	Increased RFS in premenopause and postmenopause after RT + CMF and CMF vs RT alone, increased OS after RT + CMF vs RT

Modified from Bonadonna and Valagussa (1985)
RFS, Relapse-Free Survival; OS, Overall Survival;
RT, Postoperative irradiation
Chemotherapy acronyms: PAM, melphalan; C, cyclophosphamide; M, methotrexate; F, fluorouracil; L, leukeran; A, doxorubicin.

Table 4. Reduction in breast cancer mortality following adjuvant chemotherapy: trials with untreated controls

	Reduction (%)		
	Total	< 50 years	> 50 years
Single agents	4	18	−5
Combinations		29	12
CMF	24*	34*	17
Total	14*	24*	8**

From R. Peto and Trialists 1985 (unpublished data, presented at the NIH Consensus Development Conference, September)
* $P < 0.0001$, ** $P < 0.05$ compared to controls.

f) The delivery of optimal drug doses has a major impact on treatment outcome

Assessments of the value of adjuvant chemotherapy in terms of the reduction in the odds of death, derived by pooling data from separate trials and comparing only like groups of patients, were reported by R. Peto and coworkers at the Consensus Development Conference. Data derived from this overview are illustrated in Table 4.

The value of adjuvant chemotherapy in patients with negative axillary nodes has so far been investigated in very few trials. The first two randomized studies yielded inconclusive results for a number of reasons, the most important one being patient selection. The vast majority of women with uninvolved axillary nodes can be cured by locoregional therapy alone, the 10-year relapse-free survival rate being about 75%. Consequently, treating all patients can "dilute" the treatment results, and, more important, women cured by locoregional therapy alone are unnecessarily exposed to the risk of acute toxicity and long-term sequelae. Therefore, efforts should be made to properly identify patients at high risk of relapse. The Milan group has evaluated the efficacy of adjuvant intravenous full-dose CMF vs locoregional therapy alone in a selected subset of patients with estrogen receptor-negative tumors. With a median follow-up of 5 years, the relapse-free survival was 87% following CMF and 45% for the control group ($p < 0.001$). The figures for overall survival were 90% and 65%, respectively ($p = 0.02$) (Bonadonna and Valagussa 1988, 1989).

Adjuvant Tamoxifen

In the past few years, increasing emphasis has been placed on the use of adjuvant endocrine therapy. The known heterogeneity of breast cancer cells, the possibility of selecting patients by receptor status, and the lack of severe toxicity with additive hormonal manipulations were the main factors instigating this avenue of clinical research. The vast majority of trials have utilized the antiestrogen compound tamoxifen at the daily dose of 20–30 mg for 12–60 months. Decrease in relapse rate following adjuvant tamoxifen compared to untreated controls have been reported by almost all investigators to be related to the presence of estrogen receptor positive and progesterone receptor positive tumors, and was definitely more evident in postmenopausal women (Bonadonna 1986; Bonadonna and Valagussa 1985). It is worth noting, however, that only a minority of studies included premenopausal patients. Significant reduction in mortality was documented in women aged > 50 years (18%, $P < 0.0001$). Overall survival advantage was reported in particular by the Nolvadex Adjuvant Trial Organization (1985) and the Breast Cancer Trials Committee (1987). As a consequence of these recent trial results, adjuvant tamoxifen can now be utilized in postmenopausal women with receptor-positive tumors (Bonadonna and Valagussa 1987).

Combined Chemotherapy and Endocrine Therapy

Present findings do not indicate that the concomitant administration of adjuvant chemotherapy and endocrine therapy has improved the results achieved with either modality alone (Bonadonna and Valagussa 1987). In fact, even the recent 5-year results from the NSABP study showed that improvement in relapse-free survival, if any, was restricted to a minority of patients aged over 50 years and with more than three positive axillary nodes, provided both estrogen and progesterone receptors were highly positive. Therefore, one can argue that this advantage, which was evident 2–3 years after surgery and decreased thereafter, should be ascribed to the combined treatment effect rather than to a maximum therapeutic benefit induced by tamoxifen in a particularly favorable subset.

Stage III Disease

Primary chemotherapy has been tested over the past 10 years in locally advanced breast cancer, inoperable by conventional criteria (T3b–T4 or stage III). Combined treatment was deemed necessary in this stage of the disease, since the prognosis following locoregional therapy alone is very poor (5-year relapse-free survival 5%–10%, overall survival 15%–20%). Most drug regimens utilized included doxorubicin, and primary chemotherapy was delivered for three cycles before radiotherapy and/or surgery. All investigators utilized postoperative systemic cytotoxic therapy with or without hormonal manipulations. The early studies of the combined modality approach were performed in Milan, New York, and Houston. Overall, the following conclusions can be drawn so far: (a) Primary chemotherapy induced a high response rate (65%–88%). (b) The 5-year relapse-free survival rate was improved to 20%–30%, the overall survival rate to 35%–50%. Neither the drug regimen of choice nor the optimal sequence of local and systemic therapy has yet been clearly identified (Bonadonna and Valagussa 1987).

Brain Tumors

The chemotherapy of brain tumors encounters the same difficulties as the chemotherapy of systemic cancer, i.e., lack of therapeutic specificity, presence of heterogeneous cell population leading to primary drug resistance, and excessive toxicity to normal tissue. In addition, chemotherapy must contend with problems related to drug delivery, i.e., low tumor blood flow and the blood-brain barrier.

Malignant Gliomas

Until recently, malignant gliomas, the most common of which is glioblastoma multiforme, were characterized by a rapid fatal course, with 50% mortality within 6 months and 90% mortality within 18 months. This grim picture has improved with the advent of multimodality therapy aimed at reducing tumor burden (Shapiro 1986). While most of the clinical studies carried out over the past 20 years have yielded definitive data, their results have been of limited real value. Therapies tested so far have in fact extended survival only minimally and have offered no major breakthrough. The end points used in randomized studies have included overall survival, time to recurrence or relapse-free survival, and various measurements of the size of the brain tumor itself, including CT scanning and other imaging techniques.

Controlled prospective clinical trials (Shapiro 1986) have yielded the following results:

a) Postoperative irradiation (whole-brain radiotherapy plus a focal tumor boost to a total tumor dose of 6000 rad) significantly prolongs survival. Modifying radiotherapy with the radiation sensitizer misonidazole, or splitting the daily dose into two fractions, does not improve overall survival beyond that achieved with standard radiation.
b) Postoperative chemotherapy with BCNU produces a statistically significant increase in survival; other nitrosourea derivatives (CCNU, methyl-CCNU and streptozocin) were about as effective as BCNU. The number of patients living longer than 18 months is specifically related to the use of adjuvant chemotherapy.
c) High-dose corticosteroids do not in themselves prolong survival.
d) Individual patient prognostic variables (e.g., age, histological grade of tumor, postoperative performance status, extent of tumor removal, possibly tumor location within the brain, certain neurological symptoms and signs at initial presentation) may provide guidelines to the use of available therapeutic modalities.

In conclusion, the management of malignant gliomas in adults and children should be based on the rationale of cytoreduction through multimodality therapy including surgery, irradiation, and chemotherapy. Following maximal surgical resection (which ranges from 20% to 90% of the tumor, depending on its location), patients should receive radiotherapy to a full tumor dose of 6000 rad and about 4500 rad to the remainder of the brain. Adjuvant chemotherapy with one of the nitrosourea derivatives for about 12 months should be administered. With the current empirical approach, median survival can be improved to 12 months or more and 25%–30% of patients survive 18 months or longer. The heterogeneity of gliomas is responsible in part for the development of primary drug resistance, and the blood-brain barrier represents an important but still ill-understood problem in chemotherapy. Therefore, we must learn to use the available drugs better.

Medulloblastoma

While the role of radiation therapy in the treatment of medulloblastoma is now well established, the actual role of chemotherapy is not completely clear, even if the growth characteristics of this highly malignant tumor would suggest good drug responsiveness. Chemotherapy was initially tested as single-agent treatment at first relapse. The agents more frequently selected were vincristine, nitrosourea derivatives, procarbazine, and intrathecal methotrexate. In all instances, some tumor response was observed. However, the impact of chemotherapy was limited in magnitude (partial relief of symptoms) and time (no effect on survival).

To assess the role of chemotherapy in an adjuvant setting, two important randomized trials were started in Europe and the USA in 1975 (Bloom et al. 1983; Evans 1983). The study of the SIOP investigated the use of vincristine and CCNU following surgery and radiotherapy. In patients randomized to receive chemotherapy, vincristine was administered with radiotherapy weekly for nine doses followed by pulses of CCNU and further vincristine every 6 weeks for a total of eight courses. The chemotherapy regimen utilized by members of the Children's Cancer Study Group was similar to that adopted by the SIOP group, except for the addition of prednisone. The results of the American trial failed to indicate a significant benefit from adjuvant chemotherapy in the overall patient population, while the drug regimen administered by SIOP provided a significant but marginal increase in relapse-free survival. In the SIOP study, however, a detailed analysis of patient subsets revealed that adjuvant systemic treatment significantly improved the outcome of children aged less than 2 years. Furthermore, significant improvement was also detected in patients with brainstem involvement, as well as in those in whom radical surgery was not feasible. A similar retrospective analysis carried out on the material of the American study found that chemotherapy improved the survival of patients with more advanced tumors.

Immediately following surgery the blood-brain barrier is disrupted and chemotherapeutic agents penetrate the tumor most effectively at this time. On this basis, a new European study has recently been initiated to evaluate the effectiveness of preirradiation chemotherapy. The results of this sequential approach are not yet fully available; however, available findings indicate that there is no immediate disadvantage in delaying radiation.

Head and Neck Cancer

Squamous Cell Cancer

Squamous cell carcinoma of the head and neck continues to be a problem of local control. Small stage I and stage II carcinomas have a 70% cure rate, whereas the larger primary cancers (T3 and T4), regardless of the site within the aerodigestive tract, are more difficult to eradicate by locoregional measures. The primary site of failure following surgical and/or radiotherapeutic treatment is most often local; 70% of relapses manifest only primary site or nodal failure.

Squamous cell carcinoma of head and neck is a chemoresponsive tumor to a number of anticancer drugs, in particular methotrexate, hydroxyurea, cisplatin, fluorouracil, and bleomycin. With single-agent chemotherapy, complete and partial response ranges from 20% to 40%; with various combination regimens in previously untreated patients the total response rate is increased to 70%–85% (complete remission in 25%–50%). Although several combinations are active, no combination has yet been clearly identified as the best. However, cisplatin-containing regimens, particularly cisplatin and fluorouracil infusion (Wagener et al. 1985), were reported to be associated to a high complete remission rate. Over the years it has become increasingly evident that chemotherapy given after surgery and irradiation is poorly tolerated, producing severe local toxicity. More importantly, about half the patients refuse adjuvant treatment because of toxicity and disability induced by surgery and/or irradiation. More recently, two general treatment approaches have emerged: (a) induction chemotherapy to maximal response, followed by local treatment; (b) synchronous definitive irradiation and chemotherapy, with surgery for selected cases or at time of local relapse.

Despite the general strategic similarity, differences in the number of induction chemotherapy courses, stage, resectability rates, radiation doses, and criteria for surgery make general summary statements impossible. Patients achieving complete pathological response with multiple-drug treatment courses or with synchronous chemotherapy and radiotherapy have a high probability of local control and overall survival (60%–70% at 3 years) after maximal local treatment. Conversely, patients not responding to induction chemotherapy alone fare poorly (3-year survival $\leq$ 30%) regardless of subsequent local treatment. With modern drug regimens, various clinical parameters (histological subtype, performance status, and primary tumor site) have not been significant variables affecting response to induction combination chemotherapy.

Future chemotherapy studies will focus on attaining pathological complete remission as their end points, and the optimal number of courses will be that achieving a complete response. Surgery and/or definitive radiotherapy is still essential for local control and survival. In spite of present encouraging results, the question of whether induction or synchronous chemotherapy improves the cure rate of squamous cell head and neck cancer remains unanswered (Taylor et al. 1985).

Nasopharyngeal Cancer

Results on multidisciplinary treatment including combination chemotherapy are still scanty for nasopharyngeal cancer. The recent results of a multicenter controlled trial performed in Italy are worth mentioning, partly because the study includes a large number of previously untreated patients (229 cases). Following radiotherapy of the nasopharynx, the base of the skull, and both cervical regions, patients achieving locoregional complete remission were prospectively randomized to receive either no further therapy or six monthly cycles of chemotherapy with VAC. At 44 months no significant difference was observed in relapse-free and overall survival rates between controls and chemotherapy-treated patients (Rossi et al. 1986). Most probably a more intensive form of chemotherapy is required to affect the treatment outcome.

Gastrointestinal Tumors

Esophageal Cancer

Esophageal cancer remains a highly virulent disease with a poor prognosis. Long-term survival statistics have shown no significant improvement over the last 15–20 years; currently only 5%–10% of all patients will be alive 5 years from their date of diagnosis. Several autopsy studies have demonstrated that, in symptomatic patients, epidermoid carcinomas of the esophagus are already widely disseminated at the time of diagnosis. In view of the systemic nature of the tumor, effective chemotherapy should, in theory at least, play a major role in the primary management of this neoplasm.

Bleomycin, cisplatin, vindesine, and mitomycin are the best-studied drugs, but all have no more than modest to moderate activity, with response rates in the 10%–20% range and a median response duration of 2.5–5 months. Several combination regimens have been recently tested with stringent criteria for drug response. For those patients treated preoperatively, a complete remission means that no viable tumor was found in any site sampled, including the esophageal specimens, lymph nodes and visceral organs (Kelsen 1984). Response rate with multidrug regimens range from 15%–25% for cisplatin-bleomycin to 35%–80% for other platinum-containing combinations.

Combined modality approaches for patients with locoregional disease are now under study. Several preliminary trials from a number of centers indicate that preoperative chemotherapy can be given safely with no increase in operative morbidity and mortality. In the pilot trials at Memorial Hospital (Kelsen 1984), for example, resection rates were 72% and 82% in the cisplatin-bleomycin and cisplatin-vindesine-bleomycin (DVB) studies respectively. For DVB the median duration of survival was 16 months, which appears to be significantly better than in the historical control group receiving cisplatin-bleomycin. Similarly promising results were achieved at the Wayne State University with preoperative fluorouracil plus cisplatin and radiation (Kelsen 1984). Although these encouraging early results appear to change the natural history of esophageal cancer, prospective clinical trials of primary chemotherapy plus radiotherapy (with or without subsequent surgery), as well as new drug trials, are required to better define the optimal drug regimen and schedule (Wagener et al. 1985).

Gastric Cancer

Approximately 40% of gastric cancers are resectable at diagnosis, but most of these have extensively spread within the stomach, through the stomach wall, or to regional lymph nodes. Even when patients undergo "curative" surgery about 50% die within 2 years of operation and the 5-year survival is less than 20%.

The first adjuvant treatments in gastric adenocarcinoma resected en bloc for possible cure were initiated more than two decades ago. Altogether, the results of the initial form of chemotherapy, the postoperative administration of fluorouracil alone, were at best inconclusive. Often the trial design was defective and failed to properly balance important prognostic subsets, such as lymph node status (negative vs positive), depth of tumor invasion (tumor confined to mucosa vs penetrating wall to serosa vs penetrating serosa to adjacent tissue), and location of primary tumor (cardia vs elsewhere in the stomach). Essentially, all dose regimens of fluorouracil were considered to have no significant effect on 5-year relapse-free and overall survival (Schein and Sherlock 1985).

In recent years, several cooperative research groups have tested the efficacy of postoperative combination chemotherapy through randomized and properly stratified studies. The most important combination regimens tested were fluorouracil plus methyl-CCNU and FAM (fluorouracil, doxorubicin, mitomycin). Each of these combinations was found to produce an objective response rate of about 40% in advanced cancer. The Eastern Cooperative Oncology Group (ECOG) failed to confirm the findings of the Gastrointenstinal Tumor Study Group (GITSG) with fluorouracil plus methyl-CCNU: the GITSG (Douglass and Stablein 1983) reported a significant median survival adavantage for the adjuvant therapy group (control 33 months, chemotherapy 48+ months, $P = 0.03$). The ECOG (Engstrom et al. 1985) observed no clinically meaningful relapse-free and overall survival advantage for patients with limited disease, nodal disease, or partial gastrectomy. The overall findings, i.e., absence of clinical beneficial effect, are in line with those reported by the Veterans Administration study (Higgins et al. 1985). Thus, fluorouracil plus methyl-CCNU is not currently recommended as routine adjuvant therapy for resected gastric cancer, also because of possible life-threatening toxicity, including acute non-lymphocytic leukemia (Boice et al. 1983). At present there is no clear evidence that adjuvant FAM has improved overall survival.

Colorectal Cancer

With the exception of early low rectal tumors, which can sometimes be controlled by radiotherapy, surgical resection remains the only curative treatment for colorectal cancer. However, patients with transmural extension of tumor and metastases to regional lymph nodes have a 10-year survival rate of only 15%–25% when treated by resection alone. Thus, surgical staging constitutes an accurate prognostic factor in colorectal cancer.

Members of the GITSG (1984) have recently published the results of randomized trials in colon cancer and in rectal cancer. In both these studies the Dukes staging classification proved to be the major determinant of recurrence rate, with Dukes B2 tumors (penetration to serosa but no lymph node invasion) having a recurrence rate of only 20% at 5 years, considerably lower than in historical series. On the other hand, neither adjuvant immunotherapy (MER), chemotherapy (methyl-CCNU plus fluorouracil), nor both combined proved to the beneficial. With rectal cancer the trial involved the use of postoperative radiation alone, the above chemotherapy, and the combination of both, all compared with observation alone. Again, as expected, recurrence rates paralleled the Dukes classification. The rate of recurrence over 5 years was least in the combined treatment, both local and distal recurrences occurring less frequently. Radiation exerted an effect on local recurrences. None of the treatment groups had a significant advantage in overall survival, though this may also be related to the size of the trial (only 200 evaluable patients and four separate arms to be compared). More recently, the NSABP group in the United States, utilizing adjuvant methyl-CCNU, vincristine, and fluorouracil (MOF) chemotherapy has demonstrated a significant improvement in disease-free and overall survival for both colon (Wolmark et al. 1988) and rectal cancer (Fisher et al. 1988). Also in the NSABP experience, postoperative radiation therapy reduced the incidence of locoregional recurrence in rectal cancer, but it failed to affect disease-free and overall survival rates. Nevertheless, future directions in colon cancer adjuvant therapy still depend on the demonstration of an advantage over observation alone. In formulating treatment policy for these patients, one must recognize that markers and diagnostic approaches to detect early recurrences are available and that current chemotherapies are of limited usefulness. In rectal cancer, radiotherapy has a demonstrable effect on local recurrences, and other drug combinations with systemic therapy must be evaluated.

Pancreatic Cancer

In pancreatic cancer, chemotherapy has limited efficacy, thus precluding the routine use of adjuvant treatment. Nevertheless, studies by the GITSG support the use of postoperative fluorouracil plus local radiation in patients with resectable cancer of the pancreas. More aggressive chemotherapeutic regimens are being tested, but unfortunately pancreatic cancer is seldom resectable and many years will be required to confirm their efficacy.

Lung Cancer

Surgical adjuvant treatment must be considered primarily for histologies other than small cell. Few patients with small cell carcinoma are operated on, and those in whom the disease is diagnosed at surgery receive chemotherapy as if they had disseminated disease. Studies in the past, even utilizing single-agent therapy, have indicated the soundness of this approach; significant decreases in recurrence rates were observed among patients treated with cyclophosphamide.

In other histologies grouped under the term non-small cell lung cancer, systemic adjuvant therapy has a record of claims of benefit followed by disappointments. In general, it has been unrewarding, and was even deleterious to survival in two early randomized trials employing cyclophosphamide and CCNU respectively. Subsequent to this disappointing experience, studies turned to evaluation of immunotherapy, and encouraging results were reported with levamisole, intrapleural BCG, or tumor vaccines with or without chemotherapy. Unfortunately, none of the initial reports have been confirmed.

Recent controlled trials have focused on more precise definition of staging, utilizing the TNM classification and sophisticated diagnostic procedures. It is apparent that patients with early squamous cancer have better survival than was previously believed. In fact, 5-year survival rates of 85% for T1 N0 patients and 55% for T1 N1 and T2 N0 patients have been reported. Accordingly, T1 N0 patients are excluded from adjuvant therapy programs. In regional node-positive disease, radiotherapy is regarded by many clinicians as being required, particularly if mediastinal lymph nodes are involved, and obviously if residual disease is present. These two latter groups of patients have, however, a high propensity for systemic recurrences, and therefore the effect of local therapy may be difficult to demonstrate. Chemotherapy based on cisplatin plus vinca alkaloids (etoposide or vinblastine) and occasionally additional drugs appears to have an advantage over other regimens. In fact, a recent study by the Lung Cancer Study Group (Holmes et al. 1984) utilizing a combination of cyclophosphamide, doxorubicin, and cisplatin documented a survival advantage for patients with large tumors or with nodal involvement after resection (stage II M0 and stage III M0) who have adenocarcinoma or large cell carcinoma.

In conclusion, there are persuasive arguments for beginning treatment of stage II–III lesions with systemic chemotherapy. Most probably, at present, we have no effective systemic treatment for non-small cell lung cancer. However, new prospective randomized trials should be designed to determine whether more intensive adjuvant treatments will be able to improve the overall survival in properly selected subsets of patients. New multidisciplinary approaches should also include combination chemotherapy prior to radiotherapy and surgery in patients with marginally resectable cancer (Wagener et al. 1985; Ragaz et al. 1986).

Urological Malignancies

Testicular Cancer

The most exciting development in effective chemotherapy for testicular malignancies has been the introduction of cisplatin. Data on patients with advanced (stage III) metastatic testicular cancer of the nonseminomatous type indicates a significant improvement in survival since 1977. The proportion of patients presenting in the earlier stages who achieve long-term relapse-free survival has exceeded 80% in the past decade, but additional strides have been verified recently with the systematic application of rigorous follow-up techniques and either adjuvant or early salvage chemotherapy with cisplatin-containing regimens. Studies have been ongoing to determine which of these two approaches may be more advantageous. Nevertheless, it is clear that cisplatin-bleomycin-vinblastine (PVB) given for two courses in patients with positive lymph nodes (stage II) documented at retroperitoneal lymphadenectomy is nearly 100% effective in preventing subsequent development of metastases (Weiss et al. 1986). Metastases do occur in about 50% of patients subjected only to rigorous postoperative follow-up, with the lung being the predominant site. Monthly chest X-rays and serum tumor markers such as alpha-fetoprotein, the beta subunit of human chorionic gonadotropin and lactic dehydrogenase are advised during the first 2 years of follow-up. Relapses following treatment would be expected to occur mostly within the 1st year, and in less than 1% of cases during the 2nd year if there is no residual disease detectable. The toxicity of delayed (salvage) intensive chemotherapy is expected to be more severe than that of short-term adjuvant chemotherapy (Weiss et al. 1986). Less than 15% of stage I patients (disease confined to testis) may be expected to relapse if all are subjected to retroperitoneal lymphadenectomy and close follow-up. Early detection of recurrences could be anticipated to salvage these patients. Such an approach would presumably be safe and spare more than 80% of these stage I patients the toxic effects of adjuvant chemotherapy.

Bladder Carcinoma

Chemotherapy of bladder carcinoma has only recently been recognized as achieving significant tumor responses. Thus, the pessimism concerning this form of treatment appears unwarranted. There is preliminary evidence that the earlier introduction of chemotherapy in the treatment of bladder carcinoma, without compromising the drug doses, can result in a survival benefit. It has yet to be determined whether chemotherapy can be used in place of radiotherapy in a preoperative setting or replace surgery in patients with locally invasive disease. If the latter is true, patients may in future be spared the debilitating effects on sexual function and the need for urinary diversion. Properly designed controlled studies should establish whether the effects of chemotherapy merely delay the eventual relapse or result in an increased cure fraction.

Gynecological Malignancies

Ovarian Cancer

Of all malignancies, ovarian cancer presents most frequently in advanced stages. Examination of almost all recent studies utilizing cisplatin-containing regimens reveals that a high rate of pathological complete remission occurs predominantly in patients with minimal residual disease (tumor nodules <2 cm) after staging laparotomy. In this group of patients, which represents less than 30% of all those with advanced ovarian cancer, long-term survival, even cure, seems probable for approximately 40%–70% of those obtaining pathological complete remission with current combination chemotherapy. In patients with bulky disease after laparotomy, pathological complete remission (tumor nodules >2 cm) drops sharply to 10%–20%. As this latter group represents the majority of ovarian cancer patients, it is understandable why the overall 5-year survival rates ($\leq 40\%$) have changed minimally in this disease during the past few years (Young 1984).

Prospective randomized trials with pretreatment surgical staging in women with stage I or II completely resectable disease have not revealed an advantage for abdominopelvic radiation or for intraperitoneal radiocolloids vs single-agent chemotherapy (Young 1984). Furthermore, survival in these carefully staged patients is excellent, varying from 80% to

90% at 2 years with surgery alone, rendering the study of possible benefits of adjuvant treatment quite difficult. Lacking definitive trials, physicians faced with the infrequently presenting early-stage ovarian cancer must use prognostic factors to guide them in deciding on postsurgical therapy. Patients with risk factors such as high grade, dense tumor adherences at surgery, and positive peritoneal cytology should receive adjuvant chemotherapy with one of the cisplatin-containing combinations for six cycles in a randomized treatment protocol comparing radiotherapy to chemotherapy. In the absence of such studies, therapeutic decisions between chemotherapy and radiotherapy should be based on individual and institutional experience with these methods.

Cancer of Cervix and Endometrium

Cervical cancer studies await further definition of the antitumor efficacy and tolerance of cisplatin-containing regimens when combined with radiation in stage II and III. Prospective randomized trials are ongoing. Patients with adenocarcinoma of the endometrium whose risk is assessed by clinical and pathological variables would be suitable targets for adjuvant therapy including hormones (e.g., progestins) and chemotherapy (e.g., doxorubicin). However, sufficient information is not currently available to support their use. Moreover, patients who respond to progestins are likely to be those with well-differentiated tumors, which would be least likely to recur. In fact, a trial of progestins in patients with stage I yielded no improvement in results; however, the findings indicated an overall relapse rate of less than 10%, suggesting that these favorable patients do not need any adjuvant therapy.

Malignant Lymphomas

Non-Hodgkin's Lymphomas

In lymphomas of adult patients, where stages I and II were conventionally treated with radiation therapy, the relapse-free survival at 5 years varied from 40% to 70% in the presence of clearly localized lesions and from 25% to 35% in patients with regional involvement. Refinements in staging indicated that one could detect patients destined to fail by virtue of unsuspected sites of involvement through use of lymphangiography, bone marrow biopsies, laparoscopy, laparotomy, and systematic staging procedures. Newer strategies employing chemotherapy routinely have minimized the importance of staging laparotomies. Recent studies performed at the Milan Cancer Institute (Monfardini et al. 1980) established the superiority of combined therapy with cyclophosphamide-vincristine-prednisone (CVP) and radiation over radiation alone for stages I and II non-Hodgkin's lymphoma of adult patients in terms of relapse-free survival and overall survival for both stages. More recently, the same investigators (Bajetta et al. 1988) have demonstrated a significant difference in favor of a doxorubicin-containing regimen (BACOP) over CVP, when combined with radiation, in terms of 5-year freedom from progression (BACOP 78%, CVP 62%, $P=0.02$) and total survival (BACOP 85%, CVP 73%, $P<0.07$).

The need for local radiation may be questioned in the early stages, particularly in view of very favorable results obtained with chemotherapy alone by investigators in the USA utilizing modern intensive combination regimens (Bonadonna and Valagune 1989). However, relapses on the combined treatment described above seldom occur (<10%) in the irradiated area. Since morbidity of radiation in some anatomical sites is minimal, continued use of this modality may be advisable until additional long-term information is available on regimens using chemotherapy alone.

Hodgkin's Disease

Results in Hodgkin's disease with modern irradiation alone are excellent in pathological stages I and II A. Beyond these stages, integration of chemotherapy with radiation requires long-term studies, and in some instances comparison with chemotherapy alone. Short-term results from such studies may be deceptive in Hodgkin's disease. In fact, relapse-free survival advantage may not be reflected in overall survival advantage, since salvage chemotherapy is quite successful in radiation relapses. Moreover, there has been increased concern with long-term sequelae of combined treatments (see section "Long-Term Toxicity" below).

Table 5 summarizes the results of the Stanford adjuvant studies [radiotherapy vs radiotherapy followed by six cycles of mechlorethamine, vincristine, procarbazine, and prednisone (MOPP) chemotherapy] in terms of overall survival, freedom from first relapse, and freedom from second relapse. It can be seen that the survival rates and differences more closely correlate with and parallel the rate of freedom from second relapse than the rate of freedom from first relapse (Rosenberg and Kaplan 1985). At the Milan Cancer Institute a prospectively randomized study comparing MOPP and doxorubicin, bleo-

Table 5. Results of Stanford randomized trials for Hodgkin's disease

Pathologic stage	Treatment	No. of patients	FFP %	OS %	FF_2R %
IA, IIA	RT	39	65	79	83
	RT+MOPP	39	85	80	92
IB, IIB	RT	28	73	79	88
	RT+MOPP	35	76	78	88
IIIA	RT	35	70	68	78
	RT+MOPP	24	86	92	95
IIIB	RT	23	8	28	41
	RT+MOPP	23	51	52	60

Modified from Rosenberg and Kaplan 1985
FFP, freedom from first progression; OS, overall survival; FF_2R, freedom from second progression; RT, radiotherapy; MOPP, mechlorethamine, vincristine, procarbazine, prednisone.

mycin, vinblastine and dacarbazine (ABVD) (three cycles of either regimen preceding and following extensive irradiation) in adult patients was activated in 1974. The overall results indicate that at 7 years from starting combined therapy ABVD-treated patients fared significantly better than patients given MOPP in terms of complete remission (92% vs 81%, $P<0.02$), freedom from first progression (81% vs 63%, $P<0.002$), relapse-free survival (88% vs 77%, $P=0.06$), and total survival (77% vs 68%, $P=0.03$). Moreover, analysis of iatrogenic morbidity showed that irreversible gonadal dysfunction, as well as acute leukemia, occurred only in patients subjected to MOPP, while cardiopulmonary studies failed to document significant laboratory differences between the two treatment groups (Santoro et al. 1987).

In children, treatment approaches for early and intermediate stages of Hodgkin's disease vary from center to center. Staging laparotomy is still used to limit the aggressiveness of treatment (chemotherapy or radiotherapy or both). To reduce growth impairment and late sequelae of radiation, as well as morbidity from laparotomy, current trends favor an integrated approach, with intensive chemotherapy followed by limited-field low-dose radiation, especially for prepubertal children. Present results following multidisciplinary treatment are excellent, with a cure rate of over 90% in children with early and intermediate stages of disease. Current investigations are aimed at refining combined therapy on the basis of prognostic characteristics of individual patients and the risk that sequelae will occur.

Malignant Melanoma

Melanoma is potentially a very important target for adjuvant systemic therapy. The thickness of the tumor and the status of regional lymph nodes are powerful determinants of recurrence. The patterns and frequency of recurrence also vary with site of disease, sex, and age. These prognostic factors are being increasingly delineated and should be utilized in clinical trials. Immunological modalities such as vaccines and BCG, differentiating agents such as retinoids, and biological response modifiers such as interferons and inducers have been tested clinically to prevent recurrences. Favorable results in small trials were not confirmed on more widespread testing. This was the case with single-agent chemotherapy with dacarbazine (Veronesi et al. 1982) and nitrosoureas. Since the efficacy of all drugs in melanoma has been limited to about 20% of patients, it is possible that combination chemotherapy will also be unable to significantly improve overall survival. Therefore, no one adjuvant modality can be recommended in melanoma and clinical trials including control populations should be carried out.

Long-term Toxicity

Many more patients than ever before now receive cytotoxic chemotherapy, with or without irradiation, and many more individuals, both children and adults, are cured of their tumors and survive to experience the potential late adverse effects of treatment. Two significant problems have emerged: second malignancies and gonadal dysfunctions. In addition, in children there is a spectrum of potential iatrogenic long-term effects relating to growth and development, thyroid function, and neuropsychological function.

Second Malignancies

The widely utilized alkylating agents are known to exert carcinogenic activity in animals as well as in humans. Innumerable reports have been published in the medical literature relative to an increased risk of second malignancies, especially acute leukemias, following treatment with chemotherapy, with or without irradiation, for both malignant lymphomas and solid tumors. So far, most attention has been focused on adults, especially on those with Hodgkin's disease, for whom a dramatic improvement in overall survival has been achieved. Acute nonlymphocytic leukemias (ANLL) were the most common second malignancies, with an actuarial risk ranging between 2.5% and 6.5% within 10 years from starting treatment. When intensive irradiation is delivered with

MOPP or MOPP-like regimens, the risk of ANLL can be as high as 10% within 10 years, while only one case of ANLL following treatment with irradiation and ABVD has been documented so far (Valagussa et al. 1988). More recently, also non-Hodgkin's lymphomas and a variety of solid tumors (sarcomas, lung cancer, etc.) have been documented after treatment for Hodgkin's disease. However, the exact role of treatment in inducing these second cancers remains to be fully assessed. An increasing number of reports dealing with the occurrence of new cancers, especially ANLL, following treatment with alkylating agents for ovarian carcinoma, non-Hodgkin's lymphomas, and small-cell lung cancer have been published in the medical literature (Valagussa et al. 1986). More recently, second malignancies in patients treated with nitrosourea derivatives for gastrointestinal cancer (Boice et al. 1983) and for malignant glioma have been documented.

Despite the publication of some reports, the role of adjuvant systemic chemotherapy for operable breast cancer in inducing second malignancies is still controversial. The NSABP has recently published a report on the risk of ANLL in a series of 8483 women with breast cancer treated in seven different clinical trials activated since 1971. Following adjuvant chemotherapy with melphalan-containing regimens the risk for ANLL was 1.3% at 10 years, as compared to 0.06% following surgery alone and 1.4% following postoperative irradiation (Fisher et al. 1985). No cases of ANLL have yet been observed in a series of 666 patients treated with adjuvant CMF at the Milan Cancer Institute between 1973 and 1978. In this series of patients, the risk for second solid tumors within 10 years was 4.2% as compared to 4.0% in 179 women subjected to radical mastectomy alone. Median latency periods, type of second cancers, and survival from second malignancies did not differ between the two series of patients (Bonadonna and Valagussa 1987; Valagussa et al. 1987). This observation would further suggest that second tumors documented so far cannot be entirely ascribed to treatment with adjuvant chemotherapy.

The Late Effects Study Group (Meadows et al. 1985) has recently published a report on 292 cases of second malignant neoplasms occurring in individuals who were diagnosed with their first neoplasm in childhood. Bone sarcomas were the most common second malignant tumors developing in previously irradiated sites, while acute leukemia was the most common second neoplasm unassociated with radiation.

From the data reported above, it appears evident that active prolonged follow-up is necessary to accurately determine the risk of second malignancies. Efforts should be made to better identify subsets of patients for whom cytotoxic treatments really result in a survival gain, to modify therapeutic strategies, and to design intervention programs in the attempt to prevent or minimize these unpleasant long-term sequelae. However, it should also be recognized that in the assessment of the carcinogenic activity of anticancer drugs many problems remain unsolved. In fact, the consequences of the administration of cytotoxic agents in combination and/or together with other drugs, including the possibility of metabolic interactions, as well as the combination of chemotherapy and radiotherapy and individual factors such as genetic disposition and lifestyle, are mostly not stated.

Treatment-Related Infertility

Neoplastic disease and its treatment can potentially interfere with any of the cellular, anatomic, physiological or behavioral processes that comprise normal sexual and reproductive function. Many drugs used in the treatment of malignant disease have profound and often lasting effects in the testis and ovary. Germ cell production and endocrine function may both be altered with the magnitude of the effects related to the age, pubertal status and menstrual status of the patient, as well as to the particular drug, dosage, or combination administered.

Testicular function can be adequately evaluated with a careful physical examination, semen analysis, and determination of serum gonadotropin and testosterone levels. The primary testicular lesion caused by all anticancer agents studied thus far is depletion of the germinal epithelium lining the seminiferous tubules. Alkylating agents deplete the testicular germinal epithelium in a dose-related fashion, while high-dose methotrexate may produce transient oligospermia, or maturation arrest of the spermatocyte stage of development. At least 80% of men receiving MOPP or MOPP-like regimens developed azoospermia, testicular atrophy, and elevated FSH levels, and several recent studies suggest that only about 10% of these patients will ultimately have a return of spermatogenesis (Chapman et al. 1981). By contrast, ABVD and other doxorubicin-containing regimens have been shown to produce transient testicular injury (Santoro et al. 1986). Cisplatin, vinblastine, and bleomycin therapy for testicular cancer is also associated with a high degree of reversibility of testicular dysfunction, with the majority of patients showing evidence of resumption of spermatogenesis within 2 years of discontinuation of treatment.

Unlike the sperm count, no direct measurement of the female germ cell population is readily available. Thus, evaluation of the functional status of the ovary must be based primarily on menstrual and reproductive history and on determination of serum hormone levels. Drug-induced ovarian failure results in abnormally low serum levels of estradiol and progesterone, markedly elevated levels of FSH and LH, amenorrhea, and symptoms of estrogen deficiency. Recent studies of patients receiving regimens containing alkylating agents suggest that the onset of amenorrhea and the potential for resumption of menses is related to the age of the patient during chemotherapy and the total dose administered. The frequency of amenorrhea in women over 40 years of age may be as high as 90%, and resumption of menses have been observed in only about 10% of these patients. In women younger than 40, the frequency of amenorrhea ranges from 40% to 60%, and resumption of menses can be observed in 40%–50% of these women (Schilsky et al. 1981).

Though many antineoplastic drugs are teratogenic, particularly during the first trimester of pregnancy, the information available at present suggests that the incidence of spontaneous abortion or fetal abnormalities is no greater in patients previously treated with chemotherapy than in the general population. However, more careful studies with prolonged periods of observation are required before the true risks to subsequent generations will be known.

Conclusion

This review has attempted to capture only the highlights of the application of modern adjuvant treatments. Certain principles are repetitive, the two main such being the identification of patients at high risk of recurrences, through the study of prognostic variables, and the administration of an adjuvant therapy which is not only safe but of proven efficacy in more advanced stages of disease. One can expect continuous evolution of these principles as knowledge is gained from progress in diagnostic and therapeutic clinical science. A prospective clinical trial is one of the best ways of accumulating such knowledge, and the adjuvant as well as neoadjuvant situation represents the optimal opportunity to obtain the most complete data on a disease and on our therapeutic impact on its course.

References

Bajetta E, Valagussa P, Bonadonna G et al. (1988) Combined modality treatment for stage I–II non-Hodgkin's lymphomas: CVP versus BACOP chemotherapy. Int J Radiat Oncol Biol Phys 15: 3–12

Bloom HJG, Thornoton Jones H (1983) Adjuvant chemotherapy for medulloblastoma: the multicenter controlled trial of the International Society of Pediatric Oncology. Proceedings XIII International Congress of Chemotherapy, Vienna, August 28–September 2

Boice JD Jr, Greene MH, Killen JY Jr et al. (1983) Leukemia and preleukemia after adjuvant treatment of gastrointestinal cancer with semustine (methyl-CCNU). N Engl J Med 309: 1079–1084

Bonadonna G (guest ed) (1986) Breast cancer. Semin Oncol 13: 383–449

Bonadonna G, Valagussa P (1989) Influence of clinical trials on current treatment strategy for malignant lymphomas. J Clin Oncol (in press)

Bonadonna G, Valagussa P (1985) Adjuvant systemic therapy for resectable breast cancer. J Clin Oncol 3: 259–275

Bonadonna G, Valagussa P (1987) Current status of adjuvant chemotherapy for breast cancer. Semin Oncol 14: 8–22

Bonadonna G, Valagussa P (1988) The contribution of medicine to the primary treatment of breast cancer. Cancer Res 48: 2314–2324

Bonadonna G, Valagussa P (1989) Role of chemotherapy in stage I breast cancer. In: De Vita VT, Hellman S, Rosenberg SA (eds) Important advances in oncology 1989. Lippincot, Philadelphia

Bonadonna G, Valagussa P, Rossi A et al. (1985) Ten-year experience with CMF-based adjuvant chemotherapy in resectable breast cancer. Breast Cancer Res Treat 5: 95–115

Breast Cancer Trials Committee (1987) Adjuvant tamoxifen in the management of operable breast cancer: the Scottish trial. Lancet 2: 171–175

Chapman RM, Sutcliffe SB, Malpas JS (1981) Male gonadal dysfunction in Hodgkin's disease. JAMA 245: 1323–1328

D'Angio GJ (1985) Clinical trials in Wilms' tumor. In: Veronesi U, Bonadonna G (eds) Clinical trials in cancer medicine: past achievements and future prospects. Bristol Myers Symposia, vol 6. Academic, Orlando, pp 539–546

Donaldson SS (1985) The value of adjuvant chemotherapy in the management of sarcomas in children. Cancer 55: 2184–2197

Douglass HO Jr, Stablein DM (1983) Controlled trial of adjuvant chemotherapy following curative resection for gastric cancer. Cancer 49: 1116–1122

Edmonson JH, Green SJ, Ivins JC et al. (1984) A controlled pilot study of high-dose methotrexate as postsurgical adjuvant treatment for primary osteosarcoma. J Clin Oncol 2: 152–156

Engstrom PF, Lavin PT, Douglass HO et al. (1985) Postoperative adjuvant 5-fluorouracil plus methyl-CCNU therapy for gastric cancer. Cancer 55: 1868–1873

Evans AE (1983) Therapeutic approaches to medulloblastoma and results. The trial of the Children Cancer Study Group (CCSG) and Radiation Therapy Oncology Group (RTOG). Proceedings XIII International Congress of Chemotherapy, Vienna, August 28–September 2

Fisher B, Rockette H, Fisher ER et al. (1985) Leukemia in breast cancer patients following adjuvant chemotherapy or postoperative radiotherapy: the NSABP experience. J Clin Oncol 3: 1640–1658

Fisher B, Wolmark N, Rockette H et al. (1988) Postoperative adjuvant chemotherapy or radiation therapy for rectal cancer: result from NSABP Protocol R-01. J Natl Cancer Inst 80: 21–29

Frei E III (1985) Curative cancer chemotherapy. Cancer Res 45: 6523–6537

Gastrointestinal Tumor Study Group (GITSG) (1984) Adjuvant therapy of colon cancer: results of a prospective randomized trial. N Engl J Med 310: 737–743

Goldie JH, Coldman AJ (1985) Genetic instability in the development of drug resistance. Semin Oncol 12: 222–230

Goorin AM, Abelson HT, Frei E III (1985) Osteosarcoma: fifteen years later. N Engl J Med 313: 1637–1643

Higgins GA, Amadeo JH, Smith DE et al. (1985) Efficacy of prolonged intermittent therapy with combined 5-FU and methyl-CCNU following resection for gastric carcinoma. Cancer 52: 1105–1112

Holmes EC, Eagan RT and the Lung Cancer Study Group (1984) Surgical adjuvant therapy for resectable stage II/III adenocarcinoma and large cell undifferentiated carcinoma of the lung. Proc Am Soc Clin Oncol 3: 220

Kelsen D (guest ed) (1984) Esophageal cancer. Semin Oncol 11: 1–201

Martin DS, Fugman RA, Stolfi RL et al. (1975) Solid tumor animal model therapeutically predictive for human breast cancer. Cancer Chemother Rep 5: 89–109

Maurer H, Foulkes M, Gehan E (1983) Intergroup Rhabdomyosarcoma Study (IRS) II: preliminary report. Proc Am Soc Clin Oncol 2: 70

Meadows AT, Baum E, Fossati-Bellani F et al. (1985) Second malignant neoplasms in children: an update from the Late Effects Study Group. J Clin Oncol 3: 532–538

Monfardini S, Banfi A, Bonadonna G et al. (1980) Improved 5-year survival after combined radiotherapy-chemotherapy for stage I–II non-Hodgkin's lymphomas. Int J Radiat Oncol Biol Phys 6: 125–134

Morris Jones PH, Pearson D, Johnson AJ (1978) Medical Research Council: managment of nephroblastoma in childhood. Arch Dis Child 53: 112–119

National Institutes of Health (1985) Proceedings of the Consensus Development Conference in limb-sparing treatment of adult soft tissue sarcomas and osteosarcomas. Cancer Treat Symp 3: 1–159

Noladex Adjuvant Trial Organization (1985) Controlled trial of tamoxifen as single adjuvant agent in management of early breast cancer. Analysis at six years. Lancet 1: 836–840

Norton L (1985) Implication of kinetic heterogeneity in clinical oncology. Semin Oncol 12: 231–249

Perez CA, Tafft M, Nesbit E et al. (1981) The role of radiation therapy in the management of nonmetastatic Ewing sarcoma of bone: report of the Intergroup Ewing's Sarcoma Study. Int J Radiat Oncol Biol Phys 7: 141–149

Ragaz J, Band PR, Goldie JH (eds) (1986) Preoperative (neoadjuvant) chemotherapy. Springer, Berlin Heidelberg New York Tokyo

Rosen G, Marcove RC, Huvos AG et al. (1983) Primary osteogenic sarcoma: eight-year experience with adjuvant chemotherapy. J Cancer Res Clin Oncol [Suppl] 106: 55–67

Rosenberg SA, Kaplan HS (1985) The evolution and summary results of the Stanford randomized clinical trials of the management of Hodgkin's disease: 1962–1984. Int J Radiat Oncol Biol Phys 11: 5–22

Rossi A, Molinari R, Marubini E et al. (1986) Adjuvant chemotherapy after complete response of radiotherapy in nasopharyngeal cancer: follow-up of a randomized study. Proc Am Soc Clin Oncol 5: 147

Santoro A, Bonadonna G, Valagussa P et al. (1987) Long-term results of combined chemotherapy-radiotherapy approach in Hodgkin's disease. Superiority of ABVD plus radiotherapy versus MOPP plus radiotherapy. J Clin Oncol 5: 27–37

Schein PS, Sherlock P (guest eds) (1985) Gastric cancer. Semin Oncol 12: 1–53

Schilsky RL (guest ed) (1985) Tumor cell heterogeneity. Semin Oncol 12: 201–353

Schilsky RL, Sherins RJ, Hubbard SM et al. (1981) Long-term follow-up of ovarian function in women treated with MOPP chemotherapy for Hodgkin's disease. Am J Med 71: 552–556

Shapiro WL (guest ed) (1986) Brain tumors. Semin Oncol 13: 1–122

Skipper HE, Schabel FM JR (1984) Tumor stem cell heterogeneity: implication with respect to classification of cancers by chemotherapeutic effect. Cancer Treat Rep 68: 43–61

Taylor SG IV, Applebaum E, Showell JL et al. (1985) A randomized trial of adjuvant chemotherapy in head and neck cancer. J Clin Oncol 3: 672–679

Valagussa P, Santoro A, Fossati-Bellani F et al. (1986) Second acute leukemia and other malignancies following treatment for Hodgkin's disease. J Clin Oncol 4: 830–837

Valagussa P, Tancini G, Bonadonna G (1987) Second malignancies after CMF for resectable breast cancer. J Clin Oncol 5: 1138–1142

Valagussa P, Santoro A, Fossati-Bellani F et al. (1988) Hodgkin's disease and second malignancies. Proc Am Soc Clin Oncol 7: 227

Veronesi U, Adamus J, Aubert C et al. (1982) A randomized trial of adjuvant chemotherapy and immunotherapy in cutaneous melanoma. N Engl J Med 307: 913–916

Wagener DJT, Blijham GH, Smeets JBE et al. (eds) (1985) Primary chemotherapy in cancer medicine. Liss, New York

Weiss RB, Stablein DM, Muggia FM et al. (1986) Toxicity of chemotherapy as adjuvant or salvage treatment in early stage nonseminomatous testicular cancer. Proc Am Soc Clin Oncol 5: 99

Wolmark N, Fisher B, Rockette H et al. (1988) Postoperative adjuvant chemotherapy or BCG for colon cancer: results from NSABP Protocol C-01. J Natl Cancer Inst 80: 30–36

Young RC (guest ed) (1984) Ovarian carcinoma. Semin Oncol 11: 202–332

Hormones in Cancer Treatment

F. CAVALLI

About one-quarter of all tumors are considered to be hormone-sensitive: different forms of hematologic malignancies belong to this group, since treatment with corticosteroids plays an important antitumor role in these diseases. Hormone responsiveness, which was strikingly demonstrated as early as 1898 by Beatson, who performed the first oophorectomy for breast cancer, represents an intringuing biologic phenomenon, since it opposes the often held dogma of a complete autonomy of the tumor growth. This may be more understandable today, now that our biologic comprehension of oncogenesis is rapidly evolving. We perceive that growth factors, oncogenes and receptors are very closely interrelated. The nature of hormone receptors has been partially elucidated, and most hormones may possibly act at least partly as growth factors (King 1986). It is therefore no longer surprising, that endocrinologic studies play such an important role in the current discussion about oncogenesis, which in turn has led to a revival of interest in the practical use of hormones for the treatment of cancer.

Hormone Receptors

One of the major advances in the treatment of breast cancer in the past decade has been the development and widespread use of estrogen and progesterone re-

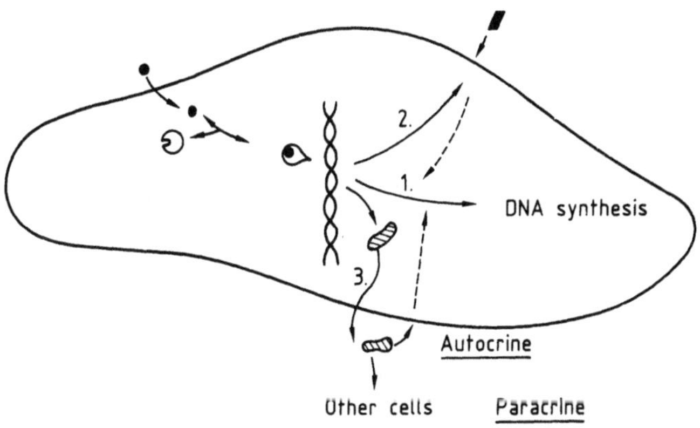

Fig. 1. Potential routes by which steroids (●) can influence cell proliferation. *1*, Direct action; *2* change in membrane sensitivity to external stimuli (cells/growth factors); *3*, production of growth factors ◌, native receptor; ◌ activated steroid receptor complex; X, chromatin

ceptor assays. In the Management of cancer of the corpus uteri, however, the role of these assays is only beginning to emerge, while the therapeutic implications of receptors in prostatic cancer are still unknown. Moreover, the presence of receptors could not be consistently ascertained in other tumors like melanomas, renal cell cancer and ovarian cancer: some of the conflicting results reported in these neoplasias may in fact be more related to methodological artifacts (Zava and Goldhirsch 1983).

Notwithstanding different practical limitations of receptor assays, which will be further discussed in the context of this chapter, it has to be recognized that these assays represent, currently, the best tool for investigating the hormone dependency of some tumors. The potential routes by which steroids can influence cell proliferation are summarized in Fig. 1. At the present time it is impossible to comment on the relative importance of each of these three pathways and it is likely that all three routes are utilized, possibly to different degrees in different tumors (King 1986).

Methodological Problems

As always in daily practice, it is of utmost importance that clinicians recognize precisely the limitations inherent in the methodology producing the results with which they are confronted. Current assays measure cytoplasmic proteins which act as receptors, binding and transferring the appropriate steroid molecule into nuclei to exert a specific hormonal function. The binding capacity is expressed as femtomoles of ^{3}H-estradiol (in the case of estrogen receptors, ER) bound per milligram of cytosol protein. Generally, values above 10 fmol/mg are considered receptor positive while < 3 fmol/mg is regarded as receptor negative. It is important to realize that biochemical assays are performed on extracts of the entire tumor sample and thus may be influenced by tumor cellularity, tumor necrosis, or stromal components. The receptor level obtained, being an average of both tumor and nontumor elements, would therefore be expected to be only a crude estimate of the actual tumor cell receptor content. This may explain why numerous investigators examining the results of simultaneous assays performed from two separate areas of the same tumor mass have reported discordant results in up to 30% of cases (Osborne 1985). Another source of errors lies in the many sensitive steps of the methodology. It is therefore not surprising that quality control studies have revealed interlaboratory differences in up to one-third of cases (Thorpe and Koenders 1986).

Another problem relates to tumor heterogeneity. Most hormone-dependent tumors are probably composed of receptor-positive and receptor-negative cells; therefore shifts in the majority cell population, due to natural selection processes or to the selective pressure of therapy, are possible. Thus, receptor status may change over time, leading the clinician to ask whether a single initial biopsy for receptors is sufficient, or whether biopsies for receptors should be repeated at the time of recurrence to optimize treatment planning. Several reports have addressed this question by analyzing patients who have had multiple sequential tumor biopsies for receptors with or without intervening therapy (Allegra et al. 1980; King et al. 1982; Hull et al. 1983). In the absence of intervening therapy, discordance rates for ER are approximately 15%–20% between sequential biopsies in breast cancer, with up to 30%–35% in the case of progesterone receptors (PgR). A similar discordance is noted for patients receiving cytotoxic chemotherapy between biopsies, indicating that chemotherapy does not selectively suppress either the receptor-positive or receptor-negative cells. Greater discordance rates have been reported with intervening endocrine therapy. However, a large study found that the discordance rate and the change in ER content for sequential assays in patients receiving endocrine therapy is no greater than in patients receiving no treatment, if those recently treated with tamoxifen are excluded (Hull et al. 1983). This antiestrogen has a prolonged half-life and can be measured in the blood many weeks after discontinuation (Fabian et al. 1980). Patients biopsied for ER within 2 months after stopping tamoxifen frequently appear falsely

ER-negative, probably due to occupancy of the receptor by the drug.

Newer methods for the detection of receptors have been developed, based on immunohistochemistry. Their exact role has still to be ascertained, even if first reports seem to hint at comparable results to the conventional steroid binding assays for the determination of receptors (McClelland et al. 1986).

Hormone Receptors in Breast Cancer

The presence or absence of ER in breast cancer is associated with several other characteristics, including patient age and menopausal status, histologic subtype of the tumor, biopsy site, and tumor size (Clark et al. 1984). About 60% of primary tumors from premenopausal women contain detectable ER. In contrast, ER can be measured in about 75% of postmenopausal women. PgR, which is probably a more accurate marker for tumor endocrine dependence, is present in about 50% of tumors from both premenopausal and postmenopausal women. Interestingly, there is no significant difference in ER concentration between premenopausal and postmenopausal women of identical age, implying that age itself, rather than endogenous estrogen concentration (menopausal status), is the major influence on ER level (Osborne 1985). However, premenopausal women have higher PgR concentrations than postmenopausal women of the same age, perhaps indicating greater estrogen-stimulated synthesis of PgR. One of the most striking variables in receptor status is the wide range of receptor concentrations observed when a large population of patients with breast cancer is examined. ER varies from 0 to >1000 fmol/mg cytoplasmic protein and PgR from 0 to >2600 fmol/mg cytoplasmic protein. The practical importance of this wide quantitative variation has still to be fully elucidated. For ER there is a certain degree of quantitative correlation, since the response rate of endocrine therapy does increase as the ER concentration increases (Allegra et al. 1980). No such correlation could be found concerning the quantitative content of PgR (Cavalli, unpublished data).

The rate of response to hormonal treatment is around 50% in ER-positive tumors and less than 10% in ER-negative tumors (McGuire 1978). Both receptors are found in 46% of cases, with a response rate to endocrine maneuvers of 77% when both receptors are considered to be positive. About 30% are ER positive but PgR negative, and this group has a poorer response to hormonal therapy (25%), underlining again the prognostic significance of PgR. Despite the presence of cytosol receptors for estrogen, at least 20% of patients fail to respond to hormonal treatment.

The current role of receptors in the management of primary breast cancer (i.e., adjuvant therapy) will be discussed later. The most important application for receptor analysis in patients with advanced breast cancer is in the selection of patients for endocrine therapy. Only about 5% of patients with receptor-negative tumors respond to endocrine therapy, and in general these patients can be spared the wasted effort of an endocrine trial and begin cytotoxic chemotherapy immediately. However, the methodological problems of these assays should be recalled. The predictive value of receptors may be useful *mainly* if their determination takes place immediately before the treatment based on their results. Otherwise the rate of spontaneous and/or therapy-induced change in the phenotypic expression of the receptors may greatly decrease their predictive value. In the case of an assay performed many years before, the clinician may therefore prefer to base his choice on the well-known prognostic factors (age of patient, free interval, tumor burden, site of metastases, etc.), particularly if these are inconsistent with the old receptor result.

Hormone Receptors in Other Tumors

Among the other hormone-responsive tumors, endometrial cancer is the only one whose management may already be influenced by the determination of receptors. Recent studies (Ehrlich et al. 1981) found the progesterone-binding affinity to correlate with the histologic grade, a finding which is consistent with the broader experience gathered in breast cancer. Although the number of patients so studied is very small, PgR content may allow more rational selection of hormonal management. Endometrial cancer with high progesterone affinity seems to respond more often than average, while only about 10% of those with "low receptors" show an objective tumor regression. However, further experience has to be accumulated before a definite assessment can be made and receptors can play in this tumor the same role they have acquired in the management of breast cancer.

The Strategic Options in the Management of Advanced Breast Cancer

Breast cancer is widely believed to encompass at least two main populations: one more chemosensitive, the other one more responsive to endocrine maneuvers (Henderson and Canellos 1980). At least three strategic options may therefore be envisaged: hormonal therapy, cytotoxic treatment and the combination of both. In the past few years the determination of hormone receptors, as well as the results of different clinical trials, have at least partially clarified the relative merit of the three options, permitting physicians to individualize treatment with considerably more accuracy than in the past.

Endocrine Treatment

The efficacy of endocrine treatment of advanced breast cancer is well established. However, only about one-third of unselected patients will respond, and this tumor regression will generally last, on average, 1 year. Even if some patients will enjoy several years of palliation with relatively nontoxic treatment, ultimately all will experience progression of the disease. As outlined above, the results of hormone receptors assays now permit partial selection of patients who are more likely to respond to endocrine therapies. More important, however, is their negative predictive value, since patients with ER and PgR negative tumors can generally be spared a hormonal trial. The outcome of the hormonal therapy is generally strongly correlated with the well-known prognostic factors: age, free interval between mastectomy and relapse, response to previous hormonal maneuvers, presence/absence of visceral metastases (besides a limited number of nodular pulmonary lesions), tumor burden. Different studies (see subsection "Combined Approach" below) have shown that endocrine therapy remains the treatment of first choice in most postmenopausal patients. Not considering menopausal status, hormonal therapy should be considered chiefly in the following situations: positive *actual* receptors, indolent disease, soft tissue and/or bony metastases. Thereby it should not be forgotten that the free interval plays a minor role in patients with skeletal involvement only, a situation with which the clinician is often confronted (Fey et a. 1981). It is also important to remember that successive response to different hormonal therapies represents the best prognostic factor, since these patients generally live 2–3 years longer than nonresponders.

Chemotherapy

The outcome of chemotherapy does not correlate with the receptor content of the tumor and is also generally less influenced by the classical prognostic factors of advanced breast cancer (Henderson and Canellos 1980). With modern chemotherapy about two-thirds of patients will show an objective tumor regression, which generally will last less than 1 year. It should also be remembered that the impact of chemotherapy upon survival has emerged clearly only in patients with an aggressive tumor; it is less evident for cases with an indolent disease. In the latter group, it has been clearly shown that a more gentle chemotherapy may elicit results similar to those achieved by more aggressive and toxic combinations of cytotoxic agents (Cavalli et al. 1983 a). Thus, chemotherapy tends to be indicated in situations in which endocrine treatment is known to be of very limited value: young patient, short free interval, visceral lesions.

Combined Approach

Since breast cancer is believed to encompass two different populations of tumor cells, it is understandable that in the last 15 years vast effort has been expended in order to demonstrate the superiority of combinations of cytotoxic agents and endocrine treatment over the use of a single modality (Brunner et al. 1977; Cocconi et al. 1983). Overall, the results have been disappointing. In postmenopausal patients at least three studies (Cavalli et al. 1983 b; Australian BCSG 1986; Taylor et al. 1986) have shown that in the majority of the cases endocrine treatments remains the approach of first choice. In our trial (Fig. 2), postmenopausal patients with an indolent disease treated first with tamoxifen alone (chemotherapy being delayed till the occurrence of relapse) lived twice as long as patients who received tamoxifen and chemotherapy from the very beginning. In premenopausal patients (Cavalli et al. 1983 a), results are more conflicting, and the same may be said about attempts to correlate the use of combinations of both modalities with tumor receptor content. Currently, therefore, no clearcut subset of patients can be defined who would certainly profit from a combined approach. Most probably the best long-term results can still be achieved by the careful use of an optimal sequence of all available treatments. In the same patient, hormonal therapy may be indicated at one time and chemotherapy at another.

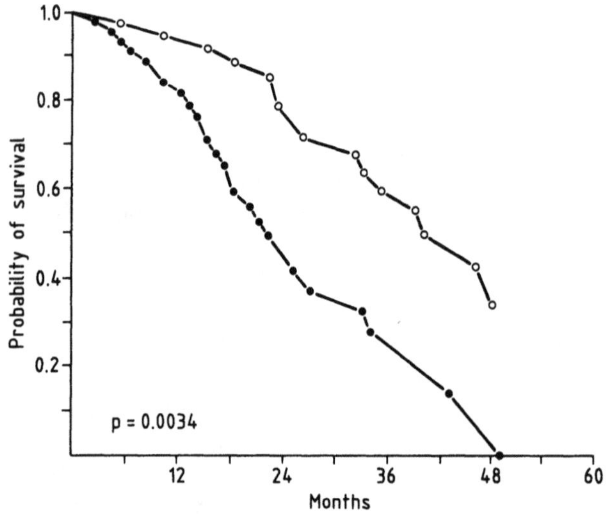

Fig. 2. Survival curve for postmenopausal low-risk patients receiving tamoxifen and either concurrent (●—●) or sequential chemotherapy (○—○)

Table 1. Endocrine therapy of breast cancer

Ablative	Oophorectomy Adrenalectomy Hypophysectomy
Additive	Estrogen Progestin Androgen
Competitive	Antiestrogen
Inhibitive	Aminoglutethimide Trilostane Danazol LH-RH analogs

Endocrine Treatment of Advanced Breast Cancer

The various endocrine therapies available for the treatment of breast cancer can be divided, according to their demonstrated or suggested mode of biological action, into four categories: ablative, additive, competitive and inhibitive (Table 1).

Ablative Therapy

The rationale for the use of ablative procedures is that hormones promote the growth of some mammary tumor cells. Thus, a decrease in the concentration of these hormones is assumed to induce tumor regression (Dao 1972). Bilateral oophorectomy in premenopausal women was the earliest form of systemic therapy for advanced breast cancer. The response rate is approximately 30%, but with appreciable variation between the different samples. Radiation (2000 rad) castration gives comparable results, but may need up to 2 months to take effect. In patients whose tumors are estrogen-dependent the procedure can be expected to induce a regression lasting 9–12 months. One of the advantages of the surgical procedure is that it may demonstrate the presence of small liver metastases, which is probably one of the few situations where early combination chemotherapy is urgently indicated. On the contrary, the presence of massive liver metastases contraindicates oophorectomy, since the expected response rate is low and the surgical procedure may accelerate liver failure.

Response rates similar to those with oophorectomy are achieved with both adrenalectomy and hypophysectomy (Robin and Dalton 1977). Only a few randomized studies have been conducted to compare different ablative treatments, and their results have been conflicting. The introduction of medical adrenalectomy, as well as the possibility to effectively control bone pain, which was the major indication for hypophysectomy, with systemic measures, have vastly reduced the necessity for these two major types of ablative surgery.

Additive Therapy

The mode of action underlying the paradoxical effect of pharmacological doses of steroid hormones such as estrogens, androgens, progestins and gluccocorticoids on tumor growth is largely unknown (Mouridsen 1986). As for ablative therapy, a wide range of response rates has been reported for additive endocrine treatment (Table 2). Apart from variations in patient selection and response criteria, some of the discrepancies may be accounted for by the different dose levels used in the individual trials. A dose-response relationship has in fact been shown, at least partially, for estrogens and androgens (Mouridsen 1986) and more recently for progestins (Cavalli et al. 1984). For progestins, however, a randomized trial has failed to demonstrate a significant impact of differences in dose upon survival (Cavalli et al. 1984). Medroxyprogesterone acetate, mainly when used in doses around 1 g daily, seems to consistently elicit many secondary responses, even in patients primarily not responding to other endocrine maneuvers. Ongoing clinical studies are trying to define the relative merit of different hormonal therapies when used as first-line treatment. Until the results of these studies

Table 2. Endocrine treatment in advanced breast cancer

Treatment	Number of patients	Response rate (%)	Range of response (%)
Oophorectomy	1674	33	21–41
Adrenalectomy	4935	32	23–58
Hypophysectomy	1890	36	24–47
Estrogen	1683	26	15–38
Androgen	2250	21	10–38
Progesterone	783	31	9–54
Tamoxifen	1269	32	16–52
Aminoglutethimide	909	32	25–50

Modified from Mouridsen (1986).

become available, progestins must still be considered an optimal second-line treatment in postmenopausal women (Ross et al. 1982), while their role in premenopausal patients remains largely undefined. Because of the introduction of tamoxifen, the other types of additive therapy have now been generally abandoned.

Competitive Therapy

The pharmacodynamics of the nonsteroidal antiestrogenic compound tamoxifen has recently been reviewed in detail (Fabian et al. 1980). The primary step is the competition with estradiol for binding to the estrogen receptor. At the chromatin level the mechanism of action is complex, ultimately leading to both partial block of the cell cycle in the early G1 phase and an increase in the concentration of the PgR protein in the tumor cells. Furthermore, it has recently been shown that tamoxifen binds to high-affinity sites that appear to be different from the ER binding sites. Tamoxifen has a prolonged half-life and can be measured in the blood up to 2 months after discontinuation. This is important not only when rebiopsy for hormone receptors assay is considered, but also if one looks for the so-called withdrawal responses which occur in about 10% in all types of systemic endocrine treatment. The average response rate with tamoxifen is 32% with a range of 16%–52% (Table 2). The most frequently used daily doses are 20–40 mg, and randomized trials have failed to demonstrate significant differences in treatment results between 20 mg and up to 90 mg daily. Some 10 trials have compared tamoxifen with estrogens, progestins, androgens and amminoglutethimide (Mouridsen 1986). In all these trials tamoxifen has yielded therapeutic results at least similar to those of the other agents, but has generally produced significantly less toxicity. This is the most important reason behind the general acceptance of tamoxifen as the treatment of first choice, at least in postmenopausal patients. Recent years have seen a number of studies on the effect of tamoxifen in premenopausal patients with advanced disease (Manni and Pearson 1980; Pritchard et al. 1980; Wada et al. 1981; Ingle et al. 1986). The response rate is close to 30% similar to that achieved with oophorectomy. This was confirmed in a small randomized comparison of the two (Ingle et al. 1986). In one study (Pritchard et al. 1980) at least, tamoxifen was shown also to be predictive of the respose to a successive oophorectomy. However, additional data are needed before the surgical procedure can be replaced by this additive therapy. Moreover, the experience of long-term treatment with tamoxifen in premenopausal women is still limited, and endocrinological data may hint at the danger of a long-term "escape" of the tumor, due to an overshoot of estradiol (Jordan 1986). Until more experience has been accumulated, caution should be employed and tamoxifen should not be regarded as equivalent to surgical castration.

Inhibitive Therapy

The mechanism of action of aminoglutethimide has recently been extensively reviewed (Santen and Wells 1980). In short, this glutethimide derivative inhibits the production of the adrenal steroid hormones and the peripheral aromatization of androstenedione to estrone. Similar mechanisms of action have been described for the synthetic steroid trilostane. The mechanism of action of danazol, a synthetic testosterone derivative, probably include binding to progesterone and androgen receptors and inhibition of the steroid synthesis in the ovaries as well (Mouridsen 1986). The LH-RH analogs lead to a striking fall in plasma steroids via interference with the secretion of hypophyseal peptides. The average response rate to treatment with aminoglutethimide supplemented by substitution with gluccocorticoids is 31% with a range of 16%–43% (Table 2). In one study, patients receiving aminoglutethimide after medroxyprogesterone acetate were found to be largely unresponsive (Alberto et al. 1985). Most studies have used a dose of 1000 mg/day aminoglutethimide supplemented by hydrocortisone. A recent study demonstrated 500–1000 mg/day to be equally effective (Bonneterre et al. 1985). For the time being aminoglutethimide is mostly indicated as a second-line treatment, mainly because of its pronounced toxicity (Smith et al. 1981). However, newer and probably less toxic analogs are just entering clinical trails and it is therefore quite possible that in a few years aromatase inhibitors will play a more important role in the management of advanced breast cancer than they do now. For the time being, the results for trilostane, danazol and the different LH-RH analogs are still too preliminary to permit any assessment of their merits.

Combination of Different Hormonal Agents

Clinicians are accustomed to seeing responses to each of a succession of endocrine agents. This, together with the differences in mode of action between the various endocrine treatments, suggests that combined use of endocrine agents might increase the therapeutic response. A number of randomized trials have been published in which one agent alone was compared to the combination of two or more drugs, and the results of these investigations have recently been reviewed (Rose and Mouridsen 1984). Most of these trials failed to show significant differences. Some differences in response rates were questionable or did not translate into differences as regards duration of response and/or survival. So far, then, the combination of different endocrine agents cannot be advised. Still unavailable, however, are the results of trials comparing oophorectomy to oophorectomy plus tamoxifen in premenopausal patients. This combination seems to be more rational than most of the combinations assessed in the past and may, therefore, elicit better results.

In recent years various other approaches have been proposed in order to optimize the results of endocrine treatment. The alternating use of cytotoxic and endocrine therapy has been viewed as a possible way of recruiting nondividing cells, creating a better environment for the effect of the cytotoxic drugs. Conversely the alternating use of tamoxifen and progestins has been proposed, since tamoxifen is sometimes believed to increase the content of PgR in the tumor tissue. Preliminary data on these approaches have been disappointing, but further and better structured clinical studies are needed in order to properly assess these theoretically attractive hypotheses.

Endocrine Aspects in Adjuvant Therapy

Despite controversy, adjuvant treatment (chemotherapy and/or hormonal therapy) has become widely used in the management of breast cancer as one possibility of improving disease-free survival and reducing mortality due to the disease (Goldhirsch et al. 1986). This area has been recently thoroughly reviewed at an important NCI consensus meeting (Lippman and Chabner 1986).

The first clinical studies investigating the possibility of curing patients via endocrine manipulation were initiated almost 40 years ago. Starting in the late 1970s, the use of tamoxifen in the adjuvant setting has been the subject of many trials in Europe and the USA.

Premenopausal Women

The most important studies related to the effect of adjuvant castration are summarized in Table 3. From these results it can been seen that adjuvant oophorectomy can elicit, at best, a survival advantage in the order of 10%. A more important benefit, at least for patients older than 45 years, was seen in the Toronto trial, where the control group was compared to radiological castration plus low-dose continuous prednisone (Meakin et al. 1983). In the Ludwig II trial, 356 premenopausal and perimenopausal patients with metastases in four or more axillary lymph nodes were randomly allocated to receive either CMF with low-dose continuous prednisone (CMFp) or surgical oophorectomy followed by CMFp (Goldhirsch et al. 1980). This trial failed to show any difference be-

Table 3. Randomized trials with adjuvant oophorectomy

Trial	No. of patients	Years of follow-up	Findings
Christie	598	15	Survival advantage for Ox: at 10 years 55% vs 48%, at 15 years 45% vs 40%
Toronto	308	15	Survival advantage for Ox + low-dose continuous prednisone in women 45 years old or older (72% vs 44%)
Saskatchewan	359	10	Survival advantage for Ox at 10 years (11% difference)
Ludwig II	327	5	No effect of addition of Ox to combination chemotherpy with CMFp

Modified from Goldhirsch et al. (1986).
Oophorectomy (Ox) was achieved either surgically or by irradiation CMFp, CMF plus low-dose continuous prednisone.

tween chemotherapy alone and the combination of chemotherapy and hormonal therapy. These data, together with information derived from other randomized trials, underscore the assumption that the effect of chemotherapy may be mediated primarily through its effect on the endocrine system. The fact that amenorrhea seems to be associated with a better outcome in the majority of the chemotherapeutic studies supports this hypothesis. However, because induced amenorrhea does not seem to improve long-term results among patients who receive full doses of chemotherapy, some direct cytotoxic activity must be postulated (Goldhirsch et al. 1986). Moreover, the overall results of adjuvant chemotherapy alone in premenopausal patients are somewhat better than those observed many years ago with oophorectomy alone (Lippman and Chabner 1986).

Postmenopausal Patients

It has become evident in recent years that the benefit in terms of disease-free survival, of the adjuvant chemotherapy in current use is less for postmenopausal than for premenopausal women. Moreover, the advantage as regards overall survival remains questionable or at best marginal. It is therefore understandable that tamoxifen was adopted for many adjuvant trials: the most important randomized trials using tamoxifen and having a surgery-alone control group are summarized in Table 4. For the time being it is evident that tamoxifen prolongs disease-free survival significantly; its impact upon overall survival has still to be clearly defined. Moreover, in some trials tamoxifen was clearly shown to decrease local recurrences, but the effect upon distant metastases was less evident (Goldhirsch et al. 1986).

Currently it seems that the combination of chemotherapy and endocrine treatment as an adjuvant modality may be more important in postmenopausal women than in premenopausal patients. In one NSABP trial, better results were achieved by adding tamoxifen to chemotherapy (Fisher et al. 1986). The combined analysis of two further trials (Ludwig III, ECOG) does, however, at least permit the hypothesis that in patients with positive receptors the addition of chemotherapy to an endocrine treatment is of little value (Goldhirsch et al. 1986). The major impact of the combined approach might therefore be in the subpopulation with ER-negative tumors.

Endocrine Treatment of Other Tumors

Even though endocrine treatment has been widely used in the therapy of other tumors such as endometrial carcinoma or prostatic cancer, its exact role in such tumors is still less clearly defined than in the management of breast cancer. This is probably mainly because these tumors often have poorly measurable parameters and the therapeutic response may, therefore, be difficult to assess with any clarity.

Table 4. The most important randomized trials with adjuvant tamoxifen in postmenopausal patients

Trial	No. of evaluable patients	Treatment duration	Findings
Copenhagen	94	2 years	DFS advantage for treated patients
Danish	1647	1 year	DFS advantage for treated patients (postoperative RT). No survival difference
Swedish	865	2 years	DFS advantage for treated patients (postoperative RT to high-risk population)
Christie	588	1 year	No survival difference for treated patients
NATO	1124[a]	2 years	DFS and OS advantage for treated patients
Toronto	366	2 years	DFS advantage for treated patients (only the series without postoperative RT)
ECOG	170	2 years	DFS advantage for treated patients
Ludwig III + IV	629	1 year	DFS advantage for treated patients (low-dose prednisone given with tamoxifen)

Modified from Goldhirsch et al. (1986).
DFS, disease-free survival; OS, overall survival; RT, radiotherapy.
[a]Including premenopausal patients.

Endometrial Adenocarcinoma

The initial treatment of endometrial adenocarcinomas is effective in a majority of patients; nevertheless, at least 40% of the women will develop advanced or recurrent disease and therefore require some type of systemic therapy. The role of adjuvant treatment with progestins in early endometrial adenocarcinoma has still to be clearly defined: such an approach can therefore not be routinely recommended. Metastatic endometrial adenocarcinoma is usually treated with either progestins or cytotoxic chemotherapy. Approximately one-third of patients have documented regression of tumor with either therapy, so that most clinicians prefer progestins because of their lower toxicity. This latter consideration is of particular importance since these patients are generally older and frequently have other medical illnesses. This approach, however, may result in an undesirable delay in instituting alternative therapy in patients not responding to one of the modalities. Historically, clinical parameters, such as age, histologic grade, and disease-free interval, have not proven clinically reliable. Recently, several investigators have shown a close correlation between the presence of PgR (and to a lesser extent ER) in the cytosol of endometrial carcinomas and tumor regression during progestin therapy (Kauppila et al. 1982). Even if additional data are needed, clinicians should, therefore, nowadays consider primarily the use of cytotoxic agents if the tumors prove to be receptor-negative (Ehrlich et al. 1981). Otherwise, treatment with progestins should remain the therapy of first choice. Whether a correlation between the dose of progestins and the antitumor effect exists in the treatment of endometrial carcinoma, as in breast cancer, has still to be defined.

Prostate Cancer

Prostate cancer is becoming a major challenge for the oncological community, at least in the developed countries (Klein 1979). It would be beyond the scope of this contribution to attempt even brief discussion of all the controversies which have arisen around this tumor, so we will limit ourselves to a few considerations.

Many patients will present with undetectable micrometastases – theoretically a population for which an adjuvant treatment would be very suitable. Overall adjuvant therapy with estrogens does not prolong survival significantly, mainly because of the negative impact of cardiovascular complications. The new LH-RH agonists have antitumor activity equivalent to that of estrogens in patients with metastatic prostate cancer, and are currently believed to elicit far fewer cardiovascular complications. Trials evaluating the role of LH-RH agonists in the adjuvant setting are therefore warranted (Torti 1984). Currently, however, no general recommendation in favor of an adjuvant treatment can be given.

Most of the controversies concerning metastatic prostate cancer are based upon inconsistent results, which in turn generally reflect the poor measurability of most metastatic lesions. Moreover, there seems to be a contradiction beween the clinical observation that hormonal manipulation may provide dramatic relief of symptoms and regression of disease and the statistical observation that survival of the prostatic cancer patient may not be enhanced by endocrine intervention. This is in contrast to the survival benefit found in patients with breast cancer responding to endocrine maneuvers. Currently, we have to admit, overall, that the therapeutic results achieved with orchiedectomy or with an additive treatment estrogens, additive or inhibitive LH-RH agonists) are similar. The choice of first-line therapy, as well as the sequence of different modalities, therefore remains mostly arbitrary. Antiandrogens may be as effective as the other forms of additive treatment, but additional data are needed. Whether drugs combining estrogens with a cytotoxic principle in their molecular structure (e. g.) estramustine phosphate) are superior to other forms of conventional systemic treatment remains to be definitely shown. Prostatic cancer, mainly in younger patients, is often sensitive to chemotherapy: the exact merits of cytotoxic drugs in the management of this disease urgently need further clarification. Completely unknown at present is whether the outcome of prostate cancer could be improved, at least for some patients, by combined use of endocrine agents and cytotoxic drugs.

References

Alberto P, Mermillod B, Kaplan E et al (1985) A clinical trial of aminoglutethimide in advanced postmenopausal breast carcinoma: low response in patients previously treated with medroxyprogesterone. Eur J Cancer Clin Oncol 21: 423–428

Allegra JC, Barlock A, Huff KK et al. (1980) Changes in multiple or sequential oestrogen receptor determinations in breast cancer. Cancer 45: 792–794

Australian and New Zealand Breast Cancer Trials Group, Clinical Oncological Society of Australia (1986) A randomized trial in postmenopausal patients with advanced breast cancer comparing endocrine and cytotoxic therapy given sequentially or in combination. J Clin Oncol 4: 186–193

Bonneterre J, Coppens H, Mauriac L, Metz M, Rouesse J, Armand JP, Fargeot P, Mathieu M, Tubiana M, Cappelaere P (1985) Aminoglutethimide in advanced breast cancer: clinical results of a French multicenter randomized trial comparing 500 mg and 1 g/day. Eur J Cancer Clin Oncol 21: 1153–1158

Brunner KW, Sonntag RW, Alberto P, Senn HJ, Martz G, Obrecht P, Maurice P (1977) Combined chemo- and hormonal therapy in advanced breast cancer. Cancer 39: 2923–2933

Cavalli F, Beer M, Martz G et al. (1983 a) Concurrent or sequential use of cytotoxic chemotherapy and hormone treatment in advanced breast cancer. Br Med J 1: 5–8

Cavalli F, Pedrazzini A, Martz G et al. (1983 b) A randomized trial of three different regimens of combination chemotherapy in patients receiving simultaneously a hormonal treatment for advanced breast cancer. Eur J Clin Oncol 19: 1615–1624

Cavalli F, Goldhirsch A, Jungi F et al. (1984) A randomized trial of low- versus high-dose medroxyprogesterone acetate in the induction treatment of postmenopausal patients with advanced breast cancer. J Clin Oncol 2: 414–419

Clark GM, Osborne CK, McGuire WL (1984) Correlations between oestrogen receptor, progesterone receptor and patients characteristics in human breast cancer. J Clin Oncol 2: 1102–1109

Cocconi G, De Lisi V, Boni C et al. (1983) Chemotherapy versus combination of chemotherapy and endocrine therapy in advanced breast cancer. A prospective randomized study. Cancer 51: 581–585

Dao TL (1972) Ablation therapy for hormone-dependent tumours. Annu Rev Med 23: 1–8

Ehrlich CE, Young PCM, Cleary RE (1981) Cytoplasmic progesterone and estradiol receptors in normal, hyperplastic, and carcinomatous endometria: therapeutic implications. Am J Obstet Gynecol 141: 539–546

Fabian C, Sternson L, Barnett M (1980) Clinical pharmacology of tamoxifen in patients with breast cancer: comparison of traditional and loading dose schedules. Cancer Treat Rep 64: 765–773

Fey MF, Brunner KW, Sonntag RW (1981) Prognostic factors in metastatic breast cancer. Am J Clin Oncol 4: 237–248

Fisher B, Redmond C, Brown A (1986) Adjuvant chemotherapy with and without tamoxifen in treatment of primary breast cancer: 5-year results from the NSABP trial. J Clin Oncol 4: 459–471

Goldhirsch A, Gelber RD, Mouridsen H (1986) Endocrine aspects in adjuvant therapy for early breast cancer. In: Cavalli F (ed) Endocrine therapy of breast cancer. Springer, Berlin Heidelberg New York Tokyo, pp 91–108 (ESO Monographs)

Henderson IC, Canellos GP (1980) Cancer of the breast. The past decade. N Engl J Med 302: 17–30, 78–90

Hull DF, Clark GM, Osborne CK et al. (1983) Multiple oestrogen receptor assays in human breast cancer. Cancer Res 43: 413–416

Ingle JN, Krook JE, Gree SJ, Kubista TP, Evanson LL, Almann DL, Chang MN, Bisel HF, Windschitl HE, Twito SI, Pfeifle DM (1986) Randomized trial of bilateral oophorectomy versus tamoxifen in premenopausal women with metastatic breast cancer. J Clin Oncol 4: 178-185

Jordan VC (1986) Tamoxifen prophylaxis: prevention is better than cure – prevention is cure? In: Cavalli F (ed) Endocrine therapy of breast cancer. Springer, Berlin Heidelberg New York Tokyo, pp 117–120 (ESO Monographs)

Kauppila A, Kujansun E, Vikko R (1982) Cytosal oestrogen and progestin receptors in endometrial carcinoma of patients treated with surgery, radiotherapy, and progestin. Cancer 50: 2157–2162

King RJB (1986) Experimental strategies for studying the development of breast cancer with special reference to hormones, growth factors and oncogenes. In: Cavalli F (ed) Endocrine therapy of breast cancer. Springer, Berlin Heidelberg New York Tokyo, pp 5–26 (ESO Monographs)

King RJB, Stewart JF, Millis RR et al. (1982) Quantitative comparison of estradiol and progesterone receptor contents of primary and metastatic breast tumors in relation to response to endocrine treatment. Breast Cancer Res Treat 2: 339–346

Klein LA (1979) Prostatic carcinoma. N Engl J Med 300: 824–833

Lippman ME, Chabner BA (1986) Editorial overview. NCI Monograph 1: 29–34

Manni A, Pearson OH (1980) Antiestrogen-induced remissions in premenopausal women with stage IV breast cancer: effects on ovarian function. Cancer Treat Rep 64: 779–785

McClelland RA, Berger U, Miller LS et al. (1986) Immunocytochemical assay for oestrogen receptor: relationship to outcome of therapy in patients with advanced breast cancer. Cancer Res [Suppl] 46: 4241–4243

McGuire WL (1978) Hormone receptors: their role in predicting prognosis and response to endocrine therapy. Semin Oncol 5: 428–433

Meakin JW, Allt WEC, Beale FA et al. (1983) Ovarian irradiation and prednisone following surgery and radiotherapy for carcinoma of the breast. Breast Cancer Res Treat 3: 45–48

Mouridsen HT (1986) Endocrine treatment of advanced breast cancer. In: Cavalli F (ed) Endocrine therapy of breast cancer. Springer, Berlin Heidelberg New York Tokyo, pp 79–90 (ESO Monographs)

Osborne CK (1985) Heterogeneity in hormone receptor status in primary and metastatic breast cancer. Semin Oncol 12: 317–326

Pritchard KI, Thomson DB, Myers RE, Sutherland DJD, Mobbs BG, Meakin JW (1980) Tamoxifen therapy in premenopausal patients with metastatic breast cancer. Cancer Treat Rep 64: 787–796

Robin PE, Dalton GA (1977) The role of major endocrine ablation. In: Stoll BA (ed) Breast cancer management – early and late. Year Book, Chicago, pp 147–156

Rose C, Mouridsen HT (1984) Treatment of advanced breast cancer with tamoxifen. Recent Results Cancer Res 91: 230–242

Ross MB, Buzdar AU, Blumenschein GR (1982) Treatment of advanced breast cancer with megestrol acetate after therapy with tamoxifen. Cancer 49: 413–417

Santen RJ, Wells SA (1980) The use of aminoglutethimide in the treatment of patients with metastatic carcinoma of the breast. Cancer 46: 1066–1074

Smith IE, Harris AL, Morgan M et al. (1981) Tamoxifen versus aminoglutethimide in advanced breast carcinoma: a randomised cross-over trial. Br Med J 283: 1432–1434

Taylor SG, Gelman RS, Falkson G et al. (1986) Combination chemotherapy compared to tamoxifen as initial therapy for stage IV breast cancer in elderly women. Ann Intern Med 104: 455–461

Thorpe SM, Koenders A (1986) Standardization of steroid receptor assays in human breast cancer. Eur J Cancer Clin Oncol 22: 939–945

Torti FM (1984) Hormonal therapy for prostate cancer. N Engl J Med 311: 1313–1314

Wada T, Koyama H, Teresawa T (1981) Effect of tamoxifen in premenopausal Japanese women with advanced breast cancer. Cancer Treat Rep 65: 728–729

Zava DT, Goldhirsch A (1983) Oestrogen receptor in malignant melanoma: fact or artefact. Eur J Cancer Clin Oncol 19: 1151–1159

Immunotherapy of Cancer

P. RÜMKE

When, in the 1960s Burnet's immunosurveillance hypotheses became common knowledge among clinicians, many of them took it for granted that human tumors carried tumor antigens which allowed the host, theoretically, to recognize and reject his or her own cancer cells. At a time when surgery, radiotherapy and chemotherapy could hardly be expected to add more to what had already been accomplished in the therapy of malignancies, and, moreover, when it was fashionable to believe that all evil could be combated by natural and nonaggressive forces, it was no surprise that immunotherapy became the new hope in the fight against cancer. After all, in many animal models, either specific or nonspecific active immunotherapy had been shown to be effective as long as the tumor burden was "microscopically" small. In spite of the fact that these models often had little in common with the situation in patients, many clinical trials were started in which all kinds of nonspecific immunostimulants were tested. Generally this was done in an adjuvant setting after radical surgery, when staging criteria predicted a high risk of micrometastasis or residual tumor. On the whole these trials have not demonstrated that immunostimulation was of much benefit to the patient. Although in some phase II studies the prognosis seemed to be improved in comparison to historical control patients, the larger prospective and randomized phase III studies were disappointing in their outcome. Therefore none of the many investigated immunostimulating substances or vaccines has found a place in standard protocols for adjuvant treatment after surgery.

However, notwithstanding the lack of substantial progress in the past decades, some clinical experiments have shown that further exploration of immunotherapeutic approaches is justified. In the following pages the human tumor models in which immunotherapy, in whatever form, has seemed to have some effect will be discussed together with some of the recent developments stemming from basic research. The emphasis will be on clinical achievements rather than experimental findings.

Specific Active Immunotherapy

In experimental animals vaccines prepared from inactivated but viable tumor cells, i.e., tumor cells that have been irradiated or treated with an alkylating agent so that they have lost the capacity to proliferate, may induce an immune response which protects the animal against the outgrowth of transplanted tumor cells of the same sort. Such vaccines could be made of virally and UV light-induced tumors, and sometimes also from chemically induced tumors, but generally not from spontaneous tumors. Consequently, a tumor is denominated "immunogenic" if vaccination leads to a 10-fold or even more than 100-fold increase in the minimum number of cells necessary to obtain a successful transplantation of a tumor. Obviously in those cases the vaccination evoked a stronger immune response than the growing tumor could by itself. A good tumor transplantation immunity appeared often to be dependent on the use of a proper adjuvant with which the inactivated tumor cells had to be admixed. Bacillus Calmette-Guerin (BCG) is renowned in this respect. As mentioned, it also became clear that only relatively small amounts of tumor cells could be rejected by an optimally immunized animal. For these reasons it was hoped that in humans, particularly in an adjuvant setting shortly after radical surgery, vaccination with autologous or allogeneic tumor cells of the same histological type would force the immune apparatus to kill residual tumor cells that would otherwise have grown out into metastases.

Clinical experiments were, in particular, carried out in patients with tumors such as melanoma and renal cancer, where the occasional occurrence of spontaneous regression of primary tumors or of metastases had raised the conjecture that natural immune responses were already in action, the more so since in some rare instances transfusion of blood plasma of such patients had caused regression of metastases in other patients with similar disease (Sumner and Foraker 1960; Hvidt and Hippe 1976). Seigler et al. (1979) vaccinated 719 primary melanoma patients with neuraminidase-treated autologous or allogeneic melanoma cells together with BCG as an adjuvant to surgery: they obtained a 5-year survival rate of 80% in patients with melanomas thicker than 1.5 mm, which seems better than historical control data from other institutions (Balch and Hersey 1985). With a Newcastle disease virus oncolysate, repeatedly vaccinated patients operated for regional lymph node metastases had an excellent prognosis, with nearly 90% still alive after 3 years (Cassel et al. 1983). Injection of irradiated allogeneic melanoma cells by the intralymphatic route in 34 patients, who received this treatment as the first-line therapy for distant metastases, resulted in two complete responses (CR) and seven partial responses (PR) (Weisenburger et al. 1982). A polyvalent melanoma antigen vaccine was used to immunize 19 patients with metastative disease. One patient with cutaneous metastases had a CR (35 + months), and in two others progression was slowed down (Bystryn et al. 1988). Intralesional injection of BCG in superficial metastases probably represents the most frequent topical or intralesional method of treating metastases. Theoretically, regression of locally treated metastases may lead to a systemic immune response. From a review of 14 publications it was concluded that 66% of 127 injected nodules may disappear, but remarkably so did 21% of 120 uninjected metastases, indicating that regression induced by intralesional BCG may indeed lead to a systemic response (Mastrangelo et al. 1982). Primary melanomas have been treated with vaccinia virus (Hunter-Craig et al. 1970; Everall et al. 1975) and with the hapten dinitrochlorobenzene (DNCB) (Illig et al. 1984). The prognosis of these patients seemed at least to be as good as that after conventional surgery, suggesting that an immune response had been induced.

Spontaneous regression of metastases of renal carcinoma after nephrectomy has been well documented, but the frequency is as low as 0.8% (Fairlamb 1982). Although there is no firm evidence that host immunity is the cause of these regressions, a number of trials were designed to investigate whether nonspecific as well as specific immunotherapy or adoptive immunotherapy could induce regression of metastases, particularly in the lung. The clinical results of various studies were reviewed by McCune (1983). With BCG as the only immunostimulator and with strict clinical criteria, in 20 patients only one partial responder was seen. Adoptive immunotherapy was carried out by preparing RNA of spleen and lymphoid tissue of animals immunized with the patient's tumor and either injecting this immune RNA directly intracutaneously into the patient or reinfusing the autologous lymphocytes after incubation with the immune RNA. In the latter case one CR and one PR of 18 and 8 months duration respectively were seen in six patients. So-called specific active immunotherapy has been performed with the use of autologous renal cancer cells mixed with various adjuvants in order to potentiate cellular immune responses to the tumor cells. Among 130 patients in five studies, 23 (18%) were claimed to respond, including some complete regressions (Tykkä et al. 1978; McCune et al. 1981; Prager et al. 1981; Neidhart et al. 1983; Kurth et al. 1987). In a recent pilot study on the use of cyclophosphamide to modulate the immune response 24 h prior to vaccination, five out of 20 evaluable patients (25%) showed a response, in one case complete. In all five there was regression of lung metastases (Sahasrabudhe et al. 1986).

Although colorectal cancer is not a malignancy known for spontaneous regressions, guinea pig models had shown that immunization with irradiated autologous tumor cells together with BCG could induce an effective immune response. Recently a prospective trial was started in which patients undergoing surgical resection are randomized either to serve as controls or to receive postoperative immunization using irradiated autologous tumor cells mixed with 10^7 BCG organisms at weekly intervals for 3 weeks. Two-thirds of the immunized patients developed a delayed type of hypersensitivity to the vaccine and a preliminary report of the study showed that during follow-up of 2–3 years recurrences occurred in only three of the 20 patients who had been immunized, none of whom had died, whereas in the 20 controls there were nine recurrences and four of these patients had died (Hoover al al. 1985). Six years after this trial started 62 patients had been randomized. With a median postoperative follow-up of 45 months there were 13 recurrences and seven deaths in the 30 control patients versus seven recurrences and two deaths in the 32 immunized patients. Moreover, 10/13 of the recurrences in the control group were diffuse and not resectable, while 5/7 of the recurrences in the immunized group were focal and surgically resectable. These interesting results will be checked in a multi-institutional phase III trial in a larger number of patients (Hanna et al. 1988).

In superficial bladder cancer, several studies have now shown that instillations of BCG into the bladder are effective in eliminating and reducing the frequency of superficial tumors (Shapiro et al. 1982; Brosman 1984; Martinez-Pineiro 1984; Pinsky et al. 1985). Since dermal scarification and oral BCG is less effective or even has no effect at all, it is likely that the contact of BCG with tumor cells in the bladder is an important factor in the induction of the supposed immunological mechanism responsible for the eradication of tumor cells or their precursors. There is evidence that intravesical BCG is as effective as, or even more effective than, various single chemotherapeutical agents (Anonymous 1988).

Although the studies in melanoma, renal cancer, colorectal cancer and superficial bladder cancer may have suggested that a specific immune response was provoked and that to a certain extent this gave protection to the patient against the outgrowth of micrometastases, or even caused regression of metastases, in none of these studies was there actual proof of a specific immune response. Antibodies to the tumor cells have not been found, nor has a specific cellular immune reactivity been detected in relation to the vaccination. Also, in randomized trials with a sufficiently great number of patients, no beneficial effect has yet been proved.

So far, from a molecular point of view, the vaccines have not been characterized. Now that monoclonal antibodies have become available and the characterization of membrane antigens of tumor cells has become possible, it can be expected that pure antigenic fractions will in the future be prepared on a scale that will permit immunization experiments. It will then become easier to measure the cellular and humoral responses of the immunized patient to the defined molecules. Monitoring of the immune response to defined vaccines is mandatory in order to gain insight into the immunogenicity of the tumor-associated antigen and the role that the particular immune response may play in the tumor-host relationship.

Inhibition of the Suppression of Tumor Immune Responses

In several animal models tumor-related immune responses are inhibited by suppressor cells which are activated during tumor progression. Even immunostimulators such as BCG and *Corynebacterium parvum* may generate suppressor cells (Klimpel and Henney 1978; Klimpel et al. 1979; Neta and Slavin 1979). Suppressor cell activity has also been demonstrated in patients with various forms of cancer. For instance, in patients with primary or regionally metastatic melanoma, suppressor T cell activity was associated with tumor growth (Werkmeister et al. 1980). Suppressor T cells can be activated by prostaglandins produced by macrophages or monocytes. This activation can be inhibited by drugs, such as indomethacin, which inhibits prostaglandin synthesis, cimetidine, which blocks the H2 receptors of the suppressor T cells, and cyclophosphamide. It is the latter chemotherapeutic agent that has been extensively studied in regard to the potentiation of immune responsiveness. By its effect on suppressor T cells, if administered in low dosage before vaccination, it may facilitate the development of cytotoxic T cells, and can therefore augment the generation of humoral and cellular immune responses. In one study 19 metastatic melanoma patients were treated with an autologous melanoma cell vaccine, either alone or 3 days after the administration of 300 mg/m^2 cyclophosphamide. Seven of the eight pretreated patients and only two of the seven patients treated with the vaccine alone developed a delayed type of hypersensitivity to the vaccine, and in two of the pretreated patients metastases disappeared completely (Berd et al. 1986). Also other cytostatic drugs may augment, rather than suppress, immune responses if administered in the proper dosages before vaccination (Mastrangelo et al. 1986). For these reasons, it can be expected that in future vaccination studies immuno-augmenting substances such as low-dose chemotherapeutic drugs and other pharmacological agents will be included.

Immunotherapy with Natural Immunomodulators

Interferons

Interferons (IFNs) are natural substances, originally described as antiviral proteins, that are induced by viral infections in various hematopoietic cells and fibroblasts. They appear to play a complex role in the immune responses, also against tumors. In vitro, IFN-alpha is mainly induced by viruses or synthetic polyribonucleotides in leukocytes or lymphoblastoid cell lines, and IFN-beta in fibroblasts. IFN-gamma is induced by stimulation with mitogens and antigens. All classes of IFN exhibit antiviral, immunomodulatory and antiproliferative activities. In vitro (and in vivo) production of IFNs can be stimulated by a variety of agents, such as bacterial and fungal extracts, mitogens, and antigens. Many of these have already been tested in clinical trials. These stimulants may also induce other substances, such as tumor necrosis factor, colony-stimulating factor and lymphotoxins, so that crude interferon extracts are possibly contaminated with other biologically active substances.

Recently, bulk production of relatively pure IFN preparations was made possible by DNA recombinant technology. Particularly, recombinant IFN-alpha became available for large clinical trials. The in vivo effects of treatment with IFN-alpha on the immune functions are complex. Depending on the dose, functions such as natural killer (NK) cell activity can be enhanced as well as decreased. Many trials have shown that occasionally patients with various sorts of tumors may show tumor regression. No clear correlation between clinical responses and changes in immunological functions have been found so far. An optimum dose for obtaining clinical responses is difficult to establish. In some studies it has been revealed that higher response rates could be achieved with higher doses. From other studies it appeared that it may take a relatively long time before responses to low dosages become evident, leaving the role of early dose escalation doubtful. Such escalation is clearly justified only when there is progression of disease. With the higher dosages toxicity can be severe, with fever, malaise, and flu-like symptoms being the most common side effects. Consistent therapeutic effects of various leukocytic or recombinant IFNs have been observed in the following malignancies (response rates in brackets): hairy cell leukemia (50%–75%) (Annotation, Lancet 1985), non-Hodgkin's lymphoma with prognostically favorable histology (30%–50%) (Foon et al. 1986), AIDS-related Kaposi's sarcoma (25%–60%) (Abrams and Volberding 1986), Philadelphia chromosome-positive chronic myelogenous leukemia (75%) (Talpaz et al. 1986), multiple myeloma (15%) (Quesada et al. 1986), cutaneous T-cell lymphoma (45%) (Bunn and Foon 1985), endocrine pancreatic cancer (75%) (Eriksson et al. 1986), renal carcinoma (15%) (Krown 1985) and melanoma (15%) (Kirkwood and Ernstoff 1986). The long and impressive improvements seen particularly in hairy-cell leukemia and in Philadelphia-positive CML make the IFNs the first-choice single agents in these diseases.

Illustrative of the different mechanisms by which the IFNs may act is that for some of the malignancies (hairy cell leukemia, CML and endocrine pancreatic cancer) relatively low doses seem to be sufficient to induce a remission, while in others (non-Hodgkin's lymphoma, Kaposi's sarcoma, cutaneous T-cell lymphoma, renal cancer and multiple myeloma) higher doses are required. Responses are also seen in patients heavily pretreated with chemotherapeutic agents.

Animal work shows that interferons may potentiate the effects of chemotherapeutic agents. Several clinical studies are underway to investigate for which human malignancies this might also be true. In addition, adjuvant trials are expected to be initiated in the near future. The difficulty remains, however, that optimal dosages are not yet known, and that side effects can be such that it is not ethically advisable to submit surgically treated patients to long periods of therapy involving constitutional side effects without certainty of the presence of residual tumor. The major obstacle in deciding which IFN in which dosage scheme is the most effective for a particular tumor is that the working mechanism of each situation may be entirely different. NK cell activity, antiproliferative activity, modulatory effects in the immune response, direct modulatory effect on the membrane of the tumor cell (so that its antigenic make-up changes, e.g., induction of transplantation antigens) and differentiation may all be involved in different proportions in different tumors.

Combinations of IFNs with other IFNs and other biological response modifiers such as tumor necrosis factor have shown synergistic activities in vitro or in animal models, warranting combination biological response modifier therapies in patients. IFNs have been shown to act as radiosensitizers, but radiation damage to normal tissue may also be enhanced (Real et al. 1985).

Interleukin-2 and Activated Killer Cells

Interleukins and other lymphokines are, like the IFNs, components of culture supernatants having effects on other cell systems. Some of them are now well characterized and have well-defined functions which have already been used in the immune manipulation of cancer patients. One of the most promising agents in immunotherapy is interleukin-2 (IL-2). IL-2 was originally known as "T-cell growth factor", since it had the capacity of maintaining clones of antigen-activated T cells in culture. IL-2 boosts the generation of antigen-specific cytotoxic T cells, but also augments NK cell activity and reverses the immune suppression induced by glycocorticosteroids. Indirectly, by its effect on T cells which are in turn producing yet other lymphokines, it enhances antibody secretion. Tumor-specific cytotoxic T cells cultured by virtue of the activity of IL-2 were shown to have therapeutic effects after adoptive transfer in tumor-bearing mice. With the cloning of the human IL-2 gene in early 1983, large-scale production of IL-2 became possible. IL-2 as a single agent has not yet been shown to be an effective anticancer drug, but it may hold promise as a reagent that can overcome immune suppression induced by chemotherapeutic agents.

A successful preliminary clinical application of IL-2 has recently attracted worldwide attention (Rosenberg et al. 1985). Leukophoresed patients were reinfused with their own leukocytes in conjunction with IL-2 after the leukocytes had been activated in vitro by coculturing with IL-2 for 3 days. The lymphokine-activated killer (LAK) cells are lymphoid cells with the ability to lyse fresh, noncultured, NK-resistant tumor cells in short-term chromium release assays. These LAK cells killed cancer cells but not normal cells, such as lymphocytes, liver or lung cells. Successful adoptive immunotherapy using LAK cells was possible in a variety of murine tumor models, provided that IL-2 was administered simultaneously. The LAK cells proliferated in the tumor-bearing hosts with retention of antitumor activity, but only in the presence of IL-2. Although in experimental animals IL-2 alone also generated LAK cells in vivo and mediated antitumor effects, optimal therapeutic effects were only achieved when the combination was given and when relatively large amounts were used. Updated results (Rosenberg 1988) show that the combined therapy is effective in renal cancer (CR 7/54, PR 10/54), melanoma (CR 3/34, PR 3/34) and marginally in colon cancer (CR 1/27, PR 2/27). With IL-2 alone effectivity was less, renal cancer being the only malignancy where CRs (4/38) were seen. Since tumor-infiltrating lymphocytes (TIL) isolated from metastases appeared 50–100 times more effective than LAK cells, a pilot study was conducted in which TIL instead of LAK cells together with IL-2 was administered to 12 patients (six with melanoma, four with renal cancer, one with breast cancer and one with colon cancer), but only two PRs were observed (Topalian et al. 1988). The toxicity appeared to be high, with water retention especially being a major problem and requiring intensive care. Studies of less toxic regimens with LAK cells (e.g., intraarterial or intraperitoneal) and IL-2 are now being conducted.

Other Cytokines

Many other cytokines, i.e., substances possessing immunoregulatory properties, have been characterized. The lymphokines are products of activated lymphocytes. In addition to the IFNs and IL-2, this group includes lymphotoxins, thymosins, macrophage-activating factor, migration-inhibition factor, tumor necrosis factor, interleukin-3, colony-stimulating factor and B-cell growth factor have to be mentioned. The monokines, secreted by macrophages, comprise interleukin-1, lymphocyte-activating factor, colony-stimulating factor, prostaglandin E and also interferons, tumor necrosis factor and B-cell growth factor. Except for those described above, no promising preliminary clinical results with any of these drugs have yet been published. Trials with tumor necrosis factor are underway.

Monoclonal Antibodies

A growing number of publications are appearing on applications of murine and recently also human monoclonal antibodies (mabs) against components of the membrane or the cytoplasm of human tumor cells. Numerous mabs have already been applied to identify and characterize tumor-associated antigens, not only in a biochemical sense but also from a functional point of view. These tumor-associated antigens are often characterized as differentiation antigens, oncofetal antigens and oncogene products. Functionally they may be receptors for growth factors, precursors of products to be secreted by the mature cell of the same lineage or they may be involved in adhesion between the cells and various substrates. Generally these antigens are not specific for tumor cells but occur also on their normal counterparts. Those antigens found in much higher density on the surface of tumor cells than on normal cells are the potential targets for immunotherapy with mabs. Ideally, these mabs should be directed at specific tumor antigens, but since the effectiveness of mabs may well depend on the amount of antibody bound by the cell, it is not an absolute prerequisite that the antibody never binds to a normal cell. Even if normal counterparts (for instance normal B or T cells in the case of leukemic cells) are equally destroyed as a result of a mab directed against a differentiation antigen, as long as the precursors of these cells do not express the differentiation antigen, recruitment of normal cells remains possible. This is comparable to the problems encountered with chemotherapy.

Several of the mabs directed against tumor-associated antigens have already found routine clinical application either in the immunohistological diagnosis of malignancies or in the follow-up of patients during and after treatment by assaying these antigens in the serum in case they are secreted or shed by the tumor cells. Carcinoembryonic antigen is an example of a marker widely used in clinical practice. For immunotherapeutic purposes the application of mabs is still in a stage of clinical pilot research.

In animal models, particularly in immunodeprived mice transplanted with human tumor xenografts, it has been shown that unmodified mabs and mabs conjugated with radio-isotopes, cytostatic drugs, plant toxins and biological response modifiers can suppress the growth of the tumors or even eradicate them.

In clinical trials, it has been shown, by biopsy of metastases, that intravenously administered mabs can accumulate in the metastases. Particularly when the mabs are of the IgG2a or IgG3 isotype, they are able to activate human complement and can activate antibody-dependent cellular cytotoxicity. In this case biopsies show evidence of inflammation, complement deposition and lymphocyte infiltration. Binding of antibodies in metastases has also been demonstrated by gamma camera imaging of mabs or their Fab fragments labeled with radio-isotopes. Considerable "background" uptake, particularly by liver and spleen, of radiolabeled mabs is often an obstacle for therapeutic application of conjugated mabs. Trials with unmodified mabs have been carried out in some human models. Patients with T-cell leukemias and lymphomas were infused with mabs against T cell antigens which are also present on normal T cells. Although tumor cell binding was demonstrated and lymphocyte counts dropped transiently in many leukemic patients, no significant sustained responses were reported (Levy et al. 1983; Foon et al. 1984; Dillman et al. 1985). Patients with B-cell lymphomas have been treated with mabs against the idiotype of the immunoglobulin expressed on the surface of the lymphoma cells. The immunoglobulin molecule has a specific configuration which allows the immunoglobulin to react with only one particular antigen and not with others. This antigen-binding site makes the immunoglobulin an antibody with defined specificity. This part of the molecule can, by itself, function as an antigen to which antibodies can be made; it is then called the idiotype. Antibodies against the idiotype are only reactive with this particular immunoglobulin molecule. Since no other lymphocytes express that idiotype, the particular idiotype of the lymphoma cells can be considered as a completely specific tumor marker. Of 11 lymphoma patients treated with anti-idiotype mabs, one has achieved a complete remission, already lasting for 5 years, while five others had partial remissions of shorter duration (1–6 months) (Meeker et al. 1985).

Administration of unconjugated monoclonal antibodies has also induced tumor regression in some patients with melanoma (Houghton et al. 1985; Cheung et al. 1987), neuroblastoma (Cheung et al. 1987) and colon carcinoma (Sears et al. 1985).

Although a few responses were observed in these studies, it is clear that passive immunotherapy with single mabs does not have much future. Several reasons for the failure of single-mab therapy have to be considered:

1. It has to be remembered that an antibody molecule itself will never kill a cell. If cell kill is the aim, it can only be by the triggering of effector mechanisms such as those mentioned above – antibody-mediated cellular cytotoxicity and complement lysis. For these mechanisms to be activated, only certain subclasses of mabs (such as mouse IgG2a and IgG3) are appropriate. Moreover, these mechanisms, particularly the cellular-mediated cytotoxicity, are limited in their capacities and can easily be exhausted, so that large numbers of tumor cells, albeit coated with mab, will not be destroyed.
2. The expression of the tumor-associated antigens to which the mabs are directed may vary. Even within

one tumor, immunohistological investigations have shown that seldom do all cells express the antigen to the same extent. Antigen-positive and antigen-negative tumor cells can even be found adjacent to each other. It is therefore likely that even with highly effective mabs, selective outgrowth of cell clones lacking the particular antigen will take place.
3. Some of the antigens can be stripped off the tumor cells by the antibody without interfering with the life of the cell. This phenomenon, called modulation, leads to the formation of immune complexes which are either internalized in the cell or expelled from it.
4. The mabs, being of murine origin, may induce the formation of antibodies to the foreign immunoglobulin. These antibodies can be directed against the binding site (idiotype) of the mabs so that binding of the mabs to the target cells becomes impossible. Moreover, the formation of immune complexes may in rare cases give rise to untoward side effects such as are also observed in serum sickness. On the other hand, if a T cell response develops against the mouse mab, this may be beneficial. These T cells may kill target cells coated with the mab (Lanzavecchia et al. 1988).
5. Some tumor-associated antigens are shed or secreted by the tumor cells. If the amounts are low, this is not a problem. The mabs may even coat the tumor cells before all free circulating antigen is removed. But if these levels are relatively high, substantial amounts of the infused mab are bound to free antigen. The immune complexes so formed are removed by the mononuclear phagocytic system and may therefore exhaust the cell systems necessary for the immune destruction of the coated tumor cells.

A number of the problems discussed so far can probably be solved. Heterogeneity and modulation of the expression of tumor-associated antigens requires the application of cocktails of mabs directed against different antigens. Not only would more malignant cells be reached, but also more antibody molecule per tumor cell would be bound. Also it is conceivable that the expression of the antigens can be enhanced by drugs such as the IFNs. It has been shown that IFN-alpha increases the expression of tumor-associated antigens recognized by specific mabs on breast and colon carcinoma cells (Greiner et al. 1984, 1985) and on melanoma (Rosenblum et al. 1988). Host mechanisms of immunodestruction may be activated by lymphokines such as the IFNs and interleukins. LAK cells administered simultaneously with mabs (the LAK cells having the appropriate receptor for the Tc part of the antibody molecule) will act synergistically. In nude mice it has been shown that human melanoma xenografts can be eradicated when mabs and killer cells are injected together (Schulz et al. 1985).

In several in vitro and animal models, great effort have been exerted to use mabs to target cytotoxic agents, such as radio-isotopes and cytostatic drugs, or biological response modifiers to the tumor cells. A major problem with the application of these conjugates is formed by the decreases in specificity and affinity of the antibodies and in activity of the drug which result from the conjugation. Antibodies partly denatured or altered by the conjugation will to a great extent be removed by the liver and spleen, so that too much of the radiation is delivered at these sites. In spite of these difficulties, some recent pilot studies have shown that this approach is possible. Tumor regression has been seen in patients with lymphoma, melanoma and colon cancer (Larson 1987), as well as in patients with leptomeningeal tumors where radiolabeled monoclonal antibodies were administered into the subarachnoid space (Lashford et al. 1988).

Conclusion

In the past two decades many, mainly adjuvant, studies have shown that immunotherapy in the form of nonspecific stimulation of the immune response has little effect on the prognosis of cancer patients in general. However, in some human tumor models, such as melanoma and renal cancer, some hope remains that vaccination procedures may improve the prognosis of patients with a low tumor burden. A better characterization of the membrane substances of these tumors is needed as well as their large-scale production, in order to investigate whether a specific immune response can be enhanced and whether this indeed improves the prognosis. The role of immune suppression and the inhibition of suppressor functions need further study in relation to vaccination experiments.

New biotechnological developments, i.e., recombinant DNA and hybridoma technology, have enabled the large-scale production of lymphokines, monokines and monoclonal antibodies. With these agents, new opportunities to manipulate the immune response – specific and nonspecific – to tumor cells and to directly influence the proliferation, differentiation and expression of oncogenes of tumor cells are opened up. A new area of biological response modifier research has begun. A single very significant first step has been made: hairy-cell leukemia can be treated better with IFN than with any other agent. Selection of the best combinations of biological response modifiers, including combinations with conventional therapies and the use of conjugated monoclonal antibodies, for different types and stages of malignancies will take time but will eventually lead to at least some improvement in cancer therapy.

References

Abrams DI, Volberding PA (1986) Alpha interferon therapy of AIDS-associated Kaposi's sarcoma. Semin Oncol 13 [Suppl 2]: 43–47

Annotation (1985) Treatment of hairy cell leukaemia. Lancet 2: 1282–1283

Anonymous (1988) Diagnostic and Therapeutic Technology Assessment (DATTA). JAMA 259: 2153–2155

Balch CM, Hersey P (1985) Current status of adjuvant immunotherapy. In: Balch CM, Milton GW (eds) Cutaneous melanoma. Clinical management and treatment results worldwide. Lippincott, Philadelphia, p 197

Berd D, Maguire HC Jr, Mastrangelo MJ (1986) Induction of cell-mediated immunity to autologous melanoma cells and regression of metastases after treatment with a melanoma cell vaccine preceded by cyclophosphamide. Cancer Res 46: 2572–2577

Brosman SA (1984) BCG in the management of superficial bladder cancer. Urology 23 [Suppl]: 82

Bunn Jr PA, Foon KA (1985) Therapeutic options in advanced cutaneous T cell lymphomas: a role for interferon alfa-2a (Roferon®-A). Semin Oncol 12 [Suppl 5]: 18–24

Bystryn JC, Oratz R, Harris MN, Roses DF, Golomb FM, Speyer JL (1988) Immunogenicity of a polyvalent melanoma antigen vaccine in humans. Cancer 61: 1065–1070

Cassel WA, Murray DR, Phillips HS (1983) A phase II study on the post-surgical management of stage II malignant melanoma with a Newcastle disease virus oncolysate. Cancer 52: 856

Cheung NV, Lazarus H, Miraldi FD, Abramowsky CR, Kallick S, Saarinen UM, Spitzer T, Strandjord SE, Coccia PF, Berger NA (1987) Ganglioside GD2 specific monoclonal antibody 3F8: a phase I study in patients with neuroblastoma and malignant melanoma. J Clin Oncol 5: 1430–1440

Dillman RO, Shawler DL, Dillman JB et al. (1985) Monoclonal antibody in patients with chronic lymphocytic leukemia and cutaneous T cell lymphoma. J Cell Biochem [Suppl] 9A: 108

Eriksson B, Alm G, Lundquist G, Wilander E, Oberg K, Karlsson A, Andersson T, Wide L (1986) Treatment of malignant endocrine pancreatic tumours with human leucocyte interferon. Lancet 2: 1307–1308

Everall JD, Ward J, O'Doherty CJ, Dowd PM (1975) Treatment of primary melanoma by intralesional vaccinia before excision. Lancet 2: 583–586

Fairlamb DJ (1982) Spontaneous regression of metastases of renal cancer. Cancer 47: 2102

Foon KA, Schroff RW, Bunn PA et al. (1984) Effects of monoclonal antibody therapy in patients with chronic lymphocytic leukemia. Blood 64: 1085–1093

Foon KA, Roth MS, Bunn Jr PA (1986) Alpha interferon treatment of low-grade B-cell non-Hodgkin's lymphomas, cutaneous T-cell lymphomas, and chronic lymphocytic leukemia. Semin Oncol 13 [Suppl 2]: 35–42

Greiner JW, Horan Hand P, Noguchi P, Fisher P, Pestka S, Schlom J (1984) Enhanced expression of surface tumor associated antigens on human breast and colon tumor cells after recombinant leukocyte α-interferon treatment. Cancer Res 44: 3208–3214

Greiner JW, Tobi M, Fisher PB, Langer JA, Pestka S (1985) Differential responsiveness of cloned mammary carcinoma cell populations to the human recombinant leukocyte interferon enhancement of tumor antigen expression. Int J Cancer 36: 159–166

Hanna MG, Hoover HC, Peters LC, Key ME, Haspel MV, McCabe RP, Pomato N (1988) Fundamental and applied aspects of successful active specific immunotherapy of cancer. In: Oldham R (ed) Cancer biotherapy: principles and practice. Raven, New York, pp 195–222

Hoover HC, Surdyke MG, Dangel RB, Peters LC, Hanna Jr MG (1985) Prospectively randomized trial of adjuvant active-specific immunotherapy for human colorectal cancer. Cancer 55: 1236–1243

Houghton AN, Mintzer D, Cordon-Cardo S et al. (1985) Mouse monoclonal IgG3 antibody detecting GD3 ganglioside: A phase I trial in patients with malignant melanoma. Proc Natl Acad Sci USA 82: 1242

Hunter-Craig I, Newton KA, Westbury G, Lacey BW (1970) Use of vaccinia virus in the treatment of metastatic malignant melanoma. Br Med J 2: 512–515

Hvidt V, Hippe E (1976) Regressor plasma treatment of patients with advanced kidney tumors. Scand J Urol Nephrol 33 [Suppl]: 17

Illig L, Paul E, Bodeker RH (1984) Epifocal dinitrochlorobenzene therapy in malignant melanoma (experience during the last eight years). Anticancer Res 4: 293

Kirkwood JM, Ernstoff M (1986) Potential applications of the interferons in oncology: lessons drawn from studies of human melanoma. Semin Oncol 13 [Suppl 2]: 48–56

Klimpel G, Henney CS (1978) BCG-induced suppressor cells. I. Demonstration of a macrophage-like suppressor cell that inhibits cytotoxic T-cell generation in vitro. J Immunol 120: 563–570

Klimpel GR, Okada M, Henney CS (1979) Inhibition of in vitro cytotoxic responses by BCG-induced macrophage-like suppressor cells. II. Suppression occurs at the level of "helper" T cell. J Immunol 123: 350–357

Krown SE (1985) Therapeutic options in renal-cell carcinoma. Semin Oncol 12 [Suppl 5]: 13–17

Kurth KH, Marquet R, Zwartendijk J, Warnaar SO (1987) Autologous anticancer antigen preparation for specific immunotherapy in advanced renal cell carcinoma. Eur Urol 13: 103–109

Lanzavecchia A, Abrignani S, Scheidegger D, Obrist R, Dorken B, Moldenhauer G (1988) Antibodies as antigens: the use of mouse monoclonal antibodies to focus human T cells against selected targets. J Exp Med 167: 345–352

Larson ML (1987) Lymphoma, melanoma, colon cancer: diagnosis and treatment with radiolabeled monoclonal antibodies. Radiology 165: 297–304

Lashford LS, Davies AG, Richardson RB, Bourne SP, Bullimore JA, Eckert H, Kemshead JT, Coakham HB (1988) A pilot study of 131 I monoclonal antibodies in the therapy of lipomeningeal tumors. Cancer 61: 857–868

Levy R, Miller RA, Stratte PT et al. (1983) Therapeutic trials of monoclonal antibody in leukemia and lymphoma: biologic considerations: In: Boss BD, Langman R, Trowbridge I et al. (eds) Monoclonal antibodies and cancer. Academic, Orlando, Fl, pp 5–16

Martinez-Pineiro JA (1984) BCG vaccine in superficial bladder tumours: eight years later. Eur Urol 10: 93

Mastrangelo MJ, Rosenberg SA, Baker AR et al. (1982) Cutaneous melanoma. In: De Vita VT Jr, Hellman S, Rosenberg SA (eds) Cancer. Principles and practice of oncology, chap 31. Lippincott, Philadelphia, p 1124

Mastrangelo MJ, Berd D, Maguire H Jr (1986) The immunoaugmenting effects of cancer chemotherapeutic agents. Semin Oncol 13 [Suppl 2]: 186–194

McCune CS (1983) Immunologic therapies of kidney carcinoma. Semin Oncol 10: 431–436

McCune CS, Schapira DV, Henshaw EC (1981) Specific immunotherapy of advanced renal carcinoma: evidence for the polyclonality of metastases. Cancer 47: 1984

Meeker TC, Lowder J, Maloney DG et al. (1985) A clinical trial of anti-idiotype therapy for B cell malignancy. Blood 65: 1349–1363

Neidhart JA, Gagen M, Young D et al. (1983) A randomized study of polymerized tumor antigen admixed with adjuvant (PTA) for therapy of renal cancer. Proc Am Soc Clin Oncol 2: 49

Neta R, Slavin SB (1979) Adjuvants in the induction of suppressor cells. Infect Immunol 23: 360–365

Pinsky CM, Camacho FJ, Kerr D et al. (1985) Intravesical administration of Bacillus Calmette Guerin in patients with recurrent superficial carcinoma of the urinary bladder: report of prospective, randomized trial. Cancer Treat Rep 69: 47–53

Prager MD, Baechtel FS, Peters PC et al. (1981) Specific immunotherapy of human metastatic renal cell carcinoma. Proc Am Assoc Cancer Res 22: 163

Quesada JR, Alexanian R, Hawkins M, Barlogie B, Borden E, Itri L, Gutterman JU (1986) Treatment of multiple myeloma with recombinant alpha-interferon. Blood 67: 275–278

Real FX, Krown SE, Nisce LZ et al. (1985) Unexpected toxicity from radiation therapy in two patients with Kaposi's sarcoma receiving interferon. J Biol Response Mod 4: 141–146

Rosenberg SA (1988) Immunotherapy of cancer using interleukin 2: current status and future prospects. Immunol Today 9: 58–62

Rosenberg SA, Lotze MT, Muul LM et al. (1985) Observations on the systemic administration of autologous lymphokine-activated killer cells and recombinant interleukin-2 to patients with metastatic cancer. N Engl J Med 313: 1485

Rosenblum MG, Lamki LM, Murray JL, Carlo DJ, Gutterman JU (1988) Interferon-induced changes in pharmacokinetics and tumor uptake of 111 In-labeled antimelanoma antibody 96.5 in melanoma patients. J Natl Cancer Inst 80: 160–165

Sahasrabudhe DM, deKernion JB, Pontes JE, Ryan DM, O'Donnel RW, Marquis DM, Mudholkar GS, McCune CS (1986) Specific immunotherapy with suppressor function inhibition for metastatic renal cell carcinoma. J Biol Response Mod 5: 581–594

Schulz G, Staffileno LK, Reisfeld RA et al. (1985) Eradication of established human melanoma tumors in nude mice by antibody-directed effector cells. J Exp Med 161: 1315–1325

Sears HF, Herlyn D, Steplewski Z, Koprowski H (1985) Phase II clinical trial of a murine monoclonal antibody cytotoxic for gastrointestinal adenocarcinoma. Cancer Res 45: 5910–5912

Seigler HF, Cox E, Mutzner F et al. (1979) Specific active immunotherapy for melanoma. Ann Surg 190: 366

Shapiro A, Kadmon D, Catalona WJ et al. (1982) Immunotherapy of superficial bladder cancer. J Urol 128: 891

Sumner WC, Foraker AG (1960) Spontaneous regression of human melanoma. Cancer 13: 79

Talpaz M, Kantarjian HM, McCredie K, Trujillo JM, Keating MJ, Gutterman JU (1986) Hematologic remission and cytogenetic improvement induced by recombinant human interferon alpha in chronic myelogenous leukemia. N Engl J Med 314: 1065–1069

Topalian SL, Solomon D, Avis FP, Chang AE, Freerksen DL, Linehan WM, Lotze MT, Robertson CN, Seipp CA, Simon P, Simpson CG, Rosenberg SA (1988) Immunotherapy of patients with advanced cancer using tumor-infiltrating lymphocytes and recombinant interleukin-2: a pilot study. J Clin Oncol 6: 839–853

Tykkä J, Oravisto KJ, Lehtonen T et al. (1978) Active specific immunotherapy of advanced renal cell carcinoma. Eur Urol 4: 250

Weisenburger TH, Jones PC, Ahn SS et al. (1982) Active specific intralymphatic immunotherapy in metastatic melanoma: evidence of clinical response. J Biol Response Mod 1: 57

Werkmeister J, Zaunders J, McCarthy WH et al. (1980) Characterization of an inhibitor of cell division in tumour cell cultures. Clin Exp Immunol 41: 487

Transplantation and Cancer

H. Pichlmaier and R. Grundmann

Association of cancer with transplantation may be seen in three situations:

1. The graft recipient is prone to development of de novo malignancies as a consequence of immunosuppression.
2. Patients who have been treated previously for cancer may plan to undergo transplantation (tumor patient as graft recipient). In this situtation the question arises whether or not the subsequent immunosuppression would promote tumor recurrence.
3. Malignancies arising in the organ itself or metastatically from other sites may be transplanted accidentally with the homograft (tumor patient as organ donor).

Malignant Diseases in Uremic Patients Treated by Dialysis

Even without renal transplantation, uremic patients are predisposed per se to malignant diseases: Matas et al. (1975) found a sevenfold higher incidence of neoplasms in patients with chronic renal failure than in the normal population, a result corresponding to the findings of Miach et al. (1976) but not confirmed by Slifkin et al. (1977).

Jacobs et al. (1981) reported tumor incidence of 8.5 per 1000 patients on dialysis treatment. They considered this risk to be acceptable when compared to the annual incidence rate in the general population of the USA, which is estimated as 3.6 per 1000. The higher incidence of cancer in uremic patients was attributed to the fact that these patients were older than those of the control group, illustrating the predominant influence of age on the tumor incidence.

These figures exemplify the increased risk of malignant disease in uremic patients, but nevertheless cancer is not a major cause of death in these patients. Siemensen et al. (1984) point out that 35% of all patients on dialysis die of cardiovascular diseases and a further 23% of cerebrovascular diseases. In contrast, death due to cancer occurred in only 11% of all patients, mainly in those of more advanced age. Furthermore, when those malignancies that were actually the cause of the terminal renal failure, such as myeloma and tumors of the kidney, were excluded from the calculation, the cancer death rate in uremic patients differed little from that in the general population, 5.6 per 1000 vs 4.4 per 1000 (Jacobs et al. 1981).

Cancer after Organ Transplantation

General Tumor Incidence

The cancer incidence in transplant patients treated with immunosuppressive agents varies as a function of geographic factors, the age of the patients, and the length of the observation period. Thus, a comparatively high frequency of tumors compared with the background population six to ninefold increase in risk was reported by Birkeland (1983a), corresponding to an incidence of cancer arising de novo after transplantation ranging from 4% to 7% (Blohmé and Bryngar 1985; Penn 1978, 1984; Sheil 1986). Kramer et al. (1984), on the other hand, found the prevalence of malignancies among patients alive on renal replacement therapy to be independent of the mode of treatment (transplantation or hemodialysis), and Jacobs et al. (1981) reported an even lower annual incidence rate of malignancies in patients with functioning grafts as compared to those on dialysis (4.0 vs 8.5 per 1000 patients), but these populations were not comparable due to the different age distributions.

Altogether, except for skin cancer, the risk of malignancy under immunosuppression can be expected to be rather low. Krueger et al. (1985) found an incidence of 2.5%, corresponding to 0.65 malignancies per 100 cumulative patient years of immunosuppression.

Incidence of Specific Types of Tumors

Tumors arising de novo in transplant patients under immunosuppression show a characteristic distribution: the malignancies over-represented, as compared to the normal population, include carcinoma of the skin and lips (38% of all cancers) (Penn 1984) and lymphomas including Kaposi's sarcoma (18%). Carcinoma of the uterine cervix affected 18% of the women in this series (Penn 1984); however, 77% of these carcinomas were in situ lesions. Other types of tumors seen in disproportionately high incidence are cancers of the vulva and anus (Penn 1986) and nasopharyngeal cancers (Blohmé and Brynger 1985). On the other hand, some of the cancers most commonly seen in the general population, including carcinomas of the lung, prostate, colon and rectum, and female breast, were not more frequent in transplant recipients (Penn 1984).

The risk of some specific types of cancer arising de novo after transplantation is given in Table 1. The incidence of tumors in our own patients is presented in Table 2.

Skin Malignancies

A direct correlation between the intensity of exposure to sunlight and the incidence of skin cancer is seen in the normal population (Boyle et al. 1984). Under immunosuppression this risk increases disproportionately (Hardie et al. 1980). Thus in Sweden the incidence of skin cancer was 3 times higher than in the general population (Blohmé and Larkö 1984), in Minneapolis 7.1 times higher, and in Queensland 20.6 times higher (Hardie et al. 1980). In Queensland a cumulative 44% incidence of skin cancer was calculated for those patients surviving 9 years with functioning grafts (Hardie et al. 1980).

The high incidence of skin cancers causes disagreements regarding the calculation of the overall tumor risk following transplantation. Hardie et al. (1980), for example, reported an overall incidence of cancer of 9.3% in renal transplant recipients; how-

Table 1. Risk of specific cancers after transplantation

Site of cancer	Risk ratio[a]
Colon	3.4
Rectum and anus	2.1
Trachea, bronchus and lung	1.4
Breast (female)	0.9
Vulva and vagina	32.5
Prostate	0.5
Kidney	6.7
Ureter	437.4
Microglioma	>1000
Thyroid	264.5
Non-Hodgkin's lymphoma	10.3
Hodgkin's disease	0
Kaposi's sarcoma	>1000

Modified from Sheil (1986).
[a] Risk ratio is observed cancer/expected cancer.

Table 2. Incidence of cancer in 501 transplant patients (Department of Surgery, University Hospital Cologne, 15.2. 68–31.3. 87)

	Total		Deaths
Skin cancer	3		0
– Squamous cell carcinoma		2	
– Melanoma		1	
Gynecological cancer	2		2
– Vulva		1	
– Cervix		1	
Non-Hodgkin's lymphoma	1		1
Colon cancer	1		1
Nasopharyngeal cancer	1		0
Total	8		4

Median follow-up: 52.2 ± 43.7 months (mean 43 months, range 0–215 months).

ever, this increase was due entirely to the high incidence of skin cancer , which was present in 93% of all cancer patients. Skin cancers following transplantation are predominantly squamous cell carcinomas, in contrast to the situation in the general population, where basal cell carcinomas are 4 times more common than squamous cell carcinomas (Sheil 1986). Squamous cell carcinomas in transplant patients tend to be more aggressive, metastasizing more frequently than skin carcinomas in the general population.

Solid Lymphomas

Lymphomas represent only 3% of the non-skin tumors in the general population but up to 25% to 29% of the non-skin neoplasms found in transplant patients (Jamieson et al. 1981; Penn 1981 b). The most common lymphomas are large cell lymphomas described as "reticulum cell sarcoma" or "microglioma," which account for 55% of these tumors (Penn 1981 b). Also surprisingly frequent Kaposi's sarcoma (16.9% of all lymphomas, Penn 1981 b), which occurs in transplant recipients with an incidence 400- to 500-fold greater than that seen in a control population (Penn 1983 a).

In the general population, Hodgkin's disease is the most common lymphoma in every age group (one-third of all lymphomas), but it accounts for only 3% of the lymphomas seen in organ transplant recipients (Penn 1984). Non-Hodgkin's lymphoma is 45–100 times more common in transplant recipients than in the general population (Penn 1981 b).

A striking feature of the lymphomas following transplantation is their localization: the most common site is the central nervous system, (ca. 40% after transplantation vs < 2% in the general population, Penn 1981 b).

Time of Onset of Cancer Following Transplantation

Treatment by transplantation and immunosuppression is perhaps the most rapidly acting oncogenic influence to which humans have been exposed: the average interval before the appearance of all malignancies is only 4–5 years (Sheil 1986).

Skin Cancer

In Queensland, skin cancer was seen in 3% of all patients only 1 year after successful transplantation, and another 5% developed it during each subsequent year of survival under immunosuppression (Hardie et al. 1980). Although skin cancer may occur as early as 4 months after transplantation (Boyle et al. 1984), in a low ultraviolet radiation area the increased risk will become apparent no earlier than 3–5 years after transplantation (Blohmé and Larkö 1984; Boyle et al. 1984).

Solid Lymphomas

Solid lymphomas may develop as little as 3–6 months after transplant, depending on the type and dosage of immunosuppression (Beveridge et al.

1984; Bia and Flye 1985; Jamieson et al. 1981). The mean time of onset of all mesenchymal tumors was 23.3 months after transplant in the study by Birkeland (1983a), while the data collected by Penn (1981b) reveal an average time of appearance of these malignancies of 28 months after transplantation. Kaposi's sarcoma appeared even more rapidly (16.5 months) (Penn 1983a).

Prognosis and Treatment of Cancer Following Transplantation

Surprisingly, overall survival rates are influenced only slightly by the incidence of tumors following transplantation. Patients developing a tumor after transplantation did not show shorter survival than a control group consisting of patients who had received the contralateral kidneys from the same donors but did not develop cancer (Birkeland 1983b). this result is explained by a look at the causes of death in these patients. In an analysis by Washer et al. (1983) infection and cardiovascular problems were the leading causes of death (41% and 20% respectively). In contrast, death due to malignant neoplasms occurred in only 4% of their patients. This corresponds to our own finding (Table 3) that malignancy was a relatively rare cause of death.

Table 3. Deaths after renal transplantation (Department of Surgery, University Hospital Cologne, 15.2.68–31.3.87)

Causes of death	No. of deaths	Immunosuppression	
		Conventional ($n=305$)	CyA ($n=196$)
Cardiovascular disease	28	24	4
Sepsis/chronic infection	17	17	0
Pneumonia	16	16	0
Gastrointestinal disease	11	11	0
Cerebrovascular disease	9	8	1
Malignancy	4	3	1
Metabolic disease	2	2	0
Pulmonary embolism	2	2	0
Operations other than transplantation	2	2	0
Pulmonary fibrosis	1	1	0
Suicide	1	1	0
Lupus erythematosus	1	0	1
Bolus	1	1	0
Total	95	88	7
Median follow-up (months)	52.2 ± 43.7	72.5 ± 44.6	20.7 ± 13.0

The findings of Sheil et al. (1979) also demonstrate that the risk of malignancy is acceptable: patients developing cancer after transplantation did not do worse in the first 7 years after transplantation than did those in a cancer-free control group. Nevertheless, it must be emphasized that malignant tumors arising de novo after transplantation are aggressive; in the Australian experience, 46% of those who developed cancer other than skin cancer died of their malignancy (Sheil 1986).

Skin Cancer

Basal Cell Carcinoma/Squamous Cell Carcinoma

Basal cell and squamous cell carcinomas are controllable and, therefore, have a favorable prognosis, at least in those countries which are not exposed to extreme ultraviolet radiation (Blohmé and Larkö 1984). But even in Australia the risk of these tumors is acceptable; in Hardie et al.'s (1980) series, the mortality from skin cancer amounted to only 2% of all post-transplant deaths.

As a consequence, skin cancer should be treated locally by conventional surgical measures; a reduction in immunosuppressive therapy is not necessary. However, when metastases spread to draining lymph nodes, block dissection and withdrawal of immunosuppression is advised (Sheil 1986).

Prophylactic measures to reduce the risk of development of these tumors are at least as important as their treatment: in areas of high risk for skin cancer, patients and staff should be educated in the early detection of such lesions and instruction should be given in the proper protection of exposed skin areas with appropriate clothing and barrier creams (Sheil 1986).

Malignant Melanomas

In contrast to most other skin cancers, which are of low-grade malignancy, malignant melanoma has an extremely unfavorable prognosis in transplant patients (Greene et al. 1981). Penn (1984) reported mortality of 46%. Patients developing these tumors should not only be treated locally, consideration should also be given to discontinuing immunosuppressive therapy when the diagnosis is established (Greene et al. 1981).

Solid Lymphomas

The mortality from lymphoma is extremely high in transplant recipients: in Penn's report only 22% of all patients found to have lymphoma after transplantation were currently alive (Penn 1981b). Patients with lymphoproliferative disorders or Kaposi's sarcoma should be treated by withdrawal or severe reduction of immunosuppressive therapy (Bia and Flye 1985; Sheil 1986; Starzl et al. 1984). It may be possible to achieve this without loss of the transplanted organ through rejection. If the lymphomas are localized, surgical intervention is indicated (Jamieson et al. 1981).

In this context it should be mentioned that the term "lymphoma" is not quite clear. "Pseudolymphoma" [seen, for example, after overimmunosuppression with antilymphocyte globulin (ALG) or antithymocyte globulin (ATG)] (Geis et al. 1978), and the lymphoproliferative disorders described by Starzl et al. (1984) and usually associated with Epstein-Barr virus infections (see "Oncogenic Viruses" below) are relatively innocuous lesions; they must not be equated with the malignant lesions (e.g., reticulum cell sarcoma or Kaposi's sarcoma, Penn 1981b).

Gynecological Tumors

The great majority of gynecological tumors are early cancers with favorable prognosis. Patients with persistent cellular dysplasia or in situ cancer should be treated by cone excision of the cervix uteri, those with invasive cancer by hysterectomy (Sheil 1986), while immunosuppressive therapy is maintained. If metastases occur, discontinuation of immunosuppression and removal of the allograft are recommended.

The rare cancers like vulval carcinoma are similar in character to squamous cell carcinoma of the skin. The appropriate treatment consists of wide local excision (Kinlen et al. 1979), possibly combined with radiotherapy (Penn 1986).

Etiology of the Increased Risk for Cancer Following Transplantation

Various factors are blamed for cancers arising de novo after transplantation

Depressed Immune Response

The primary disease necessitating transplantation may in itself reduce the cellular and humoral immune response of the patient. This applies particularly to patients with chronic renal failure (see above), but also to patients with cardiomyopathy and heart grafts. In the latter group the original heart disease may involve a defect in immune regulation causing a tenfold higher incidence of lymphomas than in renal graft recipients (Editorial, Lancet 1983).

Immune Surveillance

An increased risk of malignancies has to be anticipated when unspecific or immunologic specific defense mechanisms are diminished or even eliminated by immunosuppression. Consequently, the growth of potentially neoplastic cells arising by somatic mutation or viral infection would no longer be controlled; rather, the reduced immune surveillance allows the survival of these cells (Burnet 1971; Sodomann and Gropp 1979). The concept of diminished immune surveillance under immunosuppression has been criticized, though, as the decreased immune surveillance cannot explain the preferential appearance of specific tumors like the lymphomas.

Chronic Antigenic Stimulation

The lymphoreticular system of the recipient could be chronically stimulated by the allograft. This protracted antigenic stimulation of immunocompetent cells may permit unrestrained proliferation of lymphoid cells, giving rise to lymphoproliferative disorders after transplantation (Penn 1981a).

Oncogenic Viruses

Epstein-Barr Virus

Especially for the lymphomas, a viral role in causation of malignancy has been discussed (Klein 1975). Immunofluorescence studies revealed that over 90% of the cells of such lymphomas contained Epstein-Barr virus (EBV) nuclear antigen (Sweny et al. 1981). Whether the monoclonal B-cell lymphomas which can arise after EBV infection are true B-cell lymphomas is not quite clear, since several apparently monoclonal tumors were completely reversible by withdrawal of immunosuppression and therefore differed from true malignant lymphomas (Penn 1981a; Sheil 1986; Starzl et al. 1984).

Herpes Simplex Virus

Herpes simplex virus I (HSV-I) is believed to be oncogenic under appropriate circumstances. The high frequency of skin and lip cancers in renal transplant patients may be related to infections or reactivations of HSV-I (Rubin and Tolkoff-Rubin 1982). As these cancers usually occur in sun-exposed areas, it is of interest that ultraviolet-irradiated HSV-I causes chromosomal alterations in human cells in vitro (O'Neill and Miles 1969).

HSV-II may play a pathogenetic role in the development of human cervical carcinoma (Klein 1972), and infections with this agent may perhaps account for the high incidence of cervical carcinoma in situ (Penn 1978). A prior history of condyloma acuminatum suggests an etiologic role of this virus also in patients with carcinoma of the vulva and perineum (Penn 1984, 1986).

Papilloma Virus

Papilloma virus DNA has been demonstrated in both primary and metastatic squamous cell carcinomas, suggesting a pathogenetic role of this virus in the development of skin cancer (Penn 1981a; Rubin and Tolkoff-Rubin 1982; Sheil 1986). Papilloma virus may also contribute to the development of cervical carcinoma (Shah et al. 1980).

Hepatitis B Virus

Renal transplant patients surviving for prolonged periods with chronically active hepatitis due to hepatitis B infection are at risk of developing hepatocellular carcinoma (Rubin and Tolkoff-Rubin 1982; Ono et al. 1984).

Cytomegalovirus

Epidemiologic studies have suggested a relationship between cytomegalovirus (CMV) and the development of Kaposi's sarcoma (Penn 1983a). However, direct evidence that CMV is oncogenic in man is currently lacking (Rubin and Tolkoff-Rubin 1982).

Direct Oncogenic or Co-oncogenic Effect of Immunosuppressive Agents

Whether the commonly used immunosuppressive compounds – azathioprine, prednisolone, ALG, and cyclosporine (CyA) – exert any direct carcinogenic or cocarcinogenic effect has not been settled so far. With regard to the development of skin cancer, one possibility is that azathioprine acts as a cocarcinogen with ultraviolet radiation, photosensitizing the skin (Blohmé and Larkö 1984; Koranda et al. 1974; Sheil 1986).

It is difficult to obtain sufficient clinical data to prove or exclude the carcinogenicity of immunosuppressive compounds. Tumors that appear may be due to the carcinogenicity of a compound or to its immunosuppressive effect; alternatively, the original disease may promote tumor development. Transplant recipients under immunosuppression had a higher risk of tumor development than did a group without transplants also treated with immunosuppressive drugs (Kinlen 1985; Sodomann and Gropp 1979), demonstrating that a combination of several factors is responsible for tumor occurrence.

Types of Immunosuppression

The first clinical experience with CyA suggested that this drug increased the risk of lymphoma development (Calne et al. 1979; Sweny et al. 1981). It has, meanwhile, become evident that the frequency of lymphoma is dose dependent (Dossetor et al. 1984) and that the incidence will be higher than with conventional immunosuppression only if CyA is supplemented by other immunosuppressive agents (Calne et al. 1979; Starzl et al. 1984). Avoiding this "overimmunosuppression" (Beveridge et al. 1984; Starzl et al. 1984) tumor incidence was even lower under CyA therapy than with conventional treatment (Krupp et al. 1986). The malignancies observed are probably not specific to CyA therapy, but rather a complication of immunosuppression per se (Penn and First 1986).

Transplantation in Patients with Preexisting Malignancies

Kidney Transplantation in Patients with Preexisting Renal or Ureteric Malignancies

The prognosis of patients undergoing transplantation after previous treatment of symptomatic renal (mainly renal cell carcinoma and Wilms' tumors) or ureteric malignancies was evaluated by Penn (1977 and 1983b). The most important factor determining the prognosis was the interval between cancer treatment and transplantation: 48% of the patients who were transplanted 12 months or less after cancer treatment developed recurrences, whereas no recurrences were seen in those where the interval was over 48 months. More favorable was the outcome of those patients in whom incidental renal tumors were discovered at the time of bilateral or unilateral nephrectomy, ranging from 30 months before transplantation to the time of transplantation (average 6 months); none developed recurrences.

Thus the timing of transplantation is not determined by incidentally detected asymptomatic renal tumors; in all other cases, however, an interval of at least 1 to 2 years between cancer treatment and transplantation is advisable.

Liver Transplantation in Patients with Primary Liver Malignancies

The majority of patients treated by liver transplantation for primary malignant hepatoma (about 60%, Penn 1978) develop recurrences of cancer within the first 18 months after transplantation, others sometimes later (Sheil 1986).

Renal Transplantation in Patients with Preexisting Nonrenal Malignancies

Patients with a cancer that has a poor prognosis in general population probably should not be referred for transplantation, at least not until several years have passed since successful treatment of the malignancy (Sheil 1986). Penn (1983b) reported 119 patients with neoplasms of various internal organs before transplantation, mainly carcinoma of the uterine cervix, breast, thyroid, bladder, and colorectum. Twenty-three percent of the patients treated a year or less before transplantation developed recurrences or metastases, as did 10% of those treated more than 48 months before transplantation. Especially in patients with malignant melanoma or breast cancer, tumor recurrences have to be taken into account even years after primary tumor therapy.

Accidentally Transplanted Cancers

Cancer patients are excluded on principle from organ donation, since malignancies arising in the organ itself or metastatically from other sites could be transplanted inadvertently with the homograft (Gokel et al. 1977; Penn 1978; Peters and Stuard 1978). Nevertheless, tumor cells may be transmitted accidentally, if patients with "primary" neoplasms of the brain are accepted as organ donors, as not infrequently these tumors turn out to be cerebral metastases of an occult tumor, predominantly of the bronchus (Penn 1978). Cancer has been reported as developing in 30% of such patients who received an apparently innocuous organ from a tumor patient (Penn 1978).

Whenever there is evidence that tumor cells may have been transferred with the graft, it is advisable to remove the homograft as soon as possible in order to prevent tumor cell dissemination. Even if tumor cells have already been spread via the lymphatics or the bloodstream at the time the graft is removed, there is a possibility that they can still be eliminated when the immune system is intact and not suppressed (Gokel et al. 1977). The disappearance of widespread pulmonary metastases has been described (Krueger et al. 1985) after graft removal and cessation of immunosuppressive therapy.

Conclusions for Clinical Practice

1. Patients undergoing transplantation show an increased but acceptable risk of developing de novo cancers. The prognosis quoad vitam is not decisively influenced by tumor occurrence; deaths due to neoplasia amount to only a small fraction of all deaths following transplantation.
2. Cessation of immunosuppression and graft removal are not always necessary when malignancies develop after transplantation. If lymph node metastases are present, immunosuppressive therapy should be stopped.
3. Homografts (unwittingly) taken from cancer patients should generally be removed as soon as the diagnosis is established to avoid inadvertent transfer of tumor cells.
4. When transplantation is carried out for replacement of an organ which has been removed due to cancerous disease, tumor recurrence rates depend on the interval between treatment of the primary tumor and transplantation. If a renal or ureteric malignancy has been removed, an interval of 2 or, better, 4 years is advisable. In the case of primary liver tumors it is not possible to wait so long, and correspondingly a high incidence of tumor recurrences is seen in these patients.

5. Transplantation is rarely justified in patients with malignancies involving organs other than the organ to be replaced. Acceptable recurrence rates can only be anticipated in patients with low-grade cancer and a long interval between cancer treatment and transplantation.

References

Beveridge T, Krupp P, McKibbin C (1984) Lymphomas and lymphoproliferative lesions developing under cyclosporin therapy. Lancet 1: 788

Bia MJ, Flye MW (1985) Immunoblastic lymphoma in a cyclosporine-treated renal transplant recipient. Transplantation 39: 673–675

Birkeland SA (1983a) Malignant tumors in renal transplant patients. Cancer 51: 1571–1575

Birkeland SA (1983b) Cancer in cadaver kidney transplant patients. Surgery 93: 504–509

Blohmé I, Brynger H (1985) Malignant disease in renal transplant patients. Transplantation 39: 23–25

Blohmé I, Larkö O (1984) Premalignant and malignant skin lesions in renal transplant patients. Transplantation 37: 165–167

Boyle J, Briggs JD, MacKie RM, Junor BJR, Aitchison TC (1984) Cancer, warts, and sunshine in renal transplant patients. A case-control study. Lancet 1: 702–704

Burnet FM (1971) Immunological surveillance in neoplasia. Transplant Rev 7: 3–25

Calne RY, Rolles K, Thiru S, McMaster P, Craddock GN, Aziz S, White DJG, Evans DB, Dunn DC, Henderson RG, Lewis P (1979) Cyclosporin A initially as the only immunosuppressant in 34 recipients of cadaveric organs: 32 kidneys, 2 pancreases, and 2 livers. Lancet 2: 1033–1036

Dossetor JB, Kovithavongs T, Salkie M, Preiksaitis J (1984) Cyclosporine-associated lymphoproliferation, despite controlled cyclosporine blood concentrations, in a renal allograft recipient. Proc EDTA-ERA 21: 1021–1026

Editorial (1983) Cyclosporin and neoplasia. Lancet 1: 1083

Geis WP, Iwatsuki S, Molnar Z, Giacchino JL, Kerman RH, Ing TS, Hano JE (1978) Pseudolymphoma in renal allograft recipients. Arch Surg 113: 461–466

Gokel JM, Rjosk HK, Meister P, Stelter WJ, Witte J (1977) Metastatic choriocarcinoma transplanted with cadaver kidney. A case report. Cancer 39: 1317–1321

Greene MH, Young TI, Clark WH (1981) Malignant melanoma in renal-transplant recipients. Lancet 1: 1196–1198

Hardie IP, Strong RW, Hartley LCJ, Woodruff PWH, Clunie GJA (1980) Skin cancer in Caucasian renal allograft recipients living in a subtropical climate. Surgery 87: 177–183

Jacobs C, Brunner FP, Brynger H, Chantler C, Donckerwolcke RA, Hathway RA, Kramer P, Selwood NH, Wing AJ (1981) Malignant diseases in patients treated by dialysis and transplantation in Europe, Transplant Proc 13: 729–732

Jamieson NV, Thiru S, Calne RY, Evans DB (1981) Gastric lymphomas arising in two patients with renal allografts. Transplantation 31: 224–225

Kinlen LJ (1985) Incidence of cancer in rheumatoid arthritis and other disorders after immunosuppressive treatment. Am J Med 78: 44–49

Kinlen LJ, Sheil AGR, Peto J, Doll R (1979) Collaborative United Kingdom-Australasian study of cancer in patients treated with immunosuppressive drugs. Br Med J 2: 1461–1466

Klein G (1972) Herpes virus and oncogenesis. Proc Natl Acad Sci USA 69: 1056–1064

Klein G (1975) The Epstein-Barr virus and neoplasia. N Engl J Med 293: 1353–1357

Koranda FC, Dehmel EM, Kahn G, Penn I (1974) Cutaneous complications in immunosuppressed renal homograft recipients. JAMA 229: 419–424

Kramer P, Broyer M, Brunner FP, Brynger H, Challah S, Oules R, Rizzoni G, Selwood NH, Wing AJ, Balás EA (1984) combined report on regular dialysis and transplantation in Europe, XIV, 1983. Proc EDTA-ERA 21: 47–50

Krueger TC, Tallent MB, Richie RE, Johnson HK, MacDonell RC, Turner B (1985) Neoplasia in immunosuppressed renal transplant patients: a 20-year experience. South Med J 78: 501–505

Krupp P, Gülich A, Timonen P (1986) Treatment with cyclosporine, combination therapy. Side effects and safety of Sandimmun in long-term treatment of renal transplant patients. Transplant Proc 18: 991–992

Matas AJ, Simmons RL, Kjellstrand CM, Buselmeier TJ, Najarian JS (1975) Increased incidence of malignancy during chronic renal failure. Lancet 1: 883–885

Miach PJ, Dawborn JK, Xipell J (1976) Neoplasia in patients with chronic renal failure on long-term dialysis. Clin Nephrol 5: 101–104

O'Neill FJ, Miles CP (1969) Chromosome changes in human cells induced by herpes simplex, Types 1 and 2. Nature 223: 851–852

Ono Y, Ohshima S, Hanai S, Sugiyama S, Kano T, Suenaga M (1984) A kidney transplant patient with hepatocellular carcinoma. Transplantation 37: 620–621

Penn I (1977) Transplantation in patients with primary renal malignancies. Transplantation 24: 424–434

Penn I (1978) Malignancies associated with immunosuppressive or cytotoxic therapy. Surgery 83: 492–502

Penn I (1981a) Depressed immunity and the development of cancer. Clin Exp Immunol 46: 459–474

Penn I (1981b) Malignant lymphomas in organ transplant recipients. Transplant Proc 13: 736–738

Penn I (1983a) Kaposi's sarcoma in immunosuppressed patients. J Clin Lab Immunol 12: 1–10

Penn I (1983b) Renal transplantation in patients with preexisting malignancies. Transplant Proc 15: 1079–1082

Penn I (1984) Cancer in immunosuppressed patients. Transplant Proc 16: 492–494

Penn I (1986) Cancers of the anogenital region in renal transplant recipients. Cancer 58: 611–616

Penn I, First MR (1986) Development and incidence of cancer following cyclosporine therapy. Transplant Proc 18: 210–213

Peters MS, Stuard ID (1978) Metastatic malignant melanoma transplanted via a renal homograft. A case report. Cancer 41: 2426–2430

Rubin RH, Tolkoff-Rubin NE (1982) Viral infection in the renal transplant patient. Proc EDTA 19: 513–526

Shah KH, Lewis MG, Jenson AB, Kurman RJ, Lancester WD (1980) Papillomavirus and cervical dysplasia. Lancet 2: 1190

Sheil AGR (1986) Cancer after transplantation. World J Surg 10: 389–396

Sheil AGR, Mahoney JF, Horvath JS, Johnson JR, Tiller DJ, May J, Stewart JH (1979) Cancer and survival after cadaveric donor renal transplantation. Transplant Proc 11: 1052–1054

Siemensen H, Schlamp R, Tachezy H, Bischoff K, Rem-

mecke J (1984) Überlebenszeit und Todesursachen bei Dialysepatienten. Dtsch Med Wochenschr 109: 1833–1836
Slifkin RF, Goldberg J, Neff S, Baez A, Matto N, Gupta S (1977) Malignancy in end-stage renal disease. Trans Am Soc Artif Intern Organs 23: 34–39
Sodomann CP, Gropp C (1979) Wie groß ist die Malignomgefahr durch Immunsuppressiva? Internist 20: 571–584
Starzl TE, Porter KA, Iwatsuki S, Rosenthal JT, Shaw BW, Atchison RW, Nalesnik MA, Ho M, Griffith BP, Hakala TR, Hardesty RL, Jaffe R (1984) Reversibility of lymphomas and lymphoproliferative lesions developing under cyclosporin-steroid therapy. Lancet 1: 583–587
Sweny P, Farrington K, Younis F, Varghese Z, Baillod RA, Fernando ON, Moorhead JF (1981) Sixteen months experience with cyclosporin-A in human kidney transplantation. Transplant Proc 13: 365–367
Washer GF, Schröter GPJ, Starzl TE, Weil R (1983) Causes of death after kidney transplantation. JAMA 250: 49–54

Wound Healing and Cancer

B. ZEDERFELDT, P. BLOMQUIST, H. JIBORN, and P. UDÉN

Introduction

The ability to repair tissue injuries is essential for survival and is a prerequisite for all surgical intervention. Wound healing is influenced by many factors, quite a few of which are instrumental in cancer patients or are related to different types of oncological therapy.

This chapter begins with a short review of wound healing in general and a principal discussion of factors influencing healing. For comprehensive reviews on wound healing see, for example, Peacock and van Winkle (1976) and Hunt (1980). A more detailed discussion of cancer and wound healing follows.

Wound Healing

In man the capacity for regeneration and repair is limited. Injuries limited to epithelium can be repaired without scar (restitutio ad integrum). When other tissues are involved, continuity in deep layers is restored by nonspecific fibrous tissue and surface continuity by thin epithelium. Injury affecting tissues other than epithelium will thus leave a scar with a greater or lesser degree of functional disturbance.

Types of Healing

A surgical incision with wound edges brought into contact spontaneously, or by mechanical means, has optimal healing conditions. A minimal amount of new tissue is required, and residual functional disturbance is small. This is usually referred to as primary healing (per primam intentionem). In contrast, an open defect is more exposed to infectious agents and must be filled with granulation tissue which leaves a variable amount of scar tissue covered finally by thin and vulnerable epithelium. Such secondary healing (per secundam intentionem) often results in considerable functional disturbance but must be accepted, for instance, in the infected wound.

The biological events are essentially the same in both types of healing, differing only as regards time, amount of scar tissue and functional disturbance.

Factors Initiating and Controlling Healing

Injury with death of cells initiates a reparative process in which local, previously dormant cells proliferate, resulting in the budding of capillaries and in growth into the defect by cells from the loose perivascular fibrous tissue. Platelets and activated macrophages release substances which stimulate endothelial and fibroblastic growth. (Rutherford and Ross 1976; Leibovich and Ross 1975, 1976; Hunt 1980). Over the last few years more than 10 different growth factors have been identified and shown to influence different steps in the reparative process (For review see Laato, 1988). The healing process is controlled in that proliferation of cells ceases when the defect is filled by granulation tissue. The controlling mechanism remains unidentified but may be either passive, through cessation of stimulating factors, or active, by secretion of inhibiting factors as a result of, for example, cell contact. Hypoxia in the center of a wound defect may be one of the decisive factors as illustrated by Silwer (1980).

Phases of the Healing Process

Three main phases can be recognized in the healing process: inflammation, fibroplasia, and maturation. Although there is some overlapping between these phases, it is often appropriate to discuss them as separate entities.

Inflammation is the mechanism cleaning the injured area of cell debris, foreign body and, if present, bacteria. In a clean wound with minimal tissue injury, e.g. a surgical incision, this reaction is over in 2–3 days, but in wounds with marked tissue injury or contamination it may be greatly extended.

Fibroplasia usually can be recognized microscopically within 1–2 days after wounding, and deposition of collagen in the intercellular substance occurs at the same time. The amount of collagen (the protein responsible for structure and strength of the scar) increases rapidly up to about 2 weeks after wounding. Thereafter, the total amount of collagen remains unchanged in a sutured wound. In open wounds fibroplasia may continue for a considerable time.

Maturation of the scar continues over a period of years, and it may well be that the healing process after injury never quite comes to an end. Recent studies have shown increased collagen metabolism in 18- to 20-year-old scars. Synthesis and lysis of collagen are balanced so that total collagen remains the same. Contraction of the scar, obvious especially in open wounds, is ascribed to contractile cells in the granulation tissue, so-called myofibroblasts.

At the end of fibroplasia the scar is red due to the vascularity of the granulation tissue. With time vascularity decreases, turning the scar into a white line.

Development of Strength

During the inflammatory phase the strength of a sutured wound is dependent almost entirely on the mechanical support. Provided that adequate suture material is used and the sutures are securely tied, the strength of the tissue included in the sutures decides the wound strength. As a result of local collagenolytic processes this tissue weakens considerably during the first 2–3 days after wounding. Proteases released from polymorphonuclear leukocytes seem to be most important. The post-traumatic decrease of tissue strength is avoided in animals made neutropenic. A sutured wound, or an anastomosis, is weakest about 3 days after suturing (Jönsson et al. 1983; Högström and Haglund 1985). From then on strength increases rapidly as a consequence of bridging of the defect by new fibrous tissue and by new tissue reinforcing the tissue included in the supporting sutures.

Since fibroplasia is nonspecific development of strength, during the fibroplasia period it is virtually the same in all wounds irrespective of localization. The strength of a wound, expressed as a percentage of the original tissue strength, will, however, vary considerably, as the strength of the uninjured tissue varies with its collagen content. Two weeks after wounding an intestinal anastomosis is almost as strong as the intact intestine, while a wound in mainly fibrous tissue, such as skin or fascia, has less than 10% of the strength of the intact tissue.

During the maturation phase scars in skin, fascia and tendon undergo rebuilding, resulting in continuous increase of strength. A scar in such tissues, however, never quite reaches the strength of the intact tissue. In the intestine the increase in anastomotic strength is very limited during the maturation phase.

Factors Influencing the Rate of Healing

The rate of healing cannot be increased by any known factor. Many factors, on the other hand, delay healing.

A certain degree of inflammation is necessary for normal healing. Too little inflammation, as well as too strong or too prolonged inflammation, influences healing negatively. The factors commonly causing abnormal inflammatory reaction are listed in Table 1. Excessive inflammatory reaction can usually be avoided by adequate surgical technique, proper choice of suture material and use of prophylactic antibiotics in critically contaminated wounds. Too little inflammation as a result of medication or disease cannot be avoided. In such situations longer than normal mechanical wound support is necessary.

Many factors delay or impair the formation of new tissue which is an energy-dependent process requiring adequate oxygenation and nutrition. The most important factors influencing the period of fibroplasia are the following:

Low tissue oxygen tension
- impaired circulation
- marked anemia

Hypoproteinemia
Vitamin deficiencies
Trace metal deficiencies

Cytotoxic drugs
Radiation

Oxygen availability is mainly dependent on blood flow, but also marked anemia may lead to decreased oxygen tissue tension. As compensatory mechanisms counteract the negative effects of anemia to a certain degree, decreased tissue oxygen tension usually occurs only when the hematocrit level is below 20.

Hypoproteinemia delays healing either by causing local edema in the wound with increased diffusion distances or by a negative influence on host resistance to infection. Lack of specific amino acids is probably seldom the cause of impaired healing.

Table 1. Factors normally causing abnormal inflammatory reaction

Increased inflammation
Infection
Foreign body
Devitalized tissue
Impaired inflammation
Cortisone
Immunosuppression
Deficient leukocyte function, as in diabetes, leukemia

Vitamin C deficiency is the classical example of a factor impairing wound healing, but is hardly of significance in modern times. As regards the importance of other vitamins, knowledge is very limited.

Zinc deficiency impairs healing, probably due to changes in inflammatory reaction and to influence on fibroblastic proliferation.

Radiation and cytotoxic drugs influence healing negatively, both during the inflammatory and the fibroplasia period (see below).

Factors influencing the maturation phase are incompletely known and probably of very limited clinical importance.

Wound Dehiscence and Incisional Hernia

Dehiscence of a wound is principally due either to insufficient mechanical support during the early phase of healing or to delayed or impaired fibrous tissue formation.

Wound dehiscence often occurs within the first week after wounding and thus before true repair has influenced strength to any great extent. It therefore seems probable that decreased strength of the tissues holding the sutures is an important, possibly the most important, factor for wound dehiscence. Incisional hernias are often the consequence of a partial and undetected wound dehiscence, but may also be a consequence of delayed scar tissue formation.

Cancer and Wound Healing

In most clinical reports dealing with wound complications cancer is postulated as one important cause of impaired healing. There are no data in the literature, however, to indicate negative effects related specifically to tumour bearing. Since, however, advanced tumour disease is often associated with malnutrition and anemia, there is ample cause for such secondary factors to impair healing. Further, several treatment modalities, e.g., radiation and medication with antineoplastic drugs and cortisone, do impair healing and influence host resistance against infection. In the following paragraphs the importance of factors related to advanced tumour disease and to different treatment modalities are discussed in more detail.

Effects of Malnutrition

Malignant disease is often associated with malnutrition and anemia. Malnutrition may result either from anorexia or from inadequate food intake as a consequence of obstruction in the gastrointestinal tract. It may also be an effect of increased energy expenditure related to the tumour itself. Different treatment modalities, such as surgery, chemotherapy and irradiation, contribute to malnutrition (Shils 1979). Malnutrition can influence healing by protein and amino acid deficiency and/or by decreased immune competence with impaired defence against infection.

Protein malnutrition in experimental animals maintained for 6 to 8 weeks resulting in weight loss of 20% or more regularly impairs healing (Irvin and Hunt 1974; Irvin 1978). Some studies (Daly et al. 1972; Ward et al. 1982) have demonstrated impaired healing after as little as 1 week of protein malnutrition. Reversal of the negative effects on healing by early reintroduction of complete nutrition has been demonstrated (Steiger et al. 1971, 1973; Irvin 1978; Ward et al 1982). Local hyperalimentation in the wound has been shown to increase collagen accumulation (Niinikoski et al. 1977).

In experimental studies in the rat, 6 weeks of protein starvation resulted in total anergy (Daly et al. 1978), which was reversed by repletion of a regular protein diet. Christou and Meakins (1979a, b) have demonstrated that neutrophil leukocytes from anergic patients display increased adherence and decreased chemotaxis. These changes are brought about by a plasma factor, since normal leukocytes exposed to plasma from anergic patients exhibit the same properties.

Changes in inflammatory reaction as a consequence of altered leukocyte function may influence healing directly and/or indirectly by impaired resistance to infection. There is clear evidence of increased complication risk in malnourished surgical patients (e.g., Irvin and Goligher 1973; Mullen et al. 1979). Delayed hypersensitivity tests to reveal anergy are of value in predicting postoperative morbidity (Johnson et al. 1979).

Increased collagen formation in open wounds following parenteral nutrition has been demonstrated by Bozzetti et al. (1975).

Total parenteral nutrition for 7–10 days preoperatively reduces postoperative morbidity in high-risk patients (Williams et al. 1976; Mullen et al. 1980; Müller et al. 1982).

Short preoperative total parenteral nutrition (24–72 h) does not seem to improve healing or decrease complications (Holter and Fischer 1977; Preshaw et al. 1979).

In summary, marked malnutrition causes delay of healing and increased surgical complications. The negative effects can be reversed by preoperative total parenteral nutrition extended over 7–10 days, but shorter periods of preoperative nutrition do not seem to be effective in preventing complications.

Effects of Radiation

Radiation causes injury to all tissues exposed, but the degree of injury varies markedly for different tissues and with the size and the spacing of the radiation doses. Although much is known about the mode of action, the exact mechanism of injury to cells by radiation is not well defined. It is generally assumed that highly charged electrons and free radicals interact directly with cellular DNA. The interaction influences the reproductive mechanisms, and death of cells may occur when division is attempted. Rapidly dividing cells tend to be especially sensitive to radiation. Since rapid division is a characteristic feature of the reparative cells, a marked influence of radiation on wound healing may be anticipated (Moore 1984).

Most experimental studies have demonstrated delay in healing following radiation in therapeutic doses (see, e.g., Powers et al. 1967). The negative effects are mostly ascribed to direct effects on the reparative cells, with delay both in capillary budding and in proliferation of fibroblasts (Blythe et al. 1975) and consequently retarded deposition of collagen in the wound (Kitagawa et al. 1961; Archer et al. 1970). These morphological changes are accompanied by a slower development of wound strength, a delay which is more marked the higher the radiation dose (Zelman et al. 1969; Staije and Milanovic 1970). Administration of supplemental vitamin A has recently been described as partly counteracting these negative consequences of irradiation on anastomotic healing (Winsey et al. 1987).

A seemingly contradictory finding is that radiation in low doses (30 Gy) may have a positive effect on wound healing (Moore 1984). The plausible explanation is that a low dose of radiation causes a slight inflammatory reaction which induces a reparative process but causes no serious injury to involved cells. From other studies it is known that wounds inflicted in a tissue where a reparative process is going on gain strength faster (Sandblom and Muren 1954), as do disrupted and resutured wounds (Savlov et al. 1954). The observation of faster healing in tissues subjected to a low dose of radiation may be of clinical significance. If surgical resection is done outside the field of major radiation this mechanism may come into play, possibly explaining some of the contradictory findings in clinical studies.

Clinically, the negative effects of radiation on wound healing are not nearly as clear-cut as would appear from the experimental studies. This may be due to inability to detect even rather marked healing delay in the clinical situation. To be clinically significant, disturbances of wound healing may require not only a delay of the healing process, but in addition some other factor influencing healing, such as infection or tension over the wound. There are some indications that radiation not only causes delay in healing as such, but also renders the wound more susceptible to other negative factors such as bacterial contamination (Ariyan et al. 1980 a).

Timing of Radiation and Surgery

The most severe retardation of healing seems to occur if radiation is given either just before wounding or during the first few days thereafter, the period of most rapid proliferation of cells.

Preoperative Irradiation

It is difficult to ascertain from experimental studies the least negative period for irradiation in relation to wounding. There are, however, some indications that the healing delay is least if an interval of 2–3 weeks is allowed between irradiation and wounding (Pohle et al. 1931; Joseph and Shumrick 1973). Moderately longer intervals between irradiation and wounding do not seem to give further protection, and significantly longer intervals may have disadvantages as the chronic effects of radiation come into play.

Numerous retrospective clinical studies have tried to evaluate surgical morbidity following planned preoperative irradiation. The results are contradictory at best, many studies showing increased morbidity but an approximately equal number unable to demonstrate any such increase.

The difficulties are partly due to heterogeneity of the patients studied as regards tumour stage, dose of radiation to the wounded tissue, and type of surgical procedure.

There is no clear-cut evidence that preoperative irradiation regularly leads to increased surgical morbidity. Since, however, the potential for surgical complications certainly is increased, an optimal surgical technique is especially important. This underlines the importance of measures to minimize tissue injury and contamination and to assure mechanical support of the wound for a longer time than is customary in nonirradiated tissues. Resorbable suture materials may increase the risk of wound dehiscence, and the use of monofilament nonresorbable materials is recommended. The use of prophylactic antibiotics should be considered.

Postoperative Irradiation

Irradiation during the first few days after wounding has a markedly negative effect. With longer intervals between wounding and irradiation the degree of retardation subsides (Moore 1984). Irradiation of a surgical incision started after the end of the fibroplasia period (2–3 weeks) seems to have only an insignificant effect on wound strength development (Lawrence et al. 1953). Irradiation of open wounds causes a marked delay in wound closure, due both to a direct effect on fibroblast and epithelial proliferation and to inhibition of wound contraction.

Chronic Effects of Irradiation

Radiation leads to fibrosis in all tissues exposed. This is in fact the result of a healing process induced by tissue injury and inflammation leading to fibroblast proliferation and deposition of collagen. It remains obscure why postradiation fibrosis continues to increase long after the inflammation has subsided, but the progressive changes in microvessels with hypoxia may offer an explanation. These microvessel changes are also responsible for the typical skin changes, with atrophic epithelium and teleangiectatic capillaries. Tissue edema is usually ascribed to changes in lymphatic vessels.

Chronic changes in irradiated tissue render the tissue abnormally sensitive to trauma. "Spontaneous" wounds may occur, but ulcerations in an irradiated area should always be biopsied and histologically examined, since tumour recurrence is a frequent cause of such ulcers.

Healing of surgical wounds in previously irradiated tissues is markedly delayed due mainly to microvessel injury and hypoxia (Joseph and Shumrick 1973; Mantravadi et al. 1981). Such tissue also has poor defenses against infection (Ariyan et al. 1980 a), increasing the risk of wound complications. Incisions in irradiated tissue should always be supported for longer than normal mechanically, by sutures, and antibiotic treatment should be considered.

Especially serious are healing complications after surgery on intestine injured by irradiation. In patients with radiation enteritis, anastomotic dehiscence rates of about 50% are reported (Swan et al. 1976; Galland and Spencer 1979; Hatcher et al. 1984). This is more than 10 times the dehiscence rate in anastomoses performed on healthy intestine.

In summary, radiation causes dose-dependent delay of healing and increase of complications. Radiation given within the 2 weeks before or after wounding seems to be especially deleterious. The chronic effects of radiation likewise include serious delays in healing and increased rates of wound complications.

Effects of Antineoplastic Drugs

Antineoplastic agents exert their effect on all cells in the body. Although the mode of action is different for various drugs, they have in common an influence on DNA/RNA synthesis and mitotic activity. Rapidly dividing cells are, therefore, especially sensitive to the drugs. The cells in reparative tissue belong to this group and, consequently, a markedly negative effect on wound healing may be anticipated. The effects of antineoplastic drugs are, however, not limited to direct effects on reparative cells; secondary effects on healing may be caused by malnutrition and by impaired function of platelets, macrophages, leukocytes and lymphocytes.

Most of our knowledge about the effect of antineoplastic agents comes from animal studies. Evaluation of these studies is often difficult, due to differences in doses and routes of administration, timing of treatment in relation to wounding and possibly to species differences in dose response to the drugs. Standardization of experimental models (Hardesty 1958; Gupta et al. 1970; Cohen et al. 1975a, b; Morris et al. 1978) has, however, improved our knowledge about the functional effects of antineoplastic drugs.

Differences Between Agents

Although it may be assumed that all antineoplastic drugs have negative effects on wound healing, some agents seem to be more markedly deleterious. Nitrogen mustard, cyclophosphamide, methotrexate, doxorubicin (adriamycin) and BCNU have all been shown experimentally to impair healing. The effects of thio-TEPA, 5-fluorouracil, azathioprine and vincristine have varied (see, e.g., Shamberger 1985).

Dose Dependence

Increasing impairment with higher doses has been demonstrated for methotrexate (Calnan and Davies 1965), cyclophosphamide (Cohen et al. 1975b), and doxorubicin (Cohen et al. 1975b).

Timing in Relation to Surgery

The most sensitive period for the wound is the first 4–5 days after wounding, but preoperative administration of drugs also impairs healing. Administration of cyclophosphamide (Cohen et al. 1975a) and doxorubicin (Devereux et al. 1980) within the first 4 days after wounding impairs healing, while the same dose given 1 to 2 weeks after wounding has no or limited effect. Bleomycin, 5-fluorouracil, and *cis*-diamine dichloroplatinum (*cis*-DDP) caused reduced gain in accumulation of hydroxyproline and anastomotic strength when colonic resection was performed during the chemotherapeutic regimen, whereas chemotherapy commencing 2 days after surgery did not affect anastomotic healing (de Roy van Zuidewijn et al.1987).

Nutritional Status

Malnutrition seems to increase the negative effects of antineoplastic drugs. This has been demonstrated for 5-fluorouracil in experimental studies by Staley et al. (1961), while other drugs seem not to have been studied in this respect.

Host Resistance

The ability to handle bacterial contamination is clearly decreased after treatment with methotrexate (Ariyan et al. 1980b). This may well also be true for other antineoplastic agents, but no studies are available. If antineoplastic agents are given in close connection with surgery, antibiotic prophylaxis should be considered.

In summary, it thus appears that administration of antineoplastic drugs after the end of the fibroplasia period has very limited negative effects, and it seems advisable to delay treatment for approximately 2 weeks after surgery.

Concluding Remarks

Patients with advanced tumor disease display impairment of healing mainly due to malnutrition. Radiation therapy and antineoplastic drugs cause further impairment of healing, but these effects can be minimized by avoiding such measures in close relation to surgery. Open wounds are more sensitive than sutured surgical wounds to these therapeutic measures. Optimal surgical techniques, longer than normal mechanical support of wounds, preoperative total parenteral nutrition, and prophylactic use of antibiotics are important measures to avoid wound complications in cancer patients.

References

Archer RR, Greenwell EJ, Ware T, Weeks PM, (1970) Irradiation effect on wound healing in cats. Radiat Res 41: 104–112

Ariyan S, Marfuggi RA, Harder G, Goodie MM (1980a) An experimental model to determine the effects of adjuvant therapy on the incidence of postoperative wound infection. Plast Reconstr Surg 65: 328–337

Ariyan S, Kraft RL, Goldberg NH (1980b) An experimental model to determine the effects of adjuvant therapy on the incidence of postoperative wound infection: II. Evaluating preoperative chemotherapy. Plast Reconstr Surg 65: 338–345

Blythe JG, Buchsbaum HJ, Allen TJ (1975) The effect of delaying radiation on wound healing. Gynecol Oncol 3: 210–214

Bozzetti F, Terno G, Longoni C (1975) Parenteral nutrition and wound healing. Surg Gynecol Obstet 141: 712–714

Calnan J, Davies A (1965) The effect of methotrexate on wound healing: an experimental study. Br J Cancer 19: 505–512

Christou NV, Meakins JL (1979a) Delayed hypersensitivity in surgical patients: a mechanism for anergy. Surgery 86: 78–85

Christou NV, Meakins JL (1979b) Neutrophil function in anergic surgical patients. Ann Surg 190: 557–564

Cohen SC, Gabelnik HL, Johnson RK, Goldin A (1975a) Effects of antineoplastic agents on wound healing in mice. Surgery 78: 238–244

Cohen Sc, Gabelnik HL, Johnson RK, Goldin A (1975b) Effects of cyclophosphamide and adriamycin on the healing of surgical wounds in mice. Cancer 36: 1277–1281

Daly JM, Vars HM, Dudrick SJ (1972) Effects of protein depletion on colonic anastomoses. Surg Gynecol Obstet 134: 15–21

Daly JM, Dudrick SJ, Copeland EM (1978) Effects of protein depletion and repletion on cell-mediated immunity in experimental animals. Ann Surg 188: 791–796

De Roy van Zuidewijn DBW, Hendriks T, Wobbes T, Klompmakers AA, de Baer HHM (1987) Healing of experimental colonic anastomoses: effect of antineoplastic agents. Eur J Surg Oncol 13: 27

Devereux DF, Kent H, Brennan MF (1980) Time dependent effects of Adriamycin and X-ray therapy on wound healing in the rat. Cancer 45: 2805–2810

Galland RB, Spencer I (1979) Surgical aspects of radiation injury to the intestine. Br J Surg 66: 135–138

Gupta RC, Singh LM, Udenpor KN (1970) Effect of cyclophosphamide on the process of wound healing. Indian J Surg 32: 127–132

Hardesty WH (1958) The effect of cytostatic drugs on wound healing in rats. Cancer Res 18: 581–584

Hatcher PA, Thomson H, Ludgate S, Small WP, Smith AN (1984) Surgical aspects of intestinal injury due to pelvic radiotherapy. Ann Surg 201: 470–475

Högström H, Haglund U (1985) Postoperative decrease in suture holding capacity in laparotomy wounds and anastomoses. Acta Chir Scand 151: 533

Högström H, Haglund U (1986) Neutropenia prevents decrease in strength of rat intestinal anastomoses; partial effect of oxygen free radical scavengers and allopurinol. Surgery 99: 716–720

Holter AR, Fischer JE (1977) The effects of perioperative hyperalimentation on complications in patients with carcinoma and weight loss. J Surg Res 23: 31–34

Hunt TK (ed) (1980) Wound healing and wound infection. Appleton-Century-Crofts, New York

Irvin TT (1978) Effects of malnutrition and hyperalimentation on wound healing. Surg Gynecol Obstet 146: 33–37

Irvin TT, Goligher IC (1973) Etiology of disruption of intestinal anastomoses. Br J Surg 60: 461–464

Irvin TT, Hunt TK (1974) Effect of malnutrition on colonic healing. Ann Surg 180: 765–772

Johnson WC, Ulrich F, Meguid MM, Lepak N, Bowe P, Harris P, Alberts LH, Nabseth DC (1979) Role of delayed hypersensitivity in predicting postoperative morbidity and mortality. Am J Surg 137: 536–542

Jönsson K, Jiborn H, Zederfeldt B (1983) Breaking strength of small intestinal anastomoses. Am J Surg 145: 800–803

Joseph DL, Shumrick DL (1973) Risks of head and neck surgery in previously irradiated patients. Arch Otolaryngol Head Neck Surg 97: 381–384

Kitagawa T, Glicksman AS, Tyree EB, Nickson JJ (1961) Radiation effect on skin and subcutaneous tissue. A quantitative study on collagen content. Radiat Res 15: 761–766

Lawrence W, Nickson JJ, Warshaw LM (1953) Röntgen rays and wound healing. Surgery 33: 376–384

Laato M (1988) The effect of epidermal growth factor on granulation tissue formation in the rat. Acta Chir Scand Suppl. 546

Leibovich SJ, Ross R (1975) The role of macrophages in wound repair. A study with hydrocortisone and antimacrophage serum. Am J Pathol 78: 71

Leibovich SJ, Ross R (1976) A macrophage dependent factor that stimulates the proliferation of fibroblasts in vitro. Am J Pathol 84: 501

Mantravadi RUP, Skolnik EM, Applebaum EL (1981) Complications of postoperative and preoperative radiation therapy in head and neck cancers. Arch Otolaryngol Head Neck Surg 107: 690–693

Moore MJ (1984) The effect of radiation on connective tissue. Otolaryngol Clin North Am 17: 389–399

Morris T, Lincoln F, Lee A (1978) The effect of 5-flourouracil on abdominal wound healing in rats. Aust NZ J Surg 48: 219–221

Mullen JL, Buzby GP, Waldman MT, Gertner MH, Hobbs CL, Rosato EF (1979) Prediction of operative morbidity and mortality by preoperative nutritional assessment. Surg Forum 30: 80–82

Mullen JL, Buzby GP, Matthews DC, Smale BF, Rosato EF (1980) Reduction of operative morbidity and mortality by combined preoperative and combined postoperative nutritional support. Ann Surg 192: 604–613

Müller JM, Brenner U, Dienst C, Pichlmaier H (1982) Preoperative parenteral feeding in patients with gastrointestinal carcinoma. Lancet 1: 68–71

Niinikoski J, Kivisaari J, Viljanto J (1977) Local hyperalimentation of experimental granulation tissue. Acta Chir Scand 143: 201

Peacock EE, van Winkle W (1976) Wound repair. Saunders, Philadelphia

Pohle EA, Ritchie G, Wright CS (1931) Studies of the effect of röntgen rays on the healing of wounds. Radiology 16: 445–460

Powers WE, Ogura IH, Palmer LA (1967) Radiation therapy and wound healing delay in animals and man. Radiology 89: 112–115

Preshaw RM, Attisha RP, Hollingsworth WJ, Todd JD (1979) Randomized sequential trial of parenteral nutrition in healing of colonic anastomoses in man. Can J Surg 22: 437–439

Rutherford RB, Ross R (1976) Platelet factors stimulate fibroblasts and smooth muscle cells quiescent in plasma to proliferate. J Cell Biol 69: 196

Sandblom P, Muren A (1954) Differences between the rate of healing of wounds inflicted with short tissue interval. Ann Surg 140: 449

Savlov ED, Dunphy IE, Andersson MA (1954) The healing of the disrupted and resutured wound. Surgery 36: 362–370

Shamberger R (1985) Effect of chemotherapy and radiotherapy on wound healing: experimental studies. In: Metzger U, Largiadér F, Senn HJ Recent results in cancer research, vol 98, perioperative chemotherapy. Springer, Berlin Heidelberg New York Tokyo pp 17–34

Shils ME (1979) Nutritional effects induced by cancer. Med Clin North Am 63: 1009–1025

Silwer IA (1980) The physiology of wound healing. In: Hunt TK (ed) Wound healing and wound infection. Appleton-Century-Crofts, New York

Staije J, Milovanovic A (1970) Radiation and wound healing: evolution of tensile strength in excised skin wound of irradiated rats. Strahlentherapie 139: 87–90

Staley CJ, Trippel OH, Preston FW (1961) Influence of 5-fluorouracil on wound healing. Surgery 49: 450–453

Steiger E, Allen TR, Daly JM (1971) Beneficial effects of immediate postoperative total parenteral nutrition. Surg Forum 22: 89

Steiger E, Daly JM, Allen TR (1973) Postoperative intravenous nutrition. Surgery 73: 686

Swan RW, Fowler WC, Boronow RC (1976) Surgical management of radiation injury to the small intestine. Surg Gynecol Obstet 142: 325–327

Ward MW, Danzi M, Lewin MR, Rennie MJ, Clark CG (1982) The effects of subclinical malnutrition and refeeding on the healing of experimental colonic anastomoses. Br J Surg 69: 308–310

Williams RHP, Heatley RV, Lewis MH, Hughes IE (1976) A randomized controlled trial of preoperative intravenous nutrition in patients with stomach cancer. Br J Surg 63: 667

Winsey K, Simon R, Levenson S, Seiffer E, Demetriou A (1987) Effect of supplemental vitamin A on colon anastomotic healing in rats given preoperative irradiation. Am J Surg 153: 153

Zelman D, Song IC, Porteous DD, Bromberg BE (1969) The effect of total body irradiation on wound healing and the hematopoetic system in mice. Bull NY Acad Med 45: 293–300

Nutrition and Cancer

L. L. Moldawer and T. Schersten

Introduction

Cachexia is the most visually recognizable symptom associated with cancer. To family members and to most physicians, the loss of body weight and the wasting of host tissues indicates a very ominous outlook for the patient newly diagnosed with cancer and has been shown to be a significant negative prognostic factor in cancer treatment studies with a broad range of tumor types. The cancer cachexia syndrome, which results from the continued loss of body fat and lean tissue, ultimately involves most of the organs of the body and when severe is associated with decreased survival.

Depending upon tumor type, the incidence of cachexia in cancer varies widely. Although it is rarely observed in breast cancer and lymphomas, DeWys et al. (1980) reported weight loss in over half of the patients with metastatic disease from assorted primaries. Furthermore, numerous studies have revealed that malnourished cancer patients have increased morbidity and mortality (Harvey 1980; Harvey et al. 1981; Nixon et al. 1980; Mullen et al. 1980). Early studies revealed that 10%–20% percent of all cancer patients die with malnutrition as the primary cause (Warren 1932; Inagaki et al. 1974). Sixty-five per cent of cancer patients die from associated infections (Sickles et al. 1973), and such patients have evident immune system dysfunction.

With the widespread availability of total parenteral nutrition, including home nutrition, and continuous advances in enteral nutritional support, the physician has at hand considerable resources to improve nutritional status. Today, nutritional support has become an integral component, along with surgery, chemotherapy, radiation and immunotherapy, of a holistic approach to the treatment of the patient with cancer.

Yet aggressive nutritional therapy is not appropriate in all patients with cancer and cachexia. The indiscriminate use of invasive nutritional support places an overwhelming financial burden on health care systems with limited resources. The great challenge to clinicians today is the appropriate design of nutritional therapies for patients in whom such treatment will have demonstrable benefits. Just as it is incorrect not to support nutritionally the patient in whom benefits can be expected, it is equally wrong to undertake elaborate and expensive programs for patients in whom nutritional support will have only limited effect on outcome or quality of life. The rationale for giving the cancer patient nutrition support must be based upon a firm scientific expectation that such a therapy (1) will be effective in either offsetting or reducing the progression of cancer cachexia, and (2) will have a beneficial impact on outcome to antineoplastic therapy, or improve the patient's quality of life.

Metabolic Causes of Cancer Cachexia

The reason cancer cachexia develops is still not fully understood. There have been several excellent reviews on the metabolic causes of cachexia (Young 1977; Theologides 1979; Waterhouse 1974, 1981) and thus they will not be extensively discussed here. However, it is important to briefly review our current knowledge regarding cancer-associated cachexia, because the mechanisms behind the loss of body weight will also determine to some extent how successfully the patient will utilize exogenously administered nutrients.

The patient experiencing cachexia has distinguishable metabolic abnormalities which both reduce the desire for food intake and adversely affect nutrient utilization. It is frequently advantageous to divide the broad classification of cancer cachexia into two mechanistic groups (Nixon 1985). "Primary cachexia" is thought to result from some tumor-host interaction that leads to the progressive loss of fat and body protein, primarily from the somatic tissues, skeletal muscle and connective tissue. The underlying causes are not fully known, but metabolic abnormalities, including increased protein turnover, glucose cycling and fatty acid oxidation, all contribute. "Secondary cachexia" is a result of either mechanical obstruction of food intake or digestion by the tumor. This group also includes cachexia secondary to antineoplastic therapies, such as anorexia, malabsorption or vomiting resulting from radiation, chemotherapy or surgery. In many patients both mechanisms are operating.

The mechanisms behind reduced food intake are still unclear but both hypothalamic and extrathalamic factors are of importance (Morrison 1976; Krause et al. 1981; DeWys et al. 1981). The phenomenon of food aversion has been amply demonstrated and represents, in many cases, a learned aversion against certain components of food, especially during radiation and chemotherapy (Bernstein and Bernstein 1981). This cancer-associated anorexia is probably not a specific phenomenon unique to the tumor-bearing state. Similar responses are common in infectious diseases, inflammation, trauma, and after major surgery. The similarities among the host reactions to these various inflammatory states, including cancer, has suggested a common endogenous initiator (McCarthy 1985). Monokines and lymphokines, such as interleukin-1, tumor necrosis factor and lymphotoxin, which are synthetized and released from macrophages, lymphocytes and perhaps also from the tumor itself, have been focused on as possible etiological factors. Both biologically derived and recombinant interleukin-1, when given to experimental animals, cause a decline in spontaneous oral energy intake.

The importance of anorexia as a contributing factor to cancer cachexia is frequently unappreciated. Studies from our own laboratory have emphasized the importance of anorexia as the primary contributory factor to weight loss and tissue wasting in cancer disease (Lindmark et al. 1984; Lundholm et al. 1982). Utilizing both animal models and clinical studies, many of the host protein and substrate changes seen in an individual with a tumor could be explained by the reduced food intake (Lundholm et al. 1981; Bennegård et al. 1982). Such findings do not disregard the role of tumor-induced metabolic aberrations as contributory factors to the development of cancer cachexia. Indeed, recent preliminary studies by McRussell et al. (1984) have suggested that repletion of body protein and fat in previously malnourished cancer patients results in increased anorexia following the period of nutritional supplementation. These findings suggest that the presence of a tumor has altered the thalamic "set point" and that food intake in cancer patients is closely related to both substrate utilization and size of substrate depots.

It has been clearly demonstrated that there are characteristic differences in the metabolic response to fasting between individuals with and without tumors (Lindmark et al. 1984; Warnold et al. 1978). Tumor patients are frequently in a negative energy balance due to uncompensated elevated energy expenditure which cannot be ascribed to the energy requirements of the tumor. Although the increases are generally small – 10%–15% in several studies (Lindmark et al. 1984; Dempsey et al. 1984) – over a period of months they can explain the loss of several kilograms of body weight. Numerous investigators have attempted to identify the cause of this increased energy expenditure. It has been frequently shown that the turnover of body protein is increased in such patients (Edén et al. 1984), and the energy required to synthesize and degrade the additional protein can explain approximately one-third of this increase. In animal studies, the site of this increased protein synthesis and degradation is principally visceral and immune tissues (Kawamura et al. 1983; Ternell et al. 1985). Most patients also experience an acute-phase response similar to that seen during acute inflammatory states (Walker and Gray 1983).

Early studies investigating the causes of cancer cachexia demonstrated increased glucose turnover and recycling through lactate in patients with cancer (for review, see Young 1977). Although it was originally believed that an increase in such "futile cycling" might explain the higher energy expenditure seen in cancer, more recent studies have shown that it can, in fact, account for only a small fraction of the increase in energy expenditure (Waterhouse 1981; Edén et al. 1984). Similarly, other studies have shown augmented lipolysis and fatty acid oxidation in patients with cancer (Edén et al. 1985). However, the increase in the concentration and oxidation of fatty acids can explain only a small component of the increase in energy expenditure. In total, no one component of substrate utilization can explain the increase in energy expenditure in cancer; rather, the evidence suggests that small but significant increases in amino acid, carbohydrate and fat turnover all contribute to the increase in metabolic rate. The trigger mechanisms for the increased protein, fat and glucose turnover in cancer have not been discovered. However, the increase in energy expenditure reported in cancer patients is similar in magnitude to that seen when interleukin-1 is administered to experimental animals (Tocco-Bradley et al. 1987).

If anorexia is the primary reason why patients with cancer lose weight and lean tissue, nutritional supplementation should counteract to a major extent the development of cachexia. Similarly, if undernutrition shortens the life of cancer patients, successful nutritional intervention should prolong survival. Nutritional support should enable the patient's immune system better to combat the tumor by promoting wound repair, improving organ function and permitting the patient to tolerate more rigorous antineoplastic therapies.

In contrast, if underlying metabolic processes are altered by the tumor, as in primary cachexia, then nutritional supplementation in a cancer patient would be less effective than in similarly malnourished patients without cancer.

Nutritional Support of the Cancer Patient

Both retrospective and prospective studies have reported increased morbidity and mortality after surgical and medical therapy in malnourished patients with and without cancer (Warnold and Lundholm 1984; Symreng et al. 1983). Furthermore, Harvey et al. (1980, 1981) and Nixon et al. (1981) reported that malnutrition correlates with shorter survival in patients with cancer.

Such data would imply that if malnutrition adversely affects outcome in patients with cancer, then nutritional support in such patients should be associated with improved survival and reduced morbidity. Rather surprisingly, there has been a paucity of data demonstrating that nutritional intervention has any real impact on clinical outcome in cancer. In many cases, this highlights the almost insurmountable difficulty in properly stratifying patient populations and objectively evaluating response. Most studies have utilized too few patients, with heterogeneous forms of cancer, to obtain meaningful, statistically valid data on outcome.

In 1981, Brennan reviewed 19 controlled trials to evaluate whether total parenteral nutrition had any impact on antineoplastic therapies and ultimately outcome in patients with cancer. At that time, available data suggested that for most patients with advanced cancer, short-term total parenteral nutrition had no effect on either survival or tolerance to chemotherapy or radiotherapy. In many cases, the results were variable. Some investigators had reported improvements in nutritional status (Smales et al. 1981; Rickard et al. 1979; Cohn et al. 1981), but the clinical importance of these findings was unclear.

More recent studies in patients with advanced cancer have obtained similar results. A study of oral nutritional support in patients with advanced colon and non-oat cell lung carcinoma has revealed that aggressive oral nutritional support including supplementation with nasogastric or gastric feeding tubes was not associated with improved survival (Nixon 1984). Similarly, objective disease response and tolerance of antineoplastic therapy were unaffected. In this case, the results are not unexpected, since effective therapy is more or less lacking in progressive metastatic colorectal and advanced lung cancer.

Other controlled studies of tumor disease which is more sensitive to treatment, such as lymphomas, have also failed to find significant improvements in survival or outcome with nutrition (Popp et al. 1981; Donaldson et al. 1982). In one such study, cancer patients who "responded" to their antineoplastic therapy showed significant improvements in nutrient utilization in response to feeding. Such findings emphasize the importance of patient stratification to identify possible candidates for controlled studies in the future.

In two reports in particular, controlled metabolic balance studies were performed. A series of cachectic cancer and noncancer patients were evaluated by Nixon and colleagues (1981) before and after parenteral and enteral nutrition. It was reported that cancer patients gained less body weight and lean tissue and had smaller increases in serum protein concentrations than similar noncancer patients. Metabolic balance data revealed that mineral balances, particularly of magnesium and phosphorus, were less positive in cancer patients than in noncancer patients, despite the fact that nitrogen balances were similar. This abnormal balance in cancer patients is consistent with incomplete repletion of lean tissue mass. Similar conclusions can be obtained from the data of Bennegård et al. (1983). These investigators observed that when malnourished cancer patients received enteral feeding, there was a significant net release of amino acids from the leg, indicating net protein catabolism. In contrast, similar enteral feedings in noncancer patients resulted in significant improvement in the amino acid balance across the leg, although it was still negative. Combined, these two studies suggest that in patients with advanced cancer, there is inefficient utilization of nutrients and thus no normal repletion of lean tissue, primarily in skeletal muscle.

In many patients with advanced cancer and primary cachexia, techniques of nutritional repletion will not be successful until we have a greater knowledge of the underlying mechanisms. The key question, however, is whether nutritional support has a role as an adjunctive therapy in other cancer patients in whom the prognosis may be better.

Two more recent studies have reported prolonged survival in cancer patients who received nutritional support as an adjunctive therapy. In an often cited and highly controversial study, Müller et al. (1982) reported that preoperative intravenous nutrition decreased postoperative mortality in patients with mainly gastrointestinal cancer. Somewhat surprisingly, the authors could not demonstrate any difference in complication rates or infections, despite improved survival, between groups given nutritional support and those maintained on standard crystalloid therapies. The study can be criticized because nutritional support was not related to the degree of existing malnutrition and because the diets were devoid of fat.

In a much less frequently cited work, Yamada and colleagues (1983) studied patients with advanced gastric carcinoma who were randomized in a prospective manner to total parenteral nutrition. The patients all received a cytostatic agent, orally administered 5-fluorouracil. The authors reported improved cellular immunity in the total parenteral nutrition group, increased tolerance 5-fluorouracil and improved 3-year survival. Survival increased from 0% in the control group to 54% in the group receiving total parenteral nutrition. The authors speculated that the increased survival was due to improved tolerance of the cytostatic agent, permitting a more intensive treatment schedule.

Conclusions and Recommendations

It is clear that certain patients with cancer cachexia secondary to mechanical causes will benefit from intensive nutritional support. Those patients with gastrointestinal obstruction, difficulty in swallowing, food aversions or discontinuity of the gastrointestinal tract, but in whom host-tumor interactions are not the main reason for the cachexia, will undoubtedly benefit from such therapy. Present evidence suggests that in these individuals, aggressive nutritional support will almost always lead to better tolerance of antineoplastic therapies.

However, nutritional support should still be considered in those patients whose cachexia cannot be easily attributed to mechanical causes and who have marked weight loss and a continued inability to maintain fluid and calorie balance. Equally important is the long-term strategy for treatment of the patient. Invasive nutritional support, such as central venous alimentation, in a patient with advanced cancer where no reasonable chance of cure or remission exists is probably inappropriate. In such cases, enteral nutrition or peripheral intravenous feeding regimens are superior for supportive care since they do not restrict the patient to the hospital setting in the terminal stages of their disease.

However, when the physician and patient have decided upon an aggressive treatment plan, nutritional support should be an integral component of a combined antineoplastic therapy. In this case, preliminary evidence would suggest that a period of preoperative or pretreatment nutritional support, when possible, may improve tolerance to therapy and have a favorable impact on outcome. In such cases, up to 7 days' pretreatment nutritional support would be recommended. In many cases, this does not have to be performed in the hospital. Rather, it can frequently be achieved at home through enteral feeding via supplements or a small-bore nasogastric tube.

In the planning of nutritional supportive therapy to cancer patients, it should be emphasized that a rapid and aggressive supply of energy to the malnourished patient can induce acute metabolic disturbances. A rapid glucose infusion can give rise to the hyperosmolar syndrome with coma and dehydration. Further, an increased production of carbon dioxide because of enhanced lipogenesis from glucose may induce acute respiratory failure. The extra fluid load on the depleted heart can result in cardiac insufficiency and/or sudden death. To avoid such problems, nutritional support during the first few days must be carried out with caution. The energy supply should not exceed energy expenditure, which is often 20%–30% lower than the basal metabolic rate in normal subjects of the same age and sex. If the patients tolerate this initial nutritional support well, the energy supply, which should be balanced and contain all nutrients, can then be increased up to 20%–30% above energy expenditure to achieve positive energy balance.

Nutritional support can be a powerful adjunct to antineoplastic therapies. Expensive, labor-intensive, total parenteral nutrition is best reserved for those patients in whom the gastrointestinal tract is not functioning and who are thought to have a reasonable chance of remission or cure. Such therapies should be used only in conjunction with surgery, radiotherapy or chemotherapy in situations where oral intake is not possible. Enteral feeding regimens employing feeding tubes and oral supplements, when used appropriately, offer an effective and cost-efficient method for supporting many patients with cancer. Equally important, however, is the realization that nutritional support offers little to the advanced cancer patient who is not responding to, or is not a candidate for, effective antineoplastic therapy.

References

Bennegård K, Edén E, Ekman L, Scherstén T, Ekman L (1982) Metabolic response of whole body and peripheral tissues to enteral nutrition in weight-losing cancer patients. Gastroenterology 85: 92–99

Bernstein IL, Bernstein ID (1981) Learned food aversions and cancer anorexia. Cancer Treat Rep 65: 43–47

Brennan MF (1981) Total parenteral nutrition in the cancer patient. N Engl J Med 305: 375–381

Cohn SH, Gartenhaus W, Vartsky D, Sawitsky A, Zanzi I, Vaswani A, Yasumura S, Rai K, Cortes E, Ellins KJ (1981) Body composition and dietary intake in neoplastic disease. Am J Clin Nutr 34: 1997–2001

Dempsey DT, Feurer ID, Crosby LO, Knox LS, Buzby GP, Muller TL (1984) Energy expenditure in malnourished cancer patients. Cancer 53: 1265–1273

DeWys WD, Beggs C, Lavin PT (1980) Prognostic effect of weight loss prior to chemotherapy in cancer patients. Am J Med 69: 491–497

DeWys WD, Costa G, Henkin R (1981) Clinical parameters related to anorexia. Cancer Treat Rep 65: 49–52

Donaldson SS, Wesley MN, Ghavimi F, Shils ME, Suskind RM, DeWys WD (1982) A prospective randomized clinical trial of total parenteral nutrition in children with cancer. Med Pediatr Oncol 10: 129–139

Edén E, Edström S, Bennegård K, Scherstén T, Lundholm K (1984) Glucose flux in relation to energy expenditure in malnourished patients with and without cancer during periods of fasting and feeding. Cancer Res 44: 1718–1724

Edén E, Edström S, Bennegård K, Lindmark L, Lundholm K (1985) Glycerol dynamics in weight losing cancer patients. Surgery 97: 176–184

Harvey KB (1980) Prognostic strength of nutritional assessment. Prog Clin Biol Res 77: 689–697

Harvey KB, Moldawer LL, Bistrian BR, Blackburn GL (1981) Biological measures for the development of a prognostic index in the hospitalized patient. Am J Clin Nutr 34: 2013–2022

Inagaki J, Rodriguez V, Bodey GB (1974) Causes of death in cancer patients. Cancer 53: 568–573

Kawamura I, Moldawer LL, Bistrain BR, Blackburn GL (1982) Altered amino acid turnover in rats with progressive tumour growth. Cancer Res 42: 824–829

Knox LS, Crosby LO, Feures ID, Buzby GP, Miller CL, Muller JL (1983) Energy expenditure in malnourished cancer patients. Ann Surg 197: 152–162

Krause R, Humphrey C, Von Meyenfeldt M, Howard J, Fischer JE (1981) A central mechanism for anorexia in cancer: a hypothesis. Cancer Treat Rep 65: 15–21

Lindmark L, Bennegård K, Edén E, Ekman L, Scherstén T, Svaninger G, Lundholm K (1984) Resting energy expenditure in malnourished patients with and without cancer. Gastroenterology 87: 402–408

Lindmark L, Bennegård K, Edén E, Svaninger G, Ternell M, Lundholm K (1986) Thermic effect and substrate oxidation in response to intravenous nutrition in cancer patients who lose weight. Ann Surg 204: 628–636

Lundholm K, Karlberg I, Ekman L, Edström S, Scherstén T (1981) Evaluation of anorexia as the cause of altered protein synthesis in skeletal muscles from nongrowing mice with sarcoma. Cancer Res 41: 1989–1996

Lundholm K, Bennegård K, Edén E, Svaninger G, Emery PW, Rennie MJ (1982) Efflux of 3-methylhistidine from the leg in cancer patients who experience weight loss. Cancer Res 42: 4807–4811

McCarthy DO, Kluger MJ, Vander AJ (1985) Suppression of food intake during infection. Is interleukin-1 involved? Am J Clin Nutr 42: 1179–1185

McRussell D, Shike M, Marliss EB, Detsky A, Shepherd RA, Feld R, Evans WK, Jeejeebhoy KN (1984) Effects of total parenteral nutrition and chemotherapy on the metabolic derangements in small cell lung cancer. Cancer Res 44: 1706–1711

Morrison Sd (1976) Control of food intake in cancer cachexia: a challenge and a tool. Physiol Behav 17: 705–714

Mullen JL, Buzby GP, Matthews DC, Smale BF, Rosato EF (1980) Reduction of postoperative morbidity and mortality by combined preoperative and postoperative nutritional support. Ann Surg 192: 604–613

Müller JM, Dienst C, Brenner U, Pichlmaier H (1982) Preoperative parenteral feeding in patients with gastrointestinal carcinoma. Lancet 1: 68–71

Nixon DW (1984) Nutritional support in cancer patients. J Med Assoc Ga 73 (1): 39–40

Nixon DW (1985) Nutritional management of the medical oncology patient. Nutr Intern 1: 37–39

Nixon DW, Heymsfeld SB, Cohen AE, Kutner MH, Ansley J, Lawson DH, Rudman D (1980) Protein calorie undernutrition in hospitalized cancer patients. Am J Med 68: 683–690

Nixon DW, Lawson DH, Kutner M, Ansley J, Schwarz M, Heymsfeld S, Chawla R, Cartwright TH, Rudman D (1981) Total parenteral nutrition as an adjunct to chemotherapy in metastatic colorectal cancer. Cancer Treat Res 65: 121–127

Nixon DW, Daly JM, Jeejeebhoy KN, Ellenburg S, Hoffman FA (1982) Augmented or standard nutritional intervention in advanced colorectal and small cell lung carcinoma. Cancer Res 25: 172 A

Popp MB, Fischer RI, Wesley R (1981) A prospective randomized study of adjuvant parenteral nutrition in the treatment of advanced diffuse lymphoma: influence on survival. Surgery 90: 195–203

Rickard KA, Grossfield JL, Kirksey A, Ballantine TVN, Baehner RL (1979) Reversal of protein energy malnutrition in children during treatment of advanced neoplastic disease. Ann Surg 190: 771–781

Sickles EA, Young WM, Greene WH, Wiernik PH (1973) Pneumonia in acute leukemia. Ann Intern Med 78: 528–534

Smales BF, Mullen JK, Buzby GP, Rosato EF (1981) The efficacy of nutritional assessment and support in cancer surgery. Cancer 47: 2375–2381

Symreng T, Anderberg B, Küagedal B, et al. (1983) Nutritional assessment and clinical course in 112 elective surgical patients. Acta Chir Scand 149 (7): 657–662

Ternell M, Lönnroth C, Lundholm K (1985) Nuclear RNA polymerase activity in tumour-host livers. Am J Physiol 249: E 461–469

Theologides A (1979) Cancer cachexia. Cancer 43: 2004–2012

Tocco-Bradley R, Georgieff M, Jones CT Moldawer LL, Dinarello CA, Blackburn GL, Bistrian BR (1987) Changes in energy expenditure and fat metabolism in rats infused with interleukin-1. Eur J Clin Invest 17: 504–510

Walker C, Gray BN (1983) Acute phase reactant proteins and canceroenzymic antigen in cancer of the colon and rectum. Cancer 52: 150–154

Warnold I, Lundholm K (1984) Clinical significance of preoperative nutritional status in 215 noncancer patients. Ann Surg 199: 299–305

Warnold I, Lundholm K, Scherstén T (1978) Energy balance and body composition in cancer patients. Cancer Res 38: 1801–1807

Warren S (1932) Immediate causes of death in cancer. Am J Med 184: 610–615

Waterhouse C (1974) How tumour affects host metabolism. Ann NY Acad Sci 230: 86–93

Waterhouse C (1981) Oxidation and metabolic interconversion in malignant cachexia. Cancer Treat Rep 65: 61–66

Yamada N, Koyama YH, Hioki L, Yamada T, Yamamoto M (1983) Effect of postoperative total parenteral nutrition as an adjunct to gastrectomy for advanced gastric carcinoma. Br J Surg 70: 267–274

Young VR (1977) Energy metabolism and requests in the cancer patient. Cancer Res 37: 2336–2347

Infection in Cancer Patients

P. Dejace and J. Klastersky

Patients with cancer are at increased risk of infection. In fact, infectious complications constitute the main obstacle to more aggressive cancer chemotherapy. Infections arise in patients with cancer because of (a) their underlying disease, (b) prolonged hospitalization and (c) cancer therapy. We will review the factors that predispose to infections in cancer, their clinical manifestations, their diagnosis and treatment and finally how to prevent them.

Factors Predisposing to Infections in Cancer Patients

Many factors predispose cancer patients to infections. The most important of these are immunological and involve phagocytic defenses or cellular or humoral immunity. Others involve obstruction to natural passages, for example by solid tumors, or central nervous system dysfunction, which can result in aspiration pneumonias and urinary tract infections. Iatrogenic procedures, from the use of various catheters and respiratory devices to those associated with the treatment of cancer, may also be responsible.

Granulocytopenia

Granulocytopenia, which is usually associated with cancer therapy and concomitant damage to body barriers is certainly the most important factor predisposing patients to infections and thus limiting the aggressiveness of cancer therapy. Bacteremia is the ultimate result of granulocytopenia or impaired neutrophil function. The relationship between infections and bacteremias and the granulocyte count is well established. Nearly all patients who remain profoundly neutropenic (< 100 circulating neutrophils/ml) become infected by the 3rd week or earlier. Granulocytopenia is mainly associated with myelotoxic chemotherapy, although it can also be due to intensive radiotherapy or invasion of bone marrow by tumor cells.

Almost all cytotoxic agents are also toxic for the rapidly developing marrow cells, with few exceptions (vincristine, bleomycin, asparaginase, dacarbazine). The time-course of this toxic effect on bone marrow is very important to know. With most agents it is uniphasic and the nadir is reached in 8–10 days, but for certain drugs it may be delayed (busulfan 3–4 weeks, procarbazine 6–8 weeks) and may also be biphasic with a misleading plateau before the second nadir (BCNU, melphalan). Similarly, granulocytopenia due to X-ray irradiation of bone marrow is usually biphasic. Its intensity depends on the areas of the body that have been irradiated. It is important, in this respect, to know the contribution of different parts of the bone marrow to circulating granulocytes. Irradiation of the pelvis and lower vertebral column, for example, is more likely to lead to cytopenia. Invasion of bone marrow by tumors, or myelophtisis, occurs most frequently with metastastic carcinoma of breast, prostate, lung, kidney, adrenal or thyroid or in malignant melanoma.

Severe bone marrow involvement may occur with Hodgkin's disease and even more often with non-Hodgkin's lymphomas, with resulting neutropenia. Bacteremia in severely neutropenic patients is most often caused by *Escherichia coli*, *Klebsiella pneumoniae*, *Pseudomonas aeruginosa* or *Staphylococcus aureus*. The distribution of these infections may depend upon local hospital flora, as well as the colonization of the gastrointestinal tract and other sites before onset of bacteremia.

Invasive fungal infections caused by *Aspergillus fumigatus*, *Candida albicans*, *Candida tropicalis*, *Mucor* spp. and other agents may occur in severely neutropenic patients. These infections are associated with very high mortality and may occur simultaneously with bacterial infections or, more often, develop during antibiotic therapy for a primary bacterial infection.

Patients with profound neutropenia may have defective leukocyte mobilization, and they may not be able to limit bacterial invasion locally. Thus, they show few of the classical signs of inflammation: *rubor, calor, dolor* and *tumor;* abscess formation may be limited. Local infection may be more subtle and more easily overlooked than in otherwise normal hosts.

Radiological findings of pneumonia, for example, may not be present at the onset of infection, and a radiological infiltrate may not appear until several days after pneumonia has developed. Frequent chest X-rays should be taken in neutropenic patients with fever in order to identify pneumonia as a possible source.

Cellular Immune Deficiency

Patients with any advanced neoplasm of any type are likely to have nonspecific defects in both humoral and cellular immunity that contribute to their increased risk of serious infection.

However, more specific defects in cellular immunity may be present in some untreated neoplastic disorders. Patients with Hodgkin's disease have decreased delayed sensitivity responses to recall antigens such as mumps, candidin and purified protein derivative (PPD). Similarly, the T-lymphocyte response to phytohemagglutinin and the ability to proliferate in mixed lymphocyte cultures are depressed in these patients.

Patients with tumors of the head and neck may also manifest some defects of cell-mediated immunity.

Depressed cell-mediated immunity has similarly been reported in untreated patients with acute lymphoblastic leukemia. Patients whose cell-mediated immunity is altered are at increased risk of disseminated infections with intracellular bacteria such as *Mycobacterium tuberculosis*, atypical mycobacteria, *Listeria monocytogenes*, *Salmonella* spp. and *Brucella* spp. These patients are also at special risk of contracting DNA viruses such as cytomegalovirus (CMV), herpes simplex virus and varicella-zoster virus. Patients with T-cell defects also are at risk of acquiring fungal infections and, in particular, meningitis and pulmonary infection with *Cryptococcus neoformans* and disseminated infection with *Candida*, *Mucor* and *Aspergillus* spp.

Patients with AIDS have profound defects in cellular immunity: there is an increased incidence of Kaposi's sarcoma and central nervous system lymphoma in these patients. They are also subject to infections by opportunistic microorganisms: *Pneumocystis carinii*, herpes-viruses, CMV, *Candida albicans*, *Cryptococcus neoformans*, *Mycobacterium* spp., *Cryptosporidium* spp., *Toxoplasma gondii* etc.

Humoral Immune Deficiency

Alteration in humoral immunity is likely to occur in patients with untreated chronic lymphocytic leukemia (CLL), multiple myeloma and Waldenström's macroglobulinemia. Immunoglobulin antibody levels may be decreased, and these patients may exhibit decreased responsiveness to antigenic stimulation.

Patients with multiple myeloma have increased levels of immunoglobulin which does not react with bacterial antigens and does not protect against infection. These patients, as well as those with Waldenström's macroglobulinemia, have decreased polyclonal immunoglobulin response to bacterial antigens. Patients with defects in humoral antibodies are particularly susceptible to infections with encapsulated bacteria such as *Streptococcus pneumoniae, Hemophilus influenzae, Neisseria meningitidis* and *Klebsiella pneumoniae.*

Similarly, splenectomized patients are at increased risk of septicemia, usually with *S. pneumoniae*, occasionally with *H. influenzae* or *N. meningitidis*. The pneumococcal sepsis syndrome is much more common in splenectomized children and relatively rare in adults. However, patients in whom splenectomy has been done for staging of lymphoma, for example, seem to be at higher risk than patients who have undergone splenectomy for trauma. This syndrome of pneumococcal sepsis can have a devastating mortality (Bisno and Freeman 1970).

Local Effects of Tumor Growth and Obstruction on Natural Passages

Primary skin tumors or secondary skin lesions produce erosive or ulcerative lesions which may predispose to local infection and bacteremia. Organisms involved include group A streptococci and *Staphylococcus aureus:* They are both more common and more ominous in their consequences if the patients are immunosuppressed. In the oral cavity and nasopharynx, ulcerating tumors may predispose to local infections with streptococci, pneumococci or *Hemophilus* spp. Anaerobic infections may begin in the mouth, nose or throat.

Ulceration along the gastrointestinal tract may occur with locally invading neoplasms. This mucosal breakdown also destroys an important physical barrier to the penetration of infection.

Oropharyngeal colonization with *Candida* spp. is frequent in cancer patients, particularly those treated with antibiotics, and mucosal ulceration can certainly facilitate invasion of the blood stream by yeast cells. Actually, the source of candidemia in most patients with cancer seems to be the digestive tract rather than the skin, with occasional invasion through an indwelling catheter.

Similarly, ulcerating neoplasms of the female genital tract may result in invasive infections caused by enterococci, anaerobic or aerobic gram-negative rods or *Clostridium* spp.

Another local effect of tumor growth is obstruction at various sites: as the adage says "obstruction leads to infection." Partial obstruction of a bronchus by bronchogenic carcinoma can lead to postobstructive pneumonia, partial urethral obstruction secondary to prostatic carcinoma to urinary tract infection, obstruction of the biliary tract to ascending cholangitis. Obstruction results in retention of mucus secretions and subsequent distal infection by locally colonizing organisms that may be resistant pathogens acquired during hospitalization. Similarly, invasive and obstructing lesions in the gastrointestinal tract often result in bowel perforations with subsequent peritonitis and intra-abdominal abscess formation, which may be associated with aerobic and/or anaerobic bacteremia.

Changes in Endogenous Microflora

Much of the risk of infection in patients with cancer is associated with prolonged hospitalization and suppression of normal host defenses resulting from chemotherapy. Approximately half of these infections are the result of endogenous microflora present on admission to the hospital. The remainder are from organisms acquired during the hospital stay. Shifts in normal oropharyngeal flora toward gram-negatives have been observed with illness and hospitalization. These organisms colonize various mucosal and skin sites and are likely to be more virulent and resistant to more antimicrobial agents than the organisms present on admission (Schimpff et al. 1972b). Organisms responsible for bacteremia in profoundly neutropenic patients may be found colonizing various body sites before development of bacteremia. Colonization of the nasopharynx with potentially pathogenic gram-negative rods directly correlate with severity of illness (Johanson et al. 1969).

Iatrogenic Factors

We have alluded to many iatrogenic factors that lead to more infections in cancer patients. Cancer chemotherapy and radiotherapy can destroy the body's immune defenses in hurting immunologically important cells but also in breaking the barriers represented by skin and mucous membranes.

Also breakdown of skin by permanent catheters, and of mucosa by feeding tubes and the like, obviously facilitates access to the body by various infecting agents. The same problems arise from tubes placed for respiratory assistance: they permit direct access to the respiratory tract for pathogenic microorganisms. In addition, these devices often play the role of a "foreign body," attracting microorganisms. Similarly, it has been known since the days of Semmelweis that physicians and other medical personnel can transmit infections from patient to patient by not washing their hands after each patient contact.

Clinical Manifestations of Infections in Cancer Patients

Fever

Fever is extremely common in cancer patients and scrupulous attention should always be paid to the temperature chart. It is useful to ask the patient to actually take and document the temperature, because it can be the only symptom of infection. The first question to be answered in the case of fever is whether the patient is neutropenic or not.

This is a critical question, because neutropenic patients with disseminated infection have very high mortality, so high that it leads one to break a commonly held principle in infectious diseases: namely, to treat only obviously "septic" toxic patients or patients with a clinical or radiological focus of infection. That is why knowledge of the expected nadir of neutrophil count in patients treated for cancer is so important for physicians following them.

The white cell count is therefore one of the most helpful laboratory tests in oncology. Levels of below a total count of 1000 white cells are dangerous, levels below 100 neutrophils much more so. Actually, there is a remarkable correlation between a decreasing neutrophil count and the likelihood of infection (Bodey et al. 1966).

The attitude toward fever is thus, of necessity, fundamentally different when the patient is neutropenic: broad-spectrum empiric antibiotics should be started as soon as microbiological specimens are obtained (Schimpff et al. 1971). Regimens have varied with time and local epidemiology, but should include drugs active against *Pseudomonas aeruginosa*. In most studies, about 40% of the patients will have microbiologically documented infections, half of them bacteremia. The remainder of the patients will have no precise microbiological documentation of infection, although many will nevertheless respond to empiric treatment (EORTC 1978).

Longstanding fever without known cause is present in 1% of patients admitted to a cancer ward. In many of these patients, an infectious process will ultimately be proven, but some of them have fever attributed to the neoplastic process itself ("B" symptoms in lymphoma). Noninfectious causes are also possible: thrombophlebitis (occasionally septic) with or without pulmonary embolism, transfusion reactions, febrile reactions to cancer chemotherapy (mainly seen with bleomycin but also described with dacarbazine, mithramycin and methotrexate), allergic reactions etc.

Bacteremia

Large studies such as those of the EORTC (1978) have shown that approximately 20% of neutropenic patients with fever actually develop bacteremia. The sources of bacteremia are diverse and often difficult to find, presumably because of poor local response to infection in neutropenia. That is why, when the patient is neutropenic, broad-spectrum antimicrobial therapy should be started at once, even if no focus is identified. Sources include pneumonia, anal lesions, pharyngitis (probably often precipitated by mucositis due to chemotherapy), urinary tract and skin infections.

The greatest danger of bacteremia is obviously the development of septic shock, which can rapidly lead to death in compromised patients.

In recent years, various measures of preventing infections have been used and this could lead to a reduction of bacteremias (Pizzo et al. 1982).

The organisms involved include gram-positive cocci, such as *Staphylococcus aureus* and also, more recently, *Staphylococcus epidermidis* (Wade et al. 1982), and streptococci, including *S. pneumoniae* (Dejace et al. 1985), but gram-negatives such as *Pseudomonas aeruginosa*, *Escherichia coli*, *Klebsiella* spp. and *Enterobacter* spp. continue to represent at least 50% of the pathogens isolated from bacteremic patients. Bacteremia can also be a problem in non-neutropenic patients: the role of various breaks in natural barriers to infection is here paramount. The skin represents an important barrier which can be broken by the disease itself, in skin, head and neck and breast cancer, or even more frequently, in iatrogenic situations. The use of permanent catheters for easy administration of chemotherapy, parenteral nutrition or antibiotics can be complicated by bacteremia. Similarly the use of occlusive dressings which decreases the relative dryness of the skin, (normally a limiting factor for the growth of some organisms) also contributes.

Breakdown of the mucosal barrier by oropharyngeal or digestive tumors or by mucositis due to chemotherapy also represents an important risk factor for the development of bacteremia.

Pneumonia

Pneumonia is common in cancer patients. The spectrum of infectious agents is wide, from bacteria often present in community-acquired pneumonias, such as *Streptococcus pneumoniae* and *Legionella pneumophila*, to gram-negatives, mycobacteria, *Nocardia* spp., fungi, viruses and parasites like *Toxoplasma gondii* and *Pneumocystis carinii* (Robbins et al. 1976).

In neutropenic patients, the infection is often caused by gram-negative bacilli, such as *Pseudomonas aeruginosa, Escherichia coli, Klebsiella* spp. and/or *Staphylococcus aureus*. Because of the poor inflammatory response associated with granulocytopenia, few or no physical findings are present at examination and the chest X-ray film may be normal, so both physical examination and X-rays should be repeated often to make the diagnosis (Sickles et al. 1975). Similarly, sputum may be minimal in amount, may consist of nonpurulent material and may be of little diagnostic value because of the frequent colonization of hospitalized patients by pathogenic bacilli.

However, sputum should always be examined because important clues to a dominant pathogen can sometimes be obtained.

Staphylococcus aureus pneumonia can occur: it usually is very acute with rapid spread of necrotizing lung damage. *Legionella* pneumonia can present with associated abdominal symptoms, hypophosphatemia and hyponatremia. *Mycobacterium tuberculosis* infections are described in immunosuppressed patients, particularly those with lymphomas, lung, and head and neck cancers. Although the infection is usually subacute, a syndrome of "tuberculous pneumonia" with very high mortality has been described in such patients (Kaplan et al. 1974). In some areas, infections with atypical myocobacteria are common (Feld et al. 1976). There are many other causes of pulmonary infections in the immunocompromised host.

Infections with *Nocardia* spp. are usually rather insidious in onset, but fulminant cases have been described (Neu et al. 1967); nocardiosis can also disseminate and cause brain abscesses or soft tissue infections (Young et al. 1971).

Pulmonary infections caused by fungi, although usually subacute, can be devastating, particularly when an *Aspergillus* species is the offending agent.

Occasional pulmonary infections with *Candida* spp. *Cryptococcus neoformans* and Mucorales have been described in immunocompromised hosts. Other fungi that may cause interstitial pneumonitis include *Histoplasma capsulatum, Coccidioides immitis* and *Blastomyces dermatitidis*.

Viruses are also important agents of pulmonary infections in immunosuppressed patients. Among viruses, the most important is certainly CMV, both because of its frequency and its role in morbidity and mortality. It is a particularly striking cause of pulmonary infections in patients with hematological neoplasms and especially after bone marrow transplantation. In one study, it accounted for 44% of all histologically proven pneumonias in that setting, with 88% mortality (Meyers et al. 1975). CMV pneumonia is often insidious in onset with fever and dry cough followed by dyspnea and hypoxemia. The chest X-ray is variable but usually shows interstitial infiltrates or bilateral small nodular densities. In bone marrow transplants, the risk is maximal between 30 and 90 days after the transplant. The differential diagnosis of this syndrome of interstitial pneumonia in immunosuppressed patients is, in fact, extremely wide, and includes many other infections, some noninfectious causes and probably unknown ones.

Another important virus is herpes simplex. Herpes simplex tracheobronchitis and bronchopneumonia has been described in immunosuppressed patients (Nash 1972). Local infection might be enhanced by local trauma due to endotracheal intubation. The varicella-zoster virus may also be responsible for pneumonias, and in fact when the virus disseminates during primary varicella, the lung is the major target organ, with liver and brain involved less commonly (Ramsey et al. 1982). Visceral dissemination in adult patients with varicella-zoster virus also occurs occasionally with central nervous system, lung, heart and gastrointestinal tract involvement (Schimpff et al. 1972a).

Pneumocystis carinii is a very important pulmonary pathogen in immunocompromised patients: its prominence as an opportunistic infection in patients with AIDS has reemphasized its importance, although its incidence in cancer patients has been decreased by the widespread use of trimethoprim-sulfamethoxazole prophylaxis. The presentation of *Pneumocystis carinii* pneumonia can also be very insidious, and cases of dyspnea with profound hypoxia have been described with a normal chest X-ray. The chest X-ray picture might also be rather nonspecific, with perihilar infiltrates at the beginning.

Another protozoon responsible for pulmonary infections in immunosuppressed patients is *Toxoplasma gondii,* which is rare and usually associated with dissemination to the central nervous system (Ruskin and Remington 1976). Finally, *Strongyloides stercoralis* has been described as a cause of diffuse pulmonary infiltrates in the overwhelming strongyloidiasis syndrome seen in immunocompromised patients, especially those whose immunosuppression is the result of corticosteroids (Scowden et al. 1978).

Noninfectious causes of pulmonary infiltrates should also be borne in mind, especially those due to cancer chemotherapy agents such as bleomycin, methotrexate and busulfan.

Oral, Pharyngeal and Esophageal Infections

The most important predisposing factor to oral, pharyngeal and esophageal infections in cancer patients is undoubtedly the common occurrence of mucosal ulcerations after chemotherapy. This so-called mucositis is a frequent side effect of therapy with cyclophosphamide, 5-fluorouracil and methotrexate. Similarly, about 10% of patients receiving cytosine arabinoside, 5-azacytidine or mitomycin develop oral inflammation and ulceration.

Mouth ulceration due to bleomycin is usually associated with skin hypertrophic changes at pressure points, leading to desquamation and occasional bulla formation. It has been described in 15%–40% of patients.

Doxorubicin, daunomycin and actinomycin D often cause severe mucosal inflammation and ulceration, and the combination of doxorubicin and radiotherapy also can cause severe esophageal lesions. Stomatitis is seen in about 10% of patients treated with vinblastine but has not been described with vincristine.

Oropharyngeal colonization with *Candida* spp. is frequent in cancer patients particularly those treated with antibiotics, and mucosal ulceration can certainly facilitate invasion of the bloodstream by yeast cells. The source of candidemia in most patients seems to be the digestive tract.

With bacterial, fungal or viral pharyngitis, the patient complains of severe pharyngeal pain, dysphagia, fever and chills. The throat is erythematous and cervical adenopathy may be present. Because of the poor inflammatory response, many of these cases of pharyngitis can initially appear rather benign. Throat cultures yield multiple organisms, particularly gram-negative bacilli and *Staphylococcus aureus*, but it is often difficult to ascertain whether those organisms actually are the cause of pharyngitis. The oropharyngeal mucosa can also present the characteristic white infiltration and/or exudate of *Candida* infection. Gram staining and culturing such lesions is an easy way of making the diagnosis. Similar lesions can also be seen in candidal esophagitis, and complaints of dysphagia and odynophagia should always be taken seriously and investigated by endoscopy in immunocompromised patients.

Herpetic esophagitis has also been described frequently in those patients, and the diagnosis is also made by endoscopy.

Sinusitis, which may be caused by viruses, *Streptococcus pneumoniae, Hemophilus influenzae* and other gram-negative bacteria, as in other patients, can also be caused by unusual pathogens, like *Aspergillus* or *Mucor* spp. It should always be investigated.

Skin and Soft Tissue Infections

Our skin represents a very important physical barrier to infection. But the skin is also important because of its rich blood supply, which means that it is frequently involved in infections elsewhere in the body by blood-borne septic emboli.

Since the skin is easily accessible, it is a very important organ to examine and biopsy when establishing the presence and the cause of an ongoing infectious process (Dejace and Klastersky 1986c).

The skin is often involved in infections in immunocompromised patients: some reports state a frequency of 20%–30% (Wolfson et al. 1985).

The keratinized layers of the epidermis prevent penetration by microorganisms, and the relative dryness of the skin tends to limit the proliferation of some microorganisms requiring moisture for growth, such as gram-negative bacteria and *Candida* spp.

Bacterial cellulitis can be due to the same pathogens as in normal hosts, namely gram-positive bacteria such as group A streptococci and *Staphylococcus aureus.* But unusual pathogens are always a possibility in immunocompromised patients. A typical skin infection encountered in neutropenic patients is ecthyma gangrenosum, which is a necrotic lesion surrounded by erythema. This is almost pathognomonic of sepsis due to *Pseudomonas aeruginosa*, although similar lesions can be seen in infections due to Enterobacteriacae.

Gram staining of this lesion will establish the diagnosis. In approximately 15% of patients with candidal septicemia, typical macronodular skin lesions have been described: direct examination and/or biopsy with culture will also provide the diagnosis.

Various other rare causes of skin infections in immunocompromised patients include *Aspergillus* spp., endemic mycotic infections due to *Histoplasma capsulatum*, *Coccidioides immitis* and *Blastomyces dermatitidis*, and typical and atypical mycobacteria.

Another important cause of skin infections in immunocompromised patients are the herpesviruses. Herpes simplex virus (type I or type II) commonly causes recurrent, localized, facial or anogenital infections, but more severe infections can occur in compromised patients, particularly in patients with hematological malignancies, where large, chronic, ulcerated lesions (herpes phagenda) have been described.

Dissemination can occur in transplant patients and in leukemia or lymphoma. Similarly, varicella-zoster virus infections can cause severe infections in children with hematologic malignancies, who should be protected with zoster immunoglobulins within 72 h of exposure.

Reactivation of zoster has been described in lymphoma patients but also in solid tumors: it can even become generalized ("recurrent chickenpox").

Gastrointestinal Tract Infections and Hepatitis

We mentioned earlier the importance of the esophagus, which is often involved in the so-called mucositis secondary to cancer chemotherapy, as a portal of entry of candidal septicemia. It is likely, although there are few studies to substantiate this, that there is similar damage all along the digestive tract with similar consequences. Necrotizing lesions of the colon can occur with neoplasia or its therapy, and they can lead to bacteremia caused by bowel flora. One striking example of this is the syndrome of necrotizing ileocecal enterocolitis or typhlitis described in children with acute leukemia (Amromin and Solomon 1962).

Similarly, typical pseudomembranous colitis has been described in a few patients not receiving antibiotics but rather cancer chemotherapy (doxorubicin, methotrexate and 5-fluorouracil). Enteritis secondary to herpes simplex virus or CMV can present as colitis. Hepatitis is a frequent occurrence in patients with cancer, especially if multiple transfusions had to be used. In addition to hepatitis caused by viruses A and B, which has decreased in incidence since the introduction of blood screening, non-A, non-B hepatitis remains a problem, often difficult to distinguish from toxic hepatitis due to various chemotherapy agents (methotrexate, 6-mercaptopurine, cytosine arabinoside and asparaginase). Hepatitis due to CMV can also be associated with transfusions. Differentiation between necrosis in hepatic metastases and true bacterial hepatitis or liver abscesses as the cause of fever can be very difficult indeed. Similarly, liver involvement has been described with *Candida* spp. (Jones 1981).

Perianal abscesses occur frequently in cancer patients, particularly in acute myelomonocytic and monocytic leukemias – the clinical presentation is that of an extensive and necrotic cellulitis – and particular attention should be paid to that area in the physical examination of such immunosuppressed patients.

Urinary Tract Infections

Urinary tract infections are not a common problem in neutropenic patients, unless there is a complicating factor such as urinary tract obstruction, catheterization or another urological procedure or preceding recurrent urinary tract infection.

Dysuria and pyuria might not be present because of a decreased inflammatory response.

Central Nervous System Infections

In central nervous system dysfunction, again, symptoms and signs in patients whose host response to infection is limited by their disease or therapy can be more subtle than in normal hosts. Signs may be minimal, with fever or headache the most common presenting complaint (Hooper et al. 1982), although obviously more ominous signs of central nervous system dysfunction, such as meningeal signs, disorders of consciousness and focal neurological signs, can develop. A careful neurological examination should be made, and regularly repeated, and the use of CT scanning and/or lumbar puncture should be liberal and include, for example, unexplained headache (Rubin and Hooper 1985). The pathogens involved are numerous but depend on the immune status of the patient. Patients with impaired cell-mediated immunity (mostly those with lymphoma, especially Hodgkin's disease) are predisposed to infections by intracellular parasites: *Listeria monocytogenes*, *Cryptococcus neoformans*, *Mycobacterium tuberculosis*, *Toxoplasma gondii*, varicella-zoster virus, *Aspergillus* spp., *Nocardia* spp. etc. Patients with defective humoral immunity (CLL, multiple myeloma and lymphoma after aggressive treatment), especially if they have had splenectomy, are more susceptible to infections with encapsulated bacteria such as *Streptococcus pneumoniae*, *Hemophilus influenzae* type b and *Neisseria meningitidis* (Armstrong and Wong 1982).

Patients with a decreased number of polymorphonuclear neutrophils often have infections with *Pseudomonas aeruginosa* and other Enterobacteriacae, but infections due to fungi such as *Candida* and *Aspergillus* spp. are also prominent.

Listeria monocytogenes is the most common single agent causing bacterial central nervous system disease in the compromised host (Hooper et al. 1982). Although the epidemiology of the infection is not entirely clear, it mostly affects newborn babies and immunocompromised and/or aged patients. Several recent reports (Ho et al. 1986) have linked it to food contaminated by diseased animals. It can present in one of three ways: the most common is acute meningitis with or without bacteremia, but bacteremia alone has been described, as well as meningoencephalitis or cerebritis without concomitant meningitis (Nieman and Lorber 1980). In a large study in renal transplant recipients, 50% of the patients had meningitis, 10% parenchymal central nervous system disease, 9% parenchymal central nervous system disease and meningitis, 30% primary bacteremia and 1% urinary tract infections (Stamm et al. 1982).

Central nervous sytem infections caused by *Listeria* spp. can present in a very mild way, with fever and headache at the beginning, but because of possible parenchymal brain involvement, focal signs like cranial nerve palsies can develop later. The development of focal signs is rare in bacterial meningitis and should point toward *Listeria* spp. or *Mycobacterium tuberculosis* as the cause of infection. The CSF picture can be very variable, from near-normal in patients with cerebritis without meningitis, to the classical mononuclear predominance and, more often, a picture typical of purulent bacterial meningitis. Other causes of purulent bacterial meningitides include *Pseudomonas aeruginosa* or Enterobacteriacae, either with overwhelming sepsis or by contiguous spread from infected nasal sinuses, and *Streptococcus pneumoniae* and *Hemophilus influenzae* type b in splenectomized patients. *Nocardia asteroides* is another unusual cause of central nervous system infections in immunocompromised patients: it is usually associated with infections elsewhere, particularly in the lungs, and most frequently presents as a brain abscess (Young et al. 1971).

Tuberculosis of the central nervous system is a rather rare cause of infection in the immunocompromised patient. Fungal infections are also an important consideration: among them, infection due to *Cryptococcus neoformans* is probably the most common in this setting: the presentation can be rather mild, and the CSF picture is usually lymphocytic with positive India ink and latex tests (Kaplan et al. 1977).

Other fungi that can be responsible for central nervous system infections in immunocompromised patients include *Aspergillus* spp., mainly responsible for brain abscess, usually secondary to a pulmonary focus (Meyer et al. 1973), and *Candida* spp., usually in the setting of disseminated candidiasis (Bayer et al. 1976).

Rarer fungal causes of central nervous system infections include rhinocerebral mucormycosis (Meyer et al. 1972), and the geographically limited nonopportunistic fungi should not be forgotten: infections with *Coccidioides immitis*, *Blastomyces dermatitidis* and *Histoplasma capsulatum* can occur in anyone, but are more likely to cause disseminated infection in immunocompromised patients.

Among viruses, the most important are the herpesviruses, because of their frequency and the fact that they can be treated effectively. Varicella-zoster virus infection can disseminate, particularly in patients with depressed cell-mediated immunity, such as those with lymphoma: in such patients, symptoms of encephalitis usually begin 1–8 weeks after the cutaneous eruption (Dolin et al. 1978). Herpes simplex encephalitis can also occur, although probably not more often than in normal hosts. Finally, a syndrome of progressive multifocal leukoencephalopathy due to the papovavirus JC has been described in patients with chronic defects in cell-mediated immunity (Richardson 1974).

Parasites are also an important cause of neurological infection in immunosuppressed patients: diffuse and focal encephalitis, or brain abscess, can be due to the protozoon *Toxoplasma gondii* (Ruskin and Remington 1976).

Infections with *Strongyloides stercoralis* have already been alluded to: there can be a "hyperinfection" syndrome with massive invasion of the gastrointestinal tract and the lungs, and also a syndrome of "disseminated strongyloidiasis" with involvement of the central nervous system (Scowden et al. 1978).

Diagnostic Considerations

When one sees the number of different pathogens that can be responsible for infections in immunocompromised patients, it follows that precise diagnosis is often difficult and that all possible means of making that diagnosis should be used, including, from time to time, invasive procedures. Simple, routine bacteriological procedures should not be neglected, however, and should be repeated as often as necessary, although it is often more difficult to distinguish infection from contamination in immunocompromised patients because of the lack of inflammatory response. Any local area of possible infection should be aspirated and cultured and a biopsy done if the diagnosis is not provided by the microbiologist. The value of rather simple and relatively innocuous procedures, such as skin biopsy, or biopsy through endoscopy cannot be overemphasized (Wolfson et al. 1985).

Similarly, a lumbar puncture should be done at the slightest sign of neurological disturbance and the fluid thoroughly examined for cellular reaction, protein and glucose, bacterial antigen, cryptococcal antigen by latex agglutination etc.

In pulmonary infections, it is even more important to consider using invasive procedures to obtain a specific diagnosis, although the risk/benefit ratio has been questioned (Browne et al. 1985).

Serology is not always helpful, because immunocompromised patients have poor antibody response, but it should always be done: although the value of a negative result is often questionable, a positive test is very helpful and noninvasive.

Untreated infection is likely to progress rapidly in cancer patients, all the more so if they are neutropenic or otherwise immunosuppressed, and an aggressive diagnostic approach with institution of specific therapy can be the only chance of cure.

Therapeutic Considerations

Any specific infection documented in immunocompromised patients should obviously be treated with parenteral antibiotics, according to the results of cultures and antibiograms. But the lack of immune defenses means that an infection may pursue a relentless fulminant course unless treated promptly (Sickles et al. 1975). This has led to the use of empirical broad-spectrum antibiotics at the first sign of infection in neutropenic patients.

Recommended regimens vary with time and local hospital epidemiology: they usually include a beta-lactam active against *Pseudomonas* and an aminoglycoside. The best regimen in the latest EORTC study uses the combination of ceftazidime and amikacin (EORTC 1986). Recently, there has been renewed interest for the combination of two beta-lactams in that setting, especially in selected patients where the risk of nephrotoxicity is particularly high, e.g., those receiving other nephrotoxic agents, such as cyclosporine or amphotericin B (Dejace and Klastersky 1986a). Those regimens cannot be generally recommended at the present time, for lack of large-scale clinical trials.

For the same reason of limited experience, monotherapy with broad-spectrum agents like ceftazidime or cefoperazone, although attractive because of the lesser risk for nephrotoxicity, cannot yet be generally recommended (see, however, Pizzo et al. 1986). In the case of failure of this initial therapy regimen, which usually becomes obvious only after 72 h in immunocompromised patients but might be manifest earlier with rapid deterioration, possible causes should be carefully sought after. Potential causes of failure are as follows:

1. Ineffectiveness of the treatment regimen against the organism causing infection: the cultures taken at the onset of fever show that the causative organism is not susceptible to the drugs used in the first-line regimen. Specific therapy against the causative organism should then be initiated, using an agent shown to be active.
2. Mixed infection: infection due to more than one organism, one of which is resistant to the drugs used. In this case, an antibiotic generally known to be active against this organism should be added to the first-line regimen.
3. Superinfection: resistant gram-negative bacilli detected in surveillance cultures, coagulase-negative staphylococci associated with an IV line, fungi etc.
4. Infections not usually controlled with antibiotics alone, such as abscesses and empyemas: these should be located and surgically drained.
5. Noninfectious causes of fever: these should be considered and dealt with if possible.

Empirical use of antifungal agents, mostly amphotericin B with its attendant toxicity, in patients not responding to antibacterial agents is problematic, but should be considered, particularly in patients heavily colonized with possibly pathogenic fungi (Pizzo et al. 1982). The duration of empirical antibacterial therapy mainly depends on whether granulocytopenia subsides or not. If granulocytopenia resolves, it is generally not recommended to continue antibiotics for more than the period of 7–10 days recommended for the treatment of septicemia in nonimmunocompromised patients. However, in persistently neutropenic patients, early discontinuation of empirical antibiotics may result in recurrence of possibly lethal, microbiologically documented infections (Pizzo et al. 1979).

At the same time, viruses and parasites should be continually searched for as causes of localized or disseminated infections, even if invasive procedures are necessary for diagnosis.

The use of granulocyte transfusions is only helpful in patients with nonresponsive bacterial sepsis (Klastersky 1979), or possibly in patients with localized undrained infections.

The use of lithium carbonate to boost the leukocyte count is still investigational (Lyman et al. 1980), as are various forms of passive antibody therapy (Glauser et al. 1982).

Prevention of Infection

Since infectious complications of cancer therapy are so important in terms of morbidity and mortality, one obvious avenue of research has been the investigation of ways to prevent at least some of those complications. Various trials have been and will be done to prevent infections in immunosuppressed patients.

Most of these trials mix many different ways of preventing infection, thus complicating their evaluation. There are at least four possible approaches to infection prevention (Pizzo and Schimpff 1983). The first approach consists in bolstering host defense mechanisms by vaccination (influenza, pneumococcus), which can be hampered by the poor antibody response in those patients, by leukocyte transfusions (already alluded to above), by various immunomodulators (e.g., lithium carbonate) and by attention to proper nutrition. The second "obvious" approach is to avoid both damage to body barriers and the use of invasive procedures involving IV or urinary catheters, respiratory devices etc. unless absolutely mandatory. The third approach consists in trying to reduce acquisition of new pathogens by careful handwashing, decreased amount of microbes in food, proper housekeeping procedures and various isolation procedures, the most sophisticated of which is laminar air-flow room isolation. The fourth approach comprises trials to suppress colonizing organisms. Such trials are based on the concept that most infections in these patients are endogenous in origin (Schimpff et al. 1972b) and that the most important reservoir of potentially pathogenic microorganisms is the digestive tract (Schimpff et al. 1979).

But, since many pathogenic organisms are acquired in the hospital, many trials of "decontamination" have been associated with various measures of patient isolation, which very much complicates their evaluation.

Two general methods have been used: total and selective digestive decontamination. The total decontamination procedure consists in using nonabsorbable antibiotics in the hope of achieving near-total suppression of the digestive flora. Various regimens have been and are still being investigated. For the reasons cited above they are difficult to evaluate critically, but it seems fair to state that they seem to reduce the burden of infections (although not clearly affecting mortality figures), at least in patients with protracted and profound neutropenia (e.g., more than 20 days of granulocyte counts <100) and in conjunction with total protective isolation in laminar air-flow rooms. In addition to the selection of resistant microorganisms (Dejace and Klastersky 1986b) and fungi, these programs are expensive, psychologically difficult to bear because of the protected environment and also difficult to maintain because of compliance problems related to antibiotic bulk and taste.

Another method, called selective digestive decontamination, has been developed. It is based on the concept of resistance of the digestive tract to colonization by pathogenic microorganisms (and possibly fungi), which seems to be related to the preservation of the anaerobic flora (Van Der Waaij 1979). The use of antibiotics with systemic effect but no antianaerobic activity has therefore been investigated. Trimethoprim-sulfamethoxazole and nalidixic acid are the drugs that have been most thoroughly investigated. Although many trials are again difficult to evaluate and although there is no clear-cut incidence on mortality, it seems that the use of this selective decontamination procedure can lead to a reduction in the number of infections, at least in some settings. For example, a large study from the EORTC showed that there was no difference in the rate of bacteremia between patients receiving trimethoprim-sulfamethoxazole and placebo, unless one excluded patients with acute nonlymphoblastic leukemias from the analysis. In patients with other cancers, there was a significant reduction of the rate of infection and bacteremia (EORTC 1984).

On the other hand, these regimens are certainly easier to follow and less expensive than those aiming at total decontamination. They also have the advantage of not necessitating a totally protected environment.

Another issue for which there are no clear-cut data is the use of isoniazid (INH) prophylaxis in immunocompromised patients with a positive tuberculin reaction or a past history of tuberculosis (Kaplan et al. 1974). However, it seems reasonable to recommend INH prophylaxis in patients about to receive heavy immunosuppressive therapy, for instance those with hematological neoplasms and a positive PPD, or in patients with documented, incompletely treated tuberculosis in the past.

Various drugs have also been used in attempts to prevent fungal infections, usually in association with prophylactic antibacterial agents. As for viral infections, we have already mentioned the use of hyperimmunoglobulins in children at risk after contact with a case of varicella. Similarly, administration of immunoglobulins has been tried in the prevention of CMV infection in bone marrow transplants (Meyers et al. 1983).

Acyclovir has also been administered prophylactically to patients at risk of herpes simplex virus reactivation while receiving chemotherapy. Acyclovir prophylaxis effectively suppresses infections as long as it is used, but it does not eradicate the latent state, since in about 50% of patients virus reactivation occurred after acyclovir was discontinued (Saral et al. 1981).

Finally, prophylaxis against *Pneumocytis carinii* with trimethoprim-sulfamethoxazole has been shown to be successful in children with acute leukemia (Hugues et al. 1977).

Although there are still many questions left unanswered, the outlook for preventive approaches to infections in immunocompromised hosts thus seems hopeful.

Conclusions

Infections are still a major problem in cancer patients. We have reviewed the different ways in which cancer and, perhaps more importantly, its therapy, lead to multifactorial defects in host defenses and we have examined how to minimize them. A review of the pathogens involved and of the clinical manifestations of infection in these immunocompromised patients has emphasized the variety of possible causes and the frequently atypical presentation compared to other patients. This leads to a different, more aggressive approach toward diagnosis and especially treatment, unhappily mostly empirical, in this category of patients. Finally, possible ways of reducing the burden of infectious morbidity and mortality in these patients by preventive measures have been critically reviewed.

Overall, this review shows how much work still needs to be done in order to lessen the problems caused by infections in cancer patients: they probably constitute the most important obstacle to even more effective cancer therapy.

References

Amromin GD, Solomon RD (1962) Necrotizing enteropathy: a complication of treated leukemia or lymphoma patients. JAMA 182: 133–139

Armstrong D, Wong B (1982) Central nervous system infections in immunocompromised hosts. Annu Rev Med 33: 293–308

Bayer AS, Edwards JE, Seidel JS et al. (1976) *Candida* meningitis: report of seven cases and review of the English literature. Medicine (Baltimore) 55: 477–486

Bisno AL, Freeman JC (1970) The syndrome of asplenia, pneumococcal sepsis, renal and disseminated intravascular coagulation. Ann Intern Med 72: 389–393

Bodey GP, Buckley M, Sathe YS, Freireich EJ (1966) Quantitative relationships between circulating leucocytes and infection in patients with acute leukemia. Ann Intern Med 64: 328–340

Browne M, Wesley R, Pass H, Potter D, Cotton D, Gress J, Roth J, Pizzo P (1985) Randomized trial of early open lung biopsy vs empiric antimicrobial therapy in cancer patients with diffuse interstitial pneumonitis. ICAAC Abstract 250

Dejace P, Klastersky J (1986a) A comparative review of combination therapy: two beta-lactams versus beta-lactam plus aminoglycoside. Am J Med 80: 29–39

Dejace P, Klastersky J (1986b) Emergence of resistance as a consequence of antimicrobial prophylaxis in immuno-compromised patients. Scand J Infect Dis [Suppl] 49: 165

Dejace P, Klastersky J (1986c) Alteration of skin and mucosa leading to infections in cancer patients. Internal Medicine for the Specialist, December: 107

Dejace P et al. (1985) *Streptococcus pneumoniae* bacteremia in cancer patients. 25th ICAAC, Minneapolis. Abstr no 42

Dolin R, Reichman RC, Mazur MH, Withley RJ (1978) Herpes zoster-varicella infections in immunosuppressed patients. Ann Intern Med 89: 375–388

EORTC International Antimicrobial Therapy Project Group (1978) Three antibiotic regimens in the treatment of infection in febrile neutropenic patients with cancer. J Infect Dis 137: 14–29

EORTC International Antimicrobial Therapy Project Group (1984) Trimethoprim-sulfametoxazole in the prevention of infection in neutropenic patients. J Infect Dis 150: 372–379

EORTC Antimicrobial Therapy Cooperative Group (1986) Prospective randomized comparison of three antibiotic regimens for empirical therapy of suspected bacteremic infection in febrile granulocytopenic patients. Antimicrob Agents Chemother 29: 263–270

Feld R, Bodey GP, Greschel D (1976) Mycobacteriosis in patients with malignant disease. Arch Intern Med 136: 67–70

Glauser MP, McCutchan JA, Ziegler EJ, Braude A (1982) Adjuvant therapy for severe infections. In: Klastersky J, Staquet MJ (eds) Combination antibiotic therapy in the compromised host. Raven, New York, pp 239–244

Ho JL, Shands KN, Friedland G, Eckind P, Fraser DW (1986) An outbreak of type 4b *Listeria monocytogenes* infection involving patients from 8 Boston hospitals. Arch Intern Med 146: 520–524

Hooper DC, Pruitt AA, Rubin RH (1982) Central nervous system infection in the chronically immunosuppressed. Medicine 61: 166–188

Hugues WT, Kuhn S, Chaudhary S, Feldman S, Verzosa M, Rhomes JA, Aur RJA, Pratt C, George SL (1977) Successful chemoprophylaxis for *Pneumocystis carinii* pneumonitis. N Engl J Med 297: 1419–1427

Johanson WG, Peirce AK, Sanford JP (1969) Changing pharyngeal bacterial flora of hospitalized patients: emergence of gram negative bacilli. N Engl J Med 281: 1137–1140

Jones JM (1981) Granulomatous hepatitis due to *Candida albicans* in patients with acute leukemia. Ann Intern Med 94: 475–477

Kaplan MH, Armstrong D, Rosen P (1974) Tuberculosis complicating neoplastic disease: a review of 201 cases. Cancer 33: 850–858

Kaplan MH, Rosen PP, Armstrong D (1977) Cryptococcosis in a cancer hospital: clinical and pathological correlates in forty-six patients. Cancer 39: 2265–2274

Klastersky J (1979) Granulocyte transfusions as a therapy and a prophylaxis for infection in neutropenic patients. In: Glauser M, Klastersky J (eds) Proceedings of a symposium on therapy and prevention of infections in cancer patients. Pergamon, Oxford, pp 15–22

Lyman GH, Williams CC, Preston D (1980) Use of lithium carbonate to reduce infection and leukopenia during systemic chemotherapy. N Engl J Med 302: 257–260

Meyer RD, Rosen P, Armstrong D (1972) Phycomycosis complicating leukemia and lymphoma. Ann Intern Med 77: 871–879

Meyer RD, Young LS, Armstrong D, Yu B (1973) Aspergillosis complicating neoplastic diseases. Am J Med 54: 6–15

Meyers JD, Spencer HC Jr, Watts JC, Gregg MP, Stewart JA, Troupin RH, Thomas ED (1975) Cytomegalovirus pneumonia after human marrow transplantation. Ann Intern Med 82: 181–188

Meyers JD, Leszczynski J, Zaia JA, Flournoy N, Newton B, Snydman D, Wright G, Levin M, Thomas E (1983) Prevention of cytomegalovirus infection by cytomegalovirus immune globuline after marrow transplantation. Ann Intern Med 98: 442–446

Nash G (1972) Necrotizing tracheobronchitis and bronchopneumonia consistent with herpetic infection. Hum Pathol 3: 283–291

Neu HC, Silva M, Hazen E, Rosenheim S (1967) Necrotizing nocardial pneumonitis. Ann Intern Med 66: 274–284

Nieman RE, Lorber B (1980) Listeriosis in adults, a changing pattern: report of eight cases and review of the literature, 1968–1978. Rev Infect Dis 2: 207–227

Pizzo PA, Schimpff SC (1983) Strategies for the prevention of infection in the myelosuppressed or immunosuppressed cancer patient. Cancer Treat Rep 67: 223–234

Pizzo PA, Robichaud KJ, Gill FA, Witebsky FG, Levine AS, Deisseroth AB, Glaubiger DL, MacLowry JD, Magrath IT, Poplack DG, Simon RM (1979) Duration of empiric antibiotic therapy in granulocytopenic patients with cancer. Am J Med 67: 194–200

Pizzo PA, Robichaud KJ, Gill FA, Witebsky FG (1982) Empiric antifungal therapy for cancer patients with prolonged fever and granulocytopenia. Am J Med 72: 101–111

Pizzo PA et al. (1986) A randomized trial comparing ceftazidine alone with combination antibiotic therapy in cancer patients with fever and neutropenia. N Engl J Med 315: 552–558

Ramsey PG, Fife KH, Hackman RC, Meyers JD, Corey L (1982) Herpes simplex virus pneumonia: clinical, virological and pathologic features in 20 patients. Ann Intern Med 97: 813–820

Richardson EP Jr (1974) Our evolving understanding of progressive multifocal leukoencephalopathy. Ann NY Acad Sci 230: 358–364

Robbins JB, DeVita VT Jr, Dutz W (eds) (1976) Symposium on *Pneumocystis carinii* infection. National Cancer Institute, Washington

Rubin RH, Hooper DC (1985) Central nervous system infection in the compromised host. Med Clin North Am 69: 281–296

Ruskin J, Remington JS (1976) Toxoplasmosis in the compromised host. Ann Intern Med 84: 193–199

Saral R, Burns WH, Laskin OL et al. (1981) Acyclovir prophylaxis of herpes-simplex-virus infection: a randomized double-blind controlled trial in bone marrow transplant recipients. N Engl J Med 305: 63–67

Schimpff SC, Satterlee W, Yong VM, Serpick A (1971) Empiric therapy with carbenicillin and gentamicin for febrile patients with fever and granulocytopenia. N Engl J Med 284: 1061–1066

Schimpff SC, Serpick A, Stoler B, Rumack B, Mellin H, Joseph J, Block J (1972a) Varicella-zoster infections in patients with cancer. Ann Intern Med 76: 241–254

Schimpff SC, Young VM, Greene WH, Vermeulen GD, Moudy MR, Wiernik PH (1972b) Origin of infection in acute nonlymphocytic leukemia. Significance of hospital acquisition of potential pathogens. Ann Intern Med 77: 707–714

Schimpff SC, Aisner J, Wiernik P (1979) Infection in acute non-lymphocytic leukemia. The alimentary canal as a major source of pathogens. In: Van der Waaij D, Verhoef J (eds) New criteria for antimicrobial therapy: maintenance of digestive tract colonization resistance. Excerpta Medica, Amsterdam, pp 12–29

Scowden EB, Schaffner W, Stone WJ (1978) Overwhelming stronglyloidiasis: an unappreciated opportunistic infection. Medicine (Baltimore) 57: 527–544

Sickles EA, Greene WH, Wiernik PH (1975) Clinical presentation of infection in granulocytopenic patients. Arch Intern Med 135: 715–719

Stamm AM, Dismukes WE, Simmons BP, Glenn Cobbs C, Elliott A, Budrich P, Harmon J (1982) Listeriosis in renal transplant recipients: report of an outbreak and review of 102 cases. Rev Infect Dis 4: 665–682

Van Der Waaij D (1979) The colonization resistance of the digestive tract in experimental animals and its consequences for preventing acquisition of new bacteria and the prevention of spread of bacteria between cage mates. In: Van Der Waaij D, Verhoef J (eds) New criteria for antimicrobial therapy: maintenance of digestive tract colonization resistance. Excerpta Medica, Amsterdam, pp 43–53

Wade JC, Schimpff SC, Newman KA, Wiernik PH (1982) *Staphylococcus epidermidis:* an increasing cause of infection in patients with granulocytopenia. Ann Intern Med 97: 503–508

Wolfson JS, Sober AJ, Rubin RN (1985) Dermatologic manifestations of infections in immunocompromised patients. Medicine (Baltimore) 64: 115–133

Young LS, Armstrong D, Blevins A et al. (1971) *Nocardia asteroides* infection complicating neoplastic disease. Am J Med 50: 356–367

Psychological Aspects of Surgical Oncology

P. MAGUIRE

Introduction

Patients with cancer will gain considerable confidence if they perceive that their surgeon understands the hurdles they have to overcome if they are to adapt psychologically to their diagnosis. I will first describe these hurdles and then discuss the nature and extent of the psychological morbidity associated with cancers whose primary treatment is surgical. Finally, I will suggest ways in which this morbidity may be reduced or prevented.

Disease-Related Hurdles

Uncertainty

The most difficult hurdle cancer patients face is their worry that their illness could return at any time, metastasise, cause further physical suffering, invalidity and even premature death. These worries about recurrence and spread are likely to be activated whenever they attend for follow-up, since they realise that further cancer may be found. Indeed, the practice of continued follow-up implies that there is cause for concern and may make it hard for patients to accept that they are free of disease and will remain so. It can be especially difficult for patients to adapt to their cancer if they believe that there was an undue delay in diagnosis. If patients had asymptomatic cancers which were picked up on routine screening or during investigation of other physical conditions, they may have little confidence in their future care. For if their cancer was not evident in the first place, how can they be sure that any recurrence will be detected by themselves or their surgeon?

Undue delays in initiating treatment after primary surgery, like radiotherapy, because of problems of access to facilities will also provoke anxiety. Patients who have had an adverse experience of cancer in a close relative or friend are less likely to accept reassurance that a recurrence will not occur, especially if their relative or friend was similarly reassured but died within a short time.

Debate about the relative merits of different treatments for cancer within the mass media, together with publicity given to the deaths of famous people from the disease, serves to remind patients that they have had cancer and cause them to question whether their treatment was optimal. Because of this terrible uncertainty about outcome, many cancer patients become highly sensitised to any physical changes. If they experience symptoms like backache or headache they interpret them as evidence of recurrence and spread and become extremely worried.

Search for Meaning

With the exception of a few cancers (e.g. lung cancer) there are still no adequate scientific explanations of why individual patients develop cancer. This makes it more difficult for patients to adapt, since most cope better with adversity if they find a sensible explanation for it. Patients may fill the vacuum in two ways. First, they blame themselves by implicating some commonly professed theories. They may consider that they developed cancer because they have a type C personality, i.e. they are introverted, or because they have always 'bottled up' their feelings, particularly anger, instead of expressing them. Alternatively, they believe that they developed cancer because they were unable to cope with recent chronic (e.g. housing or financial difficulties) or acute (e.g. divorce or bereavement) stressors. If patients accept such explanations they have to cope both with having cancer and the realisation that it is their fault. This is difficult to live with if they see no way of modifying their personalities or reducing the stressors that they believe have caused the cancer.

Second, patients may blame external factors like physical traumas (e.g. a blow to the body or a car accident) or mental cruelty inflicted by a partner. If they do this they are likely to become very bitter about the person who inflicted the trauma and this will hinder their adaptation. Patients may also attribute the cancer to radiation from nuclear power stations, the excessive use of X-rays or heredity.

Controlling the Disease

A patient who suffers a heart attack can feel positive because he can adopt practical measures like dieting, exercise or giving up smoking which are thought to be effective in reducing the risk of a further attack. However, no such preventative measures have been established for cancer, so some patients feel there is nothing they can do to combat their disease or prevent recurrence. Other patients react positively and take up measures like dieting, exercise, yoga or meditation in the belief that these will delay recurrence and prolong survival. As long as such measures do not become an overriding obsession and disrupt key relationships, they are likely to facilitate adaptation.

Reappraisal

Some patients adapt to the threat of cancer by reappraising their priorities. For example, they may decide to give up their jobs so that they can make the most of what time they have left and fulfil cherished goals. Other patients feel that there is nothing they can do and begin to feel helpless. They are then likely to become depressed in the future.

Stigmatisation

Apart from AIDS, cancer is the physical illness that people fear most and it is still considered a contagious disease within many communities. So, it is not surprising that some patients with cancer feel 'unclean' and are frightened of 'passing it on' to others. These worries are rational given current medical theories which claim that some cancers are caused by viruses which trigger oncogenic transformation of normal cells. When patients feel 'contagious' they worry that other people will treat them differently and that they will be less acceptable to them. This can result in their withdrawing socially and being deprived of emotional support.

Openness

A major issue for patients with cancer is how open they should be about their illness and treatment with relatives, close friends and employers. Some patients worry that honesty could affect key relationships adversely, drive friends away and cause employers to demote or sack them. Worries about employment are well founded, since a considerable proportion of patients whose cancer has been eradicated fail to return to their former level of work. Patients also fear that if they discuss their illness and attendant worries this will cause undue concern and upset to their loved ones. If patients do not disclose their illness and worries they will not be given support by those to whom they would normally have turned. This will render them vulnerable to psychiatric breakdown.

Attitudes of Other People

When a person suffers a heart attack the crisis is usually short-lived and a good recovery evident. While relatives and friends are shocked by the initial illness they can take comfort in the obvious improvement. They can also reassure the patient that he is likely to remain well. Reassurance is much harder to give to patients with cancer. The patient may not be clear of disease despite initial treatment. Even if the cancer has been eradicated the relatives may realise that recurrence and death is still possible. Thus, some friends and relatives do not know what to say to soften the blow and reassure the patient. They may decide that this is too difficult and begin to avoid seeing the patient. This may further isolate the patient from crucial support.

Undervaluation of Medical Support

In many countries there has been a growing emphasis on treating cancer patients in specialist centres. So, it is not surprising that patients come to see these centres as the only source of knowledge and expertise. They then undervalue their own medical practitioners and no longer perceive them as having sufficient up-to-date knowledge to be of help. Such perceptions are not unreasonable. It is hard for general practitioners to keep up to date with the latest information about optimal treatments for different forms of cancer. The patients also assume, albeit wrongly, that the practitioner will be unable to provide emotional support. So, they look to the centres for support. However, the centres assume the general practitioners will cover the psychological aspects of care. Consequently, the patients fail to receive adequate support from the specialised centre or the general practitioner.

Psychological Morbidity

Breast Cancer

At least one in four women who undergo mastectomy develop a depressive illness within the first year (Morris 1979; Maguire et al. 1978; Dean 1987). The patient reports that she has felt persistently low and miserable to an extent which represents a clear and significant departure from her normal mood. She also complains that she can no longer pull herself out of this depression or be distracted by others. She may describe it, for example, in terms of 'a black cloud hanging over me'. There will be several other symptoms of depressive illness, including irritability, impairment of concentration, forgetfulness, a loss or gain of appetite, a decrease or increase in weight, loss of libido, loss of energy, repeated or early morning waking, agitation or retardation, feelings of hopelessness about the future, feelings of guilt, feelings of worthlessness, or feeling a burden to others. Some patients may have felt so low that they contemplated suicide. This depression will usually have had an adverse effect on the patient's ability to function from day to day. She will report that she is finding it an increasing effort to cope with her housework or job. The depression may have caused her to fail to return to work even though she has made a good physical recovery from the operation. She may now avoid meeting other people by staying at home.

This depression after mastectomy is usually related to an inability to adapt to the uncertainty of prognosis and/or the loss of a breast because it was crucial to her sense of physical integrity, self-esteem, or feelings of femininity and attractiveness. Moreover, the absence of a breast can remind her that she had a cancer removed. Her external prosthesis may also act as a trigger of worries about survival.

The risk of depression is increased if patients are given cyclophosphamide, methotrexate and 5-fluorouracil in combination (CMF) (Maguire et al. 1980a; Hughson et al. 1986). At least half the women studied by Hughson and his colleagues developed a depressive illness during the 12 months of treatment. Chemotherapy appears to cause depression in two ways. First, patients find it increasingly hard to adapt to unpleasant adverse effects, particularly those concerning the gastrointestinal tract (nausea and vomiting). Up to a third develop conditioned responses where any sight, sound, smell or thought which reminds them of chemotherapy causes them to feel sick or to vomit reflexively (Morrow and Morrell 1982).

Such conditioning leads patients to become increasingly miserable about the prospect of further treatments. They are terrified of further treatment, but are aware that if they stop it their chances of survival will diminish. Second, in some patients the depressive illness appears due to a direct effect of chemotherapy on the brain, since the depressive illness develops immediately in relation to infusions. Hughson and his colleagues (1986) have suggested that limiting chemotherapy to 6 months would reduce psychiatric morbidity, because the incidence of psychiatric problems markedly increased between 6 and 12 months of a 1-year course.

Radiotherapy also contributes to the development of depressive illness (Fallowfield et al. 1986) via a fatigue syndrome. Some women become extremely tired towards the end of a course of radiotherapy, fail to recover and develop biological symptoms of depression, such as early morning waking and diurnal variation of mood. Depression is more likely when a greater number of fractions are used and there are more adverse effects (Lucas et al. 1987). This may happen because the adverse effects hinder psychological adaptation to the diagnosis of cancer and breast loss. The adverse effects of radiotherapy could also explain why women who had no strong treatment preference and were randomised to wide local excision plus radiotherapy experienced as much depression as those who were randomised to mastectomy alone (Fallowfield et al. 1986).

The contribution of axillary clearance to depressive illness is not clear, but a higher proportion of women who develop pain and swelling in the arm become depressed than could be explained by chance. The pain and swelling frustrate attempts to return to normal life and functioning and remind patients of their cancer and the possibility of recurrence (Maguire 1982).

It might be expected that recurrence of disease would be associated with a greater incidence of depression, and this has been reported in one study (Silberfarb et al. 1980). However, studies of patients with advanced disease show that the incidence is not much greater (33%) than in those with early disease (Plumb and Holland 1981).

Anxiety States

A fifth of women develop an anxiety state (Maguire et al. 1978; Dean 1987) after mastectomy. They find themselves plagued by worries and cannot push these out of their minds or be distracted by others. They are unable to relax and feel on edge and tense. They have difficulty getting off to sleep and feel increasingly irritable. They find it harder to make decisions and concentrate. Physical concomitants of anxiety (like palpitations, sweating, headache, breathlessness, shakiness and trembling) may be prominent. If they suffer from hyperventilation they will also report episodes of numbness and tingling.

While anxiety usually presents in this generalised way, it can present as a phobic disorder when it is triggered by an irrational fear of specific situations. For example, a woman fears that if she goes out alone she will collapse and die. Fear may also be triggered by going into shops, particularly supermarkets, or by travelling on a bus or train. Women with such phobias will try and organise their lives to avoid these situations. There is usually a clear radius from the house beyond which they cannot go unless accompanied by someone close to them or a pet.

Anxiety can present as a social phobia. The patient panics at the thought of meeting other people, particularly in social situations like a dinner or a dance. When she attempts to socialise she feels extremely self-conscious and thinks people are noticing her every action. This causes her to become anxious, shaky, panicky and to leave. Such social phobias are especially likely when the woman has difficulty accepting her breast loss.

Patients who have difficulty adapting to diagnosis may present with cancer phobias. Although they are free of the disease they cannot believe that all the cancer has been removed and they may develop the habit of examining their breast repeatedly to check for cancer and seek reassurance frequently. Such reassurance will only last a short time before they consult again.

Phobic reactions are also likely in patients who develop conditioning on combination chemotherapy. They may panic when they begin the journey to the cancer hospital and even refuse further treatment.

Body Image Problems

As many as a quarter of women who have undergone mastectomy find that they cannot come to terms with the loss of a breast (Maguire et al. 1983). This may be because they cannot tolerate being less than physically whole, feel more vulnerable psychologically and are less able to cope with subsequent major stresses. Some women feel particularly self-conscious and believe that other people must be able to tell that they have had a mastectomy even if they hide their shape by wearing different clothes. This can lead to marked social withdrawal and social phobias. Other women are devastated by the belief that they are no longer attractive or feminine. They may use strong phrases to indicate this like 'I'm no use to anyone anymore' or 'I'm a one-breasted monster'. Avoidance behaviour is common, and women will prevent themselves catching sight of their chest wall by wearing a bra in bed, dressing and undressing in the dark, by changing the height of mirrors or covering them up. Because of their own revulsion they usually believe that their partners cannot tolerate their breast loss either, but this is usually untrue.

Body image problems following mastectomy can be intensified if radiotherapy is used to ablate the ovaries in a premenopausal woman. The premature menopause may intensify the patient's feeling that she is no longer feminine and attractive, particularly if she also puts on weight.

The provision of external breast prostheses does not prevent the development of these body image problems.

Sexual Problems

Up to a third of patients who had an active and enjoyable sex life before surgery develop sexual problems (Morris et al. 1977; Maguire et al. 1978; Jamison et al. 1978). They obtain much less enjoyment from love-making, find it harder to achieve orgasm and may avoid intercourse altogether. There is a strong link between the development of sexual problems and the inability to adapt to the breast loss. Sexual problems may also be due to a loss of libido caused by the development of a depressive illness. There is a marked increase in sexual problems when CMF is used (Maguire et al. 1980a), due to hormonal changes. There is a marked fall in oestrogen levels and an increase in follicular stimulating and luteinising hormones. Premenopausal women undergo an artificial menopause. Difficulty in lubricating the vagina may cause dyspareunia. These changes in sexuality may intensify any body image problems due to mastectomy. Sexual problems may also arise during radiotherapy because of fatigue or depression. The increasingly used agent tamoxifen also causes sexual problems in premenopausal women, as well as hot flushes which provoke distress in some patients.

Anorectal Cancer

Some 23%–33% of patients develop an anxiety state and/or depressive illness after surgery for anorectal cancer and the formation of a colostomy (Thomas et al. 1987; Devlin et al. 1971; Macdonald and Anderson 1984). The reasons are poor expectation of survival (if they have been told their diagnosis) and/or inability to adapt to the stoma and colostomy bag.

Patients fear that the bag and its contents could cause a smell, leak, burst or make a noise. Some 38% will feel 'embarrassed', 'dirty' or 'unclean', and 23% will remain preoccupied by their stoma (Macdonald and Anderson 1984). Marked social avoidance is evident in 15% or more of patients. Between a third and a half of patients will experience a loss of interest in or enjoyment of sex. In some this is due to surgical ablation of the nerve supply to the genital organs.

Cancer of the Cervix

Over a third of women with cancer of the cervix develop an anxiety state and/or depressive illness in the first year of treatment (Stewart et al. 1988).

Such morbidity is associated with feelings of stigma which are evident in over 40%. Some women cannot adapt to theories that cervical cancer is due to promiscuity or viral infections. Sexual problems are common because of vaginal soreness, dryness and atrophy caused by the use of radiotherapy implants and inadequate advice about the use of dilators after treatment. They also arise because of worries that intercourse will reactivate the cancer through trauma or the transmission of a virus. The use of external radiotherapy and associated adverse effects like nausea, vomiting, radiotherapy, diarrhoea and damage to the large bowel increases the risk of anxiety, depression and sexual problems.

Other Cancers

The adaptation of patients who have cancers which arise within other internal organs of the body and could be explained away as an 'ulcer' or 'bit of inflammation' has yet to be studied rigorously. Consequently, the psychiatric morbidity associated with surgical treatment of cancer of the uterus, ovary, larynx, oesophagus, stomach, small bowel, lung, kidney, prostate and brain has yet to be properly established through prospective studies of representative populations.

Problems of Recognition

Low Disclosure

Surgeons, like other doctors, tend to assume that patients will disclose any problems which develop as a result of diagnosis and treatment. Unfortunately, this assumption is not justified. Only one in every five patients who develop psychological problems discloses them to the clinicians involved in their aftercare. There are important reasons for this. They perceive correctly that the surgical staff are busy and they do not want to burden them further. Since the surgeons generally focus their questioning on patient's physical wellbeing and recovery, the patients believe, albeit wrongly, that surgeons are only interested in physical aspects of care. So, they do not disclose any mood disturbance, sexual or body image problems. Since few patients disclose their problems, those who develop difficulties believe they are the only ones who are not coping. They feel inadequate and ashamed and this encourages them to remain silent about their problems. When faced with direct questions they may still pretend that everything is alright. They worry that disclosure will cause them to be labelled as inadequate, uncooperative, neurotic or ungrateful. A further barrier to disclosure is their belief that their problems are an inevitable consequence of diagnosis and treatment and that nothing can be done to eradicate or ameliorate them.

Low Recognition

This problem of low disclosure is compounded by the reluctance of surgeons, nurses and general practitioners involved in aftercare to enquire explicitly about how the patients are adjusting socially and psychologically. For example, in a follow-up study of patients who had undergone mastectomy, not a single patient was asked spontaneously about whether her sex life had been affected by surgery (Maguire et al. 1978). Similarly, few patients were asked how they felt about losing a breast or how they had been feeling in themselves since surgery. So, they did not feel that it was legitimate to discuss such concerns. Consequently, most of the psychological morbidity remained hidden. Direct observation of staff interacting with cancer patients revealed that doctors and nurses try to keep them at a 'safe' emotional distance, attending selectively to cues about physical problems in preference to cues about psychological difficulties. They ignore clear signals that the patient is distressed or offer premature reassurance by saying 'It's going to be alright' without having established what the patient is worried about. Sometimes, in a bid to ease a patient's worry, they offer false reassurance by insisting that he or she will recover when they know this is unlikely. Other common distancing tactics include explaining away any emotional upset as normal ('You are bound to be upset at this stage, everybody is, but you will soon find you'll get used to your colostomy'). Alternatively, when faced with a difficult situation the doctor may simply switch the subject on to safer and neutral ground or try and jolly the patient out of it. These distancing tactics prevent doctors and nurses getting close to patients and enable them to avoid being confronted with difficult and time-consuming problems. For, if they try and establish how a patient has been adjusting they may provoke awkward questions like 'How long have I got?', 'Is treatment worth it?' and 'How will I know if it comes back?'. They also worry that routine enquiry about how patients are feeling may release strong emotions like despair, anger and worry. They fear that they will not be able to deal with these emotions constructively and might be accused of upsetting the patient. Moreover, attempting to deal with psychological aspects within busy clinics could take up too much time and prevent them giving adequate care to other patients.

This low disclosure and recognition of problems allows some surgeons to continue to argue that there are few psychological problems in patients with cancer since they have never encountered them. But much can be done to improve the recognition and management of patients who need psychological help after the diagnosis and treatment of cancer.

Improving Psychological Management

Assessment

It is important that the surgeon be prepared to enquire about the possibility of psychological problems. He can best do this by asking questions which indicate that he is interested in psychological matters and that it is legitimate for the patient to disclose any problems.

It is useful to begin the assessment with an open question which directs patients' attention to aspects other than their physical health, for example, 'So far we have been discussing how you have been getting on physically, but how have you been in yourself since your operation?' If cues about possible problems are forthcoming (for example, 'I've been very worried') it is important to follow up each cue by clarifying what the patient means ('In what way have you been worrying?' 'What have you been worrying about?' 'Just how worried do you get?'). If cues are not given it is important to screen for possible problems by asking direct questions ('How have you felt about losing a breast/having a stoma?' 'Can you look at yourself?' 'Has it made any difference to your relationship with your partner?' 'Have you at any stage felt especially low or miserable, or been on edge and unable to relax?' 'Have you been experiencing any problems with your radiotherapy/chemotherapy?').

When anxiety, depression, body image or sexual problems are present and/or other treatments are having adverse effects, the exact nature, extent and duration of the problems should be clarified and questions asked to elicit other symptoms of anxiety and depression. Such enquiry will lead the patient to disclose any subsequent problems more readily.

It is also useful to check how patients are adapting to each of the psychological hurdles posed by diagnosis. Helpful probes include 'How do *you* see your illness working out?' (to elicit if troubled by uncertainty), 'Do you feel there is anything *you* can do to combat your illness?' (control), 'Do you have any theories about why you got this trouble?' (search for meaning), 'Has your surgery made you feel different in any way?' (stigma), 'Has it affected how people regard you or behave towards you?' (social contacts), 'Have you felt able to tell other people about your illness?' (openness), and 'Do you feel you are getting support from people around you?' (support).

Other Methods of Recognition

Specialist nurses and ward nurses can be taught to assess, recognise and refer for psychological or psychiatric help those patients who develop problems (Maguire et al. 1980 b; Maguire et al. 1983; Faulkner and Maguire 1984). Their training should include video-tape demonstration of the areas to be covered and skills to be learned. They should then practice assessing cancer patients and record the conversations on audio tape so they can be discussed with a tutor who is knowledgeable about key interviewing, assessment and counselling skills.

Once trained, such staff require regular support and audit of their caseload and pattern of contact if they are to maintain a high recognition and referral rate.

Identifying Those at Risk

Recognition would be easier if those at risk of psychological morbidity could be identified. Some potentially useful markers of risk have been identified (Maguire 1982; Lucas et al. 1987; Macdonald and Anderson 1984; Stewart et al. 1988). These include an inability to adapt to the loss of a body part or function, the lack of someone to confide in, physical complications of surgery and a previous psychiatric illness. These markers of risk have the advantage that they can be identified easily by asking the appropriate questions when a patient attends for follow-up appointments.

Specialist nurses and social workers should monitor particularly closely the progress of any patient who presents with any of these markers.

Treatment

Depression

A depressive illness should be treated promptly with appropriate antidepressant medication. New-generation antidepressants like lofepramine or dothiepin cause fewer adverse side effects than the more established tricyclic antidepressants such as amitriptyline or imipramine. This is important because patients who have been treated for cancer tend to attribute any side effects to recurrence or spread of their disease. Adverse effects also cause compliance with medication to be low. Whichever drug is chosen, it should be given in an effective dosage and continued for 4–6 months to prevent relapse.

It is important to explain to the patient that the stress of the diagnosis or surgery has provoked a depressive illness which, although understandable, has persisted and warrants treatment. It is important to stress that the antidepressant is not a tranquilliser and does not promote dependence. Patients should be warned that they may experience side effects like dry mouth or drowsiness which should lessen as they adapt to the medication but could interfere with driving and other daily activities. It is important to emphasise that antidepressants take 2–3 weeks to take effect, otherwise patients may stop them prematurely. As the depressive illness lifts, it will become clear whether fears of recurrence or problems of adapting to a loss of a body part or function or to an external appliance persist and require attention.

Anxiety

If anxiety has been overwhelming and is hampering a patient's ability to function, an anxiolytic drug (e.g. a benzodiazepine) should be used to alleviate it but only for 3–4 weeks in order to forestall dependence. If somatic aspects predominate, a beta-blocker (e.g. propanolol) may be tried. If the patient is extremely agitated a major tranquilliser like thioridazine or chlorpromazine should help. But it is important to help patients to learn how to manage their own anxiety. Many benefit from being taught progressive muscular relaxation, which involves showing them how to contract and relax major muscle groups systematically and then to relax mentally (Janoun et al. 1982). Instructional audio tapes can be of assistance. Once the patients have learned how to relax they are instructed to employ these techniques whenever they begin to feel anxious or are about to confront an anxiety-provoking situation. Patients can also be taught to summon up tranquil scenes to distract themselves from their anxious thoughts.

Patients who develop agoraphobia, social or cancer phobias often benefit from desensitisation. A hierarchy is first constructed of the situations or thoughts which provoke anxiety. For instance, a woman who has undergone mastectomy is taught to relax and asked to imagine an item low in the hierarchy, for example, 'when my breast feels prickly'. If she can relax and imagine this situation without becoming anxious she moves to the next item ('pain in my breast'). If the goal is not achieved the patient is asked to try to relax again and reimagine the ideal situation. Once she has managed the particular item, she is encouraged to test it out in real life when appropriate. For example, once an agoraphobic patient is able to imagine walking from the front door to the gate without becoming anxious she is advised to relax and then actually do this. It is possible to adopt a different approach ('flooding') and start with an item high on the hierarchy, but patients are less happy with this approach. Patients with cancer phobias who develop habits of repeated self-examination also benefit from being taught techniques of relaxation, distraction and thought stopping. The therapist may also find response prevention useful. Thus, when the patient becomes anxious and wants to examine himself or herself, he or she is prevented from doing so.

Sexual Problems

Patients with sexual problems of psychological origin respond well to the Masters and Johnson conjoint approach where the patient and partner are helped together (Masters and Johnson 1970). This begins with a ban on sexual intercourse in order to lessen anxiety about intercourse. The couple are then taught to find ways of pleasuring each other other than by genital contact. As they regain confidence in each other they can proceed gradually towards full intercourse.

Body Image Problems

Body image problems can be resolved by the use of progressive muscular relaxation and desensitization to help patients look, first in imagination and then in real life. The therapist may then encourage the patient to let the partner look. In some patients body image problems remain despite such help and a 'cognitive' approach may be useful. This involves challenging patients' assumptions that they are, for example, no longer attractive or of any use to anybody. Patients are encouraged to consider positive aspects of their situation, for example, the fact that the cancer was caught early. However, both desensitization and cognitive therapy may fail to eradicate body image problems. Whenever possible, plastic surgery should then be considered.

Conditioned Responses

When conditioned vomiting develops in patients who are being treated with combination chemotherapy it is important to act promptly to prevent them opting out from treatment. Covering each major injection of infusion with an anxiolytic (e.g. lorazepan), a major tranquilliser (e.g. chlorpromazine) and an antiemetic in combination may be sufficient. Teaching anxiety-management techniques can also be effective (Burish and Lyles 1981; Redd and Andrykowski 1982; Morrow and Morrell 1982). It is important to treat any associated depressive illness with the appropriate medication.

Cognitive Therapy

When fears of recurrence persist but are unreasonable because the patient has a good prognosis, cognitive therapy is useful (Tarrier and Maguire 1984). This entails detailed examination of what is reasonable about the patient's fears and what is unreasonable. Exploration of what triggers these fears off and their consequences is also required. Teaching anxiety-management techniques may also help because the patient can then be confident of being able to combat any anxious thoughts. However, the exact contribution of antidepressant medication, anxiolytics, and cognitive therapy to psychological recovery still needs to be determined.

Who Should Treat?

The surgeon may wish to treat patients with a depressive illness himself and only refer them to a psychiatrist if the condition fails to remit or there are persisting underlying problems. Similarly, he may be prepared to treat an anxiety state in the short term to see if it remits. However, when anxiety-management training, desensitization, cognitive therapy and sexual counselling are required he will need the prompt assistance of a clinical psychologist or psychiatrist. Alternatively, he may alert the patient's general practitioner and request initiation of such help.

Prevention

As yet, there is no firm evidence (Watson 1983) that the provision of information, advice and counselling before and after surgery prevents psychological morbidity. But it has been shown to promote the recognition and referral of those who needed help (Maguire et al. 1980b) after mastectomy. Consequently, there was a threefold reduction in psychological morbidity, earlier return to work, better social recovery and greater satisfaction with breast prostheses (Maguire et al. 1983).

Providing patients with early disease with an opportunity to discuss the advantages and disadvantages of different treatment options with a counsellor, and make an appropriate choice, also appears to lessen morbidity (Ashcroft et al. 1985). However, this is only possible if a diagnosis is first established by biopsy and there is time for discussion.

It has also been claimed that self-help groups prevent psychological morbidity. However, there is no firm evidence to support this claim, and only 10% of all patients will use such groups. While they may not be preventative, they can have an important role providing they are properly led and sensibly resourced. Patients can meet other patients who understand and validate how they feel and can suggest strategies which might resolve their problems, or advice on where they can turn for help.

References

Ashcroft JJ, Leinster SJ, Slade PD (1985) Breast cancer – patient choice of treatment: preliminary communication. J Roy Soc Med 78: 43–46

Burish TG, Lyles JN (1981) Effectiveness of relaxation training in reducing adverse reactions to cancer chemotherapy. J Behav Med 4: 65–77

Dean C (1987) Psychiatric morbidity following mastectomy: preoperative predictors and types of illness. J Psychosom Res 31 (3): 385–392

Devlin HB, Plant JA, Griffin M (1971) Aftermath of surgery for ano-rectal cancer. Br Med J 3: 413–418

Fallowfield L, Baum M, Maguire GP (1986) Effect of breast conservation on psychological morbidity associated with diagnosis and treatment of early breast cancer. Br Med J 293: 1331–1335

Faulkner A, Maguire P (1984) Teaching ward nurses to monitor cancer patients. Clin Oncol 10: 383–389

Hughson AVM, Cooper AF, McArdle CS, Smith DC (1986) Psychological impact of adjuvant chemotherapy in the first two years after mastectomy. Br Med J 293: 1268–1271

Jamison KR, Wellisch DK, Pasnau RO (1978) Psychological aspects of mastectomy. 1. The women's perspective. Am J Psychiatry 135: 432–438

Jannoun L, Oppenheimer C, Gelder M (1982) A self-help treatment programme for anxiety state patients. Behav Ther 13: 103–111

Lucas D, Maguire P, Reason J, Goldberg D, Sellwood R (1987) Predicting psychiatric morbidity in women with breast cancer. Report to North West Regional Health Authority

Macdonald LD, Anderson HR (1984) Stigma in patients with

rectal cancer: a community study. J Epidemiol Commun Health 38: 284–290

Maguire P (1982) Psychiatric morbidity associated with mastectomy. In: Baum M, Kay R, Scheurlen H (eds) Clinical trials in early breast cancer. Birkhauser, Basel, pp 373–380

Maguire GP, Lee EG, Bevington DJ, Kuchemann C, Crabtree RJ, Cornell C (1978) Psychiatric problems in the first year after mastectomy. Br Med J I: 963–965

Maguire P, Tait A, Brooke M, Thomas C, Howat JMT, Sellwood RA (1980 a) Psychiatric and physical toxicity associated with adjuvant chemotherapy after mastectomy. Br Med J 281: 1179–1180

Maguire P, Tait A, Brooke M, Thomas C, Sellwood R (1980 b) Effect of counselling on the psychiatric morbidity associated with mastectomy. Br Med J 281: 1454–1456

Maguire P, Brooke M, Tait A, Thomas C, Sellwood R (1983) The effect of counselling on physical disability and social recovery after mastectomy. Clin Oncol 9: 319–324

Masters WE, Johnson VE (1970) Human sexual inadequacy. Bantam, London

Morris T (1979) Psychological adjustment to mastectomy. Cancer Treatment Rev 6: 41–61

Morris T, Greer S, White P (1977) Psychological and social adjustment to mastectomy: a two year follow-up study. Cancer 40: 2881–2887

Morrow GR, Morrell C (1982) Behavioural treatment for the anticipatory nausea and vomiting induced by cancer chemotherapy. N Engl J Med 307: 1476–1480

Plumb M, Holland J (1981) Comparative studies of psychological function in patients with advanced cancer. II. Interviewer rated current and past psychological symptoms. Psychosom Med 43: 243–254

Redd WH, Andrykowski MA (1982) Behavioural intervention in cancer treatment: controlling aversion reactions to chemotherapy. J Cons Clin Psychol 50: 1018–1029

Silberfarb PM, Maurer HL, Crouthamel CS (1980) Psychosocial aspects of neoplastic disease. 1. Functional status of breast cancer patients during different treatment regimes. Am J Psychiatry 137: 450–455

Stewart F, Maguire P, Walker A (1988) Psychiatric and social morbidity associated with cervival cancer. Report to Cancer Research Campaign

Tarrier N, Maguire P (1984) Treatment of psychological distress after mastectomy. Behav Res Treat 22: 31–35

Thomas C, Madden F, Jehu D (1987) Psychological effects of stomas. 1. Psycho social morbidity one year after surgery. J Psychosom Res 31: 311–316

Watson M (1983) Psychosocial intervention in cancer patients: a review. Psychol Med 13: 839–846

Pain Treatment in Cancer

V. VENTAFRIDDA and A. SBANOTTO

The Dimension of the Problem

World Health Organization data published in 1983 show that some 965 000 patients in the United States and 18 million people throughout the world were at that time afflicted by pain in the advanced or terminal stages of cancer diseases.

The highest incidence of pain is encountered in primary bone tumours (85%) and in cancers of the oral cavity (80%), the genitourinary tract (70%), the breast (50%), the lung (45%) and the lymphatic system (5%). Among children, 30% of those with advanced cancer suffer pain, due for the most part to neoplastic involvement of the skeleton.

The Nature of Cancer Pain

Physical Aspects

Cancer pain can be classified into pain due to the tumour, pain connected with the tumour, pain due to therapy and pain independent of both tumour and therapy (Table 1).

Other associated factors which cause a worsening of the quality of life for cancer patients include cachexia, anorexia and poor absorption. These conditions can influence the metabolization of many drugs, including analgesics. Involvement of the kidney and the lower urinary tract can cause, in addition to hyperazotaemia and hypercreatininaemia, a slowing down in the excretion of the drugs, with possible consequences. Involvement of the liver parenchyma is another source of pharmacological interference, with a reduction of the plasmatic proteins accompanied by an increase in the free quota of drugs and the lowering of hepatic catabolism, which are all factors potentiating greater toxicity of drug therapy in cancer patients.

Psychological Aspects

Pain is a two-sided phenomenon, involving on the one hand the perception of a sensation and on the other the emotional response to it.

The emotional response is multifactorial, including such things as mood, moral and religious views and previous experiences of pain. The context in

Table 1. Main causes of pain in cancer patients

Due to cancer	Connected to cancer	Due to therapies	Independent of both tumor and therapy
Bone infiltration with/ without muscle spasm	Muscle spasm	Postoperative pain	Musculoskeletal pain
Nerve compression/ infiltration	Constipation	Postoperative neuralgia	Headache (migraine, tension headache)
Visceral involvement	Decubitus	Painful phantom limb	Arthritis
Soft tissue involvement	Lymphoedema	Post-RT inflammation/fibrosis	Cardiovascular disorders
Ulceration with/without infection	Candidiasis	Post-RT myelopathy	
Raised intracranial pressure	Postherpetic neuralgia	Postchemotherapy neuropathies	
	Deep-vein thrombosis Pulmonary embolism	Aseptic necrosis of bone	

which pain makes its appearance and the significance attributed to it can considerably influence that attitude of the patient: the difference between postoperative pain and that from a bone metastasis is obvious. An all-encompassing view of pain must, therefore, be adopted, embracing the physical, spiritual, social and psychological aspects which together constitute the so-called total pain experience.

The most commonly encountered attitudes, on the part of both doctor and patient, are generally defeat and refusal. This can lead to unjustified 'overtreatment' or to abandonment of the patient; it must be remembered, however, that the principal tasks of the doctor include not only curing the disease, but also caring for the whole patient, even in the last moments of life.

Neurophysiological Aspects

The peripheral receptor is the basis of pain perception. Specific receptors of pain do not exist, but there are specialized receptors capable of responding to particular ranges of physiological variables. In particular, one can identify mechanonociceptors, thermonociceptors and polymodal nociceptors; these latter can respond to mechanical, thermal and chemical stimulation.

These receptors are connected to the posterior horn of the spinal cord by slow-conduction, unmyelinated, class C small-calibre fibres and by larger, class A delta fibres with a myelin sheath and a higher conduction velocity. The 'slow' type stimulus constituting the so-called slow pain has been attributed to the first of these fibres, while the conduction of the better-discriminated 'acute' or 'fast' pain, has been attributed to the second type.

Starting from the spinal cord, pain can be conducted not only along afferent pathways formed of specific and well-identifiable routes, but also along complex neuronal systems which terminate not only in thalamic areas, but also in the cortical and subcortical regions.

There are two fundamental nociceptor conduction systems, the neurospinothalamic system extends from the spinal cord to the ventrobasal, ventroposteromedial and ventroposterolateral nuclei of the thalamus and proceeds from there to the postrolandic parietal cortex (somatosensorial area I); this is a fast-conduction oligosynaptic route which supplies the epicritical component of the pain sensation. The other system consists of the paleospinothalamic and the spinoreticular component, both of which have important "relays" in the reticular substance and, issuing from this, in the limbic system. These latter are slow-conduction polysynaptic routes which convey the emotive and affective protopathic component of the pain sensation. An important aspect of these conduction routes is the potential on the part of the inhibitory or excitatory influences for modulation in any part of the nociception afferent pathways, from the dorsal horn of the spinal cord to the cerebral cortex.

One of the principle systems of modulation is that of the first Rexed laminae, in the posterior horn of the spinal cord, where a complex neuronal system was previously thought to give rise to the so-called gate control. This particular model of the mechanism is considered too simple today, but the basic concept is still valid: the large-calibre sensorial afferents appear to be able to inhibit the further development of the pain stimulus carried, predominantly by small-calibre fibres. This hypothesis explains the efficacy of some therapeutic procedures such as massage and electrostimulation, which, by mainly stimulating the large fibres, determine the inhibition of pain input. Another important inhibitory control is exercised by descending pathways, for example those descending directly from the periacqueductal grey matter to the nucleus of the raphe magnus and from there to the enkephalinergic nuclei of the posterior horn of the spinal cord.

Activation mechanisms arising from algogenic impulses also exist, involving structures which regulate the emotional tone, such as the hypothalamus, the rhinencephalus and the dorsomedial thalamus.

All of this explains the intense emotional colouring that pain, in particular chronic pain, can assume, together with the innumerable psychological sequelae accompanying the experience of pain.

Assessment of Cancer Pain

In order to treat cancer pain effectively, it must be correctly assessed; both the physical and the psychological factors should be considered. A fundamental premise is the existence of a trusting relationship between doctor and patient.

As well as the oncological diagnosis, one should naturally be aware of the stage of the disease, the prognosis and the life expectancy, all essential parameters in the planning of antalgic treatment.

The nociceptive stimulus should be investigated in terms of the following:

a) *Case history*
   - Site and spreading of pain
   - Temporal characteristics of pain
   - Quality of pain
   - Circumstances of onset and passing of pain
   - Alleviating and aggravating factors

b) *Intensity of pain*
   - Objective data – Scott Huskisson analogue, Keele-Dundee scale (Fig. 1)
   - McGill pain questionnaire

c) *Personality changes:* IPAT, Hamilton, Zung, MMPI, self-appraising tests

d) *Quality of life*
   - Hours of sleep, hours spent standing, sitting, lying down
   - Interference with work or hobbies
   - "Performance status" according to the Karnofsky index or the ECOG scale (Fig. 2)

A		B	
The worst pain possible		5	Excruciating
|		4	Horrible
|		3	Distressing
|		2	Discomforting
|		1	Mild
No pain		0	No pain

Fig. 1 A, B. Evaluation of pain intensity: **A** Scott-Huskisson analogue, **B** Keele-Dundee scale

e) *Previous anticancer antalgic therapies:* results and side effects

f) *Detailed objective general and neurological examination:* drawing on previous diagnostic examinations and/or planning others, bearing in mind the consequent psychophysical stress for the patient

g) *Definition of types of pain*
   Presence or absence of nerve lesions in:
   - Pain from partial or total deafferentiation of nerve trunks, accompanied by sensory or motor deficiency in the region of the damaged nerve. This dysaesthesia is described by the patient as a sensation of burning, pins and needles, shocks etc.
   - Pain due to excitement of, or damage to, the free peripheral nerve endings by endogenous chemical agents such as quinine and prostaglandin, which do not cause sensory or motor deficiency, but cramp and a piercing sensation of pain.
   - Mixed pain, in which both the above types are present; this kind of pain mostly occurs in advanced stages of disease.

A final distinction should be made between 'static' pain, which is not affected by movement, and 'incident' pain, which is correlated to movement, as, for example, in the case of load placed on metastasized bone structures.

Therapeutic Strategy

The therapy of cancer pain should *not* be of an occasional nature; the requirement should be not only the immediate relief of pain, but also the prospect of long-term control, perhaps for a very extended period and probably until the death of the patient.

There is thus a need for a real therapeutic strategy: treatment must be multimodal and not based on a single therapeutic arm (Fig. 3). Moreover, where possible, it should be administered with controls in the home environment. Therapy should be com-

Description Karnofsky	scale (%)	scale	ECOG description
No complaints; no evidence of disease	100		Normal activity
Able to carry on normal activity; minor signs or symptoms of disease	90	0	
Some signs or symptoms of disease with effort	80		Symptoms of disease, but ambulatory and able to carry out activities of daily living
Cares for self; unable to carry on normal activity or to do active work	70	1	
Requires occasional assistance but is able to care for most personal needs	60		Out of bed more than 50% of time; occasionally needs assistance
		2	
Requires considerable assistance and frequent medical care	50		
Disabled; requires special care and assistance	40		In bed more than 50% of time; needs nursing care
Severely disabled; hospitalization indicated although death not imminent	30	3	
Very sick; hospitalization necessary, requires active supportive treatment	20		Bedridden; may need hospitalization
		4	
Moribund; fatal processes progressing rapidly	10		

Fig. 2. Evaluation of quality of life: Karnofsky index and Eastern Cooperative Oncology Group (ECOG) scale

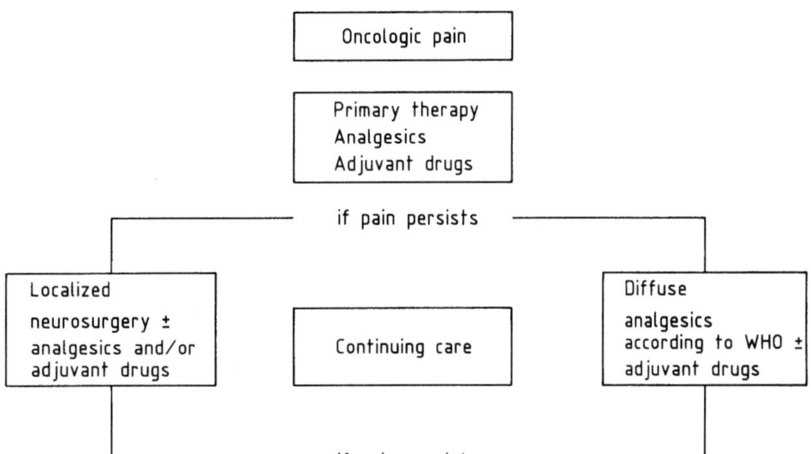

Fig. 3. Therapeutic strategy

menced with specific antitumour drugs (primary therapy) if indicated, possibly associated with analgesics or adjuvant drugs. Should the primary therapy fail or prove no longer feasible, it should be suspended and purely palliative treatment adopted.

It is useful to set oneself some practical goals to be achieved sequentially:

- Increase in hours of sleep
- increase in hours free from static pain (mobile in wheelchair)
- increase in hours free from incident pain (spontaneous ambulation and ambulation with orthopaedic devices).

It is not always possible to achieve this latter aim, particularly in the patient with advanced disease.

The basic disease must not be forgotten, a possible 'recuperation' therapy should be assessed, and some radiotherapy or surgery should be attempted, even with solely antalgic or palliative intent. In any case, the quality of life of the patient after treatment, not only long-term survival, must be borne in mind.

Whenever possible, a drug therapy should be the treatment of choice. The lesion should be removed surgically in those patients who prove refractory or intolerant of drug therapy or present obvious indications for such treatment. Surgery does not always suppress pain completely, and analgesic treatment should be continued, usually with smaller doses than before surgery.

Drug Therapies

Analgesics

There are three basic analgesics: acetylsalicylic acid, codeine and morphine. One or two alternatives to each of these substances should, however, be available for administration to those patients who are intolerance or allergic (Table 2).

It is strongly advisable to follow the sequential approach recommended by WHO, when administering drug therapy (Fig. 4).

The first step consists of non-steroid anti-inflammatory drugs (NSAID). If, despite following the advice on timing and dosage given in Table 3, pain cannot be controlled, one should proceed to weak narcotics with or without NSAID. If this fails, the third step is to administer strong narcotics, again with or without NSAID. The so-called adjuvant drugs can be associated with all the steps.

Some points must be emphasized:
- Oral administration should be preferred.
- Drug dosage should be adequate and equally strong drugs should be used whenever the regimen is changed (Table 4).
- The dosage of drugs should be 'personalized'.
- One should bear in mind the factors interfering with the metabolism and excretion of drugs: vomiting, malabsorption, surgical outcome, occlusion, hepatic and renal insufficiency etc.

Table 2. Basic analgesic drugs

Class	Main drug	Alternative(s)	Mechanism of action
Non-narcotics	Acetylsalicylic acid	Paracetamol Indomethacin Naproxen Diclofenac	Peripheral inhibition of chemical mediators of inflammation
Weak narcotics	Codeine	Dextropropoxyphene Oxycodone Buprenorphine	Inhibition of transmission of painful impulses in brain and spinal cord
Strong narcotics	Morphine	Methadone	

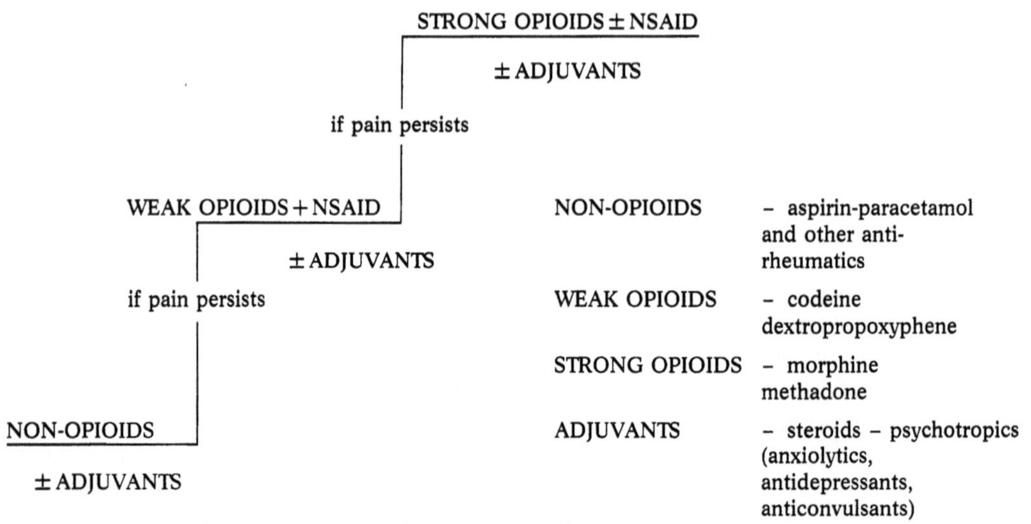

Fig. 4. Pharmacological treatment of pain according to WHO

Table 3. NSAID in cancer pain

Drug	Suggested dosage	Notes
Acetyl-salicylic acid	500 mg q 4–6 h	Associate with anti-H_2 drugs (ranidine 150–300 mg nocte) or antacids
Paracetamol	500 mg q 4–6 h	Indicated in gastropathic patients; attention in hepatopathic patients
Diclofenac	50 mg q 8 h	Retard form: 100 mg q 12 h
Naproxene	250 mg q 12 h	Perhaps less liable to cause gastric lesions; long plasma half-life

Table 4. Equipotential doses of drugs used to combat cancer pain (referred to morphine 10 mg i.m.)

Drug	Route of administration	Equianalgesic dose (mg)	Duration of action (h)	T½
Morphine	i.m.	10	4–6	2–4
	p.o.	60	4–6	
Codeine	i.m.	130	4–6	3
	p.o.	200	4–6	
Oxycodone	p.o.	30	3–5	–
Methadone	i.m.	10	–	15–30
	p.o.	20		
Buprenorphine	i.m.	0.4	4–6	–
	p.o.	0.8	4–6	

Nonsteroidal Anti-inflammatory Drugs

The NSAID are highly significant in the treatment of cancer pain, they can be used, in fact, for intense, moderate and slight pain, and in association with analgesic narcotics they can control pain deriving from bone, serosal and dermocutaneous metastases without involvement of the nerve trunks. Since the NSAID have significant antioedema and antiprostaglandin properties they are particularly effective in the treatment of pain from bone metastases and also antagonize the osteoclastic activity.

Unfortunately, the analgesic efficacy of NSAID tends to decrease with time, while the side effects, in particular those on the mucosa, tend to increase. The passage on to narcotics, or to their association, should not be delayed in these cases.

Weak Narcotics

If the NSAID no longer provide satisfactory analgesia they can be associated with weak narcotics. In this way pain symptoms can be controlled for even quite long periods of time, exploiting the synergism between these two classes of substances.

The narcotics act centrally, interacting with specific receptors lying at the encephalic and spinal levels and inhibiting the transmission of the pain impulse. The periacqueductal gray matter in the encephalic trunk seems to be the main area of action of these substances. There are two categories of weak narcotics the partial agonists and the agonist-antagonists. The first group include codeine, dihydrocodeine, dextropropoxyphene and oxycodone; recently buprenorphine has been added (Table 5). The second group of weak narcotics includes pentazocine, butorphanol and nalbuphine. These drugs should never be used in the treatment of chronic pain due to their excessive psychomimetic effects and uneven analgesic effect. It is of prime importance to remember that, because of possible antagonism, the drugs in these two categories must never be associated.

Table 5. Weak narcotics

Drug	Suggested dosage
Codeine	60 mg q 4–6 h
Dextropropoxyphene	60 mg q 6 h p.o.
Oxycodone	5 mg q 4–8 h
Buprenorphine	0.2 mg q 6–12 h

Strong Narcotics

The strong narcotics are the most important drugs in the treatment of cancer pain, due to their effectiveness, their versatility of action and mode of administration and, with correct use, their good therapeutic index.

The principal substances employed are morphine and methadone. Frequently, however, their use is impeded by the widespread misconception that they are dangerous drugs which can lead to addiction, tolerance and respiratory and circulatory collapse.

In cancer patients addiction may be only physical. It is, in any case, insignificant and, in relation to the relief from pain which can be achieved, irrelevant. Tolerance is also of little importance: after an initial increase in dosage a threshold is generally reached above which further increases in the dosage depend not on tolerance but on an increase in the intensity of pain.

Respiratory collapse is extremely rare if drugs are correctly administered. In fact, the pain and associated psychophysical stress counteract the depressive action of the narcotics.

There are some other typical side effects of narcotics which are more significant because of their greater frequency and they must be prevented (Table 6). Constipation, which is nearly always present, can be prevented by the regular use of laxatives and a high-fibre diet. Nausea, sometimes associated with vomiting, is another possible sequela; generally it can be controlled by the administration of neuroleptics, e.g. haloperidol, antihistamines, e.g. prochlorperazine, or antiemetics, e.g. metachlorproamide.

Certain basic principles should be emphasized with regard to the correct use of narcotics:

- Use agonist narcotics as first choice
- Never associate agonists and agonist-antagonists
- Whenever possible use oral route
- Avoid 'as needed' drugs as far as possible
- Prefer 'by the clock' administration
- Do not use weak narcotics for severe pain
- Titrate dosages
- If necessary use coanalgesics
- Do not forget other therapeutic resources

Morphine is the basic drug amongst the strong analgesics. Although it is only partially absorbed when taken orally, this is the most convenient and most frequently employed means of administration for chronic cancer pain. Having been absorbed after significant metabolism in the liver, it spreads rapidly and targets prevalently the parenchymal tissues, such as the liver, spleen and lungs and, after undergoing glycuroconjugation, is eliminated mostly through the urine and a partly through the faeces.

The analgesic effect and the plasma half-life of morphine coincide (ca. 4 h); it must, therefore, be administered regularly every 4 h. The initial dose on starting treatment can vary from 5–10 mg q 4 h, for patients who have already received NSAID therapy or weak narcotics like codeine, to 10–25 mg q 4 h for those patients who were receiving strong narcotics, such as buprenorphine. Should the pain recur before administration of the next dose, the dosage interval should not be shortened, but rather the dose should be increased. The initial dose should be reduced by 50% for elderly patients and for those suffering from hepatic or renal insufficiency. If there is no relief, or should pain return before the 4 h has elapsed, the subsequent dose should be increased by 50%. If the patient complains of somnolence, which is, in any case, normal during the first few days of treatment, the successive dose should be reduced by 25%. The night-time dose, which is indispensable at the beginning of therapy, can be eliminated by increasing the last prenocturnal dose by 50%–100%.

The progressive adaptation of dosage to the needs of the patient is the most important aspect of treatment with morphine p.o. and is the factor which permits side effects to be kept to a minimum. The majority of patients respond to doses from 20 mg to 60 mg q 4 h. Some may eventually need 150–200 mg, but still q 4 h. In cases of intolerance, or inability to take morphine orally, the drug can be administered in other ways.

In some cases it may be advisable to substitute methadone administered orally as previously described. Methadone is an efficacious substitute for morphine: it has a similar pharmacological action, but exhibits no coincidence between the duration of analgesic effect (ca. 4–8 h) and the plasma half-life (up to 25 h). Consequently, due to the accumulation of the drug in the organism, and since 3–5 days are required to reach the 'steady' state, overdose problems can be encountered. Methadone is not recommended for the elderly, or for patients afflicted with serious renal or hepatic dysfunction or mental instability; moreover, rifampicin accelerates its catabolization velocity. The most common dosage is ca. 5–10 mg q 8 h for the first 3 days, followed by 10–15 mg, increased according to need. In the event of overdose (confused mental state, bradypnoea), naloxone, a pure narcotic antagonist with no analgesic action, can be administered as an antidote. Since the duration of action of this drug is short, 0.4–0.8 mg can be administered subcutaneously or by intravenous injection at regular intervals. The side effects of narcotics can also be encountered during methadone therapy; they can be treated in the same way as those of morphine (Table 6).

Table 6. Main side effects of narcotics

Side effect	Remarks
Drowsiness, confusion	Review dosage; reassure patient and relatives
Nausea, vomiting	Prescribe antiemetic regularly (e.g. haloperidol 1.5 mg q 8–12 h)
Delayed gastric emptying	Metoclopramide 10 mg q 8 h
Pruritus	Skin care: crotamiton cream b.i.d. or t.i.d.; antihistaminic sedatives (e.g. chlorpheniramine 4 mg q 8–12 h)
Constipation	Prescribe laxative regularly

Alternative Methods for the Administration of Narcotics

Despite the fact that oral administration of drugs for cancer pain is the most efficacious and convenient method, some alternative procedures have to be considered because some patients may be unable to take narcotics orally:

- *Intramuscular injection:* This method is usually reserved for the treatment of acute pain. It should be used for short periods only.
- *Subcutaneous administration:* This can be a substitute for both oral and intramuscular administration. Continuous subcutaneous administration of strong narcotics (particularly morphine) can be effected by way of an infusion pump similar to those used by diabetics, connected subcutaneously by a simple butterfly type needle. This method of continuous administration of a drug has proven more useful than repeated bolus administration, which is burdened by a higher incidence of sequelae, in particular nausea and vomiting.

  Subcutaneously administered opioids represent a valid alternative for those patients who prove intolerant to oral administration of narcotics, particularly morphine and methadone, for they will often control pain with a reduced incidence of side effects. Moreover, the method can easily be taught to both the patient and his relations. Another important aspect of this method is its low cost; the pump can be reutilized after the death of the patient.

  Recently, some new devices for the administration of drugs by this route have been developed. A few of them, which have been computerized, can be employed in many ways, including bolus administration. These technological developments have made it possible to adopt a special approach to pain, patient-controlled analgesia (PACA). This method of intravenous administration 'on demand' makes analgesic care extremely personalized. As yet this approach has no great application to chronic cancer, but results are highly positive in the control of postoperative pain.
- *Peridural and subarachnoid procedures:* Following the discovery of specific endogenous and exogenous receptors for the opioids, situated in the posterior horn of the spinal cord, the effectiveness of this method has been demonstrated by several authors. The initial low dose of analgesic is advantageous: ca. 0.5 mg × 2/day for the subarachnoid method and 2 mg × 3/day for the peridural procedure using morphine hydrochloride. These doses can be further reduced by adding an infusion pump to these methods of administration. A more uniform level of analgesia is thus guaranteed, thanks to the continuous occupation of the opioid receptors. The needle used for both methods has a specially shaped tip to facilitate the introduction of the catheter and reduce the possible risk of damaging the dura mater and the spinal cord. The catheter is subsequently tunnelled under the skin up to the side and supplied with an appropriate antibacterial filter.

This system of administering drugs is called 'open' and is particularly indicated for short-term and medium-term treatments (ca. 1–3 months). For patients with a long life expectancy and with the certainty of a good analgesic response a 'closed' system can be used whereby in both the peridural and the subarachnoid methods the free end of the catheter is connected to a reservoir placed in a subcutaneous pouch and supplied by way of simple injection. It is also possible to place, subcutaneously, a small pump which can be supplied by subcutaneous injection and operated by a compressed gas expansion chamber. One of the disadvantages of the closed methods of opioid drug administration, over and above the structural complexity, is the high cost, due partly to the impossibility of reutilizing the device, except in very special cases. In any case, these methods have to be used in specifically selected patients.

Narcotic-Resistant Pain

For the most part, cancer pain can be controlled by the sequential drug approach and the administration of narcotics by alternative methods. The following types of pain, however, respond poorly to narcotics:

- Tension headache
- Post-herpetic neuralgia
- Dysaesthesias
- Gastric distension
- Muscle Spasm
- Incident pain
- Tenesmus
- Decubitus pain

In these cases the origin of the pain must be investigated, since these types of pain are more or less completely refractory to the action of opioids.

The so-called adjuvant drugs may play a very important role: these substances are not analgesic in the strict sense of the word, but if associated with analgesics, NSAID and opioids, they are able to help their action, often significantly (Table 7).

Table 7. Coanalgesics for some pain syndromes

Symptom	Coanalgesics
Raised intracranial pressure	Dexamethasone 4 mg q 8–6 h diuretic
Nerve compression pain	Corticosteroids, phenytoin
Bone pain	Acetylsalicylic acid or another NSAID
Post-herpetic neuralgia	Amitriptyline 20–100 mg q 4 h
Superficial dysaesthesia	Amitriptyline 25–100 mg nocte
Intermittent stabbing pain	Valproate 200 mg q 8 h
Gastric distension pain	Metoclopramide 10 mg q 4 h
Muscle spasm	Diazepam 5 mg q 12 h, baclofen 10 mg q 8 h
Infected malignant ulcer	Metronidazole 250–400 mg q 8 h, other antibiotics according to antibiogram
Lymphoedema	Dexamethasone 2–4 mg/day i. m., diuretics
Stomatitis	For candidiasis: nystatin 10 000 U q 6–8 h or ketoconazole 200 mg/day Mouth washes (with diluted lidocaine), artificial saliva
Reactive depression	Antidepressant (avoid benzodiazepine)
Anxiety	Benzodiazepine, phenothiazines

On the other hand, pain which has proven unresponsive to drug treatment can in some cases be controlled by neurosurgical methods.

Neurosurgical Procedures

The patient who does not respond to narcotic and non-narcotic analgesics, associated with adjuvant drugs, can often be helped by neurosurgical techniques, if the circumstances are right. The general indication is localized or unilateral pain due to compression and/or a lesion of large nerve trunks. In particular, incident pain, which is often narcotic resistant, is responsive to neurosurgery.

Some fundamental principles govern the use of neurosurgical techniques. They should:

- Be atraumatic
- Be selective of the sensitive fibres
- Cause no side effects
- Cause no pain during or after operation
- Not handicap the patient
- Be simple to carry out and of low cost
- Have the informed consent of the patient

It must be remembered that in some cases the interruption of the nervous tissues can, in time, produce some quite troublesome dysaesthesia and paraesthesia. For this reason, neurosurgery is not always feasible in patients with a long life expectancy. Neurosurgical methods must be carefully assessed for their possible morbidity, but again quality of life must be the main criterion. In many cases neurosurgery will have to be supplemented with analgesic and/or adjuvant drugs, sometimes due to the incompleteness of the intervention. This can be seen early, often due to the appearance of new pain. These patients must not be 'forgotten'.

The percutaneous, chemical or thermal techniques in current use are characteristically less invasive and have a lower morbidity than the more costly open surgery (Table 8).

Chemical techniques are based on the use of neurolytic substances, principally phenol in water or glycerine solution and variable concentrations of pure alcohol. The phenol solution is hyperbaric in relation to the cerebrospinal fluid, whereas alcohol is hypobaric. These are important considerations affecting the position the patient must assume during operation. Chemical techniques are 'blind' techniques in which it is not possible to predict the site and the entity of the lesion precisely; they are, however, procedures which are economic, only slightly invasive, can be carried out in seriously ill patients and can generally be repeated.

In thermal techniques, the tip of a needle is heated by radiofrequency and placed in the most suitable area of the lesion, causing coagulation of the surrounding tissue. Although this technique requires rather costly equipment, the procedure is favoured by the fact that it is possible to perform a trial stimulation and thus localize the site of the lesion. In general, this method can also be repeated.

The principal neurosurgical procedures used today are described below.

Chemical Lesions

Subarachnoid Chemical Rhizotomy (Fig. 5)

Indications: Pain clearly localized in the area of a few spinal nerves.

Technique: Injection into the subarachnoid space by the usual method, of a hyperbaric solution of either phenol in glycerine or a hypobaric alcohol solution.

Table 8. Main neurosurgical procedures

Operation	Results	Duration of effect	Main complications
Chemical spinal rhizotomies	30% excellent 30% good 40% poor or none	1–3 months	Paraplegia and limb weakness (5%), incontinence (15%), mortality (1%)
Coeliac gangliolysis	50% excellent 30% good 20% poor	1–3 months	Postural hypotension (50%), intestinal disturbances (10%)
Trigeminal/glossopharyngeal thermorhizotomies	70% excellent 15% good 15% poor or none	3–6 months	Swallowing difficulties (30%), sensitivity disturbances (40%), keratitis (1%)
Percutaneous anterolateral cordotomy	70% excellent 15% good 15% poor or none	1–12 months	Horner's syndrome (50%), urinary disturbances (20%), respiratory disturbances (15%), noticeable weakness (40%), paralysis (1%), severe dysaesthesia (7%), mortality (1%–4%)

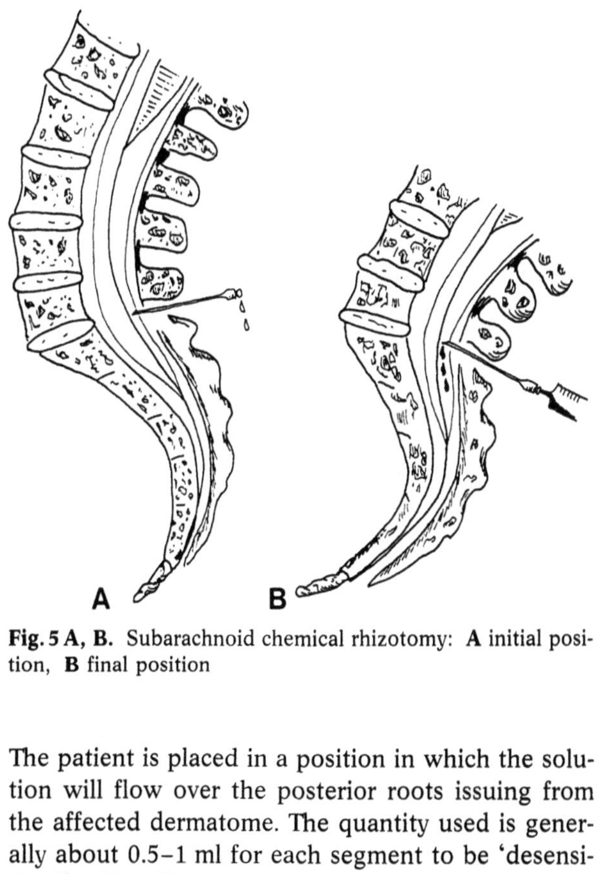

A B

Fig. 5 A, B. Subarachnoid chemical rhizotomy: **A** initial position, **B** final position

The patient is placed in a position in which the solution will flow over the posterior roots issuing from the affected dermatome. The quantity used is generally about 0.5–1 ml for each segment to be 'desensitized'. This effects a shallow, superficial and partial hypoaesthesia, extending to the corresponding metameres, which can last as little as 2–3 days or as long as a few months. Since this is a blind technique the motor tracts can become involved, causing a subsequent loss of sphinteric and muscular tone. This method is strongly indicated where sensory, motor and sphinteric deficiency already exists: a typical example is perineal pain from recurrent tumours in colostomized patients.

In patients suffering from motor and sphinteric deficiency who cannot be treated with drugs, pain in the pelvis and lower limbs can be controlled by administering 2–5 ml phenol in 10% glycerine solution distributed through the T11–T12, L2–L3 and L4–L5 interspaces.

Subdural Chemical Rhizotomy

Indications: Cancer pain at the cervical level.

Technique: Usually performed at the cervical level, where the subdural space is widest. Phenol in 5%–10% glycerine solution is used at doses varying from 0.5 to 2.5 ml. An X-ray amplifier should be used to check on the special appearance of the contrast medium which is typical of the subdural space.

Celiac Gangliosis (Fig. 6)

Indications: Pain from pancreatic, gastric, hepatic, renal and lower bowel tumours where there is no occlusion, but tumour growth along the celiac axis revealed by CT scan. This procedure can be repeated with equally satisfactory results.

Technique: A quantity of 30–60 ml pure alcohol diluted in saline solution (70%) is injected in the celiac ganglion region. A bilateral approach is used with two needles inserted at about the angles of the 12th ribs, placing the tips immediately behind T12 or L1. This intervention should be checked throughout by means of X-ray amplification. A unilateral approach by transaortic insertion has also been proposed recently.

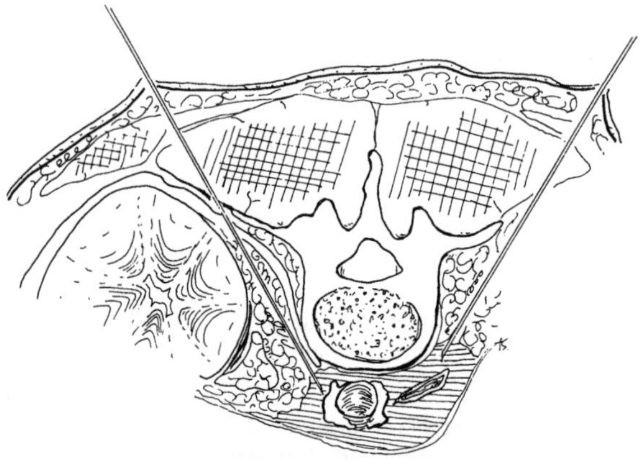

Fig. 6. Coeliac gangliolisis: final position of needles as seen from below (L1 vertebral level)

Thermal Lesions

Percutaneous Thermal Rhizotomy

Indications: Head and neck pain (rhizotomy of the first cervical roots), thoracic pain and, less frequently, pain of the shoulder and upper limb (thoracic rhizotomy), pain in the perineal and sacrococcygeal area (thermolysis of the cauda from S2–S3, sparing the root of S2 on one side in patients with good sphinteric control).

Technique: A 17-gauge guide needle is introduced through the skin and the paraspinal muscles, checked continuously by way of light amplification. On reaching the root the spindle of the guide needle is replaced with another one equipped with an electrode. Stimulation permits the exact position of the needle to be identified. Neurolesion is then effected by a radiofrequency-guided generator at temperatures of between 55 °C and 70 °C for about 120 mSec.

Trigeminal Thermal Rhizotomy

Indications: Cancer pain in the area of innervation of the trigeminus nerve. This technique can also be used in debilitated patients. The introduction of the needle may sometimes be difficult due to the tumour mass and changes in the points of reference.

Technique: A 19-gauge needle with a rigid spindle is inserted under local anaesthetic 2.5 cm lateral to the commissura labiorum. It is directed towards the oval space following two imaginary lines, one sagittal through the pupil, the other transverse passing along the upper margin of the ears. The length of the non-isolated portion of the needle tip is determined on the basis of the size of the lesion required, generally some 4–5 mm. X-rays are then taken to confirm the correct positioning of the electrode needle; one or two stimulations are performed to ensure correct functioning. Subsequently, under ultrarapid general anaesthetic, a temperature of approximately 70 °C is applied for about 1 min. According to the extension of the hypoalgesic area, brief thermal lesions can be made at other sites.

Glossopharyngeal Thermal Rhizotomy

Indications: Cancer pain of the oropharyngeal area, larynx, epipharynx, posterior tongue and external acoustic canal. This procedure is often associated with trigeminal thermal rhizotomy.

Technique: Similar to the percutaneous approach to the trigeminal ganglion. The needle is introduced about 2.5 cm lateral to the commissura labiorum, ipsilateral to the site of the lesion. It can be directed under X-ray control in two ways: one at an angle of 12° to a line passing vertically through the pupil and one at 45° to a line passing through the internal acoustic meatus and the lower margin of the orbit. The tip of the needle must be placed along the median portion of the posterior lacrimal fossa. If the needle is correctly placed, it can produce a response from cranial nerves IX, X and XI. Electrocardiac monitoring should be carried out. The lesion is made under ultrarapid general anaesthetic at a temperature of between 65 °C and 75 °C. Attention must be paid to any bradycardia. This procedure can be repeated.

Percutaneous Cordotomy

This is the most effective neurolesional approach at the present time. It consists in the interruption of the nervous structures situated in the anterolateral quadrant of the spinal cord, where the fibres responsible for the thermal and pain sensitivity of the contralateral hemicorpus lie (Fig. 7).

Three methods of percutaneous cordotomy are in use today. The most common procedure, which we shall describe in detail, consists of a lateral approach through the C1–C2 vertebral interspace. Other possible approaches are the anterior approach through the interverterbal disc and the posterior stereotaxic approach through the interspace between C1 and the base of the cranium, but these are complex techniques and their use is much less widespread.

Percutaneous lateral cordotomy is a procedure which can also be used with a debilitated patient and necessitates only a common preanaesthetic and

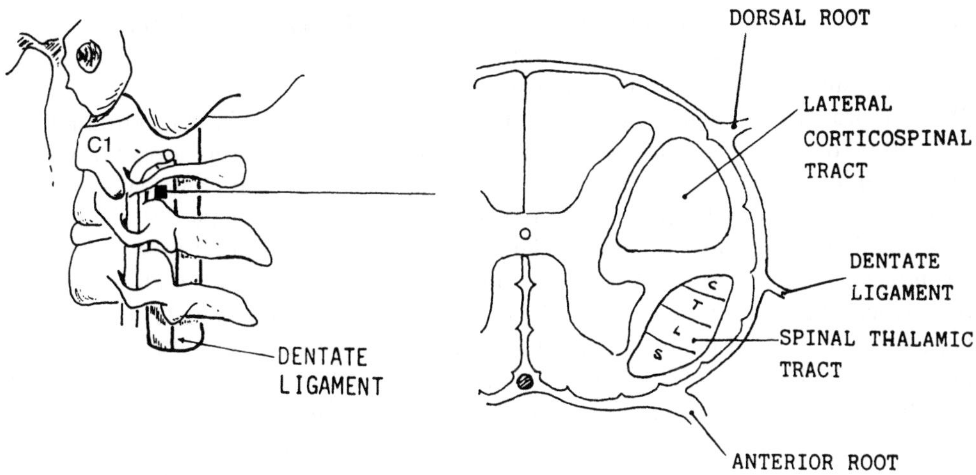

Fig. 7. Percutaneous anteriolateral cordotomy: site of lesion and somatotopic representation. *C*, cervical; *T*, thoracic; *L*, lumbar; *S*, sacral

a local anaesthetic: it can also be repeated on the same side without any great increase in risk for the patient.

Indications: Unilateral cancer pain from C5 to S5 in patients with no more than 12 months life expectancy. Due to the possible occurrence, in time, of dysaesthesia in the denervated areas, reasonably good lung function is also required [forced expiratory ventilation (FEV_1) $\geqslant$ 1 litre]. It should be borne in mind that if there are neoplastic lesions at the vertebral level, or in the half of the body not receiving the analgesic effect of the cordotomy, the treatment will have to be integrated with other methods to control the contralateral pain, which occurs in about 80% of these cases. In selected cases it is possible after a time to perform a second cordotomy on the other side to control bilateral pain which is unresponsive to drugs. If possible the second cordotomy should be performed below C5 to avoid respiratory complications, of which Ondine's syndrome is the classical example: more or less complete loss of the capacity to breathe automatically, with sometimes prolonged periods of apnea, especially at night.

Special indications for percutaneous lateral cordotomy are the following:

- Brachial plexus pain (e.g. from Pancoast's syndrome or postradiotherapy plexopathy with a recurrence of disease)
- Thoracic pain (from lung or breast cancer or from metastases)
- Left or right hypochondriac pain (primary or secondary liver or biliary tract cancer, kidney tumours)
- Hemipelvic pain (lumbosacral plexopathy from genitourinary and colorectal tumours, or as a sequela of radiotherapy with a recurrence of disease)
- Lower limb pain (e.g. from rectal cancer or pelvic bone secondaries)

Technique: With the patient in the supine position and the head flexed backwards in order to straighten the cervical column, local anaesthesia is performed about 1 cm below the contralateral mastoid apophysis. The needle is left in place and its position verified by X-ray amplification. Having localized the C1–C2 interspace, a guide needle is introduced up to the subarachnoid space. Myelography is performed with a contrast medium, the patient's CSF and air in order to identify the anterior and the posterior margin of the spinal cord and the dentate ligament. The point of insertion of the electrode through the guide needle in order to make a lesion is about 1 cm above the dentate ligament. The needle used for making the lesion is supplied with an electrode which is totally insulated except for the tip, which protrudes about 2–3 mm from the needle. It is connected to a radiofrequency apparatus by means of which both the stimulation and the microlesion can be performed. This coagulates the tissues around the tip of the needle electrode. Localization can be aided by the use of a micromanipulator, which permits precise control of the position of the tip of the needle. Whilst the needle is approaching the spinal cord the variation in the resistance of the tissues encountered can be assessed; it is slight in the fluid and increases clearly when the electrode penetrates the cord. Having placed the needle correctly, low-frequency (about 2–10 Hz) stimulation can be carried out. Stimulation must produce an ipsilateral motor response of the muscles of the neck and the trapezius muscle. Different muscular response indicates incorrect position of the needle. Subsequently, high-frequency stimulation of about 10 Hz is carried out. This will produce a tingling, cold or warm sensation. When this corresponds to the upper and lower limbs in that half of the body where the pain is localized, a small coagulation can be performed, the result assessed and, if it is positive, other coagulations effected until an analgesic area covering the side of the body where the pain is localized from C5 to S5 is obtained. The position of the needle should be checked by X-ray amplification from both the laterolateral and the posteroanterior projection during the whole operation.

Stereotaxic Myelotomy

Indications: Perineal cancer pain, 'saddle', bilateral pelvic pain.

Technique: A special surgical spinal stereotaxic instrument is required with which an electrode needle can be placed in position on the median line of the spinal cord. Having performed the usual stimulation trials to verify the position, the lesion is made, usually at about 5 cm into the posterior face of the medulla.

Stereotaxic Mesencephalic Tractotomy

Indications: Head and neck cancer pain. This procedure also requires special stereotaxic instrumentation.

Technique: The depth of the lesion is established by means of special plotting, preceded as always by precise stimulation trials. Extreme precision is required in placing the needle.

Stereotaxic Hypothalamotomy

Indications: Head and neck cancer pain, more distal cancer pain.

Technique: Following X-ray localization, the correct position of the needle is established by stimulation trials. Since this procedure is generally painful, a general anaesthetic is given. For head and neck pain ipsilateral hypothalamotomy is performed, and for pain situated more distally contralateral hypothalamotomy is carried out.

Continuing Care

Cancer pain is a continuously evolving entity which involves every aspect of the life of the person afflicted with it, physically and psychologically, socially and spiritually. To be adequate, therefore, treatment must cover all these aspects.

In the mid-1960s, first in England and then in the USA and Canada, attempts were made to solve the problems posed by advanced cancer. So-called hospices were created, either public or private institutions with about 20–40 beds staffed by medical and nursing personnel trained to assist the seriously ill and the dying. They are not modelled on the formal hospital rules, with no fixed visiting hours or meal times, and are furnished on domestic lines.

The patient can be taken in for short stays, or until death, although emphasis is placed on the care of the patient in his own home. With this aim, attempts have been made to extend the hospice network, together with home care services. These services bring all that the patient and his family needs to his home, guaranteeing a humanization of treatment and enabling the patient to live at home. A further specialization is represented by continuous care units (CCU). These take their inspiration from the philosophy of the hospice, placing emphasis on the home environment as the care unit and with the support of the technological resources of a hospital, preferably one specialized in the treatment of tumours. In this way, it is possible, whenever required, to call upon specialized personnel and services for palliative antalgic therapy. The endeavour to assist the patient as much as possible at home constitutes a real turn around in health care.

The CCU consists primarily of two services, one attached to the hospital and the other outside. The first is an outpatient service providing palliative treatment and, in particular, treatment for pain. It must have premises suitable for performing the main neurolesional interventions and must work in collaboration with a cancer psychology unit. Attached to the outpatient service there should be 5–10 beds for short stays, e.g. for neurolesional interventions or for adapting to drugs. Like the outpatient service, this department should be housed in an area which is independent of the hospital with its own entry.

Alongside this intrahospital unit there should be an extrahospital unit providing the home care service. This service should:
- Convey the patient back to his own home and enable him to stay there as long as possible
- Relieve the psychological suffering of the family

and, at the same time, include them in the work of the team
- Continue, or begin the necessary palliative therapy in the home
- Make the care of the patient more human
- Assess the need for the patient to return to hospital
- If possible, assist the family in their grief on bereavement
- Spread the care philosophy of the CCU

The patients committed to the care of the CCU are those with advanced disease, often chair- or bedridden and, above all, little cared for (patients living alone, economically underprivileged or needing treatment beyond their economic/social means).

The basis of the home care team is formed by the patient and his family. Their direct counterparts are the professional nurses and specially trained volunteers. The nurses provide the real medical care – medication, injections, administration of special antalgic therapies – as well as fulfilling an important psychosocial function, connecting the patient and his needs and the CCU. The volunteers provide the friendly support and relief of the family, making a significant contribution to the psychosocial wellbeing of the patient and his relatives. They can also maintain contact with the family following the death of the patient. The CCU doctor collaborates with the visiting nurse but remains in the background, intervening only in special cases. The doctor, however, supervises the progress of the palliative treatment through outpatients visits and also through contact with the patient's general practitioner.

The whole team meets weekly and is joined by a psychologist, who is also able to visit the patient at home. The CCU team is completed by a social assistant and a member of the clergy.

This model of patient care has produced excellent results, typified by improvement in psychoemotional parameters such as anxiety, mood and state of mind. It has given a certain stability to the quality of life and has had a positive influence on the intensity of pain, particularly in comparison with patients who are only cared for in outpatient clinics.

Selected Reading

Billings JA (1985) Outpatient management of advanced cancer. Symptom control, support and hospice-in-the-home. Lippincott, Philadelphia

Spilling R (ed) (1986) Terminal care at home. Oxford University Press, Oxford

Twycross RG, Lack SA (1983) Symptom control in far advanced cancer: pain relief. Pitman, London

Twycross RG, Lack SA (1984) Therapeutics in terminal cancer. Pitman, London

Wall PD, Melzack R (1984) Textbook of pain. Churchill Livingstone, Edinburgh

World Health Organization (1986) Cancer pain relief. WHO, Geneva

Zimmermann M, Drings P, Wagner G (eds) (1984) Pain in the cancer patient. Springer, Berlin Heidelberg New York (Recent results in cancer research, vol 89)

Terminal Care

R. Twycross

Introduction

In terminal care the emphasis moves from prolongation of life and comfort to just comfort. This shift becomes appropriate when anticancer treatment fails to prevent tumour progression. Frequently there is a period of transition rather than an abrupt change of direction in management. This is particularly true of certain cancers, such as breast cancer, in which yet another partial remission may be induced by further hormonal manipulation. The goals of terminal care are fourfold:

1. Relief for the patient from pain and other distressing symptoms
2. Psychological care for the patient
3. A support system to help patients live as actively as possible in the face of impending death
4. A support system to sustain the patient's family during the illness and bereavement

Psychological aspects of care have already been discussed by Maguire (this volume). In this chapter, the management of a number of other symptoms is discussed. Reference is also made to some of the psychological needs of the dying patient and his family.

Hospice Care

Terminally ill patients often need more care than those whose sickness is curable. Professional medical and nursing skills of a high order are called for. In a number of countries, notably Britain and North America, special teams have been established to help care for the terminally ill. These "hospice" or palliative care teams offer intensive care for the terminally ill. Some hospices offer home care only, while others have facilities for inpatients, outpatients, and day patients as well. Although the hospice philosophy is not limited by "tyranny of cure", it is, at the same time, steadfastly opposed to euthanasia. The American National Hospice Organization (1981) states:

> The purpose of hospice is to provide support and care for persons in the last phases of disease so that they can live as fully and comfortably as possible. Hospice affirms life and regards dying as a normal process. Hospice neither hastens nor postpones death. Hospice believes that through personalized services and a caring community, patients and families can attain the necessary preparation for a death that is satisfactory to them.

Hospice care is distinct from geriatric medicine and the care of the chronic sick, two specialties with which it is often compared.

> It contains many of the rewards of surgery, since it operates in a setting of crisis intervention; of internal medicine, since it calls for the fine titration of drug regimens against troublesome symptoms: and of psychiatry, since it deals with the anxious, the depressed and the bereaved (Mount 1980).

Teamwork

Terminal care is best administered by a group of people working together as a team. In addition to the patient, the team will include some or all of the following: the immediate family, friends, doctor(s), nurses, social worker, therapists, priest and other advisers. The team is collectively concerned for the total wellbeing of the patient and the family – physical, psychological, spiritual and social. In such a situation there is inevitably an overlap of roles.

It is important that everyone works together in a coordinated manner. For instance, the lead given by a doctor will be seriously undermined if other carers do not participate actively in symptom control – the nurses in hospital, and the family and community nurses at home. On the other hand, a nurse cannot raise expectations concerning greater comfort if the doctor is disinterested or inept. It is necessary, therefore, for team members to establish a common baseline of intent. From this foundation, enriched by mutual trust and respect, the possiblity of good terminal care emerges.

Appropriate Treatment

In terminal cancer the primary aim of treatment is no longer to prolong life but to make the life that remains as comfortable and as meaningful as possible (Thompson 1984). It is not a question of "To treat or not to treat?" but of "what is the most appropriate treatment?" given the patient's biological prospects and personal and social circumstances. Treatment appropriate for an acutely ill patient may be inappropriate in the dying. Nasogastric tubes, intravenous infusions, antibiotics, cardiac resuscitation, and artificial respiration are all primarily supportive measures for use in acute or acute-on-chronic illness to assist a patient through the initial period towards recovery of health. To use such measures in patients who are close to death and in whom there is no expectation of a return to health is usually inappropriate.

Medical care is a continuum, ranging from complete cure at one end to symptom control at the other. Many types of treatment span the entire spectrum of care, notably radiotherapy and, to a lesser extent, chemotherapy and surgery. It is important, therefore, to keep the therapeutic aim clearly in mind when employing any form of treatment. In deciding what is appropriate, the following must be considered:

1. The patient's biological prospects
2. The therapeutic aim of each treatment
3. The need not to prescribe a lingering death

Although the possibility of unexpected improvement or recovery should not be ignored, there are many occasions when it is appropriate to "give death a chance". All patients *must* die eventually: ultimately nature will take its course. In this respect, the art of medicine is to decide when life sustenance is essentially futile and, therefore, when to allow death to occur without further impediment. For example, antibiotics are usually appropriate for the patient with advanced cancer who develops a chest infection while still relatively active and independent. Pneumonia should, however, still be "the old man's friend". If the burden of living has become considerable, it may be more appropriate *not* to use antibiotics. When it is difficult to make a decision, the

"2-day rule" should be invoked: if after 2–3 days of straightforward symptom relief the patient is clearly holding his own, prescribe an antibiotic. If the patient is clearly much worse, do not.

As patients become bedbound, it is sensible to phase out the less important medications. Iron, multivitamins, potassium and digoxin are all medium-term supportive treatments and are irrelevent when the patient is close to death. Antihypertensive can often be phased out as weight loss and/or other medication alter the patient's need; for example, morphine reduces the cardiac preload. Continuation of pre-existing diuretic therapy may cause postural hypotension and gross debility unless the dose is reduced or stopped in the face of a poor fluid intake or repeated vomiting. Insulin reductions can be done partly by guesswork and partly on the basis of finger-prick blood glucose estimations. When the patient is stuporouse, the insulin should be stopped altogether. There is no longer any biological justification for the continued palliation of the diabetic state.

Rehabiliation

Rehabilitation is an integral part of terminal care. It means helping a patient achieve his maximum potential physically, emotionally, socially and vocationally. Many doctors, however, still do not appreciate the opportunities that exist for rehabilitation in terminal cancer. Although physical rehabilitation eventually becomes inpossible, many patients are unnecessarily restricted, often by relatives, even though capable of a greater degree of activity and independence. Control of troublesome symptoms and gentle encouragement by an attentive doctor is crucial in enabling a patient to realize his full potential.

The list of reversible causes of deterioration is long. It is important, therefore, not to assume automatically that a sudden deterioration or change relates to the inexorable progression of the disease. Is the patient exhausted because of sleepless, pain-filled nights? Has he caught influenza from another member of the family or a friend? Is he the only person with diarrhoea or is it an attack of gastroenteritis? What is needed is not a checklist but an awareness of the fact that a significant number of patients are forced into a dying role prematurely because the portents are misread.

Table 1. Corticosteroids in terminal cancer

Non-specific uses	*Other specific uses*
To improve appetite	Hypercalcaemia
To enhance sense of well-being	Carcinomatous neuropathy
To improve strength	Incipient paraplegia
	Superior vena cava obstruction
Coanalgesic	Airway obstruction
Raised intracranial pressure	Carcinomatous lymphangitis
Nerve compression	Haemoptysis
Spinal cord compression	Leucoerythroblastic anaemia
Head and neck tumour	Malignant effusion
Metastatic arthralgia	Discharge from rectal tumour[a]
	To reduce sweating

Inclusion in the list does not mean that a corticosteroid is necessarily the treatment of choice.
[a] Given rectally.

Corticosteroids

Corticosteroids are widely used in far-advanced cancer. Inclusion in the list in Table 1 does not imply that their use is the sole or most important treatment in these situations. It simply means that the use of a corticosteroid may be of benefit and should be considered as a treatment option to be tried alone or in association with other recognized measures. Dosage varies from dexamethasone 2 mg/day for appetite stimulation to 10 mg t.i.d. or more in cases of spinal cord compression. A typical starting dose for nerve compression pain is 4 mg b.i.d. Maintenance doses are usually smaller. They represent the balance between continued efficacy and a desire to avoid troublesome side effects. Prominent side effects include oral candidiasis and oedema. Some patients develop the characteristic moon-face. About 10% become overactive physically or mentally, and may develop insomnia or become hypomanic (Hanks et al. 1983). In these the need for the corticosteroid should be reviewed, and the dose reduced or completely stopped. If the corticosteroid is continued it may be necessary to prescribe a benzodiazepine as a night sedative or anxiolytic.

In the majority of patients with, for example, incipient paraplegia, superior vena cava obstruction or haemoptysis, a corticosteroid should be given in association with radiotherapy. Similarly, a corticosteroid is not generally the treatment of choice for malignant effusions but, where other measures have failed or seem inappropriate, it may be tried with or without a chemotherapeutic agent.

The use of a corticosteroid as a co-analgesic should be considered wherever there is a large tumour mass within a relatively confined space. There is often an oedematous area around a tumour, and pressure on neighbouring veins and lymphatics may lead to further local or regional swelling. In other words, total tumour mass = neoplasm + surrounding hyperaemic oedema. Corticosteroids reduce this oedema, thereby reducing the total tumour mass.

The classic situation is that of headache caused by raised intracranial pressure in association with cerebral neoplasm. There may be other central nervous symptoms or signs, and patients often show improvement for weeks or months after starting treatment. When headache is the main symptom, analgesics and elevation of the head of the bed should also be considered.

Symptom Control

A wide variety of symptoms are experienced by patients with far-advanced cancer (Table 2). No one symptom occurs in every patient. Even pain, closely associated in the popular mind with terminal cancer, is present in only about two-thirds of patients (Twycross and Lack 1983). It must be stressed, however, that the symptoms experienced are not all caused by the malignant process. Causal factors include treatment (past or present) and a concurrent second disorder. As some symptoms are caused by multiple factors, it is necessary to identify the different factors involved, and then to seek to correct those that are reversible. In this way, although the underlying pathological process remains unchanged, it is usually possible to obtain significant, sometimes complete, symptomatic relief.

If dealing with a persistent symptom for which pharmacological measures are appropriate, the drug(s) should be prescribed regularly on a prophylactic basis. This fundamental piece of advice has been increasingly adopted in relation to the use of analgesics and pain management. Its application to the use of antiemetics and laxatives is not as fully appreciated. The use of drugs "as required" instead of regularly is the cause of much unrelieved distress.

It is often not possible to predict the optimum dose of drugs used to relieve symptoms, particularly opioids, laxatives and psychotropic drugs. Moreover, side effects may jeopardize drug compliance. Adjustments will therefore be necessary, especially during the first few weeks. This should be anticipated and arrangements made for continuing close supervision.

Although many symptoms respond completely or to a large extent to a combination of drug and non-drug measures, it is sometimes necessary to compromise in order to avoid unacceptable unwanted effects. For example, anticholinergic effects such as dry mouth or visual disturbance may occasionally be limiting factors. With intestinal obstruction, it is often better to aim to reduce the incidence of vomiting to once or twice a day rather than to seek absolute control.

Table 2. Symptoms in 6677 patients admitted to St. Christopher's Hospice 1975–1984

Symptom	Percentage
Weight loss	77
Pain	71
Anorexia	67
Dyspnoea	51
Cough	50
Constipation	47
Weakness	47
Nausea, Vomiting	40
Oedema, Ascites, Pleural effusion	31
Insomnia	29
Incontinence, Catheterized	23
Dysphagia	23
Bedsore	19
Haemorrhage	14
Drowsiness	10
Paralysis	8
Jaundice	6
Colostomy	5
Diarrhoea	4
Fistula	1

From Twycross and Lack (1986).
Data collated from annual reports: *St. Christopher's Hospice – Details of Admissions and Discharges.*

Constipation

Constipation is the commonest alimentary symptom in patients with advanced cancer. Prevention is always better (and less traumatic) than the subsequent correction of impaction of faeces with or without obstructive features. The use of a laxative is usually necessary for patients receiving opioid analgesic and for those taking drugs with anticholinergic side effects. Adequate fluids, bran with breakfast cereal, fruit juice, improving appetite and mobilization all play their part in both prevention and correction. However, for many patients, some or all of these measures cannot be employed. It should, therefore, be the general rule to prescribe a laxative in patients who have been commenced on an opioid analgesic regimen. The use of co-danthrusate (danthron and

Table 3. Antiemetics in terminal cancer

Cause of nausea and vomiting	Antiemetic of choice	Comment
Drug-induced Radiotherapy Chemotherapy Metabolitic Uraemia Hypercalcaemia	Haloperidol 1.5 mg nocte or prochlorperazine 5 mg t.i.d. ↓ Haloperidol 5–20 mg/day	Side effects rare at lower dose Sometimes causes dry mouth or mild drowsiness
Raised intracranial pressure Intestinal obstruction	Cyclizine 50–100 mg t.i.d.	Anticholinergic side effects; may cause drowsiness
Oesophageal reflux Delayed gastric emptying	Metoclopramide 10 mg t.i.d.–q 4 h *or* Domperidone 10–20 mg t.i.d.–q 4 h	Do not cause anticholinergic side effects
Gastric irritation by drug	Treat gastritis, change medication	Sometimes seen with non-steroidal anti-inflammatory drugs and corticosteroids

docusate) capsules is recommended, beginning with two capsules either at bedtime or in the morning. Danthron is a peristaltic stimulant laxative similar to senna, and docusate is a surface wetting agent.

For patients who do not respond to co-danthrusate 3 capsules q.i.d., it is worth halving the dose and adding in a small bowel flusher such as magnesium sulphate (Epsom salts) or lactulose before concluding that oral laxatives are not going to work. Even so, more than a third of all terminal cancer patients will require additional rectal measures, i.e. suppositories, enemas or manual removal.

Nausea and Vomiting

Nausea and/or vomiting occurs in about 40% of patients with terminal cancer (Twycross and Lack 1986). The treatment varies according to the underlying cause (Table 3). If the symptoms are related to physical or chemical irritation of the stomach, metoclopramide is often the best antiemetic. It enhances peristalsis in the upper gastrointestinal tract, speeds gastric emptying and increases the tone of the oesophageal spincter (Gralla 1983). For nausea or vomiting of chemical origin, whether neoplastic, biochemical, or therapeutic, metoclopramide is also often efficacious. However, the anxious may respond better to a drug with sedative properties such as a phenothiazine, e.g. prochlorperazine. If the cause is intracranial, cyclizine is the drug of choice, as it acts directly on the vomiting centre (Peroutka and Synder 1982).

The author uses haloperidol for drug-induced vomiting: 1.5 mg stat and at bedtime thereafter. It is nonsedative in this dose and only rarely causes dryness of the mouth. If the patient is experiencing radiation-induced vomiting, a higher dose (e.g. 5 mg at bedtime) is indicated. If the vomiting is associated with chemotherapy, 5 mg b.i.d. or t.i.d. may be necessary. In doses of 3 mg or more a day, there is a possibility of parkinsonian side effects. If these occur, the dose should be reduced if possible. Alternatively, an antiparkinsonian agent such as orphenadrine 50–100 mg b.i.d. should be prescribed.

Intestinal Obstruction

When the gastrointestinal tract is obstructed and surgery is contraindicated, antiemetics are of less value. Cyclizine and chlorpromazine appear to be most helpful (Baines et al. 1985; Twycross and Lack 1986). It is important, however, to reduce gastrointestinal motility in order to prevent the colic which often precedes and possibly triggers obstructive vomiting (Table 4).

Unfortunately, no two obstructed patients are alike. It is necessary to consider each patient individually, weigh up the many factors relating to that patient's particular obstructive syndrome, and then proceed with a series of therapeutic trials. If the obstruction is in the pylorus, duodenum or jejunum, a nasogastric tube may be necessary. This can be aspirated before drinks and meals, and possibly left on free drainage overnight. The patient will be much relieved despite the negative fluid balance and often remains remarkably well for several days before deteriorating rapidly as a result of accumulated fluid and biochemical losses.

Table 4. Medical management of persistent partial intestinal obstruction

Explanation and dietary advice	Small meals, less roughage Eat earlier rather than later in day Eat only if want to
Relief of abdominal pain	Codeine phosphate Morphine sulphate
Control of colic[a]	Antispasmodics Mebeverine Propantheline Hyoscine butylbromide Hyoscine hydrobromide Avoid peristaltic stimulant laxatives
Antiemetics	Cyclizine 50–100 mg b.i.d. or t.i.d. Haloperidol 5 mg nocte or b.i.d. } to control chemical/toxic Chlorpromazine 25 mg t.i.d. } components of emesis if uraemic, etc.
Maintenance of defaecation	Soften bowel contents Docusate tablets 100 mg b.i.d. or t.i.d. Enemas/suppositories e.g. every 3–4 days if no spontaneous faecal evacuation
Trial of corticosteroids	Dexamethasone 4 mg b.i.d. } rarely beneficial Prednisolone 15 mg b.i.d. }

[a] Controlling visceral pain and inhibiting intestinal motility with an opioid often leads to a cessation of previously distressing colic. If the colic is very severe or recurs despite the regular use of an opioid, an antispasmodic is indicated.

Anorexia

Anorexia may be caused by the fear of vomiting; it may also be the prodrome of nausea. Careful history taking will indicate if it is the former; the latter may have to be assessed by a therapeutic trial of an antiemetic. Unrelieved pain and exhaustion from insomnia are both potent causes of anorexia. Early satiation is another cause of diminished intake. This occurs commonly in patients with gross hepatomegaly. Being offered too much or pressed to eat more by an overanxious spouse may also provoke anorexia. It is often possible to achieve an increased intake by correcting some of these contributory factors, and by offering simple dietary advice. A 7- to 10-day trial of dexamethasone 2–4 mg daily is worth considering (Hanks et al. 1983).

When the patient is close to death, giving "permission" not to eat and discouraging the family from force-feeding is often the most appropriate form of management: "Provided you are taking plenty of fluid, I shall be happy; solid food is not important at the moment".

Table 5. Squashed stomach syndrome

Definition
Dyspeptic symptoms associated with inability of stomach to distend normally because of hepatomegaly. Similar symptoms may be seen with carcinoma of stomach, linitis plastica, or post gastrectomy ("small stomach syndrome")
Symptoms
Early satiation
Epigastric fullness
Epigastric discomfort/pain
Flatulence
Hiccup
Nausea
Vomiting (especially postprandial)
Heartburn
Treatment
Explanation
Dietary advice
Antiflatulent (e.g. Asilone 10 ml *after meals* and nocte)
Metoclopramide (4-hourly if also receiving morphine) (or after meals and bedtime)

Squashed Stomach Syndrome

Epigastric pain in terminal cancer may relate to gastric distension. This occurs after partial gastrectomy or with a large inoperable or recurrent intragastric neoplasm. Relative gastric distension occurs without gastric abnormality in patients with gross hepatomegaly. The postprandial discomfort must be recognized for what it is, because explanation to the patient is most important. The aim of treatment is to prevent overdistension. This requires a combination of dietary and pharmacological measures (Table 5).

Hiccup

The most common cause of hiccup in advanced cancer is gastric distension. Most traditional remedies rely on a "gating" mechanism which is triggered by pharyngeal stimulation. The author, however, uses Asilone (Rorer, USA) as treatment of choice. This is an antacid preparation containing activated dimethicone (a defoaming agent). At other centres, drinking from the "wrong" side of the cup or the use of granulated sugar has pride of place (Table 6). It is rare to need chlorpromazine. In squashed stomach syndrome or if gastric stasis is thought to be relevant, metoclopramide is prescribed with meals and at bedtime, or with morphine every 4 h.

Dyspnoea

Careful assessment will usually indicate the main reason(s) for a patient's breathlessness. Specific causes such as heart failure benefit by traditional measures. In most patients, dyspnoea is the result of a number of factors, some of which are quite clearly irreversible, for example, chronic obstructive airways disease, anaemia and weakness. Explanation always helps, and discussion with both patient and family about ways in which the patient's pattern of living may or should be modified is an important part of treatment.

For patients with carcinomatous lymphangitis, or who are wheezing because of neoplastic pressure on one or more major bronchi a trial of corticosteroids should be instituted, for example dexamethasone 4 mg/day or prednisolone 15 mg b.i.d. In many cases dyspnoea is secondary to pleural effusion and paracentesis may be necessary. If, because of irreversible compression atelectasis, paracentesis results in little benefit, or the patient is too ill for such treatment, symptomatic measures should be used. A benzodiazepine, such as diazepam 5–10 mg at bedtime, helps to reduce the anxiety and fear that accompany dyspnoea. Morphine, with its direct depressant effect on the respiratory centre, is of particular value when the patient is markedly tachypnoeic, for example, 5–15 mg every 4 h by mouth.

Table 6. Hiccup in terminal cancer

Causes
Gastric distension
Diaphragmatic irritation
Toxic
Uraemia
Infection
CNS tumour
Phrenic nerve irritation
Treatment
Rebreathing into paper bag (or inhalations of 5% CO_2)
Pharyngeal stimulation
Drinking from "wrong" side of cup
Granulated sugar (two heaped teaspoons)
Liqueur (two glasses)
Cold key down back of neck (acts via hyperextension of neck)
Nasopharyngeal tube
Correction of gastric distension
Peppermint water (relaxes oesophageal sphincter)
Defoaming agent (e.g. Asilone 10 ml after meals and nocte)
Metoclopramide (10 mg q 6 h–q 4 h; hastens gastric emptying)
Nasogastric intubation
Drugs
Chlorpromazine 25 mg IV + 25 mg IM initially if patient distressed and other measures have failed
Chlorpromazine 10–25 mg up to q 4 h
Methylamphetamine 5–10 mg IV if (a) fails
Phenytoin 100 mg b.i.d. or t.i.d. or carbamazephine 200 mg b.i.d. to q.i.d. if related to cerebral lesion
Phrenic nerve block/crush (never necessary in terminal cancer in author's experience)

Dehydration

As the dying patient becomes weaker, he naturally drinks less. This may relate to dysphagia, nausea, anorexia, or lack of energy and interest. Also relevant is the reduced level of consciousness. As a general rule intravenous fluids are not administered to patients dying in a hospice. On the other hand, patients dying in a general hospital frequently receive intravenous fluids. This reflects, a belief that dehydration is distressing, and therefore unacceptable. This view has, however, been disputed (Editorial 1986). Indeed, in the patient close to death, dehydration may well be beneficial.

For example, in gastrointestinal obstruction, as body fluids decrease, vomiting may be reduced to only once or twice a day, even without specific symptom control measures. Intravenous fluids on the other hand, will tend to maintain secretions. This is likely to result in more copious and more frequent vomiting. A nasogastric tube is likely to become necessary, whereas this is hardly ever needed if the patient is dehydrated. Moreover, as body fluids reduce, urine output decreases. There will be fewer bedwetting episodes, and there will be less need for urinal, bedpan, commode or catheterization.

When the dying patient has a respiratory problem such as pneumonia or pulmonary oedema, pulmonary secretions are reduced by dehydration, and coughing and breathlessness are reduced. Likewise, as body secretions generally decrease, the patient who has had difficulty swallowing his saliva will gain at least partial relief from the choking and drowning sensations that accompany aspiration. (Belladonna alkaloids and anxiolytic drugs may, of course, still be needed to reduce secretions further and to control apprehension.) If intravenous fluids are given, the patient may become more dyspnoeic and the cough worsen. Suction may be required.

Perhaps the most discomforting consequence of dwindling body fluids is dry mouth. This may lead to cracking of the mucosa, inflammation and infection. Dry mouth, however, can be alleviated to a considerable extent by conscientious mouth care. Often it is possible to enlist the family's help in this. Using a bottle with a spray top allows small volumes to be introduced into the mouth at half-hourly intervals if need be. Multifocal myoclonus, secondary to electrolyte imbalance, is the other relatively common side effect of marked dehydration. Diazepam should be given to control this.

Dehydration should therefore be looked upon as a natural process in the last few days of life – a process that helps to relieve a number of symptoms. Intravenous fluids should be avoided, as they tend to exacerbate discomfort in the patient close to death and may also add to the emotional distress of the family.

Confusion

The ability of a family to cope with a death in the home depends in large measure on the doctor's ability to help patient and family understand and cope with the symptoms of confusion that ultimately occur in most cases. Confusion results from "clouding of the sensorium" which leads to the mingling of ideas. This causes a disturbance of comprehension and bewilderement. There may be associated drowsiness manifestations including:

1. Poor concentration
2. Impairment of short-term memory
3. Disorientation
4. Misperceptions
5. Paranoid delusions
6. Hallucinations
7. Rambling and incoherent speech
8. Restlessness
9. Noisy/aggressive behaviour

Confusion tends to be variable in degree and intensity. In the dying, most such states are caused by multiple factors (Table 4). In some, symptoms are never more than mild and remain intermittent (Stedeford 1978, 1984).

Unfortunately, any sort of strange behaviour or talk in an ill patient tends to be labelled "confusion." Once a patient is deemed confused, doctors, nurses, friends and family tend to shy away in embarrassment or even in fear. Precision in assessment is necessary to enable the family and other carers to continue to respond supportively to someone who happens to be very ill and who is experiencing what is often only a minor disturbance of thought.

Disorientation for time and, to a lesser extent, for place is almost the norm for the dying. Explanation and reassurance may be all that is necessary: "Most patients are like you – they lose track of time. After all, when you are not up and about and working, time is not so important, is it?" Misperceptions are common too. A similar type of explanation is generally sufficient: "You are not losing your mind/going mad; this sort of thing can happen to any of us when we are ill".

Hallucinations, misperceptions, nightmares and vivid daydreams often reflect anxiety about death. Anxiolytic medication is helpful when the content suggests this, together with continuing discussion about possible exacerbating psychological factors. Blunderbuss therapy with clorpromazine – a common medical response to this situation – may help to suppress hallucinations, for example, but may also increase the tendency to misperceive as a result of further clouding of the sensorium (Table 7).

Hope

Hope is an expectation greater than zero of achieving a desired goal. Hope tends to diminish when the patient is mentally isolated by a "conspiracy of silence"; when it is implied that "nothing more can be done"; when pain and other symptoms remain unrelieved or ignored; and when the patient feels alone or unsupported (Kubler-Ross 1970; Weisman 1979).

"Never destroy hope" is frequently cited as a reason for not informing a patient of the seriousness of the situation. Yet glib, false optimism is a potent destroyer of hope. On the other hand, an unwise catharsis by the doctor of all that is negative, either to the patient or to the family, may make the doctor feel easier, but it can irreversibly destroy hope and result in intractable anxiety and despair. It is necessary to seek to apply two parallel principles: "Never lie to a patient" and "Avoid total candour". Human

Table 7. Treatment of confusional states

Non-drug measures

Explanation to patient, family, nurses
Stress that patient is not going mad
Stress that almost always there are lucid intervals
Continue to treat patient as a sane, sensible adult
Appreciate that hallucinations, nightmares and misperceptions may reflect unresolved fears and anxiety

Drugs

Generally use drugs only if symptoms are marked, persistent and cause distress to patient and/or family. Review sooner rather than later if a sedative is prescribed, as such drugs may exacerbate symptoms
Specific
Reduction in present medication?
Oxygen if hypoxic/cyanosed
Dexamethasone (2–4 mg t.i.d. to q.i.d.) if cerebral tumour
General
Diazepam 5–10 mg by mouth or parenterally, especially if patient agitated and generally restless
Haloperidol 5 mg by mouth or intramuscularly, especially in the case of hallucinations and paranoia, and if diazepam fails

- Initial dose depends on previous medication, weight, age and severity of symptoms
- Subsequent doses depend on initial response
- Daily or b.i.d. maintenance doses are usually adequate
- Sometimes more frequent administration is necessary

Chlorpromazine, Thioridazine, Chlormethiazole } useful alternative preparations

beings – patients and doctors included – are best served when realism is tinged with optimism. Gentle, sympathetic and gradual communication of the truth, within the context of continued support and encouragement, almost always restores hope. It only does so, however, if the patient has a goal at which to aim and a direction in which to move. Good terminal care restores hope by giving the patient direction and by encouraging realistic goals. Telling the patient what you plan to do about the pain and other symptoms gives direction and helps to counter the living nightmare of never-ending unendurable pain or other physical distress.

In short, communication of painful truth does not equal destruction of hope. Despite continued physical deterioration, hope can be renewed when the patient is helped to face up to the diagnosis and prognosis. Hope of recovery is replaced by the more diffuse hope of a peaceful death, hope that one's life has been worthwhile and, possibly, the hope of immortality in some form.

Spiritual Care

When dying, many people take stock of their lives for the first time: "I have lived a good life"; "I never did anyone any harm"; "Why did it happen to me?" Although only a minority of patients discuss these issues with their doctor, the majority do so with a nurse or social worker, or with relatives and close friends. Patients are very perceptive, and they are unlikely to embarrass a doctor if they sense that communication at this level will cause discomfort.

When possible and appropriate, it is right for the doctor to alert a priest or rabbi to the fact that the patient is seriously ill and may appreciate a visit. Although regard for the patient as an individual does not allow the imposition of one's own beliefs, many patients are comforted by the discovery that their doctor has a religious faith.

As Death Approaches

When the patient becomes increasingly weak he is faced with the fact that death is inevitable and imminent. It is a time when support and companionship are of paramount importance. Although the doctor may feel powerless in the face of rapidly approaching death, the patient is often more realistic. He knows a miracle cannot be performed, he realizes that his time has come and, provided he is relatively comfortable, continued medical attentiveness is all he expects. The situation need never become totally negative and hopeless provided the doctor:

1. Continues to visit.
2. Quietly indicates that "at this stage the important thing is to keep you as comfortable as possible".
3. Simplifies medication as much as possible: "Now that your husband is not so well, we can probably manage without the heart tablets".
4. Arranges for medication to be given by suppository or injection when the patient is too weak to swallow.
5. Continues to inform the family of the changing situation: "He is very weak now, but could still go on for several days".
6. Takes steps to control on agitated confusional state even if it results in greater somnolence.
7. Listens to the nurses.

Psychological Care of the Family

The care of the family is an integral part of the care of the dying. A contented family increases the likelihood of a contented patient. Relative-doctor communication generally needs to be initiated and maintained by the doctor. It is easy to neglect the relatives as they are reluctant to bother the doctor "as he is so busy." At the time of diagnosis and later, there is much to be said for joint interviews – patient, spouse, and doctor. The doctor should also make an opportunity to see both the patient and the close relatives on their own. Further separate or joint interviews can then be arranged as necessary.

As with the patient, it is not generally necessary or wise to tell the family the whole truth (as you see it) at one time. If the family and patient are too far "out of step" in relation to knowledge about the diagnosis and prognosis, it can create a barrier between them. A common initial reaction is "You won't tell him, will you, doctor?" or "We'd prefer you not to tell him, doctor". This should be seen as the initial shock reaction and not as an excuse for saying nothing to the patient. If the family and patient are to be mutually supportive, it is necessary to help the relatives move forward from this initial reaction to a position of greater openness and trust. It is important to remember that the family cannot forbid the doctor to discuss diagnosis and prognosis with a patient.

Admission to hospital is often seen as a defeat by the family. It is necessary to emphasize that you are surprised they managed to cope for so long and that now, with the need for day and night care, it is impossible for one (or two) people to continue to cope alone without a break. Frequent visits should be encouraged, if practical. Separation anxiety may be reduced by encouraging them to help in the care of the patient – adjusting pillows, refilling a water jug, helping with a blanket bath and assisting at mealtimes. Some relatives need to be taught how to visit, to behave as they would at home, for example, sit and read a book or newspaper, knit, watch the television together. It should be emphasized that they do not have to keep up a tiring patter of conversation about trivia. Finally, if necessary, overnight accommodation should be arranged to enable a close family member to sleep nearby or with the patient in a single room.

A proportion of terminally ill patients improve following admission as a result of the control of pain and other symptoms. They become physically independent again and no longer need to be in hospital. Many relatives have fears about what will happen should the patient be discharged. A trial day out or weekend at home does much to allay their fears (or confirms that discharge is after all impractical). Clear advice should be given about whom to call in the event of a crisis.

Bereavement Support

Terminal care does not end when the patient dies; bereavement has both a morbidity and a mortality (Parkes and Weis 1983). Many relatives have false feelings of guilt: "If only I'd done this!" "Do you think if he'd gone to the hospital sooner?" etc. An opportunity should be given for such feelings to be aired and questions to be raised. It is encouraging that an increasing number of family practitioners and community nurses regard bereavement visits as time well invested. Most hospices also consider it necessary to follow up a proportion of the families with whom they have been associated (Parkes 1981). Sometimes this may be little more than courtesy. On the other hand, some relatives need skilled additional support throughout the period of their grief.

References

Baines M, Oliver DJ, Carter RL (1985) Medical management of intestinal obstruction in patients with advanced malignant disease. A clinical and pathological study. Lancet 2: 990–993

Editorial (1986) Terminal dehydration. Lancet 1: 306

Gralla RG (1983) Metoclopramide: a review of antiemetic trials. Drugs 25: 63–73

Hanks GW, Trueman T, Twycross RG (1983) Corticosteroids in terminal cancer – a prospective analysis of current practice. Postgrad Med J 59: 702–706

Kubler-Ross E (1970) On death and dying. Tavistock, London

Mount BM (1980) Hospice care. J Roy Soc Med 73: 471–473

National Hospice Organization (1981) Standards of a hospice program of care. 1901 Northfort Myer Drive, Suite 307, Arlington, Virginia 22209, USA

Parkes CM (1981) Evaluation of a bereavement service. Prev Psychol 1 (2): 179–188

Parkes CM, Weis RS (1983) Recovery from bereavement. Basic, New York

Peroutka SJ, Snyder SH (1982) Antiemetics. Neurotransmitter receptor binding predicts therapeutic action. Lancet 1: 658–659

Stedeford A (1978) Understanding confusional states. Br J Hosp Med 20: 694–704

Stedeford A (1984) Facing death: patients, families and professionals. Heinemann, London

Thompson I (1984) Ethical issues in palliative care. In: Doyle D (ed) Palliative care. The management of far-advanced illness. Croon Helm, London/Charles Press, Philadelphia, pp 461–485

Twycross RG, Lack SA (1983) Symptom control in far-advanced cancer: pain relief. Pitmans, London

Twycross RG, Lack SA (1986) Symptom control in far-advanced cancer: alimentary symptoms. Churchill Livingstone, Edinburgh

Weisman AD (1979) Coping with cancer. McGraw-Hill, New York

Emergencies in Cancer Disease

Increased Intracranial Pressure and Spinal Cord Compression

E.-O. Backlund

Introduction

The primary aim of this chapter is to familiarize the reader with the diagnostic and, above all, therapeutic implications for a patient with cancer, who presents with symptoms indicating CNS involvement of the malignant disease, often unexpectedly. The current opinion concerning indications for surgery will be described comprehensively, from the author's personal perspective but also as it is mirrored in relevant reviews from the current neurosurgical literature on metastasis to the brain (Burger and Vogel 1976; Posner and Shapiro 1976; French and Ausman 1977; Whitehouse and Kay 1979; Gamache et al. 1982; Black 1982) and to the spine (Barcena et al. 1984; Murray 1985; Overby and Rothman 1985; Siegal and Siegal 1985; Harrington 1986; Sherman and Waddell 1986; Sundaresan et al. 1986).

Brain Metastasis

Origin and Incidence

Secondary growths from malignant tumors originating outside the CNS are the cause of approximately 20% of brain neoplasias found at autopsy. On the other hand, in neurosurgical series of operated intracranial tumors, including benign forms, metastases constitute only about 4%.

Brain metastases are found in approximately 20% of patients dying from cancer most often as multiple lesions, a solitary metastasis being demonstrated in only about one case out of three. In neurosurgical practice, however, there is a common tendency to describe secondary malignancy in the brain in terms of solitary growth, which thus does not reflect the truth. This can be explained by the clinical selection made when cancer patients are referred for brain surgery, and only solitary metastases are considered suitable for removal.

Furthermore, metastatic meningeal carcinomatosis is a less frequent variant but not quite as rare as was previously thought.

Brain metastases originate from:

Lung (bronchial) carcinoma	in approximately 25%–35%
Mammary carcinoma	in approximately 20%
Malignant melanoma	in approximately 10%
Hypernephroma	in approximately 5%–10%
Gastrointestinal carcinoma	in approximately 5%

Of these primaries, the melanomas are most prone to metastasize to the brain (in 50%–90% of cases), the bronchial carcinomas less so (in 25%–40% of cases), whereas the mammary cancers are thought to seed to the brain in 15%–20% of cases.

Brain metastases from other tumors than primary lung cancer may constitute tertiary or even quarternary spread, but with the lung as the site of growth immediately proximal to the brain (Fig. 1). As brain metastases are considered blood-borne via the arterial supply, it is not surprising that their direct site of origin is the lung. The path is short from the pulmonary veins to the arterial system, thus facilitating abundant spread of neoplastic cells to the brain.

In consequence in the brain, metastases are most often found in the area supplied by the arteria cerebri media, often considered the "main stream" of the intracerebral arterial circulation. Interestingly, the cerebellum, although of a much smaller volume than the cerebrum, is nevertheless a fairly frequent site for metastases, quite out of proportion to its volume.

Symptomatology

The intracranial dynamics and thus the clinical symptoms of a brain metastasis do not differ from those of any malignant intracerebral tumor or other rapidly expanding lesion, for instance an abscess. Classically, such symptoms are divided into two categories: general symptoms due to raised intracranial pressure and focal symptoms caused by local destruction/irritation of certain specific brain areas.

Symptoms Due To Raised Intracranial Pressure

The most common pressure symptom is headache of progressive character. Typically, it is most pronounced in the mornings and not infrequently combined with nausea and sometimes vomiting. Blurred vision, diplopia, and other visual symptoms may be components in what is called "false localizing signs", a classic in this context. When the intracranial pressure becomes significantly elevated, the alertness of the patient is affected and a scale of indolence-drowsiness-sopor-coma correlates well with progressively increasing pressure. Thus, the most important parameter in the assessment of a patient with an intracranial expanding lesion is the level of consciousness. Any deviation from normal is a cause for alarm.

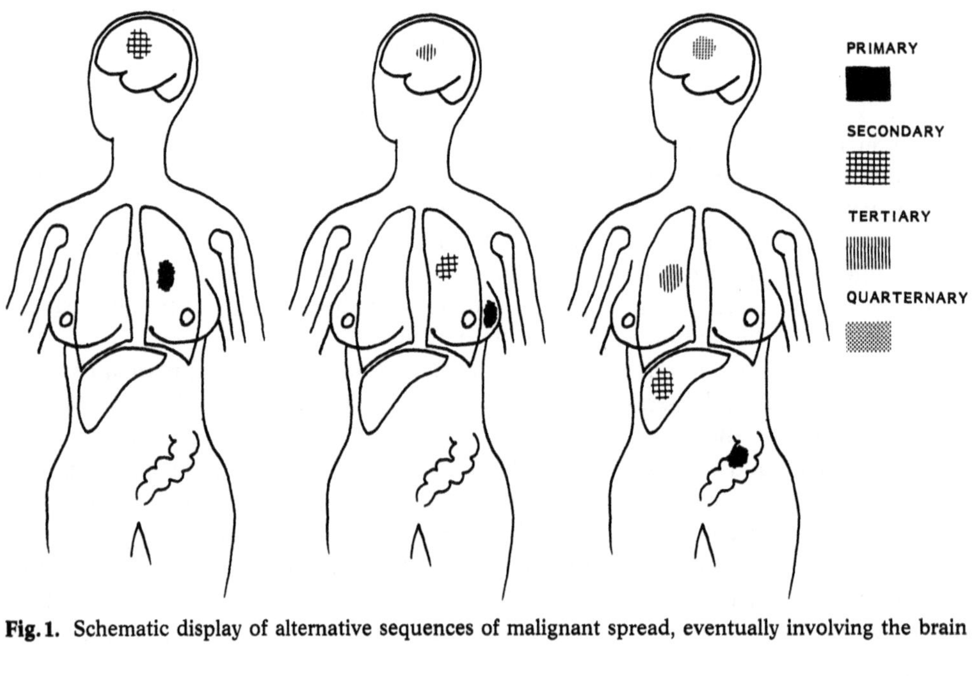

Fig. 1. Schematic display of alternative sequences of malignant spread, eventually involving the brain

The intracranial dynamics, mirrored in the clinical state of the patient, may be dramatic. The history of CNS involvement of a cancer most often is subacute or even acute and, in practice, the patient is often referred/admitted as an emergency. Under these conditions, urgent consultation with a neurosurgeon is mandatory, unless the situation is considered hopeless *a priori.*

Focal Symptoms

The so-called focal symptoms are related to the area of the brain which is involved in the local growth/expansion of the tumor. They may thus vary considerably but, when present, often indicate the location of the tumor. Typical examples are speech disturbances where the tumor influences the speech area, visual field defects when the tumor encroaches upon the calcarine area or the depth of the temporal lobe, hemiparesis concomitant upon central region involvement, etc. The focal symptoms are not always of "lesional", destructive character since epileptic manifestations may occur, in particular if the tumor (even a very small one) is located in the cortex.

Radiological Diagnosis

When secondaries in the brain are suspected clinically, the occurrence is commonly and best verified by computed tomography (CT). The tumor(s) is (are) as a role clearly seen on CT, particularly following intravenous contrast. CT is of further value for the detection of spread to the CSF pathways, indicated by dilatation of the ventricular system. Thus, even if the brain parenchyma on CT seems to be free from tumor growth, a widened ventricular system might indicate meningeal carcinomatosis.

Peritumoral Edema

An extensive edema surrounding the lesion is a constant feature in cerebral metastases. Even a small, solitary tumor may be surrounded by a formidable edematous zone. This makes any patient with secondaries in the brain an appropriate candidate for treatment with i.m. steroids (dexamethasone 4 mg × 4 daily) and/or i.v. mannitol (1.5–2.0 g/kg body weight/30–60 min), the latter as a temporary emergency treatment. A patient with impaired consciousness or other signs of raised intracranial pressure improves dramatically after such dehydration therapy, which often should be the first choice.

Surgical Treatment

The current opinion is that a *solitary* metastatic lesion in the brain should be removed whenever surgically accessible. Extirpation then must be radical. To neglect surgery most often is a terrible alternative, leaving the patient to a cruel death, caused by the gradually increasing intracranial pressure. This decision has to be the outcome when multiple brain metastases are found on CT.

Even after successful removal of a solitary metastasis, the patient's survival is limited, with an average of less than 1 year – only one case out of four survives 1 year or more. But the cause of death is then more often a general spread of the malignancy than local recurrence of the brain tumor. Nonetheless, rare instances of real long-term survival, even after spread to the brain, have surprisingly been documented in many clinical series.

Recently, systematic attempts have been made to analyze the surgical decision-making in cases of brain metastasis. The use of "risk profiles", obtained empirically, seems to be a valuable aid when the optimal answer is sought to the crucial question: surgery or not? (Pelletieri et al. 1987). In addition, the following questions should always be assessed before surgery is decided:

- Is the tumor really solitary?
- Could the lesion be another type of intracranial tumor, requiring a stereotactic biopsy as the first step?
- Is the tumor surgically accessible at reasonable cost, i.e., no risk of new neurological deficits postoperatively?
- Will removal of the tumor relieve the patient from his/her dominant current problem, for instance intractable seizures?
- With regard to the general situation of the patient, the prognosis of the primary cancer and the patient's own opinion are factors of great importance. With this in mind, is it reasonable to suggest major brain surgery in addition to the total suffering of the patient? Will the operation significantly improve the quality of his/her remaining life?

The removal of a single intracerebral metastasis is a relatively simple procedure as a rule, provided that the tumor is easily found. The main technical surgical problem is in fact most often confined to the localization of the lesion, something of a classical frustration to neurosurgeons dealing with intracranial metastases. The most illusive region is the parieto-occipital area. The surgeon must always scrutinize the preoperative films and plan the approach prudently. The use of preoperatively implanted guides, in connection with a diagnostic stereotactic biopsy, eliminates these problems, allowing a straight and safe direct approach to the metastatic lesion. This is a routine which could be better appreciated than is currently the case (Backlund 1987).

Operative Findings

A brain metastasis is often found in the white matter, adjacent to gray matter areas, be it either the basal ganglia or the cortex. Macroscopically, it may be fairly small, its significance as an expanding lesion being due to the often extensive peritumoral edema. The gross appearance of the tumor during surgery most often differs markedly from the surrounding brain and a real cleavage toward the brain parenchyma is more or less the rule. The tumor may be found either very soft, sometimes almost liquid, or more tough and substantial than the brain tissue. A central necrosis is not an uncommon finding, sometimes giving the lesion the appearance of an abscess. Melanotic metastases may have a very dark color and are often hemorrhagic. Occasionally, metastases may have the gross appearance of malignant gliomas, when even an experienced neurosurgeon may have difficulty assessing the true character of the tumor during exploration.

Additional Therapy

If surgery has been the treatment of primary choice, radiotherapy should be given in addition (Egawa et al. 1986). Cytostatic agents seem to be less effective for metastasis in the brain parenchyma, but are worth trying, combined with irradiation, especially when meningeal carcinomatosis is suspected or verified.

Spinal Cord Compression

Pathogenetic Factors

When cancer metastasizes to the skeleton, the vertebral column is the site of predilection, most commonly in the thoracic region. It is wellknown that most patients dying from cancer are seen to have malignant spread to more than one vertebra. Mammary and prostate carcinoma are common primaries, each having its predilection site in the spine, in the thoracic and lumbosacral regions, respectively.

The intimate relationship between the vertebral column and the spinal cord makes any vertebral tumor a potential threat to the medulla. The CNS can be affected in essentially one or both of two ways:

1. The tumor reduces the mechanical strength of a vertebral body, and can give rise to a reduced stability of the vertebral column following a pathological (compression) fracture. Further complications are then spinal dislocation and strain upon the medulla, in its most extreme form with a local gibbus formation.
2. The tumor tissue can penetrate the posterior longitudinal ligament at the level of the vertebral body, where the ligament is thin, in contrast to what is found at the disk level. The extradural and possibly paravertebral compartments then become occupied by tumor, progressively impinging on the spinal cord. In addition, malignant invasion of the pedicles may result in the narrowing of the root canal and bone debris formation, further encroaching upon the nervous structures. Remarkably, however, malignant growth in the spinal dura occurs very seldom, if ever.

Symptomatology

A common and early symptom from a vertebral metastasis is back pain, local, severe and continuous, and easy to provoke by percussion. In addition, segmental, radicular pain may be present, either in a belt distribution around the thorax or simulating sciatica. A common pattern is that the patient is kept awake at night by the pain, but can tolerate it better during the day. After a sometimes fairly long period of gradually increasing back pain, weakness appears in the lower extremities, often rapidly and with a short, progressive course. Such a dramatic history indicates a poor prognosis, even if maximal therapeutic measures are undertaken urgently. On the other hand, if the motor symptoms develop over a period of days or even weeks, ambitious treatment, including surgery, may result in a rather satisfactory period for the patient, sometimes with relief from paresis during the whole of the remaining life span.

From a neurosurgeon's point of view, it is disappointing to experience repeatedly the poor understanding of many collegues concerning these dynamics. Patients with short and dramatic histories are pointlessly referred as emergencies to neurosurgical departments, whereas slowly appearing weakness in the lower extremities of a cancer patient is only too often misunderstood or even neglected. Any physician responsible for patients with malignancies must develop a sensitivity for the sometimes subtle signals from a patient complaining of back pain and/or neurological symptoms from his/her feet or legs.

Impairment of sphincter functions most often is a late and hardly ever solitary symptom, indicating established and profound injury to the spinal cord/cauda equina. Sensory symptoms are even more unreliable as early diagnostic signals. They vary considerably in incidence and, particularly, in their distribution. Thus, a distinct level of sensory loss, found at examination, does not indicate with certainty the level of the pathological process.

Radiological Diagnosis

The most sensitive method of detecting vertebral metastases is bone scintigraphy. If surgical therapy is considered, however, the surgeon is not primarily interested in the distribution of occurring vertebral metastases but in the level of spinal cord compression. Thus, myelography with water-soluble contrast medium is the method of choice to obtain adequate preoperative information. In addition, it is recommendable to study the local anatomy by CT, utilizing the contrast medium left in the subarachnoidal space after myelography.

Surgical Treatment

A patient with slowly appearing neurological deficiencies in the lower part of his/her body is the typical candidate for surgery. As already mentioned, rapidly appearing and severe symptoms are a relative contraindication for surgery.

The primary aim of an operation is obvious: to eliminate the cord compression. Needless to say, an operation should also include as radical a removal of the tumor tissue as possible. Traditionally, the first of these aims has dominated the argumentation for surgery. Thus, only *decompressive* laminectomy has been the operation most often practiced.

For an effective decompression, even for a single or a few segments only, *at least* three laminae have to be removed. Any accessible tumor tissue in the extradural space should also be extirpated. Unfortunately, such tissue is most often located anterior to the spinal cord, a region which is difficult to reach via the posterior approach of a laminectomy, at least in the thoracic region.

These anatomical features and an increasing awareness of the relatively poor average results after laminectomy have directed attention to more radical and more logical surgical alternatives. Thus, a new therapeutic paradigm includes radical removal of affected vertebra(e) and subsequent fusion, using anterior or lateral approaches. A prominent advocate for this policy is Harrington (1986), whereas recently the value of laminectomy in selected cases has been emphasized by Sherman and Waddell (1986). The radical approach is quite different from laminectomy, concerning the risks and the load to the patient. For instance, when the thoracic spine is affected, thoracotomy may be necessary for removal of the tumor. The subsequent extensive reconstruction of the spine requires stabilizing rods, bone grafts, methylmetacrylate, etc. If radiotherapy is given in addition, the reconstructed area runs the risk of becoming a veritable *locus minoris resistentiae*, as callus formation and graft incorporation may be negatively influenced by the radiation. But, doubtlessly, the new and radical attitude is logical and, in essence, offers the patient a better chance of benefitting longer from the operation. And apart from surgical-technical decisions concerning choice of operative approach, the crucial factor for the patient's eventual fate is rather the alertness of the referring physician, who is responsible for observing any alarming symptoms in due time.

References

Backlund EO (1987) Stereotactic catheter insertion: a new technique. Neurol Res 9: 147–150

Barcena A, Lobato RD, Rivas JJ et al. (1984) Spinal metastatic disease: analysis of factors determining functional prognosis and the choice of treatment. Neurosurgery 15: 820–827

Black P (1982) Surgical management of intracranial metastasis. In: Schmidek HH, Sweet WH (eds) Operative neurosurgical techniques indications, methods, and results, vol 1. Grune and Stratton, New York, pp 433–446

Burger PC, Vogel FS (1976) Surgical pathology of the nervous system and its coverings. Wiley, New York

Egawa S, Tukiyama I, Akine Y (1986) Radiotherapy of brain metastases. Int J Radiat Oncol Biol Phys 12: 1621–1625

French LA, Ausman JI (1977) Metastatic neoplasms to the brain. In: Keener EB (ed) Clinical neurosurgery. Williams and Wilkins, Baltimore, pp 41–46

Gamache FW, Posner JB, Patterson RH (1982) Metastatic brain tumors. In: Youmans JR (ed) Neurological surgery, vol 5. Saunders, Philadelphia, pp 2872–2898

Harrington KD (1986) Metastatic disease of the spine. J Bone Joint Surg [Am] 68: 1110–1115

Murray PK (1985) Functional outcome and survival in spinal cord injury secondary to neoplasia. Cancer 55: 197–201

Overby MC, Rothman AS (1985) Anterolateral decompression for metastatic epidural spinal cord tumors. J Neurosurg 62: 344–348

Pelletieri L, Sjölander U, Jakobsson KE (1987) Prognostic evaluation before operative extirpation and radiotherapy of solitary brain metastasis. Acta Neurochir (Wien) 86: 6–11

Posner JB, Shapiro WR (1976) The management of intracranial metastases. In: Morley TP (ed) Current controversies in neurosurgery. Saunders, Philadelphia, pp 356–366

Sherman RMP, Waddell JP (1986) Laminectomy for metastatic epidural spinal cord tumors. Posterior stabilization, radiotherapy, and preoperative assessment. In: Urist MR (ed) Clinical orthopedics and related research, vol 207. Lippingcott, Philadelphia, pp 55–63

Siegal T, Siegal T (1985) Surgical decompression of anterior and posterior malignant tumors compressing the spinal cord: a prospective study. Neurosurgery 17: 424–432

Sundareasan N, Digiacinto GV, Hughes JEO (1986) Surgical treatment of spinal metastases. In: Little JR (ed) Clinical neurosurgery. Williams and Wilkins, Baltimore, pp 503–522

Whitehouse JMA, Kay HEM (eds) (1979) CNS complications of malignant disease. Macmillan, London

Vascular Emergencies

D. BERGQVIST and S.-E. BERGENTZ

This chapter will deal with vascular emergencies defined as vascular injuries, or diseases caused by a malignant process or its treatment, and requiring immediate care. The frequency of vascular emergencies thus defined is largely unknown. In the literature there is no systematic analysis of these problems.

Historically it may be of interest that the first report of a iatrogenic vascular injury with repair and survival was laceration of the axillary artery during removal of malignant lymph nodes (Heidenhain 1894 cited by Murphy 1897).

Local Effect of the Malignant Process

In rare cases the tumor may interfere with major arteries, causing *ischemia*. This ischemia can be due to tumor compression of the vessel (Jonsson et al. 1982) or to arterial thrombosis (Balas et al. 1981; Sharma et al. 1985). Osteogenic sarcoma is particularly known to grow invasively (van Way and Lawler 1969; Liggett and Kartchner 1979). Aortic occlusion by a thrombus composed of leukemic cells and fibrin has been described (Brinson and Garcia 1984). When an arterial or intracardiac tumor thrombus has developed, there is a prerequisite for arterial embolism (de Boer and Prillevitz 1969; Stanley and Eto 1978; Prioleau and Katzenstein 1978). The classical tumor in this respect is benign atrial myxoma (Kulkarni et al. 1969; Khan and Mujahed 1970). Endocardial metastases can give rise to large aortic saddle emboli. Another possibility for embolism is malignant invasion of the lung veins, and vein manipulation during pulmonary surgery may cause the embolization (Groth 1940; Balas et al. 1971).

The symptoms and signs of ischemia from malignancy do not differ from those seen when ischemia is caused by arteriosclerotic lesions. In patients with malignant disorders and without any other obvious cause for arterial thromboembolism it is therefore of value to send removed material for microscopic investigation. Ligation of pulmonary veins as the initial step in the resection of lung lobes with tumors seems to be recommendable.

Venous thromboembolism can be caused by direct venous invasion of the malignant process (Schechter 1985). The anatomical differences in venous drainage between the two kidneys must be considered, the right kidney largely lacking collateral venous outflow and therefore not tolerating a thrombotic occlusion.

One well-known complication of renal cancer is thrombotic occlusion of the suprarenal inferior vena cava. In a few of these cases removal of the suprarenal retrohepatic tumor and reconstruction of the vein may be of value, at least to relieve symptoms.

Hemorrhage because of erosion by the tumor is seen particularly when an infection is present. The risk of major bleeding is furthermore increased when radiation therapy has been given. Primary aortoenteric fistula, most commonly caused by aortic aneurysms, may, on rare occasions, be caused by a malignant process (Graphery et al. 1966; Geary and Walworth 1976). Kefford et al. (1981) reported that bleeding was responsible for death in 15% of the patients dying in an oncological department, 27% of these being caused by rupture of major vessels. The erosion most often involves intrapelvic or groin vessels in patients with gynecological cancer. Figge and Gaudenz (1974) reported rupture of the femoral artery in as many as 3.4% of patients with carcinoma of the vulva. The therapy is often difficult and even acute hemipelvectomy has been recommended (Malawer and Zielinski 1983). A therapeutic alternative, well known among vascular surgeons, is some form of extra-anatomical reconstruction after exclusion of the eroded vessel segment. In cases of groin vessel hemorrhage the bypass should be passed through the obturator foramen. After radical vulvectomy and groin lymph adenectomy, arterial coverage is very important, and sartorius muscle mobilization and transposition over the femoral triangle should be considered.

One very special form of local vascular engagement is the development of *arteriovenous fistulas* within some tumors, the best known being renal carcinoma (Hamilton et al. 1953; Vetto et al. 1966; Rodgers et al. 1975). In rare cases these shunts become large, giving rise to cardiac failure. Metastases from such tumors have the same inherent capacity to induce the formation of arteriovenous fistulas (Caplan et al. 1961, Howlett and Caranasos 1970). Development of renal arteriovenous fistula secondary to metastatic bronchiolar carcinoma has also been reported (Stevens et al. 1974).

Superior Vena Cava Syndrome

This syndrome is due to compression of the superior vena cava. It was first reported in 1757 in a patient with syphilitic aortic aneurysm compressing the vein (William Hunter), and in fact such aneurysms together with tuberculous mediastinitis were the most frequent causes until 1940–1950. Thereafter malignant tumors have become by far the most common etiological factor (in 97% of cases according to Rainey 1982). The most common tumors responsible are different types of lymphomas and mediastinal metastases from lung and breast cancer.

The symptoms develop acutely-subacutely with shortness of breath, head and neck edema and flush, conjunctival edema, and dilated neck veins. The diagnosis is confirmed with plain X-ray of the thorax, venography, computed tomography, and mediastinoscopy.

There is often need for acute therapy, the best being radiation. The success rate in relieving the patient's symptoms is around 75% within 3–4 days and 90% within 1 week depending on the radiosensitivity of the tumor (Davenport et al. 1978). A similar effect has been obtained with combination chemotherapy (Dombernowsky and Hansen 1978). Failure of radiotherapy may indicate invasion of the vena cava and surgery must be considered. Different types of venous bypass have been suggested but the success rate is low (Carabell and Goodman 1982).

The mean survival time in patients with superior vena cava obstruction is short; Davenport et al. (1978) reports only 20% survival after 1 year.

Thromboembolic Complications Because of Systemic Effects of the Tumor

The association between venous thrombosis/superficial thrombophlebitis and malignancy in the form of pancreatic cancer was first described by Armand Trousseau in 1865. Ironically he himself developed thrombosis and 1 year later died of gastric cancer. It is well known that malignancy is a risk factor in patients with so-called spontaneous thrombosis (Sproul 1938; Minar et al. 1982), and it is also a risk factor for the development of postoperative thromboembolic complications (for review see Bergqvist 1983). There are several changes of the hemostatic system, which can explain why patients with malignant diseases are prone to develop thromboembolic complications (for review see Bick 1978; Hasegawa and Bloomfield 1981; Peuscher 1981, Rickler and Edwards 1983). Neoplasms frequently produce and release proteolytic enzymes and thromboplastin-like material, which may also bypass several steps of the coagulation cascade, for instance by direct activation of factor X. In cases with paraneoplastic vasculitis, antigen-antibody reactions may also be involved (Fauci et al. 1978).

There are some characteristics of thrombosis which should lead to suspicion of an underlying malignancy:

- Recurrence, also with adequate therapy
- Multiple thrombi
- Atypical localization
- Venous phlegmasia or gangrene
- Migrating superficial thrombophlebitis
- Difficulty in handling anticoagulation therapy

When migrating thrombophlebitis is a paramalignant phenomenon, the majority of patients already have metastases (Sack et al. 1977). Patients presenting with superficial thrombophlebitis without having varicose veins often have a synchronous deep vein thrombosis, and they run a greater risk of developing a malignant disease within 5 years than patients with a superficial thrombophlebitis in varicose veins (Bergqvist and Jaroszewski 1986).

Patients operated on for malignant diseases must receive prophylaxis against postoperative thromboembolism. Methods effective in preventing fatal pulmonary embolism are oral anticoagulants, low-dose heparin with or without dihydroergotamine, and dextran (see Bergqvist 1987). Initial treatment of established deep vein thrombosis does not differ from that used in nonmalignant patients with thrombosis. When the prognosis of the malignant disease makes the life expectancy less than around 5 years long-term treatment with oral anticoagulants (exceeding 2 months) is of little use. These patients will never develop a postthrombotic syndrome. However, in patients with recurrent thromboembolism long-term antithrombotic treatment may be necessary.

Vascular Lesions from Radiation

As early as 1899 Gassman described microscopic vascular changes in radiodermatitis. Several experimental studies confirmed his findings. In 1959 Thomas and Forbus reported the first case of radiation damage of a large artery. The important etiological prerequisite seems to be an injury to the vasa vasorum and as a consequence larger vessels develop sclerosis and atheromatous-like changes. There is experimental and clinical evidence of a synergistic effect of hypercholesterolemia and radiation causing arterial damage (Amromin et al. 1964; Silverberg et al. 1978). Radiation causes a diminished plasminogen activator activity in endothelial cells (Åstedt et al. 1974). However, the vast majority of patients given radiation do not seem to develop arterial obstruction. So far there is no explanation for the individual variation in sensitivity. Among patients operated on for arterial disease, radiation injury is seldom the cause (Bergqvist et al. 1987). The lesions in the radiated artery may cause three types of diseases: ischemia, aneurysm, and rupture.

Ischemia is caused by an occlusive process which is known from several anatomical localizations: pelvic vessels, carotid and coronary arteries, and axillary arteries. With regard to time after radiation, there may be three types of injury:

1. Intimal damage with thrombosis within months to a few years
2. Development of vessel wall fibrosis and occlusion within about 10 years
3. Predisposition to atherosclerotic lesions, which is a long-term process

There are some characteristics which support the concept of a radiation injury:

1. The disease is limited to the radiation field.
2. The patients are younger than arteriosclerotic patients.
3. The localization is atypical.
4. There are radiation injuries to other nearby tissues, such as skin, bowel, bladder, and thyroid.

The symptoms are due to ischemia caused by the vascular lesion. Microembolization may occur. The treatment is conventional. In cases of short stenoses, percutaneous transluminal angioplasty should be considered. As the tissue around radiation-damaged vessels is often very firm and fibrous, extraanatomical reconstructions can sometimes be recommended.

Aneurysm is a rare but reported complication (Ross and Sales 1972).

Rupture after erosion of the vessel is a serious but infrequent complication. In many cases it has not been possible to isolate radiation, surgery, tumor growth, and infection as risk factors for rupture (Marcial-Rojas 1962; Fajardo-Lee 1975; McCready et al. 1983). The prognosis *quod vitam* is poor. Because of the frequent infectious component, extraanatomical reconstructions should be preferred. Radiation is a rare cause of secondary aortoenteric fistulas (Estrada et al. 1983; Bergqvist 1987b).

Iatrogenic Injury

At Operation

The frequency of iatrogenic injuries at surgery because of malignant disease is not known. In a survey among gynecological surgeons in Sweden, the frequency was 0.77/10 000 of all gynecological laparotomies, also for benign diseases (Bergqvist and Bergqvist 1987). With an increasing requirement for surgical radicality the risk of vessel injuries increases. The injury can occur in two types of tissue:

1. When the malignant tumor grows invasively into vessels.
2. In radiation-induced tissue fibrosis where there is no clear cleavage plane between the vessel adventitia and the surrounding tissue.

Principally these vessel injuries do not differ from other types of iatrogenic vascular injuries occurring during surgery. The dominating symptom is hemorrhage and there is, therefore, a need for an acute solution to the problem. Before clamping and ligation the injured vessels must be anatomically defined. When major vessels with poor collateral potential are injured, reconstruction must be aimed at. Repair with autogenous tissue is preferred.

At Intravascular Therapy

Intravenous cytostatic therapy often induces thrombophlebitis when given in peripheral veins. Administration of such drugs in a central vein is therefore preferable. A recent advance is the introduction of implantable devices for prolonged central venous infusion and injecton.

At *intraarterial* therapy via arterial catheters three types of complications can develop, all well-known side effects of angiography:

1. Thrombosis at the puncture site causing occlusion and ischemia
2. Distal embolization
3. Hemorrhage after extraction of the catheter. This can be a special problem in patients with malignant diseases, where the process itself, or treatment with radiation or cytostatics, may induce a thrombocytopenia

Lymphedema with Lymphangitis and Erysipelas

In patients with secondary lymphedema, which can be caused by the tumor itself, by surgical removal of lymph nodes, or by radiation, there is a pathophysiological prerequisite for the development of acute infection in the form of erysipelas, which may spread as lymphangitis. The incidence of lymphedema after breast cancer surgery varies from 10% to 60% (Mozes et al. 1982; Brismar and Ljungdahl 1983), but the incidence of infection is unknown. However, lymphedema predisposes to development of late cellulitis. In immunosuppressed patients the possibility of rare pathogenic organisms must be remembered (Lee et al. 1982).

References

Amromin GD, Gildenhorn HL, Solomon RD, Nadkarni BB, Jacobs ML (1964) The synergism of X-irradiation and cholesterol-fat feeding on the development of coronary artery lesions. J Atheroscler Res 4: 325–334

Åstedt B, Bergentz SE, Svanberg L (1974) Effect of irradiation on the plasminogen activator content in rat vessels. Experientia 30: 1466–1467

Balas P, Katsaras E, Zoitopoulos M (1971) Peripheral arterial embolism by malignant tumour. Vasc Surg 5: 27–29

Balas P, Delikaris P, Mizalis A, Papacharalampous N (1981) Recurrent aortic occlusion due to malignancy. J Cardiovasc Surg 22: 345–348

Bergqvist D (1983) Postoperative thromboembolism. Frequency, etiology, prophylaxis. Springer, Berlin Heidelberg New York

Bergqvist D (1987) Prophylaxis of postoperative venous thromboembolism. In: Nyhus L (ed) Surgery annual 19: 1–22

Bergqvist D (1987b) Arterioenteric fistula. Review of a vascular emergency. Acta Chir Scand 153: 81–86

Bergqvist D, Bergqvist A (1987) Vascular injuries during gynaecologic surgery. Acta Obstet Gynecol Scand 66: 19–23

Bergqvist D, Jaroszewski H (1986) Deep vein thrombosis in patients with superficial vein thrombophlebitis in the lower extremities. Br Med J 292: 658–659

Bergqvist D, Jonsson K, Nilsson M, Takolander R (1987) Treatment of arterial lesions after radiation therapy. Surg Gynecol Obstet 165: 116–120

Bick RL (1978) Alterations of hemostasis associated with malignancy: etiology, pathophysiology, diagnosis and management. Semin Thromb Haemost 5: 1–26

Brinson RR, Garcia GJ (1984) Acute lymphoblastic leukemia manifested as aortic occlusion. Am J Med 77: 385–387

Brismar B, Ljungdahl I (1983) Postoperative lymphoedema after treatment of breast cancer. Acta Chir Scand 149: 687–689

Caplan H, Sparkes R, Lemay M, Mahony D (1961) Arteriove-

nous shunt produced by metastatic hypernephroma. JAMA 177: 788–790
Carabell SC, Goodman RL (1982) Superior vena caval syndrome. In: DeVita VT, Hellman S, Rosenberg SA (eds) Cancer. Principles and practice of oncology. Lippincott, Philadelphia, pp 1582–1627
Davenport D, Ferree C, Blake D, Raben M (1978) Radiation therapy in the treatment of superior vena caval obstruction. Cancer 42: 2600–2603
De Boer HHM, Prillevitz HW (1969) Massive tumour embolism. Arch Chir Neerl 21: 223–234
Dombernowsky P, Hansen H (1978) Combination chemotherapy in the management of superior vena caval obstruction in small-cell anaplastic carcinoma of the lung. Acta Med Scand 204: 513–516
Estrada F, Tachovsky T, Orr R, Boylan J, Kram B (1983) Primary aortoduodenal fistula following radiotherapy. Surg Gynecol Obstet 156: 646–650
Fajardo LF, Lee A (1975) Rupture of major vessels after radiation. Cancer 36: 904–913
Fauci AS, Haynes BF, Katz P (1978) The spectrum of vasculitis: clinical, pathologic, immunologic and therapeutic considerations. Ann Intern Med 89: 660–676
Figge DC, Gaudenz R (1974) Invasive carcinoma of the vulva. Am J Obstet Gynecol 119: 382–395
Geary SR, Walworth EZ (1976) Aortoduodenal fistula secondary to metastatic carcinoma. Angiographic demonstration. JAMA 235: 2520–2521
Graphery A, Gupta R, Currie R (1966) Carcinoma of the head of the pancreas with aortoduodenal fistula. Am J Surg 111: 580–583
Groth KE (1940) Tumor embolism of the common femoral artery treated by embolectomy and heparin. Surgery 8: 617–632
Hamilton G, Getz R, Jerome S (1953) Arteriovenous fistula of the renal vessels: case report and review of the literature. J Urol 69: 203–207
Hasegawa DK, Bloomfield CD (1981) Thrombotic and hemorrhagic manifestations of malignancy. In: Yarbro JW, Bornstein RS (eds) Oncologic emergencies. Grune and Stratton, New York pp 141–196
Howlett S, Caranasos G (1970) Metastatic renal cell carcinoma producing arteriovenous shunt. Arch Intern Med 125: 493–495
Jonsson K, Wattsgård C, Genell S (1982) Malignant occlusion of the coeliac axis. Acta Radiol Diagn 23: 123–125
Kearney GP, Waters WB, Klein LA, Richie JP, Gittes RF (1981) Results of inferior vena cava resection for renal cell carcinoma. J Urol 125: 769–773
Kefford RF, Cooney NJ, Woods RL, Fox RM, Tattersall MHN (1981) Causes of deaths in an oncology unit. Eur J Cancer Clin Oncol 17: 1117–1124
Khan MAR, Mujahed MA (1970) Atrial myxoma producing a saddle embolus in a child. Thorax 25: 634–636
Kulkarni M, Jessiman I, French S (1969) Entire left atrial myxoma presenting as a saddle embolus. Thorax 24: 629–631
Lee WY, Corder MP, Platz CE (1982) An unusual manifestation of cryptococcal infection in a chronic lymphedematous arm. Med Pediatr Oncol 10: 397–400
Liggett C, Kartchner M (1979) Peripheral arterial tumor embolism by malignant tumor. Western J Med 130: 72–75
Malawer MM, Zielinski CJ (1983) Emergency hemipelvectomy in the control of life-threatening complications. Surgery 93: 778–785
Marcial-Rojas RA, Castro JR (1962) Irradiation injury to elastic arteries in the course of treatment for neoplastic disease. Ann Otol Rhinol Laryngol 71: 945–958
McCready, Hyde GL, Bivins BA, Mattingly SS, Griffen WO (1983) Radiation-induced arterial injuries. Surgery 93: 306–312
Minar E, Ehringer H, Marosi L, Hirschl M, Konecny U, Pollak Ch, Czembirek H, Sommer G (1982) Akute Venenthrombose. Lokalisation, Ausdehnung und Ätiologie mit besonderer Berücksichtigung der Paraneoplasie. Dtsch Med Wochenschr 107: 1303–1309
Mozes M, Papa MZ, Karasik A, Reshef A, Adar R (1982) The role of infection in post-mastectomy lymphedema. Surg Annu 14: 73–83
Murphy JB (1897) Resection of arteries and veins injured in continuity – end-to-end suture – experimental and clinical research. Med Rec 51: 73–88
Peuscher FW (1981) Thrombosis and bleeding in cancer patients. A review. Neth J Med 24: 23–35
Prioleau HG, Katzenstein AL (1978) Major peripheral arterial occlusion due to malignant tumor embolism. Cancer 42: 2009–2014
Rainey JM (1982) Oncologic emergencies. J LA State Med Soc 134: 15–20
Rickles FR, Edwards RL (1983) Activation of blood coagulation in cancer: Trousseau's syndrome revisited. Blood 62: 14–31
Rodgers M, Moss A, Hoffman M, Lipchik E (1975) Arteriovenous fistulae secondary to renal cell carcinoma. Clinical and cardiovascular manifestations: report of a case. Circulation 52: 345–350
Ross HB, Sales JEL (1972) Post-irradiation femoral aneurysm treated by iliopopliteal by-pass via the obturator foramen. Br J Surg 59: 400–405
Sack GH, Levin J, Bell WR (1977) Trousseau's syndrome and other manifestations of chronic disseminated coagulopathy in patients with neoplasms: clinical, pathophysiologic, and therapeutic features. Medicine 56: 1–37
Schechter DC (1985) Cardiovascular surgery in the management of exogenous tumors involving the vena cava. In: Bergan J, Yao J (eds) Surgery of the veins. Grune and Stratton, New York
Sharma PVP, Babu SC, Shah PM, Seirafi R, Clauss RH (1985) Arterial thrombosis and embolism in malignancy. J Cardiovasc Surg 26: 479–483
Silverberg GD, Britt RH, Goffinet DR (1978) Radiation-induced carotid artery disease. Cancer 41: 130–137
Sproul E (1938) Carcinoma and venous thrombosis: the frequency of association of carcinoma in the body on tail of the pancreas with multiple venous thrombosis. Am J Cancer 34: 566
Stanley P, Eto RT (1978) Arterial embolization of malignant tumor: report of two cases with angiographic findings. Radiology 126: 93–94
Stevens P, Lucas B, Glenn J (1974) Renal arteriovenous fistula secondary to metastatic tumor. Urology 3: 624–627
Thomas E, Forbus WD (1959) Irradiation injury to the aorta and the lung. Arch Pathol 67: 256–263
Trousseau A (1865) Phlegmatia alba dolens. Clin Med Hôtel-Dieu, Paris, 1865: 695–727
van Way CW, Lawler MR (1969) Osteogenic sarcomatous emboli to the femoral arteries. Am J Surg 117: 745–747
Vetto M, Bigelow J, Dueger W (1966) Arteriovenous fistula in pulsatile metastatic carcinoma. Report of chronic heart failure relieved by resection. Am Surg 32: 557–560

Metabolic Disorders

K. LUNDHOLM

An adequate understanding of the mechanisms behind the development of cachexia and metabolic disorders is important when considering the therapeutic and palliative treatments of cancer. Metabolic disorders in cancer disease are a composite of changes due to tumor invasion, obstruction, metastatic growth, loss of appetite, tumor cell metabolism, and activation of the immune system including cell proliferation. An important issue to consider is whether paraneoplastic changes in cancer disease represent a unique set of metabolic problems or whether such changes occur secondary to partial starvation and inflammatory reactions.

Figure 1 summarizes our present view of inducer and effector alterations in a cancer-bearing host. A malignant tumor may induce physiological changes by two different mechanisms: ectopic hormone production or presentation of unusual or unique antigens to the immune system. Ectopic hormone production is well recognized and the importance of this is probably underestimated in many patients. Such hormones may be true hormones synthesized in nonendocrine cells or hormone-like proteins with amino acid sequence homology to classic hormones. Antigen-antibody complexes may result from newly expressed plasma-membrane antigens on proliferating transformed cells or may be normal intracellular antigens that are exposed to the immune system during proliferation due to cell lysis in the tumor. Such a cell lysis may be due to specific immune cytolysis or to anoxic conditions secondary to insufficient neoangiogenesis in rapidly growing tumors. Irrespective of the underlying mechanism, antigens may elicit an acute-phase response, characterized by increased hepatic synthesis of plasma proteins, nonhepatic synthesis of immune proteins, such as monokines and lymphokines, trace metal redistribution, fever, and anorexia. The synthesis of specific and nonspecific immune proteins may then serve both to attenuate the afferent stimuli on the immune system and to prevent rapid tumor dissemination. One example of non-specific acute-phase proteins may be the synthe-

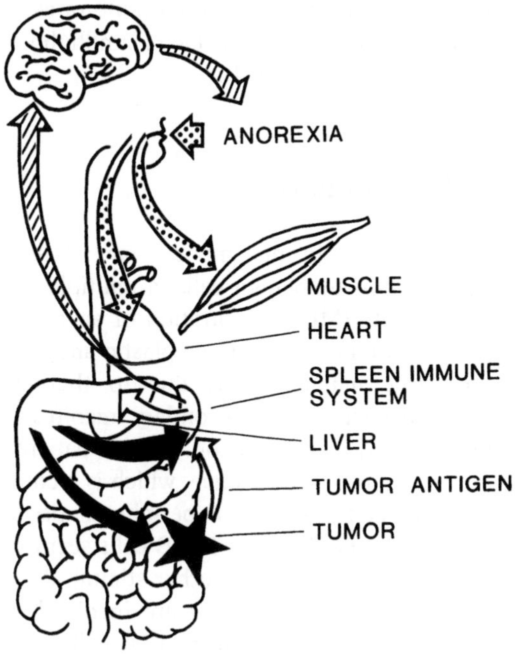

Fig. 1. Hypothetic metabolic interplay between a malignant tumor and the host. The tumor is recognized by the immune system, possibly by "tumor antigens". Immune mediators such as monokines and lymphokines are released from immune cells. The mediators elicit anorexia and an acute-phase response including the synthesis of specific and nonspecific proteins. Such proteins may modulate or attenuate the afferent signals of the immune system as well as decreasing tumor growth. Metabolic adaptation, such as is associated with negative protein balance, occurs in skeletal muscles and in the heart

sis of protease inhibitors by the liver. Other examples may be opsonins for the immune system, such as C-reactive protein.

It is currently our hypothesis that immune-associated or -derived proteins may contribute to, or elicit, the well-recognized anorexia in cancer disease. If these agents are responsible for reduced food intake in cancer, such mechanisms may also be contributory in other conditions associated with anorexia such as bacterial infections and viremia. The anorexia may then induce secondary changes in the protein metabolism of skeletal muscles, the heart, the gastrointestinal tract, and the endocrine glands, which all lead to well-recognized homeostatic disturbances (Lundholm 1985a; Lundholm 1985b). The following is a brief description of the most important metabolic alterations observed in response to growth of malignant tumors.

Anorexia

The mechanism(s) behind anorexia in cancer disease is unknown. It is likely that altered regulation of appetite is dependent upon alterations in both peripheral tissues and the CNS. It has been suggested that alterations in serotonergic neuron transmitter activity correlate with the degree of anorexia (von Meyenfeldt and Soeters 1985). Other transmitters may also be involved, although this has not been examined as closely as for serotonin. At present, however, it may be questioned to what extent neural transmitter changes are primary or secondary to malnutrition only. Acute changes in appetite during infections may be explained by other mechanisms, distinct from neurotransmitter alterations. Preliminary experiments from our and other laboratories have indicated that macrophage-derived substances, such as interleukin-1, tumor necrosis factor (TNF), and other as yet undefined material, may be potent and physiological inhibitors of appetite (McCarthy et al. 1985). Future research will clarify the importance and the relevance of such observations.

Energy Homeostasis

Loss of appetite explains a major part of the negative energy balance in cancer patients, although increased energy expenditure contributes significantly and may explain several kilos of body weight loss per month (Lundholm et al. 1982a, b; Lindmark et al. 1984). The mechanism(s) behind elevated energy expenditure is still unclear. Contributing factors may include activation of the immune system, accelerated gluconeogenesis, muscle dysfunction, or elevated adrenergic activity concomitant with increased sensitivity at the cellular level to adrenergic agonists. However, the thermic effect of food does not seem to be elevated in cancer patients. Therefore, weight loss in cancer patients is most likely explained by a less than normal adaptation to starvation rather than an abnormal dietary-induced thermogenesis.

Results regarding the alterations in intermediary metabolism during cancer may be summarized as follows: cancer growth is associated with increased turnover of plasma glucose (Lundholm et al. 1982b) and glycerol (Edén et al. 1985); the turnover of free fatty acids is probably increased, although this has not been directly assessed; and lipids are preferential substrate for oxidation (Lindmark et al. 1984). Increased whole body glucose turnover is due to increased lactate cycling (Cori cycle activity) while the intrahepatic cycling of glucose seems to be decreased. We have estimated that elevated glucose and protein turnover account for the major part of the increased energy expenditure in cancer patients (Edén et al. 1984).

Protein Metabolism

Elevated whole body protein turnover in cancer patients is a composite of depressed muscle protein synthesis and increased hepatic protein synthesis (Lundholm et al. 1981; Ternell et al. 1985). Increased synthesis in immune cells and macrophages is likely to occur but has not yet been systematically evaluated. Increased hepatic protein synthesis in itself is a composite of both increased and decreased synthesis of various proteins. It is likely that most of the proteins with increased synthesis represent acute-phase reactants.

In contrast muscle protein synthesis is depressed in tumor disease. Muscle wasting affects both myofibrillar and sarcoplasmic proteins. Although depressed food intake can explain quantitatively the reduced synthesis, the underlying mechanisms are not understood. It is likely that changes in concentrations of several hormones act in concert to inhibit muscle protein synthesis as occurs in simple starvation. However, experimental work in this laboratory has failed to demonstrate that altered insulin sensitivity and responsiveness is critical for protein synthesis in muscle tissue although insulin resistance for glucose assimilation is clearly present. Such a differentiated effect by insulin on protein and glucose metabolism at the tissue level supports the suggestion that depressed protein synthesis in muscle tissue is due to changes at both the transcriptional and translational level. We have reported that the synthesis of various muscle proteins is differentially inhibited in a tumor-bearing host, as found in animals suffering from pure starvation (Lundholm et al. 1981). This may be a teleological way to minimize detrimental effects of depressed protein synthesis in a stressed condition with insufficient protein intake. Studies on muscle protein degradation have shown that activities of proteases are increased in a tumor-bearing host (Lundholm et al. 1980). It is, however, unclear to what extent such increases reflect elevated muscle protein degradation in vivo since measurements of amino acid balances across skeletal muscles have failed to demonstrate a clearly increased efflux of amino nitrogen in vivo. Available information indicates that degradation may be high when related to the severely depressed protein synthesis, although absolute rates of degradation do not seem to be elevated (Lundholm et al. 1982 a; Bennegård et al. 1984).

Hormonal Alterations

Endocrine alterations in malignancy may include hormone production by benign cells, a multiple endocrine abnormality (MEA), infiltration of an endocrine gland by a tumor, and paraneoplastic and secondary endocrine manifestations due to therapy, infection, or cachexia. Only secondary manifestations are considered in this section. Cancer patients may early develop insulin resistance, which is a composite of both pancreatic and peripheral tissue changes (Lundholm et al. 1978). The B cells seem to be less sensitive to glucose or to other stimuli. Both receptor and postreceptor changes are involved in peripheral tissues. This alteration in islet cell function and altered peripheral tissue sensitivity may lead to hyperglycemia, but rarely results in ketosis.

Patients with cancer generally develop a low T_3 syndrome, which is characterized by decreased plasma levels of T_3, free T_4, and increased rT_3 (Persson et al. 1985). This may be viewed as a physiological means to reduce energy expenditure and preserve endogenous substrates. The secondary "hypothyroidism" may also contribute to decreased tumor growth and should not be corrected by exogenous hormone replacement. Growth hormone (GH) has been reported to be increased in several patients with nonpituitary tumors and probably supports the substrate-deficient host by stimulating gluconeogenesis and thereby promoting the breakdown of host tissues. In this sense, GH may act in concert with increased production of glucocorticoids.

Severely affected cancer patients may have a secondary hyperaldosteronism as a part of the activated pituitary-adrenal axis. This fact should be considered when treating cancer patients with intravenous infusions, which may be detrimental if high loads of electrolytes and water are given to adjust dehydration and disturbances in plasma electrolytes. Somatomedins may also be increased early in disease but tend to decrease in overt cachexia.

Hypercalcemia

Around 10% of all patients with cancer develop hypercalcemia and 10%–15% of these patients do not have evidence of bone metastases. The most common tumor types associated with hypercalcemia are breast cancer (15% generally associated with bone metastases), lung cancer (10%), and multiple myeloma (>50% usually associated with bone involvement). Mechanisms behind hypercalcemia are unknown factors induced by bone metastases, ectopic production of parathormone (PTH), primary hyperparathyroidism, excess production of prostaglandins (PGE_1, PGE_2), tumor-produced osteoclast-activating factor (OAF), and perhaps other osteolytic factors (Mundy et al. 1985). Normally, calcium balance is regulated by a series of control mechanisms. Osteolysis is promoted by PGE, PTH, OAF, thyroxine, and a monocytic-derived osteolytic-derived factor which may be interleukin-1. Inhibiting factors are calcitonin and estrogen. Intestinal absorption of calcium is regulated by PTH, GH, and vitamin D. Thus, alterations in any of these factors may disturb calcium homeostasis in cancer disease. Treatment is directed at reducing calcium resorption from bone, augmenting renal calcium excretion, and, perhaps, decreasing oral intake and intestinal absorption. The urgency requiring treatment depends upon symptoms. Intravascular fluid volume should be corrected since several of these patients presumably suffer from hypovolemia. Any medication that may increase plasma calcium should be withdrawn, i.e., thiazide diuretics, vitamins A and D, and perhaps hormonal agents in patients with breast cancer. Tumor extirpation or resection is reported to be the only effective long-term treatment. Physiological maneuvers that increase renal clearance of sodium also increase the excretion of calcium. Thus, extracellular volume restoration with saline is of utmost importance. Furosemide and ethacrynic acid promote calciuresis by decreasing reabsorption of sodium and calcium. Calcium values greater than 3.5 mmol/liter require more aggressive therapy. Glucocorticoids may be effective due to their cytotoxic effects as well as by inhibiting osteoclast-activating factor. Glucocorticoids are most useful in hematological malignancies and sometimes in association with breast cancer. Other solid tumors respond less well. The hypocalcemic effect of glucocorticoids takes several days to develop. Calcitonin is generally very effective but the effect is sometimes lost later. The therapeutic effect of calcitonin is evident within hours. The combination of glucocorticoids and calcitonin is quite effective and may prevent the "escape" effect with calcitonin alone. Mithramycin is a cytotoxic antibiotic which inhibits DNA-dependent RNA synthesis and has been proven particularly useful in hypercalcemia unresponsive to other measures. It acts by directly inhibiting osteoclastic bone resorption. Its effect is usually obvious within 36–48 h and one or two doses per week are usually sufficient. Treatment should not be repeated until hypercalcemia recurs (Percia et al. 1970; Kiang et al. 1979).

The intravenous infusion of phosphate is one of the most effective methods to decrease blood calcium. The decline in serum calcium with phosphate infusion is probably dependent on a redistribution of calcium within the body, since urinary excretion is not increased. Calcification of tissues has been reported in combination with intravenous and oral phosphate treatment. Other major complications in phosphate treatment are hypocalcemia, hypotension, renal failure, and sudden death. Therefore, its use should be reserved for cases not responding to other treatments. The incidence of side effects is reduced if the dosage is not more than 50 mmol infused over 6–8 h. Oral phosphate therapy, although less rapid in action, is often very useful for the chronic treatment of hypercalcemia. The useful dose is 1–3 g phosphorus daily. Oral therapy should not be used in patients with serum phosphate more than 1.3 mmol/liter. Sometimes dialysis may be used to control hypercalcemia (Goldsmith and Ingbar 1966; Massry et al. 1968).

Hypocalcemia

Hypocalcemia is reported in 10%–20% of patients with cancer. This may be due to tumor production of calcitonin although there is little evidence for this. No specific treatment is usually indicated except in some rare cases with tetany where calcium can be given. A paraneoplastic syndrome with unknown etiology is hypophosphatemic osteomalacia associated with mesenchymal tumors. This syndrome is characterized by adult onset, vitamin D resistant rickets with bone pain, severe phosphaturia, renal glucosuria, normocalcemia, and increased alkaline phosphatase. The symptoms are relieved when the tumor is extirpated.

Hypoglycemia

Hypoglycemia is generally caused by insulinomas. Hypoglycemia associated with non-islet cell tumors is rare but may occur in the presence of mesenchymal tumors (65%), hepatoma (20%), adrenal carcinoma (5%), and gastrointestinal (5%) and miscellaneous (5%) tumors. The tumor is generally large,

1–10 kg, and an average of 2–3 kg. The liver is often invaded. The underlying mechanisms may include ectopic insulin production, production of nonsuppressible insulin-like activity, high glucose consumption in the tumor, or massive liver infiltration impairing hepatic glucose production. Glucose infusions and glucagon or corticosteroid injections have been frequently used in treating hypoglycemia in cancer patients.

Lactic Acidosis

Lactic acidosis is usually associated with acute lymphocytic or myelogenous leukemia and Hodgkin's disease. High plasma levels of lactate are frequently seen in the tumor lysis syndrome. The pathogenesis is unclear but lactic acidosis may be due to high lactate production in tumor and nontumor tissue. However, hypoxia is not necessarily the immediate cause of increased lactate production. The coexistence of a second acid-base disturbance has been suggested and the picture is often mixed with coexistent respiratory alkalosis. Thus, the presence of an underlying lactic acidosis cannot be ruled out by a normal blood pH. Most reported cases of lactic acidosis are in lymphomas and solid tumors presumably closely associated with extensive liver involvement. Lactic acidosis may also occur as a complication of too rapid infusion of hypertonic glucose or fructose solutions to cancer patients with large tumors. Bicarbonate therapy is sometimes required (Cohen and Woods 1976; Park and Arieff 1980).

Amyloidosis

Amyloid deposition is a pathological deposition of a specific protein of fibrillar character. This protein is not found normally and can be formed by several different pathogenic mechanisms. The fibrils are very resistant to proteolytic cleavage and may therefore accumulate in tissue. The mechanical interference frequently affects vital organs such as heart, kidney, and nerves. Around 15% of patients with amyloidosis have cancer, including lymphomas and multiple myeloma. Carcinomas associated with amyloidosis include hypernephroma and bladder and renal pelvic cancer of which hypernephroma represents 25%. The signs and symptoms associated with amyloidosis include neuropathy, autonomic nervous symptoms, sexual impotence, gastrointestinal disturbances, and dyshidrosis. Weight loss is frequent and restrictive cardiomyopathy is well recognized. The patients are extremely sensitive to digitalis and several incidences of sudden death due to intoxication have been reported. Bone and skeletal system symptoms are frequent. Generally, the prognosis is poor. Effective treatment can stop further deposition of the amyloid precipitate but does not eliminate manifest deposition (Glenner 1980; Azzopardi and Lehner 1966).

Hyperuricemia

Hyperuricemia is a well-recognized metabolic disorder in malignant conditions, particularly common in lymphoproliferative and myeloproliferative disorders including lymphomas, acute and chronic myelogenous leukemia, polycytemia vera, and myelofibrosis with myeloid metaplasia. It is occasionally seen in disseminated carcinomas. In leukemias and lymphomas, hyperuricemia may occur spontaneously or secondary to treatment. Severe hyperuricemia may lead to acute renal failure, which may be a life-threatening complication. Hyperuricemia may result from increased production or decreased excretion of uric acid. Serum uric acid levels are generally increased even in patients with only a mild degree of kidney dysfunction. This mechanism accounts for most cases of hyperuricemia in patients with multiple myeloma, although increased production of uric acid due to elevated cell turnover may contribute. Certain diuretics such as thiazides, furosemide, and ethacrynic acid may aggravate and elicit hyperuricemia in borderline patients. Three types of renal disease are associated with hyperuricemia: acute hyperuremic nephropathy, uric acid nephrolithiasis, and gouty nephropathy. Acute hyperuricemic nephropathy is the most important complication of hyperuricemia in patients with bulky disease of leukemia and lymphoma. Precipitation of uric acid crystals in the distal nephrons is assumed to be the underlying mechanism, particularly in the collecting ducts, which results in obstruction. The precipitation of uric acid is promoted by acidic urine, since urate has a pK close to 5.4 and is thus less soluble than in blood at pH 7.4. Prophylaxis against hyperuricemia is mandatory when cytotoxic therapy is undertaken in patients with bulky disease of leukemia and lymphoma or treatment for recurrence. Dehydration must be prevented and corrected. Alkaline diuresis and allopurinol treatment are indicated in high-risk patients. Uric acid nephrolithiasis is a condition due to long-standing hyperuricemia. This disorder results from precipitation of uric acid in the renal pelvis to form a nidus for stones, which enlarge progressively. Pyelonephritis may develop in such patients. Treatment consists of chronic allopurinol treatment to suppress uric acid formation (Boss and Seegmiller 1979; Ultmann 1962).

Tumor Lysis Syndrome

Certain tumors with high fractional growth rates, large tumor mass, and acute sensitivity to antineoplastic drugs may lyse rapidly when treatment is started. Significant amounts of intracellular ions such as potassium and phosphate are released at a rate that may induce hyperkalemia and hyperphosphatemia, particularly when renal impairment or low diuresis occurs. Hypocalcemia may result secondary to the hyperphosphatemia. Life-threatening arrhythmias due to hyperkalemia and hypocalcemia are the most important potential complication of the tumor lysis syndrome, which has been reported most commonly in association with undifferentiated lymphomas, lymphoblastic lymphomas, and acute blastic leukemia. It may also occur in patients with small-cell anaplastic bronchogeneic carcinoma, but patients with solid tumors are generally not at risk. An association between high levels of lactate dehydrogenase and the tumor lysis syndrome has been reported (Schilsky 1982; Cohen et al. 1980).

Adrenal Failure

Destruction of the adrenal glands by secondary tumor growth is a well-recognized cause of adrenocortical insufficiency, although it is a rare complication. Adrenal metastatic growth is found in 5%–10% of autopsies performed on cancer patients. However, it is believed that more than 90% of the glandular cortex must be destroyed before hypofunction results. Metastatic growth only explains a few percent of Addison's disease. The tumors that most frequently metastasize to this organ are cancer of bronchus, breast, kidney, stomach, pancreas, and malignant melanomas. Its clinical signs should be identified, since this is a lethal disorder for which there exists a simple and effective therapy. Hyponatremia in combination with hyperkalemia perhaps in combination with modest metabolic acidosis is the classic biochemical sign of adrenal insufficiency. However, hyponatremia is frequently seen in cachectic cancer patients without adrenocortical insufficiency. Therefore, urine analysis to confirm a disproportionately high excretion of sodium and low output of potassium may strengthen the diagnosis. The diagnosis can be established by determining the patient's response to adrenocorticotrophic hormone (ACTH). The treatment consists of physiological doses of corticosteroids (Sahagian-Edwards and Holland 1954; Rosenthal et al. 1978).

References

Azzopardi JG, Lehner T (1966) Systemic amyloidosis and malignant disease. J Clin Pathol 19: 539–548

Bennegård K, Lindmark L, Edén E, Svaninger G, Lundholm K (1984) Flux of amino acids across the leg in weight-losing cancer patients. Cancer Res 44: 386–393

Boss, GR, Seegmiller JE (1979) Hyperuricemia and gout: classification, complications and management. N Engl J Med 300: 1459–1468

Cohen LF, Balow JE, Magrath IT (1980) Acute tumor lysis syndrome: a review of 37 patients with Burkitt's lymphoma. Am J Med 64: 486–491

Cohen RD, Woods HF (1976) Clinical and biochemical aspects of lactic acidosis. Oxford, Blackwell

Edén E, Ekman L, Bennegård K, Lindmark L, Lundholm K (1984) Whole body tyrosine flux in relation to energy expenditure in weight-losing cancer patients. Metabolism 33: 1020–1027

Edén E, Edström S, Bennegård K, Lindmark L, Lundholm K (1985) Glycerol dynamics in weight-losing cancer patients. Surgery 97: 176–184

Glenner GG (1980) Amyloid deposits and amyloidosis: the B-fibrilloses. N Engl J Med 303: 1283–1292, 1333–1347

Goldsmith RS, Ingbar SH (1966) Inorganic phosphate treatment of hypercalcemia of diverse etiologies. N Engl J Med 274: 1–7

Kiang DT, Loken MK, Kennedy BJ (1979) Mechanism of the hypocalcemic effect of mithramycin. J Clin Endocrinol Metab 48: 341–344

Lindmark L, Bennegård K, Edén E, Ekman L, Scherstén T, Svaninger G, Lundholm K (1984) Resting energy expenditure in malnourished patients with and without cancer. Gastroenterology 87: 402–408

Lundholm KG (1985 a) Origins of emaciation in cancer patients. Med Oncol Tumor Pharmacother 2: 183–187

Lundholm KG (1985 b) Energy and substrate metabolism in the cancer-bearing host. In: Bozzetti F, Dionigi R (eds) Nutrition in cancer and trauma sepsis. Karger, Basel, pp 78–89

Lundholm K, Holm G, Scherstén T (1978) Insulin resistance in patients with cancer. Cancer Res 38: 4665–4670

Lundholm K, Ekman L, Karlberg I, Edström S, Scherstén T (1980) Comparison of hepatic Cathepsin D activity in response to tumor growth and to caloric restriction in mice. Cancer Res 40: 1680–1685

Lundholm K, Karlberg I, Ekman L, Edström S, Scherstén T (1981) Evaluation of anorexia as the cause of altered protein synthesis in skeletal muscles from nongrowing mice with sarcoma. Cancer Res 41: 1989–1996

Lundholm K, Bennegård K, Edén E, Svaninger G, Emery PW,

Rennie MJ (1982a) Efflux of 3-methyl-histidine from the leg in cancer patients who experience weight loss. Cancer Res 42: 4807–4811

Lundholm K, Edström S, Karlberg I, Ekman L, Scherstén T (1982b) Glucose turnover, gluconeogenesis from glycerol, and estimation of net glucose cycling in cancer patients. Cancer 50: 1142–1150

Massry SG, Mueller E, Silverman AG (1968) Inorganic phosphate treatment of hypercalcemia. Arch Intern Med 121: 307–312

McCarthy DO, Kluberg MJ, Vander AJ (1985) Suppression of food intake during infection: is interleukin-1 involved? Am J Clin Nutr 42: 1179–1182

Mundy GR, Ibbotson KJ, D'Souza SM (1985) Tumor products and the hypercalcemia of malignancy. J Clin Invest 76: 391–394

Park R, Arieff AI (1980) Lactic acidosis. Adv Intern Med 25: 33–68

Percia CP, Gubisch NJ, Wolter J (1970) Mithramycin treatment of hypercalcemia. Cancer 25: 389–394

Persson H, Bennegård K, Lundberg PA, Svaninger G, Lundholm K (1985) Thyroid hormones in conditions of chronic malnutrition. A study with special reference to cancer cachexia. Ann Surg 201: 45–53

Rosenthal FD, Davies MK, Burden AC (1978) Malignant disease presenting as Addison's disease. Br Med J 1: 1591–1592

Sahagian-Edwards A, Holland JF (1954) Metastastic carcinoma to the adrenal glands with cortical hypofunction. Cancer 7: 1242–1245

Schilsky RL (1982) Renal and metabolic toxicities of cancer chemotherapy, Semin Oncol 9: 75–83

Ternell M, Lönnroth C, Lundholm K (1985) Nuclear RNA polymerase activity in tumor-host livers. Am J Physiol 12: E461–E469

Ultman JE (1962) Hyperuricemia in disseminated neoplastic disease other than lymphomas and leukemias. Cancer 15: 122–129

von Meyenfeld MF, Soeters PB (1985) Anorexia in cancer. Bozzetti F, Dionigi R (eds) Nutrition in cancer and trauma sepsis. Karger, Basel, pp 54–67

Haemorrhage, Obstruction, Perforation, and Infection in Head and Neck Cancer

I. A. McGregor

Haemorrhage

The vessels from which catastrophic haemorrhage occurs in head and neck surgery are the carotids, common and internal. Haemorrhage from these vessels is liable to be fatal not merely as a result of exsanguination, but because control of the bleeding by clamp or ligature, the methods likely to be required in the typical emergency situation, affects the cerebral circulation, frequently resulting in hemiplegia with a fatal outcome in a percentage of patients. The risk of haemorrhage is greatest following pharyngeal surgery and two striking aetiological factors are recognised – exposure of the vessels and damage to the vessel wall. The vessels become exposed as a result of wound breakdown or tissue necrosis. Exposure of the healthy carotid is remarkably well tolerated and it rarely if ever ruptures. It is the vessel in the neck which has previously been irradiated which is at risk (Marchetta et al. 1967). Breakdown of the neck wound is more likely and rupture of the exposed vessel becomes then a very real hazard. Exposure is most likely to be followed by rupture when the time lapse between radiotherapy and surgery exceeds 6 months (Briant 1975). Radiotherapy followed by elective surgery does not constitute the problem; it is the uncoordinated use of radiotherapy followed by salvage surgery which accounts for most carotid ruptures (Joseph and Shumrick 1973).

Awareness of rupture as a potential complication has resulted in the prophylactic use of transferred muscles such as levator scapulae (Staley 1961) and the scalenes to cover the arterial segment considered to be at risk, and grafts of dermis (Corso and Gerold 1963) have been used for the same purpose. More recently it has become recognised that an incidental virtue of the pectoralis major and lateral trapezius myocutaneous flaps and a reason for their selection as reconstructive methods of choice in the previously irradiated neck has been the fact that the muscle pedicle overlies the carotids and provides a protective cover for their wall.

A carotid exposed in the neck is not invariably an emergency but it does require to be watched very closely, particularly if the neck has been irradiated. Blurring and ultimate disappearance of structures initially visible on the vessel wall such as vasa vasorum with the development of granulation tissue is a favourable sign. Failure of these changes to occur should be viewed with concern and even more worrying is the development of thrombosis of the vasa vasorum. The appearance on the vessel of anything which could be construed as a slough is a sign of impending rupture. Small premonitory bleeds sometimes occur and indicate virtually certain rupture in the very near future.

It is when rupture is considered a virtual certainty that a decision requires to be made regarding elective as opposed to emergency ligation of the artery. Elective ligation carries a much better prognosis in terms of both patient survival and neurological sequelae (Moore et al. 1969), not surprising when one considers the shocked, partly exsanguinated, hypotensive subject whose carotid is being ligated as an emergency. Elective ligation is generally to be preferred, but even so its use does not eliminate the possibility of haemiplegia and even death of the patient.

Obstruction

In the context of cancer of the head and neck obstruction takes the form of dysphagia and the emergency situation which it is liable to create results from the fact that the act of swallowing is so intimately associated with the mechanism of respiration. The separation of the two in normal function is crucial to protection of the lungs from the inhalation of food during the act of swallowing. Failure of the mechanism to function properly is an element of certain of the forms which dysphagia takes following surgery of the oral cavity and pharynx. When this happens the lungs are at serious risk from the effects of the inhalation.

The act of swallowing may be made difficult or prevented entirely because the tongue is unable to carry out the initiating movements in which the bolus of saliva or food is collected by the tip, pushed against the hard palate and propelled backwards. The most frequent cause of this is tethering of the anterior free segment, but this occurring alone seldom gives rise to an inhalation hazard. It may of course exacerbate associated other causes of dysphagia and add to the probability of inhalation and the severity of its effects.

It is when the epiglottic mechanism is disturbed that the likelihood of inhalation problems becomes significant, to the extent of creating a potential emergency situation. Such problems can arise following surgery involving the posterior third of the tongue and the faucial area generally, and after conservative laryngeal surgery.

When the surgery has involved the tongue, faucial area or epiglottis, inhalation is most likely when the mechanism has been upset by loss of the epiglottis itself (Doberneck and Antoine 1974), but even when it is still present it may be prevented from acting in the proper manner by malfunction of the adjoining structures, tongue or fauces. Failure of normal function is most often caused by fixation of structures even when their position is not greatly disturbed, though fixation in a distorted position is an even more potent cause of inhalation problems.

The most effective method of managing the problem overall is by prevention. Clearly this is not always possible since the tissue resected is determined by the pathological situation, but the surgeon should avoid adding to it by the manner in which he or she closes the postexcisional defect or reconstructs it.

The principle which underlies the successful reconstruction is that it minimises distortion and displacement of structures from their normal position. This is achieved by using flaps which accurately match the defect in volume and in position within the cavity of the mouth and pharynx. An incidental virtue of such flaps is that their effective use minimises scarring and fibrosis, reducing the fixation of tissues and loss of function which results from such fibrosis. It is striking that considerable defects of the lateral and posterior pharyngeal wall can be closed directly, without producing problems of dysphagia provided the larynx and epiglottic mechanisms are not interfered with.

It is generally accepted that a major hazard of conservative laryngeal surgery is the potential one of inhalation during swallowing and it is accepted that in a proportion of patients the surgeon will have no alternative to proceeding to formal laryngectomy. It is a measure of the value placed on retention of laryngeal function that conservative surgery is still judged worthwhile when the pathological situation permits, even though it is known that it will be unsuccessful in a proportion of instances.

The final sequence of the swallowing mechanism involves a phase of relaxation of the cricopharyngeal sphincter and achalasia may unexpectedly follow an otherwise satisfactory resection-reconstruction. By itself achalasia is not regularly followed by inhalation of swallowed food, though if the dysphagia is severe problems may arise from spillover of unswallowed food accumulating in the pharynx. It can also add its quota to the other causes of dysphagia and it may require to be treated as part of the overall management in such circumstances.

In many of these clinical situations the patient will have undergone a temporary tracheostomy as part of the initial surgery and in the early postoperative phase inhalation problems are prevented by the use of cuffed tracheostomy tubes. In any case the use of nasogastric feeding also prevents inhalation from occurring. It is when the patient is weaned from his or her nasogastric tube that the problem becomes apparent.

In managing dysphagia and potential inhalation pneumonia a careful watch is essential with continuing reassessment of the seriousness of the threat. A difficulty is that encouragement of the patient is constantly needed. The patient who passively accepts the disability is less likely to overcome it than the patient who is highly motivated.

When it is decided that re-eduction is not possible a formal laryngectomy must be carried out with creation of a permanent tracheostomy. The decision is better made before the onset of bronchopneumonia, while the lungs are as normal as possible, but it is striking how the patient with bronchopneumonia can be greatly benefited by the thorough bronchial suction toilet which can be carried out in the anaesthetised patient. Even in the presence of an inhalation pneumonia it may still be safer to proceed with the laryngectomy if inhalation cannot be controlled by other means such as nasogastric feeding and cuffed tracheostomy tubes while the pulmonary state is being improved.

When achalasia is present alone or as an element of the overall clinical problem cricopharyngeal myotomy (Wilkins 1964) is the procedure of choice.

Perforation

The perforation which occurs in head and neck surgery is generally referred to as a fistula and it occurs when there is a communication between the mouth and/or pharynx and the skin surface.

A fistula is a serious complication of any head and neck procedure but the extent to which it becomes an emergency parallels the extent to which the carotids are exposed by the fistula and to what extent they are considered to be in danger of rupture (Mladick et al. 1972). The factors involved in this assessment are listed in discussing haemorrhage as a potential emergency.

The clinical situation is seldom one where a pre-emptive definitive reconstruction is likely to be successful. A flap transferred to cover the external opening of such a fistula is only likely to be effective if the internal opening is successfully closed simultaneously and this is rarely possible. All that the surgeon can do is watch the carotids carefully, ready to ligate if rupture is judged to be imminent. Progress towards granulation of the vessels indicates passing of the emergency and attention can then be concentrated on closing the fistula.

Infection

When one considers the fact that surgery is frequently carried out in the presence of a foul-smelling malignant ulcer on patients who are far from being ideal subjects for surgery because of their smoking habits and intake of alcohol, the remarkable thing is not that postoperative infection occurs but rather that it does not occur with much greater frequency.

Infection involves the chest and/or the neck, mouth and pharynx. In managing the chest, the problems vary in practice depending on whether or not a tracheostomy has been carried out. With both, however, physiotherapy and antibiotics provide the basis of treatment.

A preoperative sputum culture with sensitivities is likely to help provide a basis for selecting the appropriate antibiotic should the need arise postoperatively, and regular sampling thereafter will allow the drug chosen to be changed if necessary. It is essential however to be aware that antibiotics are only one facet of management. Even more important is the establishment of a regime of breathing exercises and effective coughing under supervision of a physiotherapist, coupled with humidification if a tracheostomy has been carried out, to prevent the sequence of blockage of the bronchi with secretions, segmental collapse and secondary infection.

The presence of a tracheostomy allows direct bronchial toilet and regular suction carried out with aseptic precautions to be added to the regime of supervised coughing.

Infection in the mouth, pharynx and neck most often follows localised haematoma or tissue necrosis with resulting wound breakdown and the organisms most often involved appear to be those which were present preoperatively in the tumour. The sites where a haematoma is prone to collect after neck dissection are the supraclavicular fossa and the submandibular area and it is in these sites that effective suction drainage provides the best prophylaxis.

When infection occurs it is usually associated with the smell typical of intraoral malignant ulcers and the antibiotics primarily of value in controlling aerobic organisms are ineffective in both preventing and eliminating these infections and in eliminating the accompanying odour. Metronidazole has been found to be extremely effective in eliminating the odour and also what appears to be the causative organisms, namely the *Bacteroides* group (Sweeney et al. 1984). The prophylactic administration of metronidazole has reduced the incidence and seriousness of postoperative infections very greatly. Its specificity and absence of side effects makes it the drug of choice in managing the problems of infection in head and neck malignancy surgery.

It is unusual for infection to create an emergency situation though it can create major problems in long-term management. The single most important potential or actual emergency in head and neck cancer management is exposure of the carotid system and where infection is responsible the addition of this factor obviously adds to the overall hazard, but its presence does not alter management significantly.

References

Briant TDR (1975) Spontaneous pharyngeal fistula and wound infection following laryngectomy. Laryngoscope 85: 829

Corso PF, Gerold FP (1963) Use of autogenous dermis for protection of the carotid artery and pharyngeal suture lines in radical head and neck surgery. Surg Gynecol Obstet 117: 37

Dorberneck RC, Antoine JE (1974) Deglutition after resection of oral, laryngeal and pharyngeal cancers. Surgery 75: 87

Joseph DL, Shumrick DL (1973) Risks of head and neck surgery in previously irradiated patients. Arch Otolaryngol 97: 381

Marchetta FC, Sako K, Maxwell W (1967) Complications after radical head and neck surgery performed through previously irradiated tissues. Am J Surg 114: 835

Mladick RA, Horton CE, Adamson JE, Cohen BI (1972) Management of catastrophic postoperative breakdown after massive oropharyngeal cancer surgery. Plast Reconstr Surg 49: 316

Moore OS, Karlan M, Sigler L (1969) Factors influencing the safety of carotid ligation. Am J Surg 118: 666

Staley CJ (1961) A muscle cover for the carotid artery after radical neck dissection. Am J Surg 102: 815

Sweeney G, Watson JD, McGregor IA, Sleigh JD (1984) Successful prophylaxis with tinidazole of infection after major head and neck surgery for malignant disease. Br J Plast Surg 37: 35

Wilkins SA (1964) Indications for section of the cricopharyngeus muscle. Am J Surg 108: 533

Obstruction, Perforation, Infection, and Haemorrhage in Thoracic Cancer

T. M. SCHEININ and P. J. ROBERTS

Obstruction

Several different primary or secondary malignancies cause significant, even life-threatening, obstruction of intrathoracic organs or structures. The lumen of hollow organs may be occluded by malignant invasion, or by external compression by malignancies, e.g. in the upper mediastinum. These obstructions may be single or multiple; there may be tracheal and oesophageal obstruction in addition to a superior vena cava syndrome. Mediastinal cancer in particular may lead to obstructions, with symptoms and signs such as stridor and dyspnoea, dysphagia, oedema, cyanosis and petechial haemorrhages. The aggressive types of thymic tumours or teratomas causing the obstructions should be surgically removed, and postoperative radiotherapy and chemotherapy may be needed. Lymphomas causing multiple obstructions should be treated with radio- and chemotherapy. The different obstructions and their common causes are presented under separate subheadings.

Tracheobronchial Obstruction

Tracheal cancer is rare, and consists of squamous cell carcinoma in most instances, followed by adenocystic carcinoma. Secondary lung carcinomas involving the trachea are not unusual, but can seldom be surgically treated. The symptoms arise from airway obstruction, and diagnosis can usually be made during tracheobronchoscopy. Computed tomography of the neck and mediastinum and tracheobronchial radiology provide information in planning the treatment.

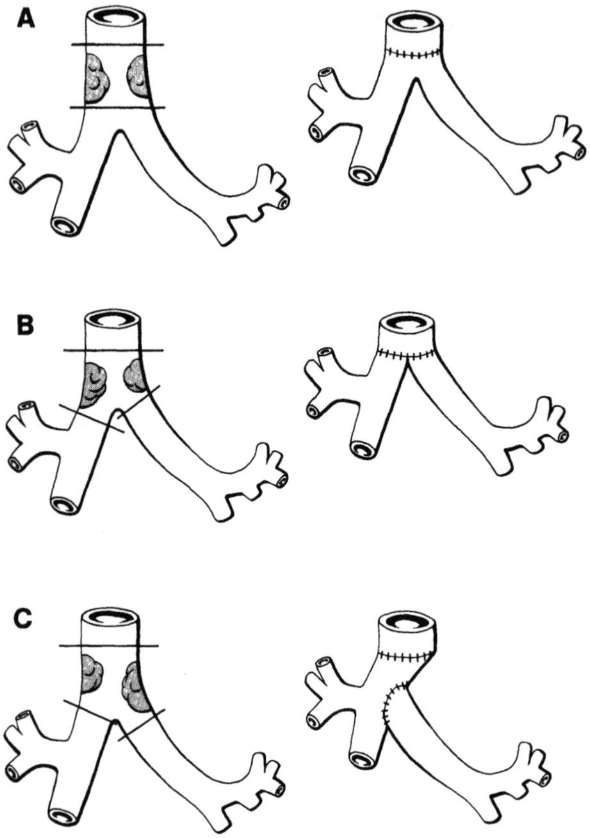

Fig. 1 A–C. Some examples of tracheal resection and reconstruction

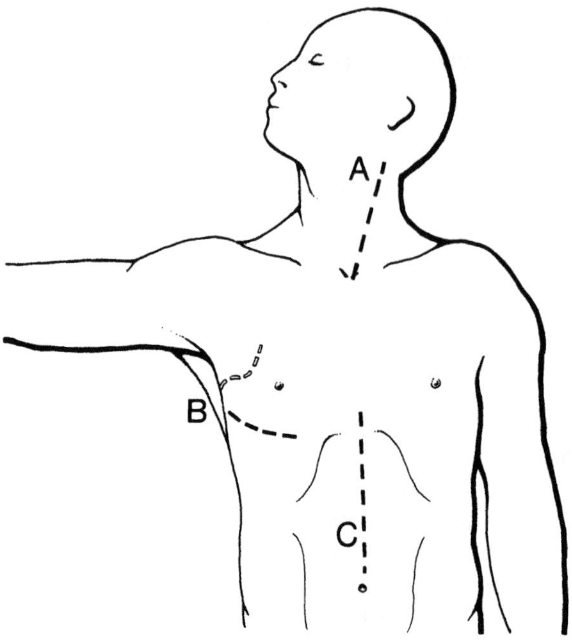

Fig. 2. Incisions for oesophageal surgery: *A*, along the anterior border of the sternocleidomastoid muscle; *B*, posterolateral thoracotomy; *C*, upper midline laparotomy

The surgical treatment for tracheobronchial obstruction is excision and reconstruction whenever possible. Endotracheal intubation prior to planned surgery may be impossible, in which case cardiopulmonary bypass may have to be used. Depending on the tumor extent and radiosensitivity, irradiation can be considered. The surgical procedures consist of different types of tracheobronchial resection with reconstruction of the remaining trachea and main bronchi (Fig. 1 A–C). It is important to gain as much as possible in tracheal length to achieve a satisfactory anastomosis. Between 3 and 6 cm can be gained by appropriate division of pulmonary ligaments, right hilar and vascular mobilization, and left main bronchus reimplantation.

Fractionated irradiation has been used for palliation with some results. It is possible to achieve good palliatation by the use of Nd:YAG laser for the treatment of obstructing tracheobronchial lesions.

Oesophageal Obstruction

The main cause of oesophageal obstruction is carcinoma. The diagnosis is usually late, delayed by lack of symptoms until pain and dysphagia occur. By then the carcinoma has invaded the paraoesophageal tissues and lymph nodes, and surgery can seldom be performed for cure.

In malignant oesophageal obstruction one must evaluate whether it can be surgically removed, bypassed or otherwise relieved. Diagnostic procedures include endoscopy of the upper digestive and tracheobronchial tract, radiological examination and computed tomography.

The tendency of oesophageal carcinoma to spread longitudinally between layers of the wall favours total or near-total removal of the oesophagus. Whenever possible ablative surgery, either radical or palliative, is performed. It consists of wide excision and oesophageal reconstruction with: (1) gastric, (2) colonic or (3) jejunal trans- or interposition. The reposition can be either in the posterior mediastinum or retrosternally. The patient is often elderly and in poor general condition and should have adequate parenteral alimentation preoperatively. The simplest and safest surgical procedure should be used for oesophageal excision and reconstruction, mostly performed in one stage. All unnecessary surgical embellishments should be omitted as being dangerous. The operation is usually carried out through a right-sided thoracotomy and laparotomy with cervical pharyngo-oesophageal mobilization in total oesophagectomy (Fig. 2). The omission of thora-

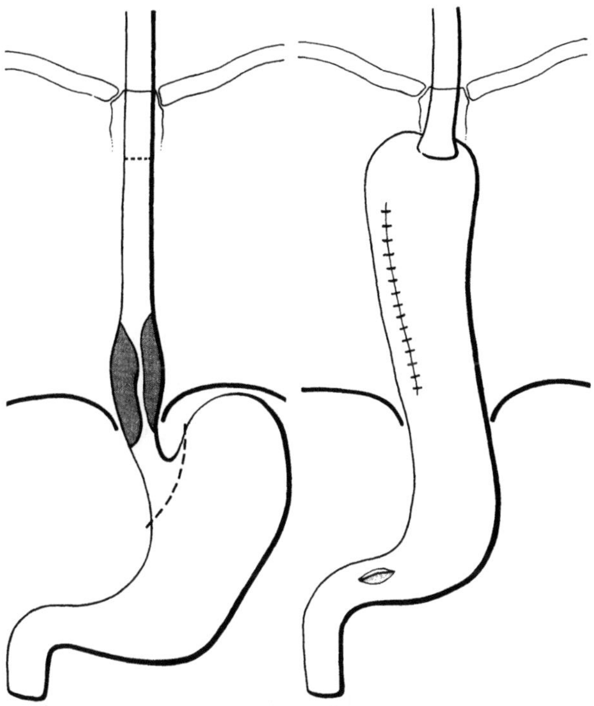

Fig. 3. Near total oesophagectomy, gastric transposition and oesophagofundostomy with pyloromyotomy (or pyloroplasty)

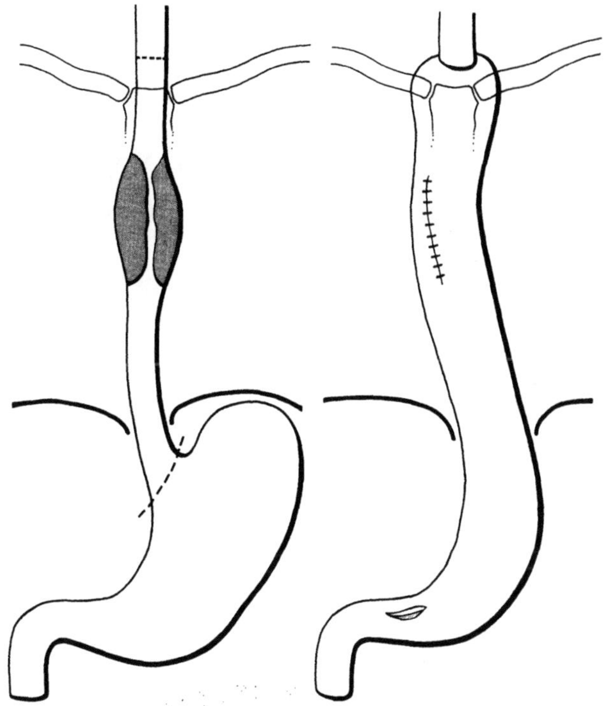

Fig. 4. Total oesophagectomy with anastomosis in the neck. Similar reconstruction as in Fig. 3

cotomy and mobilization of the oesophagus using cervical and abdominal incisions only is preferred by some surgeons. This blind technique is combined with early complications, such as bleeding, perhaps incomplete removal of the tumour and a high early mortality.

The reconstruction methods will be discussed separately.

Gastric Transposition (Figs. 3, 4)

The cardia is transected and the blood vessels of lesser and greater curvature must remain intact during mobilization of the stomach. A Kocher manoeuvre should be performed to gain some additional centimetres, and pyloromyotomy or pyloroplasty is usually added. The stomach is passed upwards through the mediastinal route. Interposition of a gastric tube from the greater curvature has also been employed.

Colonic Interposition (Fig. 5)

This method of reconstruction is suitable for oesophageal bypass in benign oesophageal stenosis. However, the simplest surgical procedure, gastric transposition, gives the best results in the treatment of oesophageal cancer. If the stomach cannot be used because of gastric disease or previous surgery, colonic interposition is a good alternative.

It is often carried out as a left colonic interposition, with the colon segment vascularized by the middle colic artery or the ascending left colic artery. However, the right hemicolon may be equally well used, based on the middle colic artery. The choice is determined by the anatomy of the colonic vasculature. The colonic segment is placed isoperistaltically, although the left colon, depending on vascularization, can be placed in an antiperistaltic direction.

Jejunal Trans- or Interposition

The main indication for jejunal transposition as a Roux-en-Y oesophagojejunostomy arises when resection of the distal oesophagus is combined with gastrectomy. The jejunum can be difficult to mobilize and is therefore best suited for short reconstructions. The use of a microsurgically revascularized free jejunal segment is seldom useful in malignant obstruction.

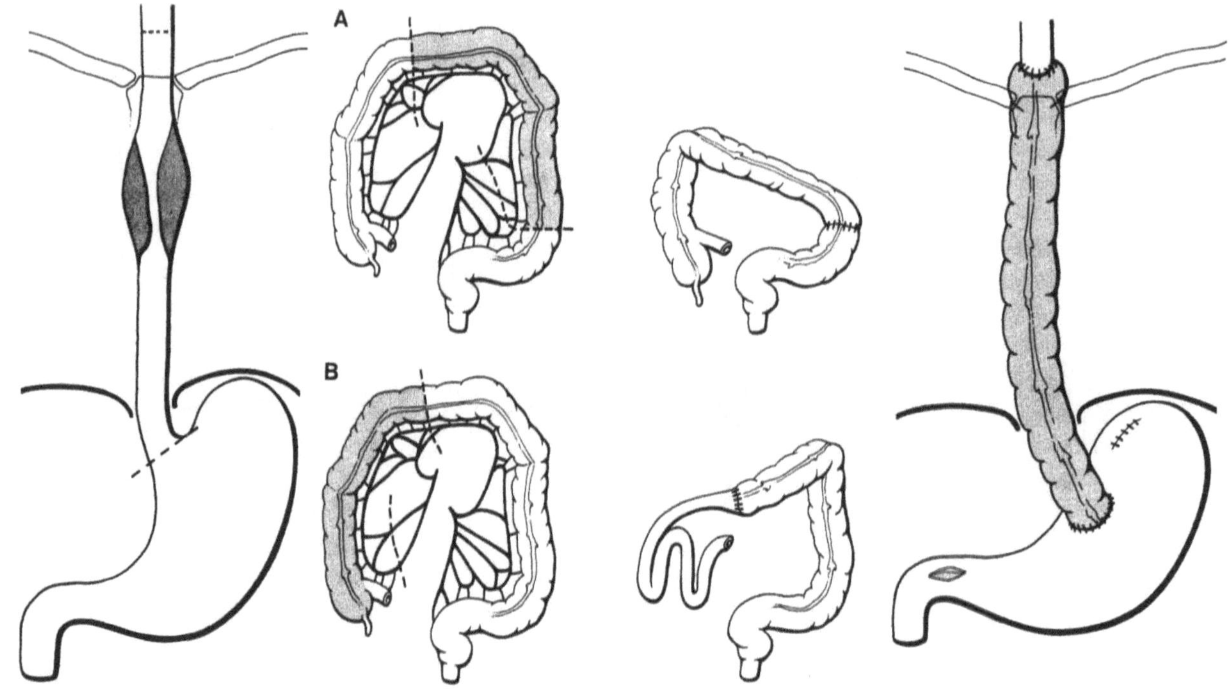

Fig. 5 A, B. Total oesophagectomy and reconstruction with: **A** interposition of antiperistaltic left colonic segment with transversosigmoideostomy; **B** interposition of isoperistaltic right hemicolon with ileotransversostomy. Pyloromyotomy (or pyloroplasty) in both reconstructions

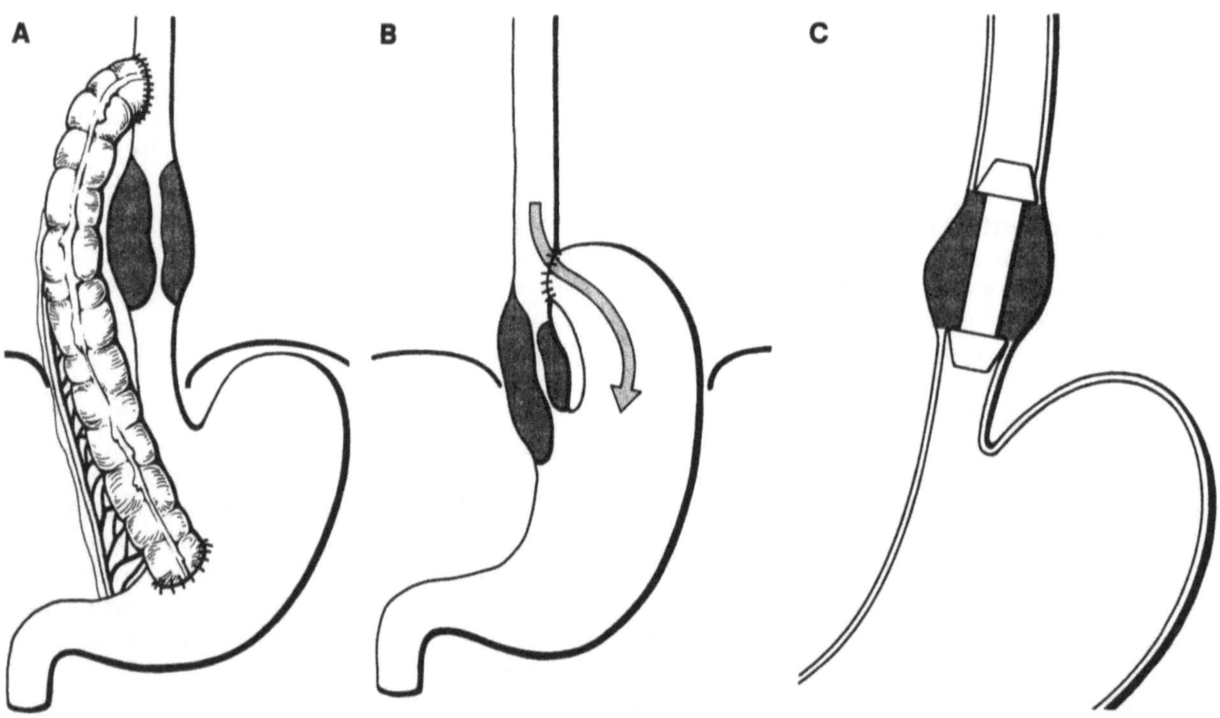

Fig. 6 A–C. Surgery for palliative purposes in malignant oesophageal obstruction: **A** bypass using interposition of colonic segment; **B** bypass with oesophagofundostomy; **C** endo-oesophageal intubation

Other Surgical Procedures To Relieve Obstruction (Fig. 6)

Inexcisable tumours of the lower oesophagus can be bypassed by a Roux-en-Y oesophagojejunostomy, or by mobilizing the stomach and performing a side-to-side anastomosis above the tumour. A segment of the left colon can also be employed to bypass a tumour and may be the best decision when the tumour is located to the upper third of the oesophagus. Relief of symptoms, particularly of dysphagia and salivation, can often be provided even when the patient is considered unsuitable for excisional or bypass surgery. There is a large selection of tubes (e.g. Celestin, Atkinson) which after dilatation of the obstruction can be placed operatively or endoscopical to achieve oesophageal patency. Nd:YAG laser therapy has proved to be useful for vaporizing the obstructive parts of the tumour and has been employed successfully in palliation of oesophageal cancer. Simple feeding gastrostomy or jejunostomy are unsatisfactory means of palliation. Sometimes, in the absence of other alternatives, repeated endoscopic dilatations gives some palliation.

Superior Vena Cava Syndrome

The superior vena cava is particularly liable to obstruction by primary lung cancer or by metastatic spread to the upper mediastinal nodes. Lung cancer causes 75% of the obstructions, with a right-to-left ratio of 4:1. The syndrome is characterized by oedema of face, neck and upper extremities, high venous pressure and petechial bleeding. Progressive dyspnoea, stridor and orthopnoea are common.

Surgical treatment including attempts at excision with or without caval bypass grafts is avoided except in selected malignancies resistant to irradiation or chemotherapy. Because lymphomas are found in 15%, irradiation is the treatment of choice. The total irradiation dose and its fractionation must be considered individually. Chemotherapy is effective only in some tumours, as in the initial treatment of some lymphomas and in small cell carcinoma of the lung.

Perforation

Perforation of the Oesophagus

Most eosophageal perforations are iatrogenic and occur during diagnostic procedures for oesophageal malignancies; they are associated with a mortality rate exceeding 20%. Indications for immediate operative treatment are the presence of pneumothorax, mediastinal emphysema or mediastinitis, pleural effusion or emphyema and sepsis. The diagnosis of oesophageal perforation is usually based on symptoms and signs presenting after oesophagogastric instrumentation or intubation. Radiological examination with water-soluble contrast medium is valuable in the diagnosis, and air or contrast medium seen in the mediastinum are diagnostic. However, in 15% the diagnosis is made after death. The treatment in perforation of the cervical oesophagus is drainage and, whenever possible, suture repair. Parenteral nutrition and antibiotic therapy are started. When the perforation is intrathoracic, suture repair should be attempted. The repair should be secured by a flap of local tissue. Many types of flaps have been used, e.g. pericardium, diaphragm, intercostal muscle, stomach wall and pleura. Usually the nearest suitable tissue is used. When carcinoma of the oesophagus causes perforation, oesophagectomy or bypass procedures can be selectively performed.

Oesophagobronchial Fistula

Oesophagotracheal and oesophagobronchial fistulas due to malignancy are not unusual. Their prognosis is poor. Usually the patients survive for some months only. The most common symptom is dysphagia and attacks of coughing. Signs point to aspiration of ingested food and aspiration pneumonia is common. The diagnosis is made by oesophagoscopy and bronchoscopy, during which a histological confirmation of the nature of the fistula can be made. A radiological examination using solutions not irritating to the lungs visualized the fistula. Treatment is different from case to case; the ideal treatment is to excise the oesophagus with the fistula. This can, however, rarely be done because of malignant invasion into surrounding tissues. Oesophageal intubation and various exclusion procedures may achieve palliation for these patients.

Inflammation and Infection

In this context only selected aspects are considered. Many cancers in the thorax are combined with infection or inflammation in surrounding tissues, organs or pleural cavity. Treatment depends on disease, condition of the patient and stage of cancer and varies according to the clinical situation. In persistent suppurative pneumonia or frank lung abscess secondary to lung cancer not amenable to surgery for cure, palliative lobectomy to remove the obstructive and/or necrotic tumour can be performed. When pleural empyema is caused by lung cancer the prognosis is poor, but thoracotomy or fenestration against infection and sepsis, and also to improve ventilation, are performed.

Pleural Effusion

Malignant pleural effusions are most commonly secondary to lung and breast cancer or lymphomas. This effusion often seriously impairs ventilatory function. Successful palliation may allow months to years of productive life. Repeated thoracocentesis is performed initially to relieve symptoms. However, effective palliation requires obliteration of the pleural space and for selected patients thoracostomy with instillation of synechia-producing agents such as tetracycline or talk suspension can be performed. Pleurectomy is the best palliative method, but is restricted to patients in otherwise good condition.

Haemorrhage

Tracheobronchial Massive Bleeding

The usual causes of massive lower respiratory tract bleeding include pulmonary cavities, bronchiectasis and aspergilloma. Only rarely is cancer found to cause massive bleeding. Preoperative localization of the bleeding site can usually be established by bronchoscopy, even during active bleeding, using fiberoptic or rigid bronchoscopes. If massive, continuing bleeding is localized to a certain lobe, it should be removed. Lobectomy may be contraindicated by advanced pulmonary disease, inability to locate the bleeding site, or inoperable carcinoma.

Pleural and Pericardial Bleeding

Whereas some degree of pleural bleeding may occur without further consequences, massive bleeding due to a malignancy associated with pleural carcinosis is unusual and a sign of poor prognosis. Thoracostomy is performed for palliation but massive bleeding may require thoracotomy for removal of clots and to relieve ventilation. Pleurectomy can be considered but can seldom be carried out. Pericardial bleeding may in exceptional cases be caused by thoracic cancer.

Oesophageal Bleeding

Only massive bleeding is discussed. Bleeding oesophageal varices may also, in addition to the usual causes, be secondary to cancer, whereas oesophageal cancer very rarely causes significant acute bleeding. The diagnosis is usually made by endoscopy, and treatment varies according to cause and site of bleeding. Small bleeding sites can be handled endoscopically by diathermy, and also Nd:YAG laser therapy has given good results.

References

Austin EH, Flye MW (1979) The treatment of recurrent malignant pleural effusion. Ann Thorac Surg 28: 190–203

Belsey RHR (1980) Palliative management of esophageal carcinoma. Am J Surg 139: 789–794

Fleischer D, Sivak MV Jr (1985) Endoscopic Nd:YAG laser therapy as palliation for esophagogastric cancer. Parameters affecting initial outcome. Gastroenterology 89: 827–831

Grillo HC (1978) Tracheal tumours: surgical management. Ann Thorac Surg 26: 112–125

Lokich JJ, Goodman R (1975) Superior vena cava syndrome. Clinical management. JAMA 231: 58–61

Lowe JE, Bridgman AH, Sabiston DC Jr (1982) The role of bronchoplastic procedures in the surgical management of benign and malignant pulmonary lesions. J Thorac Cardiovasc Surg 83: 227

Mannell A (1982) Carcinoma of the esophagus. Curr Probl Surg 14: 555–647

Michel L, Grillo HC, Malt RA (1981) Operative and nonoperative management of esophageal perforations. Ann Surg 194: 57–63

Ong GB, Kwong KH (1970) Management of malignant esophagobronchial fistula. Surgery 67: 293–301

Emergencies in Gastrointestinal Cancer

G. Willems

Emergency situations due to gastrointestinal cancers challenge the surgeon's skill as a technician as well as his or her knowledge of oncology. On the one hand complete surgical resection of the tumor is the only method for cure while on the other hand the poor general condition of the patient may prevent the required extensive surgical procedure.

Gastric Cancer

Massive bleeding causing hematemesis and/or melena occurs in approximately 5% of patients with gastric adenocarcinoma and in 10% of those with gastric sarcoma. Knowing the high mortality after emergency gastrectomies for hemorrhagic benign ulcers, the expected risk of extended gastric resections for cancer in bleeding patients is considerable. In fact, life-threatening bleeding from an operable gastric cancer is not a frequent situation. Many of these hemorrhagic cancers are relatively large tumors having reached a stage of unresectability. Whenever possible, conservative management using endoscopic coagulation is the best solution for bleeding tumors. Despite its technical feasibility, an emergency operation should be avoided when possible in such acute gastric hemorrhages.

Perforation of a gastric cancer is rare when compared with that of benign ulcers, but this emergency represents a significant problem to the surgeon because peritonitis always imposes an emergency laparotomy. Gastric perforations prove to be malignant in approximately one-third of the cases, while other perforated ulcers are usually not. Since endoscopy is contraindicated in perforation peritonitis, the preoperative diagnosis of cancer is regularly missed. Even at laparotomy the differential diagnosis between an old calloused benign ulcer and an ulcerated cancer may be extremely difficult because of the edema and inflammatory thickening of the tissues. Examination of frozen sections is not always possible in most institutions. When available, it is less reliable than that of paraffin-embedded ulcer edges because of many false-negative results. Moreover, gastric perforations are often larger and their edges are more friable than are those of duodenal or pyloric ulcers. Closing such a lesion is not always that easy and it is prone to bleed or to break down. Consequently, most authors recommend a "blind" emergency gastrectomy in patients with a gastric perforation. Only a few exceptions escape this rule, namely patients in which laparotomy is performed more than 24 h after the perforation. Perforated ulcers which are pyloric or immediately prepyloric are generally included in the group of benign duodenal ulcers.

Simple closure after wide resection of the gastric ulcer margins for biopsy may be safer for the immediate postoperative evolution of the patient. But the tight postoperative adhesions that will develop will render the curative character of a secondary elective gastrectomy much more hazardous.

Midgut Cancers

Dramatic bleeding from pancreatic adenocarcinoma is often a consequence of massive tumoral invasion of the duodenal wall in patients receiving chemotherapy. Surgery in such patients appears to be useless. Obstruction of the duodenum is another late complication of unresectable pancreatic cancers. Prevention of this complication by a gastroenterostomy at the time of an elective palliative operation for bile derivation is advocated when the tumor is not resectable. One might expect a prolonged disease-free interval from such a preventive gastrointestinal bypass, although the real benefits for the patient are still controversial.

Small intestinal cancers, though very rare, manifest themselves with acute obstruction as a first symptom in the majority of cases. Their emergency resection with the corresponding mesenterial area and adequate safety margins followed by primary restoration of the bowel continuity does not usually involve special surgical difficulties. Occasional unresectable tumors can be bypassed by latero-lateral anastomosis most of the time.

Colon Cancer

Colon adenocarcinoma is probably the cancer which is the most frequently operated on as an emergency. Mechanical *obstruction* of the large bowel, mainly in the left colon, is the commonest complication. The frequency of *perforation*, either proximal to an obstructing tumor or directly through tumoral tissue, is approximately one-half of that of obstructive ileus. Life-threatening *hemorrhage* from colon cancer is very rare and can usually be palliated by conservative therapy. The main problem of emergency colectomies is not the actual resection but the fact that colonic anastomosis without bowel preparation is forbidden by traditional surgical rules. In the past, acute obstructions of the left colon were treated by transverse colostomy and those of the right colon by cecostomy or ileotransverse anastomosis. No resection and sometimes not even an exploration of the tumor was attempted at the time of the first operation. As a rule, the tumor was resected in a second stage after several weeks of recovery. A third operation was often required to close the colostomy.

Obstruction of the Right Colon

In recent years, an increasing tendency to eradicate the cancer at the time of the primary operation has been observed (Goligher 1984). At the present time, most authors agree that obstructing cancers of the right colon ought to be treated by a primary right hemicolectomy. Preventive decompression of the cecum by transcolic aspiration before starting its dissection may sometimes be useful. Ileotransversostomy is used when the tumor is unresectable; when alarming distention or a bluish color point to an imminent cecal perforation, addition of a cecostomy may be required.

Obstruction of the Left Colon and Upper Rectum

There is still much controversy over the treatment of left-sided obstruction (Del Cimmuto et al. 1983). Three-stage operations are increasingly criticized though they were the best proposed solution 30 years ago. Yet, general progress in perioperative care is allowing for more aggressive approaches. Despite the immediate safety of primary colostomies, the cumulative morbidity of three successive operations, namely that of a colostomy closure, is high (Foster et al. 1985). Abstinence from primary resection can be deplored bitterly; for instance when infection of the initial laparotomy wound postpones the actual resection of the cancer for several weeks or when the patient obstinately refuses a second operation. Finally, there are several studies indicating that the long-term survival of obstructed cases may be better after primary resection than after initial decompression (Fielding Wells 1974; Umpleby and Williams 1984; Vidger et al. 1985). Therefore, the accumulation of arguments in favor of emergency resection is reaching a convincing critical mass.

Risky Techniques for Resection of Left Obstructing Tumors

A very audacious way to treat colon cancers in one stage is the primary resection with an immediate colocolostomy. Most of us feel that performing an anastomosis on distended and edematous colonic walls without any bowel preparation transgresses all established surgical laws. It is followed by anastomostic disruption in more than half of the cases although it may sometimes be successful in highly selected patients (Amsterdam and Krispin 1985), also without protective colostomy. But one should be careful about the initial enthusiasm for this heroic therapy because it may be rapidly tempered by some postoperative catastrophes. Moreover, when a protective colostomy is needed, many benefits of the procedure disappear.

Several methods of peroperative colonic washings have been described (Dudley et al. 1980) which may decrease considerably the risk of such primary resections with colocolostomy (Koruth et al. 1985). Recently, an ingenious method using an intracolonic bypass tube to protect a primary anastomosis without preparation has been proposed (Ravo and Ger 1985). Recent simplification of the "on table" lavage technique has made it an acceptable procedure in low-risk patients (Donaldson and Hughes 1987). One should still consider that acrobatic manoeuvers may actually lead to prolonged operations, which are best kept short in poor condition patients.

A most attractive procedure is the resection of not only the tumoral colonic segment but also that of the entire colon proximal to the tumor. Anastomosis between the ileum and the undistended empty colon distal to an obstruction has indeed appeared to be a safe procedure after right hemicolectomy in the past. Therefore, this principle has been applied also to obstructive tumors of the transverse colon, and then to cancers located more and more distally. Subtotal and even total colectomy for obstruction with primary ileosigmoid or ileorectal anastomosis is gaining interest (Deutch et al. 1983; Goligher 1984). While using this method, the manipulation of a distended colon, especially at the splenic flexure, is a dangerous manoeuver which may be factilitated by a preliminary transcolic aspiration. The immediate anastomosis between the small intestine and the empty distal colon is easy and relatively safe. Though interesting indeed, this one-stage technique should not be carried out in patients at high risk, nor by surgeons with insufficient experience of elective colon surgery.

Classical Techniques for Resection of Left Obstruction Tumors

Fortunately there are less risky alternatives for carrying out emergency resections. One of them is resection with the formation of a double colostomy, which is in fact an adaptation of the procedure of Paul Mickulicz. The free ends of the proximal and distal colon are simply brought to the skin at convenient sites separate from the laparotomy wound. This method offers the advantage of being short and safe, without any bowel suture. The necessity of subperitoneal mobilization of the rectum for bringing the distal colon end to the surface without tension may, however, lengthen the procedure when the growth lies in the mid or distal sigmoid.

Actually, the classical procedure of Hartmann seems to be a most practical alternative. Resection of the tumor, closure of the distal colonic segment with a stapler, and performing a proximal end colostomy is as quick and safe an operation as the double colostomy. This procedure can be used for resectable tumors of the mid and distal sigmoid without needing a dissection of the rectum from the sacral cavity. It is also an adequate method for obstructing high rectal tumors. Whatever the technique used, a second operation will eventually be required and the 5%–10% frequency of fecal fistulas after closure of a colostomy has to be considered (Foster et al. 1985). If the patient's condition is really very poor before the operation, a simple transverse colostomy is still useful. Finally, the only reasonable treatment of obstructing tumors which are not resectable is, of course, a diverting colostomy either on the transverse colon or on the sigmoid in the case of more distal tumors.

Perforation Peritonitis and Colon Cancer

Perforation in colon cancer may occur at the site of the tumor or proximal to an obstructive tumor, mainly in the cecum. Fecal peritonitis is still extremely lethal, ranging between 30% and 40% (Hermanek et al. 1985). Recent, though smaller, series point to a more favorable outcome when primary resection can be carried out (Day and Bates 1984; Koruth et al. 1985).

In perforated cancers of the right and transverse colon, resection and ileocolic anastomosis is advocated whenever the patient's condition and the tumoral growth permit. Primary resection with Hartmann's operation, or double colostomy, are the procedures of choice for perforated cancers of the left colon. When the tumoral growth obstructs the left colon and the perforation occurs in the cecum, a complementary cecostomy performed by inserting a Petzer tube into the perforation is a simple and expedient method. In some patients with a poor general condition a preliminary transverse colostomy with drainage may be the only reasonable possibility. However, if such a patient recovers, the secondary curative resection of the tumor several weeks later may become a challenge to oncological surgery. Tight adhesions will develop which often prevent adequate dissection of interfaces or pedicles and sectioning where it ought to be. The latter difficulty is one of the reasons why primary resection in peritonitis is generally recommended.

Postoperative Survival in Complicated Colon Cancer

The immediate postoperative mortality in obstructing cancer ranges from 20% to 25% in most unselected series of patients and this mortality is no higher in patients treated by primary resection than after staged resections (Hermanek et al. 1985; Vigder et al. 1985). The 5-year survival rate of the patients after an obstructing cancer is approximately 25%–30%, i.e., half of that of the complicated colon cancers (Ohmann 1982; Willett et al. 1985). This poor prognosis is due to several factors, namely a high incidence of advanced disease, but probably also to uselessly postponing the resection of the tumoral growth. Data indicating a twofold higher long-term survival rate after primary resection (Fielding and Wells 1974; Vigder et al. 1985) should, however, be considered with caution. Randomizing patients in such dramatic situations is difficult and may involve ethical problems, so no prospective studies on this point are available. Five-year survivals after perforation of colon cancer may reach 45% after curative resection. Increase in the proportion of cancers at a Dukes C stage may explain this outcome, but increased peritoneal seeding at the time of perforation cannot be held responsible for the observed failures (Willett et al. 1985).

References

Amsterdam E, Krispin M (1985) Primary resection with colocolostomy for obstructive carcinoma of the left side of the colon. Am J Surg 150: 558

Day T, Bates T (1984) Obstructing perforated carcinoma of the left colon treated by resection and the formation of a double colostomy. Br J Surg 71: 558–560

Del Cimmuto P, Gentile G, De Bernardinis O, De Laurentis D, Della Sciucca A, Calli T, Cellini G (1983) Il trattamento chirurgico nell' occlusione acuta da carcinoma dell grosso intestino. Chir Ital 35: 916–932

Deutch AA, Zelikovsky A, Sternberg A, Reiss R (1983) One stage subtotal colectomy with anastomosis for obstructing carcinoma of the left colon. Dis Colon Rectum 26: 227–230

Donaldson DR, Hughes LE (1987) Notes on "on table" lavage. Br J Surg 74: 465–466

Dudley HAF, Radcliffe AG, Mc Geehan D (1980) Intraoperative irrigation of colon to permit primary anastomosis. Br J Surg 67: 80–81

Fielding LP, Wells BW (1974) Survival after primary and staged resection for large bowel obstruction caused by cancer. Br J Surg 61: 16–18

Foster M, Leaper D, Williamson R (1985) Changing patterns in colostomy closure: the Bristol experience 1975–1982. Br J Surg 72: 142–144

Goligher J (ed) (1984) Surgery of the anus, colon and rectum, 5th edn. Baillère Tindall, Eastbourne, p 485

Hermanek PJ, Schweiger M, Gall FP (1985) Das colorectale Carcinom als chirurgischer Notfall. Langenbecks Arch Chir 366: 461–465

Koruth NM, Krukowski ZH, Youngeton GG, Hendry WS, Logie JRC, Jones PF, Munro A (1985) Intra-operative colonic irrigation in the management of left sided large bowel emergencies. Br J Surg 72: 708–711

Ohmann U (1982) Prognosis in patients with obstructing colorectal carcinoma. Am J Surg 143: 742–747

Ravo B, Ger B (1985) Temporary colostomy – an outmoded procedure? A report on the intracolonic bypass. Dis Colon Rectum 28: 904–907

Umpleby HC, Williamson RCN (1984) Survival in acute obstructing colorectal carcinoma. Dis Colon Rectum 27: 299–304

Vigder L, Tzur N, Huber M, Mahagna M, Amir I (1985) Management of obstructive carcinoma of the left colon. Comparative study of staged and primary resection. Arch Surg 120: 825–828

Willett C, Tepper JE, Cohen A, Orlow E, Welch C (1985) Obstructive and perforative colonic carcinoma: patterns of failure. J Clin Oncol 3: 379–384

Obstruction, Perforation, Inflammation, and Haemorrhage in Urological Cancer

R. R. Hall

Prostate Cancer

Bladder Outflow Obstruction

The commonest emergency caused by carcinoma of the prostate is retention of urine, which may be acute or chronic.

Acute retention requires immediate relief by catheterisation, per urethra or by suprapubic puncture. Histological or cytological proof of cancer is imperative before any specific anticancer treatment is commenced, so transperineal or transrectal needle biopsy is essential in all cases if transurethral resection (TUR) is not to be performed. Thereafter opinions differ about the best form of treatment.

1. Once the diagnosis has been confirmed 2 weeks of adequate hormone therapy is given while staging investigations are completed and radical prostatectomy is performed or radiotherapy commenced. If these are unsuitable and hormone treatment unsuccessful, TUR is performed as a palliative procedure.
2. An alternative treatment favoured by many urologists is to perform transurethral resection of the prostate at the earliest opportunity followed in due course by a bone scan, other staging investigations and a decision about specific anticancer treatment.

Which of these two treatment strategies is best in terms of long-term survival is unknown at the present time.

Chronic retention only requires immediate relief if it is causing impairment of renal function, in which case the patient should be catheterised and one of the two forms of treatment described above should be employed. If renal function is normal a diagnosis may be established by biopsy, the extent of the disease determined and hormone treatment or TUR performed without preliminary catheterisation, thereby minimising the infective complications associated with indwelling catheters.

Ureteric Obstruction. Prostate cancer may obstruct the lower ureters and cause oliguria or anuria and renal failure. Usually the associated hydroureter and hydronephrosis is apparent on ultrasound examination; intravenous urography is inappropriate if renal function is poor. This emergency may be relieved by percutaneous nephrostomy and the insertion of double pigtail ureteric stents introduced via the nephrostomies. Thereafter, some form of hormone manipulation will be required. Management of this situation in the past has been by cystoscopy and attempts at retrograde ureteric catheterisation or even operative ureterostomy in situ. These are no longer necessary as percutaneous nephrostomy is much easier for the patient and the clinician and avoids an anaesthetic as an emergency when the patient is most ill.

Obstruction of the Rectum. Rapidy advancing prostate cancer may obstruct the rectum. Dissimpaction of the bowel by enemas may suffice, but colostomy should be considered. This may only need to be temporary if hormone manipulation, radiotherapy or chemotherapy are successful in shrinking the obstructing prostatic growth.

Flare Phenomenon. Treatment of prostate cancer with luteinising hormone releasing hormone (LHRH) analogues may aggravate the symptoms during the first 2 or 3 weeks of treatment if an anti-androgen such as flutamide or cyproterone acetate is not given as well. Similarly, obstruction of the urinary tract may be made worse and emergency treatment may become necessary. However, this "flare" phenomenon should not occur if an anti-androgen is prescribed.

Haemorrhage. Prostate cancer may produce sudden urethral bleeding, haematuria or clot retention. The acute management of such haemorrhage is the same as for other causes of serious lower urinary tract bleeding.

Carcinoma of the Bladder

Haemorrhage. Bladder cancer may cause bleeding that requires emergency treatment in three situations:

1. As a presenting symptom with profuse haematuria and clot retention
2. Postoperative bleeding following endoscopic resection
3. Abnormal vessels or telangiectasia that develop following radiotherapy to the bladder

Profuse, spontaneous or postoperative bleeding with clot formation in the bladder can cause profound hypotension and bradycardia and requires prompt treatment. Attempts to evacuate intravesical clot with a catheter and syringe are seldom successful and many patients in this situation require urgent cystoscopy under general anaesthesia, removal of clot with a suitable evacuator and endoscopic cautery of the source of the haemorrhage. Prolonged attempts to restore the patient's general condition by intravenous transfusion and circulatory stimulants are ill advised; the circulatory shock associated with clot retetion usually improves spontaneously once the clot has been evacuated from the bladder. The bleeding usually stops as well once the clot has been removed. Bladder tumours have a good blood supply and the resection of even superficial tumours can be difficult, identification of bleeding arteries amongst the fronds of large papillary tumours can be impossible and in this situation the resection must be continued swiftly but carefully so as to reach the pedicle or base of the tumour where the vessel can be identified and haemostasis achieved.

Difficult endoscopic resection of bladder tumours is made much easier by the use of a continuous flow resectoscope sheath connected to a low-pressure suction apparatus.

Postradiotherapy bleeding can be persistent and severe and when it is life-threatening emergency cystectomy should not be discounted. However, embolisation of the internal iliac arteries can stop the bleeding provided the small branches of *both* internal iliac arteries are occluded by the procedure. Just as the operative ligation of the main internal iliac artery is usually unsuccessful, so the embolisation of the main arteries alone is of little benefit because it does not deal with the cross circulation in the pelvis that feeds the abnormal small vessels in the bladder wall that are the cause of the problem. Furthermore, some bleeding may persist because it is of venous origin.

This form of treatment is not without its complications, but should be considered if an experienced interventional radiologist is available.

For less serious postradiotherapy haemorrhage endoscopic electrocautery may be effective. For diffuse bleeding, Helmstein balloon distension within the bladder may improve haemostasis. In patients with incurable and inoperable bladder cancer, haemostasis may be achieved by the instillation of formalin in the bladder. This treatment is extremely painful and requires either general or spinal anaesthesia during which 100–200 ml 10% formalin is instilled in the bladder for 10 min, following which the bladder is washed out thoroughly with normal saline. This treatment may produce severe oedema of the bladder wall which may obstruct the ureteric orifices and cause anuria for 24–48 h, but is helpful in some patients.

Obstruction. Carcinoma of the bladder may cause acute retention but this can be relieved by catheterisation and definitive treatment instituted at subsequent cystoscopy.

A much more difficult problem is presented by the patient with invasive cancer of the base or posterior wall of the bladder that obstructs both ureters causing renal failure. The malignancy causing the problem will usually be found at cystoscopy; provided the tumour is mobile within the pelvis on bimanual examination, and is potentially operable, a deep resection biopsy should be taken and a catheter passed up each ureter. If this is not possible, percutaneous nephrostomy will allow renal function to improve as far as possible and infection to be treated while the type and extent of the underlying tumour can be established. If recovery of renal function and the general condition of the patient warrant an attempt at curative treatment, cystectomy may be undertaken with or without preoperative radiotherapy. If the latter is preferred, "flash" treatment with 20 Gy in 5 days is recommended as this shortens the duration of dependence upon percutaneous nephrostomies. If radical radiotherapy is preferred to cystectomy, bilateral ureteric stents will be required to maintain renal function during extended treatment. Because the ureteric orifices are probably obscured by tumour, these stents will have to be advanced from above via the nephrostomies.

With the advent of more effective cytotoxic chemotherapy against bladder cancer, even patients with tumours extending to the pelvic wall (T4b) may justify an attempt to improve renal function, so that one or two cycles of treatment with a drug combination including cis-platinum with methotrexate, adriamycin or vinblastine may be tried. If there is good objective evidence of tumour response, cystectomy may be possible.

Perforation. Spontaneous perforation of the bladder due to carcinoma is very rare and this complication usually arises following endoscopic resection, particularly if obturator spasm has been a problem. If *extraperitoneal* perforation occurs, there should be no problem provided it is recognised. If the resectionist is inexperienced, the resection should be stopped and a catheter inserted. However, ideally the tumour resection should be completed and then the perforation enlarged deliberately so that any extravasated fluid may drain back into the bladder from the perivesical tissues. Postoperatively, a urethral catheter should drain the bladder for 7–10 days. If an *intraperitoneal* perforation occurs, laparotomy should be performed immediately and the hole in the bladder closed by simple suture. If the possibility of an intraperitoneal perforation is suspected during tumour resection, the depth of the resection site should be probed thoroughly, even if this enlarges a small perforation, rather than run the risk of overlooking this potentially serious complication.

Carcinoma of the Renal Pelvis and Ureter

These uncommon tumours may cause acute obstruction or ureteric colic. Symptomatic treatment is all that is required immediately and subsequent investigation by ultrasound, urography and ureterorenoscopy will reveal the diagnosis.

Carcinoma of the Urethra

This malignancy is a rare cause of acute or chronic retention of urine. The presence of a mass in the perineum or the presence of a perineal fistula suggests the likely cause and in such cases suprapubic puncture is preferable to urethral catheterisation.

Carcinoma of the Kidney

Haemorrhage. Haematuria is a common presenting sympton of renal cancer but bleeding is seldom severe. Occasionally a brisk haemorrhage into the renal pelvis may cause ureteric colic during the passage of blood clot down the ureter. Opiates and bed rest are usually all that are required but ureteroscopy or ureteric catheterisation may sometimes be beneficial. If haematuria is persistently troublesome, nephrectomy is indicated as a palliative measure. Embolisation of the renal artery has been recommended as a less traumatic alternative but it may fail or be of only temporary benefit because it is impossible to embolise the whole of the parasitic circulation supplying large renal tumours.

On rare occasions a renal tumour may present as an emergency with severe loin pain due to haemorrhage within the tumour that is either spontaneous or follows mild trauma. Tenderness in the loin, a space-occupying lesion in intravenous urogram (IVU) and an intrarenal or subcapsular haematoma on ultrasound indicate the diagnosis; bed rest and analgesia relieve the symptoms pending a decision about definitive treatment. Haemorrhage occurring during nephrectomy is probably the most common cause of anxiety for surgeons dealing with carcinoma of the kidney. When operating on extensive tumours the problem arises from the numerous fragile vessels surrounding the kidney that have to be divided before the renal pedicle can be isolated. Division of these fragile vessels between metal clips is quicker and more effective than conventional ligatures or electrocautery. At the renal hilum, ligature of the renal vein before the artery can make bleeding worse and it is usually advisable to apply at least one ligature around the renal artery *before* dividing the vein. Preoperative arterial embolisation is seldom helpful in these difficult cases.

A rare but dramatic emergency during nephrectomy is the acute obstruction of the pulmonary circulation by a thrombus or tumour embolus dislodged from the vena cava or renal vein during dissection of the hilum. Immediate pulmonary embolectomy can save this situation if it is recognised and such patients have been known to enjoy a long tumour-free survival. Both of these operative problems can be anticipated and avoided by careful preoperative work-up. The site and extent of local involvement by a kidney cancer can be demonstrated clearly by ultrasound, CT scanning and angiography and these investigations are a prerequisite for safe surgery.

Cancer of the Testis

Tumors of the testis can present with acute symptoms of swelling, pain and inflammation of the scrotum, which are indistinguishable on clinical examination from epididymo-orchitis or torsion. Even after urine microscopy, scrotal ultrasound and Doppler examination of the testis, the diagnosis may still be in doubt and urgent surgical exploration is mandatory in case torsion is the cause of the problem.

If the testis is exposed through the scrotum and a tumour is found, dissemination can, and does, occur to the scrotum and inguinal lymph glands. Such spread causes major problems for effective treatment and is completely avoidable if all emergency testicular operations are performed through an inguinal incision.

Tumours of the testis may also present with a hydrocele or haematocele, sometimes following trauma, and the possibility of an underlying tumour may be overlooked. To avoid a potential rare, but real, disaster, it is safest *not* to try needle aspiration of testicular swellings in young men and to perform *all* testicular explorations in men under the age of 50 years through inguinal incisions.

Carcinoma of the Penis

Carcinoma of the penis occurs most commonly in uncircumcised men particularly when the foreskin does not retract. Because of this many men with this disease present with discharge and/or haemorrhage from under the foreskin. There may also be acute infective inguinal lymphadenopathy. Any man in this situation should be treated by dorsal slit incision of the foreskin which will reveal the underlying tumour and provide access for biopsy. Circumcision allows infection to subside and the true extent of the tumour to be determined before deciding which local treatment is most appropriate.

Following treatment of the primary tumour by partial amputation, radiotherapy or Nd:YAG laser, any inguinal lymphadenopathy should be left to subside for 4–6 weeks, helped by appropriate antibiotics. Lymphadenopathy that persists after this time is almost certainly due to metastases and needle biopsy and pelvic CT scan should be performed for confirmation followed by inguinal block dissection, radiotherapy or chemotherapy as considered appropriate.

Hemorrhage, Obstruction, Perforation, and Inflammation in Gynecological Cancer

W. H. MATTHEIEM

Hemorrhage

Hemorrhage is a frequent first symptom of gynecological cancer, in both cervical and endometrial tumors. Any abnormal bleeding necessitates immediate and adequate investigations to rule out or diagnose these conditions. Treatment consists essentially of the adequate cure of the underlying pathology by surgical or physical procedures or a combination of both.

Hemorrhage also occurs as a late complication of treated or advanced untreated gynecological tumors. In treated patients, if we exclude immediate postsurgical or radiological complications, vaginal bleeding occurring months or years later is due either to local recurrence or less frequently to late radionecrosis. Treatment will vary according to previous therapy and actual condition, especially local extension of the disease. If the bleeding reveals only a limited vaginal recurrence of either cervical or endometrial cancer, local irradiation can be useful if it can still be performed without risk of necrosis. In all other cases, surgery is the only curative or palliative measure, perhaps with some form of experimental chemotherapy. Here again, previous treatment and extent of disease will dictate the choice of procedure. In patients treated by physical therapy alone and when the lesions are still confined to the cervix, corpus uteri, and/or upper vagina, radical hysterectomy is adequate. In all other cases an exenterative procedure must be envisaged. Two conditions must be met to justify anterior, posterior, or total pelvic exenteration. The surgeon must be reasonably sure of mobilizing and removing the entire mass of tumoral tissue. Palliative incomplete surgery is unacceptable at such a price. The patient must be clearly informed before the surgeon can consider her consent as valid. In all other cases, inoperable disease, or refusal by the patient, radiation and/or chemotherapy can be considered. Nonexenterative palliative surgery has few indications when the actual or foreseeable quality of life of the patient is otherwise still acceptable.

For hemorrhage as the main disturbing complaint, ligation of the appropriate vessel(s), such as the internal iliac artery, is sometimes worthwhile, as are simple derivative procedures, digestive and/or urinary. Sudden or insidious intraabdominal hemorrhage is very rarely encountered in gynecological cancers. It occurs sometimes in partially necrotic advanced forms of cystic varieties of ovarian malignant tumors. Surgical treatment is indicated according to the stage of the disease.
External hemorrhage can occur in advanced vulvar epitheliomas, both from the primary site and from inguinal adenopathies, but are fortunately no longer seen nowadays. Treatment consists of radical surgery if possible or proximal vessel ligatures, which are preferable to attempts at superficial cauterization.

Obstruction

Digestive obstruction is frequently the first symptom of unrecognized ovarian cancer. In other gynecological tumors, it occurs as a late complication in a known disease that may or may not have been treated. Urinary obstruction is usually ignored if adequate explorations are not performed, because they are frequently unilateral and painless in the presence of very slowly progressive hydronephrosis. It occurs more frequently in cervical tumors, before or after treatment.

When intestinal occlusion, as a first symptom, leads to the diagnosis of locally advanced ovarian cancer, exploratory surgery must be planned after a complete workup. As described in the chapter on ovarian cancer, surgery must fulfill a triple mission. Complete abdominal exploration and pathological staging must deliver a definitive diagnosis and a precise description of the extension of the disease. Debulking by ascitis evacuation and resection of all extirpable tumor masses should be achieved as extensively and completely as safely possible. The site, single or multiple, of obstruction must be treated by dissection, resection, or bypass. At a first attempt in previously untreated patients, every effort should be made to avoid external stomies, and radiotherapy and/or chemotherapy, in systemic or intraabdominal form, must be given the chance to act favorably on the disease and cure or prevent obstructive lesions.

This attitude must be the same in the advanced stage or late complications after therapy failures in all gynecological cancers. Colostomy should be proposed only if it gives complete relief of symptoms and no other form of conservative therapy can be offered. If the seats of occlusion are multiple, the comfort of the patient must be ensured by gastric suction, parenteral nutrition, and adequate sedation. Further surgery in these hopeless situations only results in unjustifiable added misery.

In the presence of unilateral urinary occlusion of a functional kidney, derivation by end-to-side ureteral implantation is advisable only if active palliative treatment is possible. Bilateral ureteral obstruction in nonresectable disease necessitates at least bilateral nephrostomy or ureterostomy and preferably an ileal conduit. The first solution is simple but not very comfortable for the patient; the second constitutes major surgery. Quality of life must be very carefully considered and not just survival at those stages of ultimately incurable disease.

Perforation

Perforation is practically never a symptom in early untreated gynecological cancer if rupture of a neoplastic ovarian cystic tumor is excluded.

Ureteral fistula resulting in urinary peritonitis or leakage through a permeable vaginal suture sometimes occurs after radical hysterectomy, more often with radical lymphadenectomy, when ureteral dissection results in extended vascular suppression, or is performed in a site previously heavily radiated. Treatment must vary accordingly. If radiolesions are obvious, derivation in a healthy site by end-to-contralateral ureteral side may be performed. Sometimes the use of an ileal internal conduit offers the only solution if suitable synthetic graft material is not available. In nonradiated cases, end-to-end ureteral suture and ureterocystostomy with or without a tube-shaped bladder pediculated flap, is usually the best and simplest solution.

Vesicovaginal and rectovaginal fistulae may result from extension of the disease, mainly in cervical cancer. They are more often the consequence of late complications of radiotherapy, sometimes radical surgery, and particularly the combination of both. In the presence of residual or recurrent disease, only an adequate procedure of pelvic exenteration is able to cure the fistula and the disease. It should not be undertaken for palliation only. When no demonstrable neoplastic disease is present, closure by the simplest method must be attempted. The choice of the technique to be used depends mainly on the amount of healthy tissue available, or alternatively on the amount of necrotic damage, loss of substance, and size of the fistula. Sometimes, here again, only a form of pelvic exenteration with ileal conduit and/or terminal colostomy is a valid and definitive solution. In most of the cases, fortunately, lesser procedures are sufficient.

In all instances of rectovaginal fistulae a temporary loop colostomy must previously allow a clean operative site to be maintained. In both vesicovaginal and rectovaginal fistulae, the edge of the opening must be in a healthy condition, after spontaneous elimination of necrotic residues or by surgical trimming. The closure by tissue approximation and suture must be carried out by the easiest approach.

Laparotomy is sometimes required to separate inflammatory adhesions between the bladder, or the rectum and vagina. Closure of both defects is then performed separately and sometimes necessitates a deliberate cystostomy to visualize the fistula to be closed from the inside of the bladder. An indwelling catheter is left in place for at least 1 week when a urinary repair is performed. In the case of rectal repair, it is safe to reestablish the colonic continuity after 1 month when the lower lesion is safely healed.

Large defects can also be closed with a viable omental pediculated flap. This is sometimes difficult to perform in a previously operated, radiated, or treated abdomen. It becomes inpossible if the omentum has been removed or shows gross neoplastic spread.

When vaginal access is easy, these closures can be performed by perineal approach only, so as to avoid an unnecessary laparotomy. Technically, two procedures can be used. One consists of the section of the fused mucosae of the fistula with a sharp blade, or with a low-powered electric knife. The bladder or rectum are closed first and then the vaginal vault. Every effort should be made not to superimpose both sutures. Another useful artifice, when the fistula is fixed and its contours are clean, consists of making a circular incision around it in healthy vaginal tissue and dissecting it toward the fistula to obtain an annular flap. The distal border of this incision allows some dissection of vaginal tissue towards its external orifice. The deeper flap is sutured with its mucosa turned inside and so closes the bladder or rectal defect. The superficial flap is sutured with its mucosa turned outward and constitutes the new vaginal end. The sutures should not coincide. The indwelling catheter or colostomy should be maintained until satisfactory local healing is effected.

Small bowel fistulae, mainly ileal, are not often seen even in advanced gynecological cancers, with the exception of the sequelae of entensive pelvic exenteration when the quality of the perineal closure is compromised and when the unsupported visceral mass, without interposition of peritoneum, is allowed to adhere to thin skin flaps, poorly vascularized and often previously irradiated. At that stage, the patient is usually in poor condition and a physiological balance must first be reestablished by parenteral nutrition and continuous digestive aspiration. If no closure is obtained under these conditions, further surgery is the only solution. It is needless to say that these situations are unfortunately very precarious. Nevertheless, a cautious attempt must be made to eliminate all nonviable tissues, visceral and parietal, and to obtain the best possible closure, sometimes with synthetic reinforcing material.

Inflammation

Inflammation is not a very common symptom or complication of gynecological cancer. As an initial symptom, it occurs only in vulvar tumors, when it is first considered as an inflammatory skin condition. Biopsy should rapidly provide the correct answer. Unfortunately, in several instances, it is only the succession of failures of dermatological treatments and the extensive tendency of the disease that prompts the suspicion of a diagnosis of malignancy. It is true that superinfection is nearly always present, and inguinal nodes are often enlarged under these conditions. Before any decision is taken regarding more or less radical therapy, the pathological condition of the inguinal nodes must be assessed, by frozen sections if surgery is chosen.

Inflammation and infection complicating surgical treatment of gynecological cancer must be treated accordingly. Drainage and preventive or curative antibiotherapy must be used as the situation necessitates.

More specific inflammatory conditions are encountered in gynecological cancers as the result of the extensive use of intracavitary and external radiation therapy in areas where complete protection of adjacent organs such as the bladder, ureters, urethra, and rectum is impossible. The abdominal wall, perineum, and lower vagina are not spared either, and, when surgery is contemplated as part of a combined treatment, radiation dosage must be reduced and targetted accordingly. Salvage surgery after failure or complications of curative radiotherapy must always take into account the compromised viability of the pelvic tissues and organs.

The complications encountered are mostly described under the three other headings, hemorrhage, obstruction, and perforation. Inflammation is both cause and consequence in all the aforementioned occurrences.

Early and Late Complications of Oncological Treatment

G. C. DAVIES

Malignant tumours may be managed using one or more of several different therapeutic options. Surgery often plays a major role in primary treatment whereas irradiation, chemotherapy and hormonal manipulation may be used as adjuvant measures or for definitive treatment of the primary lesion. Palliative therapy is used in disseminated or locally advanced disease not amenable to surgical extirpation. Complications of the treatments themselves occur and may present to the surgeon. They will occasionally require surgical intervention, sometimes of an urgent nature.

Complications may occur during the administration of a course of treatment, in which case they are usually of a minor nature and usually are reasonably easily controlled without need for hospitalisation. They often subside with cessation of treatment and will not cause long-term problems. However, there may be a latent period before the onset of more severe side effects and these may be of more consequence to the patient and the surgeon.

Complications may manifest themselves as inflammatory responses with fibrosis, scarring, obstruction, gangrene or fistula formation. There may be disturbance of growth patterns of irradiated and normal tissues, impairment of repair processes and even acceleration of underlying coexistent diseases. Second neoplasms, different in nature to the primary tumour, may be induced at or near the site of the primary tumour or in a distant tissue. These complications may appear many years after the treatment of the original tumour and, indeed, the initial disease process may, erroneously, be dismissed as cured and unconnected with the subsequent presenting complaint.

The clinical picture accompanying the complication may result from a combination of factors related to the pathology of the primary tumour, its site, the mode and duration of previous treatment, the underlying pathophysiology of the complication, its site of occurrence in the body, its severity and the implications and outcome of its treatment. Paramount to the understanding of the aetiology of these complications is the need to recognise the effects of initial treatments, not only on the tumour but also on surrounding normal tissues and other elements such as the stroma within the tumour.

Antineoplastic treatment is not tumour specific but affects normal cells as well; therefore, all cancer treatments are associated with potential toxic side effects (Byrd 1985). As survival improves after cancer treatment so the frequency of long-term sequelae increases. Differences in the sensitivities of individual tissues to the various therapeutic options must be considered in determining the potential outcome of each projected treatment. These will govern which organs are to be affected and to what extent the damage to that particular organ is likely to be.

Complications of exposure to X-rays were reported within 6 months of Roentgen's discovery of ionising radiation in the Institute of Physics in the University of Wurzburg in Bavaria (Perthes 1903; Cade 1957; Dalinka and Mazzeo 1985). The first skin tumour to occur as a result of contact with these X-rays was a metastasising squamous carcinoma in an X-ray tube demonstrator within 6 years of the discovery of irradiation. Initially, complications were seen in technicians, scientists, doctors and nurses (Cade 1957). Nowadays, radiation safety procedures protect therapists and it is the patient who is at hazard. Better localisation of delivery of radiotherapy with supervoltage machines has meant the ability to deliver higher doses with increased chances of cure and an increased survival rate. Chemotherapy, which has similar effects to ionising radiation, is being more widely used, often in complex multimodal regimens, for an increasing variety of tumours, especially those of haematological, pulmonary, gastrointestinal or reproductive nature.

The recent success of combination chemotherapy for haematological malignancies, especially of a paediatric nature, has focussed attention on the long-term adverse sequelae of therapy (Byrd 1985; Matus-Ridley et al. 1985). Similar results are reported for testicular germ cell tumours where over 90% of patients expect to become long-term disease-free survivors (Oliver 1986). Adjuvant chemotherapy and hormonal treatment are being used with increasing prevalence and are likely to continue to be so used with more and varied agents becoming available. Hopefully the toxicity of these agents will continue to be reduced. However, the need for long-term studies in these patients is very obvious because of the protracted latent period that may exist between a treatment and its complications.

Many of the complications and their treatments fall within the province of the surgeon and selected examples will be discussed. The descriptions that follow are not necessarily comprehensive and take little account of the complications of surgery itself, which is, after all, still one of the major modalities of oncological treatment.

Radiation Injury to the Gastrointestinal Tract

Radiotherapy is increasingly being used to treat pelvic malignancy (Mettlin et al. 1981; MRC Working Party 1982). Encouraging results of early studies (Stearns et al. 1974; Allen and Fletcher 1982) and recent randomised trials of low-dose treatment (Roswit et al. 1975; Rider et al. 1977; Higgins 1978, 1979) have indicated higher long-term survival in irradiated patients. Increased dosage is, however, associated with a greater frequency of complications (Green et al. 1975; Palmer and Bush 1976; Piver and Lele 1976; Morganstern et al. 1977; Kinsella and Bloomer 1980; Schmitt and Symmonds 1981). Most frequently affected is the intestine.

Ionising radiation has a dose-related effect on the gastrointestinal tract by either one or both of two mechanisms. Firstly, there is a direct effect upon the intestinal epithelium (Quastler 1956; Wiernik 1966) with mucosal cell abnormalities which progress to atrophy and ulceration (Green et al. 1975) and, secondly, there is a vasculitis leading to progressive obliteration of minor and major intestinal blood vessels with consequent ischaemia, stricture formation or gangrene and perforation. The former effect tends to be an acute process occurring during treatment, whereas the latter becomes evident after a variable latent interval (Warren and Friedman 1942). The degree of damage will vary with the region of bowel irradiated and the dose of radiotherapy administered. High doses (over 4500 cGy) produce most damage, although even low-dose regimens may have potentially serious effects (Villasanta 1972; Palmer and Bush 1976). The sensitivity to irradiation seems to vary amongst individuals and it remains difficult to predict the outcome in any single patient.

Bowel complications may be expected in up to 10% of patients after pelvic irradiation (De Cosse et al. 1969; Palmer and Bush 1976), with up to one-fifth of these patients requiring surgery (Morganstern et al. 1977; Russell and Welch 1979; Schmitt and Symmonds 1981). The large bowel is most commonly affected (Hatcher et al. 1985), with the rectum being the site of injury in up to 70% of affected patients (Anseline et al. 1981; Hatcher et al. 1985). Next most commonly affected is the sigmoid colon, followed by the ileum and caecum. Multiple lesions are common. The frequency of rectal involvement may be partially accounted for by the fixity of the rectum compared with the apparent mobility of the small bowel, caecum and pelvic colon. Damage is most likely to be seen after irradiation of the uterine cervix, especially when intracavitary irradiation has been combined with external beam therapy. Injury also occurs with treatment of vesical and prostatic tumours, other reproductive organ tumours and gastrointestinal neoplasms, especially of the rectum.

Predisposing factors to intestinal damage by radiotherapy include arterial insufficiency due to hypertension, other cardiovascular diseases and diabetes mellitus (De Cosse et al. 1969), previous chemotherapy (Cassady et al. 1975) and intra-abdominal sepsis or previous operations (Localios et al. 1969; Van Nagell et al. 1974, 1977). Although, in some series, over 50% of patients with radiation injury may have undergone previous surgery for intestinal resection or staging procedures prior to radiotherapy (Schmitt and Symmonds 1981) and may have extensive adhesions (LoIudice et al. 1977), pretreatment barium studies do not, however, support the theory that tethering of the bowel predisposes to radiation injury (Green et al. 1975). Females are more likely to suffer the effects of radiation, not only because of the increased frequency of pelvic irradiation, but because they have a proportionately larger percentage of intestine within their pelvis. The presence of small bowel within the pelvis is probably the most important factor in limiting the dose of radiotherapy that can be given (Potish et al. 1979).

The median onset of symptoms has been reported as 4.2 months postirradiation and most patients who are destined to get symptoms will do so within the 1 year following radiotherapy (Kwitko et al. 1982). Occasionally the interval is longer. Presentation will vary with the type of injury and degrees of severity from trivial, easily controlled problems to life-threatening catastrophies will be encountered. There may be mucosal inflammation producing pain, nausea, diarrhoea, mucous discharge or haemorrhage. Partial or complete obstruction may occur and devitalisation of the bowel may lead to perforation and peritonitis, abscess formation or the appearance of a fistula.

Radiation Damage to the Rectum

The majority of patients undergoing pelvic irradiation develop a transient proctocolitis with diarrhoea and tenesmus. It is usually self-limiting and related to the dose and daily fractionation of radiotherapy.

Chronic lesions in the rectum may resemble inflammatory bowel disease or, especially after cervical irradiation, present as an ulcer, usually situated on the anterior wall at the level of the cervix. Differentiation from a rectal carcinoma or recurrent primary tumour is difficult, even though the margins of the ulcer are typically clean cut as opposed to the rolled edges seen in a carcinoma. Biopsy is mandatory.

Clinical features of rectal injury can be explained by mucosal damage, reduced rectal capacity and compliance combined with myenteric plexus damage and smooth muscle changes. There may be accompanying sphincter dysfunction (Varma and Smith 1984) with reduced maximal resting manometric pressure, a reduction in the length of the anal canal high-pressure zone and diminution of the rectosphincteric reflex. These effects are manifested by pain and discomfort, urgency and tenesmus and an increased frequency of bowel action. Mucus and blood may be passed with the motions leading to anaemia. Fistulae may occur into the vagina, uterus or bladder.

Patients are often in poor general condition because of prolonged illness, dehydration, anaemia, disordered nutrition, recurrent disease and other accompanying medical conditions. Management includes general measures such as correction of dehydration, blood transfusion and the improvement of nutritional status, which may necessitate a prolonged period of parenteral feeding.

Surgery may be required for resection of bowel for haemorrhage, perforation, obstruction or fistula. Some lesions may only be amenable to bypass surgery. The principles of surgery in these patients are discussed below.

Radiation and Cytotoxic Injury to the Small Bowel

Acute radiation damage to the small bowel may present as nausea, colic and diarrhoea, usually subsiding on cessation of therapy. Up to 30% of long-term survivors of childhood malignancy have been documented as developing some form of radiation enteritis (Donaldson et al. 1975). Often this develops during or soon after treatment with radiotherapy and frequently settles on conservative treatment. Cytotoxic therapy is often associated with transient disturbance of intestinal function and this may be seen even with specific chemotherapeutic agents selectively infused into hepatic arteries (Gluck et al. 1985). Symptomatic measures are often all that is required in these patients. Antispasmodic drugs, anticholinergic agents and opiates may have therapeutic effects, as may cholestyramine (Heusinkveld et al. 1978) or sulphasalazine and aspirin (Mennie et al. 1975) in selected patients.

Chronic radiation changes may be manifested by

mild to severe obstructive colicky pain, malabsorption including steatorrhoea, or features similar to those seen with large bowel disease such as haemorrhage, obstruction, perforation and fistula formation. The incidence is between 5% and 15% in patients who have received in excess of 4500 cGy (Requarm and Roberts 1956; De Cosse et al. 1969; Maruyama et al. 1974; Palmer and Bush 1976; Morganstern et al. 1977; Kinsella and Bloomer 1980). Perforations may occur in up to one-fifth of these patients (Galland and Spencer 1985). Perforations in radiation enteritis are more commonly encountered in the small bowel than in the large intestine and may present as isolated lesions or supervene on intestinal obstruction. Occasionally, they may be seen in convalescent patients after abdominal surgery for unrelated disorders. This underlines the difficulty in dealing with adhesions, of which there may be many, in these patients. Dissection is apt to produce serosal tears, more so than in the unirradiated abdomen, and these tears are more prone to perforate in ischaemic bowel.

Symptomatic treatment should be contemplated in patients who do not have absolute indications for urgent surgery, since the risk of operation in these patients is high. Improvement in symptoms has been brought about by the administration of low-residue diets which are low in gluten, fat and milk protein. Steroid therapy may be used systemically or by enema (Hatcher et al. 1985). Temporary diverting colostomy may allow inflamed rectal mucosa to return to normal (Goligher 1984) but closure of this will often lead to a recrudescence of the disease. Operation carries a high postoperative morbidity and mortality due to the frequency of anastomotic failure (Wellwood et al. 1974; Swan et al. 1976; Galland and Spencer 1979) with subsequent abscess and fistula formation. Anastomotic leakage may occur in 30%–65% of patients. It is often necessary to carry out extensive resections of large or small bowel in order to ensure using healthy bowel for anastomoses. Such bowel should be recruited from outside the confines of previous radiotherapy. Resection and primary anastomosis of involved bowel is associated with an unacceptable risk of anastomotic failure and postoperative death. Bypass may carry a lower risk to the patient and have a better outcome (Swan et al. 1976) although this has not been found to be the case by some authors (Shamblin et al. 1964; Schier et al. 1964; Swan et al. 1976). Resection and primary anastomosis has been found to carry mortality rates that may reach 20%–50%, whereas that for bypass alone may only be in the region of 10%. Bypass may be of use for total exclusion of distressing enterocutaneous and enterovaginal fistulae (Piver and Lele 1976) although resection in these instances is more favoured by some (Schmitt and Symmonds 1981). Initial treatment of rectovaginal fistula should be by defunctioning colostomy, although a definitive procedure is almost always required at a later date. Total rectal excision with colo-anal sleeve anastomosis is a useful procedure in the latter case (Parks and Percy 1982). It is imperative that healthy tissue is interposed between rectum (if it is left in situ) and vagina. Operations have been devised using muscle (Ingleman-Sundberg 1960; Graham 1965), omentum (Bastiannse 1960) and non-irradiated colon (Bricker and Johnston 1979; Bricker et al. 1981). Such operations are technically difficult although the results can be rewarding. In certain instances, for example when the viability of the bladder or ureters is in doubt, resection may not be considered a feasible option. Proximal defunctioning operations or bypass procedures with restoration of intestinal continuity have the disadvantage that they do not remove the offending area of bowel and thus will probably not manifestly contribute to the patient's symptomatic improvement. Indeed complications may continue to increase in magnitude despite these procedures.

Alterations in treatment positions during radiotherapy have been tried in order to reduce the incidence of radiation injury to the small bowel (Green et al. 1975; Morganstern et al. 1977; Caspers and Hop 1983). These include treating the patient in the prone position and Trendelenberg's position, treating the patient with a distended bladder and using a variety of fields (Kinsella and Bloomer 1980). Various surgical procedures utilising the peritoneum, omentum, bladder, uterus and broad ligaments have been tried to keep the small bowel out of the pelvis (Freund et al. 1979; Kavanah et al. 1985). These have not met with success.

Prevention of radiation-induced bowel damage has been attempted experimentally by using absorbable synthetic mesh to exclude small bowel from the pelvis (Devereux et al. 1984). This has also been tried in a preliminary series of patients and so far has prevented radiation enteritis (Kavanagh et al. 1985). Prevention using pharmacological radioprotective agents, steroids or diet although, in some instances, experimentally originally encouraging, has not been adopted into practice (Morganstern and Hiatt 1967; Morganstern et al. 1970, 1977; Rachootin et al. 1972; Phillips et al. 1973; Green et al. 1975).

Complications Affecting the Bladder

The epithelium of the bladder wall, like gastrointestinal mucosa, is extremely sensitive to ionising radiation and to one specific chemotherapeutic agent, cyclophosphamide (Editorial, British Medical Journal 1985). Cyclophosphamide has a toxic action on bladder mucosa and may be associated with increased risk of subsequent bladder tumours (Wall and Clausen 1975; Plotz et al. 1979). Haemorrhage from such epithelium damaged by X-rays or chemotherapy may be recurrent and potentially fatal. It may occur in 10% of patients who have undergone pelvic radiotherapy and up to 40% of those receiving oral or intravenous cyclophosphamide. The drug itself, the cyclic phosphamide of nitrogen mustard, is probably not toxic in the form in which it is administered but is hydrolysed to an excreted metabolite which is directly damaging to urinary epithelium, producing a sterile cystitis. Although, because of increased contact time with bladder epithelium, lesions are most likely to be produced within the bladder, cyclophosphamide also produces a focal convoluted tubule necrosis in the kidney (Phillips et al. 1961). Renal effects are considerably less likely to be encountered than the bladder problems. Damage is more likely to occur in those patients receiving larger doses of cyclophosphamide at spaced intervals rather than those on a regular small daily dose (Rubin and Rubin 1966). Both conditions may be ameliorated by maintaining high fluid intake and cystitis may be lessened by frequent voiding to reduce interaction of the drug with epithelium. Significant changes in subepithelial tissues are seen histologically and occasionally the lesion may be difficult to differentiate from recurrent tumour. Cystoscopy reveals diffuse petechiae and it may be impossible to identify the exact source of bleeding. Local treatment measures such as diathermy coagulation may not control haemorrhage, and patients, because of their age and associated medical conditions, may not be considered suitable candidates for the complex surgery that is required to stop the bleeding. Occasionally, surgeons will have to resort to proximal urinary diversion in these patients (Pomer et al. 1983) and even consider emergency cystectomy in patients who fail to stop bleeding. Recent reports have advocated the use of alum, instilled into the bladder, for the control of massive postirradiation haemorrhage (Ostroff and Chenault 1982; Kennedy et al. 1984; Goel et al. 1985). Other agents have been tried intravesically in the past but with less success and, in some cases, unacceptable toxicity. These have included formalin (Fair 1974; Rao et al. 1978), phenol (Susan and Marsh 1975), aminocaproic acid (Kumar et al. 1976), steroids, silver nitrate, vasopressin (Pyeritz et al. 1978) and the Helmstein hydrostatic technique. Angiography and embolisation may be ineffective (Ram 1970) and may lead to bladder wall necrosis and perforation.

Occasionally radiation effects, themselves, may produce necrosis of the bladder wall with perforation and formation of a vesicocolic fistula. It is often difficult to know the exact causation of this condition as usually the radiation changes coexist in both the bladder and the large bowel.

The more chronic effect of radiation on the bladder is to produce fibrosis with severe contracture and loss of volume. This will result in troublesome increased frequency of micturition. Ureteric reflux due to damage to the bladder and lower parts of the ureters may compound the problem. Ureteric diversion into the ileum is said to be preferable to ureterosigmoidostomy in this condition since the more proximal ureter and the ileum are less likely to have been affected by the radiotherapy than the distal ureter and sigmoid colon, both of which are situated in the pelvis (Ram 1970). Colocystoplasty, to enlarge the bladder, may be of use in relieving the symptoms, as may balloon dilatation using the Helmstein technique.

Lymphoedema

Secondary lymphoedema of the limbs may follow extensive dissections of the axilla, groin or pelvis (Thompson 1970; Silver and Puckett 1976) and may be worsened by postoperative radiotherapy (Miller et al. 1973; Schnur 1977) or may occur after radiotherapy alone. Infection and progressive tumour invasion of the lymphatics may aggravate the condition. Oedema of genitalia or breast may be encountered, with the former occasionally occurring after pelvic radiotherapy as sole initiating event (Ram 1970). The disorder is progressive, disabling and not curable by conventional techniques.

The disorder may decrease in incidence with present trends away from radical block dissections in management of carcinoma of the breast and malignant melanoma and more refined radiotherapeutic protocols (Savage 1985). Lymphoedema of the leg may develop in up to 30% of patients undergoing a groin dissection for melanoma, but this procedure may not nowadays be indicated as a prophylactic measure in stage 1 disease (Sim et al. 1978).

Lymphoedema is manifested by swelling of the affected limb with restriction of movements, tightness, pain and the predisposition to develop recurrent cellulitis, lymphangitis and skin ulceration. The limb is more prone to infection because of compromise of immune defences (Fergusson et al. 1985).

Management of lymphoedema is mainly by conservative measures (Savage 1985) and these produce acceptable results in the majority of patients with mild or moderate problems. Most will not require surgery. The treatments available include rest and limb elevation, weight control, graduated pressure stockings, avoidance of trauma and meticulous attention to hygiene. Antibiotics should be used early if cellulitis supervenes. Antifungal agents may be indicated at times. Diuretics are of little use as are anticoagulants. Pneumatic compression devices may bring about considerable improvement, but there are problems with patient tolerance and with recurrence of the lymphoedema on cessation of treatment.

Surgical treatments to relieve lymphoedema include the implantation of fine multifilament Teflon (PTFE) wicks which extend the length of the limb and transgress into normal subcutaneous tissues proximal to the site of lymphatic damage (Thompson 1967; Kerstein and Licalzi 1977), the use of omental flaps (Goldsmith 1974; Chavez 1977) and other more complex procedures. These include myocutaneous and intestinal flaps and direct lymphaticovenous anastomosis and nodal-venous anastomosis usually by microvascular techniques (Nielubowicz 1968). There are considerable doubts about the long-term efficacy of these procedures and their potential complications. They remain the subject of further evaluation. More readily accepted procedures include staged removal of skin and subcutaneous tissue of the affected limb (Miller 1977; Sawhney 1980) and the use of the shaved dermal flap (Thompson 1962). These operations have been used with varying degrees of success although complications can be very troublesome (Schnur 1977).

Tumours may develop in lymphoedematous limbs, especially where oedema is of long duration. The commonest tumour encountered is a lymphangiosarcoma, typically seen in the upper limb after radical mastectomy and postoperative radiotherapy (Stewart and Treves 1948; Taswell et al. 1962). Others include haemangiosarcoma, Kaposi's sarcoma, melanoma and malignant fibrous histiocytoma (Danese et al. 1967).

Tumours may develop in lymphoedematous limbs for various reasons. The limb may be immunologically compromised because of obstruction to lymphatic outflow (Olszewski et al. 1978) by surgery, postradiotherapy fibrosis or tumour involvement. Obstructed lymphatic vessels may grow autonomously under lack of normal regulatory mechanisms, or accumulation of carcinogens may occur in the obstructed lymphatics. Treatment of these tumours is difficult since metastasis may be present at the time of presentation of the primary. Where metastases cannot be demonstrated, major limb ablation may be required.

Radiation to the Breast

Radiation to the breast is increasingly used as primary treatment with conservative operation for breast carcinoma formerly treated by mastectomy. It is also used as initial therapy for larger breast tumours, considered inoperable, and for palliation of locally advanced or recurrent disease (Bostwick et al. 1984). Radiation may induce breast necrosis, radionecrosis of the chest wall with ulceration, accelerated coronary artery atherosclerosis, brachial plexus pain and paresis, lymphoedema and axillary cicatrix formation. It may induce neoplasia, especially fibrosarcoma of the chest wall and leukaemia. Osteoradionecrotic wounds are painful and malodorous and threaten major haemorrhage because of vascular or cardiac erosion. The principles of treatment include the removal of radiation-damaged tissue, stabilisation of the chest wall when necessary and closure of the wound with healthy well-vascularised tissue including omentum, muscle or myocutaneous procedures such as the latissimus dorsi and rectus abdominis flaps (Jurkiewicz and Arnold 1977; Bostwick et al. 1978; Jurkiewicz et al. 1980; Mathes and Nahai 1982).

Complications in the Cardiovascular System

Irradiation of arteries accelerates atherosclerosis and may predispose to early occlusion (Fajardo 1977). Atherosclerosis occurs within the irratiated area, is more sharply defined and may be located atypically (Lawson 1985). To date the number of cases of coronary artery thrombosis ascribed to radiotherapy remains small (Byrd 1985). Clinical and experimental studies have shown that therapeutic doses of radiotherapy can induce cardiac damage (Stewart and Fajardo 1971). This may occur during irradiation of lungs, mediastinum or breast and chest wall. The most frequent findings are pericarditis or myocardial fibrosis (Fajardo et al. 1968). Coronary artery disease distribution parallels that seen in non-irradiated individuals and correction by coronary artery bypass grafting may be appropriate. The cardiotoxic effects of anthracyclines (e.g. doxorubicin) are well known (Dana and Jones 1982). Cyclophosphamide may also cause myocardial necrosis at high doses (Buckner et al. 1972) but these side effects do not call for surgical treatment.

The effects of radiotherapy on large arteries have not been widely reported. Subclavian artery thrombosis occurs as a late complication of breast irradiation. Damage to iliac and femoral vessels accelerates atherosclerosis and poses special problems in reconstruction. Extra-anatomical bypass may be required because of previous intra-abdominal surgery for radiation enteritis or the presence of a frozen pelvis or to exclude the vascular prosthesis from the area of the irradiated tissue with its increased risk of wound infection and dehiscence. Other sites include the carotid and vertebral arteries, aortic arch, distal abdominal aorta and mesenteric and femoral arteries (Lawson 1985). An increased frequency of thromboembolism has been shown in patients with malignant disease (Lieberman et al. 1961; Miller et al. 1967). An incidence of 17.6% has been reported in advanced breast cancer patients undergoing a five-drug chemotherapy regimen, including steroids known to produce hypercoagulability (Goodnough et al. 1984). Thrombotic events tended to occur during the early phase of chemotherapy. During therapy, patients tended to have shortened prothrombin times and greater factor VIII antigen: activity ratios, suggesting hypercoagulability.

Chemotherapy often involves injection of drugs known to be toxic to endothelium of peripheral veins where blood volume is small and blood flow is low. Thus delivery via a central vein is necessary since peripheral veins will rapidly become thrombosed and extravasation of injected drugs will occur, with tissue necrosis and ulceration. Management of these injuries is difficult and may require extensive surgical procedures for reconstruction.

The thrombosis rates of bovine heterografts and arteriovenous fistulae constructed for vascular access for chemotherapy may be in the region of 30%–50% (Lempert et al. 1979; Wade et al. 1981). It is less with silicone cannulae, implanted portals and implantable infusion pumps. Central venous thrombosis has been reported in up to 30%–40% of patients with long-term indwelling catheters (Fabri et al. 1982; Lokich and Becker 1983).

Complications Affecting Bones and Cartilage

Radiation arrests chondrogenesis in epiphyses, causes defects in uptake of calcium in the bone and cartilage of the metaphysis and causes deformity of the diaphysis (Parker and Berry 1976). The effects of irradiation on bone are mainly on osteoblasts and result in decreased matrix formation. Cell death may be immediate or delayed. There may be repair with recovery or arrest of cellular division and interruption of growth. Abnormal growth may appear, giving rise to deformity, and second malignant tumours may be induced.

The sequelae of radiation therapy are most often seen in the spine after childhood treatment of Wilm's tumour, neuroblastoma or medulloblastoma. The outcome in terms of deformity is related to the length of spine irradiated, the total dosage, the age at treatment, the time interval and the medical care after the radiotherapy. The deformity is most frequently manifested as scoliosis, although shortening of the spine may occur. This is especially so after complete craniospinal irradiation for medulloblastoma (Proberts et al. 1973). The worst problems are seen when the radiotherapy is administered before the age of 6 years (Byrd 1985).

Other bones that may be involved include the ribs, clavicle and humerus (after breast irradiation), femoral neck (pelvic tumours), orbit (retinoblastoma), other long bones (Ewing's tumour, osteogenic sarcoma and secondary tumours), pelvis (Wilm's tumour and neuroblastoma) and facial skeleton.

Changes in the pelvis have become increasingly less commonly encountered with the introduction of supervoltage radiotherapy. They may occasionally involve the sacroiliac joints or the acetabulum (Dalinka and Mazzeo 1985). Ribs are most commonly fractured at their anterior angles and the fractures are usually multiple. Fractures of the femoral neck used to be fairly commonplace after treatment of pelvic disease but have now reduced to an incidence of less than one per thousand (Parker and Berry 1976).

Osteoradionecrosis is a particularly unpleasant complication that may follow irradiation of the mandible or tonsil. Radiation increases the risk of dental caries, causes gum retraction and produces xerostomia associated with a rise in the salivary pH. Aseptic osteoradionecrosis presents a more minor problem, but secondary infection produces pain, ulceration, fistula formation and cellulitis. Cartilage necrosis may be a problem after irradiation of the pinna, nasal cartilages and cartilages of the larynx.

Osteonecrosis may also, uncommonly, occur in patients with Hodgkin's and non-Hodgkin's lymphoma as a late complication of combination chemotherapy, which includes alkylating agents. Steroids are often a component of the therapy, as may be radiotherapy. The risk of developing this complication in a patient receiving combination chemotherapy and steroids is estimated at 1%–2% (Idhe and Devita 1975; Engel et al. 1981; Thorne et al. 1981; Editorial, Lancet 1982). It may be that aspects of the lymphoma, in combination with the alkylating agents, are responsible for the lesions, although such lesions are known to occur in non-lymphoma patients on steroid therapy alone. Osteonecrosis has also been reported rarely in patients receiving chemotherapy and radiotherapy (Obrist et al. 1978) in the absence of steroids and may occur in a non-irradiated site. The areas affected include the neck and head of femur, humerus, ribs and sternum (Sweet et al. 1976; Timothy et al. 1978; Blijham et al. 1985). Symptoms often appear years after the treatment (Martel and Sitterley 1969). Osteonecrotic areas in, for example, the ribs or the sternum may present as painful, red swollen areas, which may subside completely without treatment. However, lesions in the femoral head, which are weight-bearing, may be of much more consequence. X-rays reveal signs of radiolucency and subsequently segmental or wedge-shaped collapse. The appearances may be detectable as early as 24 months before the onset of symptoms.

Radiation may induce second tumours in the field of therapy (Parker and Berry 1976; Hardy et al. 1978; Dalinka and Mazzeo 1985). Benign tumours are usually seen in those patients who have had radiotherapy within the first 2 years of life and are mainly osteochondromas. Malignant tumours are sarcomas and for their diagnosis certain criteria must be fulfilled (Cahan et al. 1948). There must be microscopic or radiographic evidence that the initial bone lesion (if any was present) was either non-malignant or of a different category to the second tumour. Malignancy must arise within the irradiated area. Malignancy of the induced tumour must be confirmed histologically and a latent period (usually in excess of 2–5 years) must have existed before the development of the subsequent tumour. The latent interval is usually between 12 and 20 years (Urban 1985) and may thus make the second tumour difficult to distinguish from a spontaneously arising tumour, but makes it unlikely to be recurrent disease because of the time elapsed. Most induced tumours are in bones unavoidably irradiated during the treatment of overlying soft-tissue lesions. The sarcomas that arise are most frequently osteogenic in nature, then fibrosarcomas and chondrosarcomas. The risk of tumour induction is greatest when radiation is used in children. There is, for example, an increased incidence of osteogenic sarcomas (as well as other malignancies) in patients who have been treated for Ewing's tumour (Strong et al. 1979) and retinoblastoma (Sagerman et al. 1969).

Second Malignancies in Patients with Lymphoma

Both radiotherapy and chemotherapy are immunosuppressive in their actions and have been shown to be carcinogenic both in experimental animals (O'Gara et al. 1971) and humans (Gane et al. 1970; Martin et al. 1970; Senyszyn et al. 1970; Stewart and Kneale 1970; Pinkston et al. 1981). Induced tumours have been noted as occurring after treatment of benign disease by radiotherapy (Scanlon and Semer 1981). The use of radical radiotherapy and combination chemotherapy in patients with lymphoma has led to improvement in survival with a much reduced risk of late relapse (Editorial, Lancet 1985 a). However, this may also lead to an increased risk of developing a second tumour (Toland and Coltman 1974; Brody et al. 1977; Toland et al. 1978). Coltman and Dixon (1982), reporting the findings of the Southwest Oncology Group's 10-year follow-up of patients treated for Hodgkin's disease, found 11 solid tumours and 21 leukaemias in 659 patients. Only one solid tumour and no leukaemias occurred among 95 patients treated with radiotherapy alone. Solid tumours encountered in the other patients were situated in colon and lung predominantly. Increased prevalence has been confirmed by other studies. There is a high incidence of digestive tract involvement (Krikorian et al. 1979; Lowenthal et al. 1981, Jacquillat et al. 1984) and the risk has been estimated at 4.45% at 10 years.

The commonest malignancy complicating lymphoma is acute myeloid leukaemia (Coleman et al. 1982; Tester et al. 1984; Editorial, Lancet 1985 b). However, solid tumours may also increase in frequency by some two to four times that seen in the general population (Arsenau et al. 1972; Baccarani et al. 1980). Patients must survive a minimum latent period after treatment and thereafter the risk of developing a second tumour increases. At 5 years the cumulative risk of developing multiple primary tumours may approach 5% and is highest where combination therapy has been used.

The tumours tend to occur at a younger age than

in the population at large and have unusually malignant histological characteristics, often with a rapidly fatal course. Second tumours tend to occur in or near to the site of radiotherapy in about 60% of patients.

The usual pattern is for a course of radiotherapy for lymphoma to be followed, after a short interval, by intensive combination chemotherapy. It appears that both forms of treatment, especially in high doses, are probably necessary to induce the second neoplasm. The development of these tumours occurs more frequently in Hodgkin's disease than in other primary tumours treated in a similar fashion and probably reflects not only intensive treatment but also immunological abnormalities seen in patients with lymphoma (Aisenberg et al. 1966; Young et al. 1972).

The commonest solid tumour induced is non-Hodgkin's lymphoma (Krikorian et al. 1979; Editorial, Lancet 1985a) usually of an unfavourable histological type and with a poor prognosis. Other tumours include squamous-cell carcinomas (Berg 1967), mucin-producing tumours, fibrosarcomas (Spiegel and Bogdasarian 1985) and spindle-cell and Kaposi's sarcoma. Second tumours in children treated for Hodgkin's disease appear in different sites to those seen in adults and tend to mainly affect bone, connective tissue and the thyroid gland (Tucker et al. 1984). All patients successfully treated for lymphoma must be considered to be at risk of developing a subsequent tumour and must be subjected to long-term follow-up programmes (Spiegel and Bogdasarian 1985).

Second Tumours Induced after Treatment of Malignancies other than Lymphoma

The carcinogenic effect of irradiation has been shown in experimental animals and after accidental and therapeutic and experimental use in humans (Roswit et al. 1975; Rotmensch et al. 1986). The irradiation may occur in utero (MacMahon 1962), in childhood (Pifer and Hempelmann 1964; Sagerman et al. 1969) and in adults.

A wide variety of primary tumours, treated by radiotherapy, sometimes in combination with complex chemotherapeutic regimes, have been reported to be followed by subsequent second and even third malignancies. There is usually a long latent interval of up to 12–20 years. The development of a second tumour may be difficult to distinguish from recurrent disease. Statistically significant increases in leukaemias, lymphomas, thyroid cancer, lung and breast cancer and possibly salivary tumours have been reported in atomic bomb survivors (Pinkston et al. 1981).

Valagussa et al. (1980) found that one-third of all solid tumours developing after radiotherapy occurred within the irradiated area. The aetiology is probably multifactorial and includes impaired cellular immunity, the immunosuppressive effects of combination therapy and the direct cellular effects of radiation and chemotherapy (Canellos et al. 1975; Sieber and Adamson 1975; Casciato and Scott 1979). The cumulative rate of second neoplasms is high after orthovoltage treatment of paediatric neoplasms (Li et al. 1975), but this may have been reduced by the introduction of megavoltage irradiation (Potish et al. 1985). The knowledge that thyroid carcinoma (Hempelmann 1976; Roudebush et al. 1978), hyperparathyroidism and salivary tumours (Tisell et al. 1976, 1977; Christensson 1978; Scanlon and Sener 1981) are significantly increased in frequency after neck irradiation for either benign or malignant disease makes it reasonable to examine other sites, tumours and treatments to see the liklihood of second tumour induction.

There are many reports of induced carcinoma of the colon, although the total number of recorded cases currently is only about 70 (Rotmensch et al. 1986). In addition to displaying a latent interval, the radiation exposure to the large intestine should previously have been relatively great and radiation damage should be histologically demonstrable in and around the tumour, as suggested by subintimal foam cell plaques appearing in the walls of small arteries (Sheehan 1944; Slaughter and Southwick 1952; Black and Ackerman 1965). These tumours usually follow irradiation for gynaecological disease.

There is a significant increase in malignancies after irradiation for testicular tumours and these occur both in and outside the site of radiation. They may or may not be related to the use of alkylating agents (Reimer et al. 1977; Boivin and Hutchison 1981, Valagussa et al. 1980). The observed incidence of transitional-cell carcinomas of both upper and lower urinary tract and of skin cancers outside the irradiated area is increased in these patients. There is also a tendency towards the development of more gastrointestinal and prostatic malignancies, but the figures do not yet reach statistical significance. Curiously, there appears to be a lower than expected incidence of induced leukaemias in these patients. Isolated cases of sarcoma (Dana and Jones 1982) and retroperitoneal mesothelioma (Stock et al. 1979) have been reported.

Melphelan, cyclophosphamide and chlorambucil are the three alkylating agents which have been most frequently documented as damaging chromosomes in a manner similar to ionising radiation. They have been implicated as being carcinogenic, particularly for acute non-lymphocytic leukaemia after treatment of various primary tumours including ovarian carcinoma (Reimer et al. 1977) and multiple myeloma (Bergasgel et al. 1979). It must be expected that other solid tumours will occur at later dates after alkylating agent therapy.

Radiation of head and neck tumours, including carcinoma of the tongue, retinoblastoma and intracranial tumours, has been associated with the subsequent development of fibrosarcomas (Cruz et al. 1957; Noetzli and Malamud 1962; Gane et al. 1970). Thyroid cancer may follow irradiation of the neck for a variety of reasons, including paediatric tumours such as medulloblastoma (Raventos and Duszynski 1963; Andrew and Kerr 1965), although the sequence is probably very uncommon. There is an excess of breast cancers in patients who have had childhood malignancies treated by orthovoltage (Li et al. 1983).

Therapeutic irradiation of the cervix may be associated with an increased incidence of subsequent tumours of the bladder, endometrium, ovaries and rectum (Boice 1981; Pettersson et al. 1985). Ovarian tumour therapy may be associated with second tumour development in the bladder and colon (Bergasgel et al. 1979).

Miscellaneous Effects of Chemotherapy and Its Administration

Chemotherapy, especially with methotrexate and 6-mercaptopurine, may lead to hepatic fibrosis or cirrhosis and bleeding from oesophageal varices (Lascari et al. 1968). 5-Fluorouracil is reported to cause excessive tear loss due to damage to the tear duct. Although the condition is usually reversible, punctal-canalicular fibrosis may occur leading to epiphora, and surgical drainage may be required (Seiff et al. 1985). Chemotherapy is frequently administered via centrally placed infusion catheters. These devices and their insertion techniques carry a risk of complications (Pessa and Howard 1985) that may occur either during insertion or in the supervening period. The overall risk of complications occurring during insertion has been reported as up to 17% and includes subclavian arterial puncture, misplacement or failure of placement, pneumothorax and injury to the aorta or the brachiocephalic vein. These complications may be reduced by direct operative cannulation of the vein under local anaesthetic as opposed to using a percutaneous puncture method of insertion.

Postoperative complications include infection, thrombosis, including that of the superior vena cava, embolisation and catheter leakage. Maintenance of venous access is, in some instances, necessary for a prolonged time when long-term chemotherapy or parenteral nutrition is required. This is most commonly delivered by a tunnelled silicone catheter inserted into a central vein (Powel Tuck 1978; Vandersalm and Fitzpatrick 1981). The tunnel and the nature of the catheter are thought to be responsible for the relatively low frequency of complications, especially thrombosis and sepsis (Hoshal et al. 1971; Broviac et al. 1973; Welch et al. 1974) even though these may occur in up to 30% of patients (Thomas et al. 1980; Quigley et al. 1982; Bottino et al. 1983; Keohane et al. 1983; Martin et al. 1983; Reed et al. 1983). The necessity of a tunnelled approach has been questioned by some including Von Meyenfeldt et al. (1980) and Slater et al. (1985). A randomised trial showed no difference between the two techniques when a skilled nutrition nurse was employed in the care of the catheters (Keohane et al. 1983). Implantable portals and infusion pumps are being increasingly used in some centres in order to try and make outpatient chemotherapy a more practicable procedure, and reduce the risk of complications. Even these pumps have their complications, such as capsular leakage (Khoury et al. 1985) and pump inversion, which may make it impossible to inject drugs without repositioning the device (Seeger et al. 1985).

References

Aisenberg AC (1966) Immunologic status of Hodgkin's disease. Cancer 19: 385–394

Allen CV, Fletcher WS (1972) A pilot study on preoperative irradiation of rectosigmoid carcinoma. AJR 114: 504–508

Andrew DS, Kerr IF (1965) Carcinoma of thyroid following irradiation for medulloblastoma. Clin Radiol 16: 282–283

Anseline PF, Lavery IC, Fazio VW, Jagelman DG, Weakley FL (1981) Radiation injury of the rectum. Ann Surg 194: 716–724

Arseneau JC, Sponzo RW, Levin DL, Schnipper LE, Bonner H, Young RC, Canellos GP, Johnson RE, Devita VT (1972) Non lymphomatous malignant tumors complicating Hodgkin's disease. N Engl J Med 287: 1119–1122

Baccarani M, Bosi A, Papa G (1980) Second malignancy in patients treated for Hodgkin's disease. Cancer 46: 1735–1740

Bastiannse MA van B (1960) Bastiannse's method for surgical closure of very large irradiation fistulae of the bladder and rectum. In: Youssef AF (ed) Gynecological urology III. Thomas, Springfield

Berg JW (1967) The incidence of multiple primary cancers. 1. Development of further cancers in patients with lymphomas, leukaemias and myeloma. J Natl Cancer Inst 38: 741–752
Bergasgel DE, Bailey AJ, Langley GR, Macdonald RN, White DF, Miller AB (1979) The chemotherapy of plasma-cell myeloma and the incidence of acute leukaemia. N Engl J Med 301: 743–748
Black WM, Ackerman LV (1965) Carcinoma of the large intestine as a late complication of pelvic radiotherapy. Clin Radiol 16: 278–281
Blijham GH, Vermeulen A, De Leon DE (1985) Osteonecrosis of sternum and rib in a patient treated for Hodgkin's disease. Cancer 56: 2292–2294
Boice JD (1981) Cancer following medical irradiation. Cancer 47: 1081–1090
Boivin JF, Hutchison GB (1981) Leukaemia and other cancers after radiotherapy and chemotherapy for Hodgkin's disease. J Natl Cancer Inst 37: 751–760
Bostwick J, Vasconez LO, Jurkiewicz MJ (1978) Breast reconstruction after a radical mastectomy. Plast Reconstr Surg 61: 682–693
Bostwick J, Stevenson TR, Nahai F, Hester TR, Coleman JJ, Jurkiewicz MJ (1984) Radiation to the breast. Complications amenable to treatment. Ann Surg 200: 543–553
Bottino J, McCreadie KB, Groschel DHM, McCreadie KB, Groschel DHM, Lawson M (1983) Long-term intravenous therapy with peripherally inserted silicone elastomer central venous catheters in patients with malignant disease. Cancer 43: 1937–1943
Bricker EM, Johnston WD (1979) Repair of postirradiation rectovaginal fistula and stricture. Surg Gynecol Obstet 148: 499–506
Bricker EM, Johnston WD, Patwardhan RV (1981) Repair of postirradiation damage to colorectum. A progress report. Ann Surg 193: 555–564
Brody RS, Schottenfield D, Reid A (1977) Multiple primary cancer risk after therapy for Hodgkin's disease. Cancer 40: 1917–1929
Broviac J, Cole JJ, Scribner BH (1973) A silicone rubber atrial catheter for prolonged parenteral nutrition. Surg Gynecol Obstet 136: 602
Buckner CD, Rudolph CD, Rudolph RH, Fefer A, Clift RA, Epstein RB, Funk DD, Neimann PE, Slichter SJ, Storb R, Thomas ED (1972) High-dose cyclophosphamide therapy for malignant disease. Cancer 59: 357–365
Byrd R (1985) Late effects of treatment of cancer in children. Paediatr Clin North Am 32: 835–857
Cade S (1957) Radiation induced cancer in man. Br J Radiol 30: 393–402
Cahan WG, Woodard HQ, Higinbotham NG, Stewart FW, Coley BL (1948) Sarcoma arising in irradiated bone: report of eleven cases. Cancer 1: 3–29
Canellos GP, Devita VT, Arseneau JC, Whang-Peng J, Johnson REC (1975) Second malignancies complicating Hodgkin's disease in remission. Lancet 1: 947–949
Casciato DA, Scott JL (1979) Acute leukaemia following prolonged cytotoxic agent therapy. Medicine (Baltimore) 59: 32–47
Caspers RJL, Hop WCJ (1983) Irradiation of true pelvis for bladder and prostatic carcinoma in supine, prone or Trendelenburg position. Int J Radiat Oncol Biol Phys 9: 589–593
Cassady JR, Richter MP, Piro AJ, Jaffe N (1975) Radiation-adriamycin interactions; preliminary clinical observations. Cancer 36: 946–949
Chavez CM (1977) Understanding the therapeutic approaches to lymphedema. Vasc Surg 11: 176
Christensson T (1978) Hyperparathyroidism and radiation therapy. Ann Intern Med 89: 216–217
Coleman CN, Kaplan HS, Cox R, Varghese A, Butterfield P, Rosenberg SA (1982) Leukaemias, non-Hodgkin's lymphomas and solid tumours in patients treated for Hodgkin's disease. Cancer Surv 1: 733–744
Coltman CA Jr, Dixon DO (1982) Second malignancies complicating Hodgkin's disease: a southwest oncology group 10 year follow up. Cancer Treat Rep 66: 1023–1033
Cruz M, Coley BL, Stewart FW (1957) Postradiation bone sarcoma. Cancer 10: 72–88
Dalinka MK, Mazzeo VP Jr (1985) Complications of radiation therapy. CRC Crit Rev Diagn Imaging 23: 235–267
Dana BW, Jones SE (1982) Doxorubicin cardiotoxicity: detection and prevention. In: Jones SE (ed) Current concepts in the use of doxorubicin chemotherapy. Farmitalia Carlo Erba s. p. a., Milan, pp 155–163
Danese CA, Grishman E, Dreiling DA (1967) Malignant vascular tumors of the lymphedematous extremity. Ann Surg 166: 245–253
Devereux DF, Kavanah MT, Feldman MI, Kondi E, Hull D, O'Brien M, Deckers PJ, Mozden PJ (1984) Small bowel exclusion from the pelvis by a polyglycolic mesh sling. J Surg Oncol 26: 105–112
De Cosse JJ, Rhodes RS, Wentz WB, Reagan JW, Dworken HJ, Holden WD (1969) The natural history and management of radiation induced injury of the gastrointestinal tract. Ann Surg 170: 369–384
Donaldson SS, Jundt S, Ricour C, Sarrazin D, Lemerle J, Schweisguth O (1975) Radiation enteritis in children. Cancer 35: 1167–1178
Editorial (1982) Osteonecrosis caused by combination chemotherapy. Lancet 1: 433–434
Editorial (1985 a) Relapse in Hodgkin's disease. Lancet 2: 424–426
Editorial (1985 b) Second malignancies in lymphoma patients. Lancet 2: 1163–1164
Editorial (1985) Massive bladder haemorrhage. Br Med J 291: 1522–1523
Engel IA, Strauss DJ, Lacher M, Lane J, Smith J (1981) Osteonecrosis in patients with malignant lymphoma. Cancer 48: 1245–1250
Fabri PJ, Mirtallo J, Ruberg R, Kudsk KA, Derning DA, Ellison EC, Schaffer P (1982) Incidence and prevention of thrombosis of the subclavian vein during total parenteral nutrition. Surg Gynecol Obstet 155: 238–240
Fair WR (1974) Formalin in the treatment of massive bladder haemorrhage. Techniques, results and complications. Urology 3: 573–576
Fajardo LF (1977) Radiation-induced coronary artery disease. Chest 71: 563–564
Fajardo LF, Stewart JR, Cohn KE (1968) Morphology of radiation-induced heart disease. Arch Pathol 86: 512–519
Fergusson CM, Copeland SA, Horton L (1985) Unusual sarcoma arising in lymphoedema. J R Soc Med 78: 497–498
Freund H, Gunderson L, Krause R, Fischer JE (1979) Prevention of radiation enteritis after abdominoperineal resection and radiotherapy. Surg Gynecol Obstet 149: 206–208
Galland RB, Spencer J (1979) Surgical aspects of radiation injury to the intestine. Br J Surg 66: 135–138
Galland RB, Spencer J (1985) Spontaneous postoperative perforation of previously asymptomatic irratiated bowel. Br J Surg 72: 285–286

Gane NFC, Lindup R, Strickland P, Bennett MH (1970) Radiation-induced fibrosarcoma. Br J Cancer 24: 705–711

Gluck WL, Akwari OE, Kelvin FM, Goodwin BJ (1985) A reversible enteropathy complicating continuous hepatic artery infusion chemotherapy with 5-fluoro-2-deoxyuridine. Cancer 56: 2424–2427

Goel AK, Rao MS, Bhagwat AG, Vaidyanathan S, Goswami AK, Sen TK (1985) Intravesical irrigation with alum for the control of massive bladder hemorrhage. J Urol 133: 956–957

Goldsmith HS (1974) Long term evaluation of omental transposition for chronic lymphoedema. Ann Surg 180: 847–879

Goligher JC (1984) Irradiation proctitis and enteritis. In: Goligher JC (ed) Surgery of the anus, rectum and colon. Ballière Tyndall, London, pp 1047–1057

Goodnough LT, Saito H, Manni A, Jones PK, Pearson OH (1984) Increased incidence of thromboembolism in Stage IV breast cancer patients treated with a five-drug chemotherapy regimen. A study of 159 patients. Cancer 54: 1264–1268

Graham JB (1965) Vaginal fistulas following radiotherapy. Surg Gynecol Obstet 120: 1019–1030

Green M, Iba G, Smith WR (1975) Measures to minimize small intestine injury in the irradiated pelvis. Cancer 35: 1633–1640

Hardy TJ, An T, Brown PW, Terz JJ (1978) Post-irradiation sarcoma (malignant fibrous histiocytoma) of the axilla. Cancer 42: 118–124

Hatcher PA, Thomson HJ, Ludgate SN, Small WP, Smith AN (1985) Surgical aspects of intestinal injury due to pelvic radiotherapy. Ann Surg 201: 470–475

Hempelmann LH (1976) Thyroid neoplasms following irradiation in infancy. In: Radiation-associated thyroid carcinoma. Proceedings of a conference held at University of Chicago. Grune and Stratton, New York, pp 221–229

Heusinkveld RS, Manning MR, Aristizabal SA (1978) Control of radiation induced diarrhoea with cholestyramine. Int J Radiat Oncol Biol Phys 4: 687–690

Higgins GAJ (1978) The pros and cons of irradiation treatment of colo-rectal cancer. In: Nyhus L (ed) Surgery annual. Appleton-Century-Crofts, New York, p 175

Higgins GA Jr (1979) Adjuvant radiation therapy in colon cancer. Int Adv Surg Oncol 2: 1–24

Hoshal V, Ause R, Hoskins P (1971) Fibrin sleeve formation on indwelling subclavian central venous catheters. Arch Surg 102: 353

Ihde C, De Vita VP (1975) Osteonecrosis of the femoral head in patients with lymphoma treated with intermittent combination chemotherapy. Cancer 36: 1585–1588

Ingelman-Sundberg A (1960) Pathogenesis and operative treatment of urinary fistulae in irradiated tissue. In: Youssef AF (ed) Gynecological Urology. Thomas, Springfield

Jacquillat C, Khayat D, Desprez-Curely JP, Weil M, Brocheriou C, Auclerc G, Chamseddine N, Bernard J (1984) Non-Hodgkin's lymphoma occurring after Hodgkin's disease. Cancer 53: 459–462

Jurkiewicz MJ, Arnold PG (1977) The omentum: an account of its use in the reconstruction of the chest wall. Ann Surg 185: 548–554

Jurkiewicz MJ, Bostwick J, Hester TR, Bishop JB, Craven J (1980) Infected median sternotomy wound: successful treatment by muscle flaps. Ann Surg 191: 738–744

Kavanah MT, Feldman MI, Devereux DF, Kondi ES (1985) New surgical approach to minimise radiation-associated small bowel injury in patients with pelvic malignancies requiring surgery and high-dose irradiation: a preliminary report. Cancer 56: 1300–1304

Kennedy C, Snell ME, Witherow RO (1984) Use of alum to control intractable vesical hemorrhage. Br J Urol 56: 673–675

Keohane PP, Attrill H, Northover J, Jones BJM, Cribb A, Frost P, Silk DEA (1983) Effect of catheter tunnelling and a nutrition nurse on catheter sepsis during parenteral nutrition. Lancet 2: 1388–1390

Kerstein MD, Licalzi L (1977) Microvascular procedures in the management of lymphedema. Vasc Surg 11: 188

Khoury MD, Lloyd LR, Burrows J, Berg R, Yap J (1985) A totally implanted venous access system for the delivery of chemotherapy. Cancer 56: 1231–1234

Kinsella TJ, Bloomer WD (1980) Tolerance of the intestine to radiation therapy. Surg Gynecol Obstet 151: 273–284

Krikorian JG, Burke JS, Rosenberg SA, Kaplan HS (1979) Occurrence of non-Hodgkin's lymphoma after therapy for Hodgkin's disease. N Engl J Med 300: 452–458

Kumar APM, Wren EL, Jayalakshamma B, Conrad L, Quinn P, Cox C (1976) Silver nitrate irrigation to control bladder hemorrhage in children receiving cancer therapy. J Urol 116: 85–89

Kwitko AO, Pieterse AS, Hecker R, Rowland R, Wigg DR (1982) Chronic radiation injury to the intestine: a clinico-pathological study. Aust NZ J Med 12: 272–277

Lascari AD, Givler RL, Soper RT, Hill LF (1968) Portal hypertension in a case of acute leukaemia treated with antimetabolites for ten years. N Engl J Med 279: 303–306

Lawson JA (1985) Surgical treatment of radiation-induced atherosclerostic disease of the iliac and femoral arteries. J Cardiovasc Surg 26: 151–156

Lempert N, MacDowell RT, Karmody A et al. (1979) Vascular access for cancer chemotherapy. Cancer 43: 1934–1936

Li FP, Cassady JR, Jaffe N (1975) Risk of second tumors in survivors of childhood cancer. Cancer 35: 1230–1235

Li FP, Corkery J, Vawter G, Fine W, Sallan SS (1983) Breast carcinoma after cancer therapy in childhood. Cancer 51: 521–523

Lieberman JS, Borrero J, Urdaneta E, Wright IS (1961) Thrombophlebitis and cancer. JAMA 177: 542–545

Localios A, Stone A, Friedman N (1969) Surgical aspects of radiation enteritis. Surg Gynecol Obstet 129: 1163–1172

LoIudice T, Baxter D, Balint J (1977) Effects of abdominal surgery on the development of radiation enteropathy. Gastroenterology 73: 1093–1097

Lokich JJ, Becker B (1983) Subclavian vein thrombosis in patients treated with infusion chemotherapy for advanced malignancy. Cancer 52: 1586–1589

Lowenthal LM, Harlow RWH, Mead AE, Tuck D, Challis DR (1981) T-cell non-Hodgkin's lymphoma after radiotherapy and chemotherapy for Hodgkin's disease. Cancer 48: 1586–1589

Lynch DF, Herr HW (1981) Radiation-induced sarcoma following radiotherapy for testicular tumour. J Urol 126: 845–846

MacMahon B (1962) Prenatal X-ray exposure and childhood cancer. J Natl Cancer Inst 28: 1173–1191

Martel W, Sitterley BH (1969) Roentgenologic manifestations of osteonecrosis. AJR 106: 509–522

Martin H, Strong E, Spiro R (1970) Radiation-induced skin cancer of the head and neck. Cancer 25: 61–71

Martin JK, Beart RW Jr, Mucha P Jr, Hoagland C (1983) Hickman catheter implantation in the treatment of acute leukaemia. Arch Surg 118: 1224–1226

Maruyama Y, Van Nagell JR, Utley J, Vider ML, Parker JC

(1974) Radiation and small bowel complications in cervical carcinoma therapy. Radiology 112: 699–703
Mathes SJ, Nahai F (1979) Clinical atlas of muscle and musculocutaneous flaps. Mosby, St. Louis
Mathes SJ, Nahai F (1982) Clinical applications for muscle and musculocutaneous flaps. Mosby, St. Louis
Matus-Ridley M, Nicosia SV, Meadows AT (1985) Gonadal effects of cancer therapy in boys. Cancer 55: 2353–2363
Mennie AT, Dalley VM, Dinneen LC, Collier HOJ (1975) Treatment of radiation-induced gastro-intestinal distress with acetylsalicylate. Lancet 2: 942–943
Mettlin C, Mittelman A, Nachimuthu N, Murphy GP, Schmitz RL, Smart CR (1981) Trends in the United States for the management of adenocarcinoma of the rectum. Surg Gynecol Obstet 153: 701–706
Miller SP, Sanchez-Avalos J, Stefanski T, Zuckerman L (1967) Coagulation disorders in cancer 1. Clinical and laboratory studies. Cancer 20: 1452–1465
Miller TA (1977) A surgical approach to lymphedema. Am J Surg 134: 191–195
Miller TA, Harper J, Longmire WP (1973) The management of lymphedema by staged subcutaneous excision. Surg Gynecol Obstet 136: 586–592
Morganstern L, Hiatt N (1967) Injurious effect of pancreatic secretions on postradiation enteropathy. Gastroenterology 53: 923–929
Morganstern L, Patin CS, Krohn HL, Hiatt N (1970) Prolongation of survival in lethally irradiated dogs. Arch Surg 101: 586–589
Morganstern L, Thompson R, Friedman NB (1977) The modern enigma of radiation enteropathy: sequelae and solutions. Am J Surg 134: 166–172
MRC Working Party (1982) A trial of preoperative radiotherapy in the management of operable rectal cancer. Br J Surg 69: 513–519
Nielubowicz J, Olszewski W, Sokolowski J (1968) Surgical lymphovenous shunts. J Cardiovasc Surg 9: 262–267
Noetzli M, Malamud N (1962) Postirradiation fibrosarcoma of the brain. Cancer 15: 617–622
Obrist R, Hartmann D, Obrecht JP (1978) Osteonecrosis after chemotherapy. Lancet 1: 1316
Oliver RTD (1986) Rare cancers and specialist centres. Br Med J 292: 641–642
Olszewski WL, Loe KR, Engeset A (1978) Immune proteins and other biochemical constituents of peripheral lymph in patients with malignancy and post-irradiation lymphoedema. Lymphology 11: 174–180
O'Gara RW, Adamson RW, Kelly MG et al. (1971) Neoplasms of the hematopoietic system in nonhuman primates: report of one spontaneous tumor and two leukemias induced by procarbazine. J Natl Cancer Inst 46: 1121–1130
Ostroff EB, Chenault OW (1982) Alum irrigation for the control of massive bladder hemorrhage. J Urol 128: 929–930
Palmer JA, Bush RS (1976) Radiation injuries to the bowel associated with the treatment of carcinoma of the cervix. Surgery 80: 458–464
Parker RG, Berry MC (1976) Late effects of therapeutic irradiation on the skeleton and bone marrow. Cancer 37: 1162–1171
Parks AG, Percy JP (1982) Resection and sutured colo-anal anastomosis for rectal carcinoma. Br J Surg 69: 301–304
Perthes G (1903) Über den Einfluß der Roentgen-Strahlen auf epitheliale Gewebe. Insbesondere auf das Carcinom. Arch Clin Chir 71: 955
Pessa ME, Howard RJ (1985) Complications of Hickman-Broviac catheter. Surg Gynecol Obstet 161: 257–260
Pettersson F, Fotiou NE, Silfversward C (1985) Cohort study of the long-term effect of irradiation for carcinoma of the uterine cervix. Acta Radiol 24: 145–151
Phillips FS, Sternberg SS, Cronin AP, Vidal PM (1961) Cyclophosphamide and urinary bladder toxicity. Cancer Res 21: 1577–1589
Phillips TL, Kane L, Utley JF (1973) Radioprotection of tumor and normal tissues by thiophosphate compounds. Cancer 32: 528–535
Pifer JW, Hempelmann LH (1964) Radiation-induced thyroid carcinoma. Ann NY Acad Sci 114: 838–848
Pinkston JA, Wakabayashi T, Yamoto T, Asano M, Harada Y, Kuagami H, Takeuchi M (1981) Cancer of the head and neck in atomic bomb survivors. Hiroshima and Nagasaki 1957–76. Cancer 48: 2172–2178
Piver MS, Lele S (1976) Enterovaginal and enterocutaneous fistulae in women with gynecologic malignancies. Obstet Gynecol 48: 560–563
Plotz PH, Klippel JH, Decker JL, Grauman D, Wolff B, Brown BC, Rutt G (1979) Bladder complications in patients receiving cyclophosphamide for systemic lupus erythematosus or rheumatoid arthritis. Ann Intern Med 91: 221–223
Pomer S, Karcher G, Simon W (1983) Cutaneous ureterostomy as last resort treatment of intractable haemorrhagic cystitis following radiation. Br J Urol 55: 392–394
Potish RA, Jones TK Jr, Levitt SH (1979) Factors predisposing to radiation-related small bowel damage. Radiology 132: 479–482
Potish RA, Dehner LP, Baselow RE, Kim TH, Levitt SH, Nesbit M (1985) The incidence of second neoplasms following megavoltage radiation for pediatric tumors. Cancer 56: 1534–1537
Powell Tuck J (1978) Skin tunnel for central venous catheter: non-operative technique. Br Med J 279 i: 625
Probert JC, Parker BR, Kaplan HS (1973) Growth retardation in children after megavoltage irradiation of the spine. Cancer 32: 634–639
Pyeritz RE, Droller MJ, Bender WL, Saral R (1978) An approach to the control of massive hemorrhage in cyclophosphamide-induced cystitis by intravenous vasopressin: a case report. J Urol 120: 253–254
Quastler R (1956) The nature of intestinal radiation death. Radiat Res 4: 303–320
Quigley T, Sutherland DER, Howard RJ (1982) Use of Hickman and Broviac central venous catheters in high risk patients. Minn Med 65: 77–80
Rachootins, Shapiro S, Yamakawa T, Goldman L, Patin S, Morganstern L (1972) Potent anti-proteases derived from *Ascaris lumbricoides:* efficacy in amelioration of post radiation enteropathy. Gastroenterology 62: 796
Ram MD (1970) Complications of radiotherapy for carcinoma of the bladder. Proc R Soc Med 63: 93–94
Rao MS, Singhal PC, Bapna BC, Vaidyanathan S, Chugh KS et al. (1978) Fatal complication of intravesical formalin during control of intractable haemorrhagic cystitis. Urology 11: 588–590
Raventos A, Duszynski DO (1963) Thyroid cancer following irradiation for medulloblastoma. AJR 89: 175–181
Reed WP, Newman KA, De Jongh C et al. (1983) Prolonged venous access for chemotherapy by means of the Hickman catheter. Cancer 52: 185–192
Reimer RR, Hoover R, Fraumeni JF, Young RC (1977) Acute leukaemia after alkylating-agent therapy of ovarian cancer. N Engl J Med 297: 177–181
Requarth W, Roberts S (1956) Intestinal injuries following irradiation of pelvic viscera for malignancy. Arch Surg 73: 682–688

Rider WD, Palmer JA, Mahoney LJ et al. (1977) Pre-operative irradiation in operable cancer of the rectum: report of the Toronto Trial. Can J Surg 20: 335–338
Roswit B, Higgins GA Jr, Keehn RJ (1975) Pre-operative irradiation for carcinoma of the rectum and recto-sigmoid colon – report of a National Veterans Administration randomized study. Cancer 35: 1597–1602
Rotmensch S, Avigad I, Soffer EE, Horowitz A, Bar-Meir S, Confino R, Czerniak A, Wolfstein I (1986) Carcinoma of the large bowel after a single massive dose of irradiation in healthy teenagers. Cancer 57: 728–731
Roudebush CP, Asteris GT, Degroot LJ (1978) Natural history of radiation-associated thyroid cancer. Arch Intern Med 138: 1631–1634
Rubin JS, Rubin RT (1966) Cyclophosphamide haemorrhagic cystitis. J Urol 96: 313–316
Russel JC, Welch JP (1979) Operative management of radiation injuries of the intestinal tract. Am J Surg 137: 433–442
Sabanas AO, Dahlin DC, Childs DS Jr, Ivins JC (1956) Post-radiation sarcoma of bone. Cancer 9: 528–542
Sagerman RH, Cassady JR, Tretter P, Ellsworth RM (1969) Radiation induced neoplasia following external beam therapy for children with retinoblastoma. AJR 105: 529–535
Savage RC (1985) The surgical management of lymphoedema. Surg Gynecol Obstet 160: 283–290
Sawhney CP (1980) Lymphoedema of the extremities; a new approach to its management. Br J Plast Surg 53: 445–452
Scanlon EF, Sener SF (1981) Head and neck neoplasia following irradiation for benign conditions. Head Neck Surg 4: 139–145
Schier J, Symmonds RE, Dahlin DC (1964) Clinicopathologic aspects of actinic enteritis. Surg Gynecol Obstet 119: 1019–1025
Schmitt EH, Symmonds RE (1981) Surgical treatment of radiation-induced injuries of the intestines. Surg Gynecol Obstet 153: 896–900
Schnur PL (1977) Surgical treatment of lymphedema – a reappraisal. Vasc Surg 11: 182–187
Seeger J, Woodcock TM, Richardson JD (1985) Complications of implantable chemotherapy pump. A case of pump inversion. Cancer 56: 2428–2429
Seiff SR, Shorr N, Adams T (1985) Surgical treatment of punctal-canalicular fibrosis from 5-fluorouracil treatment. Cancer 56: 2148–2149
Senyszyn JJ, Johnston AD, Jacox HW et al. (1970) Radiation-induced sarcoma after treatment of breast cancer. Cancer 26: 394–403
Shamblin JR, Symmonds RE, Sauer WG, Childs DS Jr (1964) Bowel obstruction after pelvic and abdominal radiation surgery. Ann Surg 160: 81–89
Sheehan JF (1944) Foam cell plaques in the intima of irradiated small arteries. Arch Pathol Lab Med 37: 297–308
Sieber SM, Adamson RH (1975) Toxicity of antineoplastic agents in man: chromosomal aberrations, antifertility effects, congenital malformations and carcinogenic potential. Adv Cancer Res 22: 57–155
Silver D, Pluckett CL (1976) Lymphangioplasty: a ten year evaluation. Surgery 80: 748–755
Sim FH, Taylor WF, Ivins JC, Pritchard DJ, Soule EH (1978) A prospective randomized study of the efficacy of routine elective lymphadenectomy in management of malignant melanoma. Cancer 41: 948–956
Slater H, Goldfarb IW, Jacob HE, Hill JB, Srodes CH (1985) Experience with long-term outpatient venous access utilising percutaneously placed silicone elastomer catheters. Cancer 56: 2074–2077
Slaughter DP, Southwick HW (1957) Mucosal carcinomas as a result of irradiation. Arch Surg 74: 420–429
Soloway (1966) Radiation-induced neoplasms following curative therapy for retinoblastoma. Cancer 19: 1984
Spiegel J, Bogdasarian RS (1985) Retropharyngeal fibrosarcoma following radiation therapy for Hodgkin's lymphoma of the neck. Otolaryngol Head Neck Surg 93: 274–277
Stearns MW Jr, Deddish MR, Quan SHQ, Leaming RH (1974) Preoperative roentgen therapy for cancer of the rectum and rectosigmoid. Surg Gynecol Obstet 138: 584–586
Stewart A, Kneale GW (1970) Radiation dose effects in relation to obstetric X-rays and childhood cancers. Lancet 1: 1185–1188
Stewart FW, Treves N (1948) Lymphangiosarcoma in postmastectomy lymphoedema. A report of six cases in elephantiasis chirurgica. Cancer 1: 64–81
Stewart JR, Fajardo LF (1971) Radiation-induced heart disease: clinical and experimental aspects. Radiol Clin North Am 9: 511–531
Stock RJ, Fu YS, Carter JR (1979) Malignant peritoneal mesothelioma following radiotherapy for seminoma of the testis. Cancer 44: 914–919
Strong LC, Herson J, Osborne BM, Sutow WW (1979) Risk of radiation-related subsequent malignant tumors in survivors of Ewing's sarcoma. J Natl Cancer Inst 62: 1401–1406
Susan LP, Marhs RJ (1975) Phenolization of bladder in treatment of massive intractable haematuria. Urology 5: 119–121
Swan RC, Fowler WC, Boronow RC (1976) Surgical management of radiation injury to the small intestine. Surg Gynecol Obstet 142: 325–327
Sweet DL, Roth DG, Desser RK, Miler JB, Ultmann JE (1976) Avascular necrosis of the femoral head with combination chemotherapy. Ann Intern Med 85: 62–68
Taswell HF, Soule EH, Coventry MB (1962) Lymphangiosarcoma arising in chronic lymphedematous extremities. Report of thirteen cases and review of literature. J Bone Joint Surg [Am] 44: 277–294
Tester WJ, Kinsella TJ, Waller B, Makuch RW, Kelley PA, Glatstein E, Di Vita VT (1984) Second malignant neoplasms complicating Hodgkin's disease: the National Cancer Institute experience. J Clin Oncol 2: 762–769
Thomas JH, MacArthur RK, Pierce GE, Hermreck AS (1980) Hickman-Broviac catheters. Ann J Surg 140: 791–796
Thompson N (1962) Surgical treatment of chronic lymphoedema of the lower limb. Br Med J 2: 1567–1573
Thompson N (1967) The surgical treatment of chronic lymphoedema of the extremities. Surg Clin North Am 47: 445–503
Thompson N (1970) Buried dermal flap operation for chronic lymphedema of the extremities; ten year survey of results of 79 cases. Plast Reconst Surg 45: 541–548
Thorne JC, Evans WK, Alison RE, Fournasier V (1981) Avascular necrosis of bone complicating treatment of malignant lymphoma. Am J Med 71: 751–758
Timothy AR, Tucker AK, Park WM, Cannell LB (1978) Osteonecrosis in Hodgkin's disease. Br J Radiol 51: 328–332
Tisell LE, Carlsson S, Lindberg S, Ragnhult I (1976) Autonomous hyperparathyroidism: a possible late complication of neck radiotherapy. Acta Chir Scand 142: 367–373
Tisell LE, Hansson G, Lindberg S, Ragnhult I (1977) Hyperparathyroidism in persons treated with X-rays for tuberculous cervical adenitis. Cancer 40: 846–854
Toland DM, Coltman Ca Jr (1977) Second malignancies complicating Hodgkin's disease. Blood 46: 1013
Toland DM, Coltman CA Jr, Moon TE (1978) Second malig-

nancies complicating Hodgkin's disease: the southwest oncology group experience. Cancer Clin Trials 1: 21–33

Tucker MA, Meadows AT, Boice JD, Hoover RN, Fraumeni JF (1984) Cancer risk following treatment of childhood cancer. In: Boice JD, Fraumeni (eds) Radiation carcinogenesis: epidemiology and biological significance. Raven, New York

Urban JA (1985) Sequelae of breast irradiation. JAMA 253: 3589

Valagussa P, Santoro A, Kenda R, Bellani FF, Franchi F, Banfi A, Rilke F, Bonadona G (1980) Second malignancies in Hodgkin's disease: a complication of certain forms of treatment. Br Med J 280: 216–219

Vandersalm TJ, Fitzpatrick GF (1981) New technique for placement of long-term venous catheters. JPEN 5: 326

Van Nagell JR Jr, Maruyama Y, Parker JC Jr, Dalton WL (1974) Small bowel injury following radiation therapy for cervical cancer. Am J Obstet Gynecol 118: 163–167

Van Nagell JR Jr, Parker JC Jr, Maruyama Y, Utley J, Hager WD, Donaldson ES, Wood EG (1977) The effect of pelvic inflammatory disease on enteric complications following radiation therapy for cervical cancer. Am J Obstet Gynecol 128: 767–771

Varma JS, Smith AN (1984) Internal anal sphincter damage in radiation proctitis. Gut 25: 564

Villasanta U (1972) Complications of radiotherapy for carcinoma of the uterine cervix. Am J Obstet Gynecol 114: 717–726

Von Meyenfeldt MM, Stapert J, De Jong PC, Soeters P, Wesdorp R, Greep J (1980) TPN catheter sepsis: lack of effective subcutaneous tunneling of PVC catheters on sepsis rate. JPEN 4 or 5: 514–517

Wade JC, Newman KA, Schimpff SC et al. (1981) Two methods for improved venous access in acute leukaemia patients. JAMA 246: 140–144

Wall RL, Clausen KP (1975) Carcinoma of the urinary bladder in patients receiving cyclophosphamide. N Engl J Med 293: 271–273

Warren S, Friedman NB (1942) Pathology and pathologic diagnosis of radiation lesions of the gastrointestinal tract. Am J Pathol 18: 499–507

Welch GW, McKeel DW, Silverstein P et al. (1974) The role of catheter composition in the development of thrombosis. Surg Gynecol Obstet 138: 421

Wellwood JM, Jackson BT, Bates TD (1974) Breakdown of small bowel anastomosis after pelvic radiotherapy. Ann R Coll Surg Engl 54: 306–308

Wiernik (1966) Radiation damage and repair in the human jejunal mucosa. J Pathol Bacteriol 91: 389–393

Young RC, Corder MP, Haynes HA et al. (1972) Delayed hypersensitivity in Hodgkin's disease: a study of 103 untreated patients. Am J Med 52: 63–72

Rehabilitation Procedures

Plastic and Reconstructive Surgery in Breast Cancer Patients

H. BOHMERT

The evolution of breast reconstruction mirrors the progress in the field of reconstructive surgery in general. Early breast reconstructive attempts included migration of local and distant tubed pedicle flaps into the mastectomy defect and sharing of the opposite breast. These procedures are of historical interest only, as such methods usually fell short of a pleasing and satisfying reconstruction. With the development of new and reliable techniques, particularly rotation and advancement flaps, in combination with synthetic breast prosthesis, results have improved tremendously. Recent advances in reconstructive surgery, particularly the application of the latissimus dorsi and rectus abdominis musculocutaneous flap, have made breast reconstruction possible for virtually any patient who has had a mastectomy. Microvascular free flaps were added to these techniques and earned a role in certain breast reconstructions difficult to accomplish with convential techniques. Furthermore, tissue expanders have enriched our armamentarium, especially for immediate breast reconstruction. Now there are different ways to rebuild the breast and the development of numerous procedures have resulted in the most dramatic and impressive improvements in confidence and self-esteem that have been seen in the field of plastic surgery during the past decade.

General Considerations

Female breasts are certainly the most significant symbol of feminity. This focus is intensified by today's culture and fashion, which stress pleasing breasts as a basic aspect of a woman's attractiveness.

Therefore, one of the most devasting blows to the feminine image is radical surgical loss of the breast due to cancer. Certainly, concern for the loss of the breast should be less than concern for loss of life, but mastectomy frequently evokes a decrease in self-esteem, self-confidence, and self-assertiveness, and a general feeling of unattractiveness. This can result in a very depressing outlook for the patient. For this reason, it is most appropriate that concepts of breast reconstruction proceed hand in hand with the surgical management of primary breast cancer. In this respect, surgeons dealing with breast cancer have lagged far behind their colleagues treating head and neck malignancy and have performed other deforming operations and reconstructions. An unfounded concern has been that breast reconstruction may possibly adversely affect the natural history of the disease and mask local recurrence of disease. Therefore the general surgeon advised against the "plastic" repair of the defect. On the other hand, inadequate techniques of breast reconstruction during earlier times did little to encourage the general surgeon to change this position.

Therefore the breast could be removed with no need for concern about reconstruction. However, current techniques make successful breast reconstruction a possibility in virtually all women regardless of the extent of surgical or radiation treatment. It must also be understood and constantly remembered that local recurrence or appearance of distant metastases is a natural part of breast cancer disease and that there is no evidence that breast reconstruction affects the natural course of breast cancer. On the other hand, we do know its universally positive effect on the patient's self-esteem and general outlook on life.

Therefore, the right of the patient to have reconstruction should be the same as for reconstruction following extirpation of any other malignancy.

For this reason plastic surgeons must educate their general surgical colleagues and oncologists about what can be done for the woman who is emotionally upset following a mastectomy and also how she can be informed about immediate reconstruction. Many patients will accept mastectomy almost with a sense of relief, when immediate reconstruction can be offered because of much less emotional distress. Women after mastectomy have a double psychological problem. Not only is there a gross deformity with serious sexual and mutilative overtones, but there is also a constant reminder to the woman that she has had a dangerous malignancy, one with a high risk for recurrence at some time in her life. We are now all well aware of the emotional anguish associated with mastectomy. For this reason, there has been increasing interest in preserving, if possible, the breast form to reduce the psychological trauma accompanied by the loss of the breast.

Despite the trend for lumpectomy and radiation therapy, modified radical mastectomy will most likely continue to be used initially as the standard therapy for adequate cancer control in many patients for several years to come. As long as this remains the case, reconstruction of the breast will remain an integral part of the treatment of cancer of the breast as an important option of the rehabilitation process of these patients. The concept of breast reconstruction after mastectomy may substantially affect the psychological problem associated with mastectomy and the rehabilitive efforts must be considered in this respect.

Selection of Patients

The primary indication for breast reconstruction is the desire of a strongly motivated patient with a reasonable life expectancy for reconstructive rehabilitation.

Patients' Expectations

It is important for women to feel that they themselves have the opportunity to make the choice for reconstruction or not. The patient must decide upon whether further surgery is worthwhile to restore her personal image. Realistically, breast reconstruction necessitates one to three operations for an optimal result, including nipple-areola reconstruction. General experience has found that especially young and intelligent women with differentiated personality structure and pronounced body consciousness appreciate a reconstruction most and feel the loss of the breast as a considerable constriction on their personality.

A suitable candidate should have a realistic understanding of the possibilities and limitations of reconstruction. Detailed information must be given to the patient concerning what is to be expected and what it is not possible to achieve. Every patient must clearly understand that even the best-reconstructed breast will not match completely the natural breast and exact symmetry is rarely obtained. In many patients an excellent result is achieved, but in each individual case this depends also on the anatomical situation after the mastectomy. In general, the reconstructive surgeon can offer the patient breast contour and symmetry to the extent that under a brassiere or bathing suit the uncritical eye will observe nothing out of the ordinary, so that the patient feels comfortable.

Oncological Aspects

The ideal patient for reconstruction has a small primary tumor with minimal risk of local recurrence. Patients with a tumor less than 2 cm in diameter and with no involved axillary nodes and positive hormone receptors should have the lowest risk of developing recurrence based on available statistics. Patients with more advanced disease have a higher risk of recurrence both locally and systemically, and these factors must necessarily be considered when the surgeon and the patient decide to attempt reconstruction following mastectomy.

There is no evidence that reconstruction will mask local recurrence of disease, but an early local recurrence after reconstruction would be a tremendous disappointment to the patient. In most techniques of reconstruction the implant is placed under the pectoral muscles. Because local recurrences almost always appear in the skin or subcutaneous tissue and rarely in the pectoralis major muscle it is extremely unlikely that any local recurrence will be masked by the reconstruction. Depending on its location, even when recurrent disease is detected, removal of the breast prosthesis may not be necessary. The old concept that reconstruction has to wait until complete healing is obtained is not practical and not according to the demands of the patient. Even in the presence of documented distant metastases such as bony involvement, reconstruction may be considered, not as rule but as an exception when progress of the disease is not detectable or when the patient, in spite of the poor prognosis, urgently desires the reconstruction. Some patients have indicated that they would certainly rather spend their last days or years with two breasts than without them and wish to get a chance to feel "whole" again.

In such circumstances, the adequately informed patient should not be denied reconstruction, since it might increase the quality of life, even if only for a relatively short period. To undergo the procedure is essentially the patient's decision not a medical one. Since it is well known that women with metastatic breast cancer and more advanced disease can live many years in a fairly normal fashion, reconstruction should not be denied to patients in high-risk categories for recurrence.

Timing of Breast Reconstruction

The timing of breast reconstruction varies according to the opinion of the individual surgeon, the patient's desire, and the stage of the disease.

As the philosophy of curative breast surgery has undergone a major change with the trend to less radical procedures, and recent data indicate that reconstruction of the breast does not influence the course of the disease, a change in thinking in terms of timing of reconstruction is also taking place.

There has been increasing interest recently for immediate reconstruction to reduce the psychological trauma often accompanied by the loss of the breast. Patients with a carcinoma of the breast vary considerably in their reactions when they are faced with both the threat of cancer and the loss of the primary female symbol. There is often a feeling of panic and severe situational depression. The patient is often relieved simply by the knowledge that breast reconstruction is a possibility immediately after mastectomy, carried out at the same time as the ablative procedure. While most women would like to have their breast restored at the time of mastectomy, other patients prefer removal of the cancerous breast before they can contemplate the physical and psychological implications of breast reconstruction.

Experienced psychologists closely involved in the management of breast cancer patients reported a less traumatic event, less of a loss of feeling of attractiveness and feminity, when immediate reconstruction was performed. These patients where less self-conscious about their appearance and showed better overall adaptation to their surgery.

Nevertheless, the decision about when the reconstruction should be peformed is essentially the patient's decision. The options are immediately, at the time of the ablative operation, or to delay with reconstruction to be performed at any time after the ablative procedure. Close cooperation and meaningful dialogue between the patient, the general surgeon, and the reconstructive surgeon is mandatory, in order that the patient be able to make a well-informed, intelligent decision.

Immediate reconstruction is best reserved for a primary tumor with minimal risk of local recurrence but this concept has been recently extended also to more advanced disease. In general, the alternative treatment for the group of patients who qualify most for immediate reconstruction may be local excision of the tumor with radiation therapy as an appropriate procedure.

However, poor prognostic factors are not in themselves a contraindication to immediate breast reconstruction, but avoiding the performance of this procedure in women with locally advance disease will reduce the chance for local recurrence. It may be considered in those patients who strongly desire it. In most other patients breast reconstruction is usually delayed 3–6 months following mastectomy. Although chemotherapy is not a contraindication and reconstructions have been successfully performed between treatment cycles, in most patients it is best to wait for completion of chemotherapy and, if administered, adjunctive irradiation. In general, reconstruction is planned for maximal patient benefit and is correlated with any adjunctive chemotherapy or radiation therapy.

Types of Reconstruction

The goals of reconstruction remain the same, regardless of the timing of the reconstruction and the nature of the mastectomy procedure. These include reconstruction of a pleasing, as near normal as possible, natural, soft, and comfortable breast contour, creation of symmetry between the reconstructed and the remaining natural breast, and reconstruction of the nipple-areola complex. No single reconstruction technique is suitable for every patient and an attempt is made to show the various methods available today. The final choice is made after considering the patient's desires and her general health, the availability of local tissue, and the surgeon's personal preference. The type of reconstruction is determined particularly by the mastectomy deformity and requirements for symmetry.

Four basic techniques are available for reconstruction of most mastectomy defects.

1. A silicone breast implant alone with or without staged enlargement of local skin is placed submuscularly beneath the available tissues. This is the simplest, safest, and most straightforward procedure and is used frequently in patients following modified radical mastectomy, in whom there remains abundant skin on the chest wall, with healthy pectoral musculature.
2. The abdominal advancement flap to add flap skin to the anterior chest wall and to create a stable inframammary fold in order to achieve a better, more natural ptotic breast shape and to improve symmetrical positioning of a silicone breast implant. This is often indicated in reconstructions following modified radical mastectomy when the myocutaneous flap procedure seems more than is necessary.
3. The latissimus dorsi flap is used with a silicone implant when additional skin and/or muscle cover is needed, particularly in patients with the radical mastectomy defect, or a modified radical mastectomy defect with radiation-injured skin or inadequate local skin area. It is also helpful after radical mastectomy to supplement axillary and infraclavicular deformity.
4. The transverse rectus abdominis musculocutaneous flap (TRAM) flap. This flap utilizes excess lower abdominal tissue for reconstruction of the breast mound and upper mastectomy area with autogenous tissue.

These four methods provide a versatile spectrum of techniques to reconstruct even the most difficult radical mastectomy deformity with skin loss and radiation damage. The flap techniques require a detailed knowledge of the musculocutaneous flap principle and the specific anatomy of each system and an artistic, three-dimensional awareness of breast form shape, and contour.

Determining Factors for Selection of Procedures

A number of factors must be taken into account prior to selecting the reconstructive procedure that is most appropriate in a given situation. The type of mastectomy performed has a major bearing on the selection of a procedure. The surgeon must evaluate the adequacy of the skin cover and the presence of the pectoralis major muscle, and must also determine the proposed size, shape, and contour of the breast mound, the proposed nipple-areola reconstruction, symmetry, and potential malignancy of the opposite breast.

With preoperative planning, most women who have a modified radical mastectomy can undergo reconstruction without a major flap transfer. In these patients usually a reasonable amount of skin is available, and if no radiation treatment has been performed, these are candidates for reconstruction by simple insertion of an implant. Unfortunately following modified radical mastectomy, the lower portion of the pectoralis major muscle is often denervated and therefore the muscle has been atrophied. This leaves a relative inferior shortage of tissue cover in the area, where breast mound projection must be greatest. A decision must be made as to whether a prosthesis alone will provide adequate projection with appropriate cover in this area or whether tissue expansion or flap transfer will be necessary.

Operative Techniques

Submuscular Insertion of an Implant

Patients with adequate skin cover and a healthy pectoralis major muscle can obtain a pleasing breast contour with simple insertion of a silicone breast prosthesis beneath the skin and musculature (Fig. 1).

The implant is inserted through the mastectomy incision. The incision is deepened to the pectoral muscle and at that level the skin undermined about 2–3 cm in all directions. Access is gained to the subpectoral plane by incising or splitting the muscle fibers about 2 cm from the edge of the lateral border of the pectoralis major muscle. The subpectoral pocket is created under direct vision, with an illuminated retractor.

With finger dissection the pectoralis major muscle is easily elevated from the ribs and pectoralis minor muscle superiorly. Blunt finger dissection is continued medially and extended to the pectoralis major origins from ribs three through seven. The muscle fibers are separated from the ribs and also partially detached from the sternum by blunt finger dissection or sharp dissection with the use of a cutting cautery. While dissecting the muscle from the chest wall, one divides perforating branches of the internal mammary artery which must be coagulated.

As the dissection is continued down the lateral aspect of the pectoralis major muscle, the serratus anterior muscle fibers are elevated and separated from the chest wall. The lateral limit is usually the line between the midaxillary and anterior axillary line.

The dissection then proceeds medially and inferiorly, extending into the rectus attachments, and it must extend beneath the rectus fascia just below the pectoralis major origin on the sixth rib for 2–3 cm below the proposed inframammary crease.

The dissection is also extended inferiorly beneath the adjacent external oblique muscle, which is separated by blunt and sharp means from the chest wall down to the level of 2 cm below the inframammary crease.

The reason for creating this large pocket, particularly in its lower region, lies in the fact that an implant stretches the skin somewhat, drawing the skin up and away from the chest wall, and moves the previously marked inframammary crease superiorly. On the other hand, about 1 cm of the created pocket often becomes obliterated as the fibrous tissue capsule forms.

Preplaced sutures between the muscle edges are used to prevent damage to the implant before the prosthesis is inserted in the submuscular pocket.

The goal should always be to achieve a complete submuscular pocket. This can be easily achieved in young patients with well-developed and flexible muscles. But this may be difficult in elderly patients because the muscles are often not stretchable and disrupt very easily. In all cases tension in the lower part of the pocket must be avoided, since this prevents a natural ptotic breast shape. If the muscles are not stretchable enough, the pectoralis major muscle can be released to the desired extent to give more space and to prevent constriction. The patients are told to massage their breast beginning some 3 to 5-days after surgery in order to maintain as large a pocket as possible. This helps to prevent capsulare contracture.

Use of Expander Implants

For patients with a less generous supply of skin the use of expander implants is of wide applicability in breast reconstruction. The majority of patients who have undergone modified radical mastectomies can be reconstructed without extensive flap procedures. The expansion prosthesis greatly increases the number of patients who can be reconstructed simply with a submuscular prosthesis. This procedure is particularly useful for primary breast reconstruction. The operative technique is similar to the insertion of a silicone prosthesis in the submuscular plane, but with laterally or inferiorly placed subcutaneous satellite filler ports or valves, which gradually expand the existing chest muscle and skin. Overexpansion is desirable for an optimal result, and the expander should be left in place for about 3 months after full expansion before replacement with a smaller silicone gel implant. This technique yields a more natural breast contour with a ptotic shape, particularly when combined with an abdominal advancement flap, when the final implant is inserted.

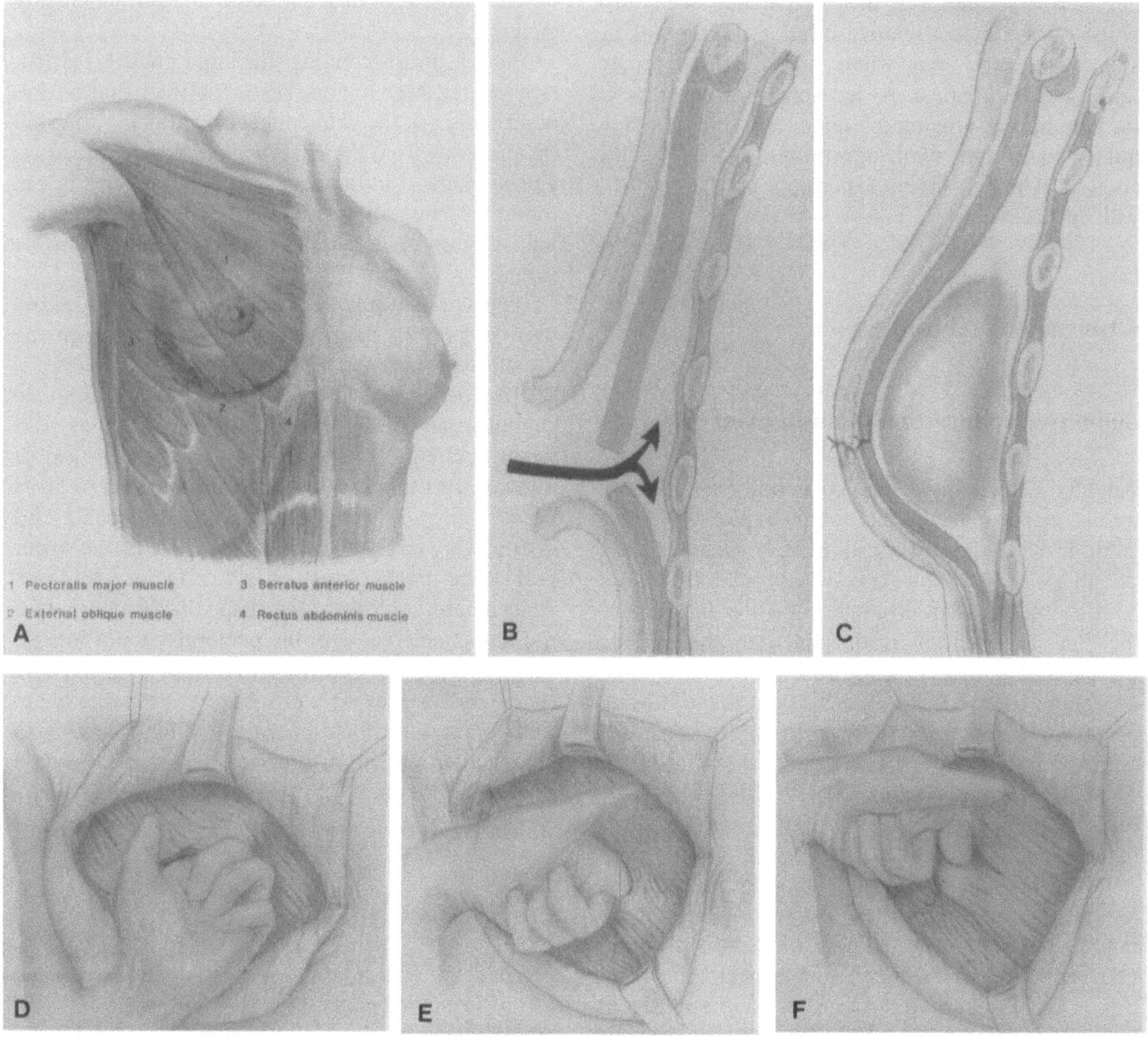

Fig. 1. **A** Musculature of the chest wall involved in the submuscular implant position. The upper medial portion of the breast is situated over the pectoralis major muscle. The lower portion covers the serratus anterior, external oblique origins and its fascia, and the fascia over the rectus abdominis muscle. **B** Submuscular implant position. The *arrow* indicates the direction of the submuscular elevation of the muscles. **C** The implant is placed totally beneath the muscles. **D** The plane beneath the pectoralis major muscle is entered through its lower border. The pectoralis major muscle is then elevated off the chest wall by blunt finger dissection up to the level of the second or third rib. **E** The pectoralis major muscle fibers are detached by blunt dissection from their sternal origins from the third rib downward to the lower extent of the submusculofascial pocket, the fascia is elevated over the rectus abdominis muscle, and dissection continues laterally beneath the fascia and some fibers of the external oblique muscle and its fascia. **F** The dissection is then continued to the fibers of the serratus anterior muscle to create a submusculofascial pocket. **G** Immediate reconstruction following modified radical mastectomy with subpectoral tissue expander implant. Intermediate stage of appearance. **H** Postoperative appearance at 1 year after insertion of a definitive silicone implant and nipple-areola reconstruction and reduction mammaplasty of the contralateral breast to achieve symmetry. **I** Profile view of the same patient preoperatively. **J** Postoperative appearance of the same patient

Advancement of Abdominal Skin

If the mastectomy was performed with a Stewart horizontal incision, or a slightly oblique incision, it is possible to compensate for the skin deficiency by advancing the abdominal skin (Fig. 2). For this purpose, the mastectomy scar is excised, and the abdominal skin undermined usually up to the level of the umbilicus. The mobilized skin cover is advanced cranially and fixed at the periosteum of the ribs at the level

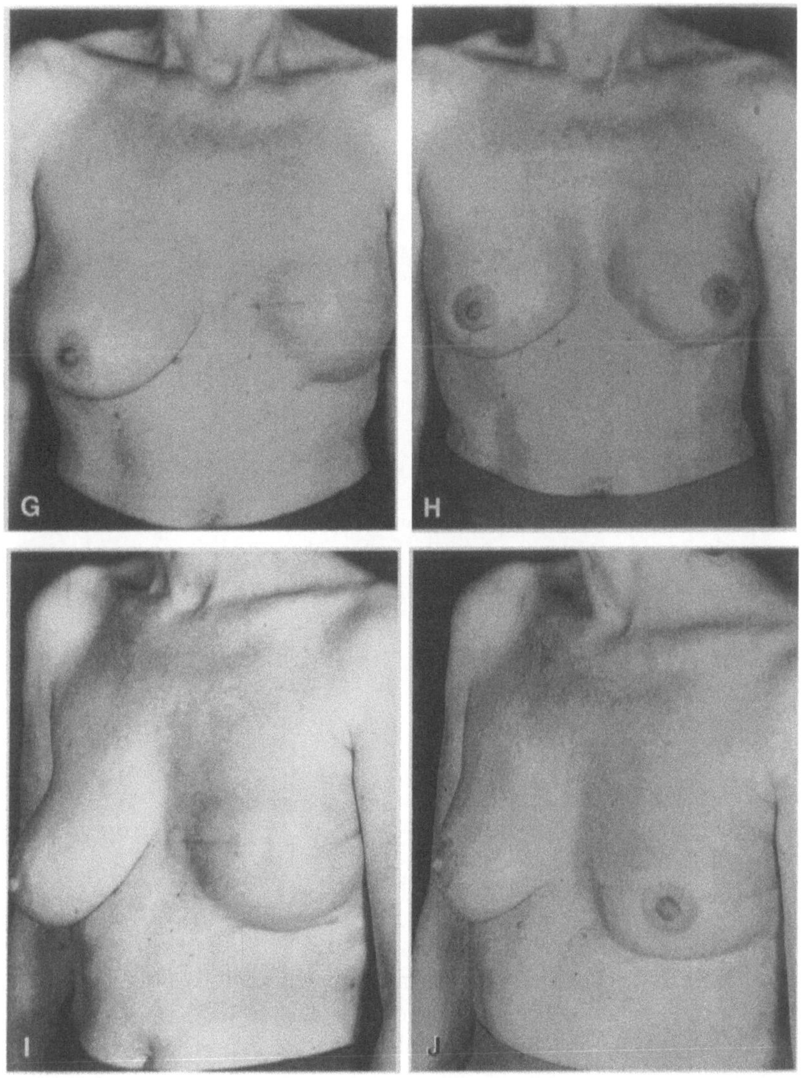

Fig. 1 G–J

of the inframammary fold. By additional undermining in the cranial direction, the pocket for the prosthesis is created.

When using the abdominal advancement technique, the submuscular implantation of the prosthesis is recommended, especially in cases of radiation-damaged skin. If the pectoral muscle is missing, reconstruction with myocutaneous flaps, particularly the latissimus dorsi flap, is to be preferred.

Thoracoepigastric Flap

The evolution of the thoracoepigastric flap has considerable merit in breast reconstruction. It was the first attractive technique to achieve a pleasing and satisfying reconstruction; and therefore changed the climate of breast reconstructions tremendously in the early seventies. The flap was developed and first described by the author in 1974 and was popularized by Cronin in 1977.

The thoracoepigastric flap, also called the upper epigastric flap, is a transverse abdominal skin flap, taken from the epigastric and lower thoracic region along the submammary fold. It is based medially on perforating vessels from the superior epigastric artery, which perforate the rectus abdominis muscle and course laterally from the epigastrium across the lower chest to the anterior axillary line, thus providing an axial pattern of vascular distribution to the main part of the flap. It has a random pattern lateral from the anterior axillary line and extends to the midaxillary line (Fig. 3).

The thoracoepigastric flap is useful for providing for lower and medial portions of the chest wall and is selected for breast reconstruction when the latissi-

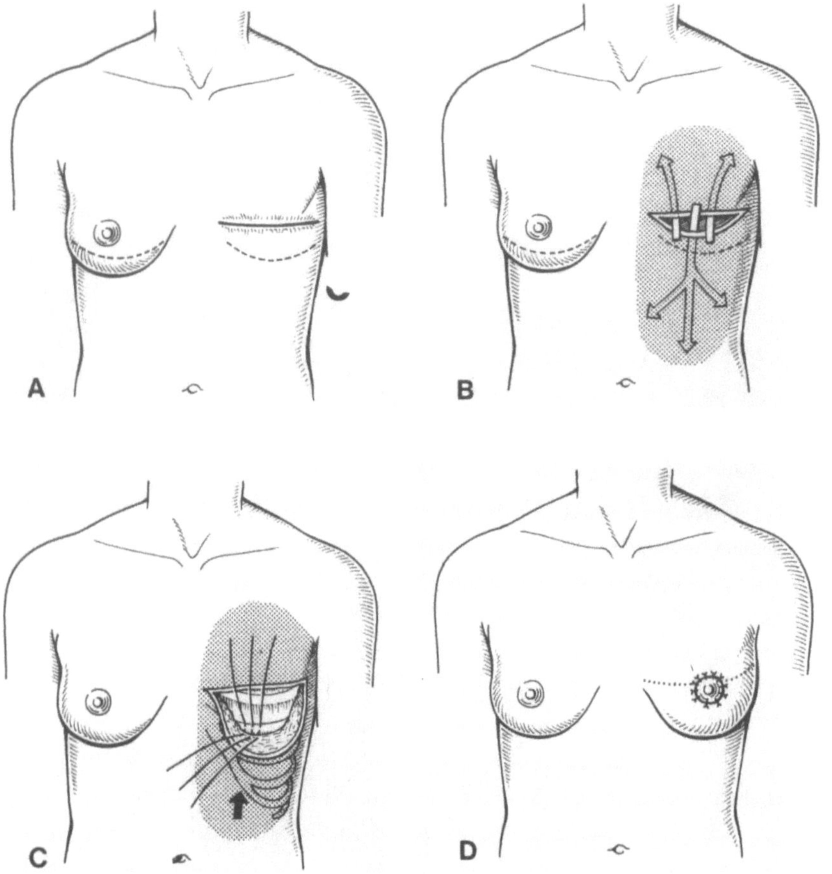

Fig. 2 A–D. Planning and markings for abdominal advancement technique. **A** Preoperative view of a left modified radical mastectomy defect with the future inframammary line. **B** Following excision of the mastectomy scar the skin and subcutaneous tissue are undermined within the *dotted* area, elevated, and pulled superiorly. **C** The *arrow* indicates the direction of advancement. The dermis and deep tissue of the flap is sutured with permanent sutures to the periosteum of the ribs and to the fascia of the serratus anterior, external oblique, and the rectus abdominis to define accurately the inframammary crease. **D** Implant in position and nipple-areola complex created

mus dorsi and rectus abdominis flaps are not available or only a minor surgical procedure is desired or advisable. It is particularly applicable when the mastectomy scar is oblique or vertical and when the chest skin is tight but not extremely thin and adherent to the chest wall. The flap substitutes for the skin area excised at mastectomy and permits a better projection by supplying additional skin to the chest wall. As the flap contains a reasonable amount of fat tissue, it offers an excellent protection for the prosthesis that even in most cases remains surprisingly soft. When a modified radical mastectomy has been performed, the presence of the pectoralis major muscle permits submuscular implantation and the flap allows a better projection by adding skin to the chest wall. The flap is not suited for a transverse mastectomy scar unless another incision is made to accommodate the flap in the medial or, even better, the lateral part of the breast. An extended thoracoepigastric flap, also called extended lateral thoracic flap, has been advocated recently for producing projection in breast reconstruction in patients with transverse mastectomy scars by insertion of the flap into the laterocaudal portion of the breast. The flap is not ideal in a radical mastectomy patient, since it cannot substitute an inadequate skin cover in the cranial breast area. The conclusive advantage in comparison with other flap techniques is that the procedure is technically simple and safe.

Technique

After having marked the flap with the average size of 10–22 cm from the middle of the rectus muscle to the midaxillary line, the flap is mobilized starting at its apex. The flap is dissected off the muscles. The fascia of the serratus and the external oblique are included in the flap, which guarantees a better circulation, since the fascia has a vascular net on both sides.

When this dissection under the fascia of the anterior serratus and external oblique abdominal muscles has reached the lateral border of the rectus sheath, it is decided whether a further dissection is necessary medially. This could be done, without any danger to the circulation, to the middle of the rectus sheath. The perforating vessels to the flap penetrate more medially and should be preserved. The postmastecto-

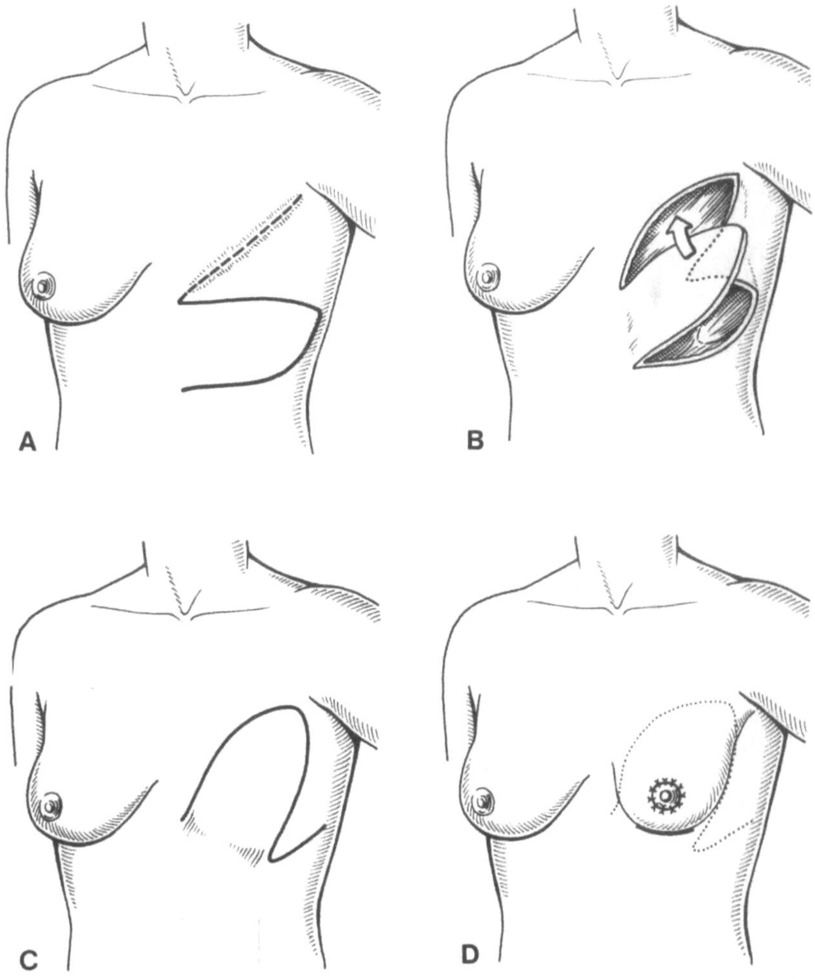

Fig. 3. **A** The thoracoepigastric flap is marked transversely across the epigastrium and lower chest with its upper line along the submammary fold, and the lower line parallels this about 10 cm caudally. The flap extends to the midaxillary line. **B** An incision is made along the markings down the fascia and the flap elevated toward the base until the medial part of the rectus sheath is reached. The mastectomy scar is excised and the skin from the chest wall elevated. The thoracoepigastric flap is rotated upwards and the lateral flap is elevated and transposed downwards. The abdominal skin is undermined down the iliac crest to allow advancement cranially. **C** The thoracoepigastric flap is transposed in the incision of the mastectomy wound. The abdominal skin is shifted upwards and sutured to the lower costal margin. **D** The prosthesis is placed under the muscle if the pectoral muscles still exist. The nipple-areola complex is reconstructed and the submammary crease determined in a second-stage procedure

my scar is excised and the wound edges are widely undermined medially to the sternum, cranially to the clavicula, laterally to the midaxillary line, and caudally to the submammary fold.

The flap can now be transposed into position. The abdominal skin is undermined often to the level of the iliac bone to make primary closure of the donor area possible. If the pectoral muscle still exists, the prosthesis is placed under the muscle. After a radical mastectomy, however, the implant is placed directly under the skin flaps in the same operation. A protruding skin surplus is often seen medially over the sternum. This dog ear cannot be excised until later, since otherwise the circulation in the base of the flap might be damaged. This correction can be done together with the nipple reconstruction. This flap will supply the extra skin and soft tissue that is needed to rebuild the breast contour with silicone implants.

The thoracoepigastric flap is a simple and safe procedure but during the past years has almost completely been replaced by the upper rectus flap technique, which is a direct extension of the concept of the thoracoepigastric flap.

Contralateral Upper Rectus Myocutaneous Flap

The contralateral upper rectus myocutaneous flap, also called contralateral thoracoepigastric flap, consists of an island of skin with the typical shape of the thoracoepigastric flap taken along the submammary fold and based on the upper part of the rectus abdominis muscle including the superior epigastric artery.

This concept was proposed and first used by Vasconez, popularized by Lejour, and improved by the author. Since this flap is directly supplied by an axial artery, in addition to several perforators from the superior epigastric artery, the design of the flap is safe in a length to width ratio of about 2 × 1. It usually

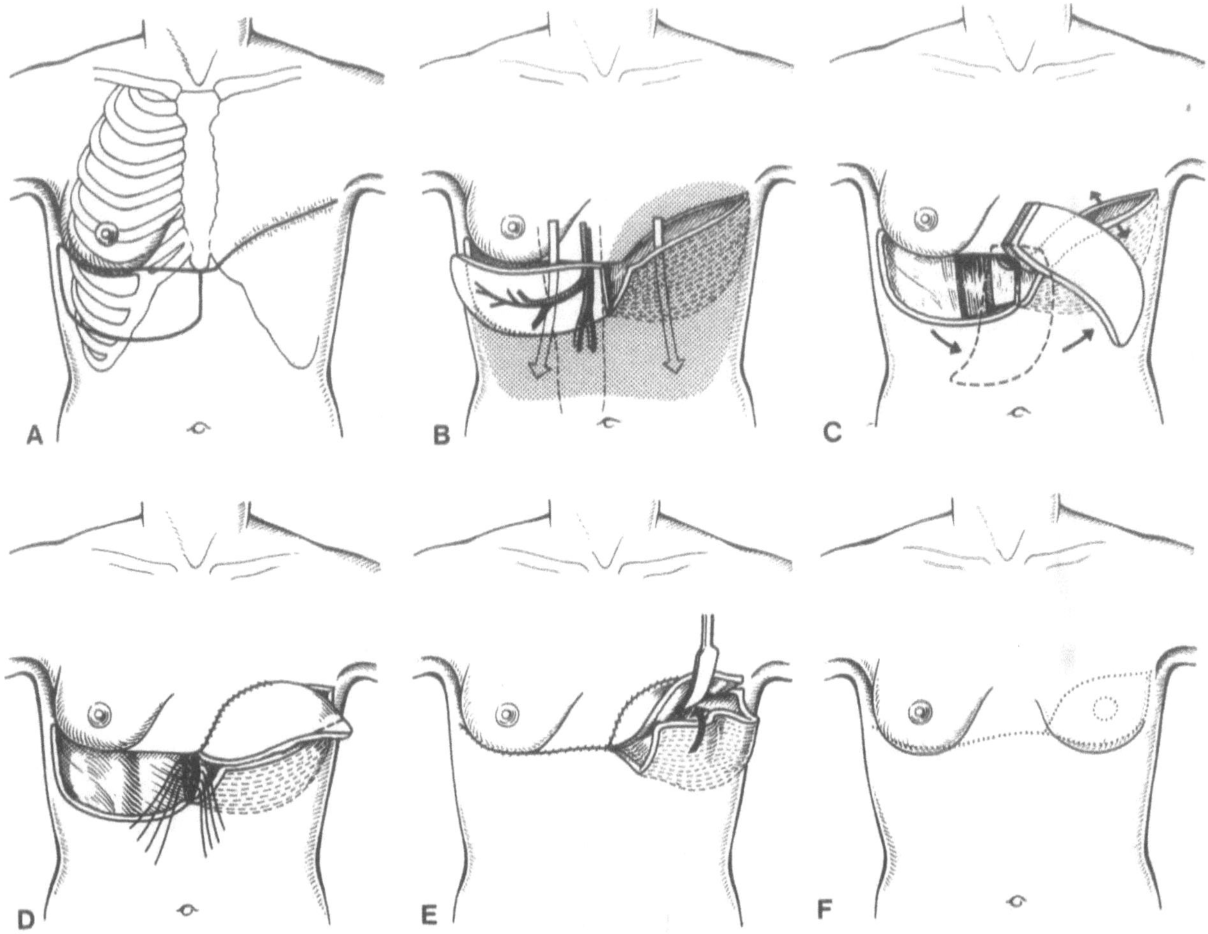

Fig. 4 A–J. Steps of operative techniques of contralateral upper rectus flap. **A** Proposed contralateral superior rectus flap on the thoracic cage. **B** Design of the upper rectus flap with vascular supply from the superior epigastric vessels. The *stippled area* is the zone which will be deepithelialized and used for volume replacement. The *arrows* indicate the extension of undermining of the abdominal wall for future advancement. **C** The flap is rotated on its vascular pedicle into the mastectomy defect. **D** The flap is sutured superiorly to the cranial border of the mastectomy wound following deepithelialization of its superior border in order to achieve an elliptical design of the flap. The anterior rectus sheath will be closed to avoid hernia. **E** Following advancement of the abdominal wall the deepithelialized area is placed beneath the upper rectus flap for contouring the breast mound. **F** Flap sutured into place and breast mound achieved with autogenous tissue. **G** Preoperative appearance in a modified radical mastectomized patient: reconstruction by contralateral upper rectus flap and reduction mammaplasty for symmetry. **H** Postoperative appearance following reconstruction by contralateral upper rectus flap. **I** Profile view of the same patient preoperatively. **J** Profile view of the same patient postoperatively

measures 22 × 11 cm. It is taken along the submammary fold from the normal side and transferred to the mastectomized side on this vascular pedicle. The donor site is closed following an upper abdominal lifting and the scar is hidden in the submammary fold (Fig. 4). Refinements to this technique, as proposed by the author, have brought excellent operative results.

According to the author's technique, the procedure is combined with an abdominal advancement flap in order to achieve volume replacement of the reconstructed breast with the patient's own tissue. Following the transfer of the contralateral thoracoepigastric flap and lifting of the upper abdominal skin, there is a large amount of surplus skin and subcutaneous fat tissue at the ipsolateral side from the mastectomy scar down to the level of the lower border of the contralateral thoracoepigastric flap in the epigastric, lower thoracic, and upper abdominal area. This large area can be deepithelialized, incised in the medial area, and doubled in order to form a breast mound. This flap is sufficient for volume replacement. Only in selected cases when the patient has hypertrophy or a large breast which she prefers not to be changed may additional volume replacement by prosthesis then be placed beneath the flap.

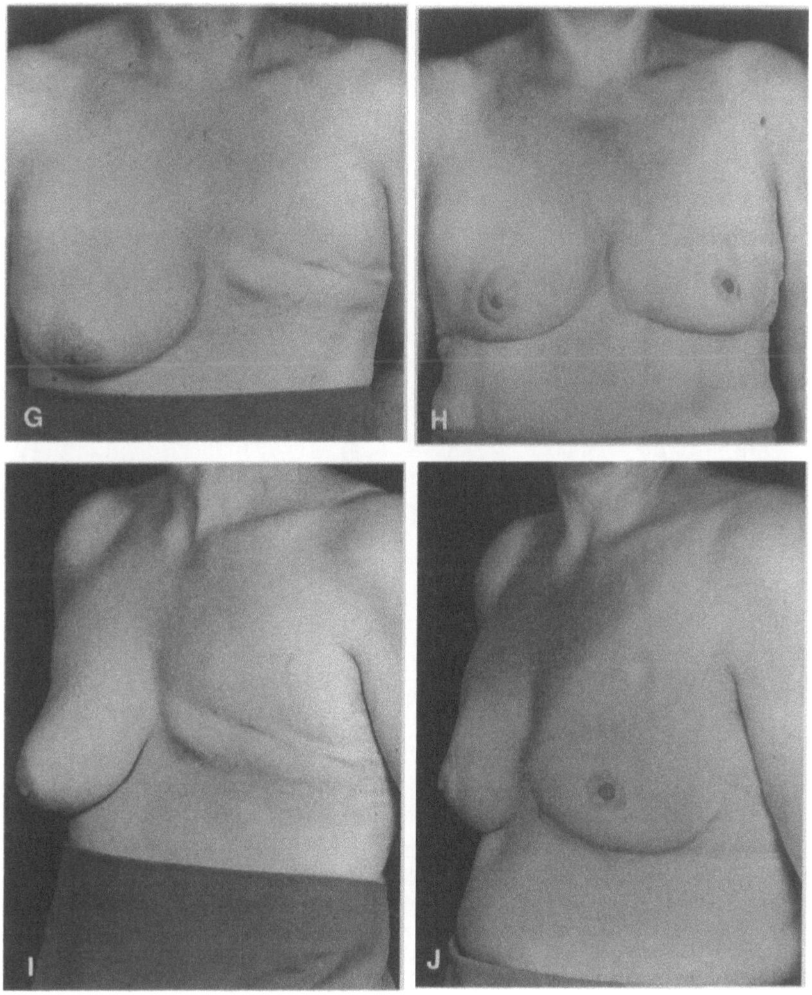

Fig. 4 G–J

In any case the breast obtained by this method is always soft and the patient is more satisfied after the reconstruction with soft tissue from her own body than with artificial material.

Technique

The flap is outlined in a length to width ratio of 22 × 11 cm along the submammary fold and incised down to the muscles. Elevation begins laterally. In respect to optimal nutrition, the aponeurosis is included in the dissection plane. The preparation is done as far as the medial part of the rectus abdominis fascia without jeopardizing the vascular nutrition. Only the medial half of the rectus muscle, which includes the blood vessels, is used for the procedure; therefore the muscle is cut through in the medial part and caudal part as well as along the midline. By means of the introduced finger, the further laterally penetrating epigastric artery is protected against damage. The vessel penetrates the muscle at the border between the medial to the mid-third.

After turning over the rectus muscle, the superior epigastric artery and vein are prepared. Only after their sure identification is the muscle cut through.

Now the myocutaneous flap is only fixed to its vascular pedicle. After turning back the flap, it becomes apparent that the vessels come out from under the costal edge. The thoracoepigastric flap can now be rotated clockwise 180° around its vascular pedicle to the other side. In the case of a small costal angle the vessel may be obturated by this. Then the rotation should be performed anticlockwise. This is usually preferable in order to prevent kinking or tension of the pedicle.

The muscle is fixed by single sutures to the subcutaneous tissue. It is necessary to spread the muscle out to avoid a medial bulk in the décolletage due to contraction and shrinkage.

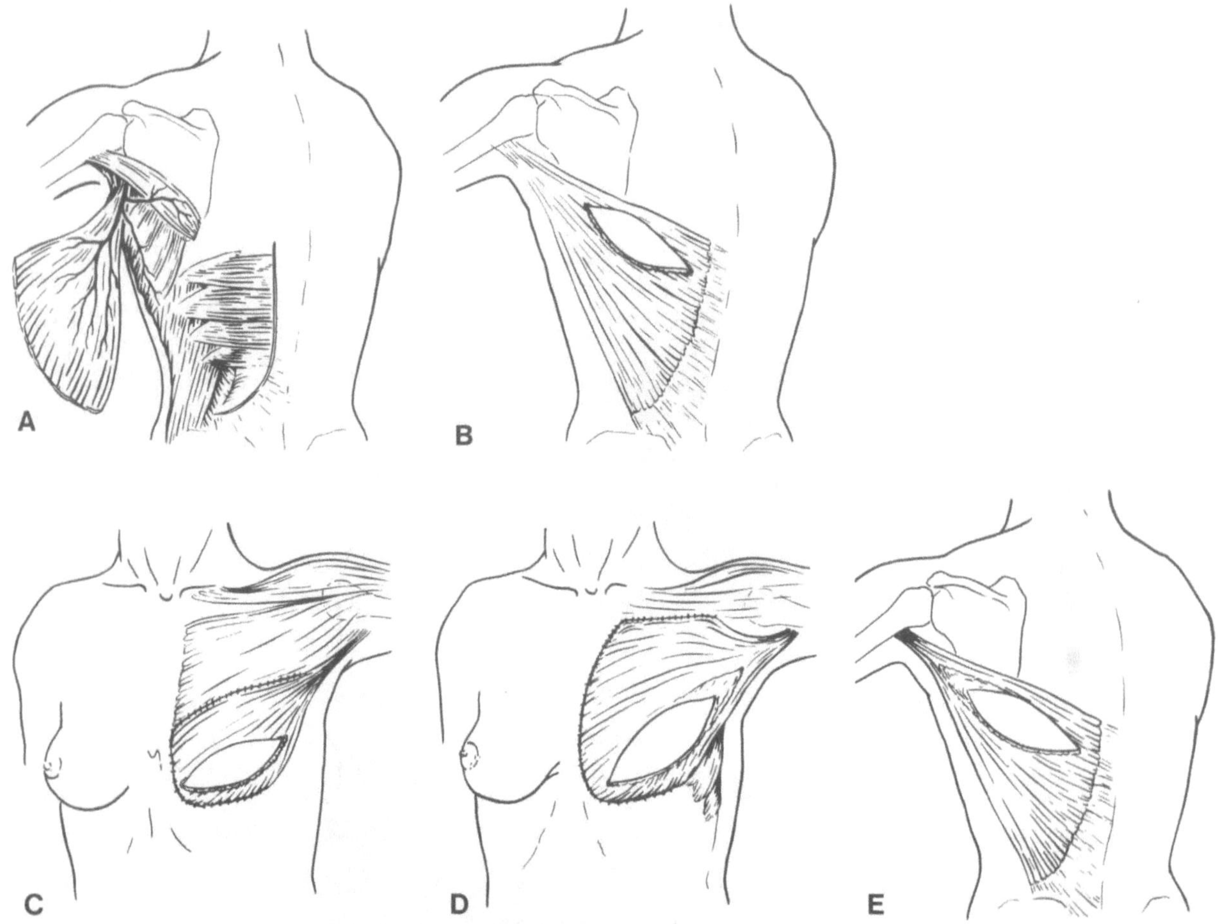

Fig. 5. **A** The latissimus dorsi flap and its vascular pedicle. **B** The latissimus muscle originates from the thoracic and lumbar vertebrae and pelvic rim and inserts on the humerus. High placement of the elliptic skin island as shown preserves as much muscle inferiorly as possible. **C** When the flap is transferred in this manner to the anterior chest, the medial portion of the skin island on the back ends up medially on the anterior chest wall, and the maximum amount of muscle is available on the chest wall following high placement of the skin island on the back. **D** For a patient who has had a radical mastectomy, high placement of the skin island is the choice generally employed whereas following modified radical mastectomy it can be placed more centrally over the latissimus muscle rather than at its edge. The cranial portion can be deepithelialized for filling of the axillary defect. **E** The maximum amount of muscle is used and the deepithelialized zone used for filling of the axillary defect following radical mastectomy. **F** Preoperative appearance in a modified radical mastectomized patient with the transverse scar: reconstruction by latissimus dorsi flap with insertion of the skin island in a horizontal direction. **G** Postoperative appearance. **H** Profile view preoperatively. **I** Profile view postoperatively. **J** Appearance following radical mastectomy with a vertical scar: reconstruction by latissimus dorsi flap with skin island insertion in a vertical direction. **K** Postoperative appearance. **L** Profile view of the same patient preoperatively. **M** Profile view postoperatively

After the rectus aponeurosis has been sutured transversely in its caudal portion, its ventral layer is cranially fixed to the costal edge. Thereby the muscular defect is totally closed and a disturbance of the contour or a functional deficiency is not to be expected.

Below the mastectomy scar the skin is marked according to the volume of the thoracoepigastric flap. This area is incised down to the dermis and then deepithelialized. After total deepithelialization the integument of the lower thoracic and abdominal wall is undermined as far the high point of the umbilicus. The extent of the mobilization on both sides to the flanks and caudally down to the umbilicus is demonstrated. The thoracoepigastric flap can then be rotated into its final position. By advancing the abdominal skin cranially the deepithelialized flap can then be buried.

For an optimal formation of the breast contour, the deepithelialized advancement flap is medially partly incised and furled back dorsally. In the medial region a sufficient contour is already produced by

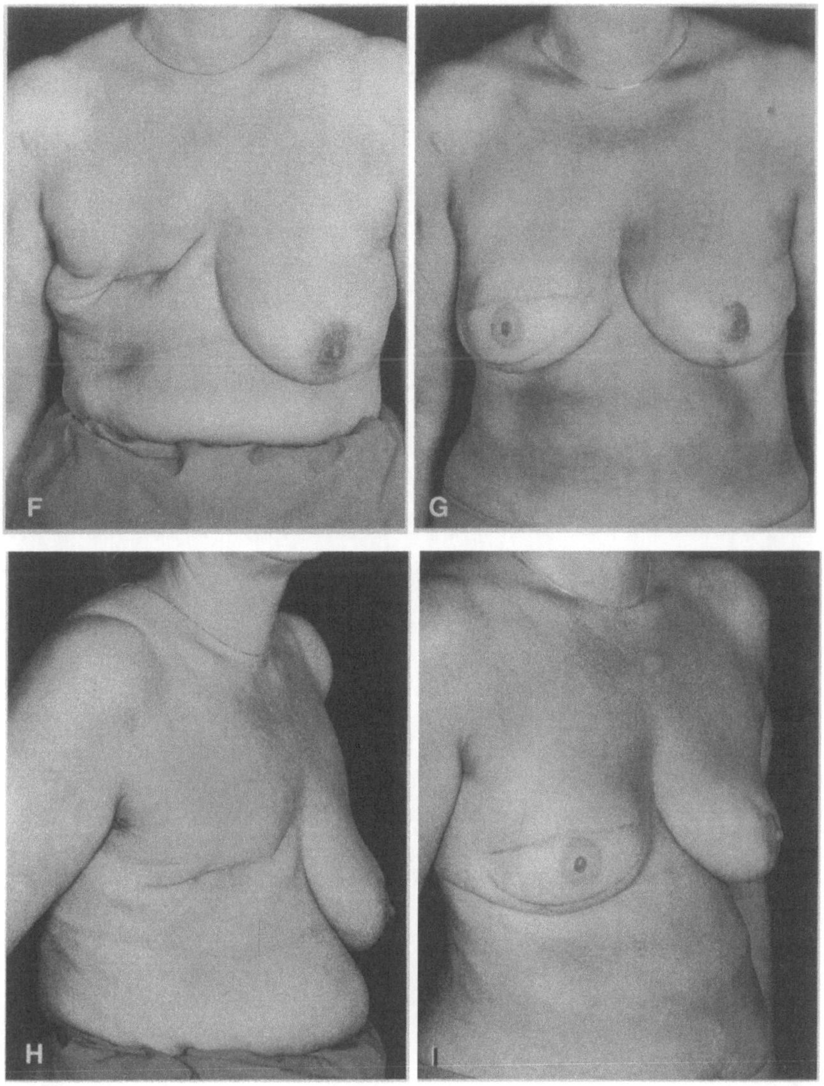

Fig. 5 F–I

the transferred rectus muscle. The central breast mound is pronounced by also doubling the lateral part.

Thus it is possible to create an appealing breast contour without any prosthesis merely by the patient's own tissue.

Latissimus Dorsi Myocutaneous Flap

The adaptation of musculocutaneous flaps for use in reconstruction surgery has had a profound impact on the field of breast reconstruction. The latissimus dorsi myocutaneous flap has become the most important technique of breast reconstruction and can be used for most mastectomy defects. It is particularly applicable when there is a deficiency of soft tissue coverage of the chest wall, with partial or complete loss of the pectoralis muscle, and a tightness of the mastectomy scar which prevents reconstruction with local tissue alone.

In 1976, Olivari described the use of the latissimus dorsi muscle to provide coverage of defects of the anterior chest wall after radiation lesions. Although this technique was actually published by Tansini as early as 1906, Olivari has to be given credit for having opened up a new area of latissimus dorsi flap techniques. The use of latissimus dorsi to provide a better cover for the implant in breast reconstruction was popularized by Mühlbauer in 1977 and especially by John Bostwick et al. 1979 (Fig. 5).

When the latissimus dorsi myocutaneous flap is employed, the latissimus dorsi muscle and varying amounts of overlying skin are transferred, in a single

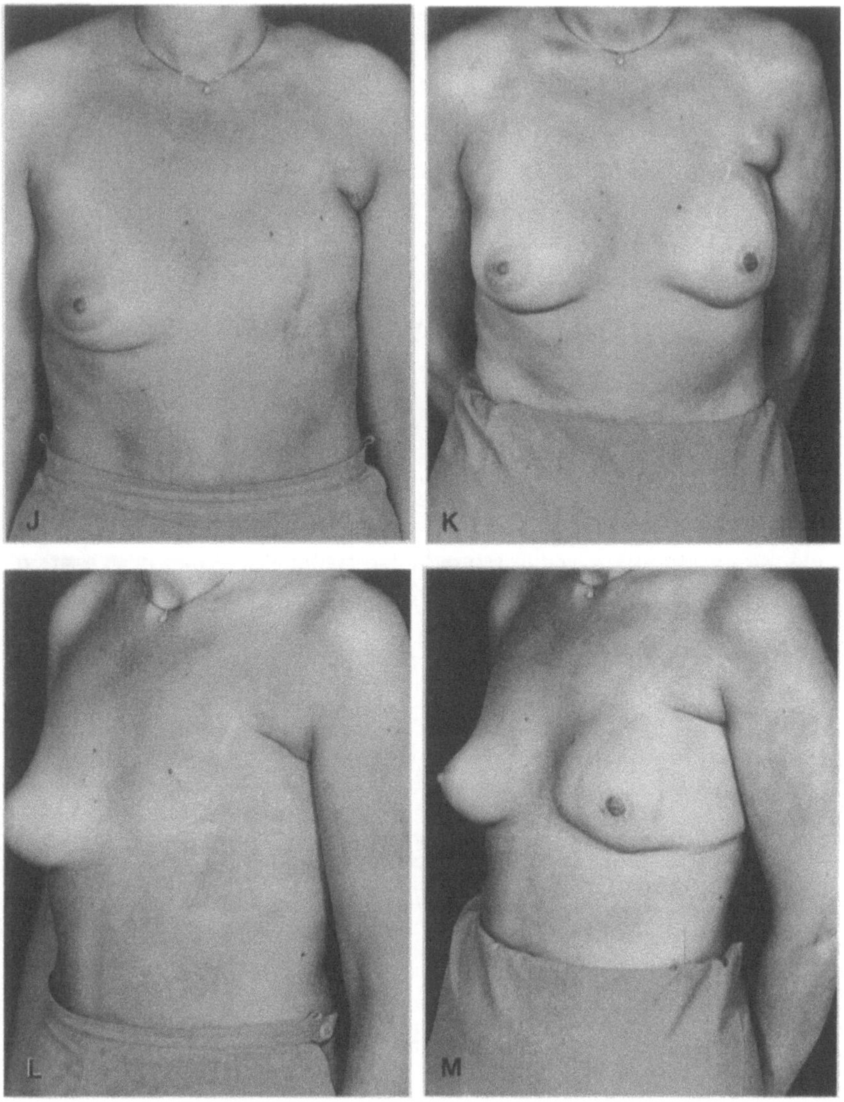

Fig. 5 J–M

operative procedure, from the back to the anterior chest wall to replace the deficient skin and pectoralis musculature. The flap is transferred, based on an intact thoracodorsal-arteriovenous system. The mastectomy scar is excised, thereby recreating the defect resultant from the mastectomy into which the latissimus dorsi myocutaneous flap is transferred. The addition of this tissue allows for the insertion of a suitably selected silicone implant to produce the breast contour projection. The donor site of the latissimus dorsi muscle on the back is repaired by direct approximation of the wound edges, resulting in a scar across the back and minimal, if any, functional deformity.

The borders of the muscle are outlined prior to surgery with the patient in the sitting position. The size and position of the skin island is designed, recognizing that the rotation point will be the posterior axillary fold. If the skin island is to be transferred to the area of an oblique mastectomy scar, the skin island will be an ellipse horizontally located below the scapula. Such a defect could be easily closed with a resulting scar being covered by the brassiere.

The operation is made with the patient in the lateral position, which gives access to both donor and recipient areas simultaneously. The skin island is circumscribed and carried down to the muscle fascia, preserving part of the surrounding subcutaneous tissue, and the rest of the skin covering the muscle is dissected free.

The anterolateral border of the muscle is identified and from here it is easy to free the deep surface of the muscle by blunt dissection. The superior border of the latissimus dorsi is dissected free and detached from the lower angle of the scapula, taking care to separate it from the serratus anterior muscle. The muscle is then cut inferiorly at a level to provide as much muscle as needed to cover the upper medial part of the chest wall. After the medial aponeurotic attachments to the spine area have been cut, the flap is made free to rotate around its neurovascular stalk in the posterior axillary fold.

The mastectomy scar is excised and a wide tunnel is made subcutaneously from the posterior axilla to the mastectomy area. The flap is brought through the tunnel to the postmastectomy wound, and the skin on the donor area is closed and the wound drained with a suction catheter. At this point in the operation, it might be more convenient to reposition the patient to have her lying on her back, though this is not necessary if one wishes to shorten the operation time.

The skin over the anterior chest wall is now undermined all the way to the clavicule, the sternum, and the submammary fold. The flap is now positioned and the cranial and medial edges are anchored to the subclacivular and sternal area respectively under the skin flap.

The inferior edge of the muscle flap is sutured to the region of the inframammary fold. The upper medial edge of the skin island is now sutured to the corresponding postmastectomy wound edge continuing with the lower edge from medial to lateral. Before the closure is completed, a prosthesis of appropriate size is introduced under the muscle flap from the lateral side, which is still open.

It is important to secure the muscle flap to the chest wall lateral to the pocket to prevent dislocation of the prosthesis into the axilla. The anterior cavity is drained with suction catheter. A soft dressing is applied, taking care not to apply any pressure on the pedicle of the flap.

Transverse Rectus Abdominis Flap

This flap, first described by Hartrampf et al. (1982), contains the amount of skin and subcutaneous tissue usually resected in a lower abdominal plasty. It is carried on the contralateral or the ipsilateral rectus muscle or both muscles nourished by the superior epigastric artery and transferred to the postmastectomy area to provide skin and tissue to build up a new breast without the use of an implant (Fig. 6).

Patients with considerable tissue defects in the mastectomy area and a fair amount of surplus skin in the lower abdomen are ideal candidates. An additional indication might be in patients refusing to have an implant, or those in whom an earlier implant has caused considerable contracture with deformation and pain.

Operative Technique

The flap is designed as a horizontal ellipse giving sufficient tissue for the reconstruction but also allowing an easy closure of the donor area. It is located in the lower abdomen with its upper border cranial to the umbilicus, which is circumscribed as a first step of the operation and left in place. The lower border of the flap is incised down to the fascia of the abdominal wall and the dissection is carried cranially until the first major perforating vessels from the rectus are reached. They are usually midway between the symphysis and the umbilicus and have to be preserved.

The upper border to the flap is now incised down to the abdominal wall, leaving some extra subcutaneous fat over the rectus sheath to save some more perforating vessels.

The lateral parts of the flap are dissected free, extending medially to the borders of the rectus, which is to carry the flap. The dissection is then extended on the rectus sheath until the perforating vessels can be seen. Now the upper abdominal skin is undermined over the deep fascia to a level above the costal margin.

Preparation of the stalk starts by incision of the rectus sheath caudal to the perforating vessels and cutting the rectus muscle at this level. The inferior epigastric artery running on the posterior surface of the muscle is ligated. The anterior rectus sheath is now incised on both sides of the perforating vessels, leaving medially and laterally as much as possible of the rectus sheath to allow good closure. The central edges of the rectus sheath are attached to the rectus muscle and could be sutured to the muscle to prevent unnecessary tearing of the perforating vessels during the preparation of the flap. The rectus abdominis muscle with its anterior sheath is then dissected free up to the costal margin. The viability of the flap has to be checked throughout the preparation. If, at an early stage, the circulation seems questionable, suture of the flap back in place could be considered, calling it a delayed procedure. If, however, the circulation becomes more than questionable at a later stage of the preparation, one might consider sacrificing the flap and converting the operation to an abdominal plasty.

With an adequate circulation, the flap is brought through a subcutaneous tunnel to the postmastectomy scar area that has been excised. If necessary, for

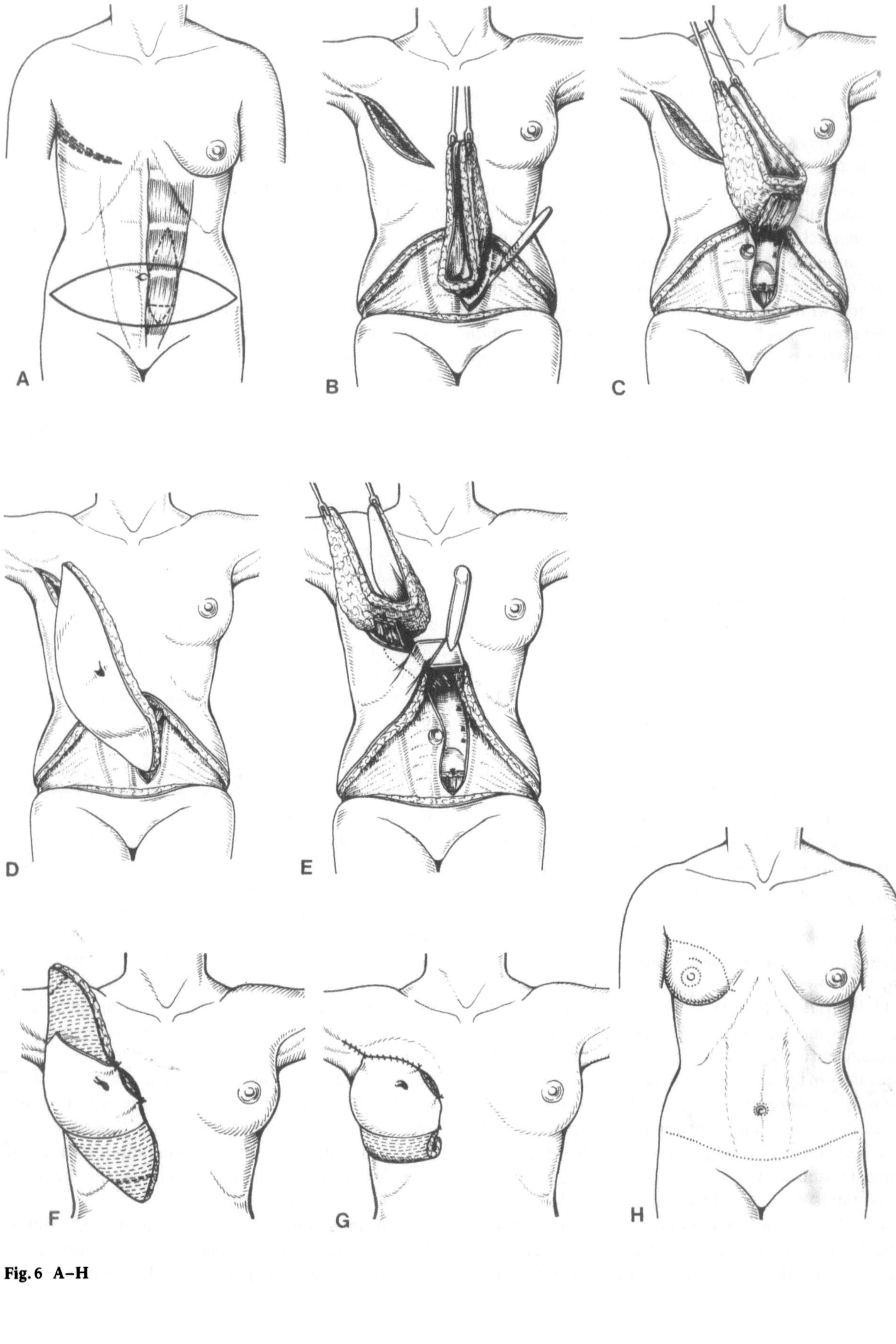

Fig. 6 A–H

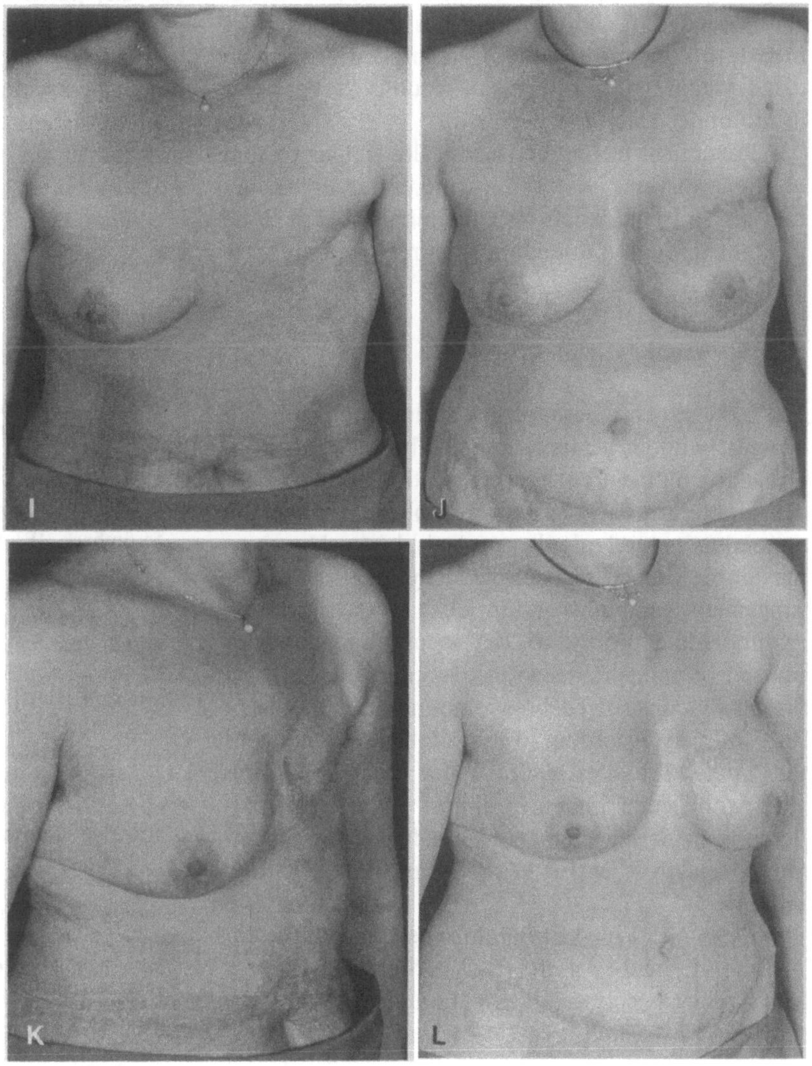

Fig. 6. A Preoperative markings of a contralateral transverse abdominal island flap. **B** The flap is raised for about 2–3 cm across the anterior rectus sheath and elevated. **C** The rectus sheath is incised and the flap elevated on the rectus abdominis muscle. **D** The flap during transfer to the breast area. **E** The anterior abdominal wall is raised above the subcostal margin and the flap is transferred through a tunnel into the mastectomy defect. **F** The flap is delivered through the mastectomy incision onto the chest wall and is deepithelialized above for filling the axillary defect and below to give filling for the breast mound. **G** The superior border of the flap is sutured in place with its deepithelialized zone under the skin in the axillary and infraclavicular region; the inferior portion will be positioned for creating the breast volume. **H** The flap is sutured in position and the nipple-areola complex created. **I** Preoperative appearance of a modified radical mastectomized patient. Reconstruction by lower rectus flap. **J** Postoperative appearance of the same patient. **K** Profile view preoperatively. **L** Profile view postoperatively

an adequate rotation, part of the upper rectus could be divided once the superior epigastric vessels have been identified. There is now a considerable amount of tissue at hand to build a breast. It has to be decided how much skin is needed and how much of the skin should be deepithelialized and brought subcutaneously to build up the anterior axillary fold, the infraclavicular groove, and the inferior bulking of the breast. This is a real challenge for a plastic surgeon to match the healthy breast.

Closure of the donor area starts with direct closure of the fascial defect of the rectus sheath, which has to be very meticulous to prevent weakness of the abdominal wall and herniation.

The abdominal wound is closed as in an abdominal plasty. The original umbilicus is often so lateralized that it has to be resected and a false umbilicus simulated. Both operative areas have to be drained.

The advantage of this procedure is the large amount of tissue offered for reconstruction; the disadvantage is that it is a major procedure with complications, and even complete loss of flaps has been reported.

Modifications to make the procedure safe include use of the both rectus muscles, to ensure optimal blood supply.

Another point is that the large amount of transposed tissue makes it impossible to detect local recurrences at an early stage. Minor areas of fat necrosis are palpated as hard lumps and may cause further worry for the patient and the oncologist.

As an alternative a vertical myocutaneous rectus abdominis flap (Robbins 1979) might be used from either the ipsilateral or contralateral side. The skin over the rectus is included in the flap. This will supply less tissue than the transverse rectus flap but is a surgically simpler procedure when not too much tissue is needed. It could make it possible to rebuild a breast contour even without an implant. The main disadvantage is the rather conspicuous vertical scar in the upper abdomen.

The surgical technique is basically similar to that of the transverse rectus flap, the difference being that a skin island is left over the rectus sheath to be brought through a tunnel into the recipient area.

Nipple-Areola Reconstruction

The reconstructed breast contour does not look like a breast without a nipple areola. The first choice of tissue for nipple-areola reconstruction is the opposite nipple areola. This is only applicable when the remaining natural nipple areola is large. However, the nipple can be reconstructed by local tissue advancement techniques and produce a very satisfactory nipple-like protusion. The areola is created by transfer of pigmented skin to the appropriate site on the newly constructed breast mound. The source of skin will vary according to the color requirements of the areola. The skin of the upper inner thigh provides good color match in almost all patients, particularly in darkly pigmented areola, whereas post-auricular skin is useful in the more lightly colored pink areola.

Nipple-areola reconstruction is usually delayed for 2–3 months and is performed at the same time as the symmetry between the natural breast and the newly reconstructed breast is created.

Conclusion

The aim of breast reconstruction is to restore body image by providing symmetry and by simulating contour and nipple-areola complex on the ablated side. Today, with the techniques that are available, every women can be offered the chance to restore her femininity. Regardless of when the mastectomy is performed, and regardless of the nature and extent of the mastectomy procedure and the resultant deformity, a very satisfactory, pleasing breast reconstruction can be obtained by one of several reconstructive techniques. Such a possibility should be presented as an option to the patient in her rehabilitation.

Since breast reconstruction does not change the course of the disease, the decision to undergo breast reconstruction is essentially the patient's decision, and any patient is a candidate for the procedure. If women are made fully aware of the possibility of reconstructive surgery following mastectomy, they may not delay seeking treatment because of fear of permanent disfigurement. Hopefully, this will mean that dreaded lumps will be reported earlier and will result in a better cure rate.

References

Argenta LC (1984) Reconstruction of the breast by tissue expansion. Clin Plast Surg 11 (2): 257

Bohmert H, Leis HP, Jackson IT (1989) Breast Cancer: Conservative and Reconstructive Surgery, Thieme, Stuttgart New York

Bohmer H (1986) Postmastectomy reconstruction. In: Strömbeck JF, Rosato E (eds) Surgery of the Breast. Thieme, Stuttgart

Bohmert H (1975) Eine neue Methode zur Rekonstruktion der weiblichen Brust nach radikaler Mastektomie. In: Bohmert H (ed) Plastische Chirurgie des Kopf- und Halsbereichs und der weiblichen Brust. Thieme, Stuttgart

Bostwick J (1983) Aesthetic and Reconstructive Breast Surgery, Mosby, St. Louis

Bostwick J, Nahai F, Wallace JG, Vasconez LO (1979) Sixty latissimus dorsi flaps. Plast reconstr Surg 63

Bostwick J, Vasconez L, Jurkiewicz MJ (1978) Breast reconstruction after radical mastectomy. Plast Reconstr Surg 61: 682

Cronin TD, Upton J, McDonough JM (1977) Reconstruction of the breast after mastectomy. Plast reconstr Surg 59, 1

Dinner MI, Labandter HP (1981) Total mammary adenectomy with histiologic evaluation and immediate reconstruction. Plast Reconstr Surg 68: 505

Hartrampf CR, Scheflan M, Black PW (1982) Breast reconstruction with a transverse abdominal island flap. Plast Reconstr Surg 69: 216

Leis HP, Jr (1979) Selective and reconstructive surgical procedures for carcinoma of the breast. Gynecol Obstet 148: 17

Lejour M (1982) Reconstruction of the breast with a contralateral epigastric rectus myocutaneous flap. Chir plast 6: 181

Mühlbauer W, Olbrisch R (1977) The latissimus dorsi myocutaneous flap for breast reconstruction. Chir plast 4 27

Olivari N (1976) The latissimus flap. Brit J plast Surg 29 126

Robbins TH (1979) Rectus abdominus myocutaneous flap for breast reconstruction. Aust NZJ Surg 49 527

Scheflan M, Dinner MI (1983) The transverse abdominal island flap. I. Indications, contraindications, results and complications. Ann plast Surg 10: 24

Tansini I (1906) Sopra il mio nuovo processo di amputazione della mammella. Riforma medica 12: 757

Tai Y, Hasegawa H (1974) A transverse abdominal flap for reconstruction after radical operations for recurrent breast cancer Plast reconstr Surg 53: 52

Vasconez LO, Psillakis J, Johnson-Gieberk R (1983) Breast reconstruction with contralateral rectus abdominus myocutaneous flap. Plast reconstr Surg 71: 668

Urban JA (1973) Reconstruction after mastectomy. In: Snyderman RK (ed) Symposium on Neoplastic and Reconstructive Problems of the Female Breast Mosby Saint Louis

Microsurgical Reconstruction of Large Defects after Tumor Surgery in the Head and Neck Region

R. G. H. Baumeister and H. Bohmert

Microsurgical methods for reconstruction in the head and neck region after tumor therapy are mostly necessary when large defects must be closed, special requirements are necessary, or when local flaps have already been used and no further local reconstruction is possible. Different conditions call for different reconstructive techniques.

In reconstructing large one- or two-layer soft tissue defects the skin and subcutaneous tissue have to be replaced. For example, the radial forearm flap, the dorsalis pedis flap, and the scapular and parascapular flap can be used (Dielert and Stock 1987; Gilbert and Teot 1982; Dos Santos 1980; Sauter et al. 1983; Yang et al. 1981). In the reconstruction of full thickness cheek defects, the mucosa has to be replaced together with skin and soft tissue. The inferior epigastric abdominal wall flap or a sandwich flap can be used. Reconstruction of larger defects within the oral cavity can be covered with free jejunal grafts (Dielert and Stock 1987; Mees et al. 1987; Reuther and Steinau 1980).

Defects of several layers or full thickness defects together with parts of the mandible can be reconstructed by composite grafts, for example, with a cortico-cutaneous flap of the inguinal region. Another composite flap is the radial forearm flap including parts of the radius (Dielert et al. 1987; Sauter et al. 1983; Yang et al. 1981).

As examples of microsurgical reconstruction, the free scapular flap and the inferior epigastric abdominal wall flap will be described in detail. The free scapular flap was designed by Dos Santos (1980) and used clinically by Gilbert and Teot (1982) for the first time in 1980. The dominant vessel of the flap is the horizontal branch of the circumflex scapular artery. The artery appears at the medial gap of the axilla and can be easily detected here during the opera-

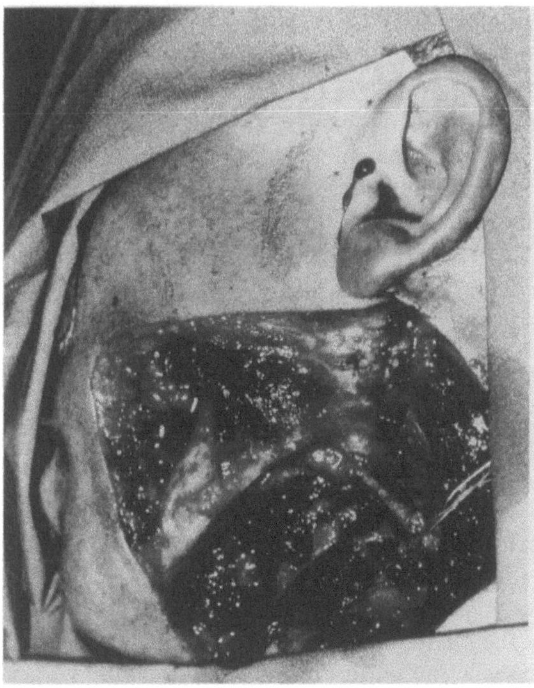

Fig. 1. Defect in a 49-year-old patient after resectional therapy of a recurrent carcinoma of the submandibular gland

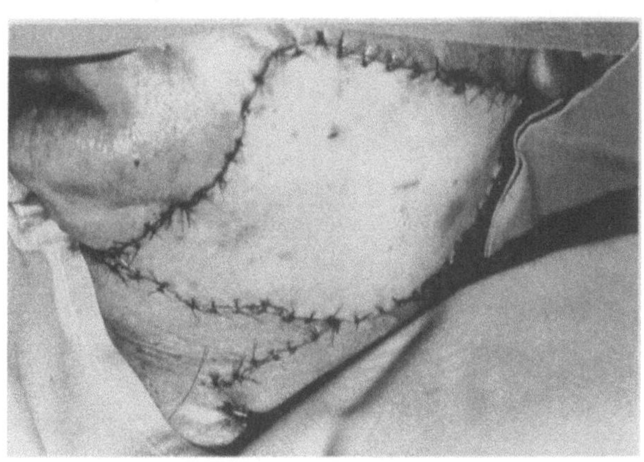

Fig. 2. Closure of the defect with a free microvascular scapular flap

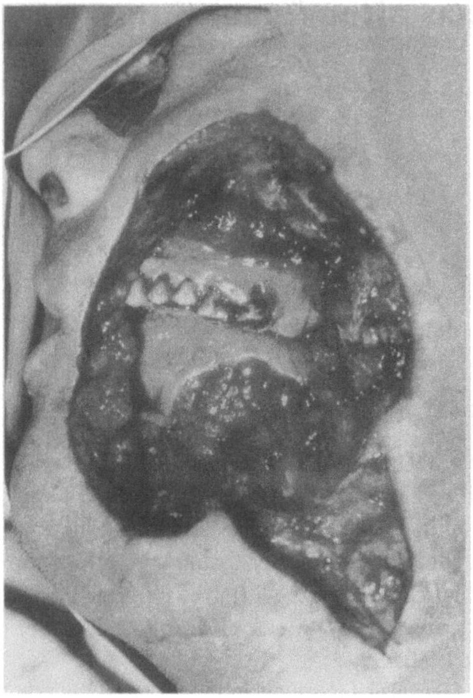

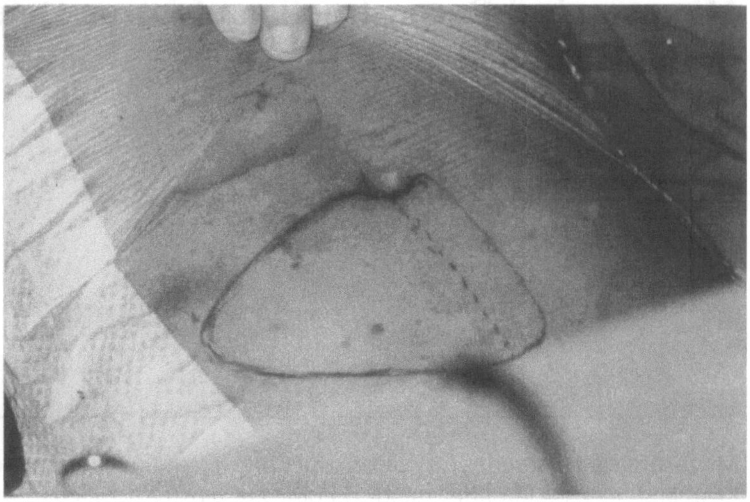

▲
Fig. 4. Extent of the inferior epigastric abdominal wall flap

◀ **Fig. 3.** Large penetrating defect of the cheek after resectional therapy in a case of recurrent alveolar cell carcinoma

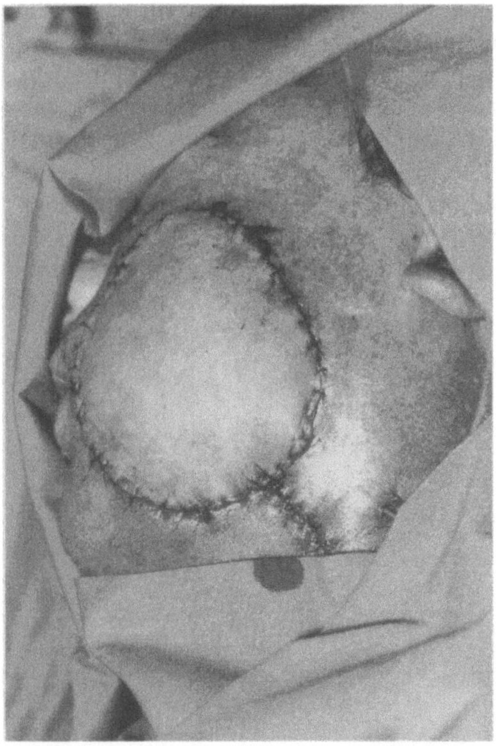

Fig. 5. Restoration of all three layers of the cheek by the free microvascular inferior epigastric abdominal wall flap

tion. The vessel lies suprafascially. The average thickness of the flap is about 1 cm. The length of the vascular pedicle is 6–7 cm. The diameter of the circumflex scapular artery is 1.5–2.5 mm.

The main advantages of the flaps are: (a) the constant anatomy of the vessels; (b) the possibility of a direct closure of the defect; and (c) the minimal morbidity of the donor side. Using this method, large defects after tumor resection procedures can be closed easily (Figs. 1, 2).

To restore large full thickness defects of the cheek, skin and mucosa should closed simultaneously. Two different flaps can be used: a flap with formation of two surfaces of the same material (sandwich-like) or – as a new development – the abdominal wall with the skin as outer surface and the peritoneum as inner surface (Mees et al. 1987).

The second possibility should be discussed in detail. The lower abdominal region is suitable as a donor area (Fig. 4). The dominant vessel is the inferior epigastric artery which arises from the external iliac artery. The vessel together with accompanying veins can be easily found during the operation. The whole abdominal wall is used as a flap. The rectus muscle is dissected distal to the insertion of the inferior epigastric vessels. The cranial cutting area lies near the navel. The vascular network around this area is used to nourish the flap. A direct closure of the donor defect is nearly always possible, even when large flaps are excised. If there are problems, a Prolene net can stabilize the abdominal wall.

When in place, the peritoneum covers the defect of the oral mucosa, the abdominal musculature restores the soft tissue of the cheek, and the abdominal skin covers the skin defect. The single-layer epithelium of the peritoneum is rapidly transformed into an epithelium with several layers.

Figures 3 and 5 show the defect and the repair using an inferior epigastric abdominal wall flap in a patient with a recurrent carcinoma of the submandibular gland.

Microsurgical procedures are of great help in the therapy of advanced stages of carcinomas in the head and neck region. The resection can be extended almost without any consideration for the demands of the secondary repair. Microsurgery provides a wide variety of possibilities to cover very large and complex defects.

Remark: The patients shown in the figures are treated in collaboration with the ENT Department, Klinikum Großhadern, University of Munich.

References

Dielert E, Stock W (1987) Neurovaskulär anastomosierter Radialislappen zum Haut-, Schleimhaut- und Nerv-Ersatz. Dtsch Z Mund Kiefer Gesichts Chir 11: 288–295

Dielert E, Stock W, Fischer-Brandies E, Wolf K (1987) Wiederherstellung der Kinnkontur mit mikrochirurgisch revaskularisiertem Osteomyokutanlappen. Dtsch Z Mund Kiefer Gesichts Chir 11: 186–194

Dos Santos LF (1980) The scapular flap: a new microsurgical free flap. Bol Chir Plast 70: 133–144

Gilbert A, Teot L (1982) The free scapular flap. Plast Reconstr Surg 69: 601–604

Mees K, Baumeister R, Kastenbauer E (1987) Mikrochirurgische Rekonstruktion großer dreischichtiger Wangendefekte. Laryngol Rhinol Otol (Stuttg) 66: 591–594

Reuther J, Steinau U (1980) Mikrochirurgische Dünndarmtransplantation zur Rekonstruktion großer Tumordefekte der Mundhöhle. Dtsch Z Mund Kiefer Gesichts Chir 4: 131

Sauter DS, Scheker LR, Tanner NSB, McGregor IA (1983) The radial forearm flap: a versatile method for intraoral reconstruction. Br J Plast Surg 63: 1

Yang G, Gao Y Chem B, Liu X, Li J, Jiang S, He S (1981) Forearm free skin flap transplantation. Natl Med J China 61: 139

Orthopaedic Procedures in the Rehabilitation of Cancer Patients

R. KOTZ and A. AZZARELLI

Introduction

In the past 10 years significant progress has been made in the management of malignant bone tumours, with improved functional results and patient survival. This fact is due to more experienced and defined conservative surgery, sophisticated endoprostheses and aggressive neoadjuvant multidrug chemotherapies. This chapter reports the current concepts and approaches widely accepted in major cancer orthopaedic institutes towards the diagnosis, treatment and rehabilitation of patients with malignant bone lesions and in particular those seen at the Orthopaedic University Clinic of Vienna and recorded in the Vienna Bone Tumor Registry (Kotz et al. 1984), which over the past 25 years has collected more than 3700 cases[1] as well as those seen at the Istituto Nazionale Tumori of Milan. In a specialised institute an interdisciplinary team should evaluate each patient, taking into account histological diagnosis, location and extent of the disease and the expected and achieved effects of therapeutic procedures and functional results. Diagnosis, symptoms, physical examination and single X-ray may provide a first indication towards appropriate diagnosis. If a malignant bone tumour is suspected the roentgenographic diagnosis must be verified with further investigation, such as bone scan, CT scan, angiography and nuclear magnetic resonance (NMR).

Finally, the biopsy is the main task in the diagnostic phase of a malignant bone tumour: it should be performed by the surgeon who will be responsible for the total and definitive surgery of the patient. The diagnosis can be ascertained by open biopsy, which should provide the pathologist with sufficient material and should not compromise limb-sparing surgery by soft tissue contamination.

In some cases large needle biopsy can be attempted first. A frozen section can establish the diagnosis immediately, or, at least, the validity of a reliable specimen. It should be stressed that the biopsy scar,

[1] Vienna Bone Tumor Registry (Head: Prof. Dr. Mechthild, Salzer-Kuntschik) at the Orthopaedic University Clinic (Head: Prof. Dr. R. Kotz) and the Institute of Pathology (Head: Prof. Dr. J. H. Holzner).

or needle way, must be removed en bloc at the time of the final operation. Having once reached a diagnosis, each case is discussed by a team of specialists and the therapeutic plan is usually determined by treatment protocols. Osteosarcoma and Ewing's sarcoma are treated in our institute with preoperative chemotherapy, in accordance with multicentric protocols: Cooperative Osteosarcoma Study (COSS) (Winkler et al. 1986), Co-operative Ewing's Sarcoma Study (CESS) (Jürgens 1981), the Consiglio Nazionale delle Ricerche (CNR) (Gasparini 1987), and at the Istituto Nazionale Tumori of Milan. Surgery is performed at the scheduled time and postoperative CT is modulated on the response to neoadjuvant treatment. Malignant histiocytomas are usually treated in the same way as osteosarcoma. In cases of chondrosarcoma, or other rare primary malignancies of the bone, surgery is performed soon after the biopsy, usually without adjuvant chemotherapy.

Definition of Surgical Adequacy

The staging system for the anatomosurgical classification of bone tumours proposed by the Muscolo Skeletal Society (Enneking 1980) combines the pathological grading and the extent of the tumours (intra- or extraosseous) and these parameters influence the choice of the surgical approach (Table 1).

In planning surgical treatment of bone tumours the choice of operation to be performed must satisfy two main requirements:

1. Achievement of radicality
2. Preservation fo the optimal functionality of the affected part of the body

The Enneking staging system provides a clear definition of what kind of operation can be considered adequate or not:

Inadequate Surgery

Intralesional surgery, with macroscopic residual tumour, can be tolerated only for some benign lesions. *Marginal resection,* which gives the impression of gross radicality, could leave residual microscopic tumour and should be avoided in the treatment of malignant tumours.

Adequate Surgery

Wide resection with removal of the tumour surrounded by normal tissue is the method of choice for intraosseous malignant tumours. Radical *compartmental resection,* resection of the whole of the involved osseous segment with surrounding soft parts, is appropriate for large and extracompartmental malignant tumours.

These definitions are independent of whether ablative or conservative surgery is performed.

Ablative Surgery

Amputation above the involved bone, i.e. above the knee amputation for tumours of the tibia, is a radical resection of the tumour in any case; in fact, the involved compartment is removed completely. Amputation through the involved bone cannot be considered a compartmental procedure because it is performed through the affected compartment. It is a wide resection if adequate distance from the tumour is respected, but can also be marginal or intralesional when the extent of the tumour into the marrow cavity is larger than expected. New technology in radiology and scintigraphy has reduced this risk, especially the nuclear magnetic resonance technique.

Exarticulation, i.e. hip disarticulation for tumours of the femur, removes the involved compartment and is considered as radical if the tumour is far enough from the joint to provide enough uninvolved

Table 1. Musculoskeletal tumour surgery (Enneking 1983 b)

	Surgical stages				
	Stage	Grade	Site		Metastases
I					
	A	Low (G_1)	Intracompartmental	(T_1)	None (M_0)
	B	Low (G_1)	Extracompartmental	(T_2)	None (M_0)
II					
	A	High (G_2)	Intracompartmental	(T_1)	None (M_0)
	B	High (G_2)	Extracompartmental	(T_2)	None (M_0)
III					
	A	Low (G_1)	Intra or Extra	(T_1–T_2)	Regional or Distant (M_1)
	B	High (G_2)	Intra or Extra	(T_1–T_2)	Regional or Distant (M_1)

skin and soft tissue to cover the cartilaginous end of the proximal bone.

Conservative (En Bloc) Surgery

The advent and perfecting of endoprostheses improved results of conservative surgery. The aforementioned principles of radicality can be respected, also, with preservation of the limb, provided that all the involved bony or soft tissue compartments are removed and that neurovascular bundles are not infiltrated. Inferior limb conservative surgery is usually completed by sophisticated and moveable endoprostheses, which, on certain occasions, may not be employed for the upper limbs.

Surgical Operations for Bone Tumours of Limbs and Girdles

In terms of rehabilitation, a great difference exists between surgery of the upper and that of the inferior limbs and girdles. In fact, the major effort in orthopaedic rehabilitation of the inferior limbs is stability of the hip and knee, whereas the major problem for the upper limb is the mobility and sensitivity of the hand, stability being of somewhat less importance. These priorities have an impact on the decision of whether to perform ablative or conservative surgery and the eventual employment of endoprostheses. The ablative and conservative operations are listed below in detail and stratified into upper and lower extremities.

Ablative Surgery of the Lower Extremities

Amputation Below the Knee Joint

The external prostheses replacing the leg and foot are so functional and aesthetic that, for bone malignancies of the distal tibia or the foot, leg amputation and modified amputation of the foot are usually still the best treatment from the oncological and rehabilitative point of view.

Mid-Thigh Amputation and Hip Disarticulation

These operations provide a severe impairment of functionality, due to the lack of one weight-bearing major articulation. Since the advent of tumour endoprostheses, this method is indicated only for large tumours involving the femur, or proximal tibia and surrounding soft tissue, vessels and nerves. When the neurovascular bundle can be spared, limb salvage procedures and also hip rotation plasty can be taken into consideration (see "Conservative Surgery for Tumours of the Upper Thigh" below) (Winkelmann 1983).

Hemipelvectomy

This operation is indicated for large lesions of the pelvic and hip region and can be recommended if different kinds of conservative surgery (so-called inner hemipelvectomy or pelvic resection with limb salvage) cannot be performed (Pack 1956; Miller 1962; Pack and Miller 1964; Nilsonne 1965; Salzer 1965). The hemipelvectomy is no more mutilating than hip disarticulation, but rehabilitation is more difficult. Given successful external prostheses, a fair deambulation and aesthetic look can sometimes be achieved (Fig. 1 a, b). The surgical technique depends on the site of the tumour. In the ventral location a dorsal flap can be used to sew the abdominal wall to the fascia lata and gluteus medius. A ventral flap is necessary to close the defect in cases of multiple scars, or a dorsal location of the tumour near to the skin (Larson and Liang 1983): the skin of the anterior thigh, if not too close to the tumour, can be used together with the quadriceps muscle to cover tissue defects (Fig. 2). The hemipelvectomy is frequently performed when circumstances demand and enables bedridden patients with severe pain or discomfort to be rehabilitated and allows for a fair possibility of cure if the procedure is radical. Eight out of the 22 hemipelvectomies performed at the Orthopaedic University Clinic in Vienna and six out of 19 at the Istituto Tumori of Milan have survived with a good quality of life score (Gennari 1981; Kotz et al. 1986).

Hemicorporectomy

This is the most demolitive surgical treatment possible. The vertebral column is divided between the third and the fourth lumbar spinal body and the caudal half of the body is removed. This operation has been performed in very few cases, usually for low-grade pelvic destructive lesions (Aust and Absolon 1962; Yancey et al. 1964; Miller et al. 1966); nevertheless, frequently large tumours of the pelvic regions could not be removed despite hemicorporectomy having been performed.

Mortality in this type of surgery is high and, in Vienna, has only been performed once, without success. Rehabilitation requires a strong personality in

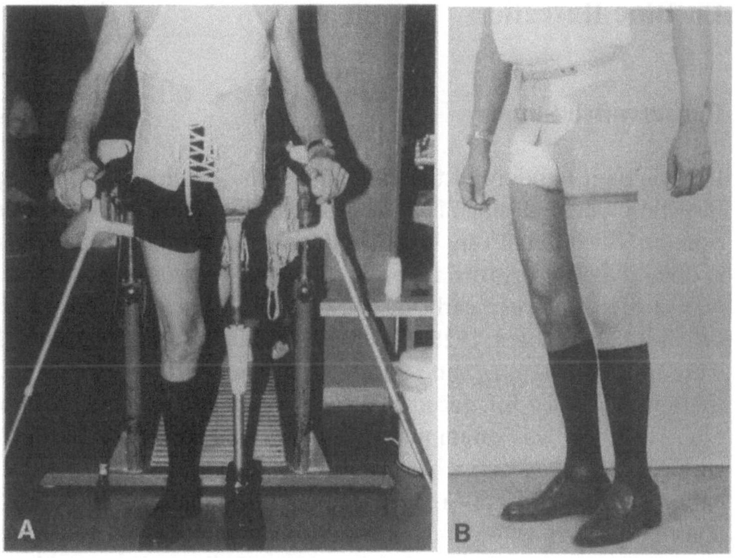

Fig. 1 A, B. Patient 2 years after hemipelvectomy for chondrosarcoma of the pelvis with different movable prostheses fitted to the trunk

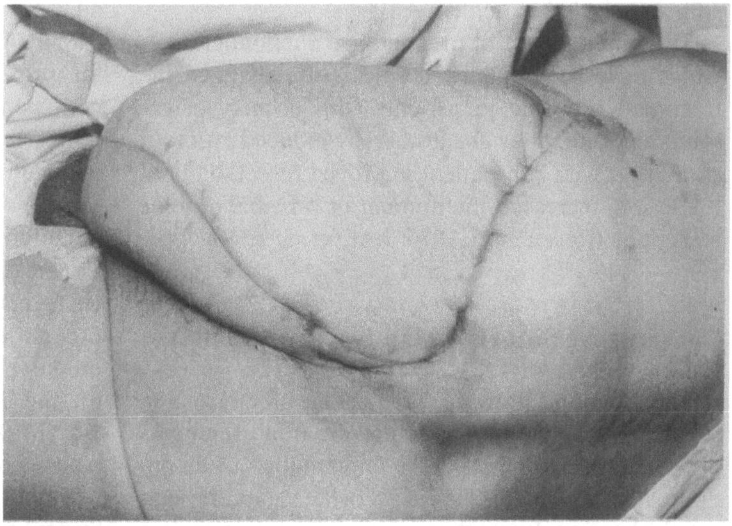

Fig. 2. Hemipelvectomy using a quadriceps muscular cutaneous flap to cover a large dorsal defect, due to primary dorsal tumour extension of a chondrosarcoma

the patient with an equally strong desire to live combined with optimal social and family circumstances (Grimby and Stener 1973).

Ablative Surgery of the Upper Extremities

The volume of soft parts surrounding the bony structure of the upper limb, especially at the elbow, wrist and hand, is low and demolitive surgery is frequently the only chance to remove a malignant tumour in these areas. The choice of the type of amputation depends on the site of the primary lesion. Therefore, amputation of the hand, amputation of the forearm (below the elbow) and amputation of the arm (above the elbow) are taken into consideration. For tumours of the proximal humerus and scapular girdle some possiblities of performing conservative procedures exist, with or without endoprostheses, so that humeral disarticulation and interscapular disarticulation are reserved for large tumours which involve vessels and nerves. The most extensive and frequently performed operation is the interscapulothoracic disarticulation which, like hemipelvectomy, is one of the major procedures of ablative surgery. Sometimes the operative field must be extended to the thoracic wall and, in these cases, muscles and cutaneous flaps are, frequently, required to cover the defect in the thoracic wall.

En Bloc Resection

Conservative Surgery

In malignant tumours of the extremities, the en bloc resection, when feasible, is an alternative to amputation, provided that a very low risk of local recurrence is obtained. Conservative resection for bone tumours was carried out very early on (Juvara 1929; Sauerbruch 1922; Linberg 1928; Troell 1931), but results were not encouraging and amputation remained the therapy of choice for decades. Twenty years ago en bloc resection was attempted again with improved surgical technique and a better rationale for its indication (Wilson and Lance 1965; Zenker 1967; Nadjafi 1970; Parrish 1973; Steiner et al. 1973; Marcove and Khafagy 1974; Kotz and Salzer 1975; Dölle and Rinecker 1975; Smith et al. 1975; Salzer and Knahr 1976; Rosen et al. 1976) and produced some good results in selected patients.

The development of preoperative chemotherapies, which have been employed since 1975, changed the treatment schedule in patients with primary osteosarcoma; and the chemotherapy-induced tumour shrinkage, with subsequent improved resectability of the lesion, increased the number of possible en bloc resections (Rosen et al. 1976; Kotz et al. 1977).

Conservative Surgery of the Lower Extremities

Reconstruction following a radical en bloc resection for malignant tumours affecting the bone segments of the lower extremities is the implantation of an endoprosthesis which should provide stability and weight bearing. In most cases, en bloc resection is a wide resection of bone and soft parts and radicality is essential in performing these operations.

With this in view, intraoperative histological control of the resection margins is advisable and, usually, only small bone tumours and others which have responded well to chemotherapy are suitable for en bloc resection and endoprosthetic replacement.

Tumour Endoprosthesis for the Knee Region

The simplest endoprosthesis after en bloc resection of the knee is a femurotibial rod with cement, which results in a stiff knee, poor functionality, but good stability and prompt rehabilitation. After adequate follow-up, according to the tumoral history, a Putti-Juvara (Juvara 1929) bony graft can consolidate the surgery. This intervention bridges the resected bone by means of autologous and homologous bone transplants and stabilizes it with nails and plates. Excellent results can be obtained with this procedure in the region of the knee, especially for tumours invading the joint, when the extensor mechanism cannot be spared (Fig. 3a, b). Of course, a moveable prosthesis could achieve a more physiological functionality of the leg: for bone tumours of the distal femur, or proximal tibia, the knee joint must be removed en bloc with all the ligament and tendon insertions; for this reason hinged prostheses with long stems and possible cement can be employed radically, different from those employed for common osteopathies.

At the Orthopaedic University in Vienna, tumour endoprostheses without bone cement were experimented on: a rough surface with plates and screws provided a primary stability and secondary anchorage for the ingrowth of bone into the rough surface.

Between 1976 and 1982 30 cases of custom-made knee endoprostheses were inserted (Ramach et al. 1987), 14 for lesions of the distal femur and 16 for the proximal tibia. There were many complications with perioperative mortality (five cases) and infections (three cases). In eight cases the prosthesis was removed and five were amputated, one recurring locally.

Different types of endoprostheses have been designed (Chao and Sim 1983), which have been specially manufactured for different sites. A new approach to the problem was the development of modular prostheses for the proximal femur as well as for the entire bones of the lower extremities (Kotz 1983b) (Fig. 4a), which also permits total femur replacement (Fig. 4b, c).

The Kotz Modular Femur Tibia Reconstruction System (Kotz 1983a) (KMFTR) (Fig. 4a) is now available for special cases and consists of 25 major sections: proximal femur (three sizes, 12, 14, 16 cm long), distal femur (three sizes × two sides), proximal (three sizes) and diaphyseal anchorage pieces (three sized and two sides) which connect the prosthesis to the diaphysis of the remaining bone. These parts are connected by means of a tapered cone which can be put together with a firm hammer blow. This modular system permits every length to be obtained from 12 cm to a total femur, ranging from 30 cm (three components), with increments of 2 cm up to more than 48 cm (five components) (Fig. 4b, c). At the University in Vienna from September 1982 to September 1985, 48 modular prostheses were implanted, 22 in the proximal femur, 15 in the distal femur, 7 in the proximal tibia, 2 total femurs and 1 femur-tibia total knee joint. These operations were

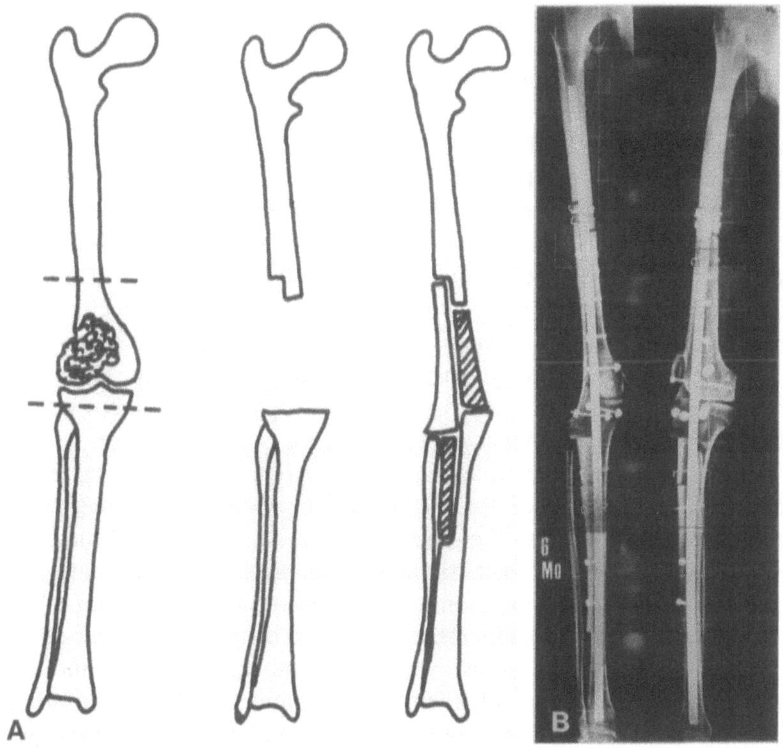

Fig. 3. **A** Putti-Juvara plasty to bridge the defect after resection of the distal part of the femur. **B** The case of an osteosarcoma of the distal femur reconstructed by this method using a long nail

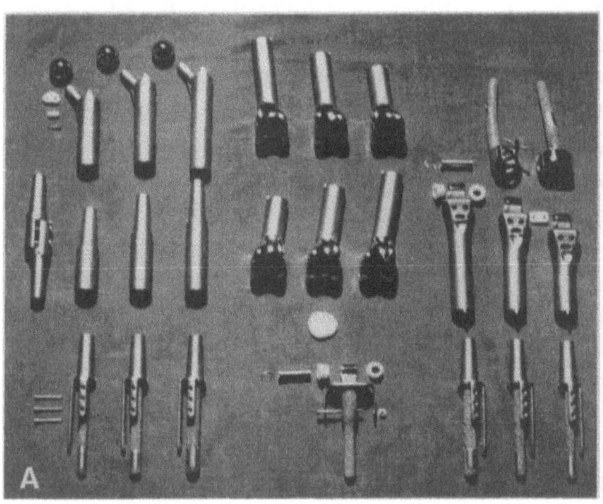

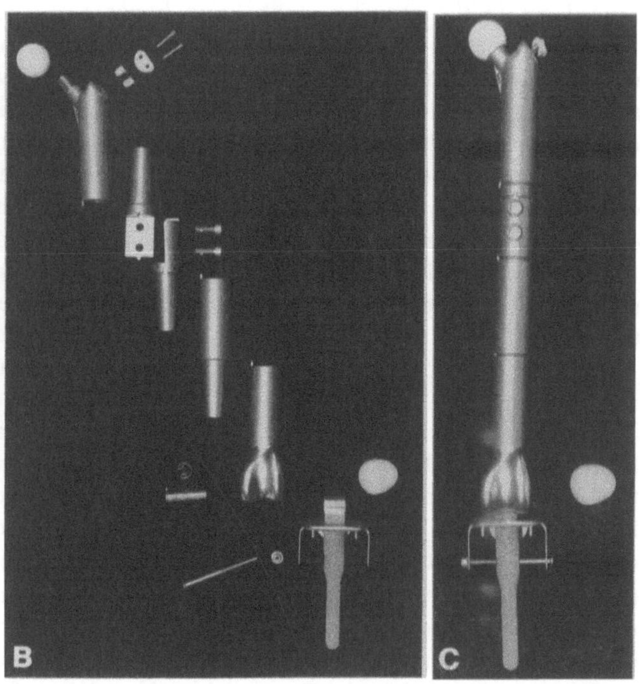

Fig. 4 A–C. Kotz Modular Femur Tibia Reconstruction System (KMFTRS): **A** 25 major parts; **B** 6 parts of the KMFTRS to form a total femur; **C** the total femur after attachment to a connecting piece and by means of tapered cones of the appropriate length

performed for bone metastases (17 cases), primary tumours (15 cases) and complications after implantation of proximal femur, or conventional hip prostheses.

Good rehabilitation of the knee joint requires strong stability: in proximal tibia endoprostheses the fixation of ligamentum patellae is important. The peroneal nerve is isolated and the fibula is osteotomized twice to bring the ligamentum collaterale fibulae in front to the ligamentum patellae and connected with it: this technique ensures strength and stability of the extensor apparatus.

Radiological postoperative evaluation showed bone ingrowth in 15 cases and no reaction in 10. Out of these 25 cases with an average follow-up of 14 months (range 6–31 months) dislocations of hip endoprostheses occurred in 4 cases. This possibility is much higher in resection of the proximal femur than with the conventional hip arthroplasty, because conspicuous muscular and ligamentous tissue are removed en bloc with the lesion.

Five cases had soft tissue complications and three of these required skin graft or muscle transplantation. One stem fracture was observed with a 10-mm stem in the femur, which following this experience is no longer recommended for the femur, the 13-mm stem fitting most cases. The fractured stem was replaced with a longer prosthesis and the clinical result of this case of osteosarcoma was excellent. Two elderly patients died postoperatively and four died of disease. Rated by the Enneking system (Enneking 1983), seven results are excellent, seven good, six fair, due to muscle weakness of the patients, and one poor with stiffness of the knee.

Special mention should be made of limb-sparing procedures in the growing child. Long bones are commonly sites of bone tumours and as an alternative to amputation several attempts have been made with expandable internal prostheses for part of the bones, or the entire bone. These prostheses are designed to be expanded periodically by way of small surgical procedures in order to maintain equality of limb length as the child grows (Lewis 1986). In appropriate patients this kind of treatment is felt to be preferable to amputation or rotation plasty.

Rotation Plasty

If the vessels and the knee joint cannot be spared, a total resection of the distal thigh and knee joint can be performed en bloc with the major femuropopliteal vessels: the lower leg, rotated 180°, will be implanted on the femural stump, so that the ankle joint replaces the function of the knee joint. This procedure, called rotation plasty, was originally mentioned by Borggreve (1930) and afterwards by Van Nes (1950); it is now performed on patients with osteosarcomas of the region of the knee (Kotz and Salzer 1982). The first case was operated on in 1974; since then rotation plasty has been indicated for tumours of the distal femur in growing children, for tumours which have contaminated the knee joint and surrounding soft parts, for tumours which have involved the major vessels and for large tumours which do not respond to chemotherapy.

The skin is incised in a rhomboid shape (Fig. 5 a, b) and first the peroneal nerve on the lateral side is exposed, as well as the tibialis and the sciatic nerve. The vessels are then prepared (Fig. 5 c). If it is planned to cut the vessels because of tumour involvement, they are exposed in the knee joint region and in the upper thigh, and are then clamped and dissected. The tibia is transresected below the knee joint and, following transresection of the muscles, the femur is resected at least 5 cm proximally to the tumour.

The whole specimen must be removed without opening the knee joint. Reconstruction is carried out after leg rotation of 180° (Fig. 5 d) with osteosynthesis of the back-facing tibia to the femur stump with a side plate (Fig. 5 e). In case of vessel dissection, vascular anastomoses provide vitality to the rotated leg. Muscles of the upper thigh are resutured to the lower leg and the skin is closed.

A plaster cast is applied for the first six postoperative weeks and the patient is mobilized a few days after the operation on crutches. We now have data from 1974 to 1985 on 31 cases who underwent surgery at the Orthopaedic University Clinic of Vienna; the median age is 14 years (average 6–36 years). Twenty patients had vessels resected. Vascular thrombosis occurred in four of them in the postoperative stage; all of the latter were operated on again, three of them had limb salvage and one had to be amputated. Other complications have been two pseudoarthroses and one transient peroneal nerve palsey. Out of these 31 patients with an average observation time of 30.5 months (3–108 months), none had local recurrence, and 6 (20%) patients died with metastatic disease.

Patients who have undergone this type of surgery have to wear external prostheses replacing the shortened leg and stand on the tips of their toes in the prosthesis (Fig. 6 a–c). After some time they get a better extension in the ankle joints and acquire 90° motion. Their proprioception is not changed and, in fact, by stretching the knee joint the ankle will stretch at the same time when walking; consequently a natural gait comes automatically and they adapt fully to the rotated foot. Patients do not get the feeling of having an amputated limb and sometimes use their legs without a prosthesis. They are able to walk without limping when wearing the prosthesis and some of them run and practice sports, such as jumping, skiing, cycling and football. The advantage of the rotation plasty is the preservation of a weight-bearing and functional lower extremity, with sensi-

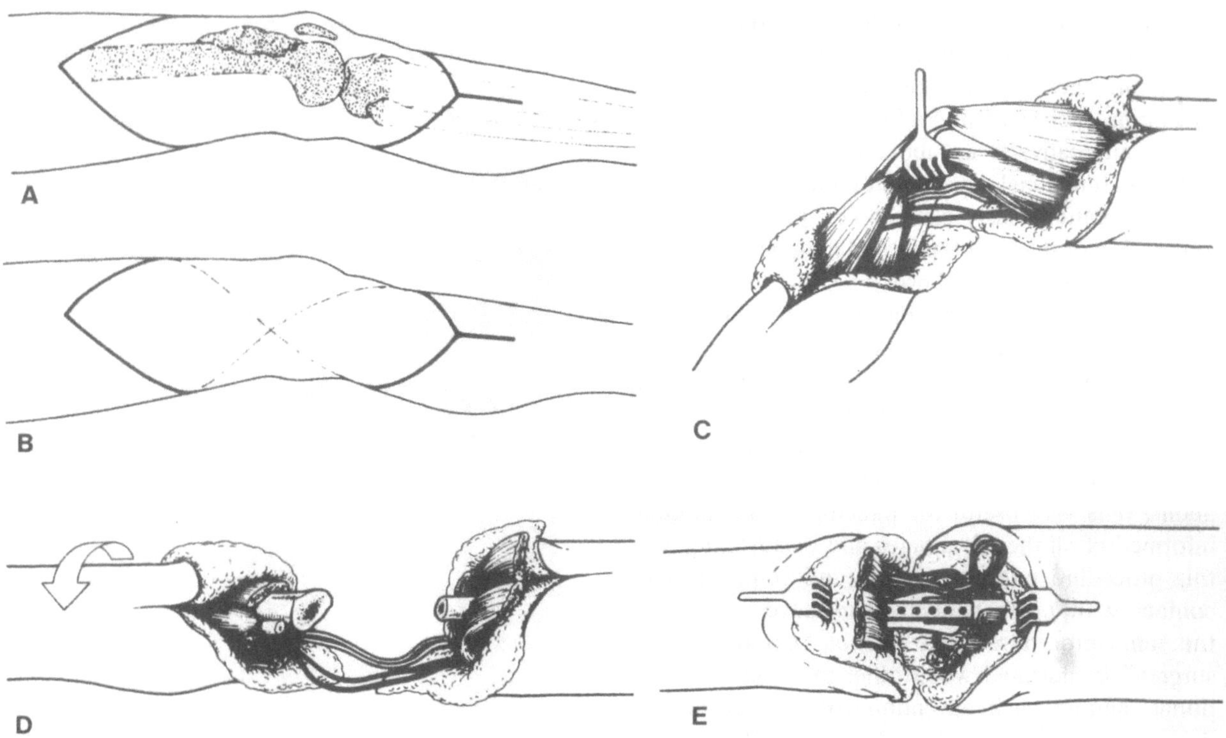

Fig. 5 A–E. Rotation plasty. (From Salzer et al. 1981)

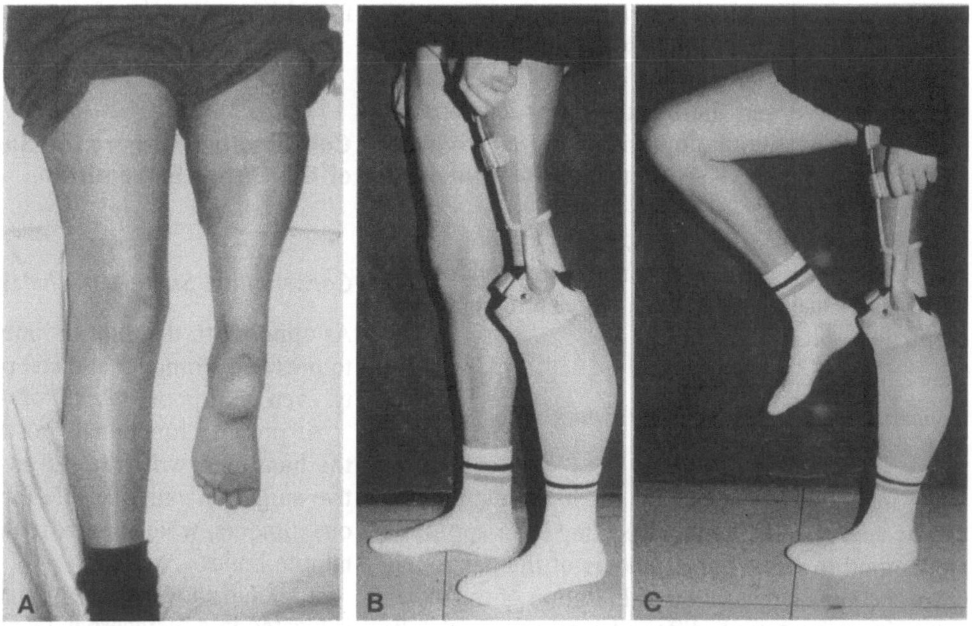

Fig. 6. A Rotation plasty in a 10-year-old boy with an overflap of the upper thigh to compensate growth inequality. **B** Prosthesis for a rotation plasty for an osteosarcoma of the distal femur. **C** The patient is standing on this prosthesis and fixing the knee joint by means of the ankle joint

tivity in the foot. The leg is greatly shortened with the ankle joint at the level of the knee joint: the active ankle joint results in a much better functioning of the prosthesis and the patient has no stump complications, such as phantom limb or neuroma pain.

The alternative is an above-the-knee amputation with less functional capacity. In femur diaphyseal tumours, rotation plasty can also be performed with extirpation of the total femur and a hip endoprosthesis inserted in the rotated proximal tibia (one case).

Due to the bizarre-looking extremity this procedure is under discussion because of the psychological problems it brings with it. It is interesting to note that none of the patients wished to have a revision of the rotation plasty or a secondary amputation, not even of the toes, as is recommended by some surgeons. It is very useful for patients to be carefully informed of all the advantages and disadvantages of this procedure prior to surgery and some form of contact with other patients who have undergone the same procedure. This type of "compartmental surgery" is indicated when other methods of resectional therapy, such as endoprostheses, or arthrodeses, are not indicated as for major II B lesions (Enneking 1980), which responded poorly to chemotherapy.

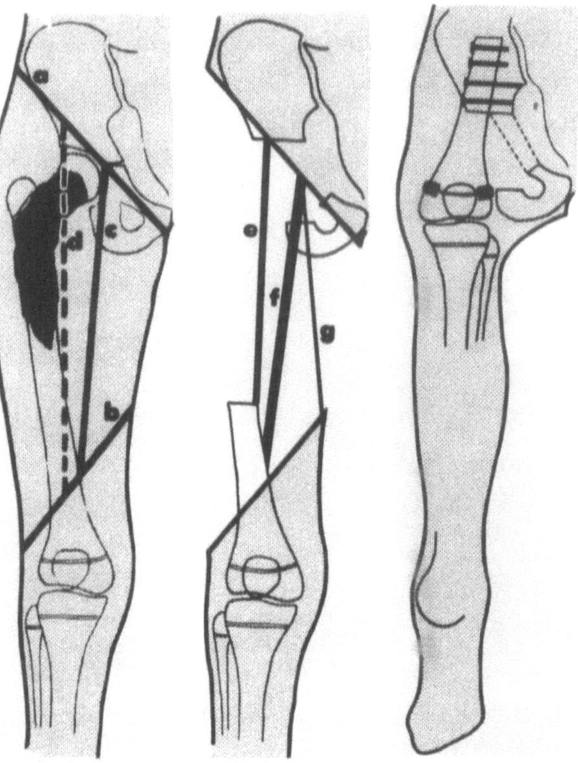

Fig. 7. Schedule of the Winkelmann (1983) hip rotation plasty. The knee joint is used as a hip joint after 180° rotation

Conservative Surgery for Tumours of the Upper Thigh

If the tumour involves the vessels, but spares the sciatic nerve, a so-called *hip rotation plasty* can be performed (Winkelman 1983), which means that part of the pelvis together with the complete upper thigh can be removed and the healthy lower leg retransplanted with vessel anastomosis after 180° rotation (Fig. 7), in a similar way to the above-mentioned knee rotation plasty.

If the vessels can be spared, an en bloc resection and replacement with a proximal femur endoprosthesis can, usually, give a much better functional and cosmetic result.

Conservative Surgery of Bone Tumours of the Pelvis

If the main nervous trunks for the lower extremities can be spared, inner hemipelvectomy is an appropriate method to resect bone tumours of the pelvis and spare the limb. Because the stabilisation of the lower extremity is important, different methods of stabilisation such as bone grafting, saddle prostheses or pelvic prostheses have to be inserted to support the body (Nieder et al. 1983). Radicality of the en bloc resection is more difficult than with the classic ablative hemipelvectomy and local recurrence is, usually, found in about 50% of the cases.

Conservative Surgery for Bone Tumours of the Upper Extremities

Conservative Surgery of the Hand and Forearm

As opposed to the inferior limb, surgical efforts tend to preserve a functional distal portion of the extremity, even with poor stability of the girdle.

At present, functional prosthetic replacements of the hand and wrist are not available and conservative surgery is only feasible for very small intraosseous tumours, which are extremely rare in this area of minute bones.

It should, however, be remarked that if a tumour is located in a metacarpal, or phalangeal ray, a longitudinal amputation of the involved and contiguous rays can preserve the first finger and, at least, one of the others, thus providing a prehensile functionality.

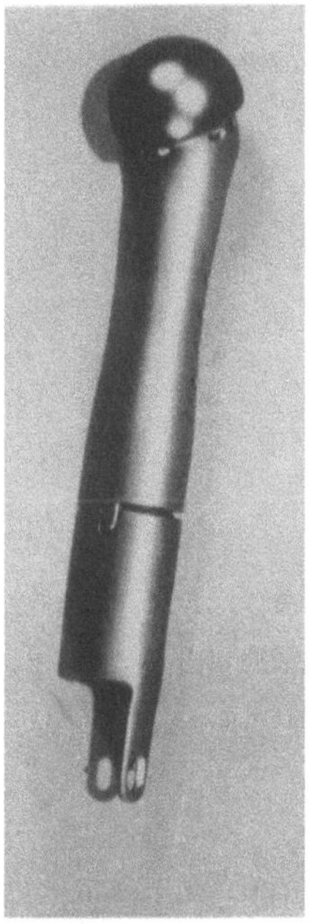

Fig. 8. Modular Salzer Humerus Endoprosthesis for bridging the defect

Conservative Surgery for Bone Tumours of the Scapular Girdle (Tikhoff-Linberg Resection)

In most cases, malignant bone tumours of the upper extremities are situated in the region of the proximal humerus and the scapula. In this location en bloc resection has a special importance, due to the efforts which have to be made to preserve the functional capacity of the hand, despite poor stability of the upper girdle.

For intraosseous tumours of the proximal humerus, en bloc resection can be performed with endoprostheses. For tumours involving the scapulohumeral articulation, or other bony structures of the scapular girdle, the most important and extensive limb salvage procedure is the operation first reported by Linberg (1928). It consists of the removal of the scapula, clavicula and proximal humerus en bloc with the soft parts, preserving the limb, providing that the neurovascular bundles are not involved. Initially, the use of endoprostheses proved difficult due to technical problems, but, even without endoprosthesis, the remaining extremity could be supported by braces (Burwell 1965; Dor 1962; Francis and Worcester 1962; Fuchs 1966; Genovesi 1962; McFarlane 1971; Meary 1970; Pack and Baldwin 1961; Packard 1973; Kotz and Salzer 1975).

More recently, with the development of modular systems for the proximal humerus (Campanacci 1983; Salzer 1979; Ungethüm 1983), these resections can be performed successfully also with internal prostheses (Fig. 8).

Bone Transplantation

Sometimes homologous bone from a bone bank can be used instead of metallic or ceramic implants (Volkow 1970; Parrish 1966; Parrish 1973; Manking et al. 1982). With the replacement of human bone and cartilage there is a high risk of infection and it requires a long period for the consolidation of the skeletal segments; in fact, patients should wear the plaster cast for up to 6 months. For these reasons, during the early postoperative period this method is less effective than endoprosthetic replacement and rehabilitation is longer: better results are expected after at least 1 year and, therefore, homologous bone transplantation is indicated for intracompartmental low-grade bone tumours, where the cure rate is high and the patient can endure a long and fatiguing rehabilitation period.

Metastatic Bone Tumours

Orthopaedic procedures are often necessary in the rehabilitation of cancer patients with secondary involvement of bones. Besides the above-mentioned methods (e.g. amputation or en bloc resection) in these particular cases, intralesional procedures are allowed in terms of palliation and are frequently necessary for stabilising the involved bone. Nailing and plating is used in pathological fractures of the long bones as well as the use of cement for large and destructive lesions. In the case of involvement of a vertebral body, ventral procedures have been performed successfully when using bone cement for the defect and for stabilising it with plates (Fig. 9a, b) (Salzer et al. 1973; Kotz and Sunder-Plassmann 1977).

Final Considerations

All the cases which undergo amputation or major exarticulation of limbs and girdles can be rehabilitated with sophisticated external devices which, for the inferior extremity, allow for as good a performance as the level of the amputation is peripheral, but with a proper external prosthesis and re-education, even after hemipelvectomy, the aesthetic appearance, deambulation and principal movements are possible without crutches (Fig. 1a, b). Naturally, conservative surgery is more and more frequently requested, but the final results should be handled with some circumspection. Conservative en bloc resection for primary malignant bone tumours should only be per-

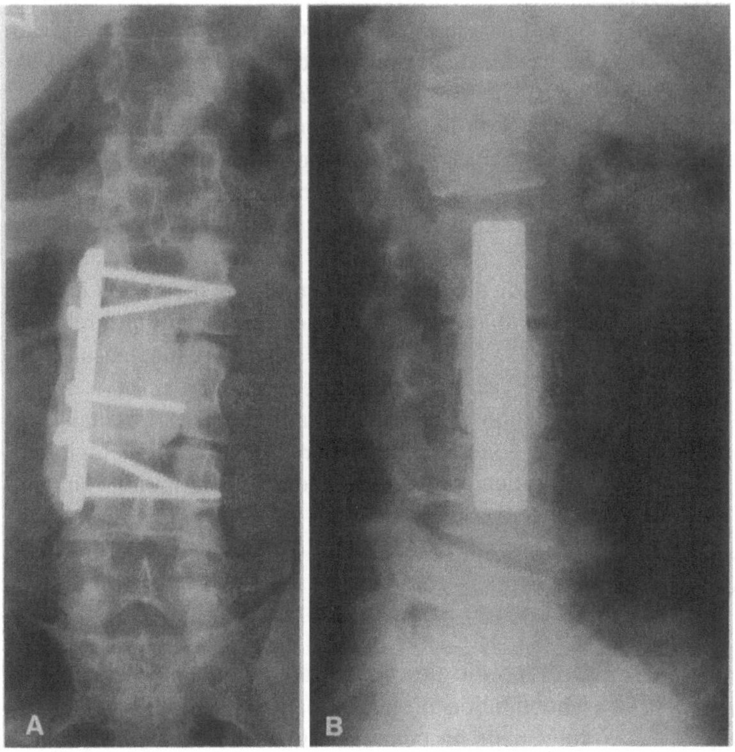

Fig. 9 A, B. Radiological views of the lumbar vertebral spine of a case with a metastatic lesion of the third lumbar vertebral body, after curettage and the filling of the defect with bone cement and stabilising the spine by means of a side plate and screws

formed in orthopaedic tumour centres and the functional result should be observed very carefully.

Implantation of endoprostheses for tumours is still fairly experimental, especially according to the results of the COSS 80-Study (Winkler 1984) and, similarly, the Italian CNR study (Gasparini 1987) reported some local recurrences after en bloc resection, and the survival of these failures is worse. The Vienna experience showed that, after a period of rehabilitation, rotation plasty gives a better performance than en bloc resection, which, on the other hand, brings about the most rapid rehabilitation and, in many instances, should be regarded as the surgical approach of choice. Furthermore, from the rehabilitative point of view, we are not enthusiastic about the internal hemipelvectomies, whereas, the Tikhoff-Linberg operation (a limb salvage scapular girdle disarticulation) is strongly suggested as an alternative to scapulothoracic disarticulation, even without endoprostheses.

Some authors report that the occurrence of lung metastases is higher in the resected cases than in the amputees (Winkler 1986), but prognosis depends, basically, on the histology and size of the tumour and on its possible response to chemotherapy, and these parameters alone will select patients for limb salvage procedures and endoprosthesis replacement in bone tumours.

References

Aust J, Absolon B (1962) A successful lumbosacral amputation hemicorporectomy. Surgery 52: 756–579

Borggreve J (1930) Kniegelenksersatz durch das in der Beinlängsachse um 180° gedrehte Fußgelenk. Arch Orthop Unfall-Chir 28: 175–178

Burwell HN (1965) Resection of the shoulder with humeral suspension for sarcoma involving the scapula. J Bone Joint Surg [B] 47: 300–303

Campanacci M, Capanna R, Cervellati C, Calderoni P (1983) Modular rotatory endoprosthesis for segmental resection of the proximal humerus: experience with 33 cases. Thieme-Stratton, New York, p 64

Chao EYS, Sim FH (1983) Tumor prostheses design: a system approach. Thieme-Stratton, New York, p 157

Dölle V, Rinecker H (1975) Die Behandlung maligner Frakturen des Femurs durch die totale Hüft-Femur-Kniegelenks-Alloplastik. Arch Orthop Unfall-Chir 83: 295–303

Dor P (1962) La resection de la ceinture scapulaire. Acta Chir Belg 61: 897–902

Enneking WF, Spanier MA, Goodmann MA (1980) Current concept review. The surgical staging of musculoskeletal sarcoma. J Bone Joint Surg 62: 1027–1030

Enneking WF (1983 a) Functional evaluation of reconstruction after tumor resection. In: Proceedings of the second international workshop on the design and application of tumor prostheses for bone and joint reconstruction. September 5–8, Vienna, pp 5–10

Enneking WF (1983 b) Musculoskeletal tumor surgery. Churchill-Livingstone, New York, p 81

Francis KC, Worcester JN (1962) Radical resection for tumors of the shoulder with preservation of a functional extremity. J Bone Joint Surg [Am] 44: 1423–1430

Fuchs G (1966) Resektion des proximalen Oberarmes und Ersatz durch eine Vitallium-Endoprothese. Chir Prax 10: 69–75

Gasparini M, Azzarelli A (1987) Chemotherapy: protocols and results at the Istituto Nazionale Tumori of Milan. In: Consensus meeting on Osteosarcoma – state of the art in Europe. Istituto Ortopedico, Rizzoli Editore, Bologna, pp 19–22

Gennari L, Bignami P, Azzarelli A, Nava M (1981) Emipelvectomie e disarticolazioni interscapolotoraciche. In: Veronesi U, Perussia A, Gennari L, Emanuelli H (eds) I tumori delle ossa e dei tessuti molli. CEA, Milano, pp 375–381

Genovesi A (1962) Resezione ed innesto osseo autoplastico per neoplasie primitive dell'estremo prossimale dell'omero. Clin Orthop 14: 233–253

Grimby G, Stener B (1973) Physical performance and cardiorespiratory function after hemicorporectomy. Scand J Rehabil Med 5: 124–129

Jürgens H (1981) Ewing-Sarkom bei Kindern und Jugendlichen: Planung einer kooperativen Therapiestudie der Gesellschaft für Pädiatrische Onkologie (CESS 1981). Klin Pädiatr 193: 253–256

Juvara E (1929) Reconstruction de la tige osseuse femore-tibiale, interrompue pour la resection d'une des extremites osseuses, qui constitute l'articulation du genu, par une greffe provenant du deboublement de l'extremity osseuse apposee. Bull Soc Chir [Paris] 55: 541

Kotz R (1983 a) A modular femur and tibia reconstruction system. In: Proceedings of the second international workshop on the design and application of tumor prostheses for bone and joint reconstruction. September 5–8, Vienna, pp 223–226

Kotz R (1983 b) Possibilities and limitations of limb-preserving therapy for bone tumors today. J Cancer Res Clin Oncol 106 [Suppl]: 68–76

Kotz R, Salzer M (1975) Resection therapy of malignant tumors of the shoulder girdle. Öst Z Onkol 2: 97–109

Kotz R, Salzer M (1982) Rotationsplasty for childhood osteosarcoma of the distal part of the femur. J Bone Joint Surg [Am] 64: 959–969

Kotz R, Sunder-Plaßmann M (1977) Ventrale Stabilisierung bei Metastasen der Hals- und oberen Brustwirbelsäule. Orthop Prax 12: 891

Kotz R, Leber H, Ramach W, Arbes H, Wolf A (1977) Erfahrungen mit der Durchführung der hochdosierten Methotrexatbehandlung beim Osteosarkom. Wien Klin Wochenschr 89: 474–479

Kotz R, Salzer-Kuntschik M, Lechner G, Immenkamp M, Kogelnik HD, Salzer M (1984) Orthopädie in Praxis und Klinik. Band III: Allgemeine Orthopädie, Teil 2: Tumore und tumorähnliche Erkrankungen. Thieme, Stuttgart

Kotz R, Ritschl P, Pongracz N, Zimmermann R (1986) Hemipelvektomie: Indikation, Operationstechnik und Ergebnisse. Acta Chir Austriaca 18: 108–109

Larson DL, Liang MD (1983) The quadrizeps musculocutaneous flap: a reliable, sensate flap for the hemipelvectomy defect. Plast Reconstr Surg 72 (3): 347–354

Lewis MM (1986) The use of an expandable and adjustable prosthesis in the treatment of childhood malignant bone tumors of the extremity. Cancer 57: 499– 502

Linberg BE (1928) Interscapulo-thoracic resection for malignant tumors of the shoulder joint region. J Bone Joint Surg 26: 344–349

MacFarlane DA (1971) Radical surgery for malignant lesions of the shoulder with upper limb preservation. Bull Soc Int Chir 30: 23–30

Mankin HJ, Doppelt SH, Sullivan TR (1982) Osteoarticular and intercalary allograft transplantation in the management of malignant tumors of bone. Cancer 50: 613–630

Marcove RC, Khafagy MM (1974) Total femur and knee replacement using a metalic prosthesis. Clin Bull 4: 69–71

Meary R (1970) Wide resections in bone-tumors (except pelvis and knee). In: Chapchal G (ed) Operative treatment of bone tumors. Thieme, Stuttgart, pp 89–91

Miller ThR (1962) Hemipelvectomy in the treatment of advanced cancer. AJR 87: 531

Miller ThR, Mackenzie AR, Randall HT (1966) Translumbar amputation for advanced cancer: indications and physiologic alterations in four cases. Ann Surg 164: 514–521

Nadjafi A (1970) The results of limb-saving plastic procedures for malignant bone sarcomas of the skelton. In: Chapchal G (ed) Operative treatment of bone tumors. Thieme, Stuttgart, p 98

Nieder E, Engelbrecht E, Steinbrink K, Keller A (1983) Modular system of the total femoral prosthesis – endo – model. In: Proceedings of the second international workshop on the design and application of tumor prostheses for bone and joint reconstruction. September 5–8, Vienna, pp 231–235

Nilsonne U (1965) Radical amputation for malignant tumours of the extremities. Acta Chir Scand 129: 150

Pack GT (1956) Major exarticulations for malignant neoplasms of the extremities: interscapulothoracic amputation, hipjoint disarticulation and interilio-abdominal amputation. A report of endresults in 228 cases. J Bone Joint Surg [Am] 38: 249

Pack GT, Baldwin JC (1961) The Tichof-Linberg resection of the shoulder-girdle, indications for its substitution for interscapulothoracic amputation, recent data on endresults of the forequarter amputation. Clin Orthop 19: 148

Pack GT, Miller ThR (1964) Exarticulation of the innominate bone and corresponding lower extremity (hemipelvectomy) for primary and metastatic cancer. J Bone Joint Surg [Am] 46: 91

Packard AG (1973) Prosthetic replacement of the proximal half of the humerus. Clin Orthop 93: 250–252

Parrish FF (1966) Treatment of bone tumors by total excision and replacement with massive autologuous and homologous grafts. J Bone Joint Surg [Am] 48: 968–990

Parrish FF (1973) Allograft replacement of all or part of the end of long bone following excision of a tumor. Report of twenty one cases. J Bone Joint Surg [Am] 55: 1–22

Ramach W, Sigmund R, Sekera J, Salzer-Kuntschik M, Kotz R, Knahr K, Salzer M (1987) Functional results of customized prosthetic devices for the knee region after resection of bone and joints. In: Enneking WF (ed) Limb Salvage in Musculoskeletal Oncology. Churchill Livingstone, New York, pp 215–220

Rosen G, Murphy ML, Huvos AG, Gutierrez M, Marcove RA (1976) Chemotherapy en bloc resection and prosthetic bone replacement in the treatment of osteogenic sarcoma. Cancer 37: 1–11

Salzer M (1965) Die Hemipelvektomie. Wien Klin Wochenschr 77: 330

Salzer M, Knahr K (1976) Resection treatment of malignant bone tumors. Recent Results Cancer Res 54: 239

Salzer M, Salzer G, Denck H, Brenner H (1973) Operative Behandlung "solitäter" Metastasen der Brust- und Lendenwirbelkörper. Arch Orthop Unfall-Chir 75: 249–254

Salzer M, Knahr K, Locke H, Stark M, Metajovsky Z, Plenk H, Punzet G, Zweymüller K (1979) A bioceramic endoprosthesis for the replacement of the proximal humerus. Arch Orthop Trauma Surg 93: 169–184

Salzer H, Knahr K, Kotz R, Kristen H (1981) Treatment of osteosarcoma of the distal femur by rotation-plasty. Arch Orthop Trauma Surg 99: 131
Sauerbruch F (1922) Die Exstirpation des Femur mit Umkipp-Plastik des Unterschenkels. Dtsch Z Chir 169: 1
Smith WS, Simon MA, Arbor A (1975) Segmental resection for chondrosarcoma. J Bone Joint Surg [Am] 57: 1097–1103
Steiner AK, Müller W, Remagen W, Rüedi Th (1973) Extremitätenerhaltende Resektion bei Tumoren der langen Röhrenknochen. Helv Chir Acta 40: 177–183
Troell A (1931) Sarkom in den langen Röhrenknochen mit besonderer Berücksichtigung ihrer Behandlung und der Bedeutung des Traumas für die Geschwulstätiologie. Langenbecks Arch Chir 163: 199–299
Ungethüm M, Knahr K, Salzer M, Blömer W (1983) Zementfrei zu implantierende Spezialendoprothesen nach dem Baukastenprinzip für den proximalen Femur- und Humerusersatz. Med Orthop Technik 4: 104
Van Nes CP (1950) Rotationplasty in the treatment of congenital defects of the femur. J Bone Joint Surg [Br] 32: 12
Volkow M (1970) Allotransplantation of joints. J Bone Joint Surg Br 52: 49–53
Wilson PD, Lance EM (1965) Surgical reconstruction of the skeleton following segmental resection for bone tumors. J Bone Joint Surg [Am] 47: 1629–1656
Winkelmann W (1983) Die Umdrehplastik bei malignen proximalen Femurtumoren. Z Orthop 121: 547–549
Winkler K, Beron G, Kotz R, Salzer-Kuntschik M, Beck J, Beck W, Brandeis W, Ebell W, Erttmann R, Göbel U, Havers W, Henze G, Hinderfeld L, Höcker P, Jobke A, Jürgens H, Kabisch H, Preusser P, Prindull G, Ramach W, Ritter J, Sekera J, Treuner J, Wüst G, Landbeck G (1984) Neoadjuvant chemotherapy of osteogenic sarcoma: results of a cooperative German/Austrian study (COSS-80). J Clin Oncol 2 (6): 617–624
Winkler K, Beron G, Kotz R, Salzer-Kuntschik M, Beck J, Beck W, Brandeis W, Ebell W, Erttman R, Göbel U, Havers W, Henze G, Hinderfeld L, Höcker P, Jobke A, Jürgens H, Kabisch H, Preusser P, Prindull G, Ramach W, Ritter J, Sekera J, Treuner J, Wüst G, Landbeck G (1986) Einfluß des lokalchirurgischen Vorgehens auf die Inzidenz von Metastasen nach neoadjuvanter Chemotherapie des Osteosarkoms. Z Orthop 124: 22–29
Yancey AG, Ryan HF, Blasingame JT (1964) An experience with hemicorporectomy. J Natl Med Assoc 56: 323–325
Zenker H (1967) Zum Problem des Knochenersatzes durch Endoprothese bei einem bösartigen Tumor am koxalen Femurende. Z Orthop 103: 539–541

Stoma Construction and Care

L. HULTÉN

Creation of an enterocutaneous stoma, permanent or temporary, forms an important part in the surgical treatment of colorectal neoplasia but is often also an adjunctive measure in urological and gynecological malignancy. Diverse manifestations of intestinal complications of radiotherapy such as sigmoid strictures, ileo- or rectovaginal fistula, or radiation proctitis with rectal ulcer and stricture may also require the formation of a diverting stoma. Although the psychological and social problems associated with a stoma in these patients treated for cancer may be similar to those with stomas in nonmalignant disease, there are important differences which have to be taken into account in their rehabilitation. Acceptance of the stoma may be more difficult and many patients have to live and cope with uncertainty, particularly those having a palliative stoma. In addition to concern of the stoma, the patient will be fearful of the underlying disease and occasionally be plagued by side effects from chemo- and/or radiotherapy. The care and rehabilitation of these patients therefore require various skills ranging from the medical staff to the stomatherapist and nursing staff, social workers, pharmacist, and dietician, i.e., on a multidisciplinary basis.

The correct selection of the type of stoma for the specific situation, and its proper construction and siting on the abdomen, forms the basis for stoma care and management. Experience and skill on the part of the surgeon will therefore be a prerequisite for the subsequent optimal rehabilitation of the patients. The importance of these measures cannot be overestimated and is convincingly reflected in the gradually increased success rate of conventional ileostomy, the most difficult stoma to manage.

Construction of the Conventional End Ileostomy

Although the major indication for this operation is ulcerative proctocolitis and Crohn's colitis, it may also be advisable in patients with familial adenomatosis and in those with multiple malignant or premalignant tumors in the large intestine. It may also be recommended as an emergency measure in combination with subtotal colectomy for an obstructive or perforated colon carcinoma, or it may be the only alternative for deviation where pelvic malignancy and/or radiation injury has caused obstruction, perforation, or fistulation.

Placement of the Ileostomy

Since an ileostomy is conveniently and best sited on the right side, many surgeons by tradition prefer to use a left paramedian laparotomy incision. Others have refrained from this traditional policy, however, and use a midline incision primarily. The advantage is that both sides of the lower abdomen are left intact should stoma revision or relocation be necessary in the future.

It is often stated that a proper ileostomy location should be at a level of 1 cm or so below the umbilicus, passing through the lateral third of the rectus sheath (Goligher 1984). However, this general rule of thumb must be tempered with the realization that the configuration of the abdomen varies considerably. The accurate selection of the optimum stoma site should therefore be best determined individually by preoperative fitting of an appliance to the abdomen in both the sitting and supine positions. In patients with a prominent belly the stoma should rather be at a somewhat higher level to allow it to be watched during its management. Previously scarred areas should be avoided and in the case of a previous appendectomy with a scar in the McBurney area it may be preferable to fashion a left-sided ileostomy.

Preparation of the Ileostomy Wound

A separate circular "trephine"-shaped opening is made in the skin (Fig. 1). The subcutaneous fat is excised or dissected aside so that the aponeurosis is completely bared. The aponeurosis is then incised in a cruciate fashion and the fibers of the rectus muscle either separated by blunt dissection or its lateral edge cut by cautery. The posterior wall of the rectus sheath is cut. The preferable size of the canal through the abdominal wall varies according to the thickness of the ileum and its mesentery, but as a working rule it is better to err on the tight side, since the exit canal can be widened if necessary. Usually, however, an opening into which two fingers can be inserted will be suitable.

Fixation of the Ileostomy

The terminal ileum is then passed through the channel in the abdominal wall so that about 6 cm of the gut projects through the skin opening (Fig. 2). The edge of the ileal mesentery is fixed to the peritoneum and the posterior rectus sheath by a few isolated sutures and the inner fixation should be reinforced by additional interrupted sutures between the anterior parietal peritoneum and the intestinal wall along its circumference. Through the skin opening a row of seromuscular sutures are similarly applied between the ileal wall and the anterior rectus sheath. Provided that the bites in the bowel wall are superficial and these sutures are tied loosely, necrosis and subsequent fistulae will be prevented. This measure should probably be omitted in patients who have had radiation, however.

Closure of the Lateral Gutter

Having drawn the ileum directly through the abdominal wall, the para-ileostomy gutter must be closed, either by a pursestring or a running suture. To lessen the incidence of lateral space hernia inherent in the above-mentioned technique, Goligher (1951) introduced an alternative technique (Fig. 3), in which the ileum is brought forward to the site chosen for the ileostomy through an extraperitoneal tunnel dissected alongside the lateral abdominal wall. This method is said to have other distinct advantages, such as a reduced incidence of stomal retraction and prolapse.

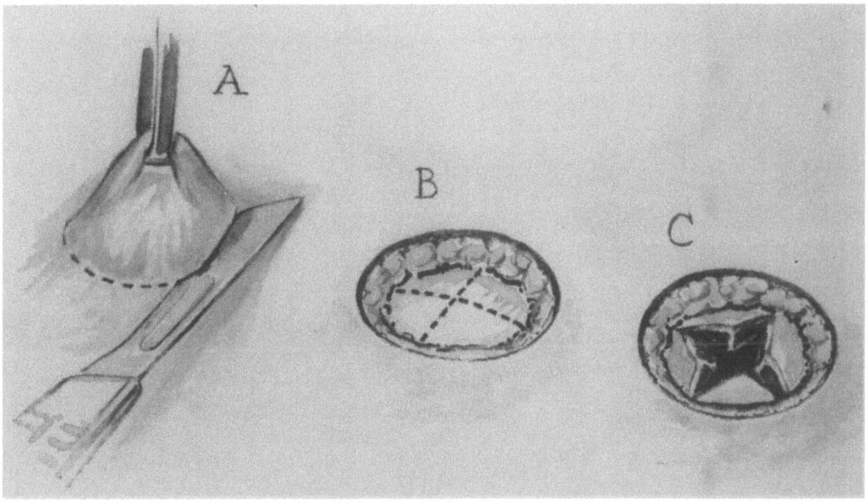

Fig. 1 A–C. Preparation of the ileostomy wound

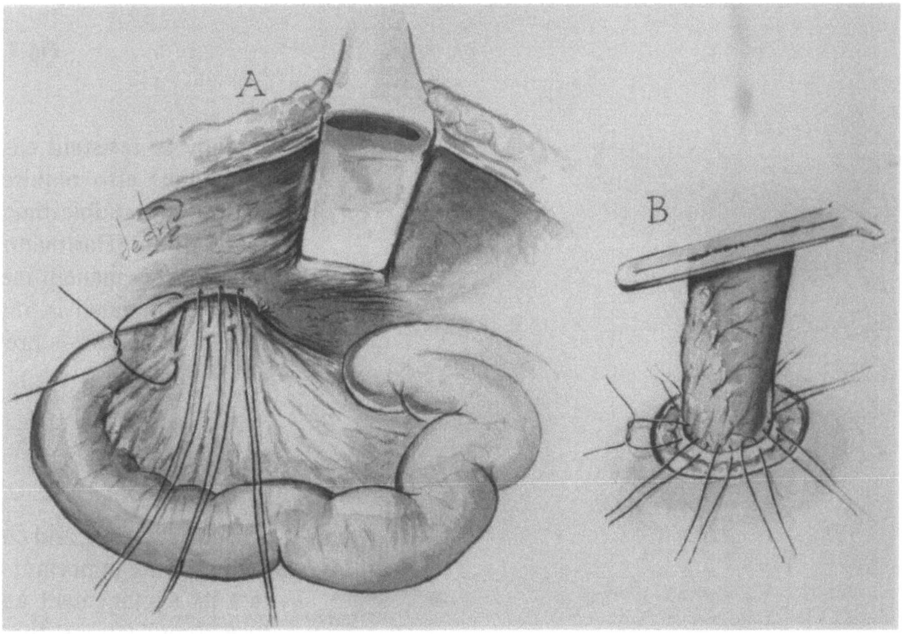

Fig. 2 A, B. Fixation of the ileostomy

Fashioning of the Ileostomy

This can be done safely and preferably before closure of the abdominal incision. The projecting ileum is trimmed and its end amputated so that the final everted spout will measure about 2–3 cm (Fig. 4). The eversion is accomplished by means of four quadrant sutures placed between the end of the ileum and the subcuticular fascia. Additional mucocutaneous sutures are placed around the entire circumference. To eliminate the bowing effect of the ileal mesentery on the terminal end of the intestine, Turnbull and Weakley (1967) suggested that it should be divided at skin level and resected. Moreover, the technique of two-directional myotomy, supposed to render the stoma aperistaltic, was also recommended by these authors. The advantages of these measures remain unproven, however. The Turnbull loop end ileostomy is an important modification, however, to be used in obese patients in whom the combination of a thickened abdominal wall and a short fat mesentery presents a particular hazard. The end of the ileum is closed in this method and a tape passed around the ileum at its point of greatest mobility. The loop is then drawn through the abdominal aperture and the tape exchanged by a supporting rod. Eversion and completion of the nipple stoma is shown in Fig. 5.

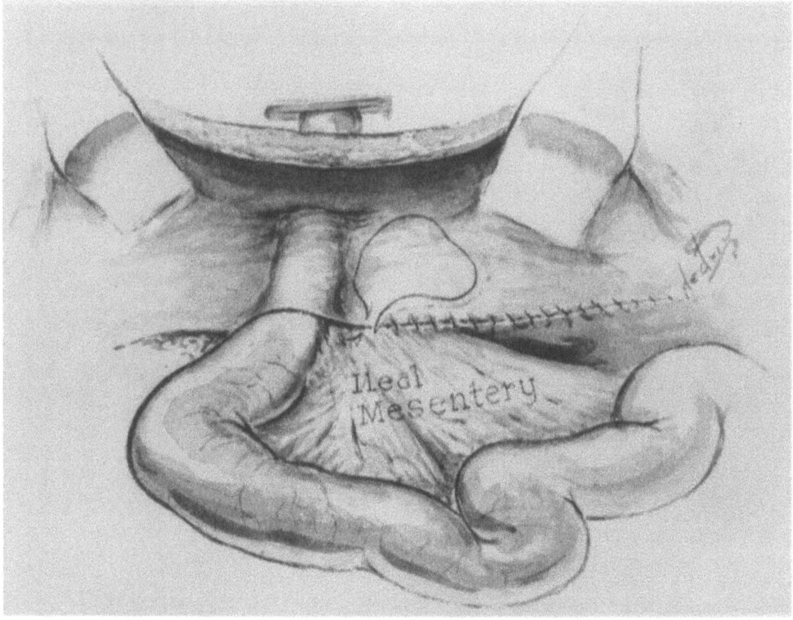

Fig. 3. Extraperitoneal ileostomy

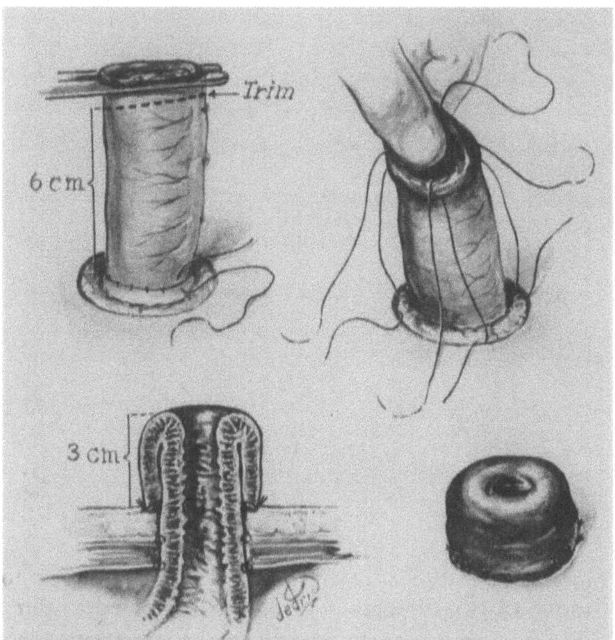

Fig. 4. Final fashioning and eversion of the ileostomy

Conventional End Colostomy – or Sigmoidostomy

This is the traditional permanent stoma used after abdominoperineal resection of a rectal or anal cancer. Patients with a rectovesical fistula after radiotherapy or resistant cases of radiation proctitis may sometimes also require an end sigmoid colostomy with a suprapubic mucous fistula or closure of the rectal stump (Hartmann's operation), as either a temporary or permanent measure, an approach that is also recommended in many other situations where a staged procedure is preferred.

Construction

The correct siting and construction of an end sigmoidostomy is as important as for an ileostomy, to facilitate its management and particularly to prevent future complications, the most distressing of which is the paracolostomy herniation.

According to traditional teaching, the sigmoidostomy should be placed in the left iliac fossa midway between the anterior superior iliac spine and the umbilicus (Goligher 1984). If this recommendation is followed, which is probably often the case, the colostomy will only occasionally by correctly sited, however. The accurate selection of the stoma site should, as for an ileostomy, be determined individually preferably by preoperative fitting of an appliance.

The common use of a left-sided paramedian incision for the laparotomy may be another error contributing to an inaccurate siting of the sigmoidostomy. To avoid interference with such an incision, the trephine wound has then to be located more laterally,

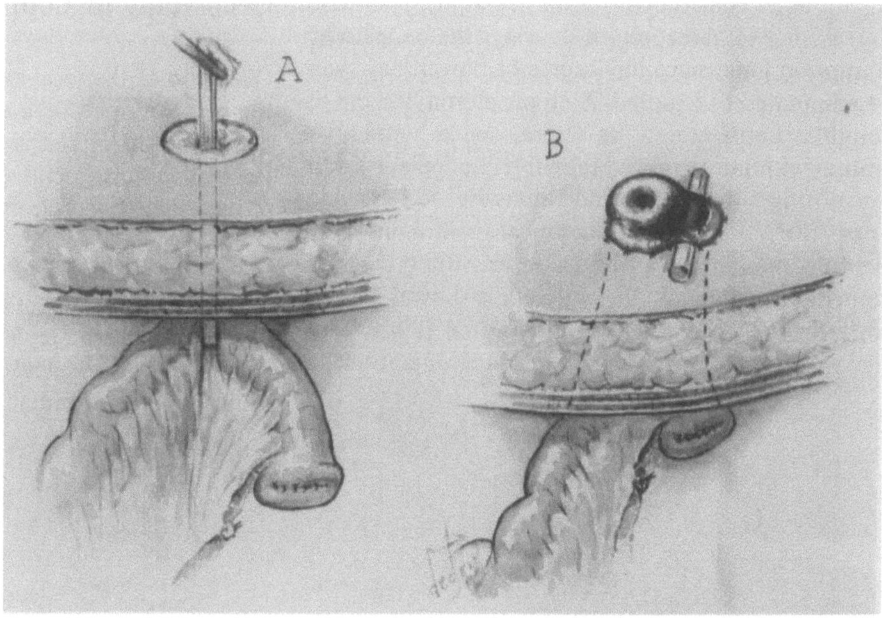

Fig. 5 A, B. Turnbull loop end ileostomy

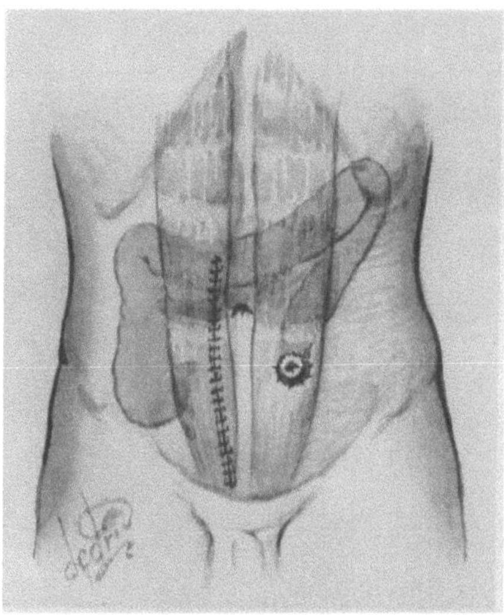

Fig. 6. Correctly placed colostomy through the rectus sheath. Note right-sided paramedian incision

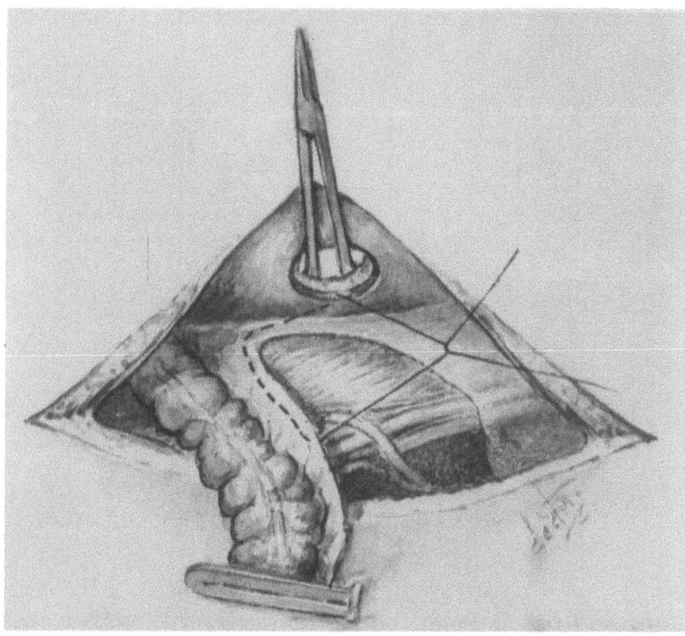

Fig. 7. Closure of paracolic gutter

through the oblique and transversalis muscles, which are often weak and thinned structures in elderly patients. This difference from the technique employed for formation of an ileostomy may well explain the reported high incidence of paracolostomy herniation. A median (or even right-sided paramedian) incision (Fig. 6) would probably be preferable since it allows the colostomy to be sited medially and to be correctly fitted in a vertical trephine through the rectus sheaths and muscle, similar to the procedure used for the creation of an ileostomy. There is evidence that this is a preventive for future herniation (Eldrup et al. 1982, Sjödahl et al. 1988). When the colon has been drawn through the abdominal opening it is important to see that there is an adequate amount of bowel projecting beyond skin level.

Again, as in construction of an ileostomy, it is wise to err in the direction of leaving the colostomy stump too long, since any excess of bowel may then be amputated as required. A nipple stoma 2–3 cm in length is satisfactory. The lateral space should be closed without tension preferably by means of a pursestring suture or should otherwise be left wide open (Fig. 7). The extraperitoneal technique may even be an alternative (Fig. 8). After wound closure, immediate suture of the end of the bowel to the edges of the skin should be performed (Fig. 9) and an appliance fitted at completion of the operation.

Cecostomy or Loop Transverse Colostomy

Diversion of the fecal stream by a temporary vent on the colon formed by a cecostomy or loop colostomy may be used either as an emergency measure for large bowel obstruction or a threatening perforation, or as a planned procedure to prepare a fecal-loaded colon for a subsequent resection. The most common indication for their use, however, is to protect a newly constructed colorectal anastomosis. It is occasionally also employed for management of perforation or fistulation in the pelvis as caused by gynecological tumor growth or radiation injuries.

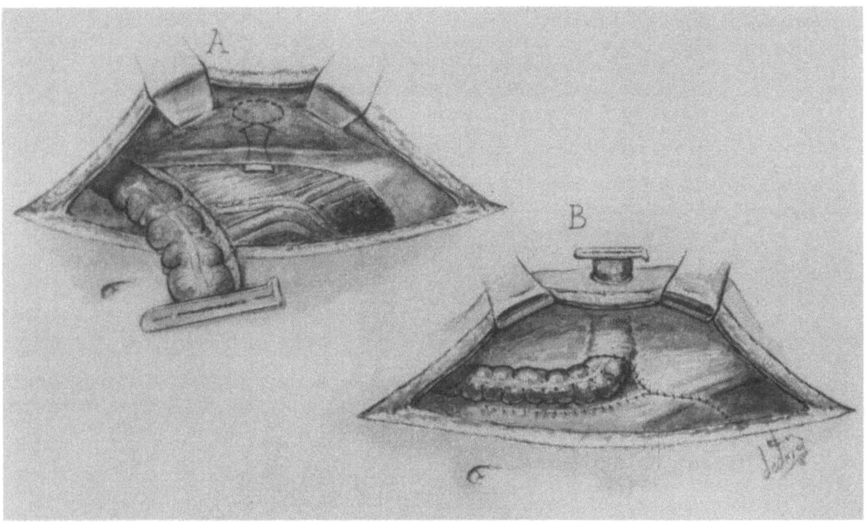

Fig. 8 A, B. Extraperitoneal colostomy

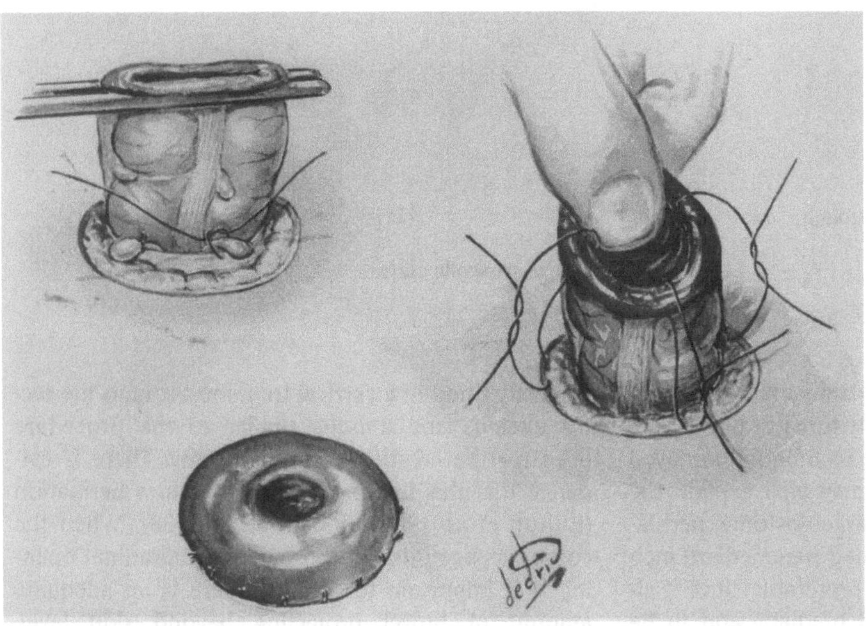

Fig. 9. Eversion and mucocutaneous suturing of colostomy

Technique of Cecostomy

There are two main techniques for the performance of a cecostomy. The exposed anterior cecal wall is sutured to the edges of the peritoneal wound, and after incision the full thickness of its wall can be sutured to the skin as a mucous fistula or a wide-bore tube may be tied into its wall. A more commonly used approach appears to be insertion of a large-bore Foley catheter, securing it according to the Witzel technique (Fig. 10). This type of tube cecostomy is more likely to close spontaneously on withdrawal, which may in some cases be an advantage, while the tendency toward spontaneous and early closure is certainly unsatisfactory in others.

Technique of Loop Colostomy

The transverse loop colostomy is traditionally sited in the right upper abdomen midway between the costal margin and the umbilicus. As with any other enterostomy, it should be placed in a separate wound and preferably be drawn through the incised rectus sheaths and muscle. Whenever possible, the site should be carefully selected preoperatively so that its suitability may be assessed with the patient wearing an appliance. Since the transverse colon is commonly mobile, or at least can be mobilized, it is an advantage to aim for the stoma to be placed low, just above the waistline.

The main laparotomy incision should be in the midline or well to the left of the planned separate incision (Fig. 11). The latter should be transverse and about 5 cm in length or less depending on the dimension of the colon, and should pass through the rectus musculature. A puncture hole for deflating gross distension may therefore sometimes be advantageous. The loop segment, freed from the attached greater omentum, is drawn through the stab wound, and a rubber tubing or a glass rod is then passed through the mesocolon to support the bowel at skin level (Fig. 12). No further attempts are needed for fixation of the stoma to the parieties. If the dimension of the opening for colostomy is properly chosen, the loop will fit snugly. Otherwise, the wound should be closed on each side of the intestine. An incision is now made on the convexity of the loop and in its long axis. The cut edges are sutured to the skin to produce a mucocutaneous apposition around the entire circumference, except where the glass rod projects on either side. On completion of the operation an adhesive two-piece appliance is immediately fitted in the theater (for details see below).

Although the cecostomy may still have its advocates and would be advantageous in occasional cases, the transverse loop colostomy has gradually replaced it and appears to be preferred by most surgeons today on the same indications. Certainly, despite its safety the cecostomy, irrespective of technique employed, is unsatisfactory since it does not provide complete diversion of feces. The transverse loop colostomy has proved to be superior in this respect.

However, a transverse colostomy has obvious disadvantages of its own. A transverse colostomy sited midway between the costal margin and waistline is inconvenient and interferes with clothing. It is often bulky, and the feces are loose, erosive, and offensive. It is sometimes difficult to fit an appliance particularly when the stoma is flush and elliptical. Modifications in technique have improved but little. It follows that although the transverse loop colostomy

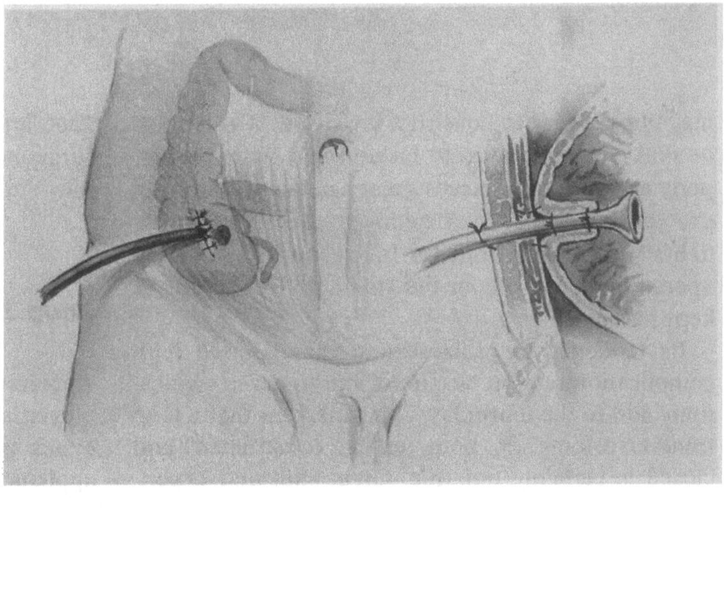

Fig. 10. Tubececostomy

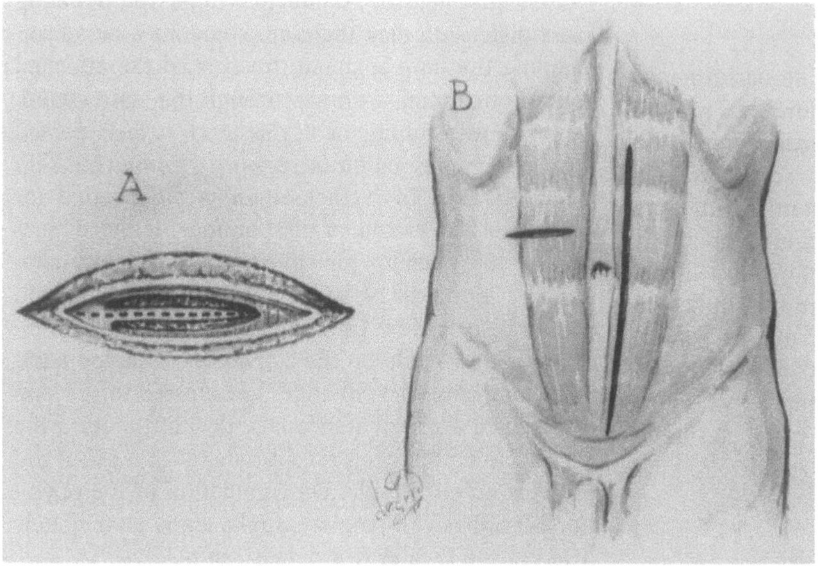

Fig. 11 A, B. Type of incision for transverse colostomy construction

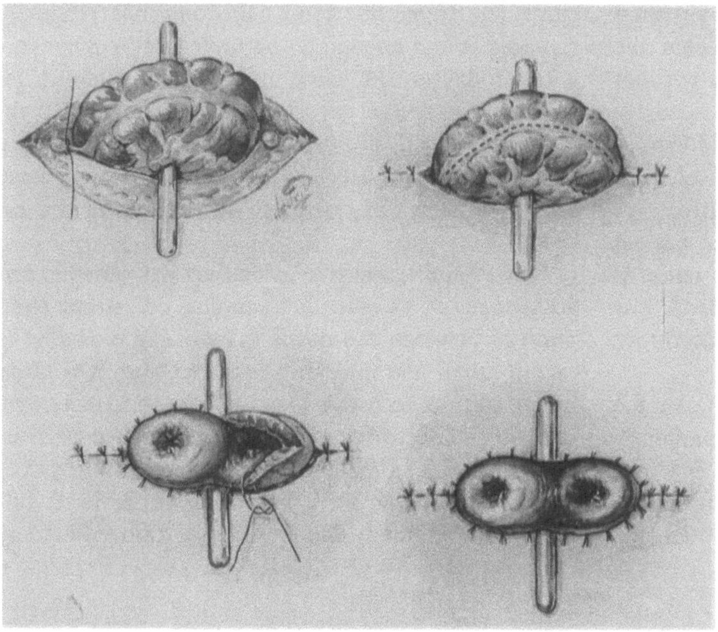

Fig. 12. Loop colostomy supported by a rod, opened, and sewn immediately to the skin

may appear easy to construct it requires a great deal of skill and experience to fashion and function properly and the stoma needs great care to prevent skin problems. It will be particularly troublesome for patients who remain unfit for the second stage of the operation and in whom the stoma will therefore be kept permanently.

Its tendency to prolapse and the reported high complication rate on closure of the transverse colostomy add to the morbidity. The statement that a loop transversostomy is both easily constructed and closed is certainly not true. Great skill and experience are needed for both procedures, and a junior surgeon should not been given the task unless carefully supervised.

Loop Ileostomy

A defunctioning loop ileostomy was originally employed as a sole procedure for treatment of an acute attack of ulcerative colitis. Difficulties in fitting an appliance and its liability to undergo retraction and/

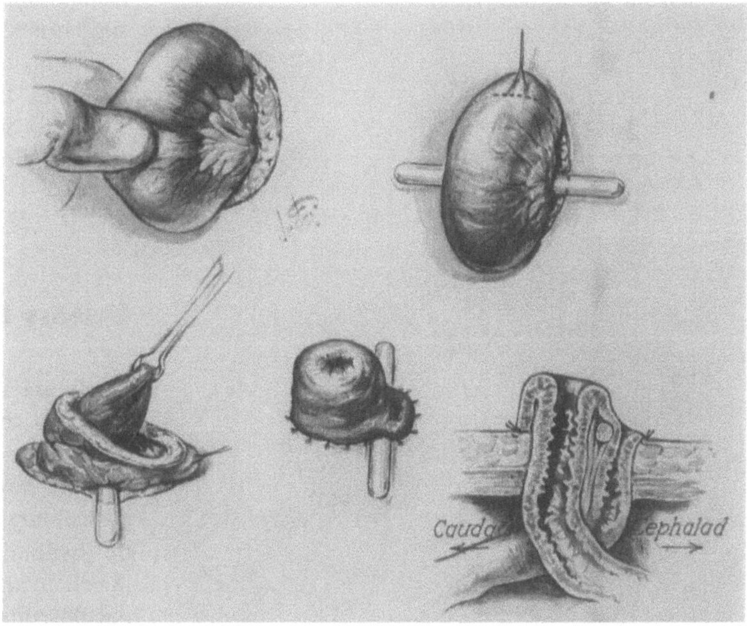

Fig. 13. Construction of a loop ileostomy. Note proximal (functioning limb) location

or prolapse caused it to disappear from surgical practice and it has until recently been employed mainly as a safety measure covering an ileorectal anastomosis. There has been a great revival of interest in the technique in recent years, however (Parks and Nicholls 1978; Hultén and Fasth 1981). It may indeed be favorably employed in many different situations where a temporary stoma is required, either for emergency or as a staged procedure, such as an obstructing cancer in the large bowel or for protection of a coloanal anastomosis. In fact it may be used in most situations where a loop colostomy is otherwise employed (Fasth et al. 1980).

Construction of the Loop Ileostomy

The stoma site is selected using the same criteria as those for a terminal and ileostomy. It should be marked preoperatively in cooperation with the stomatherapist. In the case of a previous right-sided scar, a left-sided ileostomy should be preferred.

A circular disk of skin, about 2 cm in diameter, is removed and the anterior rectus sheath is incised in a cruciate fashion. After separation of the fibers of the rectus muscle the posterior rectus sheath and peritoneum is then incised. The hole in the abdominal wall is dilated to correspond to the dimension of the intestine.

An appropriate site is then selected in the ileum as far distal as possible, usually 15–20 cm above the ileocecal valve, allowing a loop to be brought out without tension (Fig. 13). The loop is turned clockwise so that the proximal limb is located inferiorly and the distal superiorly. A glass rod is passed through the mesentery close to the intestinal wall to support the bowel at skin level. No internal or external fixation sutures are needed. A transverse incision about 1–2 cm long is made in the antimesenteric part of the distal limb, close to the skin level. The wall of the efferent active limb of the loop is peeled back and everted, forming a stoma 2–3 cm in length. Mucocutaneous interrupted silk sutures are then placed to give a good apposition between the cut edges of the bowel and the skin. In patients with colon distension due to an obstructing distal carcinoma, or in those with fecal loading, an indwelling widebore tube may preferably be introduced through the distal limb of the loop for deflation or lavage (Fig. 14). An appropriate appliance should then be immediately fitted on completion of the operation.

It has been convincingly demonstrated that a loop ileostomy presents no more problems than a conventional terminal ileostomy when it is sited, constructed, and managed according to these principles (Fasth and Hultén 1984, Williams et al. 1986). With a well-projecting spout it will in most cases be easily managed, both in the early and late postoperative phase.

Indeed with increased technical knowledge and experience on the part of the surgeon and with access of stoma therapy and modern ileostomy appliances to cope with its management, the indications

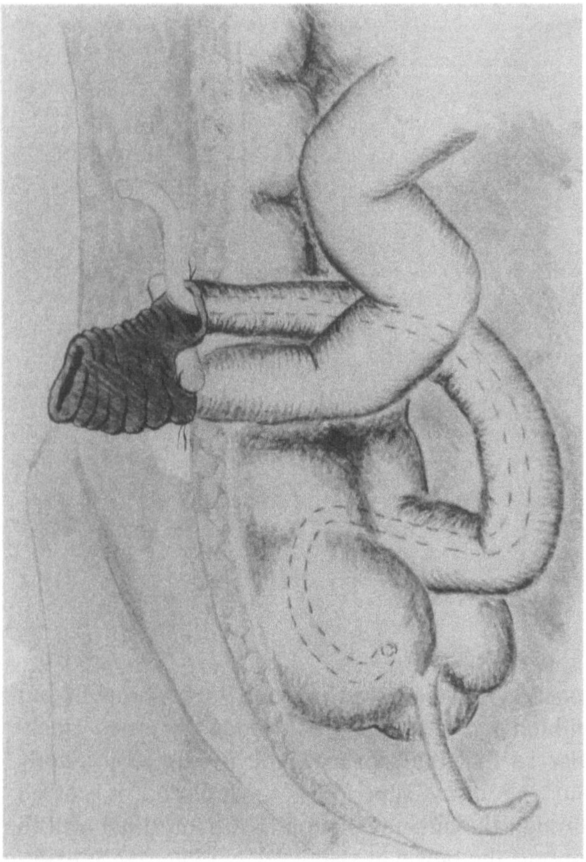

Fig. 14. Loop ileostomy with indwelling tube for deflation of the cecum

for loop ileostomy have broadened in recent years and in some units it has even replaced other ostomies previously employed for temporary deviation or for emergency situations. With careful supervision and intense parenteral support during the immediate phase after surgery, the excess saltwater losses can as a rule be managed, and once the ileostomy has been brought into steady state it is mostly easily controlled.

It is in many respects superior to the widely used temporary loop transverse colostomy. The stoma position is more convenient and interferes less with clothing. It is a relatively small stoma and is sited where the patient can see it clearly when fitting the appliance, and its effluent has little odor.

Loop ileostomy appears to provide more efficient diversion than a loop transversostomy, in which sidetracking of the fecal stream may often be incomplete. Since adequate decompression of the distended colon may not be achieved, an indwelling wide-bore tube introduced through its distal limb into the cecum is, therefore, an important measure. A loop ileostomy may sometimes be difficult both to fashion and to close, however, and only experienced surgeons should be allowed to deal with these demanding cases. Among the alternative methods available, the one should be chosen which is best suited to each individual patient, having taken into account both medical and psychosocial aspects of the case.

Urinary Diversion with an Ileal Conduit

There are many alternative forms of urinary diversion, but the ileal or colon conduits have so far remained the most consistently reliable techniques. Although the common indication in this context is cystectomy for bladder carcinoma, it may sometimes be justified for treatment of primary and recurrent gynecological cancer and for palliation in vesicovaginal postradiation fistulae as well as for other recurrent pelvic cancers. Since problems related to urostomy affect these patients most and can ruin an otherwise successful operation, it is clear that the outcome is largely dependent upon making the ileal stoma correctly. There is in fact still a high incidence of stoma-related complications (Remigailo et al. 1976), adding to the morbidity in urostomy patients – stoma complications mainly or entirely resulting from improper technique and management.

Construction

After isolation of a suitable length of ileum for the conduit to bridge the gap between the ureters and the abdominal wall without tension in the mesentery (Fig. 15) and after insertion of the ureters, attention is turned to the stoma construction. The formation of the ileostomy should be done exactly as for the conventional ileostomy, and the optimum site should have been carefully assessed and well marked beforehand.

The trephine wound is made passing through the rectus fascia and muscles and its size kept small to allow the ileum to fit snugly. As with conventional ileostomy, it is important to fix the edge of the mesentery to the peritoneum and posterior rectus sheath by firmly anchored sutures. The inner fixation should also be reinforced by interrupted sutures between the parietes and the ileal wall along its entire circumference. A row of external sutures is similarly applied between the ileal wall and the anterior rectus sheath. The bites should be superficial in the seromuscular

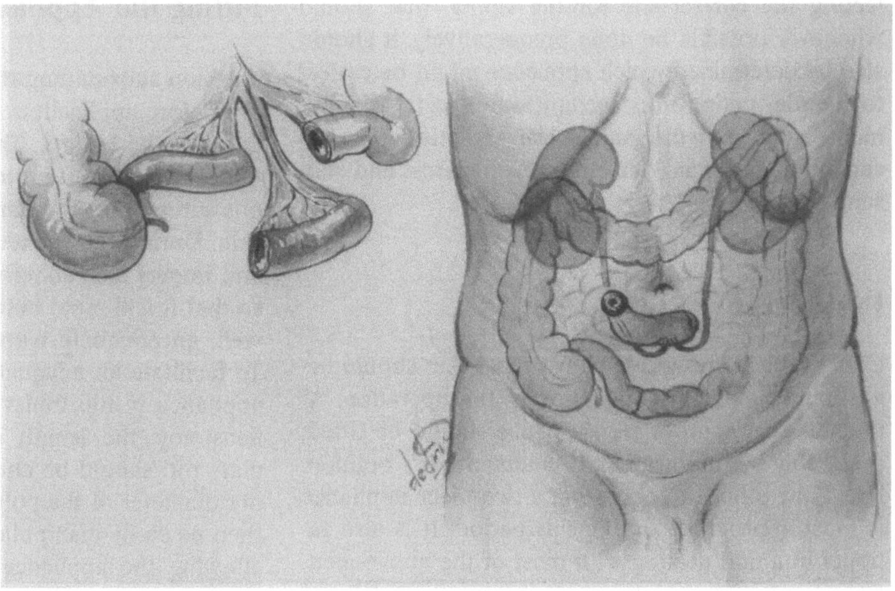

Fig. 15. Urine diversion with traditional ileal conduit

layer and the sutures tied loosely to prevent necrosis and subsequent fistula. With about 6 cm of ileum projecting above skin level, the everted stoma fashioned with primary mucocutaneous technique should measure about 3 cm in length. A nipple stoma sufficient in length is as important as in conventional ileostomy, or perhaps even more important, since, besides facilitating stoma care, it has also been shown to resist backflow into the conduit better than a flat stoma (Bergman et al. 1977). Construction of the urostomy according to the Turnbull-Hewitt technique, i.e., a loop end ileostomy (see Fig. 5) is preferred by some recent authors (Crawford 1984) and has been suggested to lessen postoperative stenosis, representing the most common reason for conduit revision.

The sigmoid conduit is preferred in several other urological units. From the technical point of view it is merely a colonic version of the ileal conduit and the construction of the nipple stoma should closely follow the principles for end colostomy (see p. 402).

Rehabilitation and Stoma Care

Preparation and construction of an entero- or urostoma irrespective of type requires attention to detail. To obtain a well-functioning oostomy the proper selection of the site, the creation of an adequate abdominal aperture for the end or loop intestinal segment, and the firm anchoring of the stoma that should be fashioned to protrude as a nipple sufficient in length are all important measures. This is also the prerequisite for an optimum stoma management and care. Any patients subjected to a stoma operation when correctly constructed may then be reassured of an almost normally active life. Carelessly or incorrectly constructed, a stoma can produce lifelong misery, however, and in such cases should be referred to an expert clinic for reconstruction.

Even the perfectly fashioned and efficient stoma makes certain demands as regards its management both on the nursing staff in the immediate postoperative course and subsequently on the patient, who has to adopt a new life-style to cope with an external appliance. With modern and adequately fitted appliances and training by a skilled stoma nurse, most patients should soon learn to manage the stoma.

Preoperative Preparation

Any surgeon performing enterostomal surgery must not only be technically competent but must also be committed to rehabilitation of the patient, and rehabilitation begins as soon as the decision has been made to perform the operation. The patients should be carefully informed about what is going to happen and should be told from the very beginning that they can return to normal living and that they are expected to learn how to manage the stoma. A positive attitude, which should also be reinforced by the ward and/or stoma nurse, can have great influence upon a patient's adaptation to the stoma operation. In selecting the correct site for the stoma, that should whenever possible be done preoperatively, it should also be determined which appliance might be easiest to handle, taking into account any special requirements such as work and social activities, physical capabilities, manual dexterity, vision status, and skin sensitivity.

Postoperative Stoma Care

Care of the stoma and the peristomal skin should begin immediately on completion of the operation. At that time an appropriate appliance should be fitted, preferably by the surgeon. It is the author's opinion, like many other surgeons, that a two-piece appliance is most appropriate during this period. It is also rational in a unit dealing with most of the above-mentioned enterostomies to rely upon one main type of appliance fitting them all. There are many such appliances available today and it is beyond the scope of this presentation to name them all, but Surgicare System II (synonym, Combihesive, Surfit) is the prototype and still the most popular in many places. This two-piece appliance consists of a skin protective and adhesive body flange, which, properly applied, will remain in situ for several days, and a bag which fits on the flange and which may be emptied or exchanged when necessary (Fig. 16).

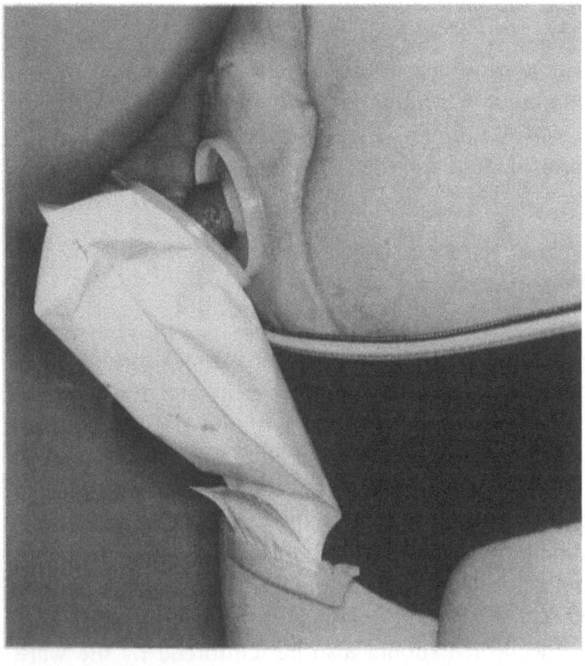

Fig. 16. A "two-piece" appliance with an adhesive skin protective body flange and snap lock fitting bag

Fitting the Appliance

The skin surrounding the stoma should be clean and dry before application. A hair dryer on the cool setting may be helpful. The flange size is selected and the central hole is cut to fit close to the mucocutaneous suture line. The flange is pressed firmly onto the skin. During this maneuver the warmth of the hands and fingers aids adherence of the flange to the skin so that it will mold better to its contours. Performed well, an adequate watertight seal can be obtained. To facilitate an adequate fitting of such a two-piece appliance in the transverse colostomy and the loop ileostomy, the length of the supporting elastic or glass rod should be chosen to correspond to the inner diameter of the polyethylene flange. The rod can then be easily manipulated through the cut aperture, allowing the appliance to stick to the skin underneath its projecting ends all around the stoma (Fig. 17). The edges of the body flange can preferably be secured by means of nonirritant adhesive tape. Properly applied, the wafer will commonly remain in position for several days, often until the sutures have to be removed on the 7th day.

Although it is usually 2 or 3 days before a colostomy discharges feces, an ileostomy may start to act earlier, even on the 1st day. At first ileostomy flow is often liquid and voluminous, about 1000–1500 ml escaping per 24 h and, due to its enzyme contents, it is corrosive to the skin. The fecal contents escaping from a colostomy, irrespective of type, are at first fluid, abundant, and irregular and the contents from a right-sided transverse colostomy will often remain liquid and corrosive permanently. It is therefore important at this stage for all types of enterostoma to rely upon a two-piece appliance with a skin-protecting adhesive wafer, allowing the bag to be changed frequently while the body flange remains firmly attached. Most of the skin troubles that previously used to occur in ostomy patients have been largely overcome by fitting such an appliance immediately in the operating theater.

Training the Patient

As soon as the patient has recovered to such an extent that he or she can be expected to take an interest in the care of the stoma, the main aim should be to teach the patient to look after the stoma entirely unaided, and this training should preferably be complete before discharge from hospital. At this stage it will be time to choose the permanent appliance.

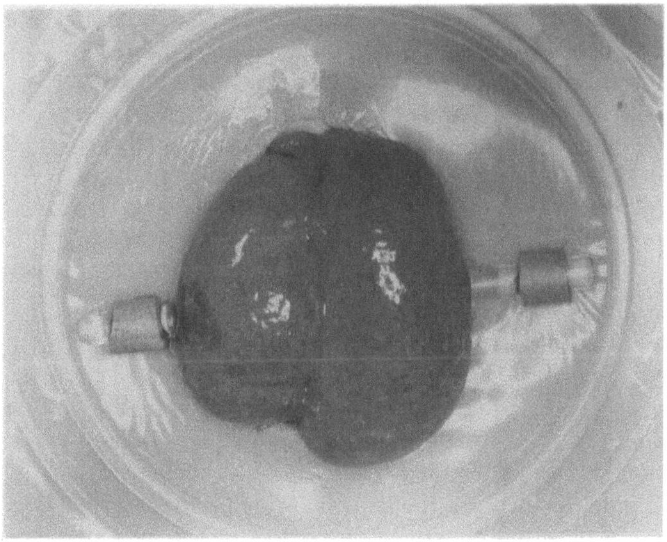

Fig. 17. The supporting rod for loop ileo- or colostomy is manipulated through the cut aperture of the body flange

There is a wide range of modern appliances to choose from, but the correct choice depends on the individual patient's need, bearing in mind the type and characteristics of the stoma, its location, the patient's work and recreational activities, and the cost and availability of the equipment. For sigmoidostomy, an adhesive disposable appliance may often be satisfactory but, on occasions, when frequent changes are needed, other alternatives should then be recommended to avoid sore skin. The use of odor-proof plastic in the pouches, together with gas-deodorizing filters, minimizes offensive smell. For proper management of an ileostomy as well as for a transverse colostomy, a skin protection barrier such as the stomadhesive wafer should be an obligatory constituent of the appliance.

Stoma care is essentially meticulous and proper care of the skin. Irrespective of appliance used, it should be carefully removed to avoid the stripping effect on the skin. The skin should then be gently cleaned and residues of the adhesive removed by bathing the skin with a tissue and lukewarm water. Solvents like ether and benzine should be avoided, the best detergent being acid unperfumed soap. Profuse hair growth around the stoma interfering with fitting of the appliance should be removed, preferably with a dry razor. Before fitting the new appliance the skin should be allowed to dry, and drying the skin with a hair dryer on the cool setting may be helpful. A suitable time should be chosen for these routines. The stoma is most productive after meals and quietest in the morning before breakfast. All these practical instructions on the care of the stoma should be carefully explained to the patients and in a well-organized surgical clinic dealing with entero- or urostomal surgery a specially educated stoma nurse or enterostomal therapist is indispensable and will be the most appropriate person to deal with both the practical and psychosocial problems in rehabilitation of these patients (Brooke et al. 1982).

Special Considerations for Ostomy Patients Undergoing Chemo- and/or Radiotherapy

The number of ostomy patients receiving chemo- and/or radiotherapy is increasing as advances are made in the use of these therapeutic methods. There is great variety of side effects related to such treatment; however, many of them cause specific problems interfering with the management of the stoma (Click 1981). Thrombocytopenia occurs to some extent in conjunction with most chemotherapeutic drugs and special caution should therefore be used when cleaning the stoma and the surrounding skin to prevent traumatizing. An erythematous skin reaction due to peristomal *Monilia* infection is common in myelosuppressed patients and may interfere with fitting the appliance. Diarrhoea of varying severity may develop with some drugs, often in combination with nausea and vomiting, and common problems in patients on chemotherapeutic agents are also their nephrotoxicity and their liability to cause urinary infection. The general side effects from radiotherapy are in many respects similar to those after chemotherapy. Others are more specific and vary depending on the area treated. The urinary bladder, rectum and pelvic colon, and a variable amount of the small intestine are all exposed in pelvic irradiation. Cystitis with increased frequency, dysuria, and nocturia are common. Symptoms due to proctitis may also be severe and frank diarrhoea is not uncommon. The skin on the lower abdomen may sometimes also be affected with erythema and skin desquamation. Some of these side effects occur at the time of treatment while others develop with time as late sequelae. With specific measures and appropriate treatment, most of these adverse reactions can be managed or even prevented but they should all be taken into account in stoma care and management. Special attention should be directed toward the care of the skin. Gentle removal of the pouch is important not to traumatize the peristomal area, and the change of the appliance should be limited to decrease skin trauma. The standard use of a skin barrier, preferably a two-piece appliance, may prevent skin problems in these patients.

References

Bergman B, Nilsson AE, Petterson S, Sundin F (1977) Backflow from urinary collecting devices into the ileal conduit. Br J Urol 49: 503–507

Brooke BN, Jeter KF, Todd IP (1982) Stomas. Clin Gastroenterolog 11: 235–419

Click C (1981) Special considerations for the ostomy patient. Cancer Bull 33: 24

Crawford ED, Davis MA (1984) New directions in urinary diversion. Ostomy Q: p 72

Eldrup J, Wied U, Bischoff N, Møller Pedersen V (1982) Parakolostomihernier. Ugeskr laeger 144/50: 3742

Fasth S, Hultén L, Palselius I (1980) Loop ileostomy – an attractive alternative to a temporary transverse colostomy. Acta Chir Scand 46: 203

Fasth S, Hultén L (1984) Loop ileostomy: a superior diverting stoma in colorectal surgery. World J Surg 8: 401

Goligher JC (1951) Extraperitoneal colostomy or ileostomy. Br J Surg 46: 98

Goligher JC (1984) Surgery of the anus, rectum and colon, 5th edn. Baillière Tindall, London

Hultén L, Fasth S (1981) Loop ileostomy for protection of the newly constructed ileostomy reservoir. Br J Surg 68: 11

Parks A, Nicholls J (1978) Proctocolectomy without ileostomy for ulcerative colitis. Br Med J [Clin Res] 2: 85

Remigailo RV, Lewis EL, Woodard JR, Walton KN (1976) Ileal conduit urinary diversion. Urology 7: 343

Sjödahl R, Anderberg B, Bolin T (1988) Parastomal hernia in relation to site of the abdominal stoma. Br J Surg 75: 339–341

Turnbull RB, Weakley FL (1967) Atlas of intestinal stomas. Mosby, St. Louis

Williams NS, Nasmyth DJ, Smith AH (1986) Defunctioning stomas: a prospective controlled trial comparing loop ileostomy with loop transverse colostomy. Br J Surg 73: 566–570

Planning and Evaluation of Cancer Treatment

Regional Treatment Programmes and Cancer Registration

T. R. MÖLLER and T. LANDBERG

Introduction

Optimal care must be uniformly available to all patients with cancer regardless of geographical location, man-power limitations, economic restrictions and variations in method of health care delivery. Modern cancer care requires a multidisciplinary approach to management, requires thorough knowledge and understanding of the particular malignant disease and puts heavy demands on highly specialized facilities and equipment for diagnostic and therapeutic use.

The specific goals in cancer management have been defined by several authorities. The ones cited here were proposed by the Committee for Radiation Oncology Studies (1981).

1. The cancer patient should be given the most favourable management to achieve cure or long-term control and palliation of the disease.
2. The organizational structure for cancer management should provide for only the optimal level of care.
3. This optimal management should be available for all patients regardless of economic, social or geographical considerations.
4. Multidisciplinary participation in diagnosis, pretreatment evaluation, treatment and follow-up must be available in any circumstance in which cancer management is undertaken.
5. Currently limited highly trained personnel, sophisticated equipment and facilities must be efficiently utilized with minimization of the cost being consistent with high-quality care.
6. Sufficient numbers of highly qualified personnel in all of the cancer-related disciplines must be adequately trained.
7. Maximum information must be derived from all patients with cancer as a basis for study of the disease and its treatment.
8. Research advances must be rapidly translated into widely used clinical applications.

In a number of countries, the realization of these goals has led to the establishment of specialized hospitals, devoted entirely to cancer care, or comprehensive cancer centres (UICC 1980). Another approach has been taken in other countries, where coordination of available resources for cancer care at already existing clinics and hospitals is promoted in various ways (WHO Regional Office for Europe 1982).

Since the majority of cancer patients will still be diagnosed and probably also have their initial treatment outside cancer centres, physicians at the primary health care level and general hospitals must be involved in the process of cancer control. Thus, there is a need for dissemination of information on diagnosis and treatment of various forms of malignant disease and agreement on patient referral. One approach to solving this problem is to implement management programmes for cancer patients within a well-defined area of appropriate size, such as the catchment area of a regional hospital or a health care region (WHO Regional Office for Europe 1985).

Definition of and Rationale for Regional Treatment Programmes

By a regional treatment programme, or rather cancer care programme, is meant an agreed means of referral, diagnosis, classification and staging, treatment and follow-up of *all* patients with a specific disease within a region. Such programmes therefore not only specify the medical management of a specific disease, but also define the appropriate health care facilities needed for carrying out specific measures.

Thus, the three main reasons for setting up a regional treatment programme are:

1. To guarantee an optimal and uniform management of all patients with a particular disease in the area.
2. To obtain maximal utilization of existing resources for cancer care.
3. To guarantee that the entire patient material is efficiently utilized in gaining information and experience on the disease and its treatment.

Treatment programmes have been used, in various forms, for many years in the management of malignant disease. The concept that will be discussed here, based on Swedish experience (Möller 1985), is implemented within a cancer care organization based on coordinating regional oncological centres. The organisational aspects of a treatment programme are illustrated in Fig. 1.

Setting Up of the Programme

The idea of starting a treatment programme for a specific disease is usually generated by the medical specialists involved in management of that particular disease. The setting up is usually a stepwise procedure, involving collection of information from the literature, evaluation of results of currently used treatment in the region, and a survey of existing routines, knowledge and diagnostic and therapeutic facilities in the region. A draft programme is then usually produced by a working committee, and this programme is discussed at meetings with representatives of all involved medical disciplines from all the participating hospitals in the region. When a final agreement on the contents and format of the treatment programme has been reached, it is submitted to the regional oncological board for approval. If relevant, approval by the research ethical committee, isotope committee, pharmacological board or similar authorities should be obtained.

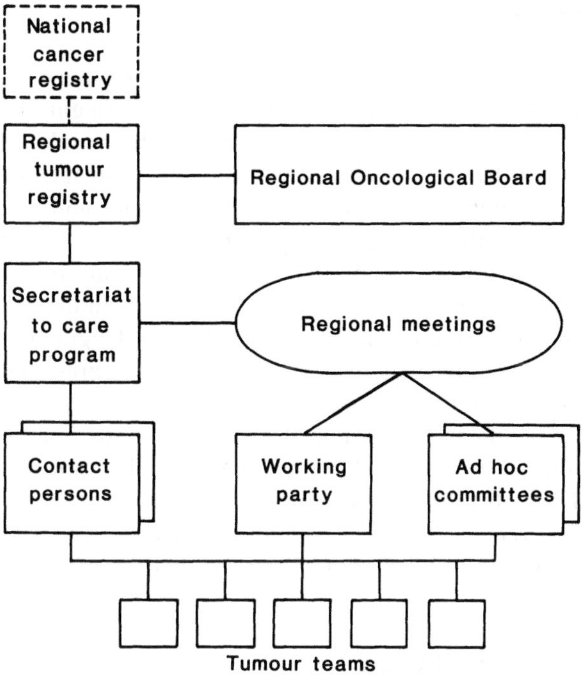

Fig. 1. Organization of a treatment programme (cancer care programme) in the Southern Swedish Health Care Region. The secretariat is closely associated with the Regional Tumour Registry, within the Oncological Centre. The Regional Oncological Board is the main authority for decisions on cancer care policy within the region, including treatment programmes. Tumour teams form the multidisciplinary approach to cancer care at all hospitals within the region. The other functions are described in the text

If the programme is multiregional or multinational, the same steps should be taken at all participating regions, preferably simultaneously.

Contents of the Treatment Programme

General Description

This is usually an abbreviated survey of the diagnostic and therapeutic procedures carried out for different stages, histologies or other subgrouping used for the particular disease. A schematic representation, like the one given in Fig. 2, or as described by Eiserman et al. (1982), may be of help as a quick reference.

Overview of the Epidemiology and General Clinical Course of the Disease and Possible Preventive Measures

Treatment programmes are often used for teaching purposes, and thus it is of great value to include a short description of the incidence and epidemiological characteristics of the disease, and its general clin-

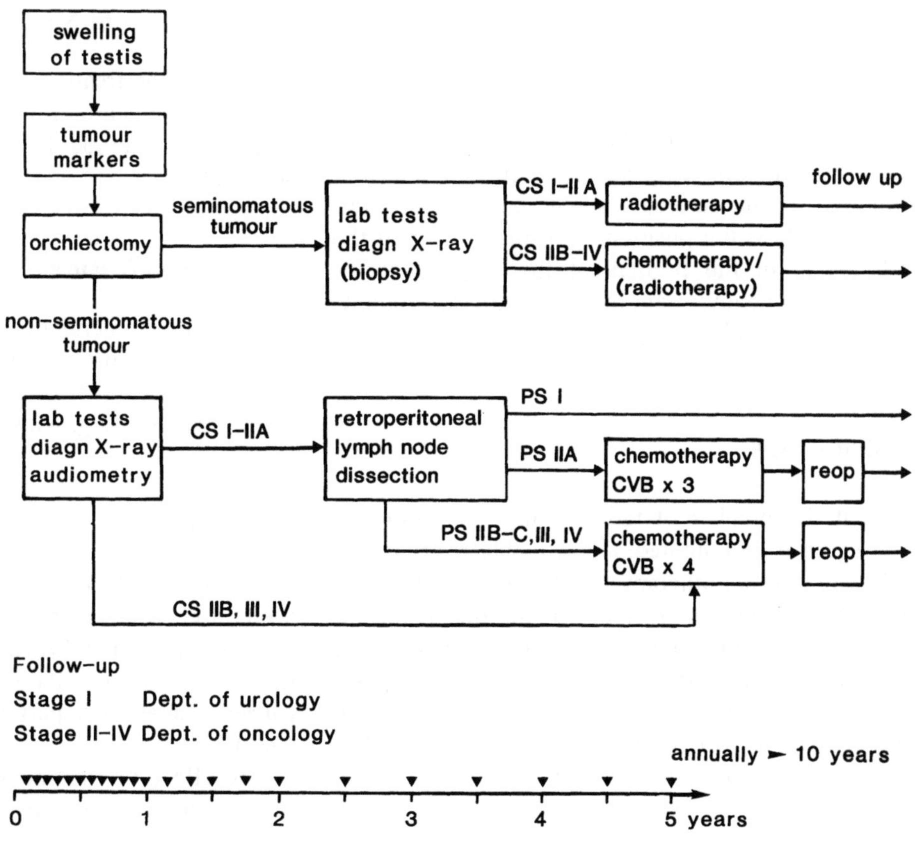

Fig. 2. Schematic representation of a treatment programme. Example taken from a joint Swedish-Norwegian testicular cancer management project, SWENOTECA (1981). All the individual steps in the procedure are fully described in the programme booklet

ical course. Treatment results in terms of remission rates and duration, as well as survival, should be given for different stages and histological subgroups. A discussion of factors of prognostic importance should be included.

Any preventive measures that could be taken or advocated should be described.

Criteria for Diagnosis and Staging

It is of utmost importance that all participating hospitals use the same criteria for establising a specific diagnosis. This leads to a definition of which histopathological classification should be used and what precautions should be taken when examining the biopsy material. The staging procedures to be carried out to map the extent of the disease should be clearly indicated and the facultative investigations mentioned.

The staging system should be defined and preferably reproduced in detail in the programme. For the majority of diagnoses, this means adopting the TNM classification as proposed by the UICC (Spiessl et al. 1982; UICC 1987) or AJCCS (1983), but in certain diseases other staging systems may be more generally accepted.

Surgery

It is usually worthwhile including a description of the recommended surgical technique in the programme. Specific reference should be made to information such as the positioning of incisions, and the delineation of the borders of the surgical cavity, which could be important in relation to, for example, postoperative radiotherapy.

Radiotherapy

Even if the number of radiotherapy institutions in the region is very limited, and possibly restricted to only one, the radiotherapy procedure should be described in detail. This includes definition of the target volume(s), the target absorbed doses and the fractionation. The patient positioning, the dose planning, the technique of irradiation and the control measures to be carried out should be indicated. Organs at risk and their dose limits should also be identified.

Chemotherapy

As for surgery and radiotherapy, there is a need for standardization of description for this treatment modality. All recommended regimes to be employed should be clearly defined, both first-line and second-line therapy, with dose reduction schedules and precautions to be taken during therapy. The description of a treatment regime includes dosage, route of administration and time schedule, for each individual drug component, and the overall cycle length. For combination regimes, the aponym (abbreviated name) should be given.

Maximum permissible doses at each administration, as well as total cumulative dose, if important, should be stated. Precautions to be taken to avoid drug-related emergencies and measures to be taken in case of accident should be described.

Endocrine Therapy

For endocrine therapy, the same requirements on the description of treatment as for chemotherapy apply.

In the case of ablative hormonal therapy, the indications and recommended technique(s) should be described.

Other Treatment Modalities

For any other treatment modality that may be employed (e.g. hyperthermia, immunotherapy), the indications and methodology should be adequately described.

Supportive Measures

General recommendations for the prevention and treatment of situations such as infections, anaemia, malnutrition, electrolyte disturbances and some acute toxicities (e.g. nausea) should be given.

Follow-up

It would be an advantage if all patients could be seen after conclusion of treatment in accordance with a specified follow-up schedule, indicating the time intervals for visits and the investigations to be carried out at each particular visit (Eiserman et al. 1982).

The effect of treatment should be measured according to the recommendations issued by WHO

(1979), although other, probably more adequate criteria have been proposed (Warr et al. 1984). The examinations that should be performed in order to establish the degree of remission should be clearly stated, as well as the criteria used for measuring response and progression of the disease.

Patient performance and quality of life should be assessed according to the scales and methods mentioned below. Treatments of recurrent or relapsing disease should be recommended.

The choice of length of follow-up of patients who stay in complete remission may vary greatly, depending on, for example, expected late toxic effects, and has to be defined.

Patient Referral

Since the treatment programme not only contains guidelines for the medical management of the patient, but also recommendations on at what level in the health care system a particular procedure should be carried out, it is important to define clearly the indications for referral.

Reporting

A treatment programme is not a static, once-and-for-all recommendation, but, instead, a dynamic tool for patient management, including evaluation of treatment outcome. To facilitate this, the reporting on specific patient characteristics and the results of different treatment regimes should be done in order to evaluate different aspects of the care. This calls for a description of the forms and routines used for reporting.

Conduct of the Programme

When a programme has been agreed upon by all participating clinics, by the regional oncological board or equivalent body, and by the research ethical committee, if necessary, the programme is ready for implementation within the region. This means that all physicians within the disciplines involved should be made aware of the programme at staff meetings or regional information meetings. The group responsible for the design of the programme should take an active part in this information process. At each department, a specific contact person should be appointed, responsible for information transfer between the working party and the department. This person should also be responsible for reporting patients to the programme secretariat (Fig. 1).

Regional meetings should be held at regular intervals, e.g. once or twice annually. Ad hoc committees should be set up if special projects, such as the evaluation of different diagnostic procedures requiring re-examination of X-ray films or microscopic slides, are to be carried out within the programme.

Reports should be issued at regular intervals to all participating clinics with a short statement on the progress of the programme, and any changes suggested. This feedback of information is one of the keys to the successful implementation of a programme.

Functions of a Secretariat to a Programme

The specific tasks of the secretariat to run a programme may be summarized as follows:
1. To coordinate the project.
2. To organize regional meetings.
3. To perform randomization in trials.
4. To collect data and perform data registration.
5. To assess the validity of data.
6. To report to participating clinics.
7. To publish results.

The personnel required for the secretarial function are determined by the number of patients entered into the study, the routine for reporting and the amount of information to be collected and processed. For programmes in which there is extensive data collection, a total of 500 patients seems to be a reasonable number that could be handled by a full-time secretary; in programmes which involve less extensive data collection more than 1000 patients could easily be dealt with by one person.

In the organization in Sweden, the secretariats to cancer care programmes are usually set up at the regional tumour registries, to benefit from the computer facilities and statistical expertise available at these institutions (Fig. 1).

The interactions between data bases created for different regional treatment programmes and a population-based cancer registry will be dealt with separately.

Data Collection

All programmes require a more or less extensive collection of data, in order to facilitate the evaluation of the programme from various aspects. This data collection may be either a continuous process, based on report forms to be sent to the secretariat at each follow-up visit, or an intermittent process, where at certain points in time, e.g. annually, reports on the patients or copies of their clinical records are requested.

The design of the data base depends on a number of factors, such as which diagnostic or therapeutic procedures should be evaluated, or whether special studies are performed within the programme. A considerable number of oncological data bases have been described in the literature and recommended (Hansluwka 1984; Mould 1984) and the one given here may be considered to fulfil most of the basic demands on data analysis in treatment programmes (Table 1).

Table 1. Suggested data base for a treatment programme. Additional parameters, relevant for specific tumour types, may be defined.

Patient identification	**Treatment**
Personal identification number Name Address Sex Date and place of birth (Marital status) (Ethnic group) (Nationality)	*Surgery* (Anaesthesia) Type of operation Radicality Major complications *Radiotherapy* Target volume(s) Technique of irradiation Target absorbed doses Fractionation Modifying agents Deviations from plan
Social and Medical History	
Occupational history Hereditary factors (Reproductive history) Relevant diseases and medication Prior antitumour therapy Concurrent malignancy (-ies) Symptoms and duration	*Chemotherapy* Regimen or drug Route of administration Dosages (including modifications) No. of cycles; overall time Toxicity
Diagnosis	*Other treatment modality*
Laboratory and radiological data Diagnostic image information Complete blood counts Renal and liver function tests Tumour markers Immune status	*Combined modality therapy* Description of each individual therapy Time relationship **Follow-up**
Tumour data Date of diagnosis Most valid basis of diagnosis Site of primary Anatomical extent of disease TNM classification and stage Size of tumour Histopathology (Tumour doubling time)	Date of follow-up/contact Patient performance Objective response of tumour Acute and subacute toxic effects Chronic and late toxic effects Date of death Cause of death State of malignancy at death Autopsy performed

Contents of the Data Base

Patient Data

This data set should include full identification of the patient, occupational history, relevant medical history, all prior antitumour therapy and actual performance status.

Tumour Data

This includes a full description of the site of the primary tumour, the anatomical extent of the disease including size and TNM stage (or equivalent) when applicable and the method used for mapping. The histopathology and any other descriptive parameter of the tumour should be recorded. When possible, tumour doubling time should be reported. Internationally accepted codes should be used, such as ICD-O (WHO 1976a) and SNOMED (Sobin et al. 1978; Rothwell 1980). The reporting forms designed by UICC (Sellers 1980) and AJCCS (1983) may be adopted.

Treatment Data

The treatment data set should include a full description of each treatment modality employed and, in multimodal therapy, the treatment sequence and its chronology.

Whenever possible, it should be indicated whether the intent of treatment was curative or palliative.

For *surgery*, the procedure could either be described by giving the appropriate code according to the WHO Classification of Procedures in Medicine (WHO 1978) or by applying the following category subdivision proposed by WHO (1979):

1. Local excision of the tumour without excision of regional lymph nodes.

2. Local excision of the tumour with excision of the regional lymph nodes.
3. Excision of the tumour with involved organ, without excision of the regional lymph nodes.
4. Excision of the tumour with involved organ, with excision of the regional lymph nodes.
5. Excision of the tumour extended to adjacent organs.
6. Partial excision of the tumour (reduction, debulking or other).
7. Excision of metastatic lesions.
8. Reconstructive surgery.
9. Surgery for alleviation of symptoms only.
10. Other surgery (i.e. exploratory, second look).

Whenever relevant, the radicality (macroscopic as well as microscopic) of the procedure should be stated. Major complications following surgery should be described.

For *radiotherapy*, the minimum specifications include a description of the target volume(s), the quality of radiation, the technique of irradiation, and the target dose(s) and its fractionation (ICRU 1978). Similar data should be given for intracavitary radiotherapy in gynaecology (ICRU 1985).

For *chemotherapy*, the precise description includes the drugs, route and duration of administration, dosages and a comprehensive schedule. Dose modifications should be indicated, as well as major complications to therapy. Similar data sets may be defined for hormonal therapy and immunotherapy.

Follow-up Data

At each follow-up visit, or annually, the effects and side effects of treatment should be assessed, as well as patient performance (see below).

Acute and subacute toxic effects of treatment should be recorded according to the five-grade system proposed by WHO (1979), and chronic and late toxic effects should be evaluated annually.

The response to treatment should at least be recorded as complete remission, partial remission, no change or progressive disease, according to the definitions issued by WHO (1979).

Finally, the date and cause of death should be recorded

Evaluation of the Programme

The basic analyses to be carried out within a programme are:

1. Tumour control and patterns of failure.
2. Survival.
3. Quality of life.
4. Economic considerations.

In addition, the design of the programme may permit studies on epidemiology, or evaluation of the diagnostic procedures, and/or the identification of prognostic factors.

1. Tumour control should be evaluated in terms of remission rate and duration of remission. The analysis of patterns of failure should include first site of failure, all sites of failure and failure attributable to a specific treatment, as well as causes of death (Cox and Kramer 1984).
2. The analysis of survival data should distinguish disease-free survival from survival with tumour and survival without complications from that with complications. Generally accepted life table methods should be employed, but in addition the calculation of relative survival for the entire treatment group or treated patients should be considered (Mould 1983).
3. Though quality of life is regarded as one of the most important measures of outcome in cancer treatment, there is still no general agreement on its measurement. The commonly used Karnofsky or Zubrod scales have been found to be difficult to reproduce, and do not take into account the self-assessment of the patient. Therefore, other scales, as for example the Linear Analogue Self-Assessment Questionnaire (Priestman and Baum 1976), the QL index (Spitzer et al. 1981), the Cancer Inventory of Problem Situations Test (Heinrich et al. 1984) or equivalent scales should be employed.
4. Since one of the basic ideas behind regional treatment programmes is the optimal utilization of existing resources for cancer treatment, considerations about the demands on resources raised by the programme and other economic implications should be analysed. This can be done by rather simple means, but may also require more sophisticated models employing, e.g. operational analysis (Liss et al. 1986).

Cancer Registration

Cancer registration has been employed for 50 years as a tool in cancer control, with the main goals of assessing the magnitude of the problem in the community, to measure the incidence, trends and geographical distributions of different malignant diseases, to monitor cancer mortality, and to assist in the evaluation of cancer control measures including different treatment modalities, mass-screening and preventive measures.

Cancer registries are usually either hospital based or population based. The hospital-based cancer registry collects data on all patients referred to a specific hospital. It is thus possible to evaluate the consumption of hospital resources, but not to measure incidence. The population-based registry, on the contrary, is mainly intended to monitor cancer incidence and trends, rather than to evaluate cancer treatment in specific detail (WHO 1976 b; MacLennan et al. 1978).

Cancer registries integrated in comprehensive cancer centres or regional oncological centres are usually able to collect much more data in a population-based setup, and thus seem to form the optimal environment for data collection and evaluation in regional treatment programmes.

Reporting of new cancer cases to a population-based cancer registry may be voluntary or compulsory, and registration may be based on specific report forms, discharge notes and death certificates. It is of advantage if the cancer registry has access to an up-to-date population register.

If the data base for a treatment programme is set up at, or can communicate with, the regional tumour registry, the population-based data on a specific tumour in the registry enables possible and actual accrual rates of patients to a regional treatment programme for that particular disease to be calculated. Further, patients not entered into the programme can be identified, and the reason for not entering could be analysed.

The up-to-date population register permits an automatic assessment of the vital status of all patients within and outside the programme, and the calculation of survival figures.

When analysing the results of a regional treatment programme, such data make it possible to extend the conclusions reached to the entire population, thus making them much more generally valid than conclusions reached within a limited clinical trial setup.

Clinical Trials Within a Treatment Programme

Standardized management of cancer patients in a treatment programme forms the ideal basis for testing, e.g. new drugs in phase I, II or III studies or for comparison of different diagnostic and/or therapeutic policies. If a clinical trial is included in the treatment programme, it should be properly described in the programme booklet. Special problems such as patient information and consent, as well as statistical considerations on sample size, end points, and methods and intervals of evaluation, must be addressed.

In such instances when a randomized trial includes the bulk of patients, care has to be taken to formulate alternative management policies for patients who do not fulfil the inclusion criteria.

The special problems related to clinical trials will be dealt with in a separate chapter.

Concluding Remarks

In Sweden, the ten most frequent forms of specified cancer in males cover 73% of all male cancer. The corresponding figure for females is 65% (National Board of Health and Welfare 1987). For both sexes, these figures correspond to 15 different diagnoses. Thus, a limited number of treatment programmes will cover a substantial part of the annual number of new cancer cases.

Both pros and cons can be formulated about treatment programmes. Critics have pointed out that therapy becomes less individually shaped, which may be of disadvantage to a number of patients. Furthermore, the space for pilot studies and other research initiatives may become more limited. On the other hand, a treatment programme may in general be considered to be the best way to fulfil the different goals in cancer management, as listed in the "Introduction". Of course, a treatment programme must never overrule the judgement made by the patient's physician.

References

AJCCS American Joint Committee on Cancer (1983) Manual for staging of cancer, 2nd edn. Lippincott, Philadelphia

Committee for Radiation Oncology Studies (1981) Criteria for radiation oncology in multidisciplinary cancer management. Report to the Director of the National Cancer Institute, National Institute of Health

Cox JD, Kramer S (1984) Strategic plan for radiologic sciences: outcome analysis. Cancer Treat Symp 1: 169–175

Eiserman B, Robinson WA, Steele G (1982) Follow-up of the cancer patient. Thieme-Stratton, New York

Hansluwka H (1984) Oncological database content: A note on international recommendations. In: Mould RD (ed) Computers in radiotherapy and oncology. Adam Hilger, Bristol, pp 109–122

Heinrich RL, Schag CC, Ganz PA (1984) Living with cancer: the cancer inventory of problem situations. J Clin Psychol 40: 972–980

ICRU International Commission on Radiation Units and Measurements (1978) Dose specification for reporting external beam therapy with photons and electrons. ICRU Report no 29. International Commission on Radiation Units and Measurements, Washington

ICRU International Commission on Radiation Units and Measurements (1985) Dose and volume specification for reporting intracavitary therapy in gynecology. ICRU Report no 38. International Commission on Radiation Units and Measurements, Washington

Liss A, Möller T, Sandblad B, Jogreus C, Olsson H (1986) A simulation based system for regional planning of care resources in oncology. In: Salamon R, Blum B, Jørgensen M (eds) MEDINFO 86 – 5th World Congress on Medical Informatics. Elsevier North Holland, Amsterdam, pp 736–740

MacLennan R, Muir CS, Steinitz R, Winkler A (eds) (1978) Cancer registration and its techniques. IARC Scientific Publication no 21. International Agency for Research on Cancer, Lyon

Möller TR (1985) Cancer care programmes: the Swedish experience. In: Parkin DM, Wagner G, Muir CS (eds) The role of the registry in cancer control. IARC Scientific Publications no 66. International Agency for Research on Cancer, Lyon, pp 109–119

Mould RF (1983) Cancer statistics. Adam Hilger, Bristol

Mould RF (1984) Review of oncologic databases with special reference to the assessment of quality of life after treatment for cancer. In: Mould RF (ed) Computers in radiotherapy and oncology. Adam Hilger, Bristol, pp 97–108

National Board on Health and Welfare (1987) Cancer incidence in Sweden 1984. National Board of Health and Welfare, Stockholm

Priestman TJ, Baum M (1976) Evaluation of quality of life in patients receiving treatment for advanced breast cancer. Lancet 1: 899–901

Rothwell DJ (ed) (1980) Systematized nomenclature of medicine – microglossary for surgical pathology. College of American Pathologists, Skokie

Sellers AH (ed) (1980) TNM classification of malignant tumours. A brochure of checklists. UICC Technical Report series, vol 51. International Union Against Cancer, Geneva

Sobin HL, Thomas LB, Percy C, Henson DE (eds) (1978) A coded compendium of the international histological classification of tumours. World Health Organization, Geneva

Spiessl B, Scheibe O, Wagner G (eds) (1982) TNM-Atlas. Illustrated guide to the classification of malignant tumours. UICC (International Union Against Cancer). Springer, Berlin Heidelberg New York

Spitzer WO, Dobson AJ et al. (1981) The QL-index. J Chron Dis 34: 585–597

SWENOTECA Swedish-Norwegian Testicular Cancer Project (1981) Treatment of non-seminomatous testicular cancer. Oncologic Cancer, Lund

UICC International Union against Cancer (1980) Guidelines for developing a comprehensive cancer centre. 2nd edn. Committee on International Collaborative Activities (CICA). UICC Technical report series, vol 53. International Union against Cancer, Geneva

UICC International Union against Cancer (1987) TNM classification of malignant tumours, 4th edn. Springer, Berlin Heidelberg New York London Paris Tokyo

Warr D, McKinney S, Tannock J (1984) Influence of measurement error on assessment of response to anticancer chemotherapy: proposal for new criteria of tumour response. J Clin Oncol 2: 1040–1046

WHO (1976a) International classification of diseases for oncology: ICD-O. World Health Organization, Geneva

WHO (1976b) WHO handbook for standardized cancer registries. WHO Offset Publication no 25. World Health Organization, Geneva

WHO (1978) International classification of procedures in medicine (2 vols). World Health Organization, Geneva

WHO (1979) WHO handbook for reporting results of cancer treatment. WHO Offset Publication no 48. World Health Organization, Geneva

WHO Regional Office for Europe (1982) Development of cancer centres and community cancer control programmes. Report on a WHO working group. WHO Regional Office for Europe, Copenhagen (ICP/CAN 007)

WHO Regional Office for Europe (1985) Cancer control programming in the European Region of the World Health Organization. Guideline Document. WHO Regional Office for Europe, Copenhagen (ICP/CAN 101)

Follow-up of Surgical Cancer Patients

H. WHITE and M. C. PARKER

General

Introduction

The outpatient follow-up of surgical patients is one of the most controversial aspects of clinical practice. Arbitrary intervals between outpatient checks are issued often without any clear rationale. In many cases a junior doctor will ask the patient to return in 3 months, purely because the last doctor did likewise, presuming it to be a reasonable time interval. The decision to discharge patients from a follow-up clinic is also difficult and may be left to a junior colleague. Decisions about follow-up are made all the more difficult in cancer patients, because of the stigma attached to the disease and patient anxiety. A doctor inexperienced in oncology may have difficulty in making these decisions and even greater difficulty in adhering to them.

What then are the correct and most suitable methods by which we, as specialists, should follow up cancer patients? How often should we see them? Should we see them at all? Should blood tests, X-rays and screening be performed routinely, or only upon the development of new symptoms? Is regular examination necessary? Do we remember that the patient is an individual rather than a 'cancer case' who may have developed neuroses, or unfounded anxieties, simply as a result of having had cancer treatment?

In this chapter the authors attempt to outline a rational approach to cancer follow-up based on their own personal experience and on the evidence of many other studies. Guidelines are put forward which the authors believe to be logical and expedient.

Although established specialists are unlikely to change their habits perhaps the more junior clinicians should begin to question the dogma of follow-up handed down by their seniors. The aim must be to give the best possible clinical service to the community within the particular economic and geographical constraints. These will clearly vary in different countries at different times in their development.

Regular follow-up after cancer surgery is almost a routine in clinics throughout the developed world. Initially, patients are seen frequently until it is established that they are thriving well, recovering physically and mentally and that they remain free of recurrent disease. Thereafter, attendances are often less frequent and after a delayed period, usually a matter of years, they may be abolished altogether. During this follow-up period patients develop confidence in the ability of clinicians to monitor their disease and the clinician begins to assess the prognosis. The frequency of follow-up and nature of the tests will to some extent depend on whether they can be assigned to a statistically good or bad group.

If early recurrence is detected or the patient is failing to recover for whatever reason, further investigation or treatment may be instigated, which demands either the same or an increased frequency of attendance. It may be expedient to readmit such patients to hospital for certain investigations as they are often in low physical and mental states. The mere fact that definite action is being taken may have a beneficial effect on morale at a time when fate appears to have dealt a cruel blow.

Objectives of Follow-up

1. To interview patients and assess their physical and mental state and establish any problems that have arisen since discharge from hospital or since the previous attendance: some patients have trouble remembering their ailments and encouragement should be given to write down problems as they occur, so that in the exacting environment of a busy follow-up clinic they will not be forgotten. It is important to ascertain the general health of the patient, as well as specific details which may have a particular bearing, depending on the extent and locality of the previous disease. There may be postoperative depression or a change in the pattern of sleep. Appetite, eating habits and bowel function are often disturbed after any form of surgery, but especially after operations on the gastrointestinal tract and careful documentation needs to be made before proceeding to any investigation. Current drug therapy should be established on each attendance, since quite often in the intervening period since the last consultation the general practitioner may have had reason to advise and treat the patient for some complication, or even for a totally different complaint. Social problems must be elicited, to ensure that the patient is managing at work and with domestic chores. The effects of surgery, as well as the disease, may make these tasks difficult, especially in an elderly person. It may be necessary to inform the district nursing services, or the general practitioner, that a patient is having difficulty with such problems, so that help can be organised quickly. An elderly postoperative patient may not feel able to go shopping soon after surgery and may, therefore, attempt to live frugally. This may well be inadequate and retard progress during convalescence. For these reasons we would advocate that the first postoperative consultation after major surgery should be made no longer than 2 or 3 weeks after discharge from hospital. In some cases, the first postoperative outpatient visit is the occasion at which the final histology report becomes available and the discussion of this is clearly of great importance.
2. To examine the patient is a necessary and vital procedure, not only to re-establish patient contact, but also for reassurance and to assess the outcome of surgery.
   If early recurrence is diagnosed on clinical examination, or if any other postsurgical complication is discovered, then, although that finding will in itself distress the patient, positive encouragement should be given to allay unnecessary fears. Early diagnosis means prompt investigation and appropriate treatment. Detailed clinical examination may be a time-consuming procedure. The extent of an examination partly depends on the disease and

the site. An experienced clinician can adjust the examination to the problem (without detriment to the patient). In a patient with a previously excised rodent ulcer of the forehead, for example, examination of the head and neck is usually all that is necessary to exclude recurrence and further examination will be unnecessary, unless something reported by the patient, or the general practitioner, requires further action. On the other hand a patient with a previously excised malignant melanoma deserves a more prolonged and critical examination, in order to be sure of eliminating local and distant recurrence. A full knowledge of the natural history of the various type of neoplasm is, therefore, mandatory.

3. To supervise follow-up treatment in the immediate postoperative period is important, as patients may be having radiotherapy, chemotherapy or some form of adjuvant treatment. Although this may involve other medical teams, it is the duty of the surgeon to take an active interest in the therapy, as well as being able to reassure the patient that the course of treatment recommended is that which is appropriate. Many surgeons and oncologists have developed combined modality follow-up clinics, where both surgeon and physician are present, so that difficult problems can be resolved together. This type of clinic can often avoid unnecessary repeat consultations for the patient, since both specialists are in attendance and thus joint discussions regarding any change in treatment may be made. It is also reassuring to the patient to know that there is no question of uncertainty between the various doctors regarding treatment.
   Radiotherapy is often advised after establishing clearly the full histopathology and the stage of the tumour, both clinically and with imaging. Once the decision is made, the fine details of the treatment, such as the field to be irradiated, dosage of radiotherapy and the number of fractions are all the responsibility of the radiotherapy department. Usually, clear guidelines have already been established for most standard postoperative radiotherapy courses. On occasion, however, something unusual in the operative procedure may influence the surgeon to request additional or modified techniques of radiation to be employed. Naturally, this must be in consultation with the radiotherapist.
   Similarly, many hospitals and surgical departments, nowadays, arrange for chemotherapy to be given under the supervision of a medical oncologist. Once again, our belief is that combined interspecialist consultation is necessary to acquire the best management of such therapy. Some institutions have implemented the introduction of specialist nursing teams, whose sole responsibility is the administration of chemotherapy. With this type of nursing assistance, interval chemotherapy can be given as an outpatient procedure, allowing doctors to devote more time to direct patient care.
4. To undertake further investigation, as after initial surgery, additional tests may be required. A typical example is that of a patient who has undergone excision biopsy of a lump which is found to be malignant. Full staging may include radiological, haematological, biochemical and screening facilities. The surgeon must be aware of the available techniques which will be most useful during follow-up. Later on, we shall try to advise on the appropriate staging techniques applicable to individual types of cancer. With such a profusion of sophisticated tests now available, care must be taken to ensure that they are not ordered unnecessarily and that a decision on management, or prognosis, can and will be taken as a result.
   If a group of patients can be identified who are at greater risk of developing a recurrent, or a metachronous tumour, by virtue of the type of tumour, or familial predisposition, they should be investigated and followed appropriately.
5. To supervise pain relief, for in many cases of cancer, particularly those of an advanced nature, pain is an accompanying symptom of the disease. If the pain results from local pressure, surgery may relieve the symptoms. Often, however, the pain is that of widely disseminated disease for which local surgery is inappropriate. If progression is suspected, investigation must be adequate, to establish that the pain is due to metastatic disease, before planning further therapy. In known advanced cancer, investigations should be kept to a minimum and early control of pain should be the prime objective. In both situations there is no reason to withhold analgesia even though definitive diagnosis of the pain has not yet been made. Initial symptomatic relief should be attempted using simple analgesia, withholding stronger drugs for intractable pain. The correct dose and frequency of administration of an analgesic used in the treatment of metastatic cancer is that which relieves the pain totally. There should be no restriction on the use of narcotic analgesia in these patients, since addiction is irrelevant and, in any case, it is of minimal consequence, as the long-term life expectancy is limited. The prime consideration in treating these patients is that of pain relief. In intractable pain the use of continuous analagesia is better than spasmodic or intermittent dosage. In certain spe-

cialist centres, pain clinics have now been developed. Such clinics prove invaluable in the management of long-term problems of pain.

6. To monitor the patient's mental state, as the realisation of life-threatening disease may cause depression and other psychiatric disturbance. Access to a psychiatrist, as well as social services and continuing care facilities, can be of great benefit.

Planning a Follow-up Clinic

The important features of such a clinic are the regularity, frequency and efficiency with which it operates. Regular checks are important both for the clinician to maintain close surveillance and also for the patient to know that his or her follow-up is thorough. As time goes by, however, and certainly if further problems are not anticipated, it is perhaps better to advise early discharge and the opportunity of self-referral if any problem occurs. Ritual annual appointments are more likely to induce paranoia and anxiety in the otherwise well patient. This may even be appropriate in those patients in whom a small but definite percentage may be expected to develop recurrence. In a recent survey by Dewar and Kerr in Edinburgh, the value of routine follow-up in women treated for early breast cancer by mastectomy with or without radiotherapy was assessed retrospectively (Dewar and Kerr 1985). They established that out of 6863 visits made by 546 patients over 8 years only 93 relapses were detected at scheduled visits. Ninety-nine relapses were discovered at unscheduled visits, after either self-examination by the patients themselves, or after re-referral by the attending general practitioner. A potentially curable relapse (local or in the contralateral breast) was detected in 66 (1%) of 6764 routine visits, but only 26 (39%) of these patients remained free of disease. They concluded that the intensity of follow-up of such patients might well be reduced without any adverse effect on prognosis, but with considerable financial and other benefits.

There is much to be said in favour of this attitude, since the vast number of unnecessary visits made are time-consuming both to the clinician and to the patient. Regular visits may incur loss of income to the patient, especially if he or she is self-employed and the cost of transport will be borne either by the patient or the State.

Reducing the frequency of attendance allows more time to be spent in consultation between physician and patient and is unlikely to alter dramatically the long-term prognosis for such patients (Clark and Morris 1981). On the other hand, if such decrease in frequency of attendance is to be achieved, then careful counselling of the patient in self-examination is necessary and encouragement must be made towards interval attendance should any symptoms or abnormal signs develop. In other words early open access to the outpatient clinic is necessary. We would estimate that in the few patients per clinic who attend after self-referral the problem is usually anxiety, or a potentially benign complication, rather than recurrent disease. Nevertheless, it is prudent to reserve such a number of appointments vacant at each outpatient clinic in anticipation of these self-referrals.

Regularity of attendance is not in question, but the frequency of attendance will differ both from clinic to clinic and from surgeon to surgeon and also for the different types of tumour. In the next section, the authors will try to issue guidelines on the frequency of attendance necessary for individual types of cancer.

There is likely to be an increase in specialist techniques in follow-up requiring the patient to be in hospital for several hours (e.g. endoscopy and various invasive diagnostic imaging). These inpatient visits on a day basis must be integrated as efficiently as possible into the normal outpatient follow-up programme.

Related Systems

Head and Neck Cancers

These tumours include those of the parotid and submandibular salivary glands, tongue, larynx, thyroid, parathyroid and carotid body. Those bony tumours of the face and jaw which fall into the realm of the specialist faciomaxillary surgeon are considered to be outside the scope of this review.

Parotid tumours constituting mainly mixed pleomorphic adenoma and rarely adenolymphoma should be completely contained by a superficial parotidectomy. Only in the case of incomplete excision, or spillage of tumour cells at operation, should it be necessary to consider postoperative radiotherapy. The rare adenocarcinoma of these glands may necessitate sacrifice of the facial nerve, in which case nerve grafting using the posterior auricular nerve should be performed. Although this will not restore perfect facial movement on the affected side, at least facial symmetry is maintained (Conley 1981). If the disease has extended to the regional nodes, a block dissection may have been performed. In any event, postoperative treatment in the form of radiotherapy will be required in these patients. The follow-up may be dependent upon the histology, reserving a longer and perhaps more intensive follow-up for those patients with adenocarcinoma. If the patient who has had a pleomorphic adenoma completely removed intact is seen to have made a complete recovery at his or her first outpatient visit, then there is little to be gained from multiple further attendances. The patient should be advised to reattend only if further problems develop. On the other hand, patients with carcinoma must be followed up regularly, both by clinical examination and, if indicated, by X-ray and CT scanning to search for early recurrence. These examinations must be frequent at least initially, until control of the disease is established, since locally advanced carcinoma may be impossible to eradicate.

Tumours of the tongue and oral cavity are rare in Europe (Harrison 1980), but much more common in parts of India and the Far East (del Regato et al. 1985, pp 226–424). Unfortunately, in the developing countries the conventional pattern of follow-up is not possible. Where practicable, however, regular and frequent follow-up in the immediate postoperative phase by clinical examination with radiological and CT survey is indicated. After partial or total glossectomy, or indeed after any major reconstruction of the face, speech therapy will be required postoperatively and the patient may have to be taught how to masticate if prosthetic implant has been performed. The patient and family will require counselling with regard to the new facial appearance, after either reconstruction or prosthetic replacement of a defect. It is not uncommon, particularly in the younger patient, for acute reactive depression to result after this sort of surgery, even if cure is obtained. It is often necessary in this situation to obtain urgent psychiatric advice to tide the patient through this difficult transition period, until he or she can readjust to their new appearance.

Pharyngeal and laryngeal tumours, when locally advanced, sometimes require major resection involving laryngectomy and oesophagectomy with formation of tracheostomy and with gastric replacement, and colonic or free jejunal interposition of the oesophagus. When fully healed, a speaking tracheostomy tube may be inserted, which can easily be covered with suitable clothing, preventing cosmetic embarrassment. Some patients prefer an open stoma, merely covering the stoma with the index finger at the time of phonation. Intensive speech therapy will be required during convalescence to produce either pharyngeal or oesophageal speech. Many weeks of training may be required to attain an adequate new voice. Group training and the formation of affinity groups of patients with a similar disability may be helpful.

The presence of local recurrence following this type of surgery constitutes a difficult therapeutic problem and its diagnosis at an early stage is imperative if locoregional control is to be achieved. This demands the use of CT scanning if accurate definition of recurrent local disease is to be obtained. If tumour is defined, confirmation can be determined by needle aspiration cytology and therapy instituted. Failure to control local disease may result in gross painful and ulcerating disease in the neck, which causes undue suffering to the dying patient. For the same reasons, if primary nasopharyngeal squamous carcinoma is treated without block dissection of the neck, then very frequent thorough examination of the neck is mandatory in the immediate follow-up period at monthly intervals to prevent the development of fixed ulcerating regional lymphatic involvement. At the slightest suggestion of cervical node involvement and after confirmation with scanning and positive cytology, immediate block dissection must be performed to regain local control.

Patients free of local and metastatic disease after the first 2 years require little or no further follow-up by the specialist and referral on a symptomatic basis by the attending general practitioner may be all that is required.

Thyroid cancer includes those patients with follicular, papillary or Hurtle cell carcinoma in whom long-term cure can be anticipated, medullary cell carcinoma in which only 50% of the patients will live over 10 years and anaplastic carcinoma which has a poor prognosis. There are a few rare lymphomas, sarcomas, teratomas, epidermoid and metastatic tumours which are of mixed aetiology and prognosis.

After adequate palliative surgery in patients with anaplastic carcinoma to relieve pressure symptoms, the follow-up is designed to prevent or alleviate discomfort in a short period, during which the patient will inevitably decline, as the tumour is well known to carry a 100% mortality.

Medullary cell carcinoma is an interesting follow-up challenge, since the diagnosis itself infers the possibility of familial involvement. Full screening of the blood relatives of the patient by clinical examination and serum calcitonin levels is vital. The individual follow-up of the patient also incorporates regular serum calcitonin estimation every 6 months. Any elevation of this marker suggests the presence of occult metastases, which must be sought urgently and appropriate treatment with streptozotocin instituted.

Adequate resection of adenocarcinoma of the thyroid will require thyroxine replacement therapy for life. It has been well established by Russell, who performed whole gland sectioning of 80 cases of thyroid adenocarcinoma, that the histology of the tumour merely represents the predominant feature of what is often a mixed follicular and papillary carcinoma and that tumour extension into the contralateral lobe occurs in 87% (Russel et al. 1963). If, at the time of initial surgery, any local lymphatic involvement is suspected, then these lymph nodes may be removed in association with the gland. Six weeks postoperatively, after cessation of thyroxine for 3 weeks, a radioactive iodine-131 scan is performed to ensure that there is no uptake in any recurrent thyroid tissue nor any local lymphatic or distant metastasis. The presence of positive uptake merely requires an ablative dose of 80 µCi radioactive iodine to be given orally. Thyroxine replacement is then reintroduced. If no uptake is apparent, no other treatment is necessary at this stage. At 6 months and 1 year diagnostic scanning is repeated using the same technique. If no uptake is found, the procedure can then be performed on a yearly basis until 5 years and then on a 5 yearly basis.

If at any time positive uptake is measured, then a further ablative dose of radioactive iodine is given and the frequency of screening resumes at 6 monthly intervals as previously described. With this regime the life expectancy of young patients with thyroid adenocarcinoma may be confidently predicted to approach that of the normal population (Smithers 1970). The only other parameters to be monitored at the same interval clinics are the clinical condition of the patient, which should include weight and resting pulse measurements, and the biochemical status of the patient. Serum thyroxine estimation indicates the chemical level of thyroid activity in the blood, but the serum TSH level gives a more accurate indication of satisfactory thyroid hormone replacement.

Primary parathyroid tumours are extremely rare and local radical resection with regional lymphadenectomy, if indicated, is the treatment of choice. Follow-up is based upon the detection of locoregional recurrence in much the same way as for thyroid adenocarcinoma.

Carotid body tumours, once excised completely, should not cause local problems, but do, on occasion, develop metastases which necessitate chemotherapy (Martin et al. 1973). The tumours are of APUD cell origin and may respond to radiotherapy (Mitchell and Clyne 1985). Thus, follow-up is required for a minimum period of 10 years, after which time secondary growth would be extremely unlikely to develop.

Oesophageal Cancer

Cancer of the oesophagus carries an extremely poor prognosis, whether or not the original lesion is resectable (Nakayama and Kinoshita 1974). The average 5-year survival rate is about 5% in a review of the recent literature (Earlam and Cunha-Melo 1980). Thus, in less than 95% of the patients the follow-up period is aimed at producing good palliation of the disease. To a certain extent this will depend on the surgery which was undertaken for the original lesion. If the tumour was resected and some manner of oesophagogastric or oesophagoenteric bypass performed, then swallowing should not be a problem, despite progression of the disease. It, on the other hand, the primary lesion was irresectable, or if advanced disease was discovered at the time of operation, many surgeons will simply insert a prosthetic tube, such as the Celestin or Nottingham tube, through the malignant stricture. This allows the patient to swallow, but by necessity restricts the diet to semisolid foods. Complications include perforation, bleeding, dislodgement, blockage and discomfort (Diamantes and Mannell 1983). Protagonists of this method report satisfactory results in patients whose general condition is poor. Others who find the tube prostheses poor palliation advise some form of surgical bypass, such as oesophagojejunostomy. These patients will require continuous supervision for the rest of their lives.

In a review of 618 patients with squamous cell carcinoma of the oesophagus, Pearson reported no difference in the survival rate and equally effective palliation in patients whose lesion was treated by radiotherapy alone compared with surgical excision (Pearson 1969). Follow-up at regular periods for both groups is essential to assess nutrition, symptoms and progressing disease.

In those patients who have undergone curative resection, radiotherapy will be necessary in the postoperative period. This can be undertaken on an outpatient basis in the majority of patients and, frequently, takes about 6 weeks, during which time the patient is seen regularly. The majority of patients who have had palliative bypass surgery or radiotherapy will inevitably die of their disease, usually with gradual deterioration due to hepatic metastases. It must be remembered that these metastases are often asymptomatic and, as long as no local problems arise at the site of the primary tumour, there is much to be said in favour of therapeutic nihilism. At the present time, there is no firm evidence to show that any benefits attributable to chemotherapy in terms of survival, or quality of life, outweigh the side effects and complications of the therapy itself. In the authors' experience, it is in the patients' interest to understand the serious clinical situation, which means honesty and integrity on the part of the clinician as well as compassion. If the patient asks if any further treatment can be given, we believe in providing full information regarding chemotherapy. At the same time we do not believe in destroying the will of our patients, merely in a humane approach to a currently incurable problem. Sometimes, this is extremely difficult to achieve and, like many other clinicians involved in this sort of care, we fall short of our ideals on many occasions. However, regular contact with the patient can be psychologically supportive.

Pain, either from the primary site of the tumour or rarely, for example, from a bleed into a hepatic deposit, is sometimes a problem in oesophageal cancer. The cause of the pain may be established by clinical examination together with ultrasound or CT scanning depending on the site of the pain. Symptomatic relief with analgesics should be used for hepatic metastases and occasionally chemotherapy. Radiotherapy may be useful at the primary site, if full dosage has not already been given. Otherwise intractable pain may be arrested by regular adequate analgesia using opiates. Some hospitals now have the benefit of pain clinics run by anaesthetists and such local problems are often susceptible to regional anaesthesia (Marks 1985). Others report the success of acupuncture (Kiser et al. 1983) and there is now much less demand, or necessity, for anterolateral cordotomy for pain relief, although it remains a recognised technique (Cowie and Hitchcock 1982).

The follow-up of patients who have had radical resection, whether it be curative or palliative, is often surprisingly uncomplicated. If the patient develops metastases without local recurrence, although he or she may require compassionate support and occasional pain relief, there is little necessary in the way of investigation once the metastases have been unequivocably confirmed. This may be performed by ultrasound or CT scanning, or, on occasion, by fine needle aspiration cytology of a palpable supraclavicular lymph node. Referral to a continuing care unit or terminal care hospice may be appropriate, although many patients prefer to live out their days at home, especially if they have good support from their relatives, general practitioner, district nursing and ancillary services.

In the "cured" patient who remains well in the postoperative period with a good appetite, steady weight and normal bowel function, little is required in terms of specialist advice, apart from reassurance and encouragement. After 18 months, if the patient is still well and trouble free, then it is likely that 'that elusive cure' has happened. In this situation, follow-up may then be necessary only if further problems are encountered. Unfortunately, at the present time these patients are too few and until earlier diagnosis is achieved the situation is unlikely to change.

Gastric Cancer

Much which has been said of oesophageal cancer pertains to gastric cancer. This disease also carries a poor long-term survival, with only 10% of all post-surgical patients surviving for 5 years (Armstrong and Dent 1985; Oschner et al. 1981; Brookes et al. 1965; Costello et al. 1977). If early recurrence occurs, or indeed if metastases are known to be present, then palliation and support are the qualities to be advocated. If, on the other hand, the patient remains trouble free, there are some long-term consequences of partial or total gastrectomy which must be anticipated by the specialist. It is inevitable that all patients who undergo total gastrectomy and, indeed, many who undergo partial gastrectomy will develop pernicious anaemia, due to loss of intrinsic factor. This should be anticipated and vitamin B_{12} supplement given, usually at a dose of 1000 µg monthly by intramuscular injection. This is mandatory in the patient who has had total gastrectomy, but it is a reasonable policy in those patients who have had partial gastrectomy to wait and observe, since not all will become vitamin B_{12} deficient. Our policy is to measure the haemoglobin and mean corpuscular volume (MCV) on an annual basis and to measure the serum vitamin B_{12} only if indicated by an abnormality of the former indices. If this shows a deficiency, then supplement therapy is given.

After any type of gastrectomy, the patient will have to learn to eat small meals regularly and this should be emphasised before the patient leaves hospital after surgery. Upper abdominal discomfort, vomiting and bloating are not uncommonly described by patients in the first few months after gastrectomy, but the vast majority soon learn to adapt to their new restricted gastric reservoir and only a very few complain persistently of postcibal problems. Occasionally, specific postgastrectomy syndromes occur, such as dumping or diarrhoea. Medical treatment is usually effective, with advice to take small dry meals to combat the former and using antidiarrhoeal agents such as codine phosphate for the latter. Most patients with these problems can be rendered asymptomatic by simple conservative measures and the indications for further surgical treatment are remote. This is all the more important in gastric cancer follow-up, in view of the limited prospects of most of the patients.

If a 'survivor' persists with either dumping, or diarrhoea, or both, despite good dietary advice and medical therapy, it is usually necessary to readmit the patient to hospital for intensive investigation to determine the exact nature of the problem before advising treatment. The patient must be observed and his or her eating habits documented, in particular, noting the timing of dumping attacks and, if any occur, to measure the blood glucose level at the time of the attack. In this manner, it is possible to distinguish between the early dumping syndrome caused by hypovolaemia following the osmotic pull of jejunal food content and the late dumping syndrome with associated hypoglycaemia induced by inappropriate insulin release in response to ingestion of small quantities of food.

The bowel habit should also be documented noting the quality and frequency of defaecation. Stool cultures must be obtained and sigmoidoscopy performed to exclude infective causes of diarrhoea. Small bowel motility studies are performed using barium-coated foodstuffs to obtain a true pattern of intestinal transit. Only in this way can it be established that the true cause of the diarrhoea is rapid transit, rather than some other complication, such as an enteroenteric fistula.

Even in these few patients with careful advice regarding food intake and employing drug therapy as described, the vast majority of patients can be controlled by medical means and surgery should be avoided at all costs. The patient who undergoes revision of a partial gastrectomy for postgastrectomy diarrhoea will inevitably return with similar problems no matter what revision procedure is performed.

Patients who progress to hepatic metastases with gastric cancer will exhibit some or all of the well-known features of disseminated cancer. Unfortunately, like oesophageal cancer there is no conclusive evidence that chemotherapy significantly prolongs life in these patients and the side effects of such therapy are not inconsiderable. Thus, the same advice ensues, that if, despite progression of the disease, the patient remains asymptomatic, then a conservative approach is perhaps the best. Indeed, it has been shown in one series that the mortality and morbidity in patients with gastric cancer undergoing chemotherapy was greater than in those who did not receive chemotherapy (Comis and Carter 1974). Thus, the situation remains controversial and a humane approach should be followed, adapting treatment to the individual needs of the patient.

Pancreatic Cancer

The 5-year survival for patients undergoing Whipple's procedure for carcinoma of the head of the pancreas is only 6%, whereas for periampullary and duodenal cancer the survival is in the region of 45% (Smith and Sherlock 1981). These results are not influenced by the extent of the pancreatic resection, although there have been some reports recently suggesting that total pancreatectomy may carry a similar survival and less operative mortality than partial pancreatectomy (Blumgart and Imrie 1979). However, the late results of total pancreatectomy are not good and, indeed, long-term complications with diabetes and malabsorption are extremely common, despite replacement therapy (Blumgart and Imrie 1979). These patients are particularly prone to hypoglycaemic attacks, possibly due to lack of pancreatic glucagon (Mallinson et al. 1977). In view of the high incidence of long-term problems and the lack of evidence regarding long-term survival benefit, the procedure of total pancreatectomy must be considered unnecessary. Palliative surgery is by far the most common surgical procedure, with double or triple bypass being standard practice. Sometimes, incorporated in the procedure is coeliac ganglion neurectomy to try and palliate pain (Blumgart and Imrie 1979).

The outlook for these patients is a short period of remission, but inevitably they will all die from metastatic disease, with a median survival time of about 2 months (Mallinson et al. 1977). Postoperative radiotherapy and chemotherapy have had protagonists suggesting significantly increased survival in those patients who undergo one or both of these adjuvant treatments, but, once again, the suggested benefits of these modes of treatment, which both carry a mortality, must be weighed against the well-known side effects. More recently, with the use of ultrasound, CT scanning and percutaneous fine needle aspiration cytology, endoscopic or percutaneous transhepatic stents to relieve jaundice have become standard practice in many centres. This is often performed prior to adjuvant radio- and chemotherapy and survival times similar to those following bypass surgery are reported.

Residual pain after either surgery or stenting may be susceptible to coeliac ganglion phenol nerve block. The results of percutaneous nerve block have been reported as better than surgical neurectomy (Falk 1982). If this procedure fails, regular analgesia will be necessary. Steatorrhoea, due to lack of pancreatic lipase activity, can be combated by the administration of pancreatic exocrine replacement therapy. Diabetes is occasionally a problem which may require diet restriction, oral hypoglycaemics or insulin.

Liver and Biliary Tree Cancer

Primary liver cancer is rare in the United Kingdom, but occurs more commonly in other areas of the world such as South Africa and China (Falk 1982; Berman 1951). Primary resection by partial hepatectomy is now a well-established procedure for solitary liver tumours and it is possible to resect up to 80% of the liver without inducing hepatic failure (Cooper and Williamson 1983). Inevitably, during the postoperative period, patients who have had such extensive resections will become jaundiced, but this is a temporary phenomenon and liver function can be expected to return to normal within 2 months (Islami et al. 1958).

Cancer of the gall bladder is also a rarity in Europe, accounting for only 2.8% of all malignancies (Illingworth 1935). The majority of cases present late and are inoperable at first presentation. Occasionally they are discovered as an incidental finding at cholecystectomy. The prognosis depends upon the histology of the lesions. If the tumour is confined to the mucosa and submucosa, then simple cholecystectomy will afford a 5-year survival reported as 65%–86% (Bergdahl 1980; Nevin et al. 1976). The problem occurs when the tumour has extended through the gall bladder wall. In this event, if no metastases are apparent at operation, the 5-year survival for patients undergoing simple cholecystectomy is zero (Bergdahl 1980). The only possibility of a cure in these patients is extended cholecystectomy, which, in effect, means an extended right hepatic lobectomy. After such surgery, occasional 5-year survivors are reported, but it should be noted that the operative procedure itself carries a reported mortality of about 20%, even in hepatobiliary centres (Smith and Sherlock 1981). Thus, the vast majority of patients who are found to have gall bladder cancer at operation are treated by either palliative bypass procedure or stenting. Once the jaundice is relieved, follow-up is restricted to pain relief and supportive measures. Radiotherapy may have a part to play in patients who have had endoprosthesis or percutaneous transhepatic stenting performed.

Bile duct cancers are operable by simple resection in the upper third in about 20% of cases (Smith and Sherlock 1981) and in the lower and middle third in approximately 60% (Tomkins et al. 1981). Irresectable lesions are treated either by biliary enteric bypass procedures or by stenting, in which case radiotherapy or chemotherapy may be appropriate after surgery. These tumours are sometimes chemosensitive but, in any case, the palliation obtained by stenting and radiotherapy is reported to be equally as effective as resection, with 2-year survival rates of 75% (Leung et al. 1983). In the upper and middle thirds resectable tumours are treated by excision and hepatodochojejunostomy, whereas in the lower third they are treated by pancreaticoduodenectomy. Good long-term survival is to be expected in these patients, with 12% 5-year survival in upper third and almost 50% 5-year survival in middle and lower third tumours (Mallinson et al. 1977; Falk 1982). In the absence of metastatic disease, these patients have very good quality of life and few problems are to be anticipated. Stenosis of hepatodochojejunostomy is an occasional long-term complication, which may require refashioning if jaundice or recurrent cholangitis becomes a problem. Complications of pancreaticoduodenectomy have already been discussed.

Palliative treatment for bile duct cancers includes endoscopic or transhepatic stenting. Both of these procedures carry a low mortality rate in experienced hands (Ring et al. 1975; Cotton 1982), but are noted to be complicated in the long term, with cholangitis occurring in 10% and recurrent jaundice in 6% (Leung et al. 1983). If either of these occur, the stent will have to be replaced. In a recent review, it has been shown that the initial hospital stay of patients undergoing stenting is only 3 days, whereas those undergoing surgery and bypass average 10 days. However, whereas those patients who have had surgery rarely need readmission for long-term complications, those who have been stented require an average of three readmissions for complications, so that the overall hospital stay is equal in both groups of patients (Bornmann et al. 1986).

Metastatic liver cancer is usually unremitting and although chemotherapy is appropriate in some tumours, such as carcinoid or lymphoma, there is little evidence to suggest that systemic chemotherapy is of any value in hepatic metastatic adenocarcinoma, which is by far the commonest problem. However, recent reports on the new technique of hepatic arterial infusion chemotherapy are claiming extended survival as a result of treatment in patients with hepatic metastases (Kemeny et al. 1986). At the present time, the expense of the technique would prohibit its use becoming commonplace.

Small Bowel Cancer

Primary tumours of the small bowel are rare, constituting only 2% of all bowel tumours (Barclay and Schapira 1983). However, the small bowel is often involved in other intra-abdominal cancers, such as colonic cancers, and extensive resection may be necessary for advanced local disease. Radical resection of the small bowel is still compatible with long-term survival, providing at least 30 cm of normal small intestine remains (Williamson 1982). Resection of the ileocaecal valve may contribute to postoperative diarrhoea if extensive small bowel resection has been performed. Diarrhoea is uncommon, however, after simple right hemicolectomy. Resection of the terminal ileum may result in vitamin B_{12} deficiency in the long term, which will require regular replacement. The short gut syndrome may produce diarrhoea and malabsorption due to rapid transit. Medical therapy to slow intestinal transit is often required as well as vitamins, iron, calcium, magnesium and zinc supplement. Dietary advice is very important and foodstuffs such as fresh fruit, salads, high roughage and milk products may well exacerbate diarrhoea and should be avoided.

In irresectable small bowel tumours, intestinal entero-enteric bypass may be performed, leaving a blind loop which may, in itself, predispose to diarrhoea induced by bacterial overgrowth of the stagnant microflora. For obvious reasons, conservative therapy is appropriate in this situation, using either metronidazole or tetracycline.

Colorectal Cancer

Resectable colorectal cancers may be treated by a variety of radical operations. The long-term prognosis in rectal cancer is well recognised as being dependent upon Dukes' staging and a similar modification of the system is applicable to colonic cancer. Thus, a patient who has had a radical resection of a Dukes' A tumour may anticipate a 90% 5-year survival (Dukes 1940). The follow-up of these patients should be planned with this in mind. Local recurrence at the site of an anastomosis following resection of colorectal tumour is a recognised complication. If it does occur, it is usually evident endoscopically at an early stage (Ekman et al. 1977). Approximately 2% of all patients who have had a primary colorectal cancer will develop a metachronous tumour (Heald and Lockhart-Mummery 1972). We believe that it is sensible to perform sigmoidoscopy, or colonoscopy, 3 months postoperatively and then to follow asymptomatic patients with regular faecal occult blood testing every 6 months for the first 2 years and then annually, thereafter reserving further investigation for those patients who are haemoccult positive. Patients who develop symptoms suggestive of recurrent bowel tumour should be investigated immediately.

The ultimate failure of surgery in colorectal cancer is local recurrence, since, in most cases, this will prove to be refractory to most forms of treatment. This is preventable by performing adequate radical surgery in the first place, avoiding cutting into tumour at all costs and removing involved adjacent structures, or part thereof, if necessary, to clear the lesion. If, during the follow-up, a recurrent local lesion is identified, then even in the presence of distant metastases and if the recurrent lesion is not clinically inoperable, a second laparotomy is totally justified to remove the local tumour. In these situations, ultrasound and CT scanning are helpful in planning surgery, but should not avert the surgeon from laparotomy, since, on occasion, metastases identified on scanning may prove to be a figment of the imagination. The point of further surgery is that, on occasion, long-term cure results and, for the other patients with metastases, better palliation is achieved (Cochrane et al. 1980).

The question of frequency of follow-up of patients who have had colorectal cancer excised is controversial, but there is much evidence to suggest that regular routine follow-up is of very little benefit. In 1980, Cochrane et al. reviewed 406 patients with large bowel cancer. One hundred and eighty of these patients were followed up at the same institution after radical surgery and were seen 2319 times from 6 months to 15 years. Seventy-one patients developed recurrent cancer, but of these 41 (58%) were diagnosed at times other than routine follow-up clinics. Only one patient with recurrence appeared to have been cured by further surgery. This study confirmed the earlier report by Ekman et al. (1977) who analysed the results of a prospective study in the follow-up of 243 colorectal cancer patients and compared them with a retrospective survey of 198 similar patients. In the prospective survey, all patients were seen every third month during the first year after operation and thereafter twice a year. Each control included a thorough clinical examination, proctosigmoidoscopy, roentgenogram of the chest, barium enema and some routine blood analyses. It was expected that recurrences occurring in the prospective survey would be discovered early, ensuring successful treatment. The results of the study proved otherwise. The 5-year survival of the retrospective group was 33%, whilst that of the prospective group, who in addition to surgery had received 5-fluoruracil, was 30%. The two groups were well matched for Dukes' classification, site of tumour, age, sex and curative operations. In the prospective group, 36 patients developed recurrence, 6 of which were discovered between regular follow-up appointments. Of these 36 patients, only 7 underwent further operation at which cure was intended. Only 3 out of the 36 were alive 3 years after initial surgery and these 3 were in the group of 7 patients who underwent second laparotomy.

We believe that there is little evidence to support the use of adjuvant radiotherapy after curative resection for colorectal cancer, but it is certainly worthwhile in palliating the irresectable advanced lesion (Cummings 1985). Chemotherapy has been singularly disappointing when given systemically, but there is some evidence to suggest increased survival in patients with hepatic metastases from colorectal cancer, treated by hepatic artery instillation of 5-fluoro-2′-deoxyuridine (FUDR) by continuous infusion. This treatment is currently undergoing scrutiny and the initial results are mildly optimistic, although the expense of the technique is perhaps prohibitive.

The value of monitoring patients following resection of colorectal cancer by means of carcinoembryonic antigen (CEA) blood levels is unproven as yet. Certainly there is a relationship between elevated levels and metastatic disease but whether the detection thereof can lead to increase in survival and lower mortality rates is still under review. Studies are underway at the present time addressing this particular question. For the time being it would seem appropriate to monitor CEA levels every 3 months, reserving ultrasound and CT scanning and even second-look laparotomy for those patients whose levels rise without overt clinical evidence of metastases. Certainly second-look laparotomy is justified in the event of recognising recurrent local disease or localised metastatic disease such as the solitary hepatic secondary deposit.

Renal Cancer

The primary treatment of adenocarcinoma of the kidney, the commonest renal tumour, is surgery, by either partial or total nephrectomy (Hendrey 1980). Transitional cell cancer is usually treated by nephroureterectomy (del Regato et al. 1985, pp 637–659) and, in children, Wilms tumour by a combination of chemotherapy, radiotherapy and surgery (Clouse et al. 1985). The follow-up of patients who have had renal cancer is important, since unlike many other cancers recurrent tumour and metastases are highly unlikely to be asymptomatic and yet, if discovered, may be eminently suitable for further curative surgery (Choksi et al. 1972; Wilkins et al. 1961). Solitary pulmonary metastases are not uncommon and 5-year survival rates of 31% and 37% have been reported following surgical removal (Stener et al. 1984; Clayman et al. 1979). Similarly, solitary metastases affecting bone and muscle may also be removed surgically with 40% 5-year survival and long disease-free intervals (Stener et al. 1984). It is also known that patients with treated renal cancer stand a 20% chance of developing a metachronous cancer in the contralateral kidney, or even in the remnant of the ipsilateral kidney, if partial nephrectomy has been performed. These may be totally asymptomatic in the early stages.

For these reasons, we believe that patients should be followed up regularly 3 monthly in the first year, biannually for the next 2 years and then annually for at least 10 years. At each attendance, the urine should be examined for microscopic haematuria and cytologically for malignant cells. Chest X-ray should be performed at each visit and the development of any isolated lump or localised pain in the musculoskeletal system should be investigated urgently. Any suspicious lump may be submitted to fine needle aspiration for cytological examination, after initial intravenous urogram and ultrasound. In the case of a renal mass, non-invasive screening and arteriography are preferable in the first instance, because of the rare, but recognised, complication of needle track seeding of tumour cells after this procedure. However, some consider the risk to be so low as not to be a contraindication to needle aspiration (Clayman et al. 1979).

Multiple pulmonary, or hepatic, metastases, or other systemic deposits may be treated palliatively with radiotherapy or chemotherapy, although the results are somewhat disappointing in the main. Thus, treatment should be reserved for patients with debilitating symptoms caused by metastases. Rarely, metastatic renal tumours have been reported to respond to hormonal therapy and of course some disappear spontaneously.

Bladder Cancer

The survival of patients with bladder cancer is directly related to the pattern and grade as well as the stage of the tumour, with 81% of patients with a papillary differentiated tumour surviving 3 years, compared with only 22% of patients with a solid anaplastic tumour (Pugh 1981). Over 25% of all bladder tumours are of the epithelial type, predominantly arising from the transitional epithelium.

Superficial bladder tumours are mostly well controlled by endoscopic resection or fulguration and, indeed, the most appropriate follow-up for these patients is by check cystourethroscopy. A sensible regimen is for the patient to return 6 weeks after the initial resection and, if this is clear, at 3 months. Unless there is recurrence, check cystoscopy is appropriate at similar intervals for 1 year. Thereafter, in the absence of disease a 6 monthly check cystoscopy is required for 2 years and then annual inspection indefinitely. Most patients are elderly at presentation, but for those who remain clear to 10 years it is quite reasonable to follow up, thereafter, with urinary cytology. Non-invasive superficial papillary tumours rarely lead to death, but at least 60% of patients develop recurrence and 5%–10% will develop such widespread growth that cystectomy has to be considered. However, in these patients intravesical chemotherapy may prevent extensive surgery (England et al. 1981).

The treatment of flat carcinoma in situ is controversial, but, since it is a high-grade tumour, chemotherapy is sometimes used in the initial stages of the disease. This may be given systemically, as well as intravesically. If the tumour progresses, radical radiotherapy and salvage cystectomy may become necessary. Follow-up, as for superficial tumours, is primarily by endoscopy, but in tumour progression the use of scanning procedures, such as ultrasound and CT, may give valuable information.

Advanced T_4 tumours carry a very poor prognosis, with less than 10% of patients surviving for 5 years (Hope-Stone et al. 1981). Many of these patients are already old and debilitated and radiotherapy provides the best method of palliation. Some patients with unremitting disease may even require urinary diversion, but surgery should be avoided if at all possible, in view of the very poor prognosis. Chemotherapy has little or no part to play in the management of these tumours.

The treatment of the remaining invasive T_2 and T_3 tumours remains under scrutiny. Accepted lines of treatment for T_2 tumours include radical external beam radiotherapy, with selective salvage cystectomy for non-responders (Yo et al. 1985), interstitial radiotherapy (Williams et al. 1981), flash radiotherapy with subsequent cystectomy (Bloom 1981), or for small tumours endoscopic resection and observation (Pryor 1981). T_3 tumours may be treated with either radical radiotherapy and selective salvage cystectomy for recurrence, or non-responders, or radiotherapy followed by elective cystectomy (Yo et al. 1985). The latter technique has not been shown to be of any extra benefit in males over 65 years of age.

The net result of all these modalities means that the follow-up of bladder cancer patients is arguably one of the most demanding for the clinician and patient. Regular cystoscopic examination is necessary in most patients and the use of radiological aids, such as lymphography, ultrasound and CT scanning, is commonplace in invasive tumours. Some patients will require specialist stoma care and advice after urinary diversion surgery and those patients who develop distant metastases need the support of long-term nursing and sometimes terminal care facilities.

Prostatic Cancer

Like many other cancers, the prognosis of patients with prostatic cancer is dependent upon the degree of histological differentiation of the tumour and the staging of the tumour at presentation (Parker et al. 1985). Tumours causing symptoms of urinary obstruction may be treated by endoscopic resection with or without local radiotherapy, by radical prostatectomy, or by radical radiotherapy. In the United Kingdom, endoscopic resection is the preferred treatment to obtain local control of early disease and the advantage of radiotherapy in early prostatic cancer is still under debate. Radical prostatectomy is still performed regularly in the United States (Veenema et al. 1977), but there is no clear evidence that this form of treatment confers any benefit over and above transurethral resection in terms of survival. Advanced local tumours are treated by radiotherapy. Metastatic prostatic cancer usually affects the skeleton and, if localised pain is a problem, radiotherapy is the treatment of choice. Hormonal therapy, either by orchidectomy or stilboestrol, causes regression of metastatic disease and is appropriate when symptomatic metastases are present. Systemic treatment of asymptomatic metastases confers no advantage in long-term survival, or disease-free interval, and delayed treatment, witholding therapy until symptoms of metastases present is equally as effective (Smith 1981). Progression of metastatic cancer after hormonal manipulation by orchidectomy or stilboestrol administration may be successfully treated, with either cyproterone acetate or luteinising hormone releasing hormone (LHRH) analogues (Smith 1981). There is rarely a place for systemic chemotherapy in metastatic prostatic cancer.

Local recurrence may be managed endoscopically, or by local radiotherapy. If the local disease progresses, despite these modes of treatment, hormonal manipulation may exert control and may be advocated, even in the absence of metastatic disease. It is only in the exceptional patient, or in the grossly debilitated patient, that an indwelling urethral, or suprapubic, catheter becomes necessary.

Most patients, therefore, can be followed up on an expectant basis, awaiting the development of symptoms. Thus, after initial treatment, outpatient follow-up may be limited to patients who develop further symptoms of either local or metastatic disease and further investigations and treatment reserved for these patients.

Testicular Cancer

Testicular cancer occurs in young and middle-aged men. The incidence of teratoma is highest in the 3rd decade, whereas seminoma is commonest in the 4th decade. In elderly patients, lymphoma of the testes and rare tumours, such as blast cell tumours, may occur. The treatment of testicular tumour, as far as the surgeon is concerned, is to establish the diagnosis by orchidectomy after taking blood samples for the relevant tumour markers, human chorionic gonadotrophin and alpha-fetoprotein. Postoperatively, intensive investigation for metastases will be necessary in the form of lymphangiography, CT scanning and further tumour marker identification. Further therapy with radiotherapy, chemotherapy, or a combination of both, will depend on the stage of the disease. Thus, the follow-up of these patients after surgery is primarily in the hands of the medical oncologists and radiotherapists. Combined follow-up clinics are very useful in such situations, so that surgeon and radiotherapist can follow the patient together. With modern combination therapy, the long-term outlook for these younger patients with stage I teratoma or seminoma is extremely good, with an overall cure rate approaching 100% (Peckham 1981). Even in patients with metastatic disease, 80% may achieve remission using combined therapy and many are potentially curable (Johnson et al. 1980). Thus, intensive follow-up of all these patients is mandatory, employing regular clinical examination, tumour marker monitoring and scanning as and when appropriate.

Ovarian Cancer

This is the second commonest cancer of women in the United Kingdom and in the United States it has become the 5th most common cause of death from cancer in women. In spite of attempts at early diagnosis and the use of sophisticated treatment modalities, the death rate from ovarian cancer is unaltered in the past 50 years (Seidmann et al. 1976). The reason for this is that ovarian cancer is classically one of the occult malignancies, often in an advanced stage at initial presentation. Some patients present with what initially appears to be localised grade I disease but, in truth, over 50% of these patients will actually turn out to be stage III after laparotomy, lymphangiography and CT scanning.

Surgery is still the mainstay of treatment for ovarian cancer, resecting all visible tumour, removing both ovaries, the greater omentum, uterus and any residual pelvic or peritoneal deposits. After full and proper surgical assessment and resection, all patients should then be staged by the laparotomy findings and the results of lymphography. CT scanning and chest X-ray. For stage I disease, radiotherapy has not been shown to have any greater benefit than surgery alone and these patients may be followed-up by regular clinical examination and also by laparoscopy. For stages II and III, combination radiotherapy and chemotherapy has been shown to improve survival and to procure better palliation of advanced disease. *Cis*-platinum is currently the most efficacious proven drug, but newer drugs such as JM8 are exhibiting great promise, being equally as effective in obtaining remission, but less likely to cause systemic side effects. However, there are no definitive data available yet in comparative trials for the latter.

For advanced disease which is found at laparotomy, or by examination and radiological staging, to be initially inoperable, chemotherapy and radiotherapy may be used preceding a further exploratory laparotomy if regression is apparent. If some response has resulted from the initial treatment, regression of tumour mass may then allow further response to subsequent courses of chemotherapy. Tumour response may be followed and documented by CT scanning and further laparoscopy.

Since most patients present with advanced disease, the postoperative task involves regular consultations, scans and laparoscopies and often-repeated courses of radiotherapy, chemotherapy and occasionally further surgery. It is undoubtedly one of the more challenging fields of cancer follow-up.

Cervical Cancer

The treatment of cervival cancer ranges from biopsy and local interstitial radiotherapy for the early disease to radical surgery, combined with interstitial and radical external beam radiotherapy, for advanced disease. Chemotherapy is generally reserved for palliation of symptomatic inoperable advanced disease. Follow-up of these patients has become easier with the advances of CT scanning and lymphangiography, but, despite the newer treatment modalities, the invasive poorly differentiated advanced cervical cancer still carries a high mortality, with no patients surviving to 5 years (Prempress et al. 1985). In a recent review of adenocarcinoma of the cervix, it was shown that stage I disease can be treated either by surgery or radiotherapy with equally good results, achieving approximately 80% 5-year survival. Stage II disease is best treated by combination of surgery and radiotherapy, with 5-year survival rates of 86%. Stage III and IV disease carry a poor prognosis, with 5-year survival of 33% and 0% respectively, despite combined modality treatment. This survey shows that adenocarcinoma, which constitutes only 5% of cervical cancers, behaves similarly to squamous cell carcinoma, which constitutes the other 95% (Prempress et al. 1985).

The prognosis in squamous carcinoma of the cervix depends upon stage of disease at presentation, tumour bulk and the presence of lymphnode metastases regardless of stage (Ingersoll and Ulfelder 1966). Therapy must be modified according to the presence of these criteria. Few series report cure rates in excess of 40% for patients with lymph node metastases, irrespective of the stage of the disease, and patients with bulky tumour carry a worse prognosis than those with small-volume primary tumour (Durrance et al. 1969). Thus, a patient with bulky stage 1 B disease (cervix greater than 6 cm diameter) may require radiotherapy followed by surgery, despite the early staging of the disease. The radiotherapy fields are based on the extent of the tumour by clinical staging, laparotomy, if this has been performed, lymphangiography, chest X-ray and CT scanning. Central, regional or distant recurrence occurs after surgery or radiotherapy in up to 75% of patients (Nelson et al. 1974), for which reason close follow-up of these patients is mandatory. Central or regional recurrence after radiotherapy may warrant radical surgery to ablate the severe problems of local pelvic disease, whereas the progression to distant metastasis, as well as insinuating a poor prognosis, will necessitate further radiotherapy and possible systemic treatment (del Regato 1954; Smith et al. 1967).

Uterine Cancer

The majority (74%) of uterine cancers are stage I and, of these patients, 90% will survive 10 years (Jones 1975). Stage II, III and IV constitute 9%, 10% and 7% respectively in a multistudy survey (MacKillop and Pringle 1985) and the 5-year survival decreases accordingly with staging, histological differentiation and distribution of locoregional and lymphatic spread. The treatment, which is primarily surgical for patients with adnexal disease, will produce long-term survival only if all tumour can be completely resected. Radiotherapy, however, is the mainstay of treatment for localised disease and for inoperable disease, using intracavitary and external beam modalities.

Follow-up of these patients is essentially similar to that previously described for cervical cancer. Postradiation complications, such as radiation proctitis and cystitis, are occasionally problematical and are notably resistant to standard anti-inflammatory drugs. In severe proctitis and in progressive disease with a frozen pelvis, the raising of an end colostomy to obviate bowel obstruction may become necessary and transurethral ureteric stents may be considered if renal dysfunction precedes the natural invevitable terminal pattern of the disease (Jones et al. 1983). Of course, if the patient is already terminal the development of uraemia may be considered to be a blessing in disguise, allowing the patient to die with little or no distress in renal failure.

Breast Cancer

The follow-up of breast cancer patients constitutes one of the most controversial and difficult subjects to analyse. At one end of the spectrum, there are specialists who believe that the patients should be followed up indefinitely, on the basis that late metastatic disease is occasionally reported some 20 years after treatment of a primary breast cancer (Cutler et al. 1969). At the other extreme, there have been recent reports which have shown the routine regular follow-up of breast cancer patients to be of very little value in terms of diagnosis of recurrent disease and certainly of no established value in survival figures (Brøyn and Frøyen 1982). One survey, assessing the effectiveness of routine outpatient follow-up in detecting recurrent disease after "curative" surgery for breast cancer, showed that recurrence diagnosed solely by the clinician in the absence of symptoms accounted for only 4 out of 1098 visits (Ormiston et al. 1985). This finding is corroborated by previous studies (L. P. Le Quesne and R. J. Faber 1977, personal communication). In a much larger survey of 546 patients who made a total of 6863 clinic visits, Dewar and Kerr (1985) found that a potentially curable relapse (local or in the contralateral breast) was detected at 66 (1%) of 6764 routine visits, but only 26 (39%) of these patients remained free of disease. Since one of the main reasons for follow-up is to detect relapse at a stage at which it can be treated successfully, it would appear that routine appointments are singularly unhelpful in this respect. It is clear from the reviews by Dewar and Kerr that more relapses are detected by the patients themselves than by the doctors, but, on the other hand, patients whose local relapse was detected at a routine visit had a significantly better survival than those whose local relapse was detected at an interval visit. This may represent the difference in the aetiology of the tumour type, however, with the more anaplastic type of tumour likely to cause symptoms earlier, provoking the patient to bring forward a routine appointment, rather than the suggested benefit of early treatment for those diagnosed whilst still asymptomatic. In any event, it appears that the intensity of follow-up of all patients who have had breast cancer treatment could be drastically reduced without incurring any adverse effect on prognosis and without harming the welfare of the patients. It may be possible to exercise some judicial common sense by assessment of the stage, tumour differentiation and age of the patient towards planning sensible follow-up.

We believe that after initial curative surgery and radiotherapy or chemotherapy, if this is necessary, one or possibly two outpatient visits at 3 monthly intervals are necessary to allow the patient the security of reassurance and to answer some or all of the questions which may have arisen as a result of treatment and patient awareness of the disease. Thereafter, if at 6 months there is no evidence of recurrence on clinical examination, a policy of open referral, on the basis of symptom development, or palpable or visible deformity, may be the best option.

There are many patients for whom repeat attendance at an outpatient clinic constitutes a considerable source of stress. Regular attendance may also be expensive in terms of travel, time off work and health resources. Of course, in our own centre as in many others, regular attendance is considered necessary purely for audit of outgoing research projects and for teaching purposes, but the truth remains that the vast majority of well patients seen in our clinics after the initial 6-month postoperative period could be seen on an "as necessary" basis.

In addition to clinical examination being required less often than is sometimes believed, the regular use of chest X-ray and bone scans as a means of monitoring patients is also unnecessary and should be reserved for symptomatic patients. In a review of 241 patients who had undergone modified radical mastectomy for early breast cancer with axillary node involvement, Chaudery and his colleagues found that of 1091 serial chest radiographs only 8 produced evidence of asymptomatic pulmonary metastases (Chaudery et al. 1983). Of 832 serial bone scans, 13 patients with asymptomatic bony metastases were discovered. They concluded that, although the use of the two factions is undisputed in the management of symptomatic disease, they cannot be recommended routinely in the follow-up of asymptomatic patients.

Well patients do not pose a problem. The question is how to follow up the patients with problems. These may range from apparently trivial points, such as slight swelling of an arm after axillary surgery, to serious disease with overt metastatic deposits. However, all problems must be treated with the same degree of patience and thoroughness, since even a minor symptom may evoke in the patient's mind the possibility of recurrent disease.

Most young and middle-aged patients with early breast cancer will have undergone some form of surgery, possibly radiotherapy, or chemotherapy, or both, and some may be on hormonal therapy. Older postmenopausal patients may also have undergone surgery, but some may have been treated with hormonal therapy only. Patients with advanced cancer may well have been treated with chemotherapy and/or radiotherapy, without the need for surgery apart from initial biopsy. What are the problems to be anticipated in the follow-up clinic?

The first question is that of the complications of treatment. Lymphoedema of the arm still occurs in some patients after axillary dissection and is known to be most common after radical mastectomy and radiotherapy (Stillwell 1977). With the results of Fisher's analysis now available, it would seem that this combined radical treatment to the axilla should now become obsolete, thus reducing the incidence of this side effect (Fisher et al. 1985). When it does occur, it is important to commence treatment early with graduated support sleeves, or by the use of the Flowtron cuff, and to advise the patient to take great notice of any distal injury or infection in the hand, since this may jeopardise the lymphatic drainage further.

Postradiation telangiectasia is also becoming less of a problem with the development of modern external beam irradiation techniques, but if it does occur full reassurance is required to allay any fears that it might represent recurrent disease.

Postradiation fibrosis is another complication which sometimes causes unfounded anxiety. In the majority of patients in whom this occurs, the presentation is that of a firm fibrous mass in the region of the supraclavicular, or infraclavicular, fossa. It is sometimes extremely difficult, on clinical grounds, to distinguish this from recurrent tumour, but with the use of CT scanning and needle aspiration cytology the diagnosis is apparent. Brachial plexus neuropathy may result from such fibrosis and may be refractory to any form of conservative therapy. Surgery to relieve the compression is occasionally required, but this is extremely difficult and hazardous, since it involves operating in irradiated fields, with all the problems of bleeding and poor tissue healing being evident. If the neuropathy is minimal, it is wiser to avoid surgery and advise the patient to accept the disability.

Many patients who have had extensive surgery, by either simple extended or radical mastectomy, may request advice on breast reconstruction and this should be given due consideration. In the absence of metastatic disease, it is quite justifiable to advise further reconstructive surgery to abolish the deformity caused by the initial surgery. At the Royal Marsden Hospital most breast lumps are now removed by wide local excision and thus the incidence of reconstruction is not so great as in hospitals where mastectomy is still the prime surgical treatment. Nevertheless, in situations where mastectomy has been necessary, either after secondary referral, or at our own instigation, the advice and help of the plastic surgeon is always available for these patients regarding reconstruction. Some patients who have had mastectomy may not desire further surgery and prefer to wear a prosthesis.

This requires the assistance of a fitter to measure and supply the article. At the Royal Marsden Hospital it has become apparent that the services of a female nurse specialist who is interested in this work is preferable to a male fitter, on surveying a large series of women in this situation (Simpson 1985). Women patients feel more comfortable when relating their problems to a fitter of their own sex and do not feel so apprehensive about describing problems which may have occurred with their prosthesis.

The major problems occur when local recurrence, or metastatic disease, are suspected. In these situations, full re-assessment of the patient is necessary by clinical examination, haematological and biochemical screening tests and intensive radiological review. This usually means liver ultrasound, bone scanning and possibly CT scanning, for which reason it is our policy to readmit the patient for a few days in order to expedite the review. With the results of all the tests available, it is then possible to advise on further therapy either for recurrent local disease or metastatic disease. For recurrent local disease in the absence of metastases, further surgery or radiotherapy may be appropriate and this can be commenced immediately the decision is made. If multiple metastases are discovered, hormonal manipulation, or chemotherapy, may be appropriate. Sometimes, a combination of all the modalities is necessary and we find it useful, in these situations, to follow the patient in a combined breast clinic with the cooperation of the medical oncologist and radiotherapist. In this manner the best palliative treatment can be planned.

We believe that the reassessment of progressive disease by sophisticated radiological and various scanning facilities to be imperative at each level of progression. We would have no hesitation in full reassessment of the patient for new symptoms, even if she had been submitted to this only 1 month or 6 weeks previously. Constant reassessment of therapeutic response is the most accurate way of planning continued palliation.

In the terminal stages of the disease, the help and advice of a specialist in continuing care is most valuable. Pain control is vital and can be established in nearly all patients by the administration of regular opiate analgesia, with extra dosage for breakthrough pain. It should be remembered that the correct dose of an analgesic is that which relieves the pain (Hanks 1985). There is no place in this situation for caution on the grounds of addiction, which is clearly irrelevant. Long-term nursing may be required and there are well-established nursing homes in many countries now which specialise in terminal care. These establishments fulfill a vital role in allowing patients to die free of pain, but maintaining their dignity at all times, a factor which is so important to the dying patient, but which is all too easily forgotten by those who claim to be administering care. In Great Britain, these institutions have developed this skill to a fine art and, although heavily overburdened with patients, an excellent service is provided to those requiring such professional care.

There are some patients who, during the course of their disease, enquire about the use of "fringe medicine" as an alternative treatment programme. We extend a policy always to encourage the patient to see such practitioners if they wish, but, if possible, to remain in contact with our own institution. It is important to reassure patients that should anything go wrong, or should further symptoms develop whilst they are undergoing such alternative medicines, that further consultation, advice and treatment is always available in the hospital service. In our experience, it is rare that these patients ever come to any harm through alternative medical practice, but at the same time we have not yet been privileged to see any benefit over and above that which may be obtained through accepted medical channels.

Skin Cancer

Skin cancers comprise basal cell and squamous cell carcinomas as well as malignant melanomas. Basal cell cancers characteristically grow very slowly and are usually situated on the face and forehead. Treatment by either surgery or radiotherapy is usually effective. Most of these tumours occur in an elderly population and after adequate therapy little follow-up is required. Recurrence, if it does occur, will inevitably be local and should be visibly or palpably obvious to the patient. It is a sensible plan to see the patient 1 month after treatment to ensure a successful outcome and then at 1 year, after which follow-up can be on an expectant basis.

Squamous cell carcinoma requires more intensive follow-up. Primary lesions may be treated by either surgery or radiotherapy, but unlike basal cell carcinoma recurrence may occur not only locally, but also in the regional lymph nodes and occasionally with systemic distant metastases. Also, if regional spread occurs, treatment is necessary to prevent local ulcerating disease. Mobile nodes may be treated by either regional lymphadenectomy or radiotherapy, and fixed nodes by radiotherapy only. The results of treatment are much the same for the two modalities in terms of long-term survival, but prevention of local recurrence is enhanced when the nodes can be removed whilst still mobile. Consequently, regular follow-up is mandatory at short intervals. We would recommend 6 weekly follow-up for the first 6 months and then 3 monthly to 1 year. Thereafter, 6 monthly for 2 years and then yearly to 5 years. After 5 years free of recurrence, there is probably no need for regular surveillance.

Malignant melanoma of the skin is increasing in incidence (Morris 1985). However, the survival rate of treated melanoma is also improving. The overall 5-year survival rate for all patients with malignant melanoma exceeds 60% (Rosin 1985). The prognosis is dependent upon several factors, the most important of which is the depth of tumour invasion (Taylor and Hughes 1985). Other parameters influencing prognosis include age, sex, coexisting disease, diameter of the lesion and cellular agressiveness (Polk and Linn 1971).

Patients presenting with a lesion less than 0.75 mm in depth may anticipate more than 95% 5-year survival, whilst, of those patients with a tumour depth in excess of 3.00 mm, less than 40% will survive 5 years (Morris 1985). The surgical excision margin necessary to obtain optimum local control has been shown to be related to tumour depth, with flat lesions (0.75 mm) requiring only 1 cm clearance. Deeper lesions still require wider excision (3–5 cms), although it is doubtful if this confers any real survival benefit. The controversial subject of malignant melanoma is the place of adjuvant therapy after surgery. There are those who advocate prophylactic regional lymph node dissection, claiming increased survival (Fortner et al. 1977). However, in a randomised trial by Veronesi et al. (1982) no significant improvement in 5-year survival was demonstrable by the use of this technique. Those who favour observation of the regional nodes, reserving surgery for those patients in whom the nodes become clinically involved, argue that the natural immune response of the patient may be compromised by the early, often unnecessary, removal of the nodes (Rosin 1985). In a series of 190 patients of whom 143 had lymph node dissection, Cox (1974) was unable to show any difference between the two groups with respect to recurrences, or time to recurrence.

The timely removal of involved lymph nodes is undoubtedly the correct approach to regional recurrence. In the United Kingdom, most surgeons adopt a watch and wait policy, removing regional nodes only where involvement is clinically apparent. However, in some instances, regional node dissection should be performed at the time of removal of the primary lesion: viz: (1) if upper limb perfusion is contemplated, since the histological assessment of the nodes after perfusion may be difficult, (2) for digital or nodular melanoma, if isolated limb perfusion is not to be performed, (3) adjacent to the regional nodes, such that one incision will allow the combined operation and (4) if follow-up is not anticipated.

Isolated limb perfusion using melphelan has been shown to be effective in improving survival rates and increasing disease-free interval in patients with poor-risk extremity melanoma (Sugarbaker and McBride 1976; Krementz et al. 1979). It should be considered in all poor-risk patients, as defined by tumour thickness (greater than 1.5 mm lesion), and lesions on the palm, sole of foot, or digit. The technique is also useful in the treatment of recurrent melanoma on an extremity (Creech et al. 1958). Limb perfusion can be used in the treatment of satellite disease, "in transit" melanoma and even nodal disease (Rosin and Westbury 1980).

Treatment of widespread metastatic disease is disappointing. Chemotherapy is not very effective, with less than 20% of patients exhibiting a response, and in those who do respond the duration is unlikely to exceed 6 months (Morris 1985). The two most useful agents are dacarbazine 200 mg/m^2 i.v. and vindesine 3 mg/m^2 i.v. weekly for 6 weeks. If tumour response occurs, the treatment can be repeated at regular intervals (Priestman 1985).

Amputation has virtually no part to play in the treatment of melanoma, except for a digital primary. Severe localised recurrence may be treated by wide excision, with removal of large areas of soft tissue and skin grafting purely to achieve symptomatic relief.

Bacille Calmette-Guérin vaccine, or vaccinia virus, injected directly into secondary tumours, are sometimes useful in palliative treatment, and cryotherapy has been reported as useful in advanced fungating lesions (Rosin 1985).

Radiotherapy is only of use in cerebral metastases using whole brain field administration, or in advanced disease for which other treatments are inappropriate. High-dose radiation is required to achieve any response. Recently, fast neutron therapy has been reported to produce a good response in patients with fixed node metastases and is certainly worthy of further assessment (Blake and Catterrall 1985).

Early melanoma is highly likely to be cured by excisional surgery and follow-up is rarely necessary after the first 2 years. During that time, however, the visits should be frequent, initially, at 6 weekly intervals, progressing to 3 monthly and 6 monthly during the 2nd year. Thereafter, the patient may be advised to return only if further symptoms or disturbing lesions arise. Patients with poor-risk melanomas should be referred after initial surgery and assessment to a team specialising in the treatment of melanoma (Rosin 1985).

Lung Cancer

Bronchial carcinoma is the commonest cause of death due to malignancy in males in Great Britain, the United States and many other countries (del Regato et al. 1985, pp 337–424). The incidence of the disease has risen since the Second World War, as has the ratio of female to male deaths from this cause (Smiddy and Cowen 1984).

Only 1% of all lung cancer occurs under the age of 40 years (Hood et al. 1965; Putnam 1977). The commonest bronchial tumours are of squamous cell origin, constituting almost 50% of all bronchial tumours. Twenty per cent are adenocarcinomas and 30% undifferentiated carcinomas, which include small cell (oat cell), large cell undifferentiated and some anaplastic tumours which are completely unidentifiable (del Regato et al. 1985, pp 337–424).

The treatment of lung cancer is usually palliative, since the vast majority of cases are inoperable at presentation, due to either local spread or widespread malignancy (Hoffmann and Ransdell 1980). A diagnosis of small (oat) cell carcinoma is also widely accepted as being unsuitable for surgery (del Regato et al. 1985, pp 337–424). Thus, surgery is generally reserved for the treatment of squamous cell or large cell carcinoma or adenocarcinoma of the lung. Despite this, only 25% of all bronchial tumours are operable at presentation and only 20% are resectable (Hoffmann and Ransdell 1980). Surgery usually involves lobectomy, or pneumonectomy, depending upon the situation, size and histology of the tumour.

Radiotherapy forms one of the mainstays of treatment, either for palliation in irresectable squamous cell tumours and adenocarcinomas, or as a definitive treatment instead of, or in conjunction with, surgery. Radiotherapy is reported as curative in certain situations and has been shown to produce greater survival in patients with proven hilar or mediastinal lymph node involvement when given postoperatively (Eisert et al. 1976; Green et al. 1975), compared with those who do not receive this treatment.

The treatment of small cell carcinoma is predominantly that of combination chemotherapy and radiotherapy, with an increase in median survival up to fourfold over the past decade. Some patients survive to 2 years or more, free of tumour after such treatment (Livingston 1980; Oldham and Greco 1980; Hansen and Roth 1983). Mathews reported a 30% 5-year survival and a 15% 10-year survival in 96 patients with small cell carcinoma after treatment (Mathews and Muggia 1980).

The overall prognosis of lung cancer is poor. Over 50% of all patients with lung cancer have metastatic disease, outside regional nodes at presentation, and metastases will develop in a further 40% following surgery (Hansen 1977). In a review of 3808 patients, Overholt et al. (1975) found a 34% 5-year survival for patients who had had a lobectomy and 19% for those who had had pneumonectomy. Of 686 patients considered cured by surgery, 48% survived 5 years, whereas 12% of the 1162 thought to have had palliative surgery survived the same length of time. Consequently, the follow-up of these patients is directed mainly towards the recognition of progressive disease and the appropriate institution of adequate palliation. Widely disseminated disease may be painful and debilitating and adequate pain control is a necessity in such patients. Local compression symptoms caused by mediastinal growth also constitutes a difficult problem. Patients with superior vena caval obstruction, due to bronchial carcinoma, constitute a medical emergency and must be admitted to hospital as a matter of urgency for treatment by either chemotherapy or radiotherapy, or both, depending on the histology of the tumour.

Stridor, due to occlusion of the main bronchi or trachea by tumour, also necessitates urgent treatment. Radiotherapy has been shown to be useful in this situation (Hansen 1977) and more recently bronchoscopic laser therapy has been reported as a method of disobliterating the lumen of the airway of tumour (Fazio et al. 1979).

Pleural effusion may complicate unremitting bronchial carcinoma, causing symptoms of pain, dyspnoea and a persistent cough. Several agents are known to be effective in the treatment of this condition, which is generally by pleural aspiration and instillation of a drug which will cause intense pleurisy. This results in dense adhesion formation between visceral and parietal pleura, thus preventing the reaccumulation of a malignant pleural effusion. Tetracycline has been shown to be as effective as any other agent (Bayly et al. 1978) and in view of its minimal side effects and low cost we would advocate its use in this situation.

Soft Tissue Sarcoma

These tumours of mesodermal origin are exceedingly rare, arising from smooth and striated muscle, connective tissue, fat, cartilage and blood vessels. Overexposure to radiation may predispose to the development of soft tissue sarcoma (Gane et al. 1970; Pettit et al. 1959; Davidson et al. 1986). They have a high prevalence in childhood and, despite being of low incidence, occur at a lower median age than the more common cancers (Benjamin et al. 1977).

The mainstay of treatment of soft tissue sarcomas is surgery. Wide local excision is always necessary and in some cases compartmentectomy is appropriate. Regional lymph node dissection is sometimes indicated, but only if histological proof of involvement is confirmed. The reason for such radical surgery is that the local recurrence rate for these tumours is very high. In a review of 251 patients with soft tissue sarcoma, Abbas et al. (1981) reported a 65% local recurrence rate in patients who had had simple excision and 36% local recurrence in those who had had wide local excision. Follow-up of these patients is thus directed mainly towards the early detection of local recurrence, since the options of treatment for distant metastatic disease are not only limited, but likely to be of little benefit. Local recurrence, however, may still be curable by further radical surgery alone, or in combination with radiotherapy and chemotherapy.

During follow-up, which should be at frequent intervals of not more than 6 weeks in the first 6 months and 3 months until 2 years, any suspicion of a local recurrence should be investigated immediately. CT scanning provides the best method of outlining the extent of the recurrent tumour in almost all situations in the body (Levine et al. 1979), although ultrasonography has been shown to be highly accurate in determining the size of soft tissue sarcomas of the extremities (Bernadino et al. 1981). Biopsy of a recurrent lesion is essential before proceeding to definitive surgery. Aspiration and incisional or excisional biopsy are all satisfactory, as long as definitive and adequate surgery is performed subsequently.

Radiotherapy and chemotherapy, long thought to be of no value in soft tissue sarcoma, both have a part to play as adjuvant therapy after surgery, or as palliative treatment in inoperable lesions. Indeed, in recurrent tumour, it is important to give chemotherapy and radiotherapy sequentially prior to further surgery, since the tumour response can be gauged both clinically and by CT scanning. Not all soft tissue sarcomas will respond, but if tumour regression is noted then the treatment may be beneficial. Radiotherapy and chemotherapy should not be offered as an alternative to surgery, unless the presenting lesion is clearly inoperable. There are certain situations in which chemotherapy has unquestionable success, notably in children with embryonal rhabdomyosarcomas (Rosenberg et al. 1981). Radiotherapy has also been shown to be of benefit in this condition, as well as in liposarcoma (Kinne et al. 1973), fibrosarcoma (Snit 1982) and epithelioid sarcomas (Martini et al. 1974). Finally, although distant metastatic disease usually heralds the inevitable decline of the sarcoma patient, solitary and even multiple pulmonary metastases have been resected with long-term benefit (Martini et al. 1974).

Acknowledgements. The authors are extremely grateful to Ms. Alida Beccaria and Miss Jane Healing for typing the manuscript.

References

Abbas JS, Holyoke ED, Moore R, Karakousis CP (1981) The surgical treatment and outcome of soft tissue sarcoma. Arch Surg 116: 765–769

Armstrong CP, Dent DM (1985) Gastric carcinoma. J R Coll Surg Edinb 30 (1): 15–20

Barclay THC, Schapira DV (1983) Malignant tumors of the small intestine. Cancer 51: 878–881

Bayly TC, Kisner DL, Sybert A, MacDonald JS, Tson E, Schein PS (1978) Tetracycline and quinacrine in the control of malignant pleural effusions: a randomised trial. Cancer 41: 1188–1192

Bengmark S, Blumgart LM, Launois B (1984) Liver resection in high bile duct tumours. In: Bengmark S (ed) Liver surgery. Churchill Livingstone, Edinburgh (Clinical surgery international)

Benjamin RS, Baker LH, O'Bryan RM, Moon TE, Gottlieb JA (1977) Advances in the chemotherapy of soft tissue sarcomas. In: Med Clin North Am 61 (5): 1039–1043

Bergdahl L (1980) Gallbladder carcinoma first diagnosed at microscopic examination of gallbladders removed for presumed benign disease. Annals Surg 191: 19–22

Berman C (1951) Primary carcinoma of the liver: a study. Lewis, London

Bernadino ME, Jing BS, Thomas JL, Lindell MM Jr, Zornoza J (1981) The extremity soft tissue lesion: a comparative study of ultrasound, computed tomography and xeroradiography. Radiology 139: 53–59

Blake PR, Catterall M (1985) The treatment of malignant melanoma by fast neutrons. Br J Surg 72: 517–519

Bloom HJG (1981) Pre-operative intermediate-dose radiotherapy and cystectomy for deeply invasive carcinoma of the bladder: rationale and results. In: Oliver RTD, Hendry WF, Bloom HSG (eds) Bladder cancer. Butterworth, London, pp 151–174

Blumgart LH, Imrie CW (1979) Tumours of the extrahepatic biliary tree and pancreas. In: Wright R, Alberti K, Karran S, Hillward-Sadler G (eds) Liver and biliary disease. Saunders, Philadelphia, pp 1495–1522

Bornmann PC, Harries-Jones EP, Tobias R, van Stiegmann G, Terblanche J (1986) Prospective controlled trial of transhepatic biliary endoprosthesis versus bypass surgery for incurable carcinoma of head of pancreas. Lancet 1: 69–71

Brookes VS, Waterhouse JAH, Powell DJ (1965) Carcinoma of the stomach: a 10 year survey of results and of factors affecting prognosis. Br Med J 1: 1577–1583

Brøyn T, Frøyen J (1982) Evaluation of routine follow-up after surgery for breast carcinoma. Acta Chir Scand 148: 401–404

Chaudery MA, Maisey MN, Shaw PJ, Rubens RD, Hayward JL (1983) Sequential bone scans and chest radiographs in the postoperative management of early breast cancer. Br J Surg 70: 517–518

Choski LB, Takita H, Vincent RG (1972) The surgical management of solitary pulmonary metastases. Surg Gynecol Obstet 134: 479–482

Clark PB, Morris DL (1981) Management of patients after mastectomy. Br Med J 282: 2095–2096

Clayman RV, Williams RD, Fraley EE (1979) Current concepts in cancer: the pursuit of the renal mass. N Engl J Med 300: 72–74

Clouse JW, Thomas PRM, Griffith RC, Perez CA, Vietti TJ, Fineberg B (1985) The changing management of Wilms' tumour over a 30 year period. Cancer 56: 1484–1489

Cochrane JPS, Williams JT, Faber RG, Slack WW (1980) Value of outpatient follow-up after curative surgery for carcinoma of the large bowel. Br Med J 280: 593–595

Comis RL, Carter SK (1974) A review of chemotherapy in gastric cancer. Cancer 34: 1576–1586

Conley J (1981) Management of facial paralysis associated with tumors of the parotid gland. In: Suen TY, Myers EN (eds) Cancer of the head and neck. Churchill Livingstone, New York, pp 524–556

Cooper MJ, Williamson RCN (1983) Surviving malignant disease. Surgical aspects. Br J Hosp Med 30: (1) 14–20

Costello CB, Taylor TV, Torrance MB (1977) Personal experience in the surgical management of carcinoma of the stomach. Br J Surg 64: 47–51

Cotton PB (1982) Duodenoscopic placement of biliary prostheses to relieve malignant obstructive jaundice. Br J Surg 69: 501–503

Cowie RA, Hitchcock ER (1982) The late results of antero-lateral cordotomy for pain relief. Acta Neurochir 64: 39–50

Cox K (1974) Regional cutaneous metastases in melanoma of the limb. Surg Gynecol Obstet 139: 385

Creech O Jr, Krementz ET, Ryan RF, Wimbled JN (1958) Chemotherapy of cancer: regional perfusion utilising an extracorporeal circuit. Ann Surg 148: 616–632

Cummings BJ (1985) Radiation therapy and rectal carcinoma: the Princess Margaret Hospital experience. Br J Surg 72 [Suppl]: 64–66

Cutler SJ, Axtell LM, Schottenfeld D (1969) Adjustment of long-term survival rates for deaths due to intercurrent disease. J Chronic Dis 22: 485–491

Davidson T, Westbury G, Harmer CL (1986) Radiation induced soft tissue sarcoma. Br J Surg 73: 308–309

del Regato JA (1954) Integral roentgen Therapy. Am J Roentgenol Radium Ther Nucl Med 71: 676–680

del Regato JA, Spjut HJ, Cox JD (1985) Ackerman and del Regato's cancer: diagnosis, treatment and prognosis, 6th edn. Mosby, St. Louis

Dewar JA, Kerr GR (1985) Value of routine follow up of women treated for early carcinoma of the breast. Br Med J 291: 1464–1467

Diamantes T, Mannell A (1983) Oesophageal intubation for advanced oesophageal cancer. The Baragwanath experience, 1977–1981. Br J Surg 70: 555–557

Dukes CE (1940) Cancer of the rectum: an analysis of 1000 cases. J Pathol Bacteriol 50: 527–537

Durrance FY, Fletcher GH, Rutledge FN (1969) Analysis of central recurrent disease in stages I and II squamous cell carcinomas of the cervix on intact uterus. Am J Roentgenol Radium Ther Nucl Med 106: 831–838

Earlam R, Cunha-Melo JR (1980) Oesophageal squamous cell carcinoma. I. A critical review of surgery. Br J Surg 67: 457–461

Eisert DR, Cox JD, Komaki R (1976) Irradiation for bronchial carcinoma: reasons for failure. Cancer 37: 2665–2670

Ekman C-A, Gustavson J, Henning A (1977) Value of a follow-up study of recurrent carcinoma of the colon and rectum. Surg Gynecol Obstet 145: 895–897

England HR, Paris AMI, Blandy J (1981) Intravesical thiotepa as adjuvant to cystodiathermy in multiple recurrent superficial bladder tumours. In: Oliver RTD, Hendry WF, Bloom HJG (eds) Bladder cancer. Butterworth, London, pp 67–74

Falk H (1982) Liver. In: Schottenfeld D, Fraumeni JF Jr (eds) Cancer epidemiology and prevention. Saunders, Philadelphia

Fazio F, Pratt TA, McKenzie CG, Steiner RE (1979) Improvement in regional ventilation and perfusion after radiother-

apy for unresectable carcinoma of the bronchus. AJR 133: 191–200
Fisher B, Bauer M, Margolese R et al. (1985) Five-year results of a randomised clinical trial comparing total mastectomy and segmental mastectomy with or without radiation in the treatment of breast cancer. Eng J Med 312: 665–673
Fortner JC, Woodruff J, Schottenfeld D, MacLean B (1977) Biostatistical basis of elective node dissection for malignant melanoma. Ann Surg 186: 101–103
Gane NFC, Lindup R, Strickland P, Bennett MH (1970) Radiation induced fibrosarcoma. Br J Cancer 24: 705–711
Green N, Kurohara SS, George FW III, Crews QE Jr (1975) Post resection irradiation for primary lung cancer. Radiology 116: 405–407
Hanks GW (1985) Drug treatment for relief of pain due to bone metastases. J R Soc Med 78 [Suppl 9]: 26–30
Hansen HH (1977) Management of lung cancer. Med Clin North Am 61 (5): 979–990
Hansen HH, Roth M (1983) Small cell carcinoma of the lung. In: Flenley DC, Petty TL (eds) Recent advances in respiratory med. Churchill Livingstone, Edinburgh, pp 193–202
Harrison DFN (1980) Treatment of tumours of the jaw. In: Taylor S (ed) Recent advances in surgery, vol 10. Churchill Livingstone, London, p 293–309
Heald RJ, Lockhart-Mummery HE (1972) The lesion of the second cancer of the large bowel. Br J Surg 59: 16–19
Hendrey WP (1980) Kidney. In: Chisholm GD (ed) Urology. Heinemann, London, pp 173–191
Hoffmann TH, Ransdell HT (1980) Comparison of lobectomy and wedge resection for carcinoma of the lung. J Thorac Cardiovasc Surg 79: 211–217
Hood RM Jr, Campbell DC Jr, Dooley BN, Dooking JA (1965) Bronchogenic carcinoma in young people. Dis Chest 48: 469–470
Hope-Stone HF, Blandy JP, Oliver RTD, England H (1981) Radical radiotherapy and salvage cystectomy in the treatment of invasive carcinoma of the bladder. In: Oliver RTD, Hendry WF, Bloom HJG (eds) Bladder cancer. Butterworth, London, pp 127–138
Illingworth CFW (1935) Carcinoma of the gall-bladder. Br J Surg 23 (89): 4–18
Ingersoll FM, Ulfelder H (1966) Pelvic exenteration for carcinoma of the cervix. N Engl J Med 274: 648–651
Islami AH, Pack GT, Hubbard JC (1958) Regenerative hyperplasia of the cirrhotic liver following partial hepatectomy. Cancer II: 663–686
Johnson DE, Hussey DH, Samuels ML (1980) Testis. In: Chisholm GD (ed) Urology. Heinemann, London, pp 247–265
Jones HW III (1975) Treatment of adenocarcinoma of the endometrium. Obstet Gynecol Surv 30: 147–169
Jones PA, Pittam MR, Moxon RA, Edwards LA (1983) Double-edged pigtail polyethylene stents in management of benign and malignant ureteric obstruction. J R Soc Med 76: 458–462
Kemeny MM, Goldberg D, Beatty JD, Blayney D, Browning J, Doroshow J, Ganteaume K, Hill RL, Kokal WA, Riihimaki DU, Terz JJ (1986) Results of a prospective randomized trial of continuous regional chemotherapy and hepatic resection as treatment of hepatic metastases from colorectal primaries. Cancer 57: 492–498
Kinne DW, Chu FCH, Huvos AG, Yagoda A, Fortner JG (1973) Treatment of primary and recurrent retroperitoneal liposarcoma. Cancer 31: 53–64
Kiser RS, Gatchel RJ, Bhatia K, Khatami M, Huang X, Altshuler KZ (1983) Acupuncture relief of chronic pain syndrome correlates with increased plasma met-enkephalin concentrations. Lancet 2: 1394–1396
Krementz ET, Carter RD, Sutherland CM, Campbell M (1979) The use of regional chemotherapy in the management of malignant melanoma. World J Surg 3: 289–304
Leung JWL, Emery R, Cotton PB, Russell RCG, Wallon AG, Mason RR (1983) Management of malignant obstructive jaundice at the Middlesex Hospital. Br J Surg 70: 584–586
Levine E, Lee KR, Neff JR, Maklad NF, Robinson RG, Preston DF (1979) Comparison of computed tomography and other imaging modalities in the evaluation of musculoskeletal tumours. Radiology 131: 431–437
Livingston RB (1980) Small cell carcinoma of the lung. Blood 56: 575–584
MacKillop WJ, Pringle JF (1985) Stage III endometrial carcinoma – a review of 90 cases. Cancer 56: 2519–2523
Mallinson CN, Rake MO, Fox CA et al. (1977) Final results of a controlled trial of chemotherapy for inoperable pancreatic cancer. Ir J Med Sci 146 [Suppl 1]: 19
Marks RL (1985) Terminal pain. Surgery 1 (24): 565–568
Martin CW, Rosenfeld L, McSwain B (1973) Carotid body tumors: a 16-year follow-up of seven malignant cases. South Med J 66: 1236–1243
Martini N, Bains MS, Huvos AG, Battie EJ Jr (1974) Surgical treatment of metastatic sarcoma to the lung. Surg Clin North Am 54: 841–848
Mathews MJ, Muggia FM (1980) Long term survivors with small cell carcinoma of the lung. Eur J Cancer 16: 527–531
Mitchell DC, Clyne CAC (1985) Chemodectomas of the neck: the response to radiotherapy. Br J Surg 72: 903–905
Monge JJ, Judd ES, Gage RP (1964) Radical pancreatoduodenectomy. A 22 year experience with the complications, mortality rate and survival rate. Ann Surg 160: 711–722
Morris A McG (1985) Malignant melanoma. Surgery 1 (26): 604–607
Nakayama K, Kinoshita Y (1974) Surgical treatment combined with preoperative concentrated irradiation. JAMA 227: 178–181
Nelson JH Jr, Boyce J, Macasaet M, Lu T (1974) The incidence and significance of para-aortic lymph node metastases in late invasive carcinoma of the cervix. Am J Obstet Gynecol 118: 749–756
Nevin JE, Moran TJ, Kay S, King R (1976) Carcinoma of the gallbladder. Cancer 37: 141–148
Oldham RK, Greco FA (1980) Small cell cancer. A curable disease. Cancer Chemother Pharmacol 4: 173–177
Ormiston MC, Timoney AG, Qureshi AR (1985) Is follow up of patients after surgery for breast cancer worthwhile? J R Soc Med 78: 920–921
Oschner A, Weed TE, Noessle WR (1981) Cancer of the stomach. Am J Surg 141: 10–14
Overholt RM, Neptune WB, Ashraf MM (1975) Primary cancer of the lung: a 42 year experience. Ann Thorac Surg 20: 511–519
Parker MC, Cook A, Riddle PR, Fryatt I, O'Sullivan J, Shearer RJ (1985) Is delayed treatment justified in carcinoma of the prostate? Br J Urol 57: 724–728
Pearson JG (1969) The value of radiotherapy in the management of esophageal cancer. Am J Roentgenol Radium Ther Nucl Med 105: 500–513
Peckham MJ (1981) Seminoma testis. In: Peckham MJ (ed) The management of testicular tumours. Arnold, London, pp 134–151
Pettit VD, Chamness JT, Ackerman LV (1959) Fibromatosis and fibrosarcoma following irradiation therapy. Cancer 7: 149–158

Polk HC Jr, Linn BS (1971) Selective regional lymphadenectomy for melanoma: a mathematical aid to clinical judgement. Ann Surg 174: 402–413

Prempress T, Amornmarn R, Wizenberg MJ (1985) A therapeutic approach to primary adenocarcinoma of the cervix. Cancer 56: 1264–1268

Priestman T (1985) Cancer treatment – chemotherapy. Surgery 19: 446–450

Pryor JP (1981) Introduction to the management of superficial bladder tumours. In: Oliver RTD, Hendry WF, Bloom HJG (eds) Bladder cancer. Butterworth, London, pp 59–61

Pugh RCB (1981) Histological staging and grading of bladder tumours. In: Oliver RTD, Hendry WF, Bloom HJG (eds) Bladder cancer. Butterworth, London, pp 3–8

Putnam JS (1977) Lung carcinoma in young adults. JAMA 238: 35–36

Ring EJ, Oleanga JA, Freiman DB et al. (1975) Therapeutic applications of catheter cholangiography. Radiology 128: 333–338

Rosenberg JA, Tepper J, Glatstein E, Costa J, Young R, Seipp C, Wesley R (1981) Adjuvant chemotherapy for patients with soft tissue sarcomas. Surg Clin North Am 61: 1415–1423

Rosin RD (1985) The treatment of malignant melanoma. Eur J Surg Oncol 11: 111–115

Rosin RD, Westbury G (1980) Isolated limb perfusion for malignant melanoma. Practitioner 224: 188–198

Russell WD, Ibanez ML, Clark RL, White EC (1963) Thyroid carcinoma. Classification, intraglandular dissemination and clinicopathological study based on whole organ section of 80 glands. Cancer 16 (11): 1425–1460

Seidman H, Silverberg E, Holleb A (1976) Cancer statistics. Cancer 26: 2–29

Simpson G (1985) Are you being served? Senior Nurse 2 (6): 14–16

Smiddy F, Cowen P (1984) Tutorials in Surgery. Surgical pathology II. Pitman, London, pp 86–92

Smith JP, Rutledge F, Burns BC, Soffar S (1967) Systemic chemotherapy for carcinoma of the cervix. Am J Obstet Gynecol 97: 800–807

Smith of Marlow, Lord, Sherlock S (1981) Surgery of the gallbladder and bile ducts. Butterworth, London

Smith PH (1981) Endocrine and cytotoxic therapy. In: Duncan W (ed) Prostate cancer. Recent results in cancer research, vol 78. Springer, Berlin Heidelberg New York, pp 154–172

Smithers D (1970) Tumours of the thyroid gland. Livingstone, Edinburgh, pp 22–51

Snit HD (1982) Soft tissue sarcomas: the role of radiation therapy. Hosp Pract 17: 114–120

Stener B, Henriksson C, Johansson S, Guntergerg B, Pettersson S (1984) Surgical removal of bone and muscle metastases of renal cancer. Acta Orthop Scand 55: 491–500

Stillwell KG (1977) Management of arm oedema. In: Stoll BA (ed) Breast cancer management. Early and late. Heinemann, London, p 213

Sugarbaker EV, McBride CM (1976) Survival and regional disease control after isolation-perfusion for invasive stage I melanoma of the extremities. Cancer 37: 188–198

Taylor BA, Hughes LE (1985) A policy of selective excision for primary cutaneous malignant melanoma. Eur J Surg Oncol 11: 7–13

Tompkins RK, Thomas D, Wile A, Longmire WP Jr (1981) Prognostic factors in bile duct carcinoma. Ann Surg 194: 447–457

Veenema RJ, Gursel EO, Lattimer JK (1977) Radical retropubic prostatectomy for cancer: a 20-year experience. J Urol 117: 330–331

Veronesi U, Adamus J, Hubert C et al. (1982) A randomised trial of adjuvant chemotherapy and immunotherapy in cutaneous melanoma. N Engl J Med 307: 913–916

Wilkins EW, Burke JF, Head JM (1961) The surgical management of metastatic neoplasms in the lung. J Thorac Cardiovasc Surg 42 (3): 298–309

Williams G, Jones MA, Trott PA, Bloom HJG (1981) Carcinoma of the bladder treated by local interstitial irradiation. In: Oliver RTD, Hendry WF, Bloom HSG (eds) Bladder cancer. Butterworth, London, pp 117–126

Williamson RCN (1982) Intestinal adaptation: factors that influence morphology. Scand J Gastroenterol 17 [Suppl 74]: 21–29

Yo WS, Sagerman RH, Chung CT, Dalal PS, King GA (1985) Bladder carcinoma. Experience with radial and preoperative radiotherapy in 421 patients. Cancer 56: 1293–1299

Clinical Trials

M. STAQUET

The acquisition of new therapeutic knowledge is based on observations and experiments which are of a different nature (Table 1) and reliability. All the conclusions emanating from these sources are basically comparative, even if the control group is only implicit, as is, for instance, the case in anecdotal reports. In Table 1, items 1–6 are essentially observational studies, where the treatment has been routinely administered with no attempt to extrapolate the results. Clearly, this type of study is not suitable for comparative evaluation of treatment policies, although its use is often favored because there is no need to collect new data. These studies, as well as nonrandomized prospective studies, can be used as pilot indicators, but, even repeated, such observations cannot in general be taken at their face value.

Table 1. Sources of therapeutic knowledge

1. Anecdotal case(s)
2. Population registry
3. Hospital registry
4. Retrospective study
5. Postmarketing study (phase IV)
6. Data bases
7. Dose-finding study (phase I)
8. Prospective study with historical controls (phase II and III)
9. Prospective study with randomized controls (phase II and III)

The main, but not the sole, reason is the lack of formal comparability between the groups of patients receiving treatments to be compared. Time is a well-known biasing factor in this situation. The passing of time produces variations in treatment indication, new forms of supportive care, improved diagnostic methods, and a variety of subtle changes which make the comparison of present therapeutic results with previous observations unreliable. It follows that the predictive power of nonrandomized studies is usually poor, unless the course of the disease is truly predictable, no other therapies have been given until the end point is reached, and the treatment effect is outstanding. Nevertheless, extreme caution and further confirmation are needed. Although dramatic results need only a few cases to be convincing, more subtle advances require prospective randomized trials to be established.

The randomized prospective trial can be defined as a scientific experiment, using methods limited by ethical considerations, undertaken to demonstrate the validity of a hypothesis. In oncology, these trials are often multi-institutional, because of the need to accrue large numbers of patients at the same stage of disease. Cooperative groups have been created all over the developed world to handle these studies.

The application of new therapeutic regimens to patients requires ethical justification by means of experimental (animal studies), historical (literature), clinical (previous experience), logical (rationale), methodological (design), and humanitarian (quality of life) arguments.

Most of the clinical studies are of one of the following types.

- Phase I trial: to determine the maximum tolerated dose for a specified mode of administration and to define the dose-limiting toxicities.
- Phase II trial: to evaluate therapeutic effectiveness to explicit toxicities and to perform various pharmacological studies.
- Phase III trial: to compare with other standard treatments, or to no treatment, if none exists.

Protocol

The protocol is a document pertaining to all aspects of the study, containing a rationale, objectives, methods, and logistics of the study. Tables 2 and 3 show the minimum protocol contents for phase I and phase II–III (EORTC 1985; Staquet et al. 1980).

Table 2. Phase I master protocol

I.	Objectives and background
II.	Eligibility and exclusion of patients
III.	Treatment
IV.	Number of patients per dose level
V.	Study parameters and serial observations
VI.	Termination of the study
VII.	Tumor response
VIII.	Records
IX.	References
Appendix I.	Performance status
Appendix II.	Surface area as a function of weight and height
Appendix III.	WHO grading of toxicity
Appendix IV, V.	As needed

Table 3. Phase II–III – Protocol contents

I.	Background and introduction
II.	Objectives of the trial and outline of materials and methods
III.	Patient selection criteria (eligibility criteria)
IV.	Trial design
V.	Therapeutic regimens, dose modification and toxicity
VI.	Required clinical evaluations, laboratory tests and follow-up
VII.	Criteria of evaluation
VIII.	Registration and randomization of patients
IX.	Forms and procedures for collecting data
X.	Statistical considerations
XI.	Administrative responsibilities
XII.	References
XIII.	Appendices

Each of the paragraphs outlined in Tables 2 and 3 must be addressed in detail and precisely worded. Usually a group of scientists representing each of the different disciplines involved in the study is organized to design the study and write the protocol.

The first step in conceiving a new study is to obtain information and data, published or not, about the new therapies being considered. Only in this manner can the trial be placed in the proper perspective. A possible starting point for phase II and III is the book edited by Slevin and Staquet in 1986, which critically reviews the published randomized trials for each cancer site. At the same time, the most important prognostic factors for the disease must be identified and their potential impact on the end point of the study considered (Staquet 1975).

A useful source of information is the series of computerized data bases[1] (Cancerline) maintained by the US National Institutes of Health. Information about phase II and III currently being conducted throughout the world (Clinprot) is available via the MEDLARS System of the US National Library of Medicine. The world's cancer literature (Cancerlit and Cancerexpress) is also available, as well as Cancerproj related to research projects. Other more general reference sources include the Science Citation Index, Index Medicus, Current Contents (Life Sciences), and Medline, the computerized medical reference file of the US National Library of Medicine. The TNM system is published by the UICC (Geneva) and regularly updated, as well as the Manual for Staging of Cancer developed by the American Joint Committee (Chicago). WHO (Geneva) has also published a number of booklets for the pathological staging.

Phase I Trial

Phase I trials are designed to determine the maximum tolerated dose (MTD) of a drug for a specified mode of administration, to characterize the most frequent toxic effects, and to define the dose-limiting toxicities.

The MTD is the highest dose which can be safely administered to a patient, i. e., producing acceptable, manageable, and reversible toxicity of WHO grade II–III. MTD varies according to the prognostic factors for toxicity, not only with regard to prior therapy (chemotherapy and/or radiation) and perfor-

[1] The R. A. Bloch International Cancer Information Center, National Cancer Institute, Bethesda, Maryland 20205, USA.

mance status, but also type of disease, age of patient, availability of supportive care, and, occasionally, impaired function of excretory organs. MTD is needed to perform phase II trials at the highest safe dose (i.e., near MTD), in order to obtain a reliable estimation of the clinical effectiveness of a new agent. It is, therefore, advisable that dose recommendations emanating from phase I trials be based on patients with a drug tolerance similar to those expected to enter the phase II trials.

All patients entered into phase I trials must have a histologically confirmed diagnosis of cancer which is not amenable to established forms of treatment. For these subjects, for whom no specific antineoplastic therapy may be recommended, the phase I trial is potentially beneficial, since the new drugs selected for the study have been chosen because of their expected antitumor activity.

In principle, patients with unfavorable pretreatment characteristics may be entered at the initiation of phase I studies. Lack of toxicity for a given dose in these high-risk patients is an important outcome when considering the magnitude of the increment of the dose for the next step. Early on in phase I trials, factors producing drug-related toxicity will be progressively identified and become exclusion criteria for higher doses. Also, investigators will be inclined to administer higher doses to patients with less prior therapy, so that, at the end of the study, it might be difficult to identify the population at risk. The recommended dose for phase II trials, which is often one step below the MTD, needs to be qualified with regard to the type of patients to be investigated in the phase II study. It is advisable to treat at least five subjects with well-defined and similar prognostic factors for toxicity at the recommended dose before starting the phase II trial. Any hints of antitumor activity are important for further studies and must be described. Responses must be defined according to standard criteria.

Phase II Trial

The purpose of a phase II study is to determine whether a therapy is sufficiently effective to warrant another trial with a larger number of patients. It is usually considered as a clinical screening designed according to a delicate compromise between the need for sufficient data weighted against the use of another agent possibly more active or less toxic.

The statistical methodology for phase II trials is constantly being developed, but the conclusions derived from phase II studies depend to a very large extent on the selection of patients entered in the study.

To answer the critical question as to whether a drug must be rejected or accepted for further study, one needs to consider a minimun response rate above which the drug will be considered as potentially active. This threshold, which varies between 10% and 40% in at least 15–20 evaluable patients, depends on the type of disease, on the prognostic stratum considered, on the amount of prior therapy, and on the performance status. Trials in a group of patients with mixed characteristics will be almost impossible to analyze unless the sample size is large enough in each prognostic stratum. Whenever possible, the phase II study must be performed in patients without prior therapy. Such a design seems ethically possible in GI tract cancer, non-small-cell carcinoma of the lung, bladder, cervix, prostate, and head and neck malignancies, as well as in malignant melanoma and other rare cancers. Phase II studies would be ethically more difficult to perform in nonpretreated patients with breast cancer and small cell carcinoma of the lung, ovary, and testis.

Many phase II studies are nonrandomized trials in which the response rate observed is compared with the threshold decided, in principle, in advance. It is well known that conclusions of non-randomized studies can be extremely misleading. Selection of patients is a critical factor in this setting, more so in that the sample sizes are often small. The patients could be so debilitated, or extensively pretreated, that they are unable to receive an appropriate dose of the new agent, or their disease is too advanced to respond. Another bias is the selection of inappropriate criteria of response, such as "minor response" or "subjective improvement" or "mixed response", which usually leads to positive conclusions even in groups of patients unlikely to respond. Also, the elimination of so-called inevaluable patients in the final assessment of the trial very often induces an artificial increase in the response rate.

In order to avoid these problems, many investigators use a design involving a randomization either between a new drug and a standard therapy, or between two new drugs when no standard therapy exists or is usable. Such a system implies a large increase in sample size, and, therefore, the organization of multicenter trials.

Phase III Trial

Phase III trials are the last step in the planned evaluation of new treatment modalities.

These studies are comparative disease-oriented studies aiming either to corroborate previous positive findings (confirmatory trials) or to modify an established regimen (explanatory trials). The confirmatory trial is an essential part of the evaluation of a new treatment since the superiority of the observed results in phase II needs to be confirmed before the use of the treatment can be recommended. Its function is to reduce the delta error (the proportion of all trials reported as positive which are false positives), especially if the sample sizes of the earlier trials were small (Staquet 1975).

In an explanatory study, the goal may be to prove an equivalence in effectiveness between two treatment modalities, one being less toxic or more convenient than the other.

The evaluation of a new treatment modality in a phase III trial is performed by comparison with a group of similar patients treated with a control therapy. It requires large sample sizes. One of the major controversies in clinical trials today is related to the selection of a control group to use as the base against which the new treatment is to be evaluated. Allocation of treatments by a random process is generally considered as the method of choice for phase III trials. This procedure guarantees the validity of the statistical comparisons between outcomes and ensures, on average, an equal distribution of the known and unknown prognostic factors between the treatment arms. Unfortunately, random allocation does not ensure that for a given trial all the prognostic factors will be equally distributed and therefore that the groups of patients will differ only by treatment. As a matter of fact, the probability that several prognostic factors are all evenly distributed between two groups of patients is low for small size trials. Imbalances between known prognostic factors which occur by chance must be corrected a posteriori.

Choice of Error Rates

It is important to consider the eventual consequences that an incorrect conclusion will have on the future treatment of the disease under study. In phase II trials it is customary to set the probability of a false-negative conclusion (type II error) at $\beta = 0.01$ or 0.05, since, if a truly effective drug is found to be inactive in a phase II trial, it is unlikely that the drug will be retested at a later date and an effective drug would be missed. In phase III trials, it is the type I error, α, or the probability of a false-positive error, which is preset at 0.05 or less. The level of α and β depends upon the type of study and type of treatments to be compared and should be reconsidered for each new trial.

If, for instance, the trial is a comparison between treatment regimens of equal toxicity and cost, it would be appropriate to fix the β error at a low level. Indeed, in this case, one wishes to maximize the probability of detecting a difference in treatment efficacy if a difference does exist. A false-positive conclusion is not too damaging, since the two treatment regimens are almost globally similar. If, on the other hand, the comparison is between a new more toxic, or more costly, regimen against a standard control treatment, one does not wish to conclude that the new treatment is more effective than the control unless it is highly probable. In this case it is the type I error, α, which must be minimized.

More generally, α and β should also be chosen so as to maintain at an accceptable level the false-positive and false-negative rates in a sequence of trials (delta and epsilon errors) (Staquet et al. 1979).

Conclusions

Controlled clinical trials are one of the means by which substantial progress in cancer therapy can be achieved. A proper methodology and a sound comprehension of the limitation and power of statistical analysis are needed to avoid false claims and dead end leads. The rise and fall of BCG immunotherapy is one among several examples of false-positive results. It was due in great part to the absence of randomization in the early investigations. Much waste of resources and needless toxicity result from the publication of false-positive results, especially if the idea is new and is supported by laboratory data. Such reports lead to other small trials which "confirm" the previous findings, piling the delta errors one upon the other (Staquet et al. 1979). It usually takes years to organize the large trials needed to evaluate the original outcome.

All scientific experiments and observations are performed in order to formulate "laws" from which the behavior of things can be deducted in the future. In the field of clinical trials, the conclusion that A is better than B is evidently intended to apply not only to the sample actually studied, but to all the subjects with the same characteristics as the ones in the sample. This generalization rests on both statistical and clinical reasoning.

It is often mistakenly thought that a proper random allocation of treatment to patients guarantees the soundness of the extrapolation. Indeed, in pure statistical science, all the tests used to evaluate the hypothesis are based on the theory of random sampling from a closed population. (More precisely, the present experiment is a random sample of a population of similar experiments.) This is not the case in clinical research, since a trial is performed with the patients who are available and suitable at a given time and place and the inference will be made for future patients whose disease might be different and/or treated with different supportive care.

Thus, true statistical random sampling is never performed in a clinical trial since the population of reference is not available. That is the main reason why automatic statistical inference should not be made in clinical research. Nonstatistical input is needed together with the statistical results in order to make sensible data analysis. The most common procedure is to examine the samples for uneven distribution of prognostic factors which might have affected the observed results.

In general, the examination of all aspects of a trial, logistic, medical, and statistical, will reveal the necessity of carrying out confirmatory studies to validate positive early results.

References

EORTC New Drug Development Committee (1985) EORTC guidelines for phase I trials with single agents in adults. Eur J Cancer Clin Oncol 21: 1005–1007

Slevin M, Staquet M (1986) Randomized trials in cancer: a critical review by sites. Raven, New York

Staquet M (1975) Cancer therapy: prognostic factors and criteria of response. Raven, New York

Staquet MJ, Rozencweig M, Von Hoff DD, Muggia FM (1979) The delta and epsilon errors in the assessment of cancer clinical trials. Cancer Treat Rep 63: 1721–1726

Staquet M, Sylvester R, Jasmin C (1980) Guidelines for the preparation of EORTC cancer clinical trial protocols. Eur J Cancer 16: 871–875

Statistical Analysis of Survival and Disease Recurrence Data

M. BUYSE

Introduction

In recent years, an enormous amount of literature has been devoted to the development of optimal techniques for the analysis of survival data. These techniques have been thoroughly investigated in the statistical literature and are almost universally used in the medical literature to report on the results of clinical trials and other medical and biological experiments.

A study of the statistical properties of these standard technqiues can be mathematically quite demanding (Kalbfleisch and Prentice 1980), but in this chapter we show through simple examples that they are easy to apply and to understand.

Recourse to appropriate statistical procedures is, however, only a first step towards a proper analysis of medical data. There are many ways, sometimes subtle ones, in which a statistical analysis done with the best intentions can be misleading or even frankly wrong. In the second part of this chapter, we illustrate and discuss some frequently encountered problems with the analysis of survival data in cancer clinical trials.

A Primer in Survival Data Analysis

"*Survival data*" is a generic name to denote the observed times between some well-defined origin, such as entry in a trial or surgery, and some well-defined event of interest, such as death or disease recurrence (Cox and Oakes 1984). It is customary to call *disease-free interval* the time between curative therapy and recurrence of the malignant process (either locally or in distant sites), and *disease-free survival* the time between curative therapy and either death or recurrence, whichever occurs first. Survival, disease-free interval, disease-free survival, and any other time-to-an-event data are analyzed using the same statistical techniques.

Survival data usually present two features that make their analysis somewhat complicated: first, they tend to be highly "skewed" (i.e., they do not comply with the assumption of normality that is required by many conventional statistical techniques) and, second, they are *"censored"* (i.e., they are not complete for all individuals in the data set).

"Censoring" of survival data typically occurs because, at the time of analysis, some patients are still

alive, so that the time observed for them is a lower bound of their actual survival time. If the event of interest is not death but disease recurrence, then two distinct mechanisms can cause censoring of the disease-free interval: first, some patients have not yet suffered a disease recurrence at the time of analysis and, second, some patients have died from nonmalignant causes before the analysis, so that their actual time to recurrence has not been and will never be observed.

Survival data analysis is concerned with three main types of problems:

a) Given the survival times (possibly censored) of a group of patients, estimate their survival distribution (see below).
b) Given the survival times (possibly censored) of two or more groups of patients, compare these groups with respect to their survival distributions (p. 453).
c) Given the survival times (possibly censored) and prognostic features for a group of patients, assess the importance of all of these features on survival (p. 454).

Estimation of Survival Curves

Suppose we have observed a group of ten patients over a period of time: four patients have died after 3, 7, 11, and 14 months, while the six patients still alive have been followed up for 9+, 10+, 12+, 13+, 15+, and 18+ months (the + sign indicates censored observations). How can we make use of these data? Simply computing their mean and variance, for instance, would be erroneous because of the six censored observations. The standard way of depicting these data is to compute the *survival curve*, which gives the probability of survival as a function of time (Kaplan and Meier 1958).

The method to compute the survival curve is as follows (Table 1):

a) Sort the observed survival times in increasing order (column a).
b) The number of patients *"at risk"*, i.e., still known to be alive, decreases at each censored time and at each death time by the number of patients lost to follow-up or dead at that time (columns b and c).
c) The probability of surviving past a death time is estimated by the number of patients at risk just after that time divided by the number of patients at risk just before that time; the probability of surviving past a censored time is 1 (column d).
d) The survival curve gives the probability of survival past the nth death time and is thus equal to the product of the probabilities of surviving the first, the second, the third, etc., until the nth death time (column e).

In our example, these computations are summarized in Table 1 and the resulting survival curve is shown as "group A" in Fig. 1. Table 1 also shows the standard error of the survival curve (column f), computed with Greenwood's formula (Peto 1984). Note that the survival curve drops only at death times; censored times are indicated by a tick mark on the curve.

The survival curve computed in Fig. 1 is also called the "Kaplan-Meier" estimate, the "product-limit" estimate, or the actuarial curve. Other methods of computing it are inappropriate (Sylvester et al. 1978). Caution should be taken in interpreting the shape of

Table 1. Calculation of the survival curve for patients with survival times 3, 7, 9+, 10+, 11, 12+, 13+, 14, 15+, and 18+ months (group A in Fig. 1)

a	b	c	d	e	f
Times (months)	Patients at risk		Probability of surviving past this time	Survival curve	Standard error
	before this time	after this time			
<3	10	10	1.000	1.000	0.000
3	10	9	0.900	0.900	0.095
7	9	8	0.889	0.800	0.126
9+	8	7	1.000	0.800	0.126
10+	7	6	1.000	0.800	0.126
11	6	5	0.833	0.667	0.161
12+	5	4	1.000	0.667	0.161
13+	4	3	1.000	0.667	0.161
14	3	2	0.667	0.444	0.211
15+	2	1	1.000	0.444	0.211
18+	1	0	1.000	0.444	0.211

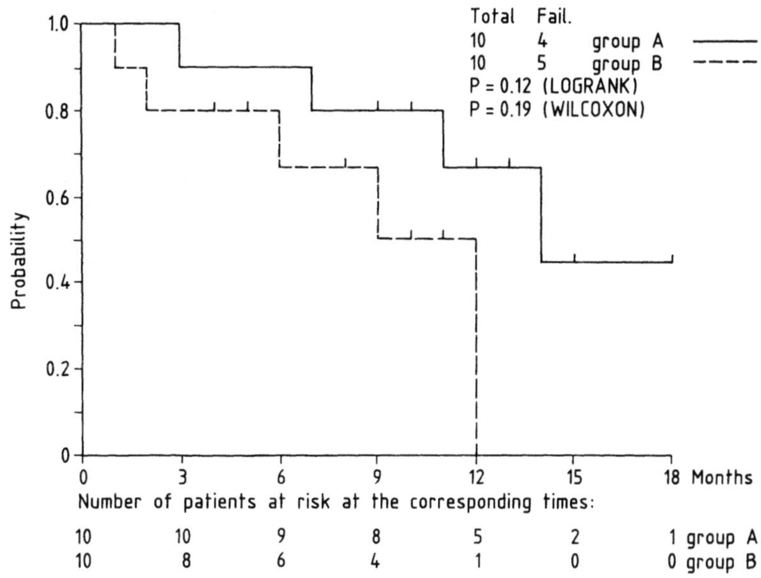

Fig. 1. Kaplan-Meier estimates of two survival curves

the survival curve, notably *"plateaus"* which can occur in the tail of the survival curve (see, for example, group A in Fig. 1). Because very few patients are usually at risk in the tail of the curve, its variability is too great to conclude that a given proportion of patients are cured and will enjoy very long survivals. Similarly, a sharp drop at the end of the curve (see, for example, group B in Fig. 1) is no cause for worry if few patients were at risk of dying at that time.

Comparison of Survival Curves

Now suppose that we have observed two groups of patients, say groups A and B, and that we have estimated their survival curves as above (Fig. 1). How can we compare these two curves, and claim that they are "significantly different" or not? The standard way of doing such a comparison is to use a nonparametric statistical test, i.e., a test that makes no assumption about the distribution of survival, and yet uses all available survival times as efficiently as possible. A test which is commonly used because it has been shown to be statistically optimal in many situations is the *logrank test*, also called the *Mantel-Haenszel test* (Mantel and Haenszel 1959; Peto and Peto 1972). Other rank tests, frequently used in situations where it is important to detect *early* differences between survival curves, are the *generalized Wilcoxon tests* (Gehan 1965; Tarone and Ware 1977; Prentice 1978). For a unifying view of these and other tests, see Harrington and Fleming (1982).

The method of computing the logrank test is as follows (Table 2):

a) Sort all observed survival times in increasing order (column a).
b) Let N be the number of patients at risk at each death time (N_A in group A, N_B in group B) and D be the number of deaths at each death time (D_A in group A, D_B in group B (columns b to d).
c) Compute the number of deaths that would be expected in group B at each death time under the null hypothesis of *no* difference between A and B by the formula:
$$E_B = D \cdot N_B / N \qquad \text{(column e)}$$
and its variance by the formula:
$$V_B = D \cdot N_A \cdot N_B \cdot (N-D) / [N \cdot N \cdot (N-1)] \qquad \text{(column g)}$$
d) Compute the difference between the *observed* and the *expected* number of deaths in group B at each death time (column f) and sum these differences over all death times: $GD = \text{sum}\ (D_B - E_B)$.
e) Sum the variances V_B over all death times: $GV = \text{sum}\ (V_B)$.
f) The logrank statistic is given by $X = GD \cdot GD/GV$. Under the *null hypothesis* of no difference between A and B, this statistic has a chi-square distribution with 1 degree of freedom, and thus a P-value can be read from a table of chi-square values.

Table 2 shows the computations for groups A and B of Fig. 1.

To compute the generalized Wilcoxon test, the method is the same with steps d and e replaced by:
d) Compute a *weighted* sum of the differences between the observed and expected number of deaths over all death times: $GD = \text{sum}\ [N. (D_B - E_B)]$.

Table 2. Computations for rank tests between two groups of patients (A and B) respectively with survival times A: 3, 7, 9+, 10+, 11, 12+, 13+, 14, 15+, and 18+ months; B: 1, 2, 4+, 5+, 6, 8+, 9, 10+, 11+, and 12 months

a	b		c		d		e	f	g
Times (months)	Group A		Group B		Total		E_B	$D_B - E_B$	V_B
	N_A	D_A	N_B	D_B	N	D			
1	10		10	1	20	1	0.500	0.500	0.250
2	10		9	1	19	1	0.474	0.526	0.249
3	10	1	8		18	1	0.444	−0.444	0.247
4+	9		8		17				
5+	9		7		16				
6	9		6	1	15	1	0.400	0.600	0.240
7	9	1	5		14	1	0.357	−0.357	0.230
8+	8		5		13				
9	8		4	1	12	1	0.333	0.667	0.222
10+	7		3		10				
11	6	1	2		8	1	0.250	−0.250	0.188
12	5		1	1	6	1	0.167	0.833	0.139
13+	4		0		4				
14	3	1	0		3	1	0.000	0.000	0.000
15+	2		0		2				
18+	1		0		1				
Total		4		5			2.925	2.075	1.765

e) Compute a *weighted* sum of the variances V_B over all death times: $GV = \text{sum}\ (N \cdot N \cdot V_B)$.

In our example, the logrank statistic is thus given by $X = (2.075) \cdot (2.075)/(1.765) = 2.44$, and a table of the chi-square distribution shows that the corresponding P-value is 0.12 as shown in Fig. 1. Using a standard alpha error rate of 0.05, we would thus say that the difference between groups A and B in Fig. 1 is not significant, since 0.12 is larger than 0.05. The reader can easily verify that the generalized Wilcoxon statistic is given by $X = (27.006) \cdot (27.006)/(418.001) = 1.74$, with a corresponding P-value of 0.19 (also nonsignificant) as shown in Fig. 1.

These computations generalize to the comparison of more than two groups, in which case either an overall test or a test for linear trend can be performed (Breslow 1984). The former would be appropriate, for example, to compare three different treatments, while the latter would be appropriate to test the effect of increasing doses of the same treatment. The tests can also be adjusted to take account of a covariate by *stratifying* the computations (Peto et al. 1977).

Multivariate Models

In some situations, the emphasis is not on stratifying the comparison between two or more groups to take account of a covariate but rather on the assessment of the importance of several covariates simultaneously on survival. Typically, this kind of problem arises when studying the predictive power of various *prognostic factors* on survival (Byar 1984). If the data were not censored, a classical way of approaching this problem would be to perform a linear regression on survival times (or some suitable transformation of them). Because of the censoring, the linear regression cannot be performed without modifications which introduce major difficulties in the analysis (Buckley and James 1979; Miller 1981).

As it turns out, a convenient way of avoiding these difficulties is to model not survival times, but *hazard functions*. The hazard function, also called the time-specific mortality rate, is simply the mortality rate at any given time among the individuals who have survived until that time (as above, this definition extends naturally to any other event than death). The hazard function can be estimated over a period by dividing the number of deaths occurring during the period by the total follow-up time in the period. Simes and Zelen (1985) argue quite convincingly that an analysis of the hazard functions usefully complements the analysis of the corresponding survival curves by revealing patterns in mortality over time.

A simple yet powerful way of modeling hazard functions to account for covariates consists of assuming that the effect of each covariate is to multiply some *baseline hazard* by a constant factor. The problem is then to estimate these multiplicative factors for all covariates, and to test their significance. It is often reasonable to assume certain parametric forms for the baseline hazard (e.g., *exponential:* Feigl and Zelen 1965; or *Weibull:* Byar 1984), but Cox showed that estimation is also possible in the more general case of a completely unspecified baseline hazard function, in which case the model is called a *proportional hazards model*, or simply *Cox's regression model* (Cox 1972). Because of its generality and mathematical elegance, Cox's model has become the preferred way of modelling survival data in the presence of covariates. Note that when there is only one covariate (say, treatment), testing the significance of that covariate in a proportional hazards model is equivalent to a logrank test.

Some Examples of Biased Survival Analyses

Exclusion of Patients and Other Pitfalls

Assume you are asked to review the following short abstract on the results of a clinical trial:

"A prospective, randomized control clinical trial was conducted to test the value of the adjuvant chemotherapy nicymotim after curative resection of colorectal cancer. Two hundred patients were randomized in the trial from 1979 to 1983, and were followed up until the analysis of the data in 1986. Patients records were reviewed by an independent committee. Six patients (3%) were considered ineligible, and three patients (1.5%) were improperly treated (Table 3). Figure 2 shows the survival curves for all eligible patients, classified by actual treatment received. Chemotherapy clearly prolongs survival, and this advantage is statistically significant ($P < 0.05$)."

Impressive as they are (perhaps too unexpectedly so), these results are worthless. Indeed, the survival times in this hypothetical trial were selected randomly from the *same* distribution to generate the survival curves of the control and of the chemotherapy groups. Technically, the common survival distribution was assumed to be exponential with a median of 5 years, and the entry of patients on trial was assumed to be uniform over a 4-year period; these assumptions approximate a plausible real-life situation. Figure 3 shows the survival curves before we "worked" on them.

How, then, can the two survival curves of Fig. 2 be so different? Because we have purposely biased the results by:

a) Excluding "ineligible" patients from the curves. Though this is generally warranted, the risk of bias must be acknowledged if the patients who are excluded from the treatment group are in a worse condition than those who are excluded from the control group (as could be the case, for example, if the chemotherapy was very toxic and

Table 3. Adjuvant chemotherapy for colorectal cancer

Patients	Control	Chemotherapy
Ineligible	3	3
Refused adjuvant therapy	–	2
Demanded adjuvant therapy	1	–
Eligible and properly treated	96	95
Total	100	100

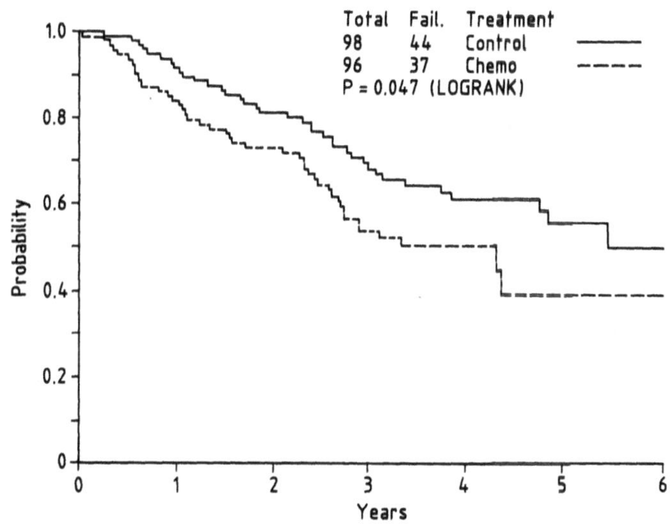

Fig. 2. Survival curves of eligible patients as treated

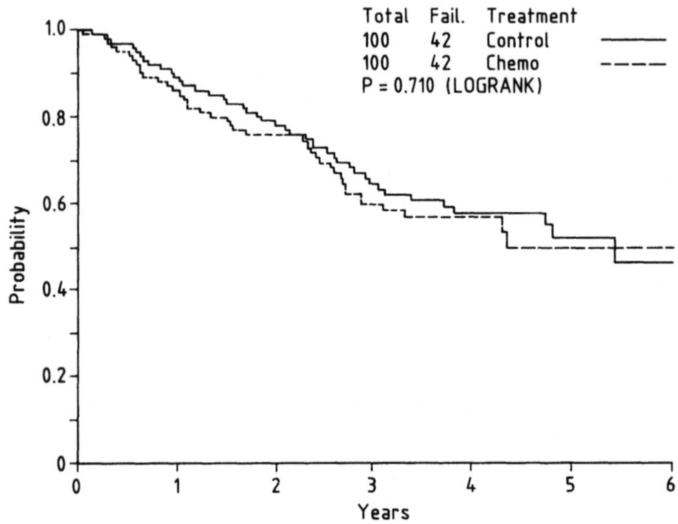

Fig. 3. Survival curves of all patients as randomized

led to suspicion of ineligibility in patients who could not tolerate it (Brown 1984)). Excluding "inevaluable" patients, i.e., patients who were eligible for the trial but somehow violated the protocol *after* randomization is almost never justifiable.

b) Grouping patients by actual treatment received, not by randomized treatment. This practice is absolutely indefensible and should be prohibited from any serious publication.
c) Censoring six observations in the control group at 3 months (as if these six patients had been lost to follow-up at that time). This could easily happen in a trial with a "no adjuvant treatment" control group, and usually remains unnoticed in the reporting of results.

The purpose of this hypothetical example is to illustrate how drastically results can be affected by apparently mundane manipulations of a few patient data.

Comparison of Responders and Nonresponders

In clinical trials testing therapies for advanced diseases, it is tempting to compare the survival of responders with that of nonresponders, and to attribute any survival advantage to a beneficial effect of therapy. This approach is utterly wrong, for it can be shown mathematically that the survival distribution conditional on having a response cannot possibly be the same as the survival distribution in the absence of a response. The basic mechanism at work here is called *length-biased sampling,* through which patients who enjoy long survivals have a higher probability of showing a response to therapy (Anderson et al. 1983; Oye and Shapiro 1984).

As an example, consider Fig. 4. The survival times come from an actual clinical trial on metastatic, measurable colon cancer treated by a combination chemotherapy. We have ignored actual response to treatment, but have generated *random* responses by a computer program that assumes a constant probability of response during every week of survival. As expected, patients with a response clearly have a better survival than those with stable disease, who in turn fare better than those with a progressive disease ($P = 0.01$)!

Conclusions and Suggestions for Further Reading

The purpose of this chapter was to provide clinical investigators with a glimpse of the techniques used in survival data analyses. It was emphasized that results can be biased if a proper statistical methodology is not strictly adhered to. Biases can easily be more important than the actual treatment effects in clinical trials with few patients or in which the difference between the effectiveness of the various therapeutic modalities is small.

For more details on the general methodology of cancer trials, see the two papers by Peto et al. (1976, 1977) or the book edited by Buyse et al. (1984). For a formal introduction to survival analysis, see the books by Cox and Oakes (1984), Miller (1981), or Kalbfleisch and Prentice (1980). For an introduction to biostatistical computer programs, see the book by Klotz and Meyer (1985).

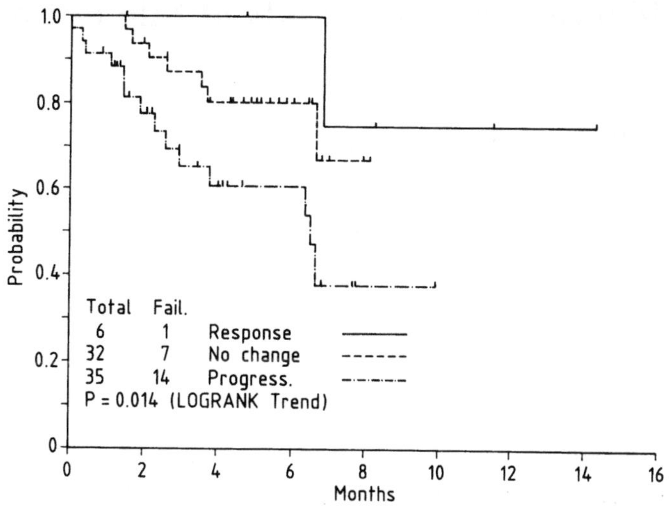

Fig. 4. Survival curves for responses, no changes and progressions.

Acknowledgements. This research is supported by PHS Grant Number 5U10 CA11488-17, awarded by the National Cancer Institute, DHHS (Bethesda, Maryland, USA) and by Contract Number MR-098-B (RS), awarded by the Commission of the European Communities.

References

Anderson JR, Cain KC, Gelber RD (1983) Analysis of survival by tumor response. J Clin Oncol 1: 710–719

Breslow N (1984) Comparison of survival curves. In: Buyse ME, Staquet MJ, Sylvester RJ (eds) Cancer clinical trials, methods and practice. Oxford University Press, Oxford, pp 381–406

Brown BW (1984) Problems related to protocol non-adherence. In: Buyse ME, Staquet MJ, Sylvester RJ (eds) Cancer clinical Trials, methods and practice. Oxford University Press, Oxford, pp 124–136

Buckley J, James I (1979) Linear regression with censored data. Biometrika 66: 429–436

Buyse ME, Staquet MJ, Sylvester RJ (1984) Cancer clinical trials, methods and practice. Oxford University Press, Oxford

Byar DP (1984) Identification of prognostic factors. In: Buyse ME, Staquet MJ, Sylvester RJ (eds) Cancer clinical trials, methods and practice. Oxford University Press, Oxford, pp 423–443

Cox DR (1972) Regression models and life-tables (with discussion). J R Statist Soc B 34: 187–220

Cox DR, Oakes D (1984) Analysis of survival data. Chapman and Hall, London

Feigl P, Zelen M (1965) Estimation of exponential survival probabilities with concomitant information. Biometrics 21: 826–838

Gehan EA (1965) A generalized Wilcoxon test for comparing arbitrarily single-censored samples. Biometrika 52: 203–223

Harrington DP, Fleming TR (1982) A class of rank test procedures for censored survival data. Biometrika 69: 553–566

Kalbfleisch JD, Prentice RL (1980) The statistical analysis of failure time data. Wiley, New York

Kaplan EL, Meier P (1958) Nonparametric estimation from incomplete observations. J Am Statist Assoc 26: 457–481

Klotz JH, Meyer RD (1985) Biostatistical microcomputing in Pascal. Rowman and Allanhed, Totowa, NJ

Mantel N, Haenszel W (1959) Statistical aspects of the analysis of data from retrospective studies of disease. JNCI 22: 719–748

Miller RG (1981) Survival analysis. Wiley, New York

Oye RK, Shapiro MF (1984) Does response make a difference in patient survival? JAMA 252: 2722–2725

Peto J (1984) The calculation and interpretation of survival curves. In: Buyse ME, Staquet MJ, Sylvester RJ (eds) Cancer clinical trials, methods and practice. Oxford University Press, Oxford, pp 361–380

Peto R, Peto J (1972) Asymptotically efficient rank invariant test procedures (with discussion). J R Statist Soc A 135: 185–206

Peto R, Pike MC, Armitage P, Breslow NE, Cox DR, Howard SV, Mantel N, McPherson K, Peto J, Smith PG (1976) Design and analysis of randomized clinical trials requiring prolonged observation of each patient. I. Introduction and design. Br J Cancer 34: 585–612

Peto R, Pike MC, Armitage P, Breslow NE, Cox DR, Howard SV, Mantel N, McPherson K, Peto J, Smith PG (1977) Design and analysis of randomized clinical trials requiring prolonged observation of each patient. II. Analysis and examples. Br J Cancer 35: 1–39

Prentice RL (1978) Linear rank tests with right censored data. Biometrika 65: 167–179

Simes RJ, Zelen M (1985) Exploratory data analysis and the use of the hazard function for interpreting survival data: an investigator's primer. J Clin Oncol 3: 1418–1431

Sylvester RJ, Machin D, Staquet MJ (1978) A comparison of the alternative methods of calculating survival curves arising from clinical trials. Biomedicine (Special Issue) 28: 49–53

Tarone RE, Ware J (1977) On distribution-free tests for equality of survival distributions. Biometrika 64: 156–160

Measurement of Quality of Life in Cancer Research

N. K. Aaronson and F. Calais da Silva

Introduction

The traditional evaluation end points employed in cancer clinical research include such biomedical outcomes as frequency of local recurrence, development of metastatic disease, length of disease-free and overall survival, and control of major physical symptoms. In recent years, however, there has been a growing recognition of the need to document the extent to which medical interventions impact on the functional, psychological, social, and economic life of the individual. Consideration of these nonmedical parameters of cancer and its treatment has been alternately termed "psychosocial," "sociomedical," or, most commonly, "quality of life" research.

While in decades past it was unusual for quality of life issues to be raised explicitly among cancer researchers, it now appears to be the rule rather than the exception. Yet, while interest in quality of life issues in cancer is clearly on the upswing, rhetoric in this area has far outpaced performance. The range of cancer types and treatments that has been evaluated from a psychosocial perspective has been relatively narrow, with most attention paid to the psychosocial sequelae of breast cancer and mastectomy (Bardelli and Saracci 1978; Fayers and Jones 1983).

Further, while the clinical trial represents the principal vehicle for the evaluation of cancer therapies, the available evidence suggests that quality of life parameters are rarely introduced into investigational protocols. For example, in a review of cancer clinical trials carried out between 1956 and 1976, Bardelli and Saracci (1978) located less than 5% of published studies in which quality of life measures were employed. Similarly, in a compliation of approximately 3000 clinical trials (US DHHS 1982), we found that only 3%–4% of studies included psychosocial assessment, with the majority of these reports limited to physicians' ratings of patients' performance status.

What might account for the failure to incorporate quality of life measures routinely into clinical trials? Perhaps the most important factor is the lack of clarity in the definition of the concept. At one level, introduction of the term "quality of life" into the medical lexicon has served an important ideological function. It points our collective attention toward a broader set of issues surrounding the human costs of disease and medical treatment. It this sense, the term "quality of life" serves a similar function to that of the World Health Organization definition of health as: "a state of complete physical, mental and social well-being, and not merely the absence of disease or infirmity.".

It is generally recognized that the WHO definition of health is intended to serve primarily an orienting function, and is not meant to be translated directly into research applications. This has not, however, always been the case with quality of life research. Rather, there is a tendency to reify the quality of life concept. This had lead to attempts at global measurement of quality of life in cancer research. For example, Gough and his colleagues (1983) suggest that a single, direct question – "How would you rate your quality of life today?" – represents a valid and reliable approach to assessing the well-being of cancer patients. The obvious difficulty with such an approach is that it provides little or no information that can be used to improve the clinical management of patients. How are we to interpret a patient reporting a low overall quality of life? Does it imply intolerable symptom levels, limitations in functional capacity, psychological morbidity, a disrupted social life, or a combination of these factors. Unless the quality of life concept is broken down into more digestible units of analysis, it is unlikely that it will achieve widespread acceptance as a legitimate, let alone routine, part of clinical research.

A second, related barrier to the introduction of quality of life parameters in clinical trials is the lack of consensus on how it should be measured. The physician interested in assessing the psychosocial impact of both routine medical care and experimental treatments is confronted with a confusing array of measurement tools. At one end of the spectrum are extensive and time-consuming interview protocols that exceed the practical limits present in the typical clinical setting. At the other end are more concise patient self-report questionnaires which, while representing a less cumbersome approach to data collection, often leave unanswered the critical questions of instrument reliability and validity.

Similarly, psychosocial research designs are often viewed by those responsible for conducting clinical trials as overly burdensome both to themselves and to their patients. Such perceived burdens may be due, in part, to a basic lack of familiarity with the nature and intent of assessing psychosocial outcomes. However, it also reflects a degree of naivité on the part of social scientists with regard to what is feasible in a clinical context. Often data collection schemes call for frequent application of lengthy questionnaires during the rush of outpatient clinics. While such procedures may be optimal in an abstract sense (i.e., they can potentially yield a maximum amount of data), they do not reconcile the practical constraints operating in clinical practice.

In this paper we will attempt to clarify a number of issues relevant to the successful application of quality of life measures in cancer clinical research. The focus will be on defining quality of life in operational terms and establishing basic guidelines for the development of quality of life measures.

A Taxonomy of Quality of Life Dimensions in Cancer Research

Just as cancer is a collective noun for some 100 forms of disease (Cairns 1985), so is quality of life a collective term representing a set of related, interacting dimensions. Further, although some instruments purported to assess quality of life are based on clinical observations (Karnofsky and Burchenal 1949; Nou and Aberg 1980; Zubrod and Schneidermann 1960), there is growing recognition that the patient him- or herself is usually the best, and sometimes the only, logical source of information about the effects of the disease and its treatment on daily living.

Working within a multidimensional framework, those aspects of quality of life that may be relevant evaluation end points in cancer research include: (1) disease symptoms, (2) side effects of treatment, (3) functional status, (4) psychological distress, (5) social interaction, (6) sexuality and body image, and (7) satisfaction with medical treatment. No claim is made as to the comprehensiveness of this taxonomy. Rather, it is intended to reflect the range of issues, both physical and nonphysical, that have been found to be of relevance to patients undergoing cancer treatment (Coates et al. 1983).

Disease Symptoms

Although each form of cancer has its own natural history and characteristic behavior, there are a number of symptoms which are present in many tumor types, particularly in advanced stages of disease. These include fatigue and malaise, dyspnea, pain, weight loss, nausea, and sleep disturbance.

Although many of these symptoms can only be assessed via clinical interviews, there is a wide range in the form and manner in which clinicians seek out such information from their patients. Thus, it may be useful to systematize the collection of such data by asking patients themselves to rate their symptom experience using standardized rather than ad hoc methods.

Each symptom can be assessed in a variety of ways, ranging from a simple dichotomous variable representing its presence or absence, to more refined measures of severity, frequency of occurrence, and duration. In general, the use of a severity or frequency rating is recommended as it can capture gradations in symptom relief which may not be noted with a cruder measure of presence/absence.

Physical Side Effects of Treatment

Each therapeutic intervention, or combination of interventions, has associated with it a certain level of toxicity. In clinical trials the monitoring of such physical side effects is essential. In those cases where there is no clear advantage for one form of treatment over another in terms of survival or disease-free interval, treatment toxicity may represent the critical factor in selecting among regimens.

In addition to the inconvenience of hospitalization and the trauma of an intensive care environment, the physical consequences of surgery can vary from transient postoperative pain to severe disfigurement with accompanying loss of function. Additionally, the psychological and social consequences of radical surgery in breast, head and neck, gynecological, and colorectal cancer have been described extensively.

The most common physical side effect of radiation treatment, regardless of site of exposure, is fatigue and malaise (Battles 1981; Haylock and Hart 1979). Other side effects depend on the site and size of the treatment field, the time-dose fractionation, and the general health condition of the patient.

The side effects of chemotherapy are also dependent on a number of factors such as dosage levels and site or mode of administration (i.e., systemically versus local instillation). Systemic cytostatic treatment can result in both acute and delayed toxic effects. Detailed descriptions of possible side effects for specific chemotherapeutic agents are available from a number of sources (Coates et al. 1983; Hubbard 1981; Medical Letter 1985). Briefly, however, those acute side effects most frequently reported include nausea and vomiting (80%–90% of all patients), appetite loss, weight loss, fatigue and malaise, alopecia, diarrhoea, soreness in the mouth, and sleep disturbances. Bone marrow depression can result in septicemia and bleeding. Delayed toxicities include organ damage (liver, kidney, and heart) and infertility (Medical Letter 1985).

Notation of treatment toxicity is typically a mandatory part of clinical trials. Again, however, it is important to stress that, due to the subjective nature of many of these side effects, direct and systematic questioning of patients is essential. Even for those symptoms that are easily observed, patient feedback may provide additional insight into their meaning and impact on daily living. For example, in assessing the extent of alopecia, what we are most interested in is not the amount of hair loss per se, but rather how the change in physical appearance affects the patient's emotional and social life. Further, direct feedback from the patient may yield information regarding unanticipated treatment side effects.

Functional Status

Functional status refers to the performance of, or the capacity to perform, a variety of activities that are normal for most people. Four categoris of such activities commonly measured are: (1) self-care activities (e.g., feeding, dressing, bathing, and using the toilet); (2) mobility (i.e., the ability to move about indoors and outdoors); (3) physical activities (e.g., walking, climbing stairs, running, etc.); and (4) role activities (i.e., the ability to carry out social roles associated with work, school, family, etc.) (Stewart et al. 1978).

The most commonly employed measures of functional status in cancer clinical trials are the Karnofsky Performance Status Scale (Karnofsky and Burchenal 1949) and the ECOG/WHO scale (Zubrod and Schneidermann 1960). Both of these scales rely on observer judgments regarding the level of functioning of the patient. While the Karnofsky scale has been found to be a useful prognostic indicator of survival (Aisner and Hansen 1981), it has been criticized on a number of grounds, the most important being its poor interobserver reliability (Hutchinson et al. 1979). Further, Hutchinson et al. (1979) found low levels of agreement (approximately 35%) between physician and patient Karnofsky ratings. Similarly, Aaronson et al. (1987) observed a weak correlation (0.36) between the ECOG/WHO scale and a patient self-report performance status measure. These findings suggest the need to incorporate a patient-based assessment of functional status into clinical trials. Such patient-based measures could also expand the scope of inquiry to include issues of social and occupational role functioning.

Psychological Distress

A number of studies have documented elevated levels of psychological distress among cancer patients as compared with rates found among primary care populations (Achute and Vauhkonen 1970; Craig and Abeloff 1974; Derogatis et al. 1983; Peck 1972; Plumb and Holland 1977). The most common symptoms reported by cancer patients are depression (Endicott 1984; Levine et al. 1978; Maguire et al. 1978) and anxiety (Gottschalk 1983; Meyerowitz 1980; Mitchell and Glicksman 1977; Peck and Boland 1977).

It should be noted that the majority of studies of the psychological status of cancer patients cannot be interpreted in terms of *pathological* states or diagnosable mental disorder. Rather, they reflect levels of more generalized, nonspecific distress. Whether reflecting generalized distress or specific disorder, such symptoms can reflect the impact of the diagnosis of cancer, reaction to the progression of the disease, and/or side effects of treatment (Greer and Silberfarb 1982; Weisman and Worden 1977).

A variety of measures are available for assessing psychological morbidity, ranging from extensive psychiatric interviews to multidimensional self-report symptom checklists to unidimensional scales. However, within the context of clinical trials, the choice of measures may be quite restricted. Clearly, lengthy, omnibus instruments designed to assess psychological status in a comprehensive sense cannot be employed for reasons of practicality. Yet, even within the narrower range of unidimensional measures certain cautions should be exercised. Of particular concern is to avoid the use of instruments that include items measuring somatic manifestations of psychological disturbance such as tiredness, decreased sexual drive, or appetite loss (Endicott 1984). In such cases it may not be possible to distinguish between symptoms of psychological disorder and physical symptoms associated with the disease or its treatment.

Social Interaction

Both clincial observation and empirical research point to the importance of social contact and social support in the life of the cancer patient (Worden and Weisman 1984; Wortman 1983; Wortman and Dunkel-Schetter 1979). Functional problems due to pain or fatigue may restrict the individuals's ability to pursue normal social activities. Similarly, the demands of treatment regimens may place serious limitations and strains on the ability to maintain social contacts (Bury 1982).

Psychological reactions of the cancer patient may also lead to restricted social interactions. Fear of being a burden to others, feelings of embarrassment about symptoms or disability, and fears of rejection may lead to avoidance of social contact and hesitancy in asking for support (Bury 1982; Maguire 1982; Strauss and Glaser 1975).

Family and friends may also reduce the level of contact with the cancer patient, or withdraw from the relationship entirely due to feelings of awkwardness or fear of inadequacy (Peters-Golden 1982; Wortman 1983). Lack of understanding of the nature of cancer and its treatment (e.g., fear of contagion) may also result in avoidance of contact.

Assessment of social interaction can be seriously hampered by an underreporting bias. Patients may be hesitant to report problems in their social sphere if questions are phrased in such a way as to imply criticism of family members and friends. By focusing on the behavioral aspects of interpersonal relationships (e.g., the ability to maintain normal social contacts) rather than on their affective dimension (e.g., feelings of love and support), such bias may be minimized.

Sexuality and Body Image

Cancer and its treatment can affect sexuality and body image both directly and indirectly. The clearest direct effect is loss of sexual function or severe change in body image due to surgical interventions such as cystectomy and mastectomy. Indirect effects (e.g., loss of libido) can result from the fatigue, pain, physical debilitation, and emotional upset associated with various treatments (Derogatis and Kourlesis 1981).

The degree of distress associated with any decrease in the ability to function sexually will, of course, vary as a function of a number of patient characteristics. Age and predisease or pretreatment levels of sexual activity are perhaps the most important of these factors, with younger patients and those with active sexual lives experiencing the greatest trauma. At the same time, it should be emphasized that sexuality remains a relevant issue throughout the life span of patients. The frequently held assumption that sexuality is of minor importance to the elderly is untenable. Decrease in the desire or ability to have sexual intercourse does not imply a parallel reduction in the desire for physical intimacy.

In assessing changes in sexuality it is important to consider both attitudinal (i.e., interest, enjoyment, satisfaction) and behavioral (i.e., capacity) dimensions. Further, because questions regarding sexual interest and behavior can be perceived as quite threatening, particular efforts should be taken to assure the strictest confidentiality, and perhaps to convey to the patient that sexual problems are not uncommon in their disease.

Satisfaction with Medical Care

The assessment of patient satisfaction with medical care is particularly salient in the cancer field. Among cancer patients, lengthy treatment procedures with concomitant dependency on the health care system are almost inevitable (Oberst 1984). Thus, the perceived quality of medical care can play a central part in the cancer patient's overall evaluation of quality of life (Locker and Dunt 1978).

In developing a measure of patient satisfaction for use in cancer research we clearly cannot assess all aspects of the phenomenon. Nevertheless, a single, global satisfaction item will probably not serve our purposes well (Locker and Dunt 1978). Rather, what is needed is a brief composite measure that will provide some specific information regarding patients' perceptions of such aspects of medical care as the interpersonal manner of physicians, the technical quality of care, the efficacy of treatment, and the adequacy of information provided both informally and formally (i.e., via informed consent).

Measurement Issues in Quality of Life Research

There are three broad categories of data collection strategies available in clinically oriented psychosocial research – clinical observations, patient interviews, and self-administered questionnaires. Structured clinical observation methods such as the Karnofsky and ECOG/WHO performance status scales represent a simple, albeit limited approach to quality of life measurement. One of the major methodological limitations of these scales – inadequate interobserver reliability – might be enhanced by supplying more specific criteria for assessing level of functional capacity (e.g., ability to work, to carry out normal activity, and to care for self) (Hutchinson et al. 1979).

Interviews, both structured and semistructured, have the advantage of yielding detailed information from patients who otherwise would be unable to complete a questionnaire (e.g., elderly, poorly educated, or physically handicapped patients). Offsetting this advantage is the fact that interviews require more commitment of staff time than is typically feasible in clinical settings.

Although self-administered questionnaires sacrifice some of the detail derived from patient interviews, they represent the most practical, efficient, and inexpensive method of obtaining patient-based information in clinical research. A particularly important advantage of questionnaires is that, if designed with simplicity in mind, they can be administered repeatedly during the course of treatment, thus yielding valuable longitudinal information regarding patterns of change in quality of life. However, careful attention must be paid to construction of such questionnaires to ensure that they have broad applicability across varying treatment settings and patient groups. Generic issues to be considered in questionnaire development include: (1) amount of patient effort required, (2) item selection, (3) time frame of the questions, (4) choice of response format, (5) psychometric properties (i.e., validity and reliability), and (6) cross-cultural applicability.

Patient Effort Required

While self-administerered questionnaires have the *potential* for minimizing the amount of staff and patient burden associated with collecting psychosocial data, this very much depends on decisions regarding the overall length of the instrument. In clinical trials, where patients may be quite ill and symptomatic, it is important to limit the number of items included in the questionnaire and the time required for its completion. While tolerance for answering questions will vary as a function of patient age, education, stage of disease, and symptom level, experience within EORTC trials has suggested that a questionnaire containing between 30 and 40 questions can be completed by the large majority of patients within 15 min. Patient compliance with questionnaires of this length has been quite high.

Item Selection

Clinicians often ask why it is desirable to include more than a single question in order to measure a particular quality of life dimension. In some cases a single item may well suffice (e.g., for measuring coughing or hair loss). Yet, we are often interested in measuring more complex sets of attitudes and behaviors. In these instances the use of a battery of questions can be recommended. To the extent that such multiple questions can be combined into summative ratings (i.e., scales or indices), they present a clear advantage over single-item measures. First, they can increase the variability (i.e., the range) of scores, an important requisite for detecting changes in health status over a period of time, and differences between patient groups. Second, they can increase score reliability by pooling information that items have in common. Third, if questions are selected carefully to provide a representative sample of information, the resulting scales will have increased validity. Fourth, by employing both positively and negatively worded questions, it is possible to reduce response bias introduced by the tendency for some individuals to agree (or disagree) with items in a questionnaire regardless of their content. Finally, the use of scales can reduce the problem of missing data by providing the option, if responses to individual questions are missing, of estimating scores based on the remaining questions comprising the scale.

In selecting items to be included in a questionnaire, every effort should be made to identify preexisiting scales that have been used with cancer patients, and that have known levels of reliability and validity. This will reduce dramatically the time and expense associated with instrument development.

Often, however, previously tested measures will not be available, and questions will have to be written to cover the topics of interest. In developing such items several general principles should be kept in mind. The wording of the questions should be as unambiguous as possible. While avoidance of uncommon words, abbreviations, and double negatives will reduce ambiguity, it is also essential to attend carefully to the potential for multiple interpretation of questions. For example, how are we to interpret responses to a question such as: "How uncomfortable do you feel today?". On the one hand, patients may respond to this question in terms of physical discomfort (e.g., pain or limitation in mobility). On the other hand, they may interpret it to mean emotional discomfort (e.g., anxiousness, self-consciousness). Similarly, it is important to avoid questions that include multiple parts (e.g., "did you feel tired or anxious during the past week?"). Such questions will confuse patients and present problems of interpretation during data analysis.

To ensure that questions are understandable, and that all relevant questions have been asked, it is useful to involve a range of individuals in the process of questionnaire development. This can include physicians, nurses, psychologists, statisticians, and, perhaps most importantly, patients themselves (Schipper 1984). Additionally, by ending a questionnaire with an open-ended question, it is often possible to pick up valuable information that would otherwise be overlooked. For example, in a study of cancer patient satisfaction with medical care, one patient complained (in response to an open-ended question) about the nauseating effect of the nurses' perfume (Huisman et al. 1987). This was a practical problem that had not been considered previously by either the research or clinical staff.

Time Frame of the Questions

In measuring psychosocial outcomes in clinical trials we may be interested in both the short-term and long-term consequences of treatment. Particularly in the case of short-term effects (e.g., during or immediately following a course of chemotherapy or radiotherpy), it is important to provide a relatively short time frame (i.e., between 1 day and 1 week) in order to assure that the patient is responding to questions in terms of the relevant period in the treatment cycle (van Dam et al. 1984). If too long a time frame is employed, or if it is left undefined, the patient may be confused as to which period he or she should report – a treatment period, a rest period, or perhaps both.

Even in the case of long-term effects, the use of a relatively short question time-frame (e.g., 1 week) can be recommended. This will minimize problems associated with memory loss, and will avoid confounding specific symptom experience with a more generalized tendency to complain (Huisman et al. 1987).

Choice of Response Format

The two major choices available for response scales are Likert-type scales and visual analog scales. The Likert-type scale is categorical, providing the patient with a set number of closed-ended response choices (e.g., "strongly agree," "agree," "disagree," and "strongly disagree"). In contrast, a visual analog scale is composed typically of a 10-cm line with descriptive anchors at each end of the line (e.g., "extreme nausea" and "no nausea"). The patient is asked to mark the point on the line that corresponds most closely to his or her experience, and the distance from the anchor points is subsequently measured.

While a number of investigators report the successful use of the linear analog approach with cancer patients (Oberst 1984; Padilla et al. 1981; Priestman and Baum 1976), others argue that the level of abstraction required by the technique is too great for many patients, and that the need physically to measure each response for purposes of coding an analysis mitigates against its routine use in clinical trials (Fayers and Jones 1983). Thus, despite the certain advantages associated with the use of linear analog scales, the Likert-type approach seems most appropriate in order to ensure that patients understand the task and can complete it without assistance.

Psychometric Properties

It is essential that the requisite psychometric tests be carried out to ensure that selected quality of life scales are both reliable and valid. Reliability refers to the consistency of the scores derived from a set of items, or the extent to which the score is free of random error. While calculation of score reliability is a fairly straightforward procedure, establishing scale validity is a much more complex task. Essentially, validity refers to whether the hypothesized scales adequately measure the concepts that they are intended to measure. There are a number of forms of validity and validity testing. At the simplest level, an examination of the form and content of questions will provide information regarding the *face* validity of a questionnaire (i.e., do the questions make sense; are the relevant subject areas covered?).

In *criterion* testing a scale is validated against some other empirical measuring procedure. For example, a self-report measure of shortness of breath could be compared with results obtained from a treadmill test. The difficulty with this type of validity testing is that, in many cases, it is difficult to find a criterion measure that is itself valid and reliable (e.g., in measuring psychological distress).

Construct validity refers to a family of procedures that provide evidence regarding not only the validity of the measuring instrument, but of the underlying theory as well (Fiske 1971). A number of multivariate statistical techniques can be used to examine the construct validity of a scale. The common denominator among these techniques is an examination of the pattern of correlations within and between various scales. To establish construct validity, one must demonstrate that the questionnaire items, and the scales formed from these items, relate to each in a predictable fashion.

While it is beyond the scope of this paper to describe the various procedures involved in reliability and validity testing in detail, it should be emphasized that such requisite psychometric analyses can be time-consuming, requiring several test runs and revisions before a satisfactory set of items is settled upon. Thus, ample time should be allocated *before* a clinical trial is activated for puposes of instrument pretesting.

Cross-cultural Validity

In many multicenter clinical trials diverse cultural groups will be represented in the patient sample. While cultural differences may have little or no effect on the measurement of biological outcomes, they can exert a significant influence when attempting to measure the subjective experiences of the patient. Thus, in constructing measures of psychosocial outcome careful attention should be paid to assuring that questions have as close to the same meaning across cultures as is possible (Sartorius 1979). The use of standard procedures for translation of questionnaires can alleviate many of the basic language problems. This involves a "forward and backward" translation process in which the questionnaire is first translated from the original into the second language ("forward") and then back again to the original language ("backward"). This is typically an iterative process, requiring several refinements in question wording before equivalence is achieved.

Standard Versus Trial-Specific Quality of Life Measures

An issue that is subject to much debate is whether it is possible to develop a standard quality of life questionnaire that has broad applicability across a range of tumor types and treatment modalites, or whether it is necessary to develop specific questionnaires for each research situation. There are currently available several omnibus measures that are designed to assess psychosocial adjustment to chronic disease in general. Examples include the Sickness Impact Profile (Bergner et al. 1981), the McMaster Health Profile (Chambers et al. 1982), and the Nottingham

Health Profile (Hunt et al. 1981). The advantage of such standard instruments is that they can potentially facilitate the comparison of results across studies. However, because these measures were not developed or validated specifically for cancer populations, their utility in cancer research has yet to be demonstrated. One barrier to their use in trial settings is their overall length, ranging from 45 questions for the Nottingham Health Profile to 136 questions for the Sickness Impact Profile.

Recently, a number of investigators have attempted to develop quality of life measures that are specific to cancer patients (Padilla et al. 1981; Priestman and Baum 1976; Schipper et al. 1984; Selby et al. 1984). Schipper and his colleagues (1984) describe the development of a 22-item instrument, the FLIC, intended for use across a range of patient groups and treatment situations. Preliminary psychometric results suggest that this instrument demonstrates adequate levels of reliability and validity, although it has yet to be tested in clinical trials. A potentially serious limitation of this questionnaire is that, as currently designed, it yields only a single, global quality of life score based on a summation of the individual items. As discussed earlier, such a global measure is unlikely to suffice in most clinical research settings where there is need for more specific information regarding the impact of treatment on various aspects of quality of life.

Selby et al. (1984) also report promising results for a 32-item measure based, in part, on the Sickness Impact Profile. While intended for use in breast cancer research, it is designed in such a way that, with some modification, it could be applied to a range of cancer populations. The available evidence indicates that it is easy to use, acceptable to patients, and displays adequate levels of reliability and validity. Its major limitation would appear to lie with the manner in which data can be summarized. While the FLIC can be criticized for yielding only a single, global score, the Selby questionnaire exhibits the opposite problem. As currently used, each of the 32 items is treated separately (i.e., no attempt is made to cluster the items into a more discrete set of scales). This could present very real problems of interpretation if the goal is to compare the relative impact of different treatments.

In summary, while there have clearly been advances made in quality of life measurement, no "gold standard" has yet to emerge that could be recommended for use as a general tool in psychosocial oncology. Rather than recommending a specific instrument, we feel that, at this time, it is more appropriate to restrict our advocacy to a certain measurement *strategy*. We would suggest that efforts be directed primarily toward developing a *modular* system for quality of life measurement. By this we mean the construction of a set of brief, multi-item measures of various quality of life dimensions. Taking the taxonomy presented earlier as a starting point, this would imply the development of modules to assess functional status, pain, fatigue and malaise, psychological distress, social interaction, sleep disorder, sexuality and body image, and satisfaction with medical care. All or a subset of these modules could form a core quality of life instrument that would have broad applicability across a range of clinical settings. Additional disease and treatment-specific symptom modules could be developed to complement the core instrument. Adoption of this approach would reconcile the two principal requirements of a quality of life measure – a sufficient degree of generalizability to allow for cross-study comparisons, and a level of specificity adequate for answering those questions of particular relevance in a given clinical research situation.

References

Aaronson NK, Bakker W, Stewart AL, van Dam FSAM, van Zandwijk N, Yarnold JR, Kirkpatrick A (1984) A multidimensional approach to the measurement of quality of life in lung cancer clinical trials. In: Aaranson NK, Beckmann J (eds) The quality of life of cancer patients. Raven, New York

Achute K, Vauhkonen ML (1970) Cancer and psyche. Kunnallispaino, Helsinki

Aisner J, Hansen HH (1982) Commentary: current status of chemotherapy for non-small cell lung cancer. Cancer Treat Rep 65: 979–986

Bardelli D, Saracci R (1978) Measuring the quality of life in cancer clinical trials: a sample survey of published trials. In: Armitage P (ed) Methods and impact of controlled therapeutic trials in cancer, part 1. International Union against Cancer, Geneva

Battles CSE (1981) Nursing management of the radiation therapy client. In: Marino LB (ed) Cancer nursing. Mosby, St. Louis, pp 250–286

Bergner M, Bobbitt RA, Carter WB, Gilson BS (1981) The sickness impact profile: development and final revision of a health status measure. Med Care 19: 787–805

Bury M (1982) Chronic illness as biographical disruption. Sociology Health Illness 41: 167–182

Cairns J (1985) The treatment of diseases and the war against cancer. Sci Am 253: 31–39

Chambers LW, MacDonald LA, Tugwell P (1982) The McMaster Health Index Questionnaire as a measure of quality of life for patients with rheumatoid arthritis. J Rheumatol 9: 780–784

Coates A, Abraham S, Kaye SB (1983) On the receiving end. Patient perception of the side-effects of cancer therapy. Eur J Cancer Clin Oncol 19: 203–208

Craig TJ, Abeloff MD (1974) Psychiatric symptomatology among hospitalized cancer patients. Am J Psychiatry 141: 1323–1327

Derogatis LR, Kourlesis SM (1981) An approach to evaluation of sexual problems in cancer patients. Cancer 31: 46–48

Derogatis LR, Morrow GR, Fetting J (1983) The prevalence of psychiatric disorders among cancer patients. JAMA 249: 751–757

Endicott J (1984) Measurement of depression in patients with cancer. Cancer 53: 2243–2248

Fayes PM, Jones DR (1983) Measuring and analysing quality of life in cancer clinical trials: a review. Stat Med 2: 429–446

Fiske DW (1971) Measuring the concept of personality. Aldine, Chicago

Gottschalk LA (1983) Measurement of mood, affect, and anxiety in cancer patients. Cancer 53 (Suppl): 2236–2240

Gough IR, Furnival CM, Schilder L, Grove W (1983) Assessment of the quality of life of patients with advanced cancer. Eur J Clin Oncol 19: 1161–1165

Greer S, Silberfarb PM (1982) Psychological concomitant of cancer: current state of research. Psychol Med 12: 563–573

Haylock PJ, Hart LK (1979) Fatigue in patients receiving localized radiation. Cancer Nurs December: 461–457

Hubbard SM (1981) Chemotherapy and the cancer nurse. In: Marino LB (ed) Cancer nursing. Mosby, St. Louis, pp 287–343

Huisman SJ, Aaronson NK, van Dam FSAM, Polak CE (1985) De mening van patienten over hun verblifj in het AVL. Internal report, Antoni van Leeuwenhoek Hospital, Amsterdam

Huisman SJ, van Dam FSAM, Aaronson NK, Hanewald GJFP (1987) On measuring complaints of cancer patients: some remarks on the time span of the question. In: Aaronson NK, Beckmann J (eds) The quality of life of cancer patients. Raven, New York

Hunt SM, McEwen J, McKenna SP (1981) The Nottingham Health Profile: subjective health status and medical consultations. Soc Sci Med 15 A: 221–229

Hutchinson TA, Boyd NF, Feinstein AR (1979) Scientific problems in clinical scales as demonstrated in the Karnofsky Index of Performance Status. J Chron Dis 32: 661–666

Karnofsky DA, Burchenal JH (1949) The clinical evaluation of chemotherapeutic agents in cancer. In: MacLeod CM (ed) Evaluation of chemotherapeutic agents. Columbia University Press, New York

Levine PM, Silberfarb PM, Lipowski ZJ (1978) Mental disorders in cancer patients – a study of 100 psychiatric referrals. Cancer 42: 1385–1391

Locker D, Dunt D (1978) Theoretical and methodological issues in sociological studies of consumer satisfaction with medical care. Soc Sci Med 12: 283–292

Maguire GP (1982) Psychological and social consequences of cancer. In: Williams CJ, Whitehouse JMA (eds) Recent advances in clinical oncology. Livingston Churchill, Edinburgh

Maguire GP, Lee EG, Bevington DJ (1978) Psychiatric problems in the first year after mastectomy. Br Med J 1: 963

Medical Letter (1985) Cancer chemotherapy. Med Lett Drugs Ther 27 (681): 13–20

Meyerowitz BE (1980) Psychological correlates of breast cancer and its treatment. Psychol Bull 87: 108–131

Mitchell GW, Glicksman HS (1977) Cancer patients: knowledge and attitudes. Cancer 40: 61–66

Nou E, Aberg T (1980) Quality of survival in patients with surgically treated bronchial carcinoma. Thorax 35: 255–263

Oberst MT (1984) Patients' perceptions of care. Measurement of quality and satisfaction. Cancer 53: 2366–2373

Padilla G, Presant CA, Grant M (1981) Assessment of quality of life in cancer patients. Proc Am Assoc Cancer Res 22: 1594–1597

Peck A (1972) Emotional reactions to having cancer. ASR 114: 591–599

Peck A, Boland J (1977) Emotional reactions to radiation treatment. Cancer 40: 180–184

Peters-Golden H (1982) Breast cancer: varied perceptions of social support in the illness experience. Soc Sci Med 16: 483–491

Plumb MM, Holland J (1977) Comparative studies of psychological functions in patients with advanced cancer. I. Self-reported depressive symptoms. Psychosom Med 39: 264–276

Priestman TJ, Baum M (1976) Evaluation of quality of life in patients receiving treatment for advanced breast cancer. Lancet 1: 899–901

Sartorius N (1979) Cross-cultural psychiatry. Springer, Berlin, Heidelberg, New York

Schipper H, Clinch J, McMurray A, Levitt M (1984) Measuring the quality of life of cancer patients. The functional living index – cancer: development and validation. J Clin Oncol 2: 472–483

Selby PJ, Chapman JAW, Etazadi-Amoli J, Dalley D, Boyd NF (1984) The development of a method of assessing the quality of life of cancer patients. Br J Cancer 50: 13–22

Stewart AL, Ware JE, Brook RH, Davies-Avery A (1978) Conceptualization and measurement of health for Adults in the health insurance study, vol 2. Physical health in terms of functioning. The Rand Corporation, R-1987/2-HEW, Santa Monica, Ca

Strauss HM, Glaser BG (1975) Chronic illness and the quality of life. Mosby, St. Louis

US Department of Health and Human Services (1982) Compilation of experimental cancer therapy protocol summaries, 6th.

van Dam FSAM, Linssen CAG, Couzijn AL (1984) Evaluating 'quality of life' in cancer clinical trials. In: Buyse M, Staquet M, Sylvester R (eds) Cancer clinical trials: methods and practice. Oxford University Press, London, pp 26–43

Weisman AD, Worden JW (1977) Coping and vulnerability with cancer patients: a research report. Massachusetts General Hospital, Boston

Worden JW, Weisman AD (1984) Preventive psychosocial intervention with newly diagnosed cancer patients. Gen Hosp Psychiatry 6: 243–249

Wortman CB (1983) Social support and the cancer patient: conceptual and methodological issues. Cancer 53: 2217–2384

Wortman CB, Dunkel-Schetter C (1979) Interpersonal relationships and cancer: a theoretical analysis. J Soc Issues 35: 120–155

Zubrod CG, Schneidermann M (1950) Appraisal of methods for the study of chemotherapy of cancer in man: comparative therapeutic trial of nitrogen mustard and triethylenethio phosphoramide. J Chron Dis 11: 7–33

Controlled Clinical Trials 1988: Ethical Considerations

H. TAGNON

Introduction

One of the most important developments in clinical medicine in this century has been the gradual introduction and strengthening of the scientific method for the evaluation of the efficacy and toxicity of old and new medical and surgical treatments. This has affected all branches of medical care, and especially the treatment of cancer. It has followed, at a distance, the tremendous progress of the biological sciences, which are transforming our conceptions of life and the world in general, as much as it has deeply modified the orientation of industrial and commercial engineering. Progress in biology always precedes progress in medicine although clinical sciences not infrequently stimulate biological research. But there has always been a lag between medical and biological research. The slower pace of clinical research is explained by several factors, among which the following are important: the length of time separating the fundamental discoveries of biology from their practical application to medical care; the socioeconomic factors of the practice of medicine, which as a profession is by nature conservative of methods and prerogatives; and finally the unique qualification of man as an object of scientific study, since man cannot be the subject of experimentation except if it is immediately useful to his health and welfare. As Kant said, every human being is to be treated as an end and never as a means to an end.

With the advent and increasing development of clinical research, it has become necessary to re-examine the fundamental principles governing the practice of medicine. Moral principles applied in a profession are usually called ethical principles or ethics, but the change in name does not change what is designated, and it really is the question of morality which is being examined here, as it arises when controlled clinical trials are contemplated and executed.

Simply expressed, the moral law of medicine is that the human being as an individual deserves first consideration, society exists for the individual and not the individual for society. This concept is acknowledged if not always applied in our civilization.

In a recent article, this author (Tagnon 1984) invoked the two principles enunciated by the philosopher Kant (1848) as the guidelines of moral behaviour: the first says "a person, yourself or someone else, should never be treated as a means to an end, but always as an end in himself." The second is as important: "Always act in every situation in such a way that your behaviour becomes a maxim of universal application." Kant stated these two principles to be "categorically imperative" and he meant that the obligation they prescribe is compelling.

In the same article, there is a reconciliation of two apparently opposite exigencies in controlled clinical research: on the one hand are the Kant principles, and on the other is the obligation for members of the medical profession, especially in institutions paid by public funds, to advance medical knowledge in order to increase our means of curing disease, and for teachers in order to provide adequate instruction for their students.

Comparative Clinical Trials

There are innumerable examples of treatments that were used for a long time even though their effectiveness was never tested. Actually they are the equivalent, for the past, of the present-day untested treatments also called "ineffective cancer therapy" (Subcommittee on Unorthodox Therapies 1983). Physicians and surgeons administered them with a good conscience, since methods of evaluation of treatment as they are available now were not practised by the medical profession, with a few exceptions. Radical mastectomy for cancer of the breast, tonsillectomy for the treatment or prevention of acute rheumatic fever, and "fixation" operations for sagging abdominal organs are a few examples of untested treatments. The same was true for medical treatments as discussed elsewhere (Atkins 1966; Center for the Study of Drug Development 1978).

Ethical preoccupation with this type of surgical or medical practice slowly gained ground with the advent in 1940–1950 of progress in therapeutic medicine, availability of new drugs, the contribution of new ancillary techniques to surgery, and the parallel development of methods of evaluation of new treatments which were also gradually extended to old untested treatments. This was accompanied by a slow awakening to the fact that the use of an untested treatment is unethical. As a result, from 1950 to 1977, the Halsted radical operation dropped from 77% to 20% of all cancer operations, while the modified radical operation, a much more limited operation during the same period, rose from 5% to 60%. These 27 years inaugurated a trend which has continued in accentuated form until today: the change in attitude is the result of a series of controlled clinical trials, based on the randomization of patients between the prevalent operation at each period with a less extensive operation. Each step was illustrated by a discussion of the ethical permissibility of exchanging a traditional for a far less mutilating surgical procedure. Since it has now become apparent that surgical removal of the tumor in breast cancer improves the prognosis, insofar as ulceration of the skin and the thoracic wall is prevented, but probably does not otherwise affect the survival (Tagnon 1986), the very considerable benefit to the patient of this evolution is the improvement in the quality of life and the reduction of the psychological shock from the dreadful mutilation of the extensive operation. This example illustrates the importance of the positive as opposed to the restraining effect of ethical principles. The ethical obligation arose in this example from an obligation to respect the quality of life as well as the ultimate survival result.

We have discussed in another publication (Tagnon 1984) the different situations which justify ethically the trial of new forms of treatment and shall not repeat it here. A confident reliance on a sterile tradition is a disservice to the patient and represents an unethical attitude.

Randomized Trials

Useful discussions of the ethical aspects of randomization are available in Atkins (1966) and also in Gehan (1978), Peto (1978) and Cochrane (1979). The essential role of randomization for the comparison of two treatments is evident when the new treatment is only slightly superior (or inferior) to the standard treatment. In this situation an unbiased evaluation can only be obtained by randomization. This is unnecessary when the new treatment is clearly superior to the traditional one: an example is given by penicillin compared with arsenicals in the treatment of syphilis.

Use of Placebo

Other ethical issues are represented by the use of placebo in the control arm of a comparative trial: the control treatment in such a trial is represented by the best available standard treatment of the disease under study. It is not permissible ethically to deprive a fraction of patients with potentially lethal or irreversibly invalidating diseases of an effective treatment. Therefore, the use of placebo as control is prohibited except under certain conditions, for instance, in research on the treatment of pain when this is not too severe and not associated with a disabling disease. It is well known that a placebo may be an efficacious treatment of certain types of pain in certain patients and this fact is a justification for its use. Finally, placebo plays an important role as control treatment when there is a strong suspicion that a treatment has a deleterious effect on the evolution of the disease for which it is used. The use of placebo may then eliminate a toxic treatment from medical practice. The use of placebo is necessary and ethically acceptable also as a control treatment in the study of adjuvant therapy in the form of chemotherapy or radiotherapy administered after the local treatment of the primary tumour.

Adjuvant Treatment

An adjuvant treatment is justified for tumours in which the primary treatment is notoriously insufficient to cure a majority of the patients. This is the case for breast cancer patients, the majority of whom eventually die of their disease, regardless of the type of primary treatment they receive (Mueller et al. 1978). But adjuvant treatment does not seem justified for tumours which are curable by the primary treatment or whose rare recurrences are easily and effectively treated when they appear: this is the case for testicular tumours at all stages. Adjuvant chemotherapy has unpleasant and potentially toxic side effects which should not be inflicted without a clear necessity and the definite hope that the patients will benefit from it. Thus adjuvant treatment consists of drugs or therapeutic procedures which have proved effective in producing regressions of established metastases of the tumour under study. For instance, the adjuvant treatment of breast cancer consists of the administration of either melphalan or the combination endoxan-methotrexate-5-fluorouracil with or without tamoxifen, because each of these two treatments is effective in the treatment of established metastatic breast disease. Untested innovative chemotherapy has no place in a programme of adjuvant therapy.

Protocol Adherence

Granted that the randomized controlled trial is more ethical there are a few questions in need of an answer. For instance, what is to be done when moderately strong, but not decisive, evidence begins to emerge in the course of the trial in favour of one treatment? Should one stop the comparative trial? Actually the investigators are not supposed to know the partial results collected during the course of the trial. On the other hand, few physicians would accept to continue giving a new treatment without having information on its favourable or unfavourable effects. The way out of this difficulty is to appoint a small committee of competent physicians not participating in the trial, but having access to the results at any time during the trial. They are given the task of ruling that the trial be continued or interrupted.

However, stopping a trial before a statistically significant result is obtained, and on the basis of a trend which could be reversed with a continuation of the trial, is not an ethically indifferent decision. The lack of a firm conclusion will lead to new trials and the involvement of more patients receiving an untested treatment. There are deplorable examples of such a chain of events (Chalmers et al. 1977), confirming the ethical obligations, with some restrictions, to conduct a comparative trial to a firm conclusion with the smallest possible number of patients.

Informed Consent

The Code of Federal Regulations (1978) entitled Protection of Human Subjects makes informed consent mandatory for all recipients or prospective recipients of DHEW (Department of Health, Education and Welfare, USA). In this area, the physician has no choice and should obey the law. However, there is no agreement among clinical investigators on the significance and value of informed consent. Patient care in a controlled clinical trial which benefits the individual patient does not, in my opinion, require a different relationship between doctor and patient than the one prevalent in ordinary medical practice; or informed consent should also be mandatory for any treatment administered in ordinary private or institutional practice. A less authoritarian and more confiding relationship is gaining acceptance in modern practice: the patients' agreement to any treatment should be informally obtained and the results explained to the patient in the course of the treatment. All novel treatments should be administered after consultation, which need not be formal, with experienced colleagues: this is true for ordinary practice and is realized by the very nature of the controlled clinical trials, which are almost always carried out by groups of clinicians. The protocol of treatment is a production of the group and the result of a group consultation: this is an additional guarantee to the patient, who should be informed of this fact. The group discussion includes ethical consideration and the final decision on the type of treatment cannot be carried out without the approval of the Ethical Committee of the hospital. These guarantees exceed those provided in the ordinary practice of medicine.

The Medical Research Council (1962) has published an excellent and short report on the responsibility in investigations on human subjects. This report also discussed the ethical and legal implications of procedures applied to an individual when not of potential benefit to him or her. It correctly points out that the benefit to humanity or posterity would afford no defence in the event of legal proceedings. There is some question in my mind whether informed consent, if obtained in this situation, makes this type of procedure ethically acceptable and whether an individual's consent gives permission to the investigator to carry out an experiment not of potential benefit to the patient. The report of the Medical Research Council suggests that it does. However, I think that if the procedure is dangerous or potentially disabling, informed consent does not relieve the investigator of his or her responsibility. Therefore, particular attention should be paid to the possible consequences of procedures not of direct benefit to the individual and abstention is advised when there is the least doubt about the consequences. The Medical Research Council does not take a firm stand on the question of informed consent. It adopts the common sense attitude that good medical practice implies a frank and open discussion of the treatment with the patient whether the treatment is experimental or not.

Other discussions on informed consent can be summarized as follows: Peto (1978) says of informed consent that "it may serve a useful purpose in warding off American lawyers, but in less litigious countries, it is not necessary unless the doctor concerned feels it to be so". Zelen (1979) thinks that if the patient has to be informed of the choice of randomization of the treatment he or she receives, he or she may interpret this as a "treatment by a computer". The patient's physician knows that randomization is ethical only if the physician believes that all treatments under study are potentially equally effective, but finds it difficult to tell the patient that he or she does not know which treatment is best. For these and other reasons Zelen thinks that "there is a serious concern that the federal regulations governing informed patient consent may be unrealistic in practice". He proposes a new way to plan randomized clinical trials. The original article should be read for the details of this new method, which does not directly concern our ethical preoccupation.

Other views on informed consent are expressed by Curran (1979) and Fost (1979).

My position is that the physician should evaluate the amount of information each individual patient can tolerate and how much responsibility in the decision the patient is able to assume without excessive anxiety and fear. Whatever the patient cannot assume should be taken by the physician him- or herself. In other words, the emotional impact of decisions about disease and treatment should not be transferred too lightly from the physician to the patient under the pretext of obtaining informed consent. The impact should be shared, and the physician's participation should be greater whenever the patient's emotional conformation lessens the possibilities of participating. This duty is exacting for the doctor but to be a physician is to accept such obligations. There are physicians of great professional competence but unable themselves emotionally to withstand the distress of their patients. These physicians should probably not participate in controlled clinical trials. Obviously, when the law or an administrative regulation requires informed consent in clinical trials, the physician has no choice and should obey the regulation.

Conclusion

The introduction of controlled clinical trials on a large scale in the past 20, and especially the past 10, years represents a revolution in clinical investigation and has altered considerably the study of clinical pharmacology and the mode of introduction of new methods of treatment. This has been striking, particularly in therapeutic oncology, but it has affected all sections of medical practice. As a result, there has developed an increasing interest in the ethical problems associated with this type of clinical investigation (Fried 1974). This is certainly a welcome development, but one may wonder why such ethical preoccupation was less prevalent in the practice of medicine before or outside controlled clinical trials. In the office or hospital practice of medicine where no research is carried out, the opportunities for ethical infractions could be more numerous than in the practice of a group of physicians carrying out a controlled clinical trial following a carefully prepared protocol and able to watch each other in open discussion. Certainly, the honest but isolated physician, by the very fact of his or her isolation, encounters less opposition to the administration of useless, if not harmful, medication than if he or she were in a group. I am not here indicting the private practice of medicine, but just mentioning that probably patients have never enjoyed as much protection and good care based on the science of medicine as the patients entered in clinical trials. Therefore, the ethical preoccupation with these trials is quite legitimate, but a similar preoccupation should be extended to the other forms of medical practice with the same interests and passions that are addressed to the controlled clinical trials, whatever the method of control is.

Clinical trials continue to be discussed in the medical literature. Some recent examples are available. For instance, castration without consent for prostatic cancer in elderly men entered into a protocol comparing castration with other treatment is extensively discussed in several letters published in the *British Medical Journal* (Hall et al. 1986). Others wonder whether informed consent influences therapeutic outcome (Dahan 1986). On the other hand, the admonition has been heeded that ethical considerations should not be confined to clinical trials of new treatments but should be observed by practising physicians in their daily routine. Administration of an unproved treatment may sometimes qualify as an unethical procedure. If so, homeopathy and other semi-magic procedures now extensively employed by the medical profession may fall under the stigma of being not only ineffective but also unethical. The appearance of a new subgroup of specialists called "medical ethicists" on the scene of medical consultation practice will further complicate matters. A question may well be: what kind of training does a physician need to be a "medical ethicist"?

Medical ethics is not a new invention. It is just the old morality applied to a situation – medical research – which is in fast evolution and presents us with puzzling circumstances. Among these are the controlled clinical trials, but they are less puzzling than many others like abortion, the new genetics, euthanasia, etc. We oncologists are lucky, our problem is relatively simple (Clouser 1975; Dunphy 1976).

References

Atkins H (1966) Conduct of a controlled clinical trial. Br Med J 2: 377

Center for the Study of Drug Development (1978) Report August 1978. University of Rochester Medical Center, Rochester, New York

Chalmers TC, Matta RJ, Smith H, Kunzler AM (1977) Evidence favouring the use of anticoagulants in the hospital phase of acute myocardial infarction. N Engl J Med 302: 351

Clouser KD (1975) Medical ethics: some uses, abuses and limitations. N Engl J Med 293: 384–387

Cochrane AL, St Léger AS, Sweetnam P (1979) Letter to the Editor. Br Med J 1: 486

Code of Federal Regulations (1978) 45 CFR 46 and certain other related laws and regulations on protection of human subjects, revised 11 January. PPR Reports, Department of Health, Education and Welfare, Washington

Curran WJ (1979) Reasonableness and randomization in clinical trials: fundamental law and governmental regulation. N Engl J Med 300: 1273–1275

Dahan R, Caulin C, Figea L, Kanis JA, Caulin F, Segrestaa JM (1986) Does informed consent influence therapeutic outcome? A clinical trial of the hypnotic activity of placebo in patients admitted to hospital. Br Med J 293: 363–364

Dunphy JE (1976) On caring for the patient with cancer. N Engl J Med 295: 313

Fost N (1979) Consent as a barrier to research. N Engl J Med 300: 1272–1273

Fried C (1974) Medical experimentation: personal integrity and social policy. North Holland, Amsterdam

Gehan A (1978) Comparative clinical trials with historical controls: a statistician's view. Biomedicine (special issue) 28: 13–18

Hall RR, Smith PH (1986) Correspondence. Br Med J 293: 389–390

Kant I (1848) Critique de la raison pratique. Lagrange, Paris, pp 58, 71

Medical Research Council Report (1962) Responsibility in investigations on human subjects. Cmnd. 2382. Medical Research Council, London, pp 21–25

Mueller CB, Ames F, Anderson GD (1978) Breast cancer in 3558 women: age as a significant determinant in the rate of dying and causes of death. Surgery 83: 123–133

Peto R (1978) Clinical trial methodology. Biomedicine (special issue) 28: 24–35

Subcommittee on Unorthodox Therapies, American Society for Clinical Oncology (1983) Ineffective cancer therapy: a guide for the lay person. J Clin Oncol 1: 154–163

Tagnon H (1984) Ethical considerations in controlled clinical trials. In: Buyse ME, Staquet MJ, Sylvester R (eds) Cancer clinical trials: methods and practice. Oxford University Press, Oxford, pp 14–25

Tagnon H (1986) Some changing concepts on the natural history of human mammary cancer and their effect on diagnosis and treatment. Eur J Cancer Clin Oncol 22: 123–128

Zelen M (1979) A new design for randomized clinical trials. N Engl J Med 300: 1242–1245

Treatment of Cancer of Different Organs

Cancer of the Head and Neck Region

G. B. Snow

Definition

Nearly every neoplastic disease may have a primary or secondary manifestation in the head and neck. Within this chapter for obvious reasons only the most frequent tumours occurring primarily in the head and neck will be discussed: squamous cell carcinomas originating in the mucous membranes. For the rarer tumour types the reader is referred to recent or classic books or reviews: for salivary gland tumours to Eneroth (1964), Conley (1975) and Spiro (1986); for non-Hodgkin's lymphoma in the upper respiratory and digestive tracts to Banfi et al. (1970), Brugere et al. (1975) and Robbins et al. (1985); for mucosal melanomas in the head and neck to Snow and van der Waal (1986 a); and for soft tissue sarcomas to Weber et al. (1986).

Epidemiology – Risk Factors

Squamous cell carcinoma can occur anywhere in the mucous membranes of the head and neck. In the Western world the following sites are most commonly involved in order of decreasing frequency: larynx, oral cavity and (oro- and hypo-) pharynx. The disease is more common in males than in females, generally with a peak incidence in the 7th decade of life. The sex ratio, however, varies considerably for the various sites. Smoking and drinking are generally considered aetiological factors, but their impact varies for the different sites. Also the patterns in incidence and mortality figures over time differ for the various sites. The two most frequently involved sites will be discussed in more detail.

Both cancer of the nasal cavity and paranasal sinuses and of the nasopharynx are rare, at least in the Western hemisphere, and their epidemiological characteristics are different from the picture which has been drawn above. Nasopharyngeal carcinoma is among the most common cancers in the Chinese. The Epstein-Barr virus (EBV) has been implicated as a factor in the aetiology of nasopharyngeal carcinoma (Pearson et al. 1983). For further information on these two cancers the reader is referred to Batsakis' book on tumours of the head and neck (1979).

Cancer of the Larynx

Cancer of the larynx occurs mainly in men. It rarely afflicts females and the sex ratio is one of the highest among malignant tumours. Cancer of the larynx rarely develops among men who do not smoke (Wynder et al. 1976) whereas non-smokers are a small proportion among the patients with laryngeal cancer (Rothman et al. 1980), implying that smoking plays a significant role in the aetiology of laryngeal cancer. In most countries there is a trend towards an increase of laryngeal cancer incidence and mortality rates, paralleling to a certain extent those for lung cancer, which can be safely related to increasing tobacco consumption (Tuyns 1982). This may indicate that smoking is also responsible for the increase in laryngeal cancer. However, the increase is much less important for larynx than for lung cancer. There is increasing evidence that alcohol consumption is also an important aetiological factor (Ramadan et al. 1982; Tuyns 1982). The considerable variation in geographical distribution within Europe – high incidence and mortality rates in the south versus low rates in the northwest – may be correlated with patterns of alcohol consumption, particularly wine, rather than tobacco smoking. In this regard it appears important to note that in southern Europe supraglottic cancer of the larynx is more common than glottic cancer, whereas the reverse is true for northwestern Europe.

Oral Cancer

Cancer of the oral cavity too is a disease of the elderly. The mobile tongue is the most frequently involved site followed by the floor of the mouth. In most parts of the world oral cancer is uncommon, with the exception of India, where the figure reaches 40% of all malignant tumours and this appears to be associated with the habit of betel nut chewing with tobacco. In the western part of the world it has been shown that both heavy smokers and heavy drinkers run a much higher risk of developing oral cancer than individuals who never smoked or drinked (Graham 1977). There seems to be a synergism between heavy smoking and heavy drinking. However, in the developed countries the incidence of oral cancer has been declining steadily over the past 4–5 decades, when cigarette smoking and alcohol consumption have increased (Pindborg 1980). This has been associated with an impressive change in the male-female ratio. In the cancer registry of the Manchester area for instance, the male-female ratio for tongue cancer was 7.8 to 1 in the 1932–1935 period, while this figure has decreased to 1.7 to 1 in the 1960–1969 period. This change was mainly due to a decrease of oral cancer in men (Easson and Palmer 1976). The role of a number of other aetiological factors has recently been reviewed by Langdon (1985). It should be noted, however, that in many patients with oral cancer, especially in females, none of the known aetiological factors appear to be present, which makes the development of oral cancer anything but completely understood.

Premalignant Lesions

Both carcinoma of the oral cavity and carcinoma of the larynx may be associated with or preceded by lesions which carry a serious risk of malignant change. These so-called precancerous lesions may precede the development of carcinoma by months or by years.

In the mouth these are leucoplakia and erythroplakia. The WHO has recommended that the term leucoplakia should carry no histological connotation, meaning a white patch in the oral mucosa that cannot be removed by rubbing and cannot be classified clinically and pathologically as any other diagnosable disease. Leucoplakia is not uncommon (Banoczy 1982). The onset is generally after the 40th year, with the peak incidence lying above the age of 50 years. The development of carcinoma from leucoplakia has been observed in somewhat older age groups. Many factors have been reported to play a role in the aetiology of oral leucoplakia. The overall risk that oral leucoplakia develops into carcinoma has been reported as between 1% and 6%. The malignant potential, however, depends on many factors, such as type and site of the leucoplakia. Although leucoplakia is most common at the commissures and the buccal mucosa, leucoplakia of the tongue and the floor of the mouth (in women) and of the lip (in men) carry the highest risk of malignant transformation. Of the three clinical types of oral leucoplakia – simple homogeneous leucoplakia, verrucous leucoplakia and erosive (speckled) leucoplakia – the erosive type bears a much greater risk of malignant transformation than the two others. Erythroplakia is a much rarer condition than leucoplakia, but has a much greater malignant potential than leucoplakia (Shafer and Waldron 1975).

A lot of uncertainty and controversy still exist about the premalignant lesions of the laryngeal mucosa. These lesions are still being described by a myriad of names, the most common of which are: leucoplakia, pachydermia, (hyper-) keratosis and dysplasia. Clinical and histological terms are used side by side. The highest incidence is found in men in the 5th and 6th decades. Smoking appears to be of aetiological importance. These lesions are almost exclusively localized on the vocal cords, the anterior third being most commonly involved; they rarely arise from the supra- or subglottic regions. Proper diagnosis is considerably hindered by the lack of an internationally accepted histopathological classification. Kleinsasser (1963) was one of the first to propose a classification based on the degree of atypical changes of the epithelium: class I simple squamous cell hyperplasia, class II squamous cell hyperplasia with atypia and class III carcinoma in situ. In North America, however, the classification proposed at the Centennial Conference on Laryngeal Cancer (Miller and Batsakis 1974) is usually used: keratosis, keratosis with atypia and carcinoma in situ. Others base their classification also on the degree of dysplasia (Hellquist et al. 1982; Michaels 1984). Although these classifications use different nomenclatures, they all distinguish three categories, which more or less coincide. Kleinsasser's classification has been demonstrated to carry prognostic significance: with increasing class there is a higher risk of malignant change (Olde Kalter et al. 1986). In routine histopathological practice, however, problems are encountered in the use of these classifications, serious interobserver and intraobserver inconsistencies in diagnoses being reported. There is a great need, therefore, for objective diagnostical methods like photometry (Hellquist et al. 1984) or morphometry (Olde Kalter et al. 1985), which may improve the reproducibility of classification.

Multiple Primary Tumours

The reported incidence of multiple primary tumours in head and neck cancer patients is high: 10%–35% (Healy et al. 1976; Gluckman et al. 1980; Hordijk and de Jong 1983). The great majority of second primary tumours occur in the respiratory tract and the upper digestive tract, including the oesophagus. They usually occur metachronously (diagnosed 6 months or more after the diagnosis of the index tumour) rather than synchronously (diagnosed at the same time as the index tumour, or within a 6-month period). The incidence and location of the second primary tumours is related to the location of the index tumour. In laryngeal cancer the second primary frequently appears in the respiratory tract, particularly the lung (de Vries et al. 1986a), while with index tumours of the upper digestive tract the second tumour is relatively frequent also in the upper digestive tract (Pasche et al. 1981). This might be explained by common aetiological factors, such as alcohol and tobacco (Wynder et al. 1969; Moore

1971). It might be that genetic factors are of importance as well. In this regard de Vries et al. (1986 b) demonstrated that head and neck cancer patients lacking immunoglobulin allotype Km(1) are more susceptible to the development of new cancers.

Wagenfeld et al. (1980; 1981) have reported a higher rate of multiple primary tumours in patients with supraglottic carcinoma of the larynx as compared with patients with glottic carcinoma. Similarly de Vries et al. (1986 c) observed that the incidence of second primary tumours in patients with oral cancer varies for the various sites of the index tumour within the mouth. Furthermore, de Vries et al. (1986 a) found that male patients with a glottic carcinoma have a statistically higher chance of developing a second primary than their female counterparts.

Histopathology

Histological Grading

It is traditionally held that the more differentiated the squamous cell cancer, the less likely it is to recur locally after treatment and to metastasize. An overall impression of the degree of differentiation is the method commonly used by pathologists (Michaels 1984). The assessment is based on the least differentiated parts of the tumour and three categories are distinguished: well-differentiated, moderately differentiated and poorly differentiated squamous cell carcinoma. For carcinoma of the larynx support for the validity of this method has been provided by McGavran et al. (1961). However, the method has serious shortcomings: it carries a large subjective element and it lacks quantitation. The well-known Broders system (Broders 1920) based on the counting of differentiated cells meets part of this criticism, but is impracticable. More refined modifications have been introduced (Jakobsson et al. 1973), but have not found wide acceptance by pathologists. Regardless of the grading system used, one should realize that there may be differences in degree of differentiation from place to place in the same tumour and that therefore the biopsy may not be representative for the whole tumour. The value of histological grading for predicting prognosis and planning treatment has remained limited.

Spread

At the Primary Site

It is not uncommon for squamous cell carcinomas of the head and neck and particularly those in the oral cavity to spread along perineural spaces (Carter et al. 1979). The site of the primary tumour is of major importance in determining the pattern of perineural spread. Once within perineural spaces tumour cells can invade axially in either direction. This may have important surgical implications. However, clinical features suggesting perineural infiltration are by no means always found. Maddox (1984) has reported that patients with a carcinoma of the mobile tongue demonstrating perineural spread are at high risk of harbouring occult nodal metastases in the neck.

A feature that has not received much attention is invasion of the microcirculation. According to a study by Poleksic and Kalwaic (1978), this is not uncommon in head and neck squamous cell carcinoma. These authors have demonstrated that microvascular invasion by carcinoma cells correlates with an increased incidence of lymph node metastases. If discovered in the initial biopsy, this may be a reason to plan more extensive treatment than would be indicated by the clinical stage alone.

When a squamous cell carcinoma invades underlying bone or cartilage, this is done by a biphasic process (Pittam and Carter 1982). At first the tumour plays an indirect role, acting mainly by stimulating local osteoclasts. It is only after the osteoclastic response wanes that carcinoma cells themselves invade the bone.

Lymph Node Metastasis

Taking into account that accurate histological examination of nodes is far more meaningful than nodal palpability in predicting prognosis, it is surprising that there is little uniformity in the way neck dissection specimens are examined by pathologists. In reporting the histological findings, it is important to mention the number and level and/or site of involved nodes and the presence or absence of extranodal spread (capsular rupture), as these factors may influence the need for further therapy.

The presence or absence of extranodal spread is of particular importance. The incidence of extranodal spread as reported in two large series of patients (Michaeu et al. 1978; Snow et al. 1982) is strikingly similar: 55% and 53.8%. Nevertheless, histological judgement in this regard may at times be difficult. In general it has been thought that extranodal spread is limited to large nodes with clinical fixation. However Cachin et al. (1979), Johnson et al. (1981) and Snow et al. (1982) have demonstrated that extranodal spread does occur in a substantial percentage of small nodes as well. This appears to be in agreement with the demonstration by Toker (1963) that primary arrest of tumour emboli within the nodal capsule or juxtacapsular tissues rather than in the subcapsular sinus may lead to extranodal spread at a comparatively early phase in the progress of the disease.

Natural History

Spread at the primary site is dictated by local anatomy and each anatomical site has its own peculiar spread patterns. Squamous cell carcinoma may extend superficially widely beneath intact mucosa. Invasion of muscle is a common feature and tumour may spread along muscle and fascial planes for a surprising distance from the visible and palpable lesion. Perineural and intravascular spread are not uncommon, as discussed under "At the Primary Site" above. Bone and cartilage invasion are usually a late event.

Squamous cell carcinomas of the head and neck have a proclivity to metastasize to regional lymph nodes rather than to spread haematogenously. It is rare to observe distant metastases in patients who never suffered from nodal metastasis in the neck. However, it is not uncommon for patients with nodal metastasis to develop distant metastases and then usually at a later stage.

The incidence of lymph node metastasis depends mainly on the site and size of the primary tumour. Degree of histological differentiation appears to play a role as well (McGavran et al. 1961). It is evident from clinical practice that lymph nodes quite often appear to be a very fertile soil for tumour growth. Everybody involved in head and neck oncology is only too familiar with patients presenting with a very small or even unknown primary tumour and huge neck node metastasis. Also, tumour deposits in lymph nodes may have a surprisingly high growth rate. This is well demonstrated by patients with an initially clinically negative neck who, after treatment of the primary tumour only, may develop nodal metastases of substantial size between two follow-up visits that lie only a few weeks apart.

The filter and barrier function of lymph nodes usually appears to be effective in the initial stage as lymphatic spread initially is generally limited to the first echelon of lymph nodes. The distribution of lymphatic metastases is for the most part explicable in mechanical and anatomical terms. Lindberg (1972) has carefully mapped the cervical metastases from the various sites within the head and neck. As a node is increasingly replaced by metastatic tumour, the local lymphatic flow will be distorted, reflected and perhaps reversed, directing new lymph-borne tumour cells to fresh nodes. The cancerous node will itself act as a focus for further "tertiary" spread (Carter 1976). This can occur via lymphatic vessels and via the blood stream, not only through the large communciations between the lymphatic and blood systems at the base of the neck but also through small lymphaticovenous shunts or through full-thickness invasion and penetration of the internal jugular vein by direct spread from adjacent nodal metastases (Djalilian et al. 1973).

It is not surprising that the rate of distant metastases correlates more with the appearance of cervical node metastasis than with the T-stage (Berger and Fletcher 1971; Merino et al. 1977). Snow et al. (1986b) found that 80% of distant metastases became manifest within 2 years after the appearance of nodal metastasis. The lungs are the most frequent site of distant metastases, accounting for 45%, followed by the skeletal system with approximately 25% (Snow et al. 1986b).

Failure to eradicate the disease above the clavicles is regarded as the major cause of death in patients with squamous cell carcinoma of the head and neck. Nearly all local and regional recurrences manifest themselves within 2 years from the date of initial treatment. However, with the employment of a treatment policy consisting of surgery followed by radiation therapy in patients at high risk for local/regional recurrence, a changing pattern of failure is being observed (Vikram 1984). Many studies report a decrease of local and regional failure rates by this type of combined therapy (Arriagada et al. 1983; Bartelink et al. 1983; Goffinet et al. 1984), but observe that this is not reflected in a proportionate increase of 5-year survival rates. As fewer patients die from uncontrolled disease above the clavicles, more are exposed to the risk of disseminated disease below the clavicles and to the appearance of second primary tumours.

Staging

In Europe the TNM classification of malignant tumours, as recommended by the International Union Against Cancer (Union Internationale contre le Cancer, UICC 1987), is used. In North America the Manual for Staging of Cancer, as developed by the American Joint Committee on Cancer (AJCC 1983), is employed, which makes use of the same symbols: T, N and M. In the past these two classification systems have differed substantially. The differences in the recommendations of UICC and AJCC, however, are gradually decreasing. With the appearance of the latest UICC classification (1987) the definitions of T-categories have become virtually identical in the UICC and AJCC classifications for all sites, only small differences remaining. Also, the definitions of the N-categories, which have been so different in the past, are now almost identical.

Staging of the Primary Tumour (T)

It appears superfluous to tabulate the T-staging of the numerous head and neck sites, as the UICC booklet and the AJCC manual are so readily available to everybody. It seems of value, however, briefly to comment on the staging procedures. In the UICC booklet it is stated that for the purpose of classification it is necessary to distinguish mandatory investigations from those which add refinement to the knowledge of the extent of disease. For all sites therefore, the minimum requirements for assessing the primary tumour are listed. The AJCC follows a similar policy, but adds to the procedures considered essential for staging a number of possibly useful procedures. Within this last category computed tomography (CT) scans are repeatedly mentioned. In the past 5 years, however, CT has been shown to be a valuable adjunct to the assessment of the extent of advanced primary tumours at various sites, such as the larynx (Hoover et al. 1984; Gerritsen et al. 1986), pharynx (Muraki et al. 1983) and paranasal sinuses (Som 1982; Tiwari et al. 1986). It is felt, therefore, that it would be appropriate to include CT scans in the investigations considered mandatory for staging of squamous cell carcinoma at the above-mentioned sites in the head and neck.

Staging of Regional Lymph Nodes (N)

Both UICC and AJCC attach importance to the size and number of involved nodes. The only difference remaining between the two classification systems regards the significance that is being attached to bilateral or contralateral nodal metastases. The parameter fixation has been dropped from the latest UICC classification because of its subjective nature. It is unfortunate that the level of involvement of cervical lymph nodes is not incorporated in the UICC and AJCC staging systems, as it has been shown that the level of nodal involvement has prognostic importance. UICC has even abandoned in its latest 1987 classification its former recommendation to use four levels of involvement of cervical lymph nodes. AJCC recommends only to indicate regional lymph nodes involved on diagrams.

Assessment of the status of the neck nodes is still based on palpation. The palpability of a lymph node depends on its location, consistency, size and type of neck. In a neck of average size and in the hands of an experienced examiner the lower limit of palpability is approximately 0.5 cm in a superficial area such as the submental and submandibular area and 1 cm in a deeper area (Sako et al. 1964). Therefore nodes containing small deposits of carcinoma may not be clinically palpable. On the contrary, not all enlarged nodes contain metastatic deposits. Moreover, large interobserver variations have been reported. It is not surprising, therefore, that the overall error in assessing the presence or absence of cervical lymph node metastasis is reported in the range of 20%–30% (Sako et. al. 1964; Spiro et al. 1974; Ali et al. 1985).

Fine needle aspiration cytology (Zajicek 1974) is an effective technique for establishing a tentative histological diagnosis in patients presenting with a neck mass without an obvious primary tumour in the head and neck, but this method is of little use in the initial workup of patients presenting with a primary squamous cell carcinoma of the upper air and food passages.

There is increasing evidence that CT scan of cervical lymph nodes is superior to the clinical examination, particularly in detecting occult metastases (Friedman et al. 1984; Stevens et al. 1985). However, the gain is modest and it is questionable whether the costs justify the results. More importantly CT scan can detect abnormal nodes beyond the range of physical examination, e.g. retropharyngeal (Mancuso et al. 1983).

Staging of Distant Metastases (M)

The minimum requirements for assessment of M categories according to the UICC classification are: clinical examination and radiography. No further specification as to the type of radiography is given. The AJCC only suggest a chest roentgenogram. In most cases investigations to be carried out for the detection of distant metastases can indeed be limited. However, it is advisable to screen thoroughly for the presence of distant metastases in lungs, skeletal system, and liver by means of CT scan of the lungs, bone scan, blood chemistries and liver scan in patients who are at high risk of harbouring distant metastases (see under "N-Factors" below).

Prognosis – Prognostic Factors

Host Factors

Age

Age may have an influence on stage. Easson and Palmer (1976) found that older patients have a higher risk of presenting with stage IV cancers of the mouth. This may mean that older patients simply delay longer in seeking advice. More importantly the same authors observed a definite influence of age on response to treatment in patients with stage I cancer of the tongue even after applying an age correction factor.

Sex

Langdon (1985) found that survival in females with oral cancer is very much better than in males and this has been confirmed by other authors (Easson and Palmer 1976). It is intruiging why this should be. Langdon (1985) could not demonstrate in his series that this is so because females present with smaller lesions, at an earlier age, with an excess of tumours at favourable sites, or with more highly differentiated tumours, and he suggests that hormonal, genetic or immunological differences could account for a better prognosis in females. Similarly Lederman (1971) has recognised a better prognosis in females with laryngeal cancer as compared with their male counterparts to such a degree that he advocated primary radiotherapy for all female patients irrespective of TNM staging.

Immunological Competence

The immune reactivity of head and neck cancer patients has been studied extensively in the past 15 years (Katz 1983; Wolf 1984). From the data it appears that cell-mediated immunity is seriously affected in these patients, as demonstrated by frequent unresponsiveness to dinitrochlorobenzene (DNCB), low T-cell numbers, diminished blastogenic responsiveness of lymphocytes and defects in the migratory capacity of macrophages. Although many investigators have found correlations between deficiencies in cellular immunity and prognosis, there have been reports to the contrary. In any event, assays of cellular immunity have found extremely limited clinical application.

It has been questioned whether the impairments in host defence mechanisms are direct reflections of tumour-host interaction. Lundy et al. (1975) have demonstrated that cell-mediated immune functions are severely impaired in individuals with alcohol abuse. Similarly Brookes and Clifford (1981) found a highly significant correlation between nutritional status and defective cellular immunity. It is well known that many head and neck cancer patients are alcohol abusers. Also malnutrition is a very common accompanying condition in head and neck cancer patients. Brookes and Clifford (1981) suggest that nutrition deficiency is of major prognostic value and that defects in immune competence are secondary phenomena. Also, it is a general clincial experience that patients who have lost considerable weight over a relatively short period carry a bad prognosis.

Tumour Factors

T-Factors

The site of the primary tumour within the head and neck and even within the same organ is of importance. This is well illustrated for patients with cancer of the larynx: patients with supraglottic carcinoma in general carry a worse prognosis than patients with glottic carcinoma.

It is generally assumed that the size of the primary tumour determines prognosis. It may well be, however, that size in itself is not all that important. Hibbert et al. (1983), for instance, found in their series of patients with oral cancer that the size of the primary tumour did not seem to affect 5-year survival, except inasmuch as the larger tumours resulted in a higher rate of cervical metastasis and in this way affected prognosis.

The degree of histological differentiation may have prognostic significance, as has been demonstrated for instance in carcinoma of the piriform sinus (Martin et al. 1980). Furthermore, lymphocytic or inflammatory infiltrate in or around tumour has been shown to correlate with a favourable prognosis in carcinomas of the larynx and hypopharynx (Bennett et al. 1971).

N-Factors

It is generally recognised that the status of the cervical lymph nodes is the single most important prognostic factor in squamous cell carcinoma of the head and neck (Spiro et al. 1974; Kalnins et al. 1977; Cachin et al. 1979). The following clinical parameters of nodal metastasis are of importance: size, number, fixation and level. The latter two are not incorporated in the UICC or AJCC staging systems (see "Staging of Regional Lymph Nodes" above). Spiro et al. (1974) and Stell et al. (1983) have shown that node level is dictated by the primary tumour and that it is a highly significant predictor of survival.

Clinical assessment of the status of the neck is far from accurate, as has been discussed under "Staging of Regional Lymph Nodes" above. It is not surprising, therefore, that retrospective clinicopathological analyses of large series of patients who underwent a radical neck dissection have demonstrated that histological parameters are of much more prognostic significance than clinical parameters (Bennett et al. 1971; Noone et al. 1974; Shah et al. 1976; Sessions 1976; Kalnins et al. 1977; Zoller et al. 1978; Cachin et al. 1979; Johnson et al. 1981; Snow et al. 1982; Grandi et al. 1985). Extranodal spread (capsular rupture) and number of histologically positive nodes are of most prognostic significance in regard to failure in the neck and failure at distant sites. Snow et al. (1986b) have demonstrated that patients who were found pathologically to have four or more positive nodes and extranodal spread have a greater than 60% likelihood of developing distant metastases. Likewise Vikram et al. (1984) have shown that the pathological extent of nodal metastasis at neck dissection is the most sensitive prognostic indicator for distant metastases. These authors attach particular importance to the level of nodal involvement in the neck.

Screening of Asymptomatic Disease

Mass Screening

Although the conditions for the early detection of cancer in the upper aerodigestive tract are extremely favourable, many patients present with advanced disease. It appears that in general the reasons for this are tumour and patient-related rather than physician related. Screening examinations thus might lead to more frequent detection of early cancers. Steiner (1984) has carried out endoscopic mass screening in the Federal Republic of Germany, using a 90°-angled magnifying laryngopharyngoscope. While in the overall group the incidence of precancerous lesions in the oral cavity and larynx was 0.4% and the incidence of early cancer 0.2%, in the group of smokers these respective percentages rose to 1.4% and 0.6%. Steiner (1984) concludes that endoscopic screening, when concentrated on high-risk groups such as heavy smokers, is feasible and economically practicable. Sputum cytology does not appear to be a very useful tool for screening of early cancer in the upper aerodigestive tract (Neel et al. 1981a).

Screening for Second Primary Tumours in Patients Presenting with Head and Neck Cancer

The incidence of multiple primary tumours in head and neck cancer patients is high (see "Multiple Primary Tumours" above). As most of these occur in the respiratory tract and the upper digestive tract, panendoscopy (laryngoscopy, nasopharyngoscopy, oesophagoscopy and bronchoscopy) is carried out by most otolaryngologists to search for second primary tumours at the initial workup of head and neck cancer patients. The incidence of simultaneous primary tumours as reported in the literature varies considerably: 2.5% (Atkins et al. 1984), 8.9% (Leipzig et al. 1985), 16% (McGuirt 1982) and 25% (Savary et al. 1984). The panendoscopy is the only source of detection of these tumours in roughly half of the cases. The reported differences in incidence might be related to endoscopic techniques. Savary's group (1984) from Switzerland routinely use vital staining with toluidine blue for screening of early second primary cancer in the pharynx and the oesophagus and indeed find the majority of second primary tumours at these sites regardless of the localisation of the index tumour (see also "Multiple Primary Tumours" above). It is not unlikely, however, that the role of the upper digestive tract as the site of second primary tumours is more important in some of the more southern European countries like Switzerland and France than it is in northwestern Europe and North America, where the lung is more important as the site of second primary tumours, particularly when the index tumour is in the larynx (see also "Multiple Primary Tumours" above). As most of the second primaries in the lung occur metachronously, regular flexible bronchoscopy during follow-up of laryngeal cancer patients could be considered.

Diagnosis of Symptomatic Disease

In Patients Presenting with a Primary Tumour

The investigations required for adequate assessment of the extent of the primary tumour vary for the different sites within the head and neck. For detailed information the reader is referred to the many excellent textbooks in head and neck cancer. The importance of palpation under general anaesthesia in advanced tumours of the oral cavity and oropharynx cannot be overemphasized. Endoscopy and radiography are important at most sites. The value of CT in advanced disease has been discussed under "Staging of the Primary Tumour" above. The role of MRI for the diagnosis of cancer in the head and neck has yet to be determined (Baker 1986). Assessment of the status of the neck has been discussed under "Staging of Regional Lymph Nodes".

A biopsy is taken to establish the diagnosis. As the great majority of lesions are ulcerating, this is easily done by taking a piece of tumour with a forceps. Taking an adequate biopsy from the margin rather than from the necrotic centre of the tumour helps the pathologist to make a proper diagnosis. In the rare case where there is no obvious ulceration, an incisional biopsy is indicated. In general, the biopsy material can be placed in a regular fixative. However, when there is doubt on clinical grounds as to the diagnosis of squamous cell carcinoma, tissue is transported immediately, while fresh, to the laboratory. Special tests can then be carried out, which can differentiate between, for instance, carcinoma and lymphoma.

In Patients with Cervical Nodal Metastases of Unknown Origin

It is important to distinguish between patients who present with nodal metastases in the upper neck and those with cervical nodes in the lower neck. In the first group the primary tumour is very likely to be found within the head and neck, whereas metastases in the supraclavicular fossa more likely originate from a primary tumour below the clavicles.

A complete history and physical examination is performed with emphasis on a thorough otolaryngological examination. If this workup is negative, aspiration cytology of the neck mass is carried out. If metastatic squamous cell carcinoma is found, panendoscopy is performed. As the nasopharynx, tonsil, base of tongue, supraglottic larynx and piriform fossa are noted to be common sites of primary tumours in this situation, special attention is paid to these areas. Palpation under general anaesthesia of the oropharynx is important. All suspicious areas should be biopsied. Selected random biopsies ("blind" biopsies) can be taken from areas of high probability based on the predictibility of lymphatic drainage or on serological evidence (Neel et al. 1981b). When a cytological diagnosis of adenocarcinoma is made, a thyroid scan and a complete radiological evaluation of the lung, the digestive tract and the genitourinary system is carried out.

Open (excisional) biopsy of the neck mass is rarely needed. The most common situation where this is indicated is when the cytology reveals malignancy, but the pathologist is not sure about its nature. The node should be sent while fresh immediately to the laboratory to allow for various techniques to be applied to the tissue (see also "In Patients Presenting with a Primary Tumour" above).

Treatment of metastatic squamous cell carcinoma to the neck of unknown primary usually consists of radical neck dissection followed by radiotherapy including full ports to presumed sites of primary disease in the pharynx from the base of skull to the pharyngeal-oesophageal junction. Patients with metastatic squamous cell carcinoma to the superior portion of the neck have a relatively favourable prognosis: >50% 3 years survival. Patients with metastatic adenocarcinoma in the neck carry a very poor prognosis (Leipzig et al. 1981).

Surgical and Combined Treatment of Locoregional Disease

Firstly, selection of patients will be considered. Management of the primary tumour and that of the neck, although often intimately associated, for reasons of clarity will be discussed separately. Then combined radiation and surgery will be discussed and, finally, complications.

Selection of Patients

During the past decade sophisticated techniques of reconstruction have become available, which allow for repair of almost every defect. Furthermore, head and neck squamous cell carcinoma is, in a small minority, only inoperable on account of its local, regional or distant spread, whereas the mortality rate for major head and neck surgery has steadily declined to 1%–3% (Beahrs 1973; McGuirt et al. 1979). However, when the magnitude of the resection is such that the patient will be left with a functional deficit resulting in a poor future quality of life, the question arises whether the patient is better off left untreated by surgery. An example of this problem is when total removal of the tongue is required to eradicate the disease. No general clues can be given to this problem; the solution should be individualised for each patient, the philosophy and psychology of both patient and doctor playing an important role.

Anaplastic carcinomas usually behave aggressively in a diffuse way and therefore should not be treated surgically but by radiotherapy. This also holds true for most of the poorly differentiated squamous cell carcinomas. Both histological types of tumours, however, are rare in the head and neck. Very rapidly progressing well or moderately differentiated squamous cell carcinomas – also an unusual situation – should probably better not be attacked by surgery as the first modality of treatment.

Finally, of course, are medical contraindications for surgery. Although, in general, biological age has to be taken into account rather than calendar age, it appears from the studies of Williams and Murtagh (1973) and McGuirt et al. (1977) that the age of 80 years marks the limit for major head and neck surgery.

Surgical Management of the Primary Tumour

A detailed account of surgical treatment relative to the site of primary tumours would exceed the scope of this chapter. Certain basic principles of surgical treatment of cancer at the most frequent sites within the head and neck will be discussed. As many excellent textbooks and atlases are available on surgical techniques, these will not be dealt with in detail.

Oral Cancer

This review will be limited to the most frequently involved sites: the mobile tongue and the floor of the mouth. Cancers of the mobile tongue and floor of the mouth particularly may spread easily along submucosal, muscular and neural planes. Except for the small (<1 cm) T_1 lesions with minimal invasion, generous margins should be taken. Westbury (1981) states that a margin of 2 cm in all three dimensions is required for all deeply invasive cancers of the tongue. Byers et al. (1978) emphasize the value of frozen section microscopic studies for the determination of the extent of the surgical margins. The author of this chapter has found electrocoagulation of the tumour before the excision has been very helpful in determining the extent of the lesion (Snow 1984).

For practical reasons management of the primary tumour will be considered first for small tumours, T_1 and T_2, less than 4 cm in greatest diameter, and then for more extensive lesions.

Small Oral Cancer

Small cancers of the mobile tongue, T_1 and T_2, situated anteriorly can be excised readily through the mouth, that is by transoral approach. The defect is usually closed primarily; this does not impair tongue mobility to a great extent, because the floor of the mouth is stretched out. Large superficial defects resulting from excision of minor invasive carcinoma or extensive leucoplakia are resurfaced with a split skin graft (McGregor and McGrouther 1978).

Large Oral Cancer

For large tumours, T_3 and T_4, commando-type surgery is needed. The cosmetic and functional loss which result from this type of surgery naturally increase directly with tumour size. However, surgical techniques of both resection and repair have improved considerably during the past 15 years and have resulted in a considerable reduction in both the functional and cosmetic difficulties which the patient faces after major surgery.

An important point in this regard is the management of the mandible, which is considered in three categories: those with gross invasion where resection is inevitable, those with a degree of involvement and those in whom there is still a measurable distance of several millimetres of normal mucosa between the gross edge of the lesion and the mandible. It has been held that the mandible, although uninvolved by tumour, should be resected in large tumours of the tongue and the floor of the mouth to obtain better access to the primary tumour and to facilitate primary closure. With the availability of adequate procedures of exposure like the mandibular "swing" approach (Spiro et al. 1981) and of the methods of reconstruction discussed below, this view is certainly obsolete. It has also been stated that the lymphatic channels draining the tongue and floor of mouth communicate with the periosteal lymphatics of the mandible and this necessitates resection of bone. This view too is to be discarded since Marchetta et al. (1971) have clearly demonstrated that involvement of the periosteum or underlying bone is by direct extension of tumour and not through periosteal lymphatics. In most patients belonging to the two last categories mentioned above, a more conservative management of the mandible, marginal mandibulectomy, can be considered and indeed has been proven feasible (Guillamondegui and Jesse 1976; Callery et al. 1984).

Many notable advances have been made in the field of reconstructive surgery in the past decade (Daniel and Taylor 1973; McGregor and Morgan 1973; McCraw et al. 1977). For oral lining and replacement of soft tissue loss, reconstructive surgeons today have a wide variety of methods available in their armamentarium, ranging from local (Cohen and Theogarj, 1975) and regional flaps (Ariyan 1979) to microvascular free flaps (Soutar et al. 1983). A major advantage of these methods over those used in the past is that they can be used as a single-stage procedure and this has considerably reduced the average stay in hospital. The pectoralis major myocutaneous flap is safe and can reach all areas of the oral cavity (Tiwari and Snow, 1983). It has the disadvantage, however, that it is a bulky flap which in general makes it less feasible when mandible has been preserved. When mandible has been resected, and it is felt that it should be replaced as in an anterior arch defect, bone can be included in a regional or free flap (Franklin et al. 1980; Panje and Cutting 1980) at the time of immediate reconstruction. Alternatively, mandibular reconstruction can be carried out as a secondary procedure, provided measures to prevent mandibular drift are taken at the initial operation (Snow et al. 1976).

Cancer of the Larynx

In western Europe traditionally small cancers of the larynx, T_1 and T_2, are in general treated by radiotherapy with good results, in terms of both cancer control and preservation of laryngeal functions, whereas large tumours, T_3 and T_4, are usually treated surgically by means of total laryngectomy. In the past 2 decades, however, the indications for, and the techniques of, so-called conservation surgery of the larynx have been delineated clearly and perfected. Also, a management policy consisting of primary radiation therapy for T_3 and T_4 carcinoma with surgery in reserve for salvage of irradiation failures has been advocated (Lederman 1970; Bryce 1979). Finally, the past 25 years have witnessed a growing interest in attempts at surgical rehabilitation of the voice after total laryngectomy. The treatment of cancer of the larynx will be considered separately for glottic carcinomas and supraglottic carcinomas.

Glottic Carcinoma

When sophisticated radiation therapy facilities are available, radiotherapy is to be preferred as initial management of T_1 and T_2 glottic carcinomas. However, local recurrent or residual tumour growth is found after radiotherapy in approximately 10% and 30% respectively (Harwood et al. 1980). Once a recurrence has been confirmed by histological examination, the salvage procedure may include total or partial laryngectomy. Total laryngectomy has been the most frequent operation for radiation failure. It provides wide tumour margins, avoids the surgical exposure of irradiated cartilage and may simplify the problem of further follow-up of a larynx altered by radiation and surgery. In a number of these patients, however, a vertical partial laryngectomy may be carried out if strict criteria are observed (Kirchner 1975; Ogura et al. 1975). A prerequisite for this type of surgery is a limited extent and infiltration of the recurrent local tumour. Croll et al. (1985) have demonstrated excellent results of this operation under such conditions.

The generally accepted treatment for T_3 and T_4 glottic carcinomas is total laryngectomy. Preferably the operation is begun with a tracheostomy under local anaesthesia, following which general anaesthesia is maintained through the tracheostomy site. It is mandatory to include the thyroid lobe on the side of the lesion as well as the isthmus in the specimen. Also, it is advisable, certainly when there is subglottic extension, to include both paratracheal lymph node chains in the specimen.

The methods of surgical voice restoration after total laryngectomy can be classified basically into two groups: one that is exclusively directed at the restoration of voice and the other which attempts to preserve the respiratory function of the larynx as well (Arslan and Serafini 1972). The last group of procedures has not gained much application. On the contrary, the techniques of the first group have been used widely in the past decade. The object of these methods is to create a communication between the air and food passages in order to facilitate the expiratory volume of air to enter the pharynx, thereby bringing it into vibration. Firstly there is Staffieri's method (1973), where a so-called neoglottis is created immediately following total laryngectomy. The long-term experiences with Staffieri's procedure as reported in the literature vary considerably (Vuyk et al. 1985), probably reflecting differences in patient selection. The problems encountered with Staffieri's procedure are mainly a high rate of postoperative pharyngocutaneous fistulas and late aspiration problems. More promising are techniques which rely on a prosthesis which is placed in a tracheo-oesophageal fistula with the object of overcoming the problems of salivary leakage through the fistula and stenosis of the fistula. The prosthesis serves as a "oneway valve", permitting the entry of air from the lungs into the pharynx only (Singer and Blom 1980; Panje 1981; Nijdam et al. 1982).

Supraglottic Carcinoma

The site of predilection of supraglottic carcinoma is the laryngeal surface of the epiglottis. These lesions usually spread bilaterally or superiorly while remaining entirely above the ventricles rather than extending downwards to the glottis (Kirchner and Som 1971) and can then be removed by horizontal supraglottic laryngectomy with excellent results in terms of tumour control (Bocca et al. 1983). A prerequisite is precise preoperative radiological and endoscopic evaluation of the extent of the tumour. Furthermore, the importance of adequate pulmonary status cannot be overemphasized, as these patients are in danger of postoperative aspiration pneumonia (Stell et al. 1984).

Surgical Management of Neck Nodes

Clinically Positive Neck

For any patient who has clinical evidence of cervical node involvement, a radical neck dissection is carried out. When nodal metastasis is present on admission, the neck operation is performed in continuity with the excision of the primary tumour because viable tumour cells may be present in the lymphatics between the primary and the regional nodes. The question whether the spinal accessory nerve may be preserved deserves special attention, if only for the fact that the most disabling alteration of function following the classical radical neck dissection is the "shoulder syndrome", resulting from the sacrifice of the spinal accessory nerve. This syndrome is characterized by a weakened, deformed and often painful shoulder with a considerable decreased range of motion. The degree of discomfort varies considerably, but in general patients feel more handicapped than is commonly believed (Carenfelt and Eliasson 1981). Obviously, patients in whom the site and size of the primary tumour do not favour spread to lymph nodes adjacent to the course of the nerve would be considered candidates for preservation of the nerve. The feasibility of preservation of the spinal accessory nerve in each individual case, however, has to be carefully evaluated by the surgeon during the dissection. Interestingly, preservation of the nerve does not preclude impaired shoulder function. For those patients in whom the spinal accessory nerve has to be removed, Jones and Stell (1985) developed a modified technique of radical neck dissection preserving the cervical spinal nerves to the trapezius muscle. Comparison of patients undergoing this modified radical neck dissection with patients undergoing a classical radical neck dissection shows them to have better shoulder function. Physical therapy rehabilitation programs can minimize shoulder problems in selective patients in whom the nerve has been sacrificed.

Clinically Negative Neck

Controversy has remained regarding the treatment policy of the NO neck. Longstanding, continuing discussion as to the indications for elective neck dissection is furthermore complicated by the more recent publications that elective irradiation of the neck might be equally effective in eliminating microscopic nodal disease (Fletcher 1972; Mendenhall et al. 1980). In general, elective treatment of regional neck nodes is considered indicated when there is a high likelihood of occult nodal metastasis, when the status of the cervical nodes cannot be adequately assessed as in patients with short muscular necks, when the patient will not be available for regular follow-up visits or when the neck must be entered for access to and/or resection of the primary tumour.

The likelihood of occult nodal metastasis, amongst other factors, depends on the site of the primary tumour within the head and neck (Ali et al. 1985). Furthermore, it has been reported that the incidence of false-negative neck nodes depends on the extent of the primary tumour (Mendenhall et al. 1980). However, others (Hibbert et al. 1983; Ali et al. 1985) could not find any relationship between the T-stage of the primary tumour and the incidence of false-negative nodes. For instance, even patients who have a T_1 lesion of the mobile tongue and whose nodes are initially disease free will have a nodal metastasis develop in the neck in 20%–30% (Spiro and Strong 1971; Mendelson et al. 1976). Nodal conversion rates for T_2 and T_3 lesions of the mobile tongue are equally high. Treatment of late-onset cervical metastasis carries a poor prognosis: not more than 35% of these patients can be cured (Johnson et al. 1980). Based on this indirect evidence, an aggressive management policy as to the clinically negative neck is being carried out for oral, oropharyngeal and hypopharyngeal cancer in most institutions.

To the author's knowledge, a randomized prospective trial comparing elective neck dissection to elective irradiation of the neck has not been carried out. Both modalities have their morbidity. If an 11th nerve-sparing operation is performed (Bocca et al. 1980; Jesse 1981), morbidity is minimal. Elective irradiation avoids initial tissue loss, but is associated with xerostomia. An important advantage of surgery over radiotherapy is that surgery allows for histopathological examination and staging of the neck nodes (see also "N-Factors", above, and "Combined Radiation and Surgery", below).

Combined Radiation and Surgery

Combined radiation and surgery became popular in the 1960s for advanced head and neck cancers at certain sites, such as in the oral cavity, oropharynx and hypopharynx. These advanced lesions pose, primarily, a locally recurrent or regionally metastatic problem. This multimodality approach attempts to increase the effectiveness of therapy to these problem areas. The philosophy behind this type of treatment is that surgery fails at the periphery and radiotherapy at the poorly oxygenated centre of the tumour and that, hopefully, a combination of the two might do better than either alone.

Radiotherapy can be administered either preoperatively or postoperatively; both methods have their advantages and disadvantages (Cachin and Eschwege 1975). Most experience has been gained with preoperative radiation therapy. Regarding retrospective studies the evidence is conflicting. More importantly, all three randomized prospective clinical trials (Strong et al. 1978; Hintz et al. 1979; Terz et al. 1981) failed to demonstrate any higher survival for those patients receiving preoperative radiation when compared with control groups treated by surgery alone. The question regarding the role of preoperative radiotherapy in the management of head and neck cancer finally appears to have been answered by the outcome of these randomized trials.

An increasing number of reports advocate postoperative radiation therapy rather than preoperative irradiation (Vandenbrouck et al. 1977; Vikram et al. 1980; Bartelink et al. 1983; Mantravadi et al. 1983). The histopathological information on the resected specimen can be used to select the patients who are most likely to benefit from combined treatment, that is, those patients with a significant probability of local and/or regional failure after surgery only. Patients with tumour close to or at the surgical resection margins are at high risk of recurrent malignancy. Looser et al. (1978) reported a 71% tumour recurrence rate in patients with inadequate margins as compared with 32% in patients with tumour-free margins. Similarly, Byers et al. (1978) found a local recurrence rate of only 12%–18% in patients with tumour-free margins as compared with 80% of patients in whom free margins could not be achieved. With the addition of immediate postoperative radiotherapy in patients with tumour at surgical margins, a significant decrease in relapse rates is reported (Vikram et al. 1980; Mantravadi et al. 1983).

The value of postoperative irradiation therapy has been demonstrated particularly in regards to failure in the neck. The reported recurrence rate in the neck after radical neck dissection alone varies from 14% to 30% (Jesse and Fletcher 1977). Such recurrences depend directly on the extent of metastatic disease present at the time of surgery. Particularly when extranodal spread and multiple histologically positive nodes are present there is a high risk of recurrence in the neck (see also "N-Factors" above). In these cases surgery should be followed by radiotherapy, as it has been demonstrated that postoperative radiation therapy is effective in reducing the number of recurrences in the neck (Jesse and Fletcher 1977; Vikram et al. 1980; Bartelink et al. 1983; Arriagada et al. 1983; Goffinet et al. 1984; Snow et al. 1986 b).

If irradiation is given postoperatively, it must cover the entire operated area that is at risk of having been infested. When there is a substantial risk of contralateral neck node metastasis, postoperative radiation is given to the opposite side of the neck as well. An important point in postoperative radiotherapy is that it preferably should be started within 3–4 weeks after the surgical procedure and not later than after 6 weeks, as it has been demonstrated that further delay in the start of postoperative radiation therapy might indeed affect the results adversely (Vikram 1979; Mantravadi et al. 1983). It should be realized that radiation therapy adds significantly to the patient's permanent disability (Schuller et al. 1983).

Complications of Surgical Treatment

Operations for cancer of the head and neck can be limited, but often they are major procedures. The anatomy of the region is complex, involving many important structures. Many and serious complications may result. Adequate knowledge concerning possible complications and their avoidance can prevent or reduce the seriousness of complications. Many details require constant and careful attention.

Many patients are of advanced age and have a variety of other disease, chronic pulmonary problems being most frequent. It is of paramount importance that the general condition of the patient is at its most favourable state before instituting surgical treatment. A majority of patients are heavy smokers and many use alcohol excessively. Some have associated liver disease. Identification of the alcoholic patient is important so that appropriate measures can be taken to lessen the postoperative withdrawal syndrome.

It would be going too far within the scope of this chapter to discuss complications of surgical treatment in detail. The reader is referred to the excellent textbook by Conley (1979) on complications of head and neck surgery.

Adjuvant Treatments

The concept of integration of chemotherapy into combined modality treatment for the primary management of advanced head and neck cancer is increasingly being applied. The rationale of this approach is the recognition that surgery and radiotherapy have reached a plateau in their ability to cure head and neck cancer. There are three theoretical mechanisms whereby chemotherapy as an adjuvant to surgery and/or radiotherapy may be effective: initial tumour shrinkage, sensitisation of radiotherapy and the irradication of micrometastases. The use of adjuvant chemotherapy in its various settings will be briefly discussed.

Induction chemotherapy aiming at initial tumour shrinkage has been reported in many studies regarding patients with advanced head and neck cancer to have a favourable influence in terms of both tumour volume reduction and survival (Weaver et al. 1982; Taylor 1983). However, the few prospective randomized studies on the value of induction chemotherapy so far carried out have not shown this type of adjuvant chemotherapy significantly to alter overall survival, disease-free survival or patterns of relapse (Kun et al. 1984; Taylor et al. 1984; Wolf et al. 1984).

The objectives of combining chemotherapy with radiotherapy are to improve local complete responses to radiotherapy and to decrease local recurrences. Although improved response rates have been reported, no differences in survival have been observed, except for the combination of 5-fluorouracil (5-FU) and irradiation in patients with oral cancer (Lo et al. 1976). Recently there has been much interest in the use of cisplatin as a radio-enhancer.

Adjuvant chemotherapy following surgery and/or radiotherapy – i.e. adjuvant chemotherapy *sensu strictu* – aims at irradication of micrometastases or microresidual tumour. In the few studies in which this type of chemotherapy has been attempted, only a small percentage of patients, for a variety of reasons, were able to complete the chemotherapy programmes. Lack of patient compliance was an important factor. A more basic problem associated with the design of studies of this type is the present lack of accurate knowledge of the prognostic factors that put patients with head and neck cancer at high risk for distant metastasis.

Follow-up

Follow-up should be well organized. A minimal requirement is an active tumour registry, which alerts both doctor and patient that the time for checkup is due. In principle, follow-up should be lifelong, taking into account the risk of second primary tumours (see "Multiple Primary Tumours" above). As most local or regional recurrences become manifest within the first 2 years after initial treatment, intensive follow-up is mandatory during that period. Except for patients with small glottic cancers, the neck must be examined, at least once a month during the 1st year after treatment. When a year has elapsed, the follow-up intervals can be extended regularly. Most lymph-node metastases occur in the 1st year and any becoming manifest later are likely to be slow-growing, so that there is a decreasing risk of failure to detect neck disease at a curable stage. The question remains how aggressive one should screen for second primary cancers (see also "Screening for Second Primary Tumours" above). This appears of particular importance in those individuals who continue their smoking and drinking habits.

Treatment of Recurrent or Disseminated Disease

The treatment of locally recurrent tumour depends on its site and extent as well as on the original extent of the tumour and the type and extent of initial treatment. Locally recurrent tumour after treatment of T_1 and T_2 lesions can, in many cases, be treated again curatively. The situation is different with residual or recurrent tumour after treatment of advanced, T_3 and T_4, lesions. In general, it can be said that a proportion of patients with advanced lesions in whom radiotherapy fails can be treated successfully surgically. The reverse is not true: radiotherapy rarely cures a patient who develops a recurrence after initial major surgery. This also holds true for the neck: recurrence in the neck after radical neck dissection invariably carries a very poor prognosis (Pearlman 1979).

There is a wide choice of options for palliative treatment, ranging from modern techniques of cryosurgery and CO_2 laser, which can be used to debulk obstructing tumour or control haemorrhage, to drugs, acting upon the nervous system, for relief of pain. Shaw (1985) has recently discussed the various options for palliation in an excellent review. His comments on palliative chemotherapy should be taken to heart: without exceptionally strong evidence of a likely response, no cytotoxic agent with toxic side effects should be used for palliation. Methotrexate as a single agent is probably still the best chemotherapy in this situation. This is not to say that new drugs or combinations of known drugs should not be attempted. If progress is to be made, new chemotherapy regimens have to be tested. However, this should be carried out within the framework of well-designed prospective studies (Snow et al. 1986c; Stell and McCormick 1986).

Disease-Free Survival

Five-year survival rates for head and neck cancer patients vary considerably with the site and the stage of disease and also with the type of treatment. The overall 5-year survival figures are best for larynx – over 60% – and worst for pharynx – 35% – with oral cavity taking an in-between position (Brugere 1986). It should be noted that these figures, particularly for laryngeal cancer patients, give a more unfavourable impression of the curative potential of treatment than is actually the case, as a substantial proportion of these patients die within 5 years after treatment from intercurrent diseases or second primary tumours. More detailed information on the results of treatment according to site and stage of disease and type of treatment can be found in the references cited in this chapter.

Rehabilitation

Head and neck cancer and its treatment often threaten almost every aspect of the patient's life. The loss of certain senses – like taste, smell and vision – and functions – such as voice, articulation and ability to swallow – occurs through either treatment or the tumour itself. In addition, the organs involved are publicly exposed, which results in an extra burden for the patient to bear. The implications of head and neck cancer for the patient and his or her family are so complex that the time has long since passed that one individual physician can manage the entire problem. An integrated team is required. Team members always include the head and neck surgeon, radiotherapist, medical oncologist, nurse and social worker. The team may include other experts, e.g. in maxillofacial rehabilitation, speech and hearing problems, nutritional problems or psychiatry.

It is essential that the patient is seen and discussed by the team on admission. It is important to appraise the defect which will result after excision in terms of its several components, so that a general outline of the ensuing reconstructive procedure can be made if necessary. Also, the role of the non-surgical members of the team, both in the treatment and in the rehabilitation process, will then be outlined. The treatment and the rehabilitation plan should be discussed with the patient and his or her family. Adequate psychological preparation prior to treatment is mandatory.

Although much remains to be desired, it can be said that the head and neck patient today is better rehabilitated than in the past. The possibilities of reconstructive surgery have improved considerably, as has been discussed under "Large Oral Cancer" above, and these find their applications mainly in the restoration of defects after major surgery for oral and oropharyngeal cancer. Also, prosthetic rehabilitation of facial and intraoral defects after surgical intervention has improved tremendously in the past decades. The development in recent years of surgical-prosthetic methods of voice restoration after total laryngectomy (see also "Glottic Carcinoma" above) has contributed equally to the rehabilitation of laryngectomees. Other developments, like special training programmes in head and neck oncology nursing care, have equally contributed to improvements in rehabilitation. Rehabilitation naturally continues after discharge from hospital in the home situation. The social worker should work closely together with the general practitioner. The ultimate goal is to help the patient maintain his or her morale and return to as meaningful a life as possible.

Future Developments

It is to be expected that further developments and refinements in diagnostic methods will lead to more accurate assessment of the extent of locoregional disease. It is hoped that sensitive tests for "early" detection of distant metastases will become available.

It is unlikely that major developments in surgery, such as we have witnessed in the past 2 decades, will occur in the forthcoming decade, although further sophistication of reconstructive techniques resulting in superior rehabilitation is to be expected. The role of postoperative radiation therapy in advanced disease is to be further determined. In the past 2 decades many of us have hoped for a breakthrough in cytotoxic treatment of head and neck cancer, but this has not occurred. However, some of the available drugs are effective in head and neck cancer patients and their role in combined treatment programmes is to be evaluated. This can be done only by means of randomized prospective studies. Taking into account the relatively low incidence of these tumours in most Western countries, multi-institutional and international cooperation is required for such studies.

Finally, it is emphasized that more efforts should be directed towards the prevention of these cancers. The public should be better informed about the risks of smoking and drinking in regard to the development of head and neck cancer. These efforts should focus particularly on young people.

References

Ali S, Tiwari RM, Snow GB (1985) False positive and false negative neck nodes. Head Neck Surg 8: 78–82

American Joint Committee on Cancer (1983) Manual for staging of cancer. Lippincott, Philadelphia

Ariyan S (1979) The pectoralis major myocutaneous flap. A versatile flap for reconstruction of the head and neck. Plast Reconstr Surg 63: 73–81

Arriagada R, Eschwege F, Cachin Y, Richard JM (1983) The value of combining radiotherapy with surgery in the treatment of hypopharyngeal and laryngeal cancers. Cancer 51: 1819–1825

Arslan M, Serafini I (1972) Restoration of laryngeal function after total laryngectomy: report of the first 25 cases. Laryngoscope 82: 1349–1360

Atkins JP, Keane WM, Young KA, Rowe LD (1984) Value of panendoscopy in determination of second primary cancer. Arch Otolaryngol Head Neck Surg 110: 533–534

Baker HL (1986) The application of magnetic resonance imaging in otolaryngology. Laryngoscope 96: 19–26

Banfi A, Bonadonna G, Carnevani G, Molinari R, Monfardini S, Salvini E (1970) Lymphoreticular sarcomas with primary involvement of Waldeyer's ring. Clinical evaluation of 225 cases. Cancer 42: 1096–1104

Banoczy J (1982) Oral leukoplakia. Nijhoff, The Hague

Bartelink H, Breur K, Hart G, Annyas AA, van Slooten EA, Snow GB (1983) The value of postoperative radiotherapy as an adjuvant to radical neck dissection. Cancer 52: 1008–1013

Batsakis JG (1979) Tumors of the head and neck. Clinical and pathological considerations. Williams and Wilkins, Baltimore

Beahrs OH (1973) Factors minimizing mortality and morbidity rates in head and neck. Am J Surg 126: 443–451

Bennett SH, Futrell JW, Roth JA, Hoye RC, Ketcham AS (1971) Prognostic significance of histologic host response in cancer of the larynx or hypopharynx. Cancer 28: 1255–1265

Berger DS, Fletcher GH (1971) Distant metastasis following local control of squamous cell carcinoma of the nasopharynx, tonsillar fossa and base of tongue. Radiology 100: 141–143

Bocca E, Pignataro O, Sasaki C (1980) Functional neck dissection. Arch Otolaryngol Head Neck Surg 106: 524–527

Bocca E, Pignataro O, Oldini C (1983) Supraglottic laryngectomy: 30 years of experience. Ann Otol Rhinol Laryngol 92: 14–18

Broders AC (1920) Squamous cell epithelioma of the lip. JAMA 74: 656–664

Brookes GB, Clifford P (1981) Nutritional status and general immune competence in patients with head and neck cancer. J Soc Med 74: 132–136

Brugère J (1986) Cancers des voies aerodigestives superieures. In: Brugere J (ed) Progres en cancerologie. Doin Editeurs, Paris

Brugère J, Schlienger M, Gerard-Marchant R, Tubiana M, Pouillar P, Cachin Y (1975) Non-Hodgkin's lymphomata of upper digestive and respiratory tract. Natural history and results of radiotherapy. Br J Cancer 31 Suppl 2: 435–440

Bryce DP (1979) The management of laryngeal cancer. J Otolaryngol 8: 105–126

Byers RM, Bland KI, Borlase B, Luna M (1978) The prognostic and therapeutic value of frozen section determinations in the surgical treatment of squamous carcinoma of the head and neck. Am J Surg 136: 525–528

Cachin Y, Eschwege F (1975) Combination of radiotherapy and surgery in the treatment of head and neck cancers. Cancer Treat Rev 2: 177–191

Cachin Y, Sancho-Garnier H, Micheau Ch, Marandas P (1979) Nodal metastasis from carcinoma of the oropharynx. Otolaryngol Clin North Am 12: 145–154

Callery CD, Spiro RH, Strong EW (1984) Changing trends in the management of squamous carcinoma of the tongue. Am J Surg 148: 449–454

Carenfelt C, Eliasson K (1981) Radical neck dissection and permanent sequelae association with spinal accessory nerve injuries. Acta Otolaryngol (Stockh) 91: 155–160

Carter RL (1976) Metastasis. In: Symington T, Carter RL (eds) Scientific foundations of oncology. Heinemann, London

Carter RL, Tanner NSB, Clifford P, Shaw HJ (1979) Perineural spread in squamous cell carcinomas of the head and neck: a clinopathological study. Clin Otolaryngol 4: 271–281

Cohen IK, Theogarj SD (1975) Nasolabial flap reconstruction of the floor of the mouth after extirpation of oral cancer. Am J Surg 130: 479–485

Conley JJ (1975) Salivary glands and the facial nerve. Thieme, Stuttgart

Conley JJ (1979) Complications of head and neck surgery. Saunders, Philadelphia

Croll GA, Tiwari RM, Manni JJ, Snow GB (1985) Vertical partial laryngectomy for recurrent glottic carcinoma after irradiation. Head and Neck Surg 7: 390–393

Daniel RK, Taylor GI (1973) Distant transfer of an island flap by microvascular anastomosis. Plast Reconstr Surg 52: 111–117

de Vries N, Snow GB (1986a) Multiple primary tumours in laryngeal cancer. J Otol Laryngol 100: 915–918

de Vries N, de Lange G, Drexhage HA, Snow GB (1987) Immunoglobulin allotypes in head and neck cancer patients with multiple primary cancers. Acta Otolaryngol (Stockh) 104: 187–191

de Vries N, van der Waal I, Snow GB (1986c) Multiple primary tumors in oral cancer. Int J Oral Maxillofac Surg 15: 85–87

Djalilian M, Weiland LH, Devine KD, Beahrs OH (1973) Significance of jugular vein invasion by metastatic carcinoma in radical neck dissection. Am J Surg 126: 566–569

Easson EC, Palmer MK (1976) Prognostic factors in oral cancer. J Clin Oncol 2: 191–202

Eneroth CM (1964) Histological and clinical aspects of parotid tumors. Acta Otolaryngol [Suppl] (Stockh): 191: 1–99

Fletcher GH (1972) Elective irradiation of subclinical disease in cancers of the head and neck. Cancer 29: 1450–1454

Franklin JD, Shack RB, Stone JD, Madden JJ, Lynch JB (1980) Single-stage reconstruction of mandibular and soft tissue defects using a free osteocutaneous groin flap. Am J Surg 140: 492–498

Friedman M, Shelton VK, Mafee M, Bellity P, Grybauskas V, Skolnik E (1984) Metastatic neck disease. Evaluation by computed tomography. Arch Otolaryngol Head Neck Surg 110: 443–447

Gerritsen GJ, Valk J, Velzen DJ van, Snow GB (1986) Computed tomography – a mandatory investigational procedure of the T-staging in advanced larnygeal cancer. To be published in Clin Otolaryngol 11: 307–316

Gluckman JL, Grissman JD, Donegan JO (1980) Multicentric squamous cell carcinoma of the upper aerodigestive tract. Head Neck Surg 90–96

Goffinet DR, Fee WE jr, Goode RL (1984) Combined surgery and postoperative irradiation in the treatment of cervical lymph nodes. Arch Otolaryngol Head Neck Surg 110: 736–738

Graham S (1977) Dentition, diet, tobacco, and alcohol in the epidemiology of oral cancer. JNCI 59: 1611–1618

Grandi C, Alloisio M, Moglia D, Podrecca S, Sala L, Salvatori P, Molinari R (1985) Prognostic significance of lymphatic spread in head and neck carcinomas: therapeutic implications. Head Neck Surg 8: 67–73

Guillamondegui OM, Jesse R (1976) Surgical treatment of advanced carcinoma of the floor of the mouth. AJR Roentgenol 126: 1256–1259

Harwood AR, Hawkins NV, Keane T, Cummings B, Biel FA, Rider WD, Bryce DP (1980) Radiotherapy of early glottic cancer. Laryngoscope 70: 465–470

Healy GB, Strong MS, Uchmahli A, Vaughan GW, Di Troia JF (1976) Carcinoma of the palatine arch. Am J Surg 131: 498–503

Hellquist H, Lundgren J, Olofsson J (1982) Hyperplasia, keratosis, dysplasia and carcinoma in situ on the vocal cords – a follow-up study. Clin Otolaryngol 7: 11–27

Hellquist H, Olofsson J, Lundgren J, Grontoft O (1984) Photometric studies on nuclear DNA content and area in different laryngeal epithelia. Cancer Detect Prev 7: 275–277

Hibbert J, Marks NJ, Winter PJ, Shaheen OH (1983) Prognostic factors in oral squamous carcinoma and their relation to clinical staging. Clin Otolaryngol 108: 197–203

Hintz B, Charynler K, Chandler JR, Surarasnam A, Garciga C (1979) Randomized study of control of the primary tumor and survival using preoperative radiation, radiation alone, or surgery alone in head and neck carcinomas. J Surg Oncol 12: 75–85

Hoover LA, Calcaterra ThC, Walter GA, Larrson SG (1984) Preoperative CT scan evaluation of laryngeal carcinoma: correlation with pathologic findings. Laryngoscope 94: 310–315

Hordijk GJ, de Jong JMA (1983) Synchronous and metachronous tumours in patients with head and neck cancer. J Laryngol Otol 97: 619–621

Jakobsson PA, Eneroth CM, Killander D (1973) Histological classification and grading of malignancy in carcinoma of the larynx. Acta Radiol Ther 12: 1–8

Jesse RH (1981) Modified neck dissection with and without radiation. In: Kagan AR, Miles JW (eds), Head and neck oncology, controversies in cancer treatment. Hall, Boston, pp 247–254

Jesse RH, Fletcher GH (1977) Treatment of the neck in patients with squamous cell carcinoma of the head and neck. Cancer 39: 868–872

Johnson MJT, Leipzig B, Cummings CW (1980) Management of T_1 carcinoma of the anterior aspect of the tongue. Arch Otolaryngol Head Neck Surg 106: 249–251

Johnson JT, Barns EL, Myers EN, Schramm VL, Borochovitz D, Sigler BA (1981) The extracapsular spread of tumors in cervical node metastasis. Arch Otolaryngol Head Neck Surg 107: 725–729

Jones TA, Stell PM (1985) The preservation of shoulder function after radical neck dissection. Clin Otolaryngol 10: 89–92

Kalnins IK, Leonard AG, Sako K, Razack MS, Shedd DP (1977) Correlation between prognosis and degree of lymph node involvement in carcinoma of the oral cavity. Am J Surg 134: 450–454

Katz AE (1983) Immunobiologic staging of patients with carcinoma of the head and neck. Laryngoscope 93: 445–463

Kirchner JA (1975) Growth and spread of laryngeal cancer as related to partial laryngectomy. Laryngoscope 85: 1516–1521

Kirchner JA, Som ML (1971) Clinical and histological observations on supraglottic cancer. Ann Otol Rhinol Laryngol 80: 638–645

Kleinsasser O (1963) Die Klassifikation und Differentialdiagnose der Epithel Hyperplasien der Kehlkopfschleimhaut auf Grund Histomophologischer Merkmale. Z Larnygol Rhinol 42: 339–362

Kun LE, Toohill RJ, Ritch PS, Duncavage JA, Hoffman RG, Cox JD, Malin TC (1984) Effect of induction chemotherapy in advanced cancers of the upper aerodigestive tract (UAD): a prospective, randomized trial. Proc Int Conf on Head and Neck Cancer. Baltimore, p 43

Langdon JD (1985) Epidemiology and aetiology. In: Henk JM, Langdon JD (eds). Malignant tumours of the oral cavity. Arnold, London, pp 1–13

Lederman M (1970) Radiotherapy of cancer of the larynx. J Laryngol Otol 84: 867–896

Lederman M (1971) Cancer of the larynx, part I: natural history in relation to treatment. Br J Radiol 44: 569–578

Leipzig B, Winter ML, Hokanson JA (1981) Cervical nodal metastasis of unknown origin. Laryngoscope 91: 593–598

Leipzig B, Zellmer JE, Klug D (1985) The role of endoscopy in evaluating patients with head and neck cancer. A multi-

institutional prospective study. Arch Otolaryngol Head Neck Surg 111: 589–594
Lindberg RD (1972) Distribution of cervical lymph node metastasis from squamous cell carcinoma of the upper respiratory and digestive tract. Cancer 29: 1446
Lo TC, Wiley AL, Ansfield FJ, Brandenburg JH, Davis HL, Gollin FF, Johnson RO, Ramirez G, Vermund H (1976) Combined radiation therapy and 5-fluorouracil for advanced squamous cell carcinoma of the oral cavity and oropharynx. A randomized study. AJR 126: 229–235
Looser KG, Shah J, Strong EW (1978) The significance of "positive" margins in surgically resected epidermoid carcinomas. Head Neck Surg 1: 107–111
Lundy J, Raaf JH, Deakins S, Wanebo HJ, Jacobs DA, Tsung-Dao L, Jacobowitz D, Spear C, Oettgen HF (1975) The acute and chronic effects of alcohol on the human immune system. Surg Gynecol Obstet 141: 212–215
Maddox WA (1984) Vicissitudes of head and neck cancer. Am J Surg 148: 428–432
Mancuso AA, Harnsberger HR, Muraki AS, Stevens MH (1983) Computed tomography of cervical and retropharyngeal lymph nodes: normal anatomy, variants of normal, and applications in staging head and neck cancer. Radiology 148: 715–723
Mantravadi RVP, Haas RE, Liebner EJ, Skolnik EM, Applebaum EL (1983) Postoperative radiotherapy for persistent tumor at the surgical margin in head and neck cancer. Laryngoscope 93: 1337–1340
Marchetta FC, Sako K, Murphy J (1971) The periosteum of the mandible and intraoral carcinoma. Am J Surg 122: 711–713
Martin SA, Marks JE, Lee JY, Bauer DC, Ogura JH (1980) Carcinoma of the piriform sinus: predictors of TNM relapse and survival. Cancer 46: 1974–1981
McCraw JB, Dibbel G, Carraway JH (1977) Clinical definition of independent myocutaneous vascular territories. Plast Reconstr Surg 60: 341–352
McGavran MH, Bauer WC, Ogura JH (1961) The incidence of cervical lymph node metastases from epidermoid carcinoma of the larynx and their relationship to certain characteristics of the primary tumor. Cancer 14: 655–666
McGregor JB, Morgan G (1973) Axial and random pattern flaps. Br J Plast Surg 26: 202–213
McGregor IA, McGrouther DA (1978) Skin graft reconstruction in carcinoma of the tongue. Head Neck Surg 1: 47–51
McGuirt WF (1982) Panendoscopy as a screening examination for simultaneous primary tumors in head and neck cancer: a prospective sequential study and review of the literature. Laryngoscope 92: 569–576
McGuirt WF, Loevy S, McCabe BF, Krause CJ (1977) The risks of major head and neck surgery in the aged population. Laryngoscope 87: 1378–1382
McGuirt WF, McCabe, Krause CJ (1979) Complications of radical neck dissection: a survey of 788 patients. Head Neck Surg 1: 481–487
Mendelson BC, Woods JE, Beahrs OH (1976) Neck dissection in the treatment of carcinoma of the anterior two-thirds of the tongue. Surg Gynaecol Obstet 143: 751–80
Mendenhall WM, Million RR, Cassisi NJ (1980) Elective neck irradiation in squamous cell carcinoma of the head and neck. Head Neck Surg 3: 15–20
Merino OR, Lindberg RD, Fletcher GH (1977) An analysis of distant metastases from squamous cell carcinoma of the upper respiratory and digestive tracts. Cancer 40: 145–151
Michaels L (1984) Pathology of the larynx. Springer, Berlin Heidelberg New York
Micheau C, Sancho H, Gerard-Marchant R (1978) Prognostic des adenopathies cervicales metastatiques en fonction des facteurs anatomo-pathologique. Nuovo Arch Ital Otol VI 1: 5–14
Miller AH, Batsakis JG (1974) Premalignant laryngeal lesions, carcinoma in situ, superficial carcinoma – definition and management. Can J Otolaryngol 3: 573–757
Moore C (1971) Cigarette smoking and cancer of the mouth, pharynx and larynx. JAMA 218: 553–558
Muraki AS, Mancuso AA, Harnsberger HR, Johnson LP, Meads GB (1983) CT of the oropharynx, tonguebase and floor of the mouth: normal anatomy and range of variations, and applications in staging carcinoma. Radiology 148: 725–731
Neel HB III, Sanderson DR, Fontana RS, Taylor WF, Woolner LB (1981 a) Sputum cytology, diagnosis of upper respiratory tract cancer: second report. Ann Otol Rhinol Laryngol 90: 312–315
Neel HB III, Pearson GR, Weiland LH (1981 b) Immunologic detection of occult primary cancer of the head and neck. Otolaryngol Head Neck Surg 89: 230–234
Nijdam HF, Annyas AA, Schutte HK, Leever H (1982) A new prosthesis for voice rehabilitation after laryngectomy. Arch Otorhinolaryngol 237: 27–33
Noone RB, Bonner H, Raymond S, Brown AS, Graham WP, Lehr HB (1974) Lymph node metastases in oral carcinoma. A correlation of histopathology with survival. Plast Reconstr Surg 53: 158–166
Ogura JH, Sessions DG, Gershon JS, Alonso WA (1975) Roles and limitations of conservation surgical therapy for laryngeal cancer. Can J Otolaryngol 4: 400–402
Olde Kalter P, Lubsen H, Delemarre JFM, Alons CL, Veldhuizen RW, Meijer CJLM, Snow GB (1985) Morphometry of squamous cell hyperplasia of the larynx. J Clin Pathol 38: 489–495
Olde Kalter P, Lubsen H, Delemarre JFM, Snow GB (1986) Squamous cell hyperplasia of the larynx (clinical follow-up study). J Laryngol Otol 101: 579–588
Panje WR (1981) Prosthetic vocal rehabilitation following laryngectomy – the voice button. Ann Otol Rhinol Laryngol 90: 116–120
Panje WR, Cutting C (1980) Trapezius osteomyocutaneous island flap for reconstruction of the anterior floor of mouth and mandible. Head Neck Surg 3: 66–71
Pasche R, Savary M, Monnier PH (1981) Multifocalite du carcinome epidermoide sur les voies digestives superieures et respiratoires distales: technicite du diagnostic endoscopique. Acta Endosc 11: 277–291
Pearlman NW (1979) Treatment outcome in recurrent head and neck cancer. Arch Surg 114: 39–42
Pearson GR, Weiland LH, Neel HB, Taylor W, Earle J, Mulroney SE, Goepfert H, Lanier A, Talvot ML, Pilch B, Goodman M, Huang A, Levine PH, Hyans V, Moran E, Henle G, Henle W (1983) Application of Epstein-Barr virus (EBV) serology to the diagnosis of North American nasopharyngeal carcinoma. Cancer 51: 260–268
Pindborg JJ (1980) Oral cancer and precancer. Wright, Bristol
Pittam MR, Carter RL (1982) Framework invasion by laryngeal carcinomas. Head Neck Surg 4: 200–208
Poleksic S, Kalwaic HJ (1978) Prognostic value of vascular invasion in squamous cell carcinoma of the head and neck. Plast Reconst Surg 61: 234–240
Ramadan MF, Morton RP, Stell PM, Pharoah, POD (1982) Epidemiology of laryngeal cancer. Clin Otolaryngol 7: 417–428
Robbins KT, Kong JS, Fuller LM, Goepfert H (1985) A comparative analysis of lymphomas involving Waldeyer's ring

and the nasal cavity and paranasal sinuses. J Otolaryngol 14: 7–13
Rothman KJ, Cann CI, Flanders D, Fried MP (1980) Epidemiology of laryngeal cancer. Epidemiol Rev 2: 195–209
Sako K, Pradier RN, Marchetta FC, Pickren JW (1964) Fallibility of palpation in the diagnosis of metastasis to cervical nodes. Surg Gynaecol Obstet 118: 989–990
Savary M, Passche R, Monnier P (1984) Endoscopic screening for multiple squamous cell carcinoma of the upper digestive and respiratory tracts (Oncologically oriented upper aero-digestive pan-endoscopy). In: Wigand ME, Steiner W, Stell PM (eds) Functional partial laryngectomy. Conservation surgery for carcinoma of the larynx. Springer, Berlin Heidelberg New York, pp 51–59
Schuller DE, Reiches NA, Hamaker RC (1983) Analysis of disability resulting from treatment including radical neck dissection or modified neck dissection. Head Neck Surg 6: 551–558
Sessions DG (1976) Surgical pathology of cancer of the larynx and hypopharynx. Laryngoscope 86: 814–839
Shafer WG, Waldron CA (1975) Erythroplakia of the oral cavity. Cancer 36: 1021–1028
Shah JP, Cendon RA, Farr HW (1976) Carcinoma of the oral cavity (factors affecting treatment failure at the primary site and neck). Am J Surg 132: 504–507
Shaw HJ (1985) Palliation in head and neck cancer. J Laryngol Otol 99: 1131–1142
Singer MI, Blom ED (1980) An endoscopic technique for restoration of voice after laryngectomy. Ann Otol Rhinol Laryngol 89: 529–533
Snow GB (1984) Surgical treatment of malignant tumors of the oral cavity. In: van der Waal I, Snow GB (eds) Oral oncology. Nijhoff, Boston
Snow GB, van der Waal I (1986 a) Mucosal melanoma. Otolaryngol Clin North Amer 19: 537–547
Snow GB, Kruisbrink JJ, van Slooten EA (1976) Reconstruction after mandibulectomy for cancer. Arch Otolaryngol Head Neck Surg 102: 207–210
Snow GB, Annyas AA, van Slooten EA, Bartelink H, Hart AAM (1982) Prognostic factors of neck node metastasis. Clin Otolaryngol 7: 185–192
Snow GB, Balm AJM, Arendse JW, Karim ABMF, Bartelink H, van der Waal I, Tiwari RM (1986 b) Prognostic factors in neck node metastases. In: Larson DL, Guillamondequi OM, Ballantyne AJ (eds) Cancer in the neck: evaluation and treatment. McMillan, New York, pp 53–63
Snow GB, Vermorken JB, Pinedo HM (1986 c) Adjuvant chemotherapy – the EORTC trials. Bloom HJ (ed) Head and neck oncology. Raven, New York, pp 83–92
Som PM (1982) The role of CT in the diagnosis of carcinoma of the paranasal sinuses and nasopharynx. J Otolaryngol 11: 340–348
Soutar DS, Scheker LR, Tanger SB, McGregor IA (1983) Radial forearm flap: a versatile method for intraoral reconstruction. Br J Plast Surg 36: 1–8
Spiro RH (1986) Salivary neoplasms: overview of a 35-year experience with 2807 patients. Head Neck Surg 1: 177–184
Spiro RH, Strong EW (1971) Epidermoid carcinoma of the mobile tongue: treatment by partial glossectomy alone. Am J Surg 122: 707–710
Spiro RH, Alfonso AE, Farr HW, Strong EW (1974) Cervical node metastasis from epidermoid carcinoma of the oral cavity and oropharynx. A critical assessment of current staging. Am J Surg 128: 562–567
Spiro RH, Gerold FP, Strong EW (1981) Mandibular "swing" approach for oral and oropharyngeal tumors. Head Neck Surg 3: 371–378
Staffieri M (1973) Functionelle totale Laryngektomie. Monatsschr Ohrenheilkd Wien 107: 77–89
Steiner W (1984) Prevention and early detection of cancer of the upper aerodigestive tract. Results of endoscopic mass screening. In: Wigand ME, Steiner W, Stell PM (eds) Functional partial laryngectomy. Conservation surgery for carcinoma of the larynx. Springer, Berlin Heidelberg New York, pp 44–48
Stell PM, Mccormick MS (1986) The design of phase III palliative chemotherapy trials in head and neck cancer. Clin Otolaryngol 11: 21–29
Stell PM, Morton MP, Singh SD (1983) Cervical lymph node metastases: the significance of the level of the lymph node. J Clin Oncol 9: 101–107
Stell PM, Morton MP, Singh SD (1984) Functional complications after supraglottic laryngectomy. In: Wigand ME, Steiner W, Stell PM (eds) Functional partial laryngectomy. Conservation surgery for carcinoma of the larynx. Springer, Berlin Heidelberg New York, pp 301–305
Stevens MH, Harnsberger HR, Mancuso AA, Davis RK, Johnson LP, Parkin JL (1985) Computed tomography of cervical lymph nodes. Arch Otolaryngol Head Neck Surg 111: 735–739
Strong MS, Vaughan CW, Kayne HL, Aral IM, Ucmakli A, Veldman M, Healy G (1978) Randomized trial preoperative radiotherapy in cancer of the oropharynx and hypopharynx. Am J Surg 136: 494–500
Taylor SG (1983) Head and neck cancer. In: Pinedo HM (ed) Cancer chemotherapy. The EORTC cancer chemotherapy annual V. Excerpta Medica. Amsterdam, pp 237–256
Taylor SG, Applebaum E, Caldarelli D, Showel J, Hutchinson W, Holingern L, Murthy A (1984) A randomized trial of methotrexate with leucovorin as adjuvant treatment of patients with head and neck squamous cancer. Proc Int Conf on Head and Neck Cancer, Baltimore, p 43
Terz JJ, King ER, Lawrence W jr (1981) Preoperative irradiation for head and neck cancer. Results of a prospective study. Surgery 89: 449–453
Tiwari RM, Snow GB (1983) Role of myocutaneous flaps in reconstruction of the head and neck. J Laryngol Otol 97: 441–458
Tiwari RM, Gerritsen GJ, Balm AJM, Snow GB (1986) A critical evaluation of the role of CT scanning in ethmoidal cancer. J Laryngol and Otol 100: 421–428
Toker C (1963) Some observations on the deposition of metastatic carcinoma within cervical lymph nodes. Cancer 16: 364–374
Tuyns AJ (1982) Incidence trends of laryngeal cancer in relation to national alcohol and tobacco consumption. In: Magnus K (ed) Trends in cancer incidence. Hemisphere, Washington
Union Internationale Contre le Cancer (1987) In: Hermanek P and Sobin LH (ed) TNM classification of malignant tumours, 4th edn. Springer, Berlin Heidelberg New York Tokyo
Vandenbrouck C, Sancho H, Le Fut R, Richard JM, Cachin Y (1977) Results of a randomized clinical trial of preoperative irradiation vs postoperative in treatment of tumors of the hypopharynx. Cancer 39: 1445–1449
Vikram B (1979) Importance of the time interval between surgery and postoperative radiation therapy in the combined management of head and neck cancer. Int J Radiat Oncol Biol Phys 5: 1837–1840
Vikram B (1984) Changing patterns of failure in advanced

head and neck cancer. Arch Otolaryngol Head Neck Surg 110: 564–565
Vikram B, Strong EW, Shah J (1980) Elective postoperative radiation therapy in stages III and IV epidermoid carcinoma of the head and neck. Am J Surg 140: 580–584
Vikram B, Strong EW, Shah JP, Spiro R (1984) Failure at distant sites following multimodality treatment for advanced head and neck cancer. Head Neck Surg 6: 730–733
Vuyk HD, Tiwari RM, Snow GB (1985) Staffieri's procedure revisited. Head Neck Surg 8: 21–27
Wagenfeld DJH, Harwood AR, Bryce DP (1980) Second primary respiratory tract malignancies in glottic carcinoma. Cancer 746: 1883–1886
Wagenfeld DJH, Harwood AR, Bryce DP (1981) Second primary respiratory tract malignant neoplasms in supraglottic carcinoma. Arch Otolaryngol Head Neck Surg 102: 135–137
Weaver A, Felming S, Vandenberg H (1982) Cisplatinum and 5-fluorouracil as initial therapy in advanced epidermoid cancers of the head and neck. Head Neck Surg 4: 370–373
Weber RS, Benjamin RS, Peters LJ, Ro RY, Achon O, Goepfert H (1986) Soft tissue sarcomas of the head and neck in adolescents and adults. Am J Surg 152 (4): 386–392
Westbury G (1981) Carcinoma of the tongue. In: Rob C, Smith R Wilson JSP (eds) Operative surgery, head and neck. Butterworths, London, pp 664–671
Williams RG, Murtagh GP (1973) Mortality in surgery for head and neck cancer. J Laryngol Otol 87: 431–440
Wolf GT (1984) Tumor immunology, immune surveillance and immunotherapy of head and neck squamous carcinoma. In: Wolf GT (ed) Head and neck oncology. Nijhoff, Boston, pp 375–411
Wolf GT, Jacobs C, Makucj RW, Vikram B (1984) Cisplatin (DDP) and bleomycin (BLM) adjuvant chemotherapy in head and neck cancer. Results of the head and neck contracts program, Proc Int Conf on Head and Neck Cancer, Baltimore, p 43
Wynder EL, Dodo H, Bloch DA, Gantt RC, Moore OS (1969) Epidemiologic investigations of multiple primary cancer of the upper alimentary and respiratory tract. Cancer 24: 730–739
Wynder EL, Covey LS, Mabuchi K, Mushinski M (1976) Environmental factors in cancer of the larynx. A second look. Cancer 38: 1591–1601
Zajicek J (1974) Monographs in clinical cytology, vol 4. Aspiration biopsy cytology, part 1. In: Cytology of supradiaphragmatic organs. Karger, Basel, pp 90–124
Zoller M, Goodman ML, Cummings CW (1978) Guidelines for prognosis in head and neck cancer with nodal metastasis. Laryngoscope 88: 135–40

Cancer of the Respiratory Tract, Pleural Cavity, Mediastinum, and Chest Wall

P. GOLDSTRAW

This chapter covers the whole of thoracic surgical oncology with the exception of oesophageal cancer. Lung cancer will be dealt with in some detail, but when dealing with the less common tumours the emphasis will be placed on newer developments in treatment.

Tumours of the Lung

Lung Cancer

The association between cigarette smoking and lung cancer is now firmly established. Since the original work by Doll and Peto (1976) many studies have been undertaken throughout the world, demonstrating an increasing risk of lung cancer with increasing cigarette consumption. This association may be influenced by the pattern of inhalation, the age at which the patient commenced smoking and the type of cigarettes smoked. The risk of lung cancer for pipe and cigar smokers is also increased, but less markedly so.

Other environmental factors influence the pathogene sis of lung cancer, some markedly so, such as asbestos, chromium and uranium, but there must also be more subtle and more widespread influences since the incidence of lung cancer varies from country to country, even amongst groups with similar cigarette consumption. It has been suggested that these influences are related to atmospheric pollution from industrial processes. Where antismoking campaigns are proving effective and smoking trends are improved there is evidence that the rate of increase in the incidence of lung cancer is decreasing. In the United Kingdom the incidence of lung cancer amongst males has now plateaued and for men in the United States the incidence is now falling. Unfortunately there is no such improvement amongst female smokers, where the incidence continues to rise. Consequently the sex ratio for lung cancer is steadily reducing. It has been estimated that in 1986 lung cancer deaths amongst women in the United States exceeded those for breast cancer, placing lung cancer at the top of the league table for cancer deaths in both sexes. Amongst female smokers the cell type would appear to be increasingly adenocarcinoma (Bringel 1985). There is increasing interest in the influence of passive smoking, and great excitement created by studies from Greece (Trichopoulos et al. 1983) and Japan (Hirayama 1981) suggesting that non-smoking wives may have as much as twice the risk of lung cancer if married to smokers. However, these studies are subject to statistical criticism and the review by Lee et al. (1986) suggests that any additional risk created by passive smoking is small.

The World Health Organization classification for lung cancer is now widely used (1981). This classification recognises four major types of lung cancer – squamous carcinoma, adenocarcinoma, large cell undifferentiated carcinoma, and small cell carcinoma. Whilst there are differences in the natural history of each of these cell types, there are profound differences in prognosis between small-cell lung cancer (SCLC) and the first three categories, which for management purposes may be grouped as non-small-cell lung cancer (NSCLC). The prognosis for lung cancer depends upon the cell type, the degree of local invasion, the extent of regional lymphatic metastases and the presence or absence of distant metastases. These features are recognised in the TNM staging system as set out in Tables 1 and 2 (Hermanek and Sobin 1987).

Table 2. Stage grouping of TNM subsets

Occult carcinoma	TX	N0	M0
Stage 0	Tis	N0	M0
Stage I	T1	N0	M0
	T2	N0	M0
Stage II	T1	N1	M0
	T2	N1	M0
Stage IIIA	T1	N2	M0
	T2	N2	M0
	T3	N0, N1, N2	M0
Stage IIIB	Any T	N3	M0
	T4	Any N	M0
Stage IV	Any T	Any N	M1

Table 1. TNM clinical classification

T – Primary Tumor

TX	Primary tumour cannot be assessed, *or* tumour proven by the presence of malignant cells in sputum or bronchial washings but not visualized by imaging or bronchoscopy
T0	No evidence of primary tumour
Tis	Carcinoma in situ
T1	Tumour 3 cm or less in greatest dimension, surrounded by lung or visceral pleura, without bronchoscopic evidence of invasion more proximal than the lobar bronchus (i.e. not in the main bronchus)[1]
T2	Tumour with *any* of the following features of size or extent: More than 3 cm in greatest dimension Involves main bronchus, 2 cm or more distal to the carina Invades visceral pleura Associated with atelectasis or obstructive pneumonitis which extends to the hilar region but does not involve the entire lung
T3	Tumour of any size which directly invades any of the following: chest wall (including superior sulcus tumours), diaphragm, mediastinal pleura, parietal pericardium; or tumour in the main bronchus C less than 2 cm distal to the carina[1]) but without involvement of the carina; or associated atelectasis or obstructive pneumonitis of the entire lung
T4	Tumour of any size which invades any of the following: mediastinum, heart, great vessels, trachea, oesophagus, vertebral body, carina; or tumour with malignant pleural effusion[2]

Notes: 1. The uncommon superficial spreading tumour of any size with its invasive component limited to the bronchial wall which may extend proximal to the main bronchus is also classified T1.

2. Most pleural effusions associated with lung cancer are due to tumour. However, there are a few patients in whom multiple cytopathological examinations of pleural fluid are negative for tumour, the fluid is non-bloody and is not an exudate. Where these elements and clinical judgement dictate that the effusion is not related to the tumour, the effusion should be excluded as a staging element and the patient should be classified T1, T2 or T3.

N – Regional Lymph Nodes

NX	Regional lymph nodes cannot be assessed
N0	No regional lymph node metastasis
N1	Metastasis in ipsilateral peribronchial and/or ipsilateral hilar lymph nodes, including direct extension
N2	Metastasis in ipsilateral mediastinal and/or subcranial lymph node(s)
N3	Metastasis in contralateral mediastinal, contralateral hilar, ipsilateral or contralateral scalene or supraclavicular lymph node(s)

M – Distant Metastasis

MX	Presence of distant metastasis cannot be assessed
M0	No distant metastasis
M1	Distant metastasis

The category M1 may be further specified according to the following notation:

Pulmonary	PUL	Bone marrow	MAR
Osseous	OSS	Pleura	PLE
Hepatic	HEP	Peritoneum	PER
Brain	BRA	Skin	SKI
Lymph nodes	LYM	Other	OTH

For any patient the TNM stage will evolve as investigations and treatment continue and follow-up becomes available. The clinical/diagnostic stage (cTNM) is formulated once all investigations are completed. This may include invasive procedures such as bronchoscopy, mediastinoscopy and needle biopsy. If treatment entails thoracotomy and resection, then considerable additional staging information becomes available and a postsurgical treatment/pathological staging (pTNM) can be made. At any stage thereafter, if relapse occurs and further investigations are undertaken, a retreatment stage (rTNM) may be formed. If death occurs and an autopsy is undertaken, then a final stage (aTNM) is possible.

It can be seen that for an individual patient proceeding through this system, several TNM stages will be formulated, but as additional information becomes available original classifications should not be altered.

It is unfortunately true that for the majority of patients suffering from small cell lung cancer the TNM stage has little practical value and staging is usually restricted to limited or extensive disease. Limited disease is defined as tumour confined to one hemithorax and the ipsilateral supraclavicular fossa. Even such "limited" disease is far beyond surgical resection, but occasional resectable small cell tumours are encountered.

Despite refinements in investigation and treatment the prognosis for lung cancer remains dismal and 90% of patients who develop this disease will die of their tumour within 5 years. Much enthusiasm and expense has been expended on screening programmes in the hope that early detection will improve survival. A major study has been instituted by the National Cancer Institute of the United States involving the Johns Hopkins Medical Institutions, the Mayo Clinic and The Memorial Sloane Kettering Cancer Centre. These three institutions enrolled over 31 000 men at high risk of developing lung cancer and subjected them to periodic chest X-ray and sputum cytology analysis. The results of the initial screen have been published (Berlin et al. 1984) and results on the incidence study are now becoming available (Sanderson 1985; Tockman 1985; Martini 1985). Following the initial negative screening examination the Mayo Lung Project identified 4.9 cases of lung cancer per 1000 patients per year. Despite encouraging statistics regarding resectability rate, postsurgical staging and 5-year survival rates, the overall lung cancer mortality in the screened and control groups was not significantly different. Improvements in 5-year survival are largely explained by a lengthening of the lead time during which tumours may remain asymptomatic. We are forced to conclude that these elaborate and expensive studies are not cost effective.

This conclusion should cause us little surprise. If we accept the theory of exponential growth, then NSCLC has a doubling time of 80–160 days (Geddes 1979). Such tumours will have been present and able to metastasize for 6–8 years prior to diagnosis, and diagnosing such tumours some months earlier cannot radically alter chances of cure.

Evaluation and Management of Non-Small-Cell Lung Cancer

In the treatment of lung cancer the only reliable prospect of cure lies in pulmonary resection. Therefore once the diagnosis is established or strongly suspected the patient should be evaluated for surgery. This process essentially asks two questions: a) is the patient's general fitness good enough to undergo major surgery, and is lung function adequate to withstand pulmonary resection, and b) is the patient's tumour sufficiently localised to offer a prospect of cure by pulmonary resection. After completing the evaluation the answer to the first question will provide the surgeon with a risk factor which can be balanced against the benefit factor derived from answering the second question. Whilst these answers will provide the surgeon with statistics, such as the percentage risk of operative death and the percentage chance of cure, these statistics have no relevance for an individual patient. However, they represent the only means by which a decision can be made. Evaluation of these two factors proceeds concurrently, but for discussion can be best considered as independent aspects of evaluation.

The assessment of patient fitness will take into account the presence of concurrent disease such as diabetes, cardiovascular disease and renal impairment, the patient's age and the patient's psychological approach to major surgery. It hinges fundamentally, however, on the patient's respiratory reserve and the lung function which can be expected following resection. Whilst a battery of sophisticated lung function tests is available to physicians (Tisi 1979), the only ones which have been shown to have a bearing on perioperative mortality are (a) an elevated pCO_2 at rest and (b) assessments of peak flow and spirometric measurement of forced vital capacity (FVC) and forced expiratory volume in 1 second (FEV1). Whilst the significance of the former is self evident – if the patient is in respiratory failure preoperatively he or she will not do well after removal of appreciable portions of lung tissue – the relevance of the latter may at first sight be obscure. It is probable that forced expiratory measurements predict the patient's ability to expectorate following surgery, thus avoiding sputum retention and consequent chest infection. The postoperative FVC can be derived from the preoperative FVC using isotope ventilation scans but in practice a satisfactory assessment can be made knowing the proposed extent of resection and assessing the function of the lung tissue to be removed clinically and on chest radiographs. Overall the risks of pulmonary resection should now be less than 5%. The mortality for pneumonectomy remains higher than that of lobectomy but should not exceed 10% (Ginsberg et al. 1983). It may be necessary to explain to the relatives and the patient that for any individual the risks of course will be 0% or 100%!

For the tumour to be suitable for pulmonary resection it should be confined to the lung and its intrapulmonary and hilar lymph nodes, stage I or II in the TNM classification. It is occasionally justified to resect stage III tumours in unusual circumstances. Stage IIIa squamous cancers involving the lateral chest wall can be resected in the absence of nodal metastases (T3N0) with good survival figures (53.7%) (Piehler et al. 1982). The chest wall resection entailed, however, adds appreciably to the operative mortality (15%–16%) (Piehler et al. 1982) (Jamieson et al. 1979) and the surgeon should take this into consideration before undertaking such resections. Stage IIIa squamous tumours with limited involvement of mediastinal glands detected at mediastinoscopy have been resected by Pearson et al. (1982) with a 9% overall survival figure rising to 15% for those tumours which can be completely resected. I have found this a difficult preoperative assessment to make, and even in the hands of Pearson et al. (1982) complete resection was possible in only 65% of this group, with an operative mortality of 16%. These authors used adjuvant irradiation to the mediastinum prior to surgery, and although this may seem prudent there is no proof that it influenced survival figures following resection of this specific subgroup. More recently there has been the suggestion that patients with isolated cerebral metastases may still benefit from surgical treatment of the primary provided surgical control of the metastases has proved or proves feasible. Early studies have shown survival figures of 35% at 3 years in these unusual circumstances (Mussi et al. 1985) (Magilligan et al. 1986). In general, however, the surgeon is restricted to operating on patients with stages I and II disease, and in the preoperative evaluation should seek to identify patients with (a) extrathoracic metastases or (b) mediastinal involvement by direct extension (T3 and T4) or mediastinal node metastasis (N2 and N3).

Extrathoracic metastases may be evident clinically, in the patient's history or on examination. The recent onset of bone pain may be dismissed by the patient as due to degenerative conditions and the surgeon must actively enquire to elucidate such symptoms. Neurological deficit may be apparent, but brain secondaries are often accompanied by subtle changes in personality which will not be evident to the clinician. The patient's relatives, if asked, may readily provide such information. Clinical examination may reveal other evidence of dissemination with palpable supraclavicular lymph nodes or irregular hepatomegaly. Non-specific evidence of metastases may be evidenced by unexplained weight loss of more than 3 kg in 6 months, and here also the patient may often rationalise, discounting his or her weight loss as due to recent attempts at dietary restriction. Other non-specific features of occult metastases are unexplained anaemia (haemoglobin $<$ 11 g%), elevated alkaline phosphatase or serum calcium estimation. In the absence of these organ-specific or non-specific features to suggest metastasis, Hooper et al. (1978) have shown routine isotope scans of bone, brain and liver to confer no advantage. In their study, isotope scans of the brain and liver were always negative, and such scans of the bones were falsely positive in half of the cases where unexpected abnormalities were demonstrated. Where these organ-specific or non-specific features existed, however, bone scans were positive in 36% of patients. As these indicators are often non-specific, metastases should also be sought within the brain and abdomen. Ultrasound of the liver has been shown to be superior to isotope scanning (Snow et al. 1979). CT scanning is more sensitive in the assessment of brain metastases (Lucins et al. 1980), is as effective as ultrasound in assessment of the liver (Snow et al. 1979) and provides a wealth of additional information. Computerised tomography allows evaluation of the brain, liver, adrenals, kidneys and retroperitoneal lymph nodes and provides additional information as to the intrathoracic extent of disease. For these reasons its routine use has become popular in the search for distant metastases prior to surgery, but its cost-effectiveness has not been proven. In a recent study (Grant et al. 1986) we undertook routine CT scans of the brain, chest and abdomen in 114 patients coming to surgery for non-small-cell lung cancer (Fig. 1). Whilst evidence suggestive of metastasis was seen in nine scans of the abdomen and ten of the brain, in only two scans of the abdomen and one of the brain was this an isolated contraindication to surgery. Whilst

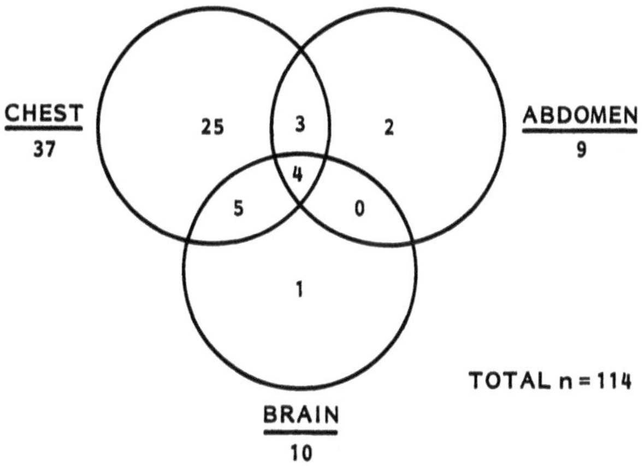

Fig. 1. Computerised tomographic detection of distant metastases in NSCLC: preoperative screening

for these three patients the scans were highly significant and prevented futile resections, this CT expenditure represents a considerable financial burden to any institution.

The assessment of the mediastinum seeks to evaluate whether a tumour is physically resectable and whether its resection is desirable, offering the patient a substantial improvement in survival over alternative treatments. Intrathoracic staging is a steplike process (Spiro and Goldstraw 1984) and many patients need proceed no further than clinical examination. There may be the fixed distension of jugular veins indicating superior vena caval obstruction. The patient may be hoarse, with the bovine cough characteristic of recurrent laryngeal palsy. The patient may complain of dysphagia and barium examination should be undertaken to exclude coincident disease such as reflux oesophagitis and to confirm the indentation and compression of the oesophagus at the level of the main carina due to extensive mediastinal gland deposits. On occasions the chest radiograph may show unequivocal mediastinal gland enlargement. The sensitivity of this test is relatively low and its specificity high, such that confirmation of glandular metastases need not be pursued histologically (Swett et al. 1982). If a pleural effusion is evident on the chest radiograph, it should be aspirated, and if cytology is positive or if the effusion is heavily blood stained, the patient is best considered inoperable (T4). Where clinical or radiographic features of mediastinal involvement are absent, or where the mediastinal contour is obscured on chest radiographs by adjacent tumour or atelectatic lung, further scrutiny of the mediastinum should be undertaken as in 25% of such cases significant gland involvement will be identified (Goldstraw et al. 1983; Pearson et al. 1972). Since its introduction by Carlens in 1959, the gold standard in this respect has become mediastinoscopy. Pearson et al. (1972) have demonstrated in a retrospective study that the routine use of mediastinoscopy will improve the resectability rate from 77% to 94% by detecting superior mediastinal invasion or gross involvement of superior mediastinal glands. Debate continues, however, as to whether more subtle degrees of mediastinal involvement at mediastinoscopy should contraindicate resection. This confusion is largely based upon comparison of surgical results containing heterogeneous groups of N2 disease. Several papers report 5-year survival figures following resection of N2 disease of 0%–30% (Kirsh et al. 1971; Abbey Smith 1978), and the latter figure is used by many surgeons as a justification not to undertake routine mediastinoscopy. In many of these studies only those patients surviving complete resection are included in the study, and frequently surgical staging is undertaken by a retrospective review of pathology reports, a notoriously inaccurate assessment. Closer scrutiny of the literature suggests that N2 disease may exist in several patterns and this point has been eloquently addressed by Pearson et al. in a keynote paper (Pearson et al. 1982). It is probable that the surgeon should recognise at least four categories of N2 disease in potentially resectable patients:

1. Mediastinoscopy may disclose extensive involvement of the superior mediastinal glands, and survival following complete resection in this group is unlikely to be above 0% (Gibbons 1972; Viikari et al. 1974; Fosburg et al. 1974).
2. Mediastinoscopy may disclose limited involvement of the lower paratracheal glands in the ipsilateral chain. Overall survival figures following thoracotomy in this group are 9% rising to 18% for those with squamous carcinoma successfully undergoing complete resection (Pearson et al. 1982).
3. Mediastinoscopy may be negative and yet at thoracotomy glands (beyond the reach of the mediastinoscope) may be found to be extensively replaced by metastases or there may be less extensive but macroscopic involvement of glands within the reach of the mediastinoscope. In this group Pearson et al. (1982) have found a 24% 5-year survival for patients proceeding to thoracotomy, rising to 41% for those undergoing complete resection.
4. There will be a further subgroup of patients where mediastinoscopy and thoracotomy find the glands macroscopically normal but routine nodal dissection will reveal micrometastases. This group represents 8% of the patients in my practice, and as yet we have no details as to the 5-year survival, but one would expect it to be in excess of 40%.

It can be seen that for any surgeon not undertaking mediastinoscopy a heterogeneous group of postsurgical N2 patients will be obtained and the overall survival of all four categories could well approach the 30% reported (Kirsh et al. 1971; Abbey Smith 1978). Mediastinoscopy does not identify all patients who have N2 disease, nor should we seek to deny surgery to all patients found to have N2 disease. Mediastinoscopy, however, does allow us to identify extensive superior mediastinal involvement where resection is futile. It may be justified in a small select subgroup to proceed to thoracotomy despite positive findings at mediastinoscopy.

The lymphatic drainage of the left upper lobe is altered by the interposition of the aortic arch and it has been shown that for tumours in this location left anterior mediastinotomy is a useful adjunct to cervical mediastinoscopy. Left anterior mediastinotomy may disclose direct invasion or mediastinal gland involvement beyond the reach of the cervical approach in as many as 36% of patients with left upper lobe tumours (Bowen 1978) and may even supplant the cervical approach (Jolly et al. 1980) for patients with tumours in this location. The alternative approach of extended cervical mediastinoscopy to explore the subaortic fossa is being evaluated (Ginsberg et al. 1987). Preoperative exploration of the mediastinum by cervical mediastinoscopy, supplemented by left anterior mediastinotomy in the case of left upper lobe tumours, remains a valuable assessment prior to surgery. These techniques, however, require a great deal of experience in their undertaking and evaluation and are attended by a small risk of rather irksome complications (Pearson 1967; Foster et al. 1972). There has been a great deal of interest in the evaluation of non-invasive methods of assessing the mediastinum. Some authors have successfully used gallium scanning of the mediastinum and the literature suggests a sensitivity of 50%–60% with a specificity of 95% (Hirleman et al. 1980; Richardson et al. 1980; DeMeester et al. 1979). This technique, however, has not proved reproducible in the hands of many people and is not widely utilised. Radiographic imaging techniques are more widely available but assume an association between gland size and microscopic pathology. All surgeons are aware that large glands may be reactive whilst small glands may contain metastases. There is no absolute size above which glands are certain to be malignant, nor below which they are certain to be benign. In several studies utilising histological examination of lymph nodes by mediastinoscopy and thoracotomy, glands less than 1 cm in diameter have been found to be malignant in 8%–36% and glands larger than 2 cm have been found to be benign in 45%–55% of cases (Friedman et al. 1984; Brion et al. 1985). Despite this basic flaw, radiographic imaging of mediastinal node size may be of value in selecting patients for mediastinal exploration prior to thoracotomy. Many surgeons place their reliance on conventional tomographic imaging and 55° oblique tomography. These techniques can identify involved glands with a sensitivity of around 50% and a specificity of about 95% (Osbourne et al. 1982). Such conventional tomographic techniques have largely become obsolete with the development of computerised axial tomography. Although its assessment of the mediastinum may be no more accurate than conventional tomography, it provides a plethora of additional information on intrathoracic extent and extrathoracic disease which renders it vastly superior. The literature contains many studies using second, third and fourth generation computerised scanners to assess the presence of mediastinal node metastases. The accuracy of this assessment varies, depending upon the speed of the scanner, its resolution, the size criteria used to determine abnormality, and the care with which histological confirmation of abnormality has been taken. This subject has been reviewed at length (Goldstraw 1986). It would appear that as one reduces the size criteria for abnormality the sensitivity with which the CT scan can detect such glands will rise at the expense of a falling specificity. CT scanning cannot, however, achieve 100% specificity, and it has therefore come to be used as a screening procedure to detect those patients with enlarged glands which must be checked histologically by mediastinal exploration prior to thoracotomy. It is most unusual for CT scanning to disclose irrefutable evidence of mediastinal involvement such that thoracotomy is contraindicated. A reasonable summary of the present state of CT scanning in the preoperative assessment of non-small-cell lung cancer would appear to be:

1. If the CT scan of the mediastinum shows no lymph nodes larger than 1 cm in diameter, mediastinal exploration will not disclose a contraindication to surgery and the surgeon may proceed to thoracotomy directly.
2. If CT scanning discloses lymph nodes larger than 1 cm in diameter or suggests mediastinal invasion, this requires to be evaluated at mediastinal exploration prior to thoracotomy.
3. In approximately 5% of cases CT scanning will disclose extrathoracic metastases which are not clinically suspected and thus contraindicate resection.

If the mediastinal abnormalities on CT scanning are beyond the reach of the mediastinoscope it is still reasonable to undertake mediastinoscopy to exclude more proximal extension. If this proves negative then the surgeon must weigh the CT evidence of invasion very carefully against the desire not to deny the patient the one hope for cure. We have found resection possible in half the patients in this dilemma (Goldstraw et al. 1983).

At thoracotomy the surgeon should check the preoperative evaluation of resectability and undertake routine dissection of mediastinal lymph nodes even if they are macroscopically normal. We have found that such routine dissection, although tiresome, will reveal metastases in 24% of glands, which might materially influence the decision regarding resection or postoperative adjuvant treatment (Goldstraw and Gaer 1986, unpublished data). Incomplete resection of macroscopic disease is rarely justified or "palliative" (Pearson et al. 1972; Rocmans 1981). Additionally, no survival advantage has been shown for undertaking resections more extensive than that necessary to remove the primary growth with its involved lymphatic drainage (Bignall et al. 1967; Kirsh et al. 1981). Indeed the trend is one of increasing conservatism. In node-negative tumours where involvement of the main bronchus is the only contraindication to lobectomy, bronchoplastic procedures have been shown to carry a lower operative risk than pneumonectomy without compromising the chances of cure in these, often localised, tumours (Jensik et al. 1972; Firmin et al. 1983). The logic of this argument would suggest that for small peripheral tumours without nodal metastases segmentectomy would prove an adequate resection. This approach is reasonable in patients with limited pulmonary reserve (Bennett and Abbey Smith 1979) and it has proved a desirable substitute in patients able to tolerate lobectomy (Jensik et al. 1979; Hoffman and Ransdell 1980).

It is customary to assess the results of treatment in lung cancer in 5-year survival statistics. Whilst this is a convenient statistical measure, it does not equate with cure, and relapses can be expected to 10 years following surgery and beyond (Abbey Smith 1981; Kirsh et al. 1981). Large series report an overall 5-year survival figure for surgery in non-small-cell lung cancer of 28%–33% (Kirsh et al. 1981; Shields et al. 1972). These crude figures incorporate the results of surgery for all cell types other than small cell, at all stages, and by all resections. We are often given few details as to the extent of preoperative staging evaluation. The results of surgery appear more favourable, and some might say more realistic, if we consider specific cell types and TNM subgroups identified at postsurgical staging. Whilst pTNM may provide the most accurate staging available for postsurgical subgroups, it does not always correlate with the cTNM categories on which decisions are based. If we consider only squamous carcinoma, Wilkins et al. (1978) have found a 40% 5-year survival figure for all stages of disease and Immerman et al. (1981) a 65% disease-free 5-year survival in stages 1 and 2. If one concentrates on the most favourable postsurgical category (T1N0), then survival figures of 80% at 5 years have been reported (Naruke et al. 1978; Williams et al. 1981). Naruke et al. (1978) has eloquently demonstrated the progressive fall in 5-year survival figures with advancing T and N subgroups. Even better results can be obtained with stage I tumours identified in a screening programme (Melamed et al. 1981), but this may be fallacious and the results favourably affected by the lead time prior to development of symptoms (VS). Pancoast tumours present a special and extremely difficult problem. These apical non-small-cell lung cancers presenting with radicular pain involve the first and second ribs and adjacent structures such as the sympathetic chain, the subclavian vessels and the brachial plexus. Cure in such situations is unlikely and the symptoms distressing and difficult to palliate. Some optimism has been produced by the work of Paulson (1975). He has a reported 34% 5-year survival figure for "superior sulcus tumours" by the combined approach of preoperative radiotherapy and en bloc resection. The use of the term "superior sulcus tumours" is confusing as it undoubtedly includes patients with apical pulmonary tumours as well as the classical Pancoast variant. The difference is important since the former is a peripheral tumour whose concentric growth invades the chest wall on one arc and where the results of surgery are favourable, and the latter represents a tumour whose growth pattern almost suggests an extrapulmonary origin and where invasion into the chest wall often grossly exceeds the superficial involvement of the lung parenchyma. The use by Paulson of preoperative radiotherapy further obscures the issue since it will undoubtedly affect postsurgical staging and the histological appearances. Paulson noted that in 4% of his patients no histological diagnosis had been obtained preoperatively and no tumour was visible in the resection specimen. One must wonder if they indeed had a neoplasm originally! It would appear from the work of Paulson (1975) and Miller et al. (1979) that some hope can be offered to patients with non-small-cell lung cancer at the apex of the lung invading the chest wall where these patients have no nodal metastases. Logic would suggest, however, that radiotherapy following surgery would be more effective in dealing with the reduced tumour bulk and where the residue has been tagged at the time of thoracotomy.

As surgeons we are incapable of improving the results of our treatment in cancer by extending the scale of our operations. Improved results must come by (a) more accurately identifying those patients whose disease is localised sufficiently to permit surgical cure or (b) effective adjuvant treatment which can deal with residual disease after surgery has excised the bulk of the tumour. The first approach will not increase the number of surgical cures, merely improve the surgical statistics by the avoidance of surgery in patients with little prospect of cure. In this respect the major advance in the past 30 years has been the routine use of mediastinoscopy, although some slight additional benefit has been gained from isotope scanning, gallium scanning and computerised axial tomography. It would appear that at present we can expect little further advance in this aspect of preoperative evaluation unless and until labelled monoclonal antibodies become available. The second approach is inherently more satisfactory as it will increase the number of patients cured of lung cancer. For adjuvant therapy to be effective we must identify the patterns of relapse at various stages and in various cell types, and then develop adjuvant treatments effective at these sites. Relapse patterns may be judged by: (a) autopsy studies; (b) clinical evidence of relapse; and (c) intensive surveillance imaging to detect occult relapse. The autopsy study by Matthews et al. (1973) studied 183 patients dying within 1 month of "curative" resection for non-small-cell lung cancer. These patients included all postsurgical staging and we have not details as to the methods used in preoperative evaluation. It is unlikely that mediastinoscopy or isotope scanning was routinely undertaken. In no less than one-third of patients macroscopic residual disease was determined at autopsy. In two-fifths of these patients, the residual tumour was intrathoracic and in three-fifths residual disease was found at distant sites. The most detailed autopsy examination must represent only a crude assessement of surgical "curability". Using the more critical test of time, Immerman et al. (1981) documented the relapse patterns of patients following resection of stage I and II non-small-cell lung cancer. Forty-four per cent of patients relapsed within 5 years, a figure higher than that found in the autopsy study of Matthews et al. (1973), but the ratio of intrathoracic to distant relapse remained surprisingly similar at two-fifths and three-fifths of the total number. Both autopsy and clinical studies may underestimate the number of sites of residual disease since patients may relapse clinically at one site but have occult metastases elsewhere. Clinically there is little to be gained in intensively investigating patients at relapse, but from a research standpoint it would be valuable to submit such patients to intensive scanning with isotope bone scans and whole body computerised tomography and autopsy. We have one such study continuing (Goldstraw et al. 1985). Of 45 patients presently entered in the study, 12 patients were postsurgical N2 and of these eight have so far relapsed. It is somewhat depressing that even in this subgroup only one of these relapses has been found to be isolated to the mediastinum; in the remainder distant metastases have either presented clinically or have been occult and detected on scanning. From the foregoing it will be evident that one can expect little improvement in surgical results by the addition of adjuvant radiotherapy limited to the mediastinum. Even if mediastinal irradiation can sterilise 20%–30% of patients with residual disease (Katz 1983), only 3%–4% of patients can expect to have their cure completed by the addition of such treatment.

There have been many studies utilising adjuvant radiotherapy in operable non-small-cell carcinoma. Many of these studies have been retrospective and non-randomised. Many could be criticised on the grounds that preoperative evaluation and perioperative staging would be judged inadequate by present standards such that groups would be heterogeneous, possibly containing patients with bulky residual disease. Early studies showed no survival advantage for adjuvant radiotherapy given preoperatively (Shields et al. 1970) or postoperatively (Paterson and Russell 1962). More recent studies have shown no survival advantage for adjuvant radiotherapy in patients with favourable staging after "curative" resection (Israel et al. 1979; Van Houtte et al. 1980). Other authors have suggested in retrospective studies that with higher dose levels the results of surgery in more advanced stages may be improved (Green et al. 1975; Chung et al. 1982) by postoperative adjuvant radiotherapy. The North American Lung Cancer Study Group prospectively assessed postoperative radiotherapy in stage II and III squamous carcinoma and found no improvement in time to recurrence or overall survival (Ginsberg 1985). Despite these gloomy precedents the British Medical Research Council and the Lung Cancer Group of the European Organization for Research on Treatment of Cancer (EORTC) are both pursuing investigations into the value of adjuvant radiotherapy in different postsurgical subgroups.

Clearly what is necessary is an effective systemic treatment which can deal with the occult micrometastases which presently elude our preoperative staging. Kennis (1980) has succinctly summarised the results in early studies utilising single-agent chemotherapy as an adjunct to surgical resection. The bulk of these studies have shown no survival difference. Some have shown a detrimental effect, and only two have shown any apparent benefit. The North American Lung Cancer Study Group are presently studying, in their protocol 772, the value of postoperative polychemotherapy following resection of stage II and III adenocarcinoma and large cell undifferentiated carcinoma. Early results suggest there may be a survival advantage for this adjuvant chemotherapy, but unfortunately their control group has received intrapleural bacille Calmette-Guérin (BCG) and oral levamisole and one cannot exclude the possibility that this is adversely influencing survival in the control group (Ginsberg 1985). Adjuvant immunotherapy has been disappointing. The initially encouraging results utilising intrapleural BCG (McKneally et al. 1976; McKneally et al. 1981) have not been substantiated by other studies (Mountain and Gail 1981; Bakker et al. 1981). Reports have appeared detailing the considerable morbidity of such intrapleural therapy (Law et al. 1981; Bakker et al. 1982).

We are forced to conclude that at present we are gaining increasing information on relapse patterns following surgery for non-small-cell lung cancer but that we lack any effective therapy which can deal with microscopic residual disease at distant sites. The use of adjuvant treatment in association with surgery for non-small-cell lung cancer at present should be restricted to prospective, randomised clinical trials.

Evaluation and Treatment of Small Cell Lung Cancer

Small cell anaplastic carcinoma accounts for 20% of all cases of lung cancer. The World Health Organization reclassification (1981) acknowledges the subdivision into the classical oat cell carcinoma and intermediate cell type. Whilst there may be differences in the response rates to chemotherapeutic regimens between these two varieties, their natural history is in most respects similar. Small cell lung cancer is a highly malignant, rapidly dividing tumour with a strong predisposition to disseminate early. In the vast majority of patients the disease is extensive by the time it presents, and survival is often measured in weeks. The pTNM staging system outlined for non-small-cell lung cancer has little application when dealing with small cell carcinoma, as 85% of patients will be stage III at presentation (Hansen 1984). Staging is usually restricted to the separation of patients with limited disease from those with extensive disease (Roswitt et al. 1968). At presentation 40% of patients will have limited disease as assessed by clinical examination, chest radiographs and bronchoscopy. More intensive evaluation will often show tumour to be more widespread (Harper et al. 1981). For the vast majority of patients presenting with small cell carcinoma of the lung, chemotherapy provides the best treatment, and median survival times can be doubled from 9 months to 18 months for those with limited disease, and from 4½ to 9 months for those with extensive disease. Combination chemotherapy using three or four drugs can be expected to produce a response in 70% of patients with limited disease (Greco and Oldham 1979). It is not yet clear whether mediastinal irradiation adds to the effectiveness of chemotherapy in small cell lung cancer. There is the suggestion, however, that it prevents local relapse, increasing the number of long-term survivals (Salazar and Creech 1980; Osterlind et al. 1986). The situation regarding prophylactic cranial irradiation (PCI) is even more confused. PCI has not been shown to improve median survival figures (Cox et al. 1978; Hansen et al. 1980). It may, however, delay the onset of cerebral relapse with its devastating consequences (Felletti et al. 1985). At present it would seem reasonable to add mediastinal irradiation and PCI to those patients with limited disease who achieve complete response following chemotherapy (Aroney et al. 1983). High-dose chemotherapy with or without autologous bone marrow transplantation has improved response rates in selected favourable subgroups but has not improved long-term survival figures (Smith et al. 1983; Souhami et al. 1985a). Disease-free survival to 2 years remains stubbornly about 20% (Ginsberg et al. 1979; Smith et al. 1981). In the absence of any dramatically more effective new agent, improved survival will depend on innovative approaches, possibly involving adjuvant surgery. The current thrust of chemotherapy research seems to be: (a) an attempt to maintain the present results with less toxic regimens or shorter treatment schedules; and (b) to identify prognostic indicators for more favourable groups who may have most to gain from aggressive therapy (Souhami et al. 1985b). The British Medical Research Council are currently exploring the effectiveness of three cycles of chemotherapy versus six, and the EORTC Lung Cancer Study Group studied five versus 12.

A number of studies are presently assessing the role of pulmonary resection in those patients with limited disease who achieve complete response. The approach has been shown to be practical but as yet its influence on survival and relapse patterns is unknown. This topic has been addressed by the North American Lung Cancer Study Group in their protocol 832, and the EORTC Lung Cancer Group have recently joined in this study.

Approximately 5% of patients with small cell lung cancer will present with extremely limited disease where surgery should be considered as primary treatment. The majority of these patients will be asymptomatic and present with a small peripheral opacity. In this small, highly selected subgroup, conventional TNM staging has some relevance. The largest study is that of Higgins et al. (1975), who accumulated 148 patients with small cell lung cancer from a group of 3133 asymptomatic patients presenting with a solitary pulmonary nodule. The overall 5-year survivorship of small cell lung cancer was 23% with figures of 59.5% for T1N0 tumours, 31% of T1N1 tumours, 28% for T2N0 tumours and 9% for T2N1 tumours. T3 or N2 lesions had a 5-year survivorship of 3.6%. Adjuvant treatment was not applied methodically in this study and such chemotherapy as was given would not now be considered to be effective. In a study from the Brompton Hospital, Shore and Paneth (1980) obtained a 25% 5-year survival figure in 41 patients retrospectively assessed. These studies suggest that small cell lung cancer may be occasionally found in a localised form by serendipity. With the increasing scope of fibreoptic bronchoscopy and the popularity of fine needle aspiration biopsy these peripheral localised tumours are now often appreciated to be small cell lung cancer and this fact should not automatically exclude the prospect of surgery. Certainly, intensive staging is necessary in such lesions. In addition to the staging procedures suggested for non-small-cell lung cancer, we would recommend that these patients undergo routine CT scanning of the brain, chest and abdomen, mediastinal exploration irrespective of the CT assessment of the mediastinum, and bone marrow biopsy. In my experience half of the patients with localised tumours successfully completing this intensive staging manoeuvre and proceeding to resection will subsequently be shown to have non-small-cell tumours. For those tumours still classified as small cell lung cancer following resection the benefit of adjuvant chemotherapy is unproven. Early trials utilising obsolete chemotherapy protocols showed no benefit (Shields et al. 1982). For postsurgical stage II patients adjuvant chemotherapy would appear reasonable, but for those with pTNM categories T1N0, T1N1 and T2N0 a prospective study is necessary (Goldstraw 1985 a) and such a study is presently being undertaken by the EORTC Lung Group in conjunction with the British Medical Research Council.

Other Primary Malignancies

Most remaining primary malignancies of the lung were historically grouped as bronchial adenoma. This misnomer reflects the previous false impression of their benignity (Dick 1950). Several large studies have now clearly demonstrated the malignant nature of these tumours (Goodner et al. 1961; Turnbull et al. 1972; Goldstraw et al. 1976). Carcinoid tumours arise from the Kulchitsky's cells between the columnar epithelial cells. They are the commonest of these malignancies and most major thoracic units will see examples of this tumour annually. The tumour may remain localised for many years, and in the majority of patients cure may be expected following surgical excision. There may be some justification for considering benign "typical" and malignant "atypical" variants of this tumour (Lawson et al. 1976). Carcinoid tumours often extend for some distance as an endobronchial polyp. This and their low degree of malignancy makes more conservative resections and bronchoplastic resections feasible and justified (Okike 1978). The position of the tumour and distal suppuration contraindicate the use of bronchoplastic operations in 10%–20% of resections (Brandt et al. 1984). It is often difficult to decide on the presence of local invasion as carcinoid tumours tend to insinuate between the bronchial cartilages, mimicking true invasion. In large series of carcinoid tumours the assessment of local invasion appears to vary between 20% and 50%. Regional node metastases have been found in 10%–25% of cases, whilst distant lymphatic or haematogenous metastases are rare, occurring in about 5% of reported cases. The carcinoid syndrome is rarely associated with pulmonary primaries, only being reported with extensive metastatic disease. Rarely hypertrophic pulmonary osteoarthropathy has been reported with the malignant variant of this tumour (Bradford et al. 1984 a).

Adenoid cystic carcinoma was previously termed cylindroma. Similar tumours occur within the salivary glands. Those within the chest usually affect the trachea or main bronchi. These tumours are obviously malignant and local invasion is always present. A marked feature of these tumours is their extensive microscopic extension along the tracheobronchial tree for some distance away from the macroscopic margins of the tumour. This feature greatly adds to the technical difficulty of resection, and frozen section analysis of resection margins is crucial in assessing tumour clearance. Most reported series (Goodner et al. 1961; Goldstraw et al. 1976) contain less than ten examples of this type of tumour. Regional node metastases are present in 25%–50% of cases and distant metastases are predominantly lymphatic, although occasional haematogenous metastases have been reported. These tumours are frequently inoperable and respond little to radiotherapy. Their palliation is discussed further in the section on tumours of the trachea and major bronchi.

Mucoepidermoid carcinoma is rare. The only reported series is that of Turnbull et al. (1972), who reported their experience with 12 such cases. In 75% of their cases metastases were present, and average survival in ten treated patients was only 5.3 months.

Secondary Malignancies

It is not uncommon for thoracic surgeons to excise a pulmonary mass only to find on histology or by subsequent events that the lesion was metastatic from an occult primary. This remains a cost-effective method of establishing the diagnosis and may have some therapeutic benefit. The excision of known metastatic lesions from the thorax is much in vogue, and several large series have been reported recently (Takita et al. 1981; Wilkins 1982; Mountain et al. 1984). We have recently reviewed our experience at the Brompton Hospital, removing metastatic deposits within the lungs, chest wall, mediastinal lymph nodes and even heart (Goldstraw 1987) from a large variety of extrathoracic primary tumours. We have shown this approach to be safe, with low mortality and morbidity. However, our large personal experience and the enormous experience already reported in the literature still leaves many unanswered questions in this area of surgical endeavour. The post-chemotherapeutic resection of intrathoracic deposits from testicular germ cell tumours can provide useful information on the effectiveness of chemotherapy, help define prognosis and identify those patients requiring further chemotherapy (Tait et al. 1984). Very occasionally the excision of metastatic deposits may be justified to relieve symptoms, but usually palliation can be achieved by non-surgical treatment. In the vast majority of patients thoracic metastasectomy is undertaken with curative intent. Thoracic surgeons are being encouraged in this approach by better long-term control of the primary tumour by aggressive combined modality treatment, and the persisting difficulty in treating pulmonary deposits by non-surgical means. Many of the carcinomas and sarcomas having a predeliction for pulmonary metastases are resistant to chemotherapy, and radiotherapy may damage large areas of lung tissue around the metastasis whilst failing to control metastatic deposits. Thoracic metastases from testicular germ cell tumours may be controlled by chemotherapy, but late relapse may occur from bulky residual deposits (Tait et al. 1984). Anecdotal reports abound of long-term survival following thoracic metastasectomy, but it is unlikely that we will ever be able to demonstrate a statistically significant survival advantage to this approach because of the highly individual nature of each patient's problem, the justifiable selection that occurs prior to surgery and the difficulty in mounting prospective randomised studies of such patients. An autopsy study by Farrell in 1935 suggested that 15% of patients dying with carcinoma and 25% of those dying with sarcoma may have metastatic disease limited to the lungs. Whilst this study provides some encouragement it is a far cry from suggesting that the removal of pulmonary deposits has any influence on survival.

In selecting patients for thoracic metastasectomy a number of guidelines may be proposed, but statistical support for many of these is lacking.

1. One must expect reliable control of the primary tumour. This will usually have been achieved by surgical excision with clear microscopic margins. Where other treatment is claimed to have controlled the primary a long period of observation must support this contention.
2. Extrathoracic metastatic sites should be excluded, using the most sensitive tests available such as hepatic ultrasound and computerised tomography. If extrathoracic metastases are known to be present, their control by surgical excision must be assured.
3. The interval from treatment of the primary to the presentation with metastases will reflect the tumour doubling time. Those patients with the longer intervals will do better with all forms of treatment, and even without treatment. There is no statistical evidence to justify any arbitrary interval being imposed prior to undertaking thoracic metastasectomy.
4. There is much to be gained by a period of observation once metastases are recognised. This will give time for other presently occult deposits to become visualised, thus demonstrating the futility of a surgical approach, or allowing a more effective clearance of metastatic deposits. Many patients cannot accept this philosophical approach. There is the theoretical possibility of tertiary deposits developing and some statistical evidence to favour early surgery once metastases have been identified (Mountain et al. 1984).

5. The decision to operate and the surgical approach must be based on the best intelligence available. In my experience computerised tomography with contiguous cuts through both lung fields is mandatory. The choice of surgical approach will depend upon the number of metastases, their size, their proximity to hilar structures, and the texture of individual metastatic deposits. If all factors are favourable, bilateral pulmonary metastases may be excised through median sternotomy (Johnston 1983).

We are increasingly returning to staged bilateral thoracotomies when tumour deposits are numerous, particularly if posterior, where tumour masses approach the hilum and may necessitate segmental or lobar resection, and in tumours such as synovial sarcoma where the consistency of deposits is so close to that of lung tissue as often to make even large deposits difficult to palpate. A combined surgical approach may be feasible if computerised tomography shows lesions within the chest and abdomen which can be approached through midline or lateral thoracoabdominal incisions. Where multiple deposits are to be excised from several sites the construction of a "scanagram" may provide a useful aide memoire in the operating theatre. Such scanagrams are constructed from computerised tomograms by the radiologist imposing metastatic deposits on posteroanterior and lateral chest radiographs (Fig. 2). At thoracotomy each deposit predicted on the CT scan must be sought and identified with a stay suture. The surgeon should carefully palpate the lung, inflated and collapsed, for additional lesions, and each is excised by wedge excision in the most conservative manner appropriate. Metal staples and clips should be avoided since they will produce scatter on subsequent computerised tomograms, adding to the difficulty of postoperative assessment. We have removed up to 16 deposits from one lung, but clearly the chances of surgical cure fall as the number of deposits increase, particularly if a substantial proportion of these have not been predicted on preoperative CT scans. In our early experience (Goldstraw 1983), 38% of metastatic deposits removed at thoracotomy had not been predicted on the preoperative CT scan. Some surgeons would use this to argue for a bilateral approach in all cases (Johnston 1983). Whilst this argument may have statistical support in patients with metastatic sarcoma we have avoided this approach since a misguided exploration may produce pulmonary atelectasis and scarring which would obscure subsequent assessment, and increase the difficulty of further explorations.

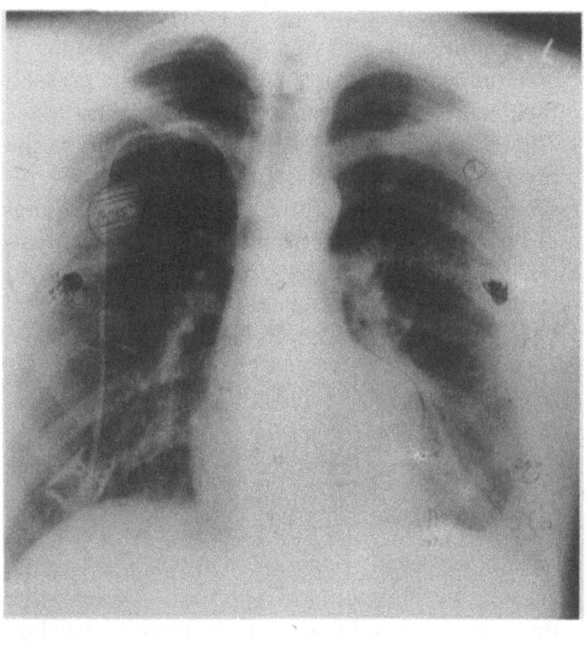

Fig. 2. "Scanagram" showing metastatic deposits in both lungs and mediastinum, superimposed on chest radiograph

Despite the lack of statistical survival advantage there can be no doubt that thoracic metastasectomy is a valuable modality in the treatment of disseminated disease. Pulmonary metastasectomy for carcinomatous deposits has led to 25%–40% 5-year survival, and for sarcomatous deposits, 20%–40% 5-year survival. We must be cautious not to allow our oncological colleagues to encourage us into an over-optimistic approach which will lead to this modality falling into disrepute.

Tumours of the Trachea and Major Bronchi

Primary tumours of the trachea, squamous carcinoma and adenoidcystic carcinoma are rare and the principles governing their surgical treatment are well established (Grillo 1973; Grillo 1982). Solitary metastatic deposits within the bronchus and trachea are even rarer, but a surgical approach to these may be feasible. Extensive irresectable primary tumours and metastatic deposits obstructing the trachea or main bronchi represent a commoner problem and the surgeon may have a valuable role in alleviating obstruction and impending asphyxia. Such tumours may have an endobronchial component but there is often a major and dominant extrabronchial component. The endobronchial lesions may be treated in a variety of ways depending on the techniques available locally. The bronchoscopic removal of bronchial deposits with large biopsy forceps or the diathermy loop may produce short-term but dramatic improvement. Laser resection is a more elegant, far more expensive, and possibly no more effective method of dealing with this endobronchial component (Toty et al. 1981; Hetzel.et al. 1985; Parr et al. 1984). Laser photoresection may relieve asphyxia, allowing a more careful and measured assessment of operability (George et al. 1986). The extrabronchial component of tracheal or main bronchus obstruction is primarily treated by external irradiation. Relief may, however, be partial and short lived, and further external irradiation may be contraindicated because of the tolerance of surrounding normal tissues. In such circumstances bronchoscopic implantation of radioactive gold grains has been shown to produce good symptomatic and radiographic improvement (Law et al. 1985). This useful technique, however, implies the usual precautions in handling radioactive materials and requires the coordinated assistance of surgeon, anaesthetist, radiotherapist and physicist. When all else fails, the insertion of a silastic hollow stent may produce worthwhile palliation of the distressing symptoms of asphyxiation. The T tube described by Montgomery (1968) and Grillo (1982) can relieve obstruction of the whole tracheal length and the bifurcated stent described by Westaby (Westaby 1983) can also deal with obstruction to one or both main bronchi (Fig. 3). The insertion of these stents requires only minor surgery and the performance of a tracheotomy, but anaesthesia may be difficult in the presence of critical airway narrowing.

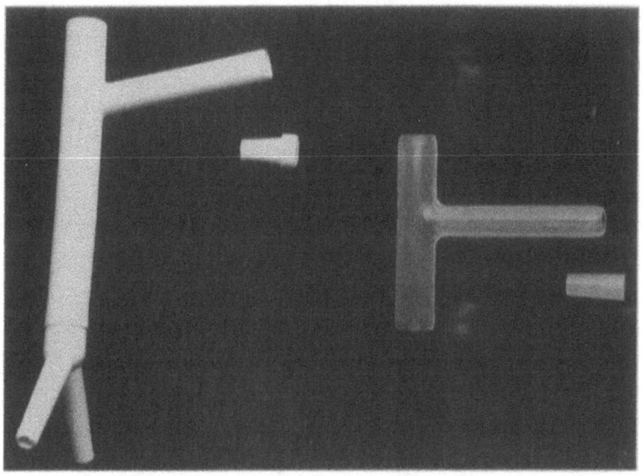

Fig. 3. Hollow stents for the tracheobronchial tree, *on the left* the Westaby pattern, and *on the right* the Montgomery tube

Tumours of the Pleura

There has been no progress in the past decade in the treatment of primary or secondary malignancies affecting the pleura. No chemotherapeutic agent has been proven to be effective, and their use should be limited to prospective phase II studies. A phase II study of mitoxantrane in mesothelioma is presently being conducted by the Lung Cancer Group of the EORTC. Radiotherapy given in high doses to a limited area may be valuable in alleviating pain. Inevitably oncologists are turning once more to the surgeon in a desperate hope for long-term palliation. Very occasionally a mesothelioma may present as a localised tumour deposit and prove amenable to surgical excision. More usually, however, such tumours are widespread and extensive, and surgical removal by pleuropneumonectomy and excision of the diaphragm carries a high mortality and morbidity (Butchart et al. 1976). There is no proof that such a radical approach extends survival or improves the quality of life. Pleural adenocarcinoma may lead to troublesome and frequent reaccumulations of effusion, and pleurodesis by pleurectomy or the insufflation of pleural irritants may prevent such reaccumulations and produce significant palliation. Pleuroperitoneal shunts are as yet unproven. The surgeon's major role in this distressing group of malignancies is usually confined to providing conclusive and accurate histology.

Tumours of the Mediastinum

The classic subdivision of mediastinal masses on radiographic appearances into anterior, middle and posterior remains valid, providing a useful differential diagnosis (Crofton and Douglas 1969). As in many areas of thoracic oncology the impact of computerised tomography of the mediastinum has been considerable, although perhaps of more diagnostic value than therapeutic. Computerised tomography can unravel the complex overlapping shadows which comprise the mediastinal outline on conventional radiography. The construction of a differential diagnosis based on anatomical localisation is not without fault, particularly within the angle formed by the sternum, the diaphragm and the pericardial outline (Fig. 4). In this area the anterior and middle mediastinal areas merge with the radiographic outline of the diaphragm, and masses in this area may arise from the diaphragm or below, or either of these mediastinal compartments (Bradford et al. 1984b).

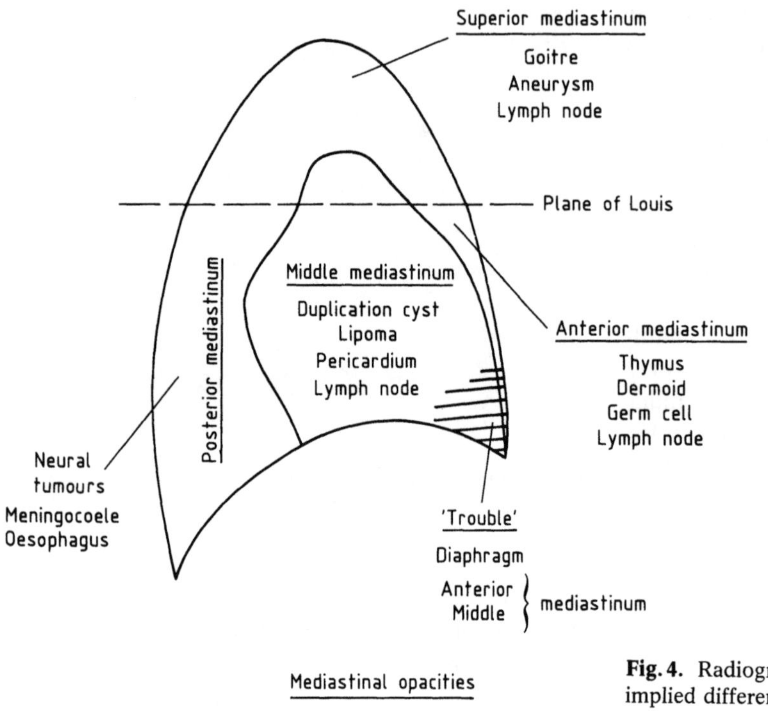

Fig. 4. Radiographic subdivision of the mediastinum and the implied differential diagnosis of opacities

Posterior Mediastinal Masses

Neural tumours are the commonest of all mediastinal masses, the majority being benign (Le Roux et al. 1984). They are often discovered on routine chest radiographs or those taken whilst investigating other ailments.

Computerised tomographic scanning may more accurately localise the tumour, predicting its immediate relationships. From time to time it will show the intraspinal extension of such tumours, allowing the thoracic surgeon to plan the operation in combination with a neurosurgeon. Surgical biopsy of posterior mediastinal masses is difficult. Needle biopsy may provide the diagnosis but is usually unnecessary as all such lesions should be resected if possible.

Middle Mediastinal Masses

Computerised tomographic scanning may accurately define the relationships of any mass located in the middle mediastinum on routine radiographs. The CT scan may prove diagnostic in the case of aortic aneurysms or diaphragmatic herniae. If the opacity is adjacent to the pericardium and has a water density (0–10 Houndsfield units) on CT scanning, then it may well be a pleuroperitoneal cyst. If translucent "spring-water" is obtained on needle aspiration and cytology of this fluid is negative, then such lesions may be left without surgery. All other middle mediastinal masses are best dealt with surgically, and the CT scan may help the surgeon in planning the approach and anticipating difficulties.

Anterior Mediastinal Masses

Anterior mediastinal tumours consist of benign and malignant tumours best treated by primary surgery, and other malignant tumours best treated initially by chemotherapy or radiotherapy. For this reason initial biopsy is usually undertaken and this can be performed with ease through a short anterior mediastinotomy incision. CT scanning may allow this step to be omitted in certain unusual circumstances (vide infra).

Thymomata are malignant in 30% of cases (Maggi et al. 1986). Malignancy may be suspected clinically by the presence of superior vena caval obstruction or shown radiographically by the presence of pleural deposits. Usually, however, the definition of malignancy will depend upon the surgeon's findings of pleural metastases or local invasion or on microscopic evidence of extracapsular extension following resection. When thymomata are malignant complete excision should be attempted. Where complete excision proves possible the relapse rate of malignant thymoma is no higher than that of benign variant (4%) (Maggi et al. 1986). It is at present unproven whether adjuvant radiotherapy is of use following complete excision of malignant thymoma, but clearly if excision is incomplete residual deposits should be tagged at surgery to facilitate postoperative radiotherapy. A CT scan is valuable in planning surgical excision and may occasionally show extensive involvement of vital structures such as to make any attempt at excision futile. A phase II study of combination chemotherapy in recurrent or metastatic thymoma is currently being conducted by the Lung Cancer Group of the EORTC.

Hodgkin's lymphoma and non-Hodgkin's lymphoma of B- and T-cell types may involve the anterior mediastinum as part of a regional involvement or be restricted to the region of the thymus (Marchevsky and Kaneko 1984). Such tumours should be initially treated by chemotherapy and radiotherapy, but we have had a small number of Hodgkin's lymphomas and B-cell lymphomas return for surgical excision of bulky residual disease following such treatment. If a prebiopsy CT scan therefore shows the lesion to be circumscribed such that it could be removed with ease, it is justifiable to proceed to excision biopsy via a median sternotomy.

Malignant germ cell tumours may arise in the anterior mediastinum. Although these tumours are rare they form an important differential diagnosis in young males since the diagnosis can be established without biopsy by detecting elevated blood levels of one or both of the tumour markers, beta human chorionic gonadotrophin and alpha-fetaprotein. Our experience with 11 such cases leads us to recommend initial chemotherapy with *cis*-platinum-based combinations. If markers normalise then surgical excision of bulky residual disease is of value and the planning of such difficult surgery is greatly facilitated by CT scanning (Goldstraw 1985b).

Computerised tomographic scanning is at its most useful in aiding the surgeon in the management of anterior mediastinal masses. It may disclose the characteristic cystic appearance of thymic and dermoid cysts, thus allowing biopsy to be avoided and excision to be undertaken. If the mass is seen to be circumscribed, excision biopsy may be undertaken with value even if subsequent histology discloses a lymphoma and adjuvant chemotherapy is considered. It may on occasion show that any attempt to excise malignant tumours would be impractical, but in the majority of cases will help the surgeon plan the surgical attack more effectively.

Tumours of the Chest Wall and Diaphragm

Primary malignancies of the chest wall are rare and one should take care to exclude metastatic deposits or intrathoracic tumours directly invading the chest wall. Chondrosarcoma is the most common of such primary tumours, but osteoblastoma, fibrosarcoma, rhabdomyosarcoma and haemangiosarcoma may occur. Malignant fibrous histiocytoma is a term increasingly used for tumours previously described as various types of spindle cell malignancy (Venn et al. 1986). The primary treatment of all such tumours is wide surgical excision if possible, usually necessitating prosthetic replacement of the chest wall (Le Roux and Sharma 1983). Such extensive surgery should not be undertaken without prior tissue diagnosis. Needle biopsy is often inconclusive or misleading, and open biopsy should be undertaken, siting the incision so that it can be excised at any subsequent resection. Many chest wall prostheses have been suggested, indicating the unsatisfactory nature of any one prosthetic material. At present the best available material would appear to be a Marlex mesh sandwich filled and rendered rigid by methyl methacrylate paste. Local relapse will follow surgical excision in 50% of chondrosarcomata and adjuvant radiotherapy is advisable in all but the most localised, well-differentiated sarcoma. The value of adjuvant chemotherapy is as yet unproven.

References

Abbey Smith R (1978) The importance of mediastinal lymph node invasian by pulmonary carcinoma in selection of patients for resection. Ann Thorac Surg 25: 5–11

Abbey Smith R (1981) Evaluation of the longterm results of surgery for bronchial carcinoma. J Thorac Cardiovasc Surg 82: 325–333

American Joint Committee of Cancer – Task Force on Staging of Lung Cancer (1979) American Joint Committee on Cancer, Chicago

Aroney RS, Aisner J, Wesley MN, Whitacre MY, van Echo PA, Slawson RG, Wiernik PH (1983) Value of prophylactic cranial irradiation given at complete remission in small cell lung carcinoma. Cancer Treat Rep 67: 675–682

Bakker W, Nijhuis-Heddes JM, Wever AM, Brutel de la Riviere A, van der Velde EA, Dijkman JA (1981) Postoperative intrapleural BCG in lung cancer: lack of efficacy and possible enhancement of tumour growth. Thorax 36: 870–874

Bakker W, Nijhuis-Heddes JMA, Brutel de la Riviere A, Dijkman JH (1982) Complications of postoperative intrapleural BCG in lung cancer. Ann Thorac Surg 33: 267–272

Bennett WF, Abbey Smith R (1979) Segmental resection for bronchogenic carcinoma: a surgical alternative for the compromised patient. Ann Thorac Surg 27: 169–172

Berlin NI, Buncher CR, Fontana RS, Frost JK, Melamed MR (1984) The National Cancer Institute Cooperative Early Lung Cancer Detection Program (CIC): results of the initial screen (prevelance). Am Rev Respir Dis 130: 545–549
Bignall JR, Martin M, Smithers DW (1967) Survival in 6086 cases of bronchial carcinoma. Lancet 1: 1067–1070
Bowen TE (1978) The value of anterior mediastinotomy in bronchogenic carcinoma of the left upper lobe. J Thorac Cardivasc Surg 76: 269–271
Bradford R, Griffith M, Goldstraw P (1984a) Hypertrophic pulmonary osteoarthropathy in association with a bronchial carcinoid tumour. Br J Dis Chest 78: 275–281
Bradford R, McLlelland J, Cohen SL, Goldstraw P (1984b) Thymoma presenting as a middle mediastinal mass. Postgrad Med J 60: 41–42
Brandt B, Heintz SE, Rose EF, Ehrenhaft JL (1984) Bronchial carcinoid tumours. Ann Thorac Surg 38: 63–65
Bringel C (1985) Sex characteristics in resected lung cancers. Fourth world conference on lung cancer, 25–30 August 1985, Toronto (Abstr 468)
Brion JP, Depauw L, Kuhn G, de Francquen PL, Friberg J, Rocmans P, Struyven J (1985) The role of computed tomography and mediastinoscopy in the preoperative staging of lung carcinoma. J Comput Assist Tomogr 9: 480–484
Butchart EG, Ashcroft T, Barnsley WC, Holden MP (1976) Pleuropneumonectomy in the management of diffuse malignant mesothelioma of the pleura. Thorax 31: 15–24
Carlens E (1959) Medistinoscopy: a method of inspection and tissue biopsy in the superior mediastinum. Dis Chest 36: 343–352
Chung CK, Stryker JA, Oneill MO, Demuth WE (1982) Evaluation of adjuvant postoperative radiotherapy for lung cancer. Int J Radiat Oncol Biol Phys 8: 1877–1880
Cox JD, Petrovich Z, Paig C, Stanley K (1978) Prophylactic cranial irradiation in patients with inoperable carcinoma of the lung. Preliminary report of a cooperative trial. Cancer 42: 1135–1140
Crofton J, Douglas A (1969) Respiratory diseases. Blackwell, Oxford
Demeester TR, Golomb HM, Kirchner P, Rezai-Zadeh K, Bitran JD, Streeter DL, Hoffman PC, Cooper M (1979) The role of gallium-67 scanning in the clinical staging and preoperative evaluation of patients with carcinoma of the lung. Ann Thorac Surg 28: 451–464
Dick B (1950) Bronchial adenoma. Edin Med J 57: 265–269
Doll P, Peto R (1976) Mortality in relation to smoking: 20 years observations on male British doctors. Br Med J [Clin Res] 2: 1525–1530
Farrell JT (1935) Pulmonary metastases: a pathological, clinical, roentgenologic study based on 78 cases at necropsy. Radiology 24: 444–451
Felleti AR, Souhami RL, Spiro SG, Geddes DM, Tobias JS, Mantell BS, Harper PG, Trask C (1985) Social consequences of brain or liver relapse in small cell carcinoma of the bronchus. Radiother Oncol 4: 335–339
Firmin RK, Azariades M, Lennox SC, Lincoln JCR, Paneth M (1983) Sleeve lobectomy (lobectomy and bronchoplasty) for bronchial carcinoma. Ann Thorac Surg 35: 442–449
Fosburg RG, O'Sullivan MJ, Ah-Tye P, Gibbons JA, Oury JH (1974) Positive mediastinoscopy: an ominous finding. Ann Thorac Surg 18: 346–356
Foster ED, Munro DD, Dobell ARC (1972) Mediastinoscopy: a review of anatomical relationships and complications. Ann Thorac Surg 13: 273–286
Friedman PJ, Feigin DS, Liston SE, Alazraki NP, Haghigi P, Young JA, Peters RM (1984) Sensitivity of chest radiography, computed tomography and gallium scanning to metastases of lung carcinoma. Cancer 54: 1300–1306
Geddes DM (1979) The natural history of lung cancer: a review based on tumour growth. Br J Dis Chest 73: 1–17
George PJM, Garrett CPO, Goldstraw P, Hetzel MR, Ramsay AD (1986) Resuscitative laser photoresection before elective surgery. Thorax 41: 812–813
Gibbons JRP (1972) The value of mediastinoscopy in assessing operability in carcinoma of the lung. Br J Dis Chest 66: 162–166
Ginsberg RJ (1985) The Lung Cancer Study Group experience. Proceedings of the mini symposia of the fourth world conference on lung cancer. 25–30 August 1985, Toronto
Ginsberg RJ, Comis RL, Gottlieb AJ, King GB, Goldberg J, Zamkoff K, El Badawi A, Meyer JA (1979) Longterm survivorship in small cell anaplastic lung carcinoma. Cancer Treat Rep 63: 1347–1349
Ginsberg RJ, Hill ID, Eagan RT, Thomas D, Mountain CF, Deslauriers J, Fry WA, Butz RO, Goldberg M, Water PF, Jones DP, Pairolero P, Rubenstein Z, Pearson FG (1983) Modern 30-day operative mortality for surgical resection in lung cancer. J Thorac Cardiovasc Surg 86: 654–658
Ginsberg RJ, Rice TW, Goldberg M, Water PF, Schmocker BJ (1987) Extended cervical mediastinoscopy: a single staging procedure for bronchogenic carcinoma of the left upper lobe. J Thorac Cardiovasc Surg 94: 673–678
Goldstraw P (1983) Workshop on pulmonary metastasectomy. E.S.S.O. Workshop, 2 November 1983, Amsterdam
Goldstraw P (1985a) Is there a place for surgery in small cell lung cancer? Journal Belge de Radiologie 68: 191–193
Goldstraw P (1985b) Thoracic surgery for germ cell tumours. In: Jones OG, Ward AM, Anderson CK (eds): Germ cell tumours II. Proceedings of the 2nd germ cell tumour conference, 15–19 April 1985, Leeds. Pergamon, Oxford
Goldstraw P (1986) CT scanning in the preoperative assessment of non-small cell lung cancer. In: Hansen HH (ed) Lung cancer: basic and clinical aspects. Nijhoff, Boston, pp 183–199
Goldstraw P (1987) Surgical management of pulmonary metastases. In: Slevin (ed) Clinical oncology, vol 1. Ballière, London, pp 601–621
Goldstraw P, Lamb D, McCormack RJM, Walbaum PR (1976) The malignancy of bronchial adenoma. J Thorac Cardiovasc Surg 72: 309–314
Goldstraw P, Kurzer M, Edwards D (1983) Preoperative staging of lung cancer: accuracy of computed tomography versus mediastonoscopy. Thorax 38: 10–15
Goldstraw P, Grant D, Edwards D (1985) Surveillance CT scans of brain, chest and abdomen following resection for non-small cell lung cancer: relapse patterns: implications for adjuvant therapy. Fourth world congress on lung cancer, 25–30 August 1985, Toronto (Abstr 315)
Goodner JT, Berg JW, Watson WL (1961) The non-benign nature of bronchial carcinoids and cylindromas. Cancer 14: 539–546
Grant D, Edwards D, Goldstraw P (1986) Preoperative CT staging in lung cancer. Annual meeting, Royal College of Radiologists, Sheffield, England (Abstr 155)
Greco FA, Oldham RK (1979) Current concepts in cancer: small cell lung cancer. N Engl J Med 301: 355–357
Green N, Kurohara SS, George FW, Crews QE (1975) Post-resection irradiation for primary lung cancer. Radiology 16: 405–407
Grillo HC (1973) Reconstruction of the trachea: experience in 100 consecutive cases. Thorax 28: 667–679
Grillo HC (1982) Primary reconstruction of airway after resec-

tion of subglottic laryngeal and upper tracheal stenosis. Ann Thorac Surg 33: 3–18

Hansen H (1984) Treatment of small cell carcinoma of the lung. Jpn J Cancer Chemother 11: 171–185

Hansen HH, Dombernowsky P, Hirsch FR, Hansen M, Rygard J (1980) Prophylactic irradiation in bronchogenic small cell anaplastic carcinoma. A comparative trial of localised versus extensive radiotherapy including prophylactic brain irradiation in patients receiving combination chemotherapy. Cancer 46: 279–284

Harper PG, Houang M, Spiro SG, Geddes D, Hodson M, Souhami RL (1981) Computerised axial tomography in the pretreatment assessment of small cell carcinoma of the bronchus. Cancer 47: 1775–1780

Hetzel MR, Nixon C, Edmonstone WM, Mitchell DM, Millad FJC, Nanson EM, Woodcock AR, Bridges CE, Humberstone AM (1985) Laser therapy in 100 tracheobronchial tumours. Thorax 40: 341–345

Higgins GA, Shields TW, Keehn RJ (1975) The solitary pulmonary nodule. Ten year follow-up of Veterans Administration Armed Forces Cooperative Study. Arch Surg 110: 570–575

Hirayama T (1981) Non-smoking wives of heavy smokers have a higher risk of lung cancer: a study from Japan. Br Med J [Clin Res] 282: 183–185

Hirleman MT, Yiu-Chiu VS, Chiu LC, Shapiro RL (1980) The resectability of primary lung carcinoma: a diagnostic staging review. J Comput Tomogr 4: 146–163

Hoffman TH, Ransdell HT (1980) Comparison of lobectomy and wedge resection for carcinoma of the lung. J Thorac Cardiovasc Surg 79: 211–217

Hooper RG, Beechler GR, Johnston MC (1978) Radioisotope scanning in the initial staging of bronchogenic carcinoma. Am Rev Respir Dis 118: 279–286

Immerman SC, Vanecko RM, Fry WA, Head LR, Shields TW (1981) Site of recurrence in patients with stages I and II carcinoma of the lung resected for cure. Ann Thorac Surg 32: 23–27

Israel L, Bonadonna G, Sylvester R and members of the EORTC Lung Cancer Group (1979). Controlled study with adjuvant radiotherapy, chemotherapy, immunotherapy and chemoimmunotherapy in operable squamous carcinoma of the lung. In: Muggia F, Rosenzweig M (eds) Lung cancer: progress in therapeutic research. Raven, New York, pp 443–452

Jamieson MPG, Walbaum PR, McCormack RJM (1979) Surgical management of bronchial carcinoma invading the chest wall. Thorax 34: 612–615

Jensik RJ, Faber LP, Milloy FJ, Amato JJ (1972) Sleeve lobectomy for carcinoma: a ten year experience. J Thorac Cardiovasc Surg 64: 400–412

Jensik RJ, Faber LP, Kittle CF (1979) Segmental resection for bronchogenic carcinoma. Ann Thorac Surg 28: 475–483

Johnston MR (1983) Median sternotomy for resection of pulmonary metastases. J Thorac Cardiovasc Surg 85: 516–522

Jolly PC, Li WI, Anderson RP (1980) Anterior and cervical mediastinoscopy for determining operability and predicting resectability in lung cancer. J Thorac Cardiovasc Surg 79: 366–371

Katz HR (1983) The effect of resection on local failure in irradiated non oat-cell carcinoma of the lung. Int J Radiat Oncol Biol Phys 9: 1793–1805

Kenis Y (1980) Surgical adjuvant chemotherapy in non-small cell carcinoma of the lung. Int J Radiat Oncol Biol Phys 6: 1075–1077

Kirsh MM, Kahn DR, Gago O, Lampe I, Fayos JV, Prior M, Moores WY, Haight C, Sloan H (1971) Treatment of bronchogenic carcinoma with mediastinal metastases. Ann Thorac Surg 12: 11–21

Kirsh MM, Rotman H, Argenta L, Bove E, Cimmino V, Tashian J, Ferguson P, Sloan H (1981) Carcinoma of the lung: results of treatment over ten years. Ann Thorac Surg 21: 371–377

Law MR, Spiro SG, Geddes DM, Hodson ME (1981) Side effects of intrapleural BCG. Thorax 36: 236

Law MR, Henk JM, Goldstraw P, Hodson ME (1985) Bronchoscopic implantation of radioactive goldgrains into endobronchial carcinomas. Br J Dis Chest 79: 147–151

Lawson RM, Ramanathan L, Hurley G, Hinson KW, Lennox SC (1976) Bronchial adenoma: review of an 18-year experience at the Brompton Hospital. Thorax 31: 245–253

Lee PN, Chamberlain J, Alderson MR (1986) Relationship of passive smoking to risk of lung cancer and other smoking-associated diseases. Br J Cancer 54: 97–105

Le Roux BT, Sharma DM (1983) Resection of tumours of the chest wall. In: Ravitch MM (ed) Current problems in surgery, vol 20, no 6. Year Book, Chicago, p 7

Le Roux BT, Kallichurum S, Shama DM (1984) Mediastinal cysts and tumours. In: Current problems in surgery, vol 21, no 11. Year Book, Chicago, p 21

Lucins JO, Chayes Z, Nakagawa H (1980) Computed tomography and radionuclide brain scanning: comparison in evaluating metastatic lesions to brain. NY State J Med 80: 185–189

McKneally MF, Maver CM, Kausel HW (1976) Intrapleural BCG immunostimulation in lung cancer. Lancet 1: 377–379

McKneally MF, Maver C, Lininger L, Klausel HW, McIlduff JB, Older TM, Foster ED, Alley RD (1981) Four year follow-up on the Albany experience with intrapleural BCG in lung cancer. J Thorac Cardiovasc Surg 81: 485–492

Maggi G, Giaccone G, Donadio M, Ciuffreda L, Dalesio O, Leria G, Trifiletti G, Casadio C, Palestro G, Mancuso M, Calciati A (1986) Thymomas: a review of 169 cases with particular reference to results of surgical treatment. Cancer 58: 765–776

Magilligan DJ, Duvernoy C, Malik G, Lewis JW, Knighton R, Ausman JI (1986) Surgical approach to lung cancer with solitary cerebral metastases – twenty-five years experience. Ann Thorac Surg 42: 360–364

Marchevsky AM, Kaneko M (1984) Surgical pathology of the mediastinum. Raven, New York

Martini N (1985) Results of the Memorial Sloan-Kettering study in screening for early lung cancer. Proceedings of the mini-symposia of the Fourth world lung cancer conference, 25–30 August, Toronto

Matthews MJ, Kanhouwa S, Pickren J, Robinette D (1973) Frequency of residual and metastatic tumour in patients undergoing curative surgical resection for lung cancer. Cancer Chemother Rep 4(2): 63–67

Melamed MR, Flehinger BJ, Zaman MB, Heelan RT, Hallerman ET, Martini N (1981) Detection of true pathologic stage I lung cancer in a screening program and the effect on survival. Cancer 47 (Suppl 5): 1182–1187

Miller JI, Mansour KA, Hatcher CR (1979) Carcinoma of the superior pulmonary sulcus. Ann Thorac Surg 28: 44–47

Montgomery WW (1968) The surgical management of supraglottic and subglottic stenosis. Ann Otol Rhinol Laryngol 77: 534–546

Mountain CF (1986) A new international staging system for lung cancer. Chest Suppl 89 (4): 225–233

Mountain CF, Gail MH (1981) Surgical adjuvant intrapleural BCG treatment for stage I non small-cell lung cancer: pre-

liminary report of the National Cancer Institute Lung Cancer Study Group. J Thorac Cardiovasc Surg 82: 649–657
Mountain CF, McMurtrey MJ, Hermes KE (1984) Surgery for pulmonary metastases: a 20 year experience. Ann Thorac Surg 38: 323–330
Mussi A, Janni A, Pistolesi M, Ravelli V, Buonaguidi R, Angeletti CA (1985) Surgical treatment of primary lung cancer and solitary brain metastasis. Thorax 40: 191–193
Naruke T, Suemasu K, Ishikawa S (1978) Lymph node mapping and curability at various levels of metastasis in resected lung cancer. J Thorac Cardiovasc Surg 76: 832–839
Okike N, Bernatz PE, Payne WS, Woolner LB, Leonard PF (1978) Bronchoplastic procedures in the treatment of carcinoid tumours of the tracheobronchial tree. J Thorac Cardiovasc Surg 76: 281–291
Osborne DR, Korobkin M, Ravin CE, Putman CE, Wolfe WG, Sealy WC, Young WG, Breiman R, Heaston D, Ram P, Haiber M (1982) Comparison of plain radiography, conventional tomography and computed tomography in detecting intrathoracic lymph node metastases from lung carcinoma. Radiology 142: 157–161
Osterlind K, Hansen HH, Hansen HS, Dombernowsky P, Hansen M, Rorth M (1986) Chemotherapy versus chemotherapy plus irradiation in limited small cell lung cancer. Results of a controlled trial with 5 years follow-up. Br J Cancer 54: 7–17
Parr GVS, Unger M, Trout RG, Atkinson WG (1984) One hundred Neodymium-YAG laser ablations of obstructing tracheal neoplasms. Ann Thorac Surg 38: 374–381
Paterson R, Russell M (1962) Clinical trials in malignant disease: Lung cancer. Value of postoperative radiotherapy, part IV. Clin Radiol 13: 141–144
Paulson DL (1975) Carcinomas in the superior pulmonary sulcus. J Thorac Cardiovasc Surg 70: 1095–1104
Pearson FG (1967) An evaluation of mediastinoscopy in the management of presumably operable bronchial carcinoma. J Thorac Cardiovasc Surg 55: 617–625
Pearson FG, Nelems JM, Henderson RJ, Delarue NC (1972) The role of mediastinoscopy in the selection of treatment for bronchial carcinoma with involvement of superior mediastinal lymph nodes. J Thorac Cardiovasc Surg 64: 382–390
Pearson FG, Delarue NC, Ilves R, Todd TRJ, Cooper JD (1982) Significance of positive superior mediastinal nodes identified at mediastinoscopy in patients with resectable cancer of the lung. J Thorac Cardiovasc Surg 83: 1–11
Piehler JM, Pairolero PC, Weiland LH, Offord KP, Spencer Payne W, Bernatz PE (1982) Bronchogenic carcinoma with chest wall invasion: factors affecting survival following en bloc resection. J Thorac Cardiovasc Surg 34: 684–691
Richardson JV, Zenk BA, Rossi NP (1980) Preoperative noninvasive mediastinal staging in bronchogenic carcinoma. Surgery 88: 382–385
Rocmans P, Defrancquen P (1981) Résultats du traitement chirugical du cancer bronchique. Rev Med Brux 2: 107–113
Roswitt B, Patno ME, Rapp R (1968) The survival of patients with inoperable lung cancer: a large scale randomised study of radiation therapy versus placebo. Radiology 90: 688–697
Salazar OM, Creech RH (1980) The state of the art toward defining the role of radiation therapy in the management of small cell bronchogenic carcinomas. Int J Radiat Oncol Biol Phys 6: 1103–1107
Sanderson DR (1985) Lung cancer screening: the Mayo study proceedings of the mini-symposia of the fourth world conference on lung cancer, 25–30 August 1985, Toronto
Shields TW, Higgins GA, Lawton R, Keilbrunn A, Kreehn RJ (1970) Preoperative X-ray therapy as an adjunct in the treatment of bronchogenic carcinoma. J Thorac Cardiovasc Surg 59: 49–61
Shields TW, Higgins GA, Keehn RJ (1972) Factors influencing survival after resection for bronchial carcinoma. J Thorac Cardiovasc Surg 64: 391–399
Shields TW, Higgins GA, Matthews MJ, Keehn RJ (1982) Surgical resection in the management of small cell carcinoma of the lung. J Thorac Cardiovasc Surg 84: 481–488
Shore DF, Paneth M (1980) Survival after resection of small cell carcinoma of the bronchus. Thorax 35: 819–822
Smith IE, Sappino AP, Bondy PK, Gilby ED (1981) Longterm survival five years or more after combination chemotherapy and radiotherapy for small cell lung cancer. Eur J Cancer Clin Oncol 17: 1249–1253
Smith LE, Evans BD, Harland SJ, Millar J (1983) Autologous bone marrow rescue is necessary after very high dose cyclophosphamide. Lancet 1: 76–77
Snow JH, Goldstein HM, Wallace S (1979) Comparison of scintography, sonography, and computed tomography in the evaluation of hepatic neoplasms. AJR 132: 915–918
Souhami RL, Finn G, Gregory WM, Burkehead BG, Buckman R, Edwards DE, Goldstone AH, Harper PG, Spiro SG, Tobias JG, Geddes DM (1985 a) High dose cyclophosphamide in small cell carcinoma of the lung. J Clin Oncol 3: 958–963
Souhami RL, Bradbury I, Geddes DM, Spiro SG, Harper PG, Tobias JS (1985 b) Prognostic significance of laboratory parameters measured at diagnosis in small cell cancer of the lung. Cancer Res 45: 2878–2882
Spiro SG, Goldstraw P (1984) The staging of lung cancer. Thorax 39: 401–407
Swett HA, Nagel JS, Sostman HD (1982) Imaging methods in primary lung carcinoma. Clin Chest Med 3: 331–351
Tait D, Peckham MJ, Hendry WF, Goldstraw P (1984) Postchemotherapy surgery in advanced non-seminomatous germ-cell testicular tumours: the significance of histology with particular reference to differentiated (mature) teratoma. Br J Cancer 50: 601–609
Takita H, Edgerton F, Karakousis C, Douglas HO, Vincent RG, Beckley S (1981) Surgical management of metastases to the lung. Surg Gynaecol Obstet 152: 191–194
Tisi GM (1979) Preoperative evaluation of pulmonary function. Am Rev Respir Dis 119: 293–310
Tockman MS (1985) Survival and mortality from lung cancer in a screened population: the Johns Hopkins study. Proceedings of the mini-symposia of the fourth world conference on lung cancer, 25–30 August, Toronto
Toty L, Personne C, Colchen A, Vourch G (1981) Bronchoscopic management of tracheal lesions using the neodymium-yttrium aluminium garnet laser. Thorax 36: 175–178
Trichopoulos D, Kalandidi A, Sparros L (1983) Lung cancer and passive smoking: conclusion of Greek study. Lancet 2: 677–678
Turnbull AD, Huvus AG, Goodner JT, Beattie EJ (1972) The malignant potential of bronchial adenoma. Ann Thorac Surg 14: 453–464
Van Houtte P, Rocmans P, Smets P, Goffin JC, Lustman-Marechal J, Vanderhoeft P, Henry J (1980) Postoperative radiation therapy in lung cancer: a controlled trial after resection with curative design. Int J Radiat Oncol Biol Phys 6: 983–986
Venn GE, Gellister J, Dacosta PE, Goldstraw P (1986) Malignant fibrous histocytoma in thoracic surgical practice. J Thorac Cardiovasc Surg 91: 234–237

Viikari SJ, Inberg MV, Puhakka H, Linna MI, Vantitinen E (1974) The role of mediastinoscopy in the treatment of lung carcinoma. Bull Soc Int Chir 2: 119–126

Westaby S (1983) A silasic stent for palliation of extensive tracheal compression and unresectable obstruction. Br J Surg 70: 259–263

Wilkins EW (1982) Consideration of ten-year survivors following pulmonary resection for metastases. J Thorac Cardiovasc Surg 84 (3): 457

Wilkins EW, Scannell JG, Craver JG (1978) Four decades of experience with resections for bronchogenic carcinoma at the Massachusett's General Hospital. J Thorac Cardiovasc Surg 76: 364–368

Williams DE, Pairolero PC, Davis CS, Bernatz DE, Spencer Payne W, Taylor WF, Uhlenhopp MA, Fontana RS (1981) Survival of patients surgically treated for stage I lung cancer. J Thorac Cardiovasc Surg 82: 70–76

World Health Organisation (1981) Histological typing of lung tumours, 2nd edn. World Health Organisation, Geneva

Cancer of the Oesophagus

R. Giulì

There are still no unanimous opinions, or even a general consensus, among those in various specialties in different parts of the world who have to treat patients with cancer of the oesophagus. However, for the time being, surgical therapy seems to be recognized as the treatment of choice whenever feasible. Attempts to improve the results currently involve the association, before, sometimes during and often after surgery, of other modes of treatments.

There is at least unanimity among surgeons and others on the anatomically rather "antisurgical" character of the oesophagus, which stretches from the pharynx to the stomach, and passes, on its long journey, through vital regions which can be invaded by carcinoma without the possibility of extending the surgical resection, in contrast to the situation with most of the other visceral cancers.

The great uncertainty persisting in the domain of lymphatic drainage (Sarrazin et al. 1984) is one reason for the therapeutic difficulties which are still the subject of so much discussion and for the often unpredictable character of the spreading of oesophageal cancers. The lymphatic system of the three regions through which the oesophagus passes drains a number of viscera, and there is no lymphatic system specific to the oesophagus: large collecting channels leave the epi-oesophageal nodes and cross the adventitia to appear beyond the pneumogastric nerves or in contact with vessels which they follow. They join the para-oesophageal nodes or more distant nodes which belong to the common mediastinal system – the nodes of the triangular ligament of the lung, the laterotracheal nodes or the nodes of the cardia. This explains the disconcerting patterns of drainage which are often observed.

Any form of drainage is possible, locally by means of short collecting channels or at a distance by means of long channels. There are long direct pathways which drain both the lower lobes of the lungs and the lower oesophagus by passing through the oesophageal hiatus, and indirect pathways which, by simple relay in an epi-oesophageal node, drain into either coeliac nodes or the nodes of the root of the lung. Finally, once the lymph reaches certain cross-road nodes, it can reach distant channels by simple pathways.

It is, however, striking that despite Sarrazin's work, direct injection of the thoracic duct has never been possible, and that the function of a Troisier's node can still be considered unknown.

Because of such anatomical peculiarities, division of the oesophagus into upper, middle and lower thirds and specification of a form of treatment for each level nowadays seems useless, or perhaps helpful only in a first, very approximate anatomical classification of the lesions. In addition, the vagueness surrounding the exact determination of the limits of a tumour, the frequent occurrence of areas of neoplastic repermeation above it, and the obvious existence of border-zone lesions involving two levels simultaneously render ineffectual any therapeutic classification which depends on the location of the tumour.

In fact, a relative degree of unity in these cancers can be found histologically in that epidermoid tumours are by far the most frequently encountered. It thus seems logical, whenever possible, to treat all tumours in a comparable way, as extended as possible.

Therefore, in this report we will deliberately leave aside adenocarcinomas of the oesophagus and glandular cancers of the cardia, even though the need for oesophageal resection as extended as possible could justify their inclusion in a chapter on oesophageal cancers (Giuli 1988 a).

The opinions that we may have today about the complex elements of gastrointestional pathology are based on the data of several successive studies: The first one, in 1979, collected 2400 resected tumours of the oesophagus from 22 different centres in Europe. This first *retrospective* study (Giuli and Gignoux 1980) formed the basis for the creation of the Organisation Internationale d'Etudes Statistiques pour les Maladies de l'Oesophage (OESO) to set up a certain number of multicentre statistical studies on oesophageal diseases.

With the enlightened help of an internationally renowned centre, the Department of Statistics of the Institut Gustave Roussy (Villejuif), where a specialized team headed by Dr. H. Sancho-Garnier was formed specifically to analyse the data furnished by the members of the OESO group, a second study, *prospective* in nature, was started. It seemed necessary to give proper consideration to all the problems of a patient with cancer of the oesophagus, from the time of diagnosis up to return to work; to involve in this study specialists of all disciplines conerned (endoscopy, gastroenterology, surgery, ENT, pathology, anaesthesia, nutrition); and to establish a series of very detailed questionnaires, available in five languages, which could be easily used by specialists in the 20 countries participating in the study. A total of 790 patients were involved in this study, which ended in 1984 (Giuli and Sancho-Garnier 1986).

At this stage we realized that our efforts should no longer be limited to the original members of the OESO group, and thus organized the first OESO international Congress to focus on all the problems brought up by this study (Giuli 1984 a).

For this conference we adopted an original approach, aiming for greater efficiency: rather than planning for a number of papers to be given on a specific theme, we decided to elaborate a list of 135 questions, the aim being to cover all the points concerning the diagnosis and treatment of a patient suffering from oesophageal cancer. For answers to these questions, we turned to the most renowned specialists in the world, asking each one to give as succinct an answer as possible.

As well as the results of our retrospective and prospective studies, this chapter covers the setting up by the OESO group of an international *randomized* therapeutic trial and the large-scale organization of a system for detecting precancerous lesions of the oesophagus.

Epidemiology and Natural History

H. SANCHO-GARNIER

Epidemiological studies have shown that while the incidence of carcinoma of the oesophagus is low in most countries throughout the world, there are a number of regions of relatively high incidence but with different etiological conditions.

France and Uruguay have the highest mortality for men (13.55 and 15.56 per 100 000 respectively). Within some countries with generally low incidence, some regions show a particularly high rate of oesophageal cancer, such as the Gonbab area in Iran, the state of Kazakhstan in the Soviet Union, the district of Linxian and the mountains of Taihung in China, the Transkei in South Africa, Brittany and part of Normandy in France.

The sex ratio also varies widely from country to country from 15:1 (France) to 1:1 (Iran, China, Transkei).

The striking contrasts inherent in the geographic pattern have been a challenge to epidemiologists for some 20 years. It has been believed that the causative factor(s) must have a similarly contrasting distribution, but although the etiological role of alcohol and/or tobacco has been clearly demonstrated in some countries, this is not the case for others.

Complex ideas have been tested, including diet deficiency with consequent build-up of gastric nitrite or, conversely, vitamin deficiency (riboflavin), silicates in the water supply or in the soil, mycotoxins in the diet and fumes from indoor open cooking fires. To date, no convincing explanation has been provided for all these factors.

Benign diseases of the oesophagus are considered to increase the risk of developing a cancer – caustic oesophagitis, mega-oesophagus, Kelly-Patterson syndrome etc. – but this hypothesis has still to be supported by epidemiological studies. In Iran and China, oesophagitis has to be considered as precancerous, with a high rate of transformation to invasive cancer (50% after 10 years' follow-up).

Screening for Asymptomatic Cancers

It was stated by Huang (1984a) during the OESO Congress that even patients with early oesophageal carcinoma are by no means symptom-free or to be considered as in the presymptomatic stage: in a study of the symptomatology of 196 patients with stage I (superficial) carcinoma of the oesophagus, only 11% were free of symptoms, while all the remaining 89% had mild but definite symptoms related to swallowing, which may come and go for a certain time before becoming more and more conspicuous and eventually persistent. The important point is that these symptoms should not be confused with those of chronic non-specific or fungal oesophagitis, which is also common is places where carcinoma of the oesophagus is prevalent.

It has been known for a long time that abrasive cytology, i.e. the examination of material obtained by scraping, can provide a positive diagnosis of cancer in a large percentage of cases, and that, in particular, a proportion of false-negative biopsies can be revealed by cytology. The non-endoscopic technique of cytology as developed by the Chinese seems very interesting in high-incidence areas, but requires, of course, the collaboration of especially well trained cytologists to affirm not as much the anomalies as the normal nature of the biopsied cells.

According to Huang (1984b), for superficial carcinoma, which is usually not detected by X-ray and may not be detected by fibre esophagoscopy, balloon cytology provides a very simple, efficient, and relatively non-invasive means of detection. It has been used in China in mass screenings of over 150 000 people with no serious complications.

Among oesophageal carcinomas of all stages, the rate of accurate diagnosis by balloon cytology is over 90%, comparable to the results of X-ray, endoscopy and endoscopic biopsy. Among superficial lesions (stage 1), balloon cytology has a positive diagnostic rate of 95.2%, which is superior to the other techniques.

The diagnosis of an asymptomatic cancer often corresponds to that of a superficial cancer, even "in situ": since the oesophageal mucosa is of a squamous, i.e. stratified, nature, carcinoma in situ in fact corresponds to an intraepithelial carcinoma, and in order to diagnose such a lesion, two criteria must therefore be fulfilled, that of malignancy and that of perfect integrity of the basal membrane.

Under such precise conditions, histological diagnosis of intraepithelial carcinoma implies the need for a specimen big enough to contain the tumor wall in its entirety, as well as the portion of the tissue *adjacent to the epithelium*, in order to confirm that it has not been involved: in other words, with a large operative specimen the diagnosis is easy, whilst with a much more limited biopsy obtained by endoscopy, the diagnosis may be difficult or impossible, since the material provided is inadequate (Chomé 1984a). In fact, at least in the western world, the tumour is unfortunately most often detected when it has already, in apparently total functional silence, developed macroscopically, making X-ray and endoscopic diagnosis easy.

On the other hand, in the overall context of medical gastroenterological practice, the endoscopic detection of superficial carcinoma of the oesophagus is still unsuccessful: taking into account the respective incidence, the rate of endoscopic detection of superficial carcinoma would seem, in Europe, to be 10 times lower for the oesophagus than for the stomach.

By contrast, panendoscopy of the upper respiratory/digestive tract, when routinely used in the pretherapeutic assessment of patients with an ENT carcinoma, is highly successful: Savary et al. (1984) detected a second simultaneous malignant site in 30% of their ENT carcinoma sufferers, and in three of every 10 cases the second carcinoma was in the oesophagus. The great majority of these second carcinomas were superficial ones.

Whatever the type of cancer, it is essential to look above the tumour for areas of neoplastic repermeation (Chomé 1984 b). This term is used to describe insidious spread of tumour cells along the lymph or blood vessels without any evidence of such spread being revealed by macroscopic examination. The meticulous and extremely reliable Savary technique, after toluidine blue staining and thorough washing with acetic acid, enables detection, then biopsy, of suspicious areas. At the level of such areas it is common to find either severely dysplastic lesions or true neoplastic invasion, allowing better determination of the necessary level of surgical resection.

Preoperative Elements of Prognosis

Within the framework of the preparation of patients for a procedure thought of as curative, respiratory function tests are not always considered capable of predicting the nature of the postoperative course: traditionally such tests can only exclude a patient from surgery in the case of very low values. On the other hand, they enable better evaluation of the risks of morbidity provided the following prerequisites are met:

- All of the parameters based on forced expiration must be taken into account: forced expiratory volume in 1 s, vital capacity, expiratory flow (litres/s) and mean expiratory flow/s between 25% and 75% vital capacity.
- The maximal voluntary ventilation, the retention volume, the functional residual capacity and the DLCO in smokers, elderly patients and patients with chronic obstructive airways disease must be investigated.
- The difference between alveolar and arterial pO_2 must be taken into account in interpretation of the blood gases (Elman et al. 1984).

Our prospective study of 790 patients (Giuli 1984 a) did not enable us to confirm the usefulness of respiratory function tests, since with regard to pulmonary complications, the clinical finding of chronic bronchitis would seem more valid: consumption of more than 40 g tobacco per day has a significant influence upon operative mortality (Table 1).

Endoscopic examinations are part of the routine work-up of a patient suffering from cancer of the oesophagus. They enable determination of the level of the upper pole of the tumour, and detection, at the level of the respiratory tree, of a neoplastic invasion which would demonstrate the impossibility of resection or show that only a palliative procedure can be carried out.

Our statistics (Table 2) show that the operative findings revealed an error rate of approximately 20% in terms of the site of the upper pole of the tumour, measured from the dental arches or even from the theoretically more accurate marker of Killian's foramen. Moreover, operative evaluation (Table 3) shows the limitations of bronchoscopy prior to surgery: 7% of cases described as normal, and 20% of cases of "simple compression", were found to exhibit true invasion on surgical exploration. It now seems to be recognized that CT scanning offers better reliability.

Teams with broad experience (Lebas et al. 1984) may very often be able to demonstrate tracheobronchial invasion. Deformities of these structures can be due to simple displacement by the tumour mass, but when there is marked reduction in their calibre or a "cuffing" of their wall, and particularly when there are irregularities in the wall, there is a very strong suspicion of tumour spread.

Invasion of the aorta is less common and often more difficult to evaluate. The absence of fatty fascia between the tumour and the aorta is not significant (indeed, almost universal in the middle third of the oesophagus), but the presence of such fascia is very reassuring.

Table 1. Preoperative respiratory condition and postoperative course

	Chronic bronchitis		Tobacco consumption		Restrictive syndrome		Obstructive syndrome	
	+	–	+	–	+	–	+	–
	77	252	266	60	85	254	131	205
Pulmonary complications	65%	46	61%	55	47%	53	54%	54
	$P<0.004$		NS		NS			
Fistula	17	14	17	10	19	14	17	15
	NS		NS		NS		NS	
Death	17	14	35	15	16	15	19	15
	NS		$P<0.05$ >40 g		NS		NS	

Table 2. Oesophagoscopy

Operative findings					
Distance from dental arches			Distance from Killian's foramen		
0–24 cm	25–34 cm	> 34 cm	0–24 cm	25–34 cm	> 34 cm
71	68	2	17	2	
35	245	35	6	3	1
15	84	112	4	1	1
	2	17			
Mistakes: 138 (20%)			Mistakes: 6 (17%)		

Table 3. Bronchoscopy

			Invasion (operative)	
	n	%	n	%
Normal	396	86	28	7
Compression	62	13	13	20
Invasion	4	1		

On the basis of surgical and autopsy findings, Picus (1983) shows that a more accurate method is to measure the arc of the aorta in contact with the tumour masses in multiples of 15°: in over 80% of cases, invasion is absent when this arc is less than 45° but present when it is greater than 90°. This criterion seems to be very reliable.

Lymph node shrouding of a mediastinal, subdiaphragmatic, peritumoral or distant region cannot usually be mistaken on the CT scan. However, neoplastic invasion of the mediastinum without lymph node enlargement is more difficult to evaluate, especially in very wasted subjects. It can usually be detected at the level of the prevertebral space, the superior mediastinum and the posterior inframediastinal space, where it causes the disappearance of the cell-fat planes which are normally present at this level, or the fairly characteristic appearance of "dirty fat".

As for lymph nodes, there are very few false positives, contrary to what one would expect from histological data, which demonstrate that a large node is not necessarily metastatic. In this case, CT probably greatly underestimates the size of large non-metastatic nodes. However, there are a certain number of false negatives, consisting of invaded lymph nodes which are not detected on CT or which are not judged to be pathological for one of the following reasons:

- Because they are too small (less than 8 mm) or the CT sections are too widely spaced.
- Because, although moderately enlarged (8 mm to 15 mm), they are at a site which is sometimes difficult to explore (aortopulmonary window).
- Because they are confused with the tumour mass, especially with its upper or lower part. This is the most frequent situation.

In practice, although CT scanning may not diagnose small adenopathies, the preoperative diagnosis of these nodes does not generally have a great influence on the decision as regards surgery. From the histological point of view, CT obviously cannot claim to have a sufficient degree of reliability, but in most cases, it also provides useful information which helps to define the best surgical strategy. Since the preparation of this paper (1986), the current development of endoscopic ultrasonography has now proved this examination to be the most useful in this field. It provides a precise morphological survey which is rapid, non-invasive and perfectly comprehensible, and can spare the surgeon from unpleasant surprises by predicting the difficulties in dissection. It can help in the choice of the most appropriate tactic, but is, however, unable to conclusively determine the resectability of the tumour in every case. This also depends, of course, on the ability of the surgeon.

It is tempting to seek, in the results of biological tests, factors which would show in advance that radical surgery cannot be carried out. Immune depression seems attractive in this respect, both from the physiopathological and the practical point of view.

In fact, Blackburn (1984) has shown that it is not so much the catabolism itself, but the absence of compensation by an anabolic reaction that causes anergia and associated disorders. Besides, there are two different factors each capable of provoking an immune reaction – malnutrition and the presence of the malignant tumor itself. The nutritional state of the cancer patient can therefore fall under two different headings, according to the importance of the metabolic stress: thus, a state of malnutrition is often found, due solely to the mechanical consequences of the stenosis. In spite of the weight loss, serum albumin and the immune function will not be disturbed. But, as soon as metabolic stress occurs, catabolism and nutritional needs are increased, and a rearrangement of the cellular mass will take place, causing hypoalbuminaemia and anergia.

Mullen et al. (1980) developed a predictive model for the risk of operative morbidity or mortality by gathering various preoperative nutritional data on 161 patients undergoing major intra-abdominal or intrathoracic surgical procedures and monitoring the clinical course until death or discharge. These data

Table 4. Lymphocyte response to phytohaemagglutinin (stimulated disintegrations per minute minus unstimulated desintegrations)

	Resectable tumours		Unresectable tumours
	Node negative ($n = 14$)	Node positive ($n = 52$)	($n = 20$)
Mean	14700	9782	10177
SD	4949	3277	4186
	$P < 0.05$		NS

Table 5. Weight loss

Average loss (kg)		Percentage of normal weight
8.4%		12%
	$P = 0.003$	
7		10%
7.3		10
	NS	
8.2		11

were used to develop a computer-based, stepwise regression to select the most important predictive variables. The authors called the result the Prognostic Nutritional Index (PNI), and followed up 145 patients, 50 of whom received preoperative total parenteral nutrition and the remaining 95 no preoperative nutritional support. The benefit was strongly correlated with PNI risk group: in the high-risk group, preoperative nutrition had a major impact, with decreases in all complications (from 56% to 23%), septic complications (from 35% to 14%), major sepsis (from 33% to 5%) and morbidity (from 47% to 9%).

These results are not supported by all studies, and Angorn and Haffejee (1984a), for instance, found that nutritional status, though reflecting the extent of the disease, could not define resectability of the tumour. Their results for lymphocyte response to phytohaemagglutinin are shown in Table 4: "transformation scores" in patients with node-positive resectable tumours, were significantly lower than in patients with node-negative resectable tumours. Transformation in patients with unresectable tumours was similar to that in patients with node-positive resectable tumours.

According to the same authors (Angorn and Haffejee 1984b), patients with oesophageal carcinoma in negative nitrogen balance have compromised non-specific cellular immunity. With the achievement of positive nitrogen balance, some aspects of non-specific cellular immunity are improved without any reduction in tumour bulk: total lymphocyte numbers and T lymphocyte numbers increase, and the mitogenic response to phytohaemagglutinin improves. However, the dinitrochlorobenzene skin test remains non-reactive.

The dissociation between in vivo skin testing and in vitro lymphocyte transformation may be explained by these functions being subserved by different subsets of T lymphocytes which may be unequally compromised in cancer patients: immunoglobulin concentrations remain unaltered, but C_3, C_4 and C_3PA concentrations increase significantly. A similar increase in complement component concentrations to levels above normal has been reported following correction of protein calorie manutrition.

Finally, it seems that immune depression will be found in 40% of malnourished patients and this does not represent, in itself, as bad a prognostic element as could be expected. It is rather the negativation of the test at the time of renutrition that is detrimental.

Moreover, certain teams (Balzola et al. 1984) maintain that the best predictive factor regarding tumour resectability is variation in body weight, as Studley, as far back as 1936, showed a relationship between body mass and operative risk.

In our own study, we verified the observation made by Ribet (1984) who was able to demonstrate neither a statistical correlation between malnutrition and anergy, nor relationship between this anergy and postoperative morbidity. In fact, we saw curative operations with an uncomplicated postoperative course in two-thirds of the small number of anergic patients in whom we studied these parameters. By contrast, the degree of weight loss seemed to be statistically related to the operability of the tumour (Table 5).

Staging

The classification of oesophageal cancers is not always as simple as one might imagine, even when the only aim is to determine their exact histological nature. Regarding epidermoid cancers of the oesophagus, the tumours as a rule present a certain, even if very low, degree of differentiation.

However, classification into the three conventional categories – well differentiated, intermediate, poorly differentiated – is not easy. The description of a lesion as "undifferentiated" carcinoma may, however, because of the very close similarity to "poorly differentiated" carcinoma, depend on the pathologist doing the examination, and there are often a certain number of "borderline" cases.

As for the small cell undifferentiated carcinomas of the lung, certain elements of endocrine differentiation can be found in the tumours. Different immunohistochemical procedures can be used to determine very fine distinctions between the types of differentiation (mucin, cytoplasmic keratin, secretory endocrine granules, carcinoembryonic antigen etc.). The abundance of these techniques, and their complexity, demonstrate the difficulty of achieving absolute uniformity in the interpretation of large series.

Generally (Chomé 1984 c), a cell is said to be differentiated when study of its morphology leads to easy recognition of the family to which the cell belongs. The progressive gradual loss of this morphology conceals the origin of a cell and the family to which it belongs, making it lose its differentiation. Therefore when different parts of a given lesion have different appearances, it is obvious that priority should be given to the more severe forms, evaluating the proportion they form of the total tumour volume.

The classification seems yet more complex, when one considers that even postoperative examination of the resection specimen and its lymph nodes may not always give exact information as to the degree of lymphatic invasion. When the lymph nodes are massively invaded with malignant cells surrounded by their connective tissue stroma, macroscopic examination is sufficient, and frozen section will also determine whether or not the lymph node capsule is intact. In other cases, however, the lymph nodes may contain groups of cells in the sinuses which have not formed a daughter tumour. These cells are migrating; they can cross the lymph node without leaving a trace and move on to another more distant node. This casts doubt on certain morphological concepts about the integrity of a lymph node group.

In any case, if, through a common international language of convention, it were possible to define the various parameters of macroscopic appearance, histology and spread, histoprognosis would imply that knowledge is available as to the pejorative or unpejorative nature of each of these features taken in isolation. Usually several parameters are present simultaneously, making it impossible to isolate the prognostic value of each of them.

In the first retrospective study published by the OESO group (Giulì and Gignoux 1980), it had already been shown how difficult the histological classification of the various tumours could be. Well-differentiated squamous cell lesions, the most numerous ($n = 1155$), were associated with the lowest long-term life expectancy (16%; confidence intervals 19%–12%). Furthermore, the prognostic value of the macroscopic aspect of the oesophageal tumour was already clearly evident at this time. The prognosis was most favourable with fungating tumours (22%; 30%–15%), intermediate in the case of ulcerated tumours (19%; 24%–14%) and poorest when the tumour was infiltrating (12%; 18%–7%).

It seemed that the macroscopic aspect was often the determining factor in deciding whether to give postoperative radiation. Infiltrating tumours were those in which radiotherapy was given the most frequently (270 patients), and were also the only lesions in which the favourable effect of such treatment could be detected (21%; 29%–13%).

A number of very surprising findings had emerged from the analysis of these 2400 patients. The first was the observation that, in all sites, the prognosis was poorer for small tumours than for large lesions. The same feature was revealed when combining tumours of equivalent size according to histological type. For those tumours with a diameter of between 1 and 3 cm, there were no postoperative survivors at 5 years, regardless of type. As the size increased, long-term survival rates also increased. For tumours up to 4 cm, the figure was 21% (30%–12%), and invariably higher for adenocarcinomas (53%; 75%–32%). For tumours larger than 5 cm in diameter, the prognosis regularly worsened, but the long-term survival rate remained markedly greater than that of small tumours (13%; 19%–7%).

A partial explanation of this phenomenon may be provided by a comparison with elements of the TN classification, which seems obviously insufficient for cancers of the oesophagus. In this comparison, which involves not the size of the tumour but its spread in terms of depth into the oesophageal wall, it may be noted that, while the influence of the criterion N was negligible for stage T3 [long-term survival rate 13% (19%–7%) if N+ and 36% (47%–6%) if N−], it became significant for tumours scored T1 [0% at 4 years if N+, and 39% (64%–14%) if N−].

Analysis of histological data provided by our second, prospective study (Giulì and Sancho-Garnier 1985), enabled us to confirm the insufficiencies of the present classification of tumours of the oesophagus. Although invasion of lymph vessels is rarer than that of blood vessels, and occurs principally in moderately differentiated or relatively undifferentiated tumours, such invasion is found in 10% of "superficial" tumours: 14% of purely mucosal tumours are associated with lymph node invasion, and more than a quarter of those classified T3 are free of such involvement. Moreover, an absence of node invasion may coexist with macroscopic tracheobronchial invasion (32%) and with invasion of the lymph vessels (14%).

Finally, observations in this series grouping 71 superficial tumours of the oesophagus (15 T1a and 56 T1b), all confirmed the uncertainties remaining for their treatment, as lymph node dissection was carried out in the majority of cases (94% of T1b), and almost half of these patients with a purely mucosal tumour (7/15) underwent total oesophagectomy.

All these insufficiencies led us to try to elaborate, for a randomized therapeutic trial organized by the OESO group which we will discuss at the end of this chapter, a new histological classification. This classification, elaborated by Appelman and Chomé within the OESO group, includes different pathological and clinical elements, each one given a numerical value increasing according to its intensity. This combination of values will allow the establishment of a global index of malignancy, which may contribute significantly to the establishment of the prognosis. The index includes seven graduations for each of 12 different criteria covering both macroscopic and microscopic aspects of the tumour.

The evaluation of this index will be made directly by the staff of the Statistical Centre. By combining the different numerical elements in a quantitatively increasing manner, a global index of malignancy may be established after the independent analysis of each factor separately. Thus, we hope to propose, at the completion of this therapeutic trial, a new classification system of tumours of the oesophagus, with the objective of a more accurate assessment of prognosis. Since the preparation of this paper (Feb 1986), some preliminary results of the OESO Malignancy index have been obtained. (Diseases of the Esophagus, (1988) Vol 1 No 3, in press).

Surgery

Surgery remains the principal treatment for cancer of the oesophagus. The real question is whether surgery will be performed with the aim of cure or simply of palliation, a decision which should ideally be made preoperatively.

The inaccuracies that persist in reports on the nature of the lymph drainage of the oesophagus explain the reports of T2 or T3 tumours remaining N0. Knowing the longitudinal nature of the spread of cancer of the oesophagus, most surgeons believe it legitimate to carry out radical subtotal resection of the oesophagus: "curative" limited resection can be justified neither from the carcinological nor the anatomical nor the embryological point of view (joint origin of oesophagus and respiratory tree, Del Genio et al. 1984).

Table 6. Operative approach

	Right 494 (66.7%)	Left 156 (21%)	Blunt 91 (12.2%)
Alone		63%	
With abdominal	86%	25%	
With cervical	14%	12%	

Table 7. Operative approach and upper limit of tumour

	Distance from dental arch				
Approach	0–14 cm	15–19 cm	20–24 cm	25–34 cm	>35 cm
Right	18	8	41	297	83
Left	3	7	9	73	67
				51%	
Blunt	15	10	8	28	16
				36%	
With cervical		36%	55%	33%	16%

The best approach is still under discussion. The OESO study (Table 6) shows that more than one patient in five is still operated on by a left thoracic approach, and that more than half of the left approaches are for tumours situated between 20 and 34 cm from the dental arches (Table 7). In addition, dissection has been made possible in most cases of aortic invasion (14/19) by use of a left approach.

Although the right thoracic and abdominal approach is the one most commonly used, for carcinomas located below the aortic arch or at the gastric cardia, in China most surgeons prefer a left posterolateral thoracotomy; right thoracotomy, whether posterolateral or anterolateral, is restricted to carcinomas at or above the aortic arch (Huang 1984 c). The advantages of left posterolateral thoracotomy are numerous:

- Only one incision is needed, so the wound is less traumatizing and less painful postoperatively.
- There is no need to change the position of the patient during operation.
- It can readily be extended into a combined thoracoabdominal incision if further exposure for an enlarged operation or a colonic interposition is needed.
- It gives excellent exposure to the oesophagogastric junction and the left upper abdomen.
- It provides good exposure to the aorta, the left main bronchus and the left upper abdomen for accurate assessment of resectability and for easy repair of the aorta in case of injury.

This is also our own attitude: we prefer the left thoracic approach for tumours localized in the middle and lower portions of the oesophagus, usually using an oblique laparotomy or a subcostal approach, rather than a phrenotomy, for the abdominal dissection. It also seems that a much smaller proportion of tumours appear unresectable when this approach is used.

Lymph node dissection is, still now, usually extended, systematic and systematized; this represents the only hope of surgical cure of slightly advanced tumours.

The number of lymph nodes necessary to resect is, however, difficult to specify (Siewert 1984), because it is impossible to define the situation as clearly for cancer of the oesophagus, as, for example, for breast surgery, where the paths of drainage are perfectly known.

There is therefore no general agreement in this field. Akiyama (1984 a) states that systematic dissection should include the superior mediastinal nodes on the innominate artery, the para-oesophageal nodes, the paratracheal nodes, and the nodes around the aortic arch. The middle mediastinal lymph nodes, consisting of the tracheobronchial, para-oesophageal or para-aortic and diaphragmatic nodes, should also be removed. Complete thoracic excision of the oesophagus should usually be associated with inframediastinal, intertracheobronchial and superior retro- and laterotracheal mediastinal lymphadenectomy.

The situation seems clearer with regard to lymph node dissection of the upper abdomen. One should attempt en-bloc resection of the lymph channels along the left gastric and coeliac arteries, including the hepatoduodenal ligament and the hilus of the spleen, i.e. all of the lymph nodes located on the superior border of the pancreas.

In this area, CT scanning cannot miss massive lymph node invasion in any region explored. In comparison with other radiological or endoscopic investigations, CT provides essential information for the surgical decision and the choice of tactics (Moraldi et al. 1984).

Others have a very different systematic approach. Orringer (1984) is among those who think that surgical intervention, from the moment the diagnosis is made, can only be palliative. He believes that the vast majority of oesophageal carcinomas are incurable when they are operated upon, and that the additional morbidity of extended mediastinal and abdominal lymph node dissection is simply unjustified. According to him, transhiatal oesophagectomy without thoracotomy achieves excellent palliation and occasional cure. Accessible subcarinal and para-oesophageal lymph nodes, as well as coeliac axis nodes, are sampled for the purpose of staging, but no attempt is made to perform en-bloc resection of the oesophagus and its contiguous lymph node-bearing tissues.

On the other hand, we know above all that diagnosis on the basis of peroperative biopsy of a node of a given group is uncertain, since it has been established that migrating cells can cross lymph nodes without trace (Chomé 1984 b).

The OESO study (Table 8) shows that this attractive approach without thoracotomy has often been adopted (90 blunt dissections, compared to 491 right and 69 left approaches), but the mortality in the OESO material was not as low as that seen by Orringer. Surprisingly, perioperative incidents, overall postoperative complications and general complications occur significantly more frequently with oesophagectomy without thoracotomy. The pulmonary complication rate is no lower than with other techniques. The incidence of fistula and of postoperative mortality is also higher, although not significantly so.

However, the statistics recorded by Orringer (1984), who has the greatest experience in this technique, must be taken into consideration: 6% operative mortality among 100 patients operated on, and, of those surviving, 17% still alive after 4 years.

Oesophageal cancer may directly invade adjacent organs in the neck, thorax or upper abdomen. As long as the extension from the wall of the oesophagus is limited to the envelope of tissues normally removed in an en-bloc resection, removal of such tissues is routine practice and does not exclude the possibility of long-term cure.

Table 8. Operative approach and complications

	Peroperative incidents (%)	Postoperative complications (%)				
		None	Fistula	Pulmonary	General	Death
Right (n = 491)	4.7	55	14	22	12	13
Left (n = 169)	4.1	56	10	34	7	17
Blunt (n = 90)	12.4	38	19	24	20	19
p	0.05	<0.005	NS	NS	<0.001	NS

According to Skinner (1984), invasion outside the oesophagus to the pleura, pericardium, membranous portion of trachea, aortic adventitia, diaphragm muscle, omentum, stomach, splenic hilum or azygos vein and thoracic duct remains within the boundaries of complete excision. Although extension beyond the oesophageal wall to these structures is one of the poor prognostic signs, curative surgery is not impossible, especially if the lymph nodes are all negative.

This en-bloc resection includes all tissues dorsal to the oesophagus as far as the vertebral bodies, and the aorta including the azygos vein and thoracic duct system with all adjacent lymphatics. Laterally the pleural surfaces are excised where they abut on the oesophagus, and anteriorly the pericardium is resected where it lies adjacent to the oesophagus.

This operation, with 10-cm margins, can be performed with mortality similar to that of standard or palliative oesophagectomy, approximately 9%.

Regarding the extension of these operations upwards, Richelme (1984) concluded that cervical anastomosis, involving the removal of about 3 cm more of oesophagus, is of only limited value, given that multicentricity is present in 10%–15% of patients, but in only one case in eight is the satellite lesion above the initial tumour. High thoracic anastomosis therefore seems perfectly legitimate in the treatment of cancers in the middle and lower portions of the oesophagus under two conditions:

- Preoperative endoscopic examination of the oesophagus above the tumour, using vital dyes and guided biopsies,
- Oesophageal resection 4–5 cm above the tumour, accompanied by extemporaneous pathological examination of the sections of the oesophageal specimen

Akiyama (1984) analysed the frequency of metastases in each group of lymph nodes along the first to fifth branches of the left gastric artery, the first branch going into the cardiac portion of the stomach and the fifth into the area around the gastric angle. The rates of positive lymph nodes from the first to fifth branches of the left gastric artery decrease from 25.1% to 0%, and it seems safe to remove the fifth branch of the left gastric artery.

The stomach remains, of course, the most commonly and simply used for replacement of the oesophagus, bearing in mind certain strict rules for construction of a gastric tube. The upper portion of the lesser curvature is removed together with the neoplastic nodes present.

The colon, however, is also widely used, and certain problems connected with the use of the stomach can be avoided. Apart from the serious bronchial regurgitation with flooding which is seen exclusively in gastroplasties, bilateral vagotomy has been claimed to create problems to do with the slowing down of the gastric drainage (Mignon et al. 1984). The colon is a non-secreting organ of satisfactory length. It represents a mode of replacement of the oesophagus which is technically more difficult but presents advantages that justify its selection.

Manometric and radiocinematographic data are completely superimposable. The colonic contents progress along the whole length of the graft to the gastric cavity, even when the patient is lying flat, when the colon has been inserted in an isoperistaltic position. In the case of antiperistaltic coloplasty, however, the motor response occurs from the distal segment towards the proximal segment. It would thus seem that the colonic transplant does not merely behave as an insert conduit, influenced only by the laws of gravity, but possesses true peristaltic activity (Mignon et al. 1984). Furthermore, the reduction in intraluminal pH in the coloplasty stimulates the onset of peristalsis by decreasing the threshold volume necessary to produce a motor response, which could have an important role in preventing anastomotic ulcers in the graft.

On the other hand, it is possible that, with time, the direction of the function of the colic transplant becomes less important, with emptying essentially effected by gravity. Finally, discussion of the functional value of the transplant takes no account of three other aspects which may be just as important as the direction of peristalsis (Bourgeon and Richelme 1984): the location of the plasty (mediastinal or retrosternal); the site of implantation of the plasty (anterior or posterior surface of stomach, antral region or greater tuberosity); and, above all, the extent to which the length of the plasty is inappropriate, with creation of a siphon or of a preanastomic cuff.

In spite of the present popularity of suturing devices, most of the surgeons in our study (Giuli 1988 b) continue to favour anastomoses performed by hand (Table 9). Especially for cervical anastomo-

Table 9. Type of anastomosis

Manual	*n*	%
Single layer	209	
Two layers	305	73
Continent	27	
Mechanical	201	27

sis, although the stapling technique can be used in the wide surgical field left after an antethoracic approach, manual anastomosis still plays a very important role in the majority of cases: in addition to the adaptation of the mucosa, adaptation of the two diameters can be achieved satisfactorily only by careful manual suture (Akiyama 1984 c).

The superficial nature of the tumour in no case permits prediction of lymph node integrity. This justifies the distinction made by some (Endo 1984) between "superficial" and "early" carcinomas. In both these categories, however, vascular invasion is possible and is likely to cause recurrences.

The uncertainties still persisting in the treatment of these tumours are reflected in the OESO statistics (Table 10), on 71 superficial tumours of the oesophagus. It can be noticed that lymphatic involvement has been found in 14% of purely mucosal tumours, and almost half of these patients underwent total oesophagectomy. Moreover, the rate of dysplasia associated with these superficial tumours is high (11% and 22%), and it seems logical to consider their systematic treatment in the light of the impressive numbers reported by very experienced workers (Huang 1984 d). In a population of 530 patients who were followed up for several years for severe dysplasia of the oesophagus, Huang's team found that the percentage of true neoplastic degeneration reached 66% among those followed up for 9–12 years after diagnosis.

For genuine intramucosal carcinomas (but is it possible to affirm this state at the time of biopsy?), the trend seems to be in favour of laser destruction. In this field, photodynamic treatment with derivatives of haematoporphyrin, already used in gastric cancer, has the advantage of a large degree of selectivity. According to the radiance used, this technique permits the localization of malignant cells and their destruction by a ray of red light.

Table 10. Superficial carcinomas

	T1a			T1b	
Interval from first consultation	$n = 15$			$n = 56$	
to operation <6 months	12			48	
Lymph nodes positive		14%	NS	31%	
Oesophageal resection	None	Limited	Total	Limited	Total
	1	7	7	41	15
Lymph node excision	Yes		No	Yes	No
	14%		86%	94%	6%
Preoperative radiotherapy		2			3
Preoperative chemotherapy		1			2
Associated dysplasia		11%			22%

As soon as the tumour is no longer completely limited in size (all surgeons are aware of the existence of superficial sheets extending over a very long segment of the oesophagus), surgical resection with complete lymph node excision becomes essential, with no attempt to adapt the operation to the apparently limited nature of the lesion. Some teams think it logical to combine chemotherapy and radiotherapy, in order to improve the patient's chances as far as possible.

The 5-year survival rate among these cases (Huang 1984 e) is 90%, and it is not evident that improvement on this high figure would be achieved with systematic chemotherapy. Treatment exclusively by chemotherapy would be of interest in the T1, N0 cases but once again, in spite of information yielded by CT, it is impossible to determine the exact state of the lymph nodes and define this group of patients.

There is currently no unanimity on the treatment of definitely non-resectable tumours. Retrosternal plasties, gastric or colic, have a mortality that seems acceptable and achieve good palliation of dysphagia. However, even after careful preoperative evaluation, some tumours prove to be technically non-resectable at operation. A palliative procedure may then be indicated, but such procedures should be selected with care, with preference given to those associated with minimum morbidity (Ellis 1984). The intubation technique by pulsion (Angorn and Haffejie 1984 c; Girault 1984) is associated with very low mortality when the surgeon has sufficient experience (0.5% for 580 patients in Girault's statistics). However, intubation is most effective when the mechanical obstruction causing the dysphagia, rather than the anorexia associated with disseminated cancer, is the major component of the malnutrition.

It is perhaps in such cases that the use of laser could be considered, without general anaesthesia, but bearing in mind the risk of perforation.

Associated Therapy

Radiotherapy

During the multidisciplinary OESO congress in Paris in 1984 (Giuli 1984 a), the problem of radiotherapy was the subject of numerous discussions. The opinions expressed do not appear to be conducive to making the various teams adopt a uniform approach.

The findings reported by Pearson (1984) do not seem to be corroborated by other statistics. Pearson believes that initial treatment by radiotherapy should only be considered for patients with no demonstrable distant metastases, a tumour involving no more than 9 cm of the oesophagus and no invasion of the trachea or bronchi. He states that irradiation of a cylindrical volume 15 cm long and 6.5 cm in diameter would include more tissue than could be removed by oesophagectomy. A minimum tumour dose of 50 Gy should be given in 20 fractions over 28 days.

In a randomized study presented at the same congress, Husemann (1984) compares a control group, radiation alone and radiation associated with chemotherapy. In this study, the postoperative mortality was 31% in the control group, 40% for radiation and 47% in the combined treatment, the most frequent reason for such high mortality being a functional lung disorder.

The Chinese experiment presented by Huang (1984 f) was important because of the large number of patients included (Giuli 1984 a). In a first study of 408 patients given preoperative irradiation, it was shown that the incidence of anastomotic leak was not significantly different from that in the group treated by surgery alone, even if the oesophageal anastomotic site was located within the field of preoperative irradiation. However, the 5-year survival rate was not statistically different from that of the control group.

To further verify the effects of preoperative irradiation, Huang (1984 f) presented a randomized study, started in 1977, on 160 patients under 65 years with middle-third oesophageal carcinoma not exceeding 7 cm in length. The subjects were randomized into two groups, one treated with preoperative irradiation and surgery, the other with surgery alone. The resectability rate was 95.2% in the irradiation group compared to 89.6% for surgery alone. The 5-year survival rate was 45.5% for the radiation group (10/22), and 25% for the surgery group ($p = 0.1$).

The earliest OESO study, embracing 2400 cases and published by Giuli and Gignoux in 1980, was only retrospective, and did not enable us to draw definite conclusions. The results showed that infiltrating tumours were those in which radiotherapy was given the most frequently (270 patients). They were also the only lesions in which the favourable effect of such treatment could be detected (21%; confidence intervals 29%–13%).

Comparison of the rates of histologically confirmed lymph node metastasis showed that while the overall invasion rate in squamous cell carcinomas was high (63% in 1882 patients), preoperative irradiation did not yield any notable improvement (61% in 589 patients).

The effects of radiotherapy were studied according to other surgical parameters. Radiotherapy before surgery did not appear to imply any modification in its course, the percentage of excision with macroscopic invasion being the same as in those cases which had not undergone radiotherapy (44% in 254 patients).

Concerning the influence of irradiation on the carcinoma according to its site, the following conclusions may be drawn: in the upper third of the oesophagus, radiotherapy was widely used (72 patients) and appeared to possess a certain degree of efficacy. However, the improvement was tangible only in the very small number of patients (14%) who received preoperative and postoperative treatment, in whom the 5-year survival rate was 46% (confidence intervals 84%–8%). Preoperative (25%; 49%–0%) or postoperative (35%; 63%–6%) radiotherapy had no evident effect.

Table 11. Preoperative radiotherapy and postoperative complications

Complications	XR + ($n = 103$)[a]		XR − ($n = 627$)
None	32	$P < 0.0001$	57
Fistula	20	$P < 0.005$	12.6
Alveolar syndrome	50	$P < 0.0001$	25.5
Interstitial syndrome	15	$P < 0.05$	6
Overall pulmonary complications	32	$P < 0.005$	20
Assisted ventilation	85.5	$P < 0.0005$	50

[a] Average dose 36 ± 22 Gy, number of sessions 15.

Table 12. Preoperative radiotherapy: tumour stage and differentiation

Stage	n	XR + ($n = 92$)	XR − ($n = 642$)
T1a	15	13%	87%
T1b	56	5%	95%
T2	206	14.5%	85.5%
T3	457	12%	88%
		NS	
Squamous cell, well differentiated	258	8%	92%
Squamous cell, moderately differentiated	147	27%	73%
Squamous cell, poorly differentiated	127	19%	81%
Adenocarcinoma	173	1%	99%
		$P < 0.001$	

Table 13. Preoperative radiotherapy and survival

	Survival (%)			
	6 months	12 months	18 months	24 months
XR+ (n = 56) Median: 5.6 ± 1.1	46 (60–32)	26 (38–13)	15.5 (26–4)	12 (22–1)
XR− (n = 102) Median: 6 ± 1.6	50 (61–38)	35 (48–21)	22 (36–8)	13 (29–0)

Table 14. Preoperative radiotherapy and occurrence of fistula

	XR	No XR
Patients (n)	103	651
Fistulas %	20	12.6

$P < 0.005$.

Our second, prospective study included 790 patients (Giulì and Sancho-Garnier 1985). In this study, 103 patients treated with radiotherapy before surgery were compared with 627 non-irradiated patients. The risk of fistula development or pulmonary complications under radiotherapy were confirmed, the percentages in both cases being highly significant (Table 11). Neither the tumour stage nor the histological differentiation of squamous carcinomas played any role in the indication for preoperative radiotherapy (Table 12). Finally, with a follow-up period of 18 months, there was no statistical difference in favour of preoperative radiotherapy. Survival medians are the same (Table 13).

To see whether any conclusions on the consequences of preoperative radiotherapy could be drawn from this study, we investigated whether a statistical bond might exist between this treatment and the subsequent development of an anastomotic fistula. Among the various parameters analysed in this search, (type of anastomosis, organ used for replacing oseophagus, location of tumour, surgical approach, location of anastomosis etc.), preoperative radiotherapy was the only one displaying a percentage of fistulae significantly greater than in the control group (Table 14).

Two relatively recent randomized studies also seem to attest to the difficulty in forming an opinion on the importance of preoperative radiotherapy. The first one, published by Launois et al. in 1981, involved 124 patients treated between 1973 and 1976. The preoperative radiation regimen was 40 Gy administered over 8–12 days, surgery being performed within 8 days following completion of radiation. Only patients with middle-third and distal-third lesions were included in this study. The resection rates of those receiving preoperative radiation and those going directly to surgery were similar (67% vs 70%). There were also no differences in operative mortality, which was substantial in both arms of the trial. Most disappointing was the mean and long-term survival: excluding operative mortality, the average survival was only 4.5 months for patients receiving preoperative radiation and 8.2 months for those treated with surgery alone. Long-term (5-year) survival was also similar, 11.5% for the surgical arm and 9.5% for those receiving preoperative radiotherapy.

Another randomized study, sponsored by the European Organization for Research and Treatment of Cancer (EORTC), was started in 1976. The treatment plan involved randomization to either 33 Gy of radiation given on 12 days and followed by surgery, or surgery alone. At the time of the preliminary report, 160 patients had been followed up for at least 1 year. The resection rate was similar for the two groups at 74.5%. The operative mortality was also similar at 19.5%. At the time of this analysis there was no difference in survival (Gignoux et al. 1985).

It seems, therefore, although a number of studies have suggested that radiotherapy has a beneficial effect on the resection rate and the short-term survival, that these hypotheses have not been confirmed by these two recent randomized trials.

Furthermore, in the studies using higher doses (Doggett and Guernsey 1970), there is an increased risk to life: in addition to the operative mortality, four of the 40 patients in this series died after receiving 50–60 Gy over 7 weeks.

This is why, when the OESO group decided to start an international randomized therapeutic trial on the advantages of treatments associated with surgical resection, it seemed preferable to turn towards the possible advantages of *postoperative* irradiation of tumours of the oesophagus. Such irradiation is designed to improve survival by reducing the frequency of locoregional recurrence, which occurs in 30%–50% of patients and is responsible for death, since there is no effective salvage treatment. In order for postoperative radiotherapy to have the maximum chance of success, an adequate prophylactic dose is required, neither too high, because of the risk of complications, nor too low, because of the risk of ineffectiveness.

Experience with other carcinomas shows that the adequate dose is 45 Gy fractionated in a classical manner, i.e. over 20–25 sessions at a rate of five sessions per week. The volume irradiated and the technique must also be appropriate, with minimal irradiation of the mediastinum, anteroposterior beams and the use of each beam at each session.

Chemotherapy

In theory at least, effective systemic therapy delivered at the time of diagnosis would allow the physician to treat both the primary tumour and its metastases simultaneously. However, until recently, few chemotherapy studies had been performed and even fewer had shown activity in this disease. The currently available chemotherapy data base has been reviewed by Kelsen (1984).

These trials indicate that single-agent activity for a variety of drugs is modest (10%–20%), with most responses being only partial and of brief duration (3–6 months). Combination chemotherapy, primarily based on cisplatin, appears to lead to higher response rates (30%–60%), but it must be emphasized that there are currently no randomized trials comparing, single agents to a combination. However, because of the dismal results seen after standard therapy for locoregional oesophageal cancer, the apparently more effective combinations have now been moved into multimodality studies.

The problem of the toxicity of the drugs used is a real one, and it appears that serious pulmonary toxicity may occur in 2%–8% of patients who receive bleomycin. This toxicity may occur at very small doses but is generally thought to be dose dependent, with a high incidence at cumulative doses greater than 450 mg/m^2 (Krakoff et al. 1985). The histological appearance is that of alveolar epithelial damage and intra-alveolar edema progressing to interalveolar fibrosis. There is no therapy which can regularly prevent pulmonary fibrosis, although it may sometimes be modified or reversed by the administration of adrenal corticosteroids.

Intratracheal administration of bleomycin to anaesthetized rats produces progressive pulmonary fibrosis identical in every respect with that seen in humans or rats given bleomycin systemically; intratracheal administration, however, produces the abnormality accompanied by an increase in angiotensin-converting enzyme in the pulmonary lavage fluid, a marked increase in prolyl hydroxylase, one of the enzymes required for assembly of the collagen molecule, and a marked decrease in pulmonary compliance. This is accompanied by a marked increase in collagen content. It is the increase in collagen deposition which leads to reversible fibrosis.

Studies have shown that all of these abnormalities can be prevented by the administration of a proline analogue, L-3,4-dehydroxyproline (DHP). Rats given bleomycin intratracheally and treated 2 weeks later with DHP exhibit none of the abnormalities characteristic of bleomycin toxicity. In addition, Krakoff et al. (1985) showed that DHP does not inhibit the antitumour activity of bleomycin.

For inoperable patients, certain combinations of chemotherapeutics have shown some efficacy. Kolaric et al. (1985), for instance, used a combination plus radiotherapy (36–40 Gy) for 51 patients divided into two groups. Their results showed that the combination of 5-FU with doxorubicin (64%), and particularly with bleomycin (75%), given concurrently with lower radiation dosage, was an effective palliative treatment for inoperable oesophageal cancer.

Some teams (Yamada et al. 1984) have published results of treatment associating, bleomycin with radiotherapy, without surgical treatment, in 121 patients; however, one must note that the radiation dose was 70 Gy and that the tumours treated were apparently of moderate extension, type T1 or T2.

The most frequent approach hitherto has consisted of combining surgery and chemotherapy. All the series published, however, concern only a very limited number of patients, too limited to draw conclusions about the effects. The Heidelberg team (Herrmann et al. 1985) has assembled a series of 21 patients who received two preoperative cycles of cisplatin, vindesine and bleomycin (DVB), 11 of whom were then able to undergo a so-called curative resection. Desai et al. (1985), associating cisplatin and methotrexate in 48 patients, observed eight preoperative complete clinical responses, confirmed in four instances by surgical exploration. After 3 years, 10 patients in this series were alive without further neoplastic development.

A conclusion may be drawn from the experience of Kelsen and colleagues: In a group of 68 patients (1983a), they obtained an objective response rate of 53%, with a resectability rate of 82% for localized lesions. Operative mortality (5.6%) did not seem affected by the association of DVB, and the median survival for the preoperative chemotherapy group was 16.2 months, superior to that of a historical control group ($p = 0.023$). In another series of 39 patients (Kelsen et al. 1983 b), objective responses were observed in 60% of the cases, but a residual tumour persisted on surgical exploration in nine patients, despite complete radiographic regression. For patients with extensive disease, treated primarily with chemotherapy alone, the median duration of response was 7 months, and drug toxicities were in general well tolerated.

These results seem to indicate that the investigational combination of cisplatin, vindesine and bleomycin can induce major regressions in a substantial proportion of patients with oesophageal cancer. Complete radiographic regressions should be confirmed by *repeated* endoscopy or by surgery. Downstaging of the primary tumour is commonly noted in the responding patients, but it is too soon to determine whether or not this will affect their long-term prognosis.

A number of other studies are presently in progress, but the very small numbers of patients do not enable any conclusions: trials have been made of oral oil bleomycin combined with sodium for the treatment of oesophageal cancer (Kamano et al. 1983) in 12 patients. In nine of them, bleomycin levels in the tumour, in the normal tissue of the resected oesophagus and in the regional lymph nodes were determined: the average level in the normal tissue was 1.2 μg/g, while the tumour level tended to be higher (4.4 μg/g). Bleomycin was also found to be efficiently transferred into the regional lymph nodes.

A combination of hyperthermia, chemotherapy and radiotherapy has also been tried by certain teams. In eight patients (Sugimachi et al. 1983), histological study of the resected specimens showed a marked effect in two cases, a moderate effect in four, and a slight effect in two. In those with a marked effect, there were no viable neoplastic cells, and severe necrosis and complete destruction were evident on the mucosal surface.

The same team (Sugimachi et al. 1982) devised two intraoperative supplemental treatments for carcinoma of the oesophagus: one is local application of bleomycin to the posterior mediastinum, where the carcinoma may possibly remain unresected. The other is intraoperative transnodal administration of bleomycin to the lymph nodes at the tracheal bifurcation, through which the agent can perfuse the upper mediastinal lymph nodes. No lymph node recurrence was encountered within 12 months after surgery in the transnodal injection group, whereas in the control group there was a high incidence of lymph node recurrence: 8.9% in 6 months, 10.6% in 9 months and 12.2% in 12 months. The incidence tended to be higher in the control group ($0.05 > p > 0.1$).

A similar trial was carried out by Watanabe (1983) in 80 patients treated from 1974 to 1981: he devised a slow-release, solid-form bleomycin tube through which the drug is given locally and absorbed slowly through the surrounding tissue possibly containing minimum residual disease. This tube was placed near the area (upper mediastinum and upper abdomen) of dissected metastatic lymph nodes at the time of surgery. In stage IV, all 27 patients of the control group died within 2 years after the operation, while in the therapy group, 11.8% of 36 patients survived for 5 years.

Randomized trials are underway comparing DVB chemotherapy plus surgery to surgery alone (National Cancer Institute, Bethesda, Maryland) or to preoperative radiation therapy (Memorial Sloan Kettering Cancer Center). Both trials have had very slow recruitment of subjects, indicating that single-institution studies will not allow assessment of this type of approach in a reasonable time frame. In addition to these randomized studies, Schlag et al. (1985) reporting an EORTC trial, have piloted a single-arm study using DVB chemotherapy.

Preliminary evaluation of the NCI data and those of Schlag et al. confirm a response rate to DVB chemotherapy of 50%, but in all these studies it is too early to assess survival rates.

Overall, the poor results obtained with single-modality treatments and the encouraging results of preliminary trials of surgery and preoperative chemotherapy emphasize the need for large-scale randomized trials. The toxicity of systemic cisplatin-based chemotherapy is substantial, but tolerable: if this drug can improve overall resection rates and survival, it is certainly worth using, but more extensive trials need to be conducted.

For this reason, the OESO group decided to set up an international randomized therapeutic trial, which we will discuss in more detail at the end of this chapter, to assess the value of perioperative chemotherapy in comparison to surgery alone, or followed by radiotherapy (Giulì 1988 c).

Postoperative Complications

Anastomotic fistulas are still significantly associated with postoperative mortality (Table 15), and punctiform fistulas would also seem to play a notable role (Table 16). In addition, almost half of all mediastinal abscesses have a cervical anastomosis as their origin.

The fistula rate remains high (Table 17), and there is no difference in subsequent fistula rate between mechanical anastomosis and manual anastomosis in

Table 15. Fistulas and postoperative mortality

	Mortality (%)	
Fistula	32	
		$P < 0.0001$
No fistula	12	

Table 16. Fistulas and postoperative mortality

	Punctiform ($n = 63$)	Large ($n = 20$)	Loose separation ($n = 14$)
Postoperative mortality (%)	19	55	71
	$P = 0.0001$		

Table 17. Fistulas (103/769 = 13.4%) and type of anastomosis

Fistulas	Single layer 225 9%	Two layers 321 19% ($P = 0.002$)	Mechanical 200 10%
Punctiform	72%	65%	62%
Large	17%	19%	24%
Loose separation	11%	16% NS	14%
Average time lapse (days)	8.1	8.8 NS	7.7
Early fistula (<5 days)	22%	50%	27%

Table 18. Fistulas related to type of oesophageal replacement, tumour site and approach

	Oesophageal replacement			Tumour site				Approach		
	Stomach	Colon	Small bowel	Upper third	Middle third	Lower third	Cardia	Right	Left	Blunt
Patients (*n*)	624	56	29	54	210	430	20	490	170	90
Fistulas (%)	15	5	10	18	13	12	10	14	10	19
		NS				NS			NS	

Table 19. Preoperative radiotherapy and occurrence of fistula

	XR	No XR
Patients (*n*)	103	651
fistulas (%)	20	12.6

$P < 0.005$.

a single layer. In the OESO series (Tables 18, 19) the only statistically significant feature concerning the aetiology of fistulas is preoperative radiotherapy.

Placing the zone of anastomosis in the cervical region does not necessarily prevent serious septic diffusion: about one half of the mediastinal abscesses observed in association with a fistula were, in our series, derived from cervical anastomoses (10 of 22).

The peculiar anatomic features of the oesophagus have been implicated in the genesis of complications, which would thus be beyond the control of the operator. Chiefly maligned has been the "oesophageal blood supply". In fact, the blood supply to the oesophagus is excellent (Payne 1984), and factors other than poor innate perfusion can be responsible for postoperative oesophageal leak and fistula formation. From autopsy and intraoperative observations on patients with oesophageal leak, it seems that the ischaemic slough of structures anastomosed to the oesophagus, rather than failure of the oesophageal blood supply, should, in most cases, be blamed for the genesis of leak after oesophageal reconstruction.

However, the major complications of oesophagectomy remain pulmonary, some of them possibly related to small undiagnosed fistulae. They have been discussed elsewhere (Elman and Giuli 1988) and will not be detailed here.

Long-term Prognosis

The basic problem in assessing the long-term prognosis is related to the fact that although the adequacy of surgical resection is evaluated clinically at operation by palpation of the resection margin, secondary mucosal lesions – distant mucosal metastases or multicentric primaries – are found in 16% of specimens examined (Wong 1984).

Furthermore, there is a discrepancy between the in situ specimen length and the length of the apparently normal oesophagus above the level of tumour. This is expected from contraction of the oesophageal musculature: the normal oesophagus shrinks to half its in situ length when resected. Tumour shrinkage, however, is virtually non-existent, reflecting transmural spread of tumour in all these patients.

In the retrospective OESO study (Giulì and Gignoux 1980), histological study of the site of oesophageal section revealed the following: a totally healthy appearance of the remaining oesophagus was seen most often (53%) after section of the oesophagus more than 4 cm from the tumour, but equally frequently for all margins ranging from 4 cm to less than 1 cm.

In 29% of cases in which histological examination revealed complete invasion, the section had nevertheless been made in an apparently healthy area more than 4 cm from the tumour. The corresponding figure for invasion after section of the oesophagus immediately adjacent to the carcinoma was 24%. Similar differences were found in intermediate cases of isolated areas of neoplastic repermeation (40% at more than 4 cm, 18% at less than 1 cm).

Recurrence of the tumour is the most obvious criterion of insufficient treatment. We have specifically studied this problem (Giuli 1984b), taking into account all the possible circumstances of recurrence, in 163 (16%) of the 1020 patients in the retrospective study. Some 131 (more than 80%) had initially undergone reconstruction of the oesophagus using the stomach, and 72 (55%) showed evidence of involvement of coeliac nodes at the time of operation.

Certain retrospective numerical data may usefully be emphasized: The presence of invaded coeliac nodes is a frequent finding (on average 28%), and is associated with 32% of recurrences. Furthermore, it is remarkable that, even when lymph nodes are healthy, a recurrence occurs in 27% of patients. Such recurrences are most often situated in the mediastinum (47%) or the oesophagus (31%). The absence of lymph node involvement does not exclude the possibility of a secondary tumour site in the neck (6%) or the ENT area (7%).

Among the recurrences in a histologically healthy oesophagus, 55 of 58 (95%) occurred in patients who had previously undergone a gastroplasty. Almost three-quarters of those patients (40/55) had evidence of involvement of coeliac nodes at the time of operation.

An attempt may be made to explain this fact, on the basis of the results of anatomical studies of the lymph vessels of the stomach carried out by Pissas et al. (1979), both in cadavers and in patients undergoing operation:

- The lymph vessels of the stomach are fully anastomosed with those of the oesophagus.
- The gastric coronary drainage territory includes, in addition to the lesser curvature, the upper two thirds of the horizontal portion of the stomach, and is anatomically superimposed in this area with the hepatic drainage territory, which, in particular, covers the greater part of the anterior and posterior surfaces of the greater curvature of the stomach (Fig. 1).
- Study of the direction of lymph drainage in the gastric wall has also shown an orientation of the valvules directing the current towards the nodes of the lesser curvature for the right-hand side of the gastric surfaces, and towards those of the greater curvature for the left-hand side. However, neoplastic invasion of the gastric coronary nodes may be responsible for reversal of lymph flow at this site, the reflux which then occurs heading towards the greater curvature of the stomach. This is facilitated by the existence of a non-valvular lymphatic zone (Fig. 2).

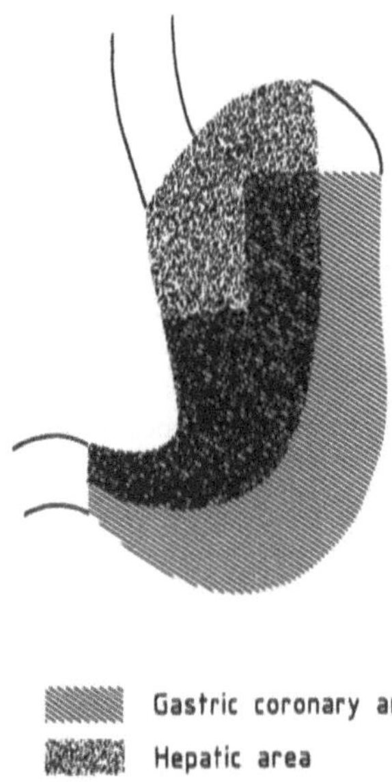

Fig. 1. Lymph drainage of the stomach. (From Pissas et al. 1979)

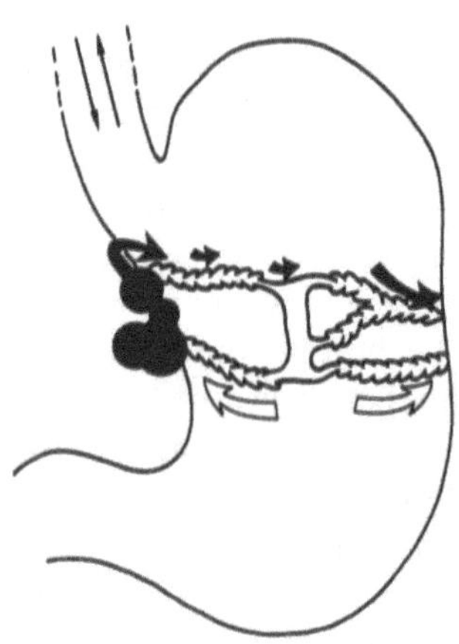

Fig. 2. Reversal of lymph flow after invasion of gastric coronary nodes

When regional dissection of the coeliac nodes is necessary because of evidence of neoplastic involvement, and the stomach is used to replace the oesophagus, one may have to check that the gastric antrum and greater curvature are completely free of tumour. In addition, the numerous anatomical communications which exist between the various lymph node groups draining the stomach are such that it is not possible to be certain of the complete absence of lymphatic emboli along the course of the vascular arcades (pyloric or gastroepiploic) around the gastric tube and in the satellite nodes of the gastric area which may have been left in place (e.g. at the hilum of the spleen).

In cases of marked coeliac lymph node involvement (remembering that these nodes were involved in 28% of the patients in this series), rather than resecting only the area of the lesser curvature and part of the surfaces of the stomach, it would appear legitimate to perform, as in the case of carcinoma of the cardia, total excision of the stomach extended to the spleen and the omenta. The time required for dissection is scarcely longer than for extended gastrolysis, but lymph node excision without any need for caution concerning preservation of vascular supply may be much more satisfactory and more radical.

The digestive reconstruction can, if necessary, be carried out at a later stage. The separation of the colon and omentum, already carried out during the total gastrectomy, is the first stage of transposition of the colon. Freeing of the transverse colon, extended towards the right or left according to the anatomical conditions encountered, its insertion in the bed left by the removal of the oesophagus, and its anastomosis, in the neck, to the residual oesophagus or the pharynx presents numerous advantages. Anastomosis of the upper end of the colonic transplant in the neck also eliminates the risk of intrathoracic anastomotic leakage during the postoperative period.

Follow-up

The consequences of recurrences or metastases on patient survival emphasize the need for a marker which can predict their development, and classical markers do not allow an accurate surveillance of oesophageal cancer. Particularly, determinations of carcinoembryonic antigen are less reliable than in colorectal carcinomas.

In contrast, sequential determination of blood histamine levels provide a valuable measure of tumour progression in oesophageal cancer. It has been shown (Burtin et al. 1984) that blood histamine levels are significantly decreased in patients with solid malignant tumours, and increased to almost normal values after successful resection. As blood histamine is a marker of carcinoma progression, sequential measurements are essential: whatever the initial value, stability of blood histamine is associated with stability of disease. By contrast, a progressive fall in blood histamine levels precedes the detection of metastases by 2–8 weeks. The OESO therapeutic trial is planned to include large-scale control of this data, which could represent a major advance in the evaluation of neoplastic development after treatment.

Long-term Survival

Factors affecting long-term survival have been selected from the OESO retrospective study (Giulì and Gignoux 1980) involving 2400 patients who underwent resection. One of the first observations was that tumours of the upper third of the oesophagus were no longer almost systematically avoided: in 106 cases, the overall postoperative mortality was 31% and the 5-year survival rate was 14% (confidence intervals 24%–4%) and 21% (32%–6%) when postoperative mortality was excluded. In the case of tumours of the middle third of the oesophagus, comparison of the results in a total of 997 resections with oesophagogastric anastomosis revealed the following 5-year survival rates: low subaortic anastomosis, 8% (16%–0%) in 177 patients; anastomosis above the aorta, 13% (16%–0%) in 736 patients; anastomosis in the neck, 24% (40%–8%) in 84 patients. Postoperative mortality is excluded. A two-stage procedure after subtotal oesophagectomy also results in 5-year survival of about a quarter of the patients.

For tumours of the lower third of the oesophagus ($n = 789$), the mean 5-year survival rate (including postoperative mortality) was 17%. As in the case of the higher tumours, the 5-year survival rates of various operations differed: The worst results (13%; 20%–11%) were found in association with low resections ($n = 289$). The prognosis was better (20%; 27%–13%) when the anastomosis was made above the level of the aorta ($n = 230$) and best (32%; 49%–14%) with subtotal excision of the oesophagus and colonic plasty and anastomosis in the neck ($n = 61$).

Furthermore, as specified by Belsey (1984) in his analysis of these statistics:

- Absence of lymph node involvement was nevertheless associated with a local recurrence rate of 27% (52% mediastinal and 35% oesophageal).

- With cervical lymph node involvement, paradoxically 33% of those who survived surgery were alive 5 years later.

Attempted curative surgery of some of the earliest carcinomas recorded has been followed by the return of the patient within 9 months riddled with metastases.

Those are the anomalies which led us to reconsider, in the OESO randomized therapeutic trial, the clinical classification of these patients as well as the histological classification of their tumour.

Stenoses occurring after 6 months are of a completely different origin and may be considered to be complications of peptic oesophagitis. Their recurrent nature is then much more marked, and instrumental dilatation is necessary.

Finally (Couraud et al. 1984), the best yardstick of the sequelae of oesophageal resection is the patient's opinion of the results:

- Delight – when operated upon for dysphagia and benefitting from surgery,
- Disappointment – when operated upon without dysphagia and complications ensue.

Mode of Survival

Diarrhoea immediately following return to oral feeding affects almost 50% of patients. However, prescription of medication and an appropriate diet quickly resolves the problem, to the extent that only 5% of patients still complain of diarrhoea after 3 months of follow-up.

In the long term, distension or progressive adaptation of the gastric pouch always results in restoration of normal alimentary rhythm within a few months, and it is unusual for a patient still to complain of small stomach syndrome at the end of the first year.

Pylorospasm, on the other hand, may severely accentuate nutritional disturbances associated with small stomach syndrome, with persistent pain, late vomiting and impaired general condition. However, pyloroplasty is not performed systematically by all authors: Wong (1985) demonstrated that whether pyloroplasty was performed or not, problems which occurred in the first weeks following surgery disappeared progressively, so that at 24 months nearly all of the 68 patients encountered no difficulty in feeding.

The technique of mechanical anastomosis was not adopted by all teams (200 of 746 in the prospective OESO statistics), and does not prevent the occurrence of anastomotic stenoses postoperatively. On the contrary, Wong (1985) showed that these were slightly more frequent (19%) after mechanical anastomosis (19%) than after manual anastomosis (8%), sometimes being due to technical problems such as poor apposition of the mucosa, hypertrophic anastomotic granulomas or anastomotic fistula. The greater frequency of such stenoses in patients treated by younger surgeons, and after technically difficult operations, emphasizes the importance of the contribution of mechanical anastomosis to early postoperative stenoses.

Future Projects

The general mediocrity of the results reported by individual centres at a time of increasing incidence of oesophageal cancer legitimizes a multidisciplinary approach to the very peculiar problems encountered in these patients.

Efficacy in such a project can be ensured only by careful statistical analysis of a multicentric study. This is indispensable in order to delineate tendencies, eliminate hypotheses and properly evaluate the correlations among the findings. It is within this context, and with the particular approach to these problems emerging from the daily experience of an entire team, that the OESO group was created in 1979 to organize a number of multicentric statistical studies on cancers of the oesophagus. Four successive studies steps were planned, of which the last two are still in progress. The first in time, and the least restrictive for the participants, was the *retrospective* study already discussed above. It was the subject of a communication during the September 1979 meeting of the European Societies of Surgery and, thereafter, a publication in the journal *Annals of Surgery* (Giulì and Gignoux 1980). This study assembled the largest number of resected tumours of the oesophagus to date, involving 2400 patients. Teams from 10 different countries shared the tedious task of compiling statistical data from questionnaires in five languages, and therefore contributed to the second stage of our programme, the realization of a *prospective* study of operated patients. This second study, embracing surgery, anaesthesia, nutrition, pathology and non-surgical treatment, was the subject first of a presentation at the world congress of the OESO group in Paris, in 1984, then a publication in a book issued shortly after congress (Giulì 1984a) and in the journal *Surgery* (Giulì and Sancho-Garnier 1985).

The collective impetus was accelerated by the international and multidisciplinary structure of the established OESO group, benefitting progressively throughout the years from the inclusion of renowned teams from various countries who gradually became accustomed to the rules of collective work. Against the background of this experience, the third stage of the programme, a study not only prospective but also *randomized*, became feasible. In order for this study, started in 1985, to have from the outset the best chances of success it was necessary, that it benefit from all the knowledge acquired over the previous years during the realization of the preliminary programme of the OESO group. The invaluable assistance in computerization of statistical data provided by a world-renowned centre, the Department of Medical Statistics of the Institut Gustave Roussy in Villejuif, was reinforced by the participation of the statistical team of another renowned international centre, the Memorial Sloan Kettering Center in New York. This ambitious project, presently in progress, covers 17 different countries and proposes to analyse simultaneously a large amount of data from patients allocated randomly to one of three different arms: surgery alone, surgery followed by radiotherapy, or surgery preceded and followed by chemotherapy. Cancer must still be considered today as a disease for which surgical treatment represents the therapeutic basis, and for this reason surgical resection has been selected as the reference arm of the study.

Postoperative radiotherapy at prophylactic doses of 45 Gy should reduce the locoregional recurrence rate and be very effective against residual disease, as observed in other tumours. The effects of such treatment, performed under precise and reproduceable conditions, are not known in cancer of the oesophagus, but should be beneficial, as the dose of 45 Gy is not toxic. This radiotherapy arm is headed by Prof. Baillet of Paris. Treatment begins 6–8 weeks after surgery and continues for 5 weeks, with five sessions of 1.8 Gy per week.

The third arm of the trial is perioperative chemotherapy. In this area the experience of large centres such as the Memorial Sloan Kettering Center in New York has been outstanding, and the protocol selected was the one developed in that centre, especially by Dr. Kelsen. It consists of the association of two cycles of cisplatin, seven of vindesine and eight of bleomycin during the 2 months preceding surgery. Then, 6–8 weeks after surgical resection, 22 weeks of treatment comprising three cycles of cisplatin and 12 of vindesine. This combination seems to meet the requirements of efficacy (50% responses on average, with improvement of surgical resectability) and acceptable tolerance which does not aggravate the morbidity or the mortality of the surgical procedure.

The experience of the Memorial Sloan Kettering Center, however, important though it is, includes only a few patients despite the Center's large recruiting capabilities. We are alluding here to a major problem in any study of this kind: the results are only fragmentary and never definitive because of the small number of cases available for a trial in a single therapeutic centre. In the OESO group, however, this problem is overcome by the number and the quality of the teams participating.

The aim is to show that one of the treatments associated with surgery improves the 2-year survival rate by at least 10% (from 15%–25%) for an α risk of 5% and a β risk of 20%. Each arm must include 100 patients, making a total of 300 patients.

The rapid recruitment of patients is an additional benefit expected from this cooperation. Depending on the recruiting capabilities of the various centres participating, it may be possible to assemble this large number of patients in less than 3 years.

The constraints of such a trial are numerous and strict. Every member of each team involved must completely accept every detail of the protocol and must be scrupulous in recording all the information required. Despite these difficulties, explicit agreement for participation has been obtained from 39 teams representing 17 different countries of Europe (Germany, Belgium, Spain, France, Hungary, Italy, Poland, Turkey, Yugoslavia), America (United States, Brazil, Argentina, Chile), the Middle East (Saudi Arabia) and Asia (India, Japan, China). The randomization of the patients is done at the Institute Gustave Roussy, where a team of five specialists was formed. This team works daily, analysing the statistical forms as they are received, verifying them and feeding the data into the computer.

As shown in the retrospective and the prospective OESO preliminary studies, the uncertainties in the field of oesophageal cancers relate as much to the nature of the appropriate treatment as to classification of the patients and their disease. For that reason, it seemed essential to set up two prognostic indices which will be tested as the various observations are received.

The first involves evaluation of the different clinical and nutritional parameters of each patient, in an attempt to elaborate a system enabling the assignment of a score. Reading the main publications, one notes that the percentages of postoperative complications, global mortality and long-term survival often vary greatly from one country to another, and even from one team to another, with no clear explanation for such variations.

The use of such an index will enable the classification of patients into precise groups within which valid statistical comparisons can be carried out. We hope then to be able to achieve a genuinely valid evaluation, from one country to another, of the differences in prognosis which can exist for a disease that undoubtedly, is not strictly the same everywhere.

The inclusion in our group of Chinese, Japanese, American and European teams allows for comparisons of the clinical and nutritional condition of the patients operated on in these different parts of the world. Uniform analysis may reveal correlations, as yet unsuspected, between the patient, the disease and the treatment given.

Our previous studies have also shown, as mentioned above, the obviously insufficient nature of the present TNM classification, which is still regularly used for cancers of the oesophagus. It seems indispensable to include not only histological criteria but macroscopic factors more directly associated with the long-term prognosis of a given tumour. For this reason, within the OESO group Professor Appelman, a world authority, and the international group of pathologists he is heading, were charged to elaborate a histological prognostic index. Again, the goal is to establish for each patient a global score which will enable, for each type of tumour operated on, the determination of a prognosis based on real data.

This index includes three to seven graduations of each of 12 different macroscopic and microscopic aspects of the tumour. The evaluation of this index will be made directly by the OESO Statistical Center, and we hope to be able to propose, at the completion of this therapeutic trial, a new classification system for tumours of the oesophagus.

To achieve perfect consistency in the exact histological typing of the tumours, Professor Appelman is centralizing the histological data for all patients in his Ann Arbor laboratory, receiving about 12 slides per patient. There will always be cases where classification is difficult, and we anticipate discussing these every 6 months during a special meeting of pathologists within the OESO group.

A first evaluation of the results of this randomized trial could be done when the randomization of the patients is completed. Since the preparation of this paper (Feb 1986) the first preliminary results of the OESO Malignancy index were published. (Diseases of the Esophagus, (1988) Vol 1 No 3, in press)

Specialists agree that the solution to the problems posed by oesophageal cancers resides mainly in their prevention. It has been clearly demonstrated by Chinese teams, who have the greatest experience, that 66% of severe dysplasias of the oesophagus are followed in 9–12 years by malignant degeneration (Huang 1984a). On the other hand, experiments have shown that treatment with carotenoids, substances of very little toxicity originating from vitamin A, is likely to reduce dysplastic lesions or make them disappear altogether.

The Group OESO has therefore set up another therapeutic trial, reserved for large gastrointestinal endoscopy centres, to test randomly the effect of simple supervision and of *treatment by carotenoid substances* (Etretinate) on dysplastic lesions found after a systematic search. This trial is presently in progress in the digestive endoscopy centres of countries from the five parts of the world, under the patronage of OMGE (Organisation Mondiale de Gastro Enterologie-World Association of Gastro Enterologie). The evolution of the oesophageal dysplasias will be observed regularly for a minimum of 2 years.

The surest guarantee of efficiency is given by the coming together, within the OESO group, of specialists in numerous disciplines, whose common objective is the improvement of the existing knowledge concerning the genesis and the therapy of the most frequent diseases of the oesophagus. The joint work already carried out for several years, the quality of the results recorded in the previous studies, and the importance of the results which may emerge from the studies presently in progress, provide each of the teams participating with the necessary motivation and enthusiasm.

The questions asked can be answered only by statistical analysis, carried out by high-level professional groups, of carefully selected data containing correlations which are not immediately evident. Only large numbers enable such research, and only multicentric studies can assemble sufficient patients. The presence within the OESO group of teams from Europe, Asia, America and Australia enables, for the first time, real comparisons which will hopefully yield interesting explanations and, especially, indisputable therapeutic conclusions.

References

Akiyama H (1984a) Which groups of lymph nodes draining the esophagus could be usually excised during operation? In: Giuli R (ed) Cancer of the esophagus in 1984. Maloine, Paris, p 90

Akiyama H (1984b) What are the rules for tubulisation of the stomach to be possible? In: Giuli R (ed) Cancer of the esophagus in 1984. Maloine, Paris, p 146

Akiyama H (1984c) Are there still indications for manual anastomosis in esophageal surgery? In: Giuli R (ed) Cancer of the esophagus in 1984. p 67

Angorn IB, Haffejee AA (1984a) May contra-indications be nutritional or immunological? Is there a relationship between these two factors? In: Giuli R (ed) Cancer of the esophagus in 1984. Maloine, Paris, p 21

Angorn IB, Haffejee AA (1984b) Do nutritional and immunological factors have prognostic value in carcinoma of the esophagus? In: Giuli R (ed) Cancer of the esophagus in 1984. Maloine, Paris, p 370

Angorn IB, Haffejee AA (1984c) At what time should intubation of the esophagus be considered, and according to what technique? In: Giuli R (ed) Cancer of the esophagus in 1984. Maloine, Paris, p 43

Balzola F, Schimenti P, Possamai D (1984) Are there immunological or nutritional arguments which may be used to predict inoperability? In: Giuli R (ed) Cancer of the esophagus in 1984. Maloine, Paris, p 106

Belsey R (1984) Is it possible to talk of cure of carcinoma of the esophagus? In: Giuli R (ed) Cancer of the esophagus in 1984. Maloine, Paris, p 382

Blackburn G (1984) Is it possible to reverse the catabolism of a patient? In: Giuli R (ed) Cancer of the esophagus in 1984. Maloine, Paris, p 67

Bourgeon A, Richelme H (1984) The direction of peristalsis would not seem to play a predominant role in the function of a colonic transplant. In: Giuli R (ed) Cancer of the esophagus in 1984. Maloine, Paris, p 271

Burtin C, Noirot C, Scheinmann P (1984) Biological factors as markers of progression in oncology. In: Giuli R (ed) Cancer of the esophagus in 1984. Maloine, Paris, p 298

Chomé J (1984a) Is the diagnosis of superficial carcinoma always possible? In: Giuli R (ed) Cancer of the esophagus in 1984. Maloine, Paris, p 325

Chomé J (1984b) The problem of neoplastic repermeation. In: Giuli R (ed) Cancer of the esophagus in 1984. Maloine, Paris, p 325

Chomé J (1984c) How to classify certain unequal aspects of histological differentiation? In: Giuli R (ed) Cancer of the esophagus in 1984. Maloine, Paris, p 213

Couraud L, Meriot S, Haffez A (1984) Functional sequelae of esophageal resections. In: Giuli R (ed) Cancer of the esophagus in 1984. Maloine, Paris, pp 276–279

Del Genio A, di Martino M, Amato G, Fei L (1984) Many prognostic factors cannot be investigated surgically. In: Giuli R (ed) Cancer of the esophagus in 1984. Maloine, Paris, p 200

Desai PB, Advani SH, Dinshaw KA, et al. (1985) The long term impact of front-loading chemotherapy in advanced esophageal cancers. A report of 88 patients treated with cisplatin methotrexate. In: Abstracts of the 1st International Congress on Neo-Adjuvant Chemotherapy. Paris (under the patronage of the UICC, INSERM and French National League against cancer)

Doggett R, Guernsey J (1970) Combined radiation and surgical treatment of the thoracic esophagus: final report. Front Radiat Ther Oncol 5: 147–154

Ellis F Jr (1984) Should palliative operations still be considered? In: Giuli R (ed) Cancer of the esophagus in 1984. Maloine, Paris, p 49

Elman A, Giuli R (1988) Immediate complications following esophageal surgery. In: Delarue NC, Eschapasse H (eds): International trends in general thoracic surgery. Saunders, Toronto

Elman A, Boudinet A, Flamant Y, Metrot-Magny C, Levy D (1984) Contra-indications related to respiratory function. In: Giuli R (ed) Cancer of the esophagus in 1984. Maloine, Paris, p 20

Endo M (1984) Should surgical treatment of superficial cancers be limited? In: Giuli R (ed) Cancer of the esophagus in 1984. Maloine, Paris, p 336

Gignoux M, et al. (1985) Pre-operative radiotherapy for carcinoma of the esophagus. Results of a prospective multicentric study (EORTC) in esophageal disorders: pathophysiology and therapy. In: DeMester TR, Skinner DB (eds) Raven, New York

Girault F (1984) At what time should intubation of the esophagus be considered, and according to what technique? In: Giuli R (ed) Cancer of the esophagus in 1984. Maloine, Paris, p 45

Giuli R (ed) (1984a) Cancer of the esophagus in 1984. Maloine, Paris

Giuli R (1984b) Gastric resection in esophageal cancer. In: Giuli R (ed) Cancer of the esophagus in 1984. Maloine, Paris, p 288

Giuli R (1988a) Viewpoint on the association of radiotherapy and surgery. In: Wilkins EW Jr, Delarve NC (eds) International trends in general thoracic surgery; vol 4, Esophageal cancer. Saunders, Toronto

Giuli R (1988b) Surgery for squamous carcinoma of the oesophagus. An overview. In: Jamieson GG (ed) Surgery of the oesophagus. Churchill Livingstone, Edinburgh

Giuli R (1988c) Surgical involvement in cooperative study protocols: experience of the OESO international group. In: Wilking EW, Delarve NC (eds) International trends in general thoracic surgery; vol 4, Esophageal cancer. Saunders, Toronto

Giuli R, Gignoux M (1980) Treatment of carcinoma of the esophagus. Retrospective study of 3400 patients. Ann Surg 192: 44–52

Giuli R, Sancho-Garnier H (1986) Diagnostic, therapeutic and prognostic features of cancers of the esophagus. Results of the international prospective study conducted by the OESO group (790 patients). Surgery, 99: 614–622

Herrmann R, Schlag P, Manegold C, et al. (1985) Preoperative chemotherapy in esophageal cancer. Results of a phase II pilot study. In: Abstracts of the 1st International Congress on Neo-Adjuvant Chemotherapy. Paris (under the patronage of the UICC, INSERM and French National League against cancer)

Huang GJ (1984a) Is it possible to define correlation between the pre-symptomatic period and the stage of carcinoma? In: Giuli R (ed) Cancer of the esophagus in 1984. Maloine, Paris, p 324

Huang GJ (1984b) What is the value of abrasive cytology? In: Giuli R (ed) Cancer of the esophagus in 1984. Maloine, Paris, p 325

Huang GJ (1984c) Is the type of thoracic approach of importance? In: Giuli R (ed) Cancer of esophagus in 1984. Maloine, Paris, p 89

Huang GJ (1984d) What is the value of abrasive cytology? In:

Giuli R (ed) Cancer of the esophagus in 1984. Maloine, Paris, p 320

Huang GJ (1984e) How to treat superficial carcinoma? In: Giuli R (ed) Cancer of the esophagus in 1984. Maloine, Paris, p 331

Huang GJ (1984f) In other cases, surgery can be envisaged. Pre-operative radiotherapy or chemotherapy. In: Giuli R (ed) Cancer of the esophagus in 1984. Maloine, Paris, p 56

Husemann B (1984) In other cases, surgery can be envisaged. Pre-operative radiotherapy or chemotherapy. In: Giuli R (ed) Cancer of the esophagus in 1984. Maloine, Paris, p 56

Kamano T, Kishino H, Kidokoro T, et al. (1983) Oral administration of oil bleomycin combined with sodium polyacrylate for the treatment of esophageal cancer. Am J Med 75 (4): 104

Kelsen D (1984) Chemotherapy of esophageal cancer. Semin Oncol 11: 159

Kelsen D, Hilaris B, Coonley C (1983a) Cisplatin, vindesine, and bleomycin chemotherapy of local-regional and advanced esophageal carcinoma. Am J Med 75 (4): 645–652

Kelsen D, Heelan R, Coonley C, et al. (1983b) Clinical and pathological evaluation of response chemotherapy in patients with esophageal carcinoma. Am J Med 75(4): 103

Kolaric K, Roth A, Dujmovic I (1985) The value of two combined chemoradiotherapy approaches in the treatment of inoperable esophageal cancer. In: Abstracts on cancer chemotheray. Nippon Kayaku, Tokyo, p 136

Krakoff IH, Newman RA, Hacker MP (1985) Modification of bleomycin pulmonary toxicity by inhibitors of collagen synthesis. In: Abstracts on cancer chemotherapy. Nippon Kayaku, Tokyo, p 180

Launois B, et al. (1981) Pre-operative radiotherapy for carcinoma of the esophagus. Surg Gynecol Obstet 153: 690–692

Lebas JF, Sarrazin R, Coulomb M, Geindre M (1984) How dependable is computerized tomography in determining contra-indications? In: Giuli R (ed) Cancer of the esophagus in 1984. Maloine, Paris, p 29

Mignon M, de Mestier P, Zielinski B (1984) The problem of remaining gastric acidity. In: Giuli R (ed) Cancer of the esophagus in 1984. Maloine, Paris, p 280

Moraldi A, Zerilli M, Iascone C, Schillaci A, Stipa S (1984) Can the scanner supply sufficient elements to specify the state of the detected lymph nodes? In: Giuli R (ed) Cancer of the esophagus in 1984. Maloine, Paris, p 92

Mullen JL, Buzby GP, Matthews DC, et al. (1980) Reduction of operative morbidity and mortality by combined preoperative and postoperative nutritional support. Ann Surg 102: 604–613

Orringer MB (1984) Is it illusory to envisage extended lymph node dissection? In: Giuli R (ed) Cancer of the esophagus in 1984. Maloine, Paris, p 138

Payne WS (1984) The role of esophageal blood supply. In: Giuli R (ed) Cancer of the esophagus in 1984. 135 questions. Maloine, Paris, p 222

Pearson JG (1984) Should radiotherapy be considered? In: Giuli R (ed) Cancer of the esophagus in 1984. Maloine, Paris, p 33

Picus D (1983) Computed tomography in the staging of esophageal carcinoma. Radiology 146: 433–438

Pissas A, Dyon JF, Sarrazin R, Bouchet Y (1979) Le drainage lymphatique de l'estomac. J Chir (Paris) 116: 583–590

Ribet M (1984) What immune studies should be undertaken in cancer of the oesophagus? In: Giuli R (ed) Cancer of the esophagus in 1984. Maloine, Paris, p 26

Richelme H (1984) Does sub-total resection necessarily require a cervical approach to the esophagus? In: Giuli R (ed) Cancer of the esophagus in 1984. Maloine, Paris, p 134

Sarrazin R, Voilin C, Bacle B, Dyon JF (1984) Lymph node anatomy and physiology of the oesophagus. In: Giuli R (ed) Cancer of the esophagus in 1984. Maloine, Paris, p 5

Savary M, Monnier P, Anani P (1984) What should the attitude be in the presence of esophageal dysplasia or healthy esophagus? In: Giuli R (ed) Cancer of the esophagus in 1984. Maloine, Paris, p 335

Schlag P, et al. (1985) Cis-platin, vindesine and bleomycin chemotherapy prior to surgery in esophageal carcinoma. International Symposium on Chemotherapy Prior to Surgery or Radiation. February, Valkenberg, (in press)

Siewert JR (1984) Quality of resection: invasion of lymph nodes or neighbouring organs. In: Giuli R (ed) Cancer of the esophagus in 1984. Maloine, Paris, p 198

Skinner DB (1984) Is it legitimate to envisage the combined excision of an organ invaded by contact with the tumour? In: Giuli R (ed) Cancer of the esophagus in 1984. Maloine, Paris, p 101

Sugimachi K, Inokuchi K, Kai H, et al. (1983) Hyperthermo-chemo-therapy for carcinoma of the esophagus. Am J Med 75 (4): 103

Sugimachi K, Inokuchi K, Natsuda Y, et al. (1982) Intraoperative local adjuvant cancer chemotherapy for carcinoma of the thoracic esophagus. Jpn J Surg 12: 105–110

Watanabe H (1983) Adjuvant chemotherapy combined with surgical treatment for cancer of the esophagus. In: Abstracts on cancer chemotherapy. Nippon Kayaku, Tokyo, p 1

Wong J (1984) What are the methods available to assess the quality of surgical resection? In: Giuli R (ed) Cancer of the esophagus in 1984. Maloine, Paris, p 198

Wong J (1985) Progress in esophageal surgery. Congrès de l'Association Française de Chirurgie, Sept 26, Paris

Yamada S, Asakawa H, Matsumoto K, et al. (1984) Combination therapy with radiation and bleomycin for esophageal carcinoma with special reference to the prognostic aspect. In: Abstracts on cancer chemotherapy. Nippon Kayaku, Tokyo, p 86

Cancer of the Cardia: The Role of Extended Esophagogastrectomy

E. M. González, M. Gomez, J. M. Jover, J. Calleja, I. Landa, J. Arias, F. Escudero, and I. Garcia

The cardia is the orifice or tunnel, 1.5–2 cm in length, joining the esophagus with the gastric cavity (Dodge 1961; McPeak and Warren 1948). Its cephalad limit is the transition between stratified esophageal squamous epithelium and columnar gastric epithelium. Tubuloacinar glands are distributed irregularly between 25 mm above this limit and 20 mm below it. Based on description of early cancer at this level (Kraus and Cain 1979; Kyoichi et al. 1966; Li et al. 1982), we can affirm that cancer of the cardia is an adenocarcinoma that originates in the columnar epithelium of the cardia (Ellis 1976; Humphrey and Kerstens 1976; Kobayashi et al. 1970), although epithelial carcinomas originating in the stratified layer of the esophageal mucosa can distally infiltrate the cardiac surface (Appelquist 1972; Humphrey and Kerstens 1976).

This carcinoma should be distinguished from gastric carcinoma (Hanklins et al. 1974; Kata et al. 1978), epidermoid carcinoma of the esophagus (Talerman and Woo-Ming 1962; Welwaart and Zwaveling 1980) and, particularly, the adenocarcinomas that can appear on areas of the esophagus affected by reflux and Barrett's ulcer (Hawe et al. 1973; Schafer 1971). Differentiation is very difficult in this region (Raphael et al. 1966)

Contributory Factors

Diverse factors have been evaluated of polyps (Morson et al. 1980; Schade 1977).

Gastroesophageal Reflux

The presence of gastric metaplasia, ulceration and pseudopolyps has been demonstrated to have a significance similar to that of atrophic gastritis and intestinal metaplasia in gastric cancer (Morson et al. 1980; Pinotti and Rilke 1977; Schafer 1971).

Chronic Peptic Ulcer. While exceptional, malignant transformation of chronic peptic ulcers has been demonstrated (Kyoichi et al. 1966; Murkami 1972; Tanai et al. 1981).

Polyps. The location for their possible contribution to the genesis of cancer of the cardia, resembling the situation with gastric cancer in the cardia is exceptional, making it difficult to affirm their role on the presentation of carcinoma (Sporn 1976).

Atrophic Gastritis. The frequent appearance of intestinal metaplasia in zones of gastritis and its existence on the tumoral margin, together with the demonstrated importance of atypical hyperplastic colonic metaplasia, have been shown to contribute to the histogenesis of gastric cancer (Cheli et al. 1973; Crespi et al. 1978), but the role of these factors in cancer of the cardia is debated.

Lymphatic Dissemination

Transmural dissemination throughout the submucosal space of the esophagus and stomach produces tumoral foci at a distance which are hard to differentiate from multicentric carcinomas (Morson 1961). In our experience (Moreno Gonzalez et al. 1986, 1987), the lymph nodes most commonly affected are the paracardiac, coronary and splenic hilar groups (Fig. 1). The lower mediastinal periesophageal group is involved in 25% and the subcardiac group in 8% of cases.

Surgical Treatment

The characteristics of lymph node invasion, transmural submucosal dissemination and long-distance lymphatic dissemination must be considered. Exeresis thus entails removal of 6–8 cm of normal gastric wall distal to the lower tumoral margin and 6–9 cm of esophagus, extended abdominally to the distal half of the pancreas, the spleen, the major and minor omenta, and the lymphadipose tissue surrounding the celiac trunk and the main hepatic artery in its trajectory over the upper edge of the residual pancreas (Payne and Bernatz 1976).

The remnants conserved are the gastric antrum, the antrocorporal dissection surface and the upper thoracic esophagus, sectioned at about the height of the tracheal carina. Both section surfaces can be used to reestablish intestinal transit, although there are several disadvantages: (a) the duodenum and pancreas must be mobilized – in order to move the residual stomach to the posterosuperior mediastinum. (b) pyloroplasty or extramucosal pyloromyotomy to be added in order to prevent postvagotomy pylorospasm. (c) left or right posterolateral thoracotomy must be performed for esophagogastric anastomosis. (d) an antireflux mechanism is needed to prevent passage of the duodenal contents into the upper thoracic esophagus. This procedure conserves lymph node groups affected by neoplastic involvement in 18%–40% of cases (Papachristou and Fortner 1980), and leaves an intrathoracic anastomosis that, in the event of a fistula forming would lead to serious complications with an important increase in mortality, neoplasms being more frequent on the esophageal or gastric remnants (Papachristou et al. 1979).

At present, the practice of total gastrectomy has gained support among those interested in making exeresis more radical and prolonging long-term survival. Digestive continuity is restored by a long Roux-en-Y loop or a segment of transverse descending colon in isoperistaltic position interposed between the proximal esophagus and duodenum. This procedure has the advantage of avoiding pyloroplasty and alkaline esophageal reflux while being more radical. However, it has the disadvantage that separate thoracotomy, or thoracophrenolaparotomy, and an intrathoracic anastomosis are needed, with the attendant risk of thoracic and mediastinal contamination, which are frequent during manual or instrumental anastomosis. On the other hand, it is not always easy to obtain a Roux-en-Y loop to move into the upper abdomen without tension or alteration of the arterial blood supply or venous drainage of the tracheal carina.

In 1978 we (Moreno González et al. 1981 b) began to treat cancer of the cardia by total gastrectomy extended to both omenta, distal hemipancreas and spleen, including the diaphragmatic edge of the esophageal hiatus, the periesophageal lymphadipose tissue and the entire thoracoabdominal esophagus (Moreno González 1988; Moreno González et al. 1981 b, 1986, 1987). The main advantages of this procedure are the following:

a) Use of two incisions, a median supraumbilical laparotomy and an oblique left lateral cervical incision, avoiding opening the chest wall
b) The fact that the patient can remain in the supine position throughout the intervention
c) Maximum radicality by prolongation of the exeresis cranially and caudally to its furthest limits
d) The ease and facility of esophageal anastomosis using the left lateral cervical approach
e) Avoidance of anastomosis in the middle third of the posterior mediastinum
f) The use of the terminal ileum and right colon, which have been demonstrated to provide the best assurance of nearly physiological deglutition (Moreno González 1988)
g) The fact that two surgical teams can work simultaneously, thus reducing operating time.

Total Extended Esophagogastrectomy Without Thoracotomy

Technique

The patient is placed on the operating table in supine position. The prepared surgical field extends to the anterior abdomen and left lateral surface of the neck. Through a medial supraumbilical laparotomy, the abdominal cavity is explored, with special inter-

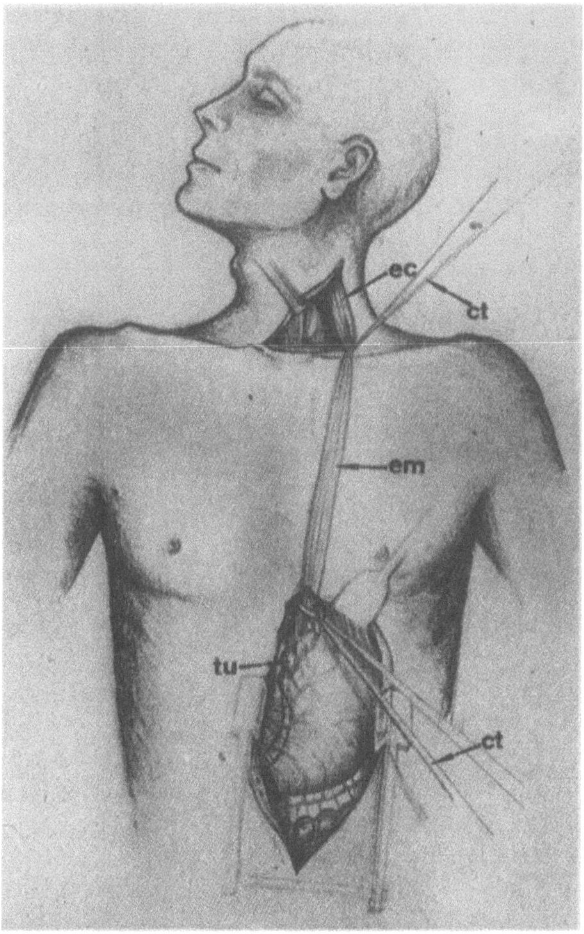

Fig. 1. Technique of esophagectomy without thoracotomy. Middle line laparotomy and cervical incision have been performed. *ec*, cervical esophagus; *ct*, ligature of esophagus; *em*, mediastinal segment of esophagus; *tu*, tumor of cardia; *ct*, ligature of abdominal segment of esophagus

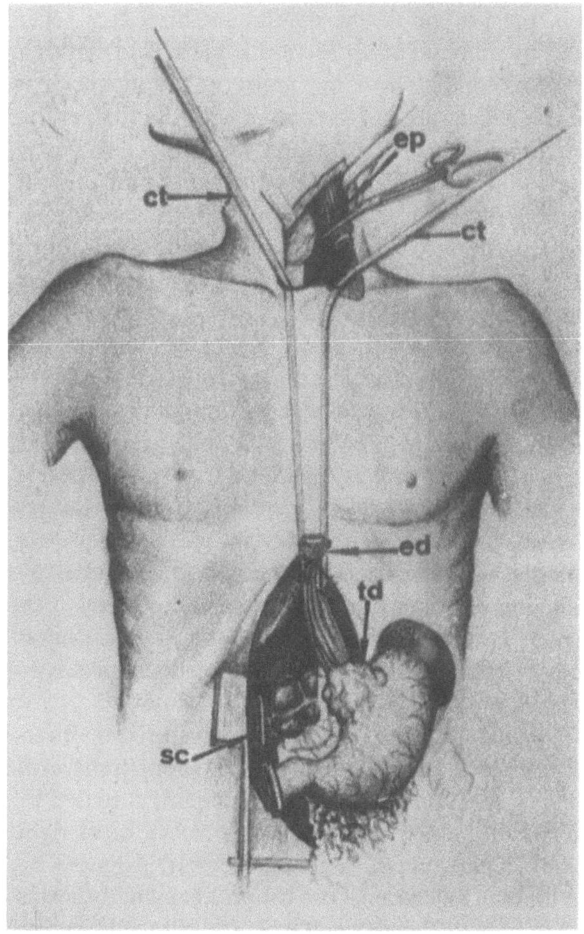

Fig. 2. After section of cervical esophagus and performing traction of it from the abdominal incision, the esophagus has been extracted. *ep*, upper remnant of cervical esophagus; *ct*, vascular tapes sutured to lower cervical esophagus *(ed)* introduced into posterior mediastinum by means of traction from tumor *(td)*; *sc*, transverse colon sectioned

est in excluding regional dissemination that might contraindicate radical exeresis.

The diaphragmatic surface is resected around the esophageal hiatus at a distance of 1–2 cm to include in the operative specimen the area of diaphragmatic contact with the tumoral surface, as neoplastic infiltration is frequently observed at this location.

This is followed by separation of the major omentum on the surface of the transverse colon, ligation and section of the right gastroepiploic artery and vein, section of the duodenum between portions I and II, and section of the pyloric artery at its origin from the hepatic artery and of the pyloric vein at its confluence with the portal vein. The stomach and portion I of the duodenum can then be moved cranially, exposing the pancreatic surface.

The common hepatic artery, its branches and the portal vein are dissected at the level of the hepatoduodenal ligament, and the lymphadipose tissue arround it is excised. The main hepatic artery is dissected at the suprapancreatic level, and the lymph nodes surrounding it are removed together with those around the celiac trunk. The splenic artery and left gastric artery are occluded between ligatures and sectioned at their celiac point of origin.

After sectioning the colosplenic and parietosplenic ligaments, the spleen and the distal half of the pancreas are freed from the retroperitoneal space. The splenic vein is occluded between ligatures and sectioned at the same level using the TA55 4.8-mm stapler.

When the operative specimen is freed in the abdomen, the portion of the diaphragmatic hiatus separated by diaphragmatic section is mobilized through this large orifice, avoiding injury to the mediastinal pleurae if they are not in contact with the tumor. The subcarinal thoracic esophagus is dissected under visual control and all periesophageal lymphadipose tissue is removed with the esophagus. Since esophageal dissection cannot be visually controlled above the carina, the upper thoracic segment is freed by blunt dissection (Fig. 1).

The cervical esophagus is dissected through an oblique incision. The inferior thyroid artery is sectioned and the periesophageal lymphadipose tissue and the transverse cervical lymph node group are excised. The esophagus is separated from the posterior wall of the trachea, taking care not to injure the recurrent nerve. Finally, the cervical esophagus is sectioned and the operative specimen is extracted by pulling the stomach through the laparotomy incision. Two vascular tapes affixed to the cervicothoracic esophagus are drawn into the mediastinal cavity by traction (Fig. 2).

Esophagoduodenal continuity is restored by interposition of a long segment of left colon (transverse colon, splenic flexure, descending colon) supplied by the cranial branch of the left colic artery, or of right colon (ileum, cecum, ascendant colon) irrigated by the middle colic artery. The cervical anastomosis was end-to-end to the left colon and end-to-side to the treminal ileum (Figs. 3, 4).

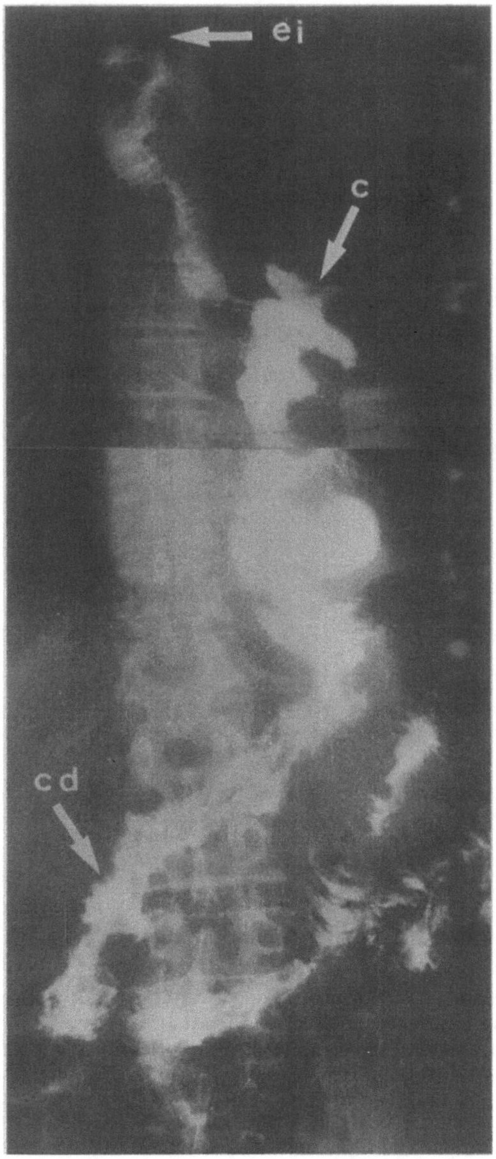

Fig. 3. Postoperative X-ray barium meal. Replacement by right colon (ileocecocoloplasty). *ei*, end-to-side esophagoileal anastomosis; *c*, cecum; *cd*, end-to-end coloduodenal anastomosis

Results

From November 1978 to June 1987, 59 patients underwent the procedure described above (Table 1). In six patients, splenopancreatectomy was not performed because of their precarious physical condition and advanced age. In the other 53 patients, the procedure included splenopancreatic exeresis, three times extended to include the left hepatic lobe. In one patient, exeresis was extended to a segment of the transverse colon due to tumoral infiltration.

The tumor was more than 4 cm in diameter in 48 patients (81.3%) (Table 2). Infiltration of the gastric serosa was observed in almost all the patients (94.9%) and affected more than 6 cm in 33%–38% of cases, similar to submucosal infiltration at a distance (27.1%). In three patients, lymphatic metastases were detected outside the lymphatic region included in the operative specimen. In four patients adjacent viscera were involved (Table 3).

Only one tumor displayed characteristics of lymphoma. Almost all were adenocarcinomas (Table 4),

Table 1. Surgical procedures

Procedure	No of patients
Total esophagogastrectomy	6
Total extended esophagogastrectomy	53
Splenectomy and distal pancreatectomy	49
Left liver resection (stages II and III)	3
Transverse colectomy	1
	59

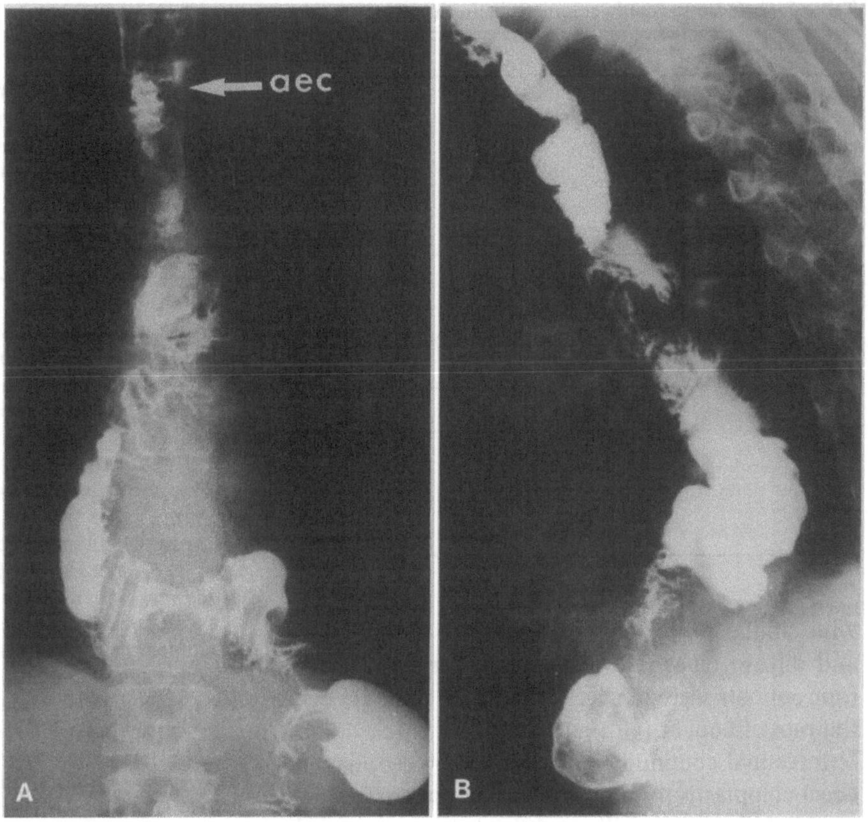

Fig. 4 A, B. Postoperative barium meal. Left isoperistaltic colon replacement after total extended esophago-gastrectomy. **A** Anteroposterior view. *aec*, end-to-end esophagocolonic anastomosis: peristaltic waves of colon can be shown. **B** Lateral view: colon has been placed through posterior mediastinum

Table 2. Tumor characteristics

Characteristics	*n*	%
Diameter > 4 cm	48	81.3
Serosa infiltration	58	98.3
Esophageal infiltration > 3 cm	56	94.9
> 6 cm	20	33.8
Submucosal infiltrations	16	27.1
Distant esophageal metastasis	3	5.0
Distant infiltration	4	6.7
Left lobe liver	3	
Transverse colon	1	

Table 3. Positive lymph nodes

Site	*n*	%
Paracardial	58	98.3
Left gastric artery	47	79.6
Right gastric artery	8	13.5
Gastroepiploic	15	25.4
Hilum of spleen	20	33.8
Right suprapancreatic	13	22.0
Left suprapancreatic	9	15.2
Celiac axis	23	38.9
Hepatoduodenal ligament	8	13.5

Table 4. Tumor type

Pathology	*n*	%
Adenocarcinoma, intestinal type	30	50.9
Adenocarcinoma, diffuse type	26	44.3
Undetermined	1	1.6
Adenoepithelial	1	1.6
Lymphoma	1	1.6

Table 5. Tumor stage

Stage	*n*	%
I	4	6.8
II	21	35.5
III	29	49.3
IV	5	8.4

Table 6. Right colon substitution: complications

Complication	*n*	%
Mortality (hospital)	1/38	2.6
Esophageal leakage	1/38	2.6
Coloduodenal leakage	–	–
Ileotransverse leakage	–	–
Subphrenic abscess	1/38	2.6

Table 7. Left isoperistaltic colonic substitution: complications

Complication	*n*	%
Mortality (hospital)	3/21	14.2
Esophagocolic leakage	2/21	19.5
Coloduodenal leakage	–	–
Colocolic leakage	1/21	4.7
Subphrenic abscess	1/21	4.7
Pericarditis	1/21	4.7

Table 8. Six-year survival after surgery related to stage of disease

Stage	Survivors	%
I	4/5	80
II	7/11	63.6
III	3/15	29
IV	0/5	0

with similar proportions of intestinal (Lauren 1965) and diffuse types (Nevalainen and Jarvi 1977). Only four patients were in stage I (Table 5), stage III being the most frequent (49.3%).

Intestinal continuity was restored by esophagoileocecocoloplasty (right colon) in 38 patients and by isoperistaltic interposition of the transverse and descending colon (left colon) in 21 patients (Tables 6, 7).

The mortality was significantly higher in the patients in whom the left colon was used. These patients had a higher frequency of anastomosis fistulas, but the inmediate cause of death was unrelated to these complications: one patient died of acute respiratory failure and the other probably as the result of an acute vascular accident (Table 8). However, the duration of hospitalization, parenteral nutrition, antibiotic therapy etc. increased significantly.

We found that survival improved with these operations: 80% of the patients corresponding to stage I and 63% of those in stage II survived more than 6 years. It is note-worthy that with other operations, no stage III patient survived 4 years, whereas with extended esophagogastrectomy, three of 15 stage III patients (20%) surpassed 6 years. As could be expected, none of the stage IV patients survived more than five years after surgery.

In spite of these figures, survival findings were not statistically significant in all groups. Time is needed for more objective evaluation. In any case, these findings and the fact that we have had no deaths in the 3 months immediately following operation in the last 32 patients suggest that this operation should continue to be performed.

References

Appelquist P (1972) Carcinoma of the esophagus and gastric cardia. Acta Chir Scand [Suppl] 430: 1–92

Cheli R, Santi L, Ciancamerla G, et al. (1973) A clinical and statistical blow-up study of atrophic gastritis. Am J Dig Dis 18: 1061–1066

Crespi M, Casale V, Garssi A, Maggio C (1978) Results and prospective of a mass screening for gastric cancer and precancerous conditions of the stomach. Act Edos 8: 73–85

Dodge OG (1961) Tehs. Surgical pathology of gastroesophageal carcinoma. Br J Surg 49: 121–125

Ellis FH JR (1976) Carcinoma of the lower thoracic esophagus and esophagogastric junction. In: Gibbon's surgery of the chest. Saunders, Philadelphia, pp 709–714

Hanklins JR, Cole FN, Attar S, Frost JL, McLaughilin JS (1974) Adenocarcinoma involving the esophagus. J Thorac Cardiovasc Surg 68: 148–152

Hawe A, Payne WS, Weiland LH, et al. (1973) Adenocarcinoma in the columnar epithelial lined lower (Barrett) oesophagus. Thorax 28: 511–514

Humphrey ED, Kerstens TE (1976) Adenocarcinoma of the gastroesophageal junction. In: Varco RL, Delancy JP (eds) Controversy in surgery. Saunders, Philadelphia, pp 603–608

Kata Y, Sugano H, Wada J, et al. (1978) Histogenesis of cardiac carcinoma (adenocarcinoma) in comparison with that of antral carcinoma. Stomach Intestine 13: 1509–1515

Kobayashi S, Prolla JC, Winans CS, et al. (1970) Improved endoscopic diagnosis of gastroesophageal malignancy, combined use of direct vision brushing cytology and biopsy. JAMA 212: 2086–2089

Kraus B, Cain H (1979) Is there a carcinoma in situ of gastric mucosa? Pathol Res Pract 164: 342–355

Kyoichi N, Haruao S, Kunio T, Ariya F (1966) Histopathological study on early carcinoma of the stomach. Criteria for diagnosis of atypical epithelium. Gan 57: 613–620

Lauren P (1965) The two histological main types of gastric carcinoma diffuse and so-called intestinal type carcinoma. Acta Pathol Microbiol Scand 64: 31–49

Li L, Pna GL, Shen Q (1982) A pathologic study of early carcinoma of gastric cardia. Chin J Oncol 4: 93–97

McPeak E, Warren S (1948) Histological features of carcinoma of cardioesophageal junction and cardia. Am J Pathol 24: 971–991

Moreno González E (1988) Indication, technique and results of transhiatal esophagectomy without thoracotomy. In: Japanese esophageal week. Excerpta Medica, Amsterdam (in press)

Moreno González E, Garcia Garcia JI, Rico Selas P, Moreno Azcoita M, Landa Garcia JI, Seoane González J (1981a) Extended esophagogastrectomy as surgical treatment for carcinoma of the cardia. Jpn J Surg 11(5): 311–316

Moreno González E, Hidalgo Pascual H, Moreno Azcoita M, Garcia Garcia I, Garcia Blanch G, Rico Selas P, Jelavic D, et al. (1981b) Indicaciones técnica y resultados de la esofaguectomía transhiatal digital sin toracotomía. Rev Esp Enferm Apar Dig 60 (6): 533–588

Moreno González E, Gomez Gutierrez M, Calleja Kemin J, Garcia Alvarez A, Jover Navalón JM, Gándara Adan N, Arias Dias J (1986) Tratamiento quirurgico del cancer de cardias. Jarpyo, Madrid, pp 1–56

Moreno González E, Gomez Gutierrez M, Calleja Kempín J, Landa Garcia I, Arias Diaz J (1987) Extended total esophagogastrectomy as surgical treatment of cancer of the cardia.

In: Siewert JR, Hölscher AH (eds) Diseases of the Esophagus. Springer, Berlin Heidelberg New York, pp 585–594
Morson BC (1961) The spread of carcinoma of the oesophagus. In: Tanner NC, Smiters DV (eds) Tumors of the esophagus. Livingstone, Edinbourgh, pp 136–146
Morson BC, Sobin LH, Grundmann E, et al. (1980) Precancerous conditions and epithelial dysplasia in the stomach. J Clin Pathol 33: 711–721
Murkami TA (1972) Pathomorphological diagnosis, definition and gross classification of early gastric cancer. Gan 11: 54
Nevalainen TJ, Jarvi OH (1977) Ultrastructure of intestinal and diffuse type gastric carcinoma. J Pathol 122: 129–136
Papachristou DN, Fortner JG (1980) Adenocarcinoma of the gastric cardia. Ann Surg 192: 5864–5871
Papachristou DN, Karas M, Fortner JG (1979) Anastomotic recurrence in the esophagus complicates gastrectomy for adenocarcinoma of the stomach. Br J Surg 66: 609–612
Payne WS, Bernatz PE (1976) One stage resection and reconstruction for carcinoma of the esophagogastric junction. In: Varco RL, Delaney IP (eds) Controversy in surgery. Saunders, Philadelphia, pp 579–602
Pinotti HW, Rilke F (1977) Atypical epithelium of the protuberant lesions in the stomach. Acta Cytol (Baltimore) 21: 1–2
Raphael HA, Rllid GH Jr, Dockerty MB (1966) Primary adenocarcinoma of the esophagus. 18 year review and review of literature. Ann Surg 164: 785–796
Schade ROK (1977) The pathology of precancerosis of the gastric mucosa. In: figus AI, Simon L (eds) Gastric precancerosis. Akademiai Kiado, Budapest, p 24
Schafer RB (1971) Adenocarcinoma in Barrett's columnar-lined esophagus. Arch Surg 103: 411–414
Sporn MB (1976) Approaches of prevention of epithelial cancer during the preneoplastic period. Cancer Res 36: 2699–2702
Talerman A, Woo-Ming MO (1962) The origin of squamous cell carcinoma of the gastric cardia. Cancer 22: 1226–1232
Tanai J, Toshimoto Y, Takagi H, et al. (1981) A statistical analysis of detecting risk factors for stomach cancer patients. In: Lindberg DA, Kalhara S (eds) Medifo 80. Elsevier North-Holland, Amsterdam, pp 974–978
Welwaart K, Zwaveling A (1980) Carcinoma of the esophagus and gastric cardia. Clin Oncol 6: 203–212

Cancer of the Stomach

F. Mazzeo, N. Mozzillo, and P. Forestieri

Definitions

Polyps are the most frequent benign tumours, being found in 3% of symptomatic patients subjected to upper gastrointestinal endoscopy. Hyperplastic polyps are the most common form (85%). Adenomatous polyps account for less than 5% and mesenchymal ones constitute 10% of the total. Multiple or diffuse polyps are unusual.

Among malignant tumours, adenocarcinoma is by far the most common (93%–97%) and will be the specific subject of this chapter. Lymphomatous, mainly non-Hodgkin's, tumours constitute 2.5%–6.5%, either as isolated (primary) disease or as

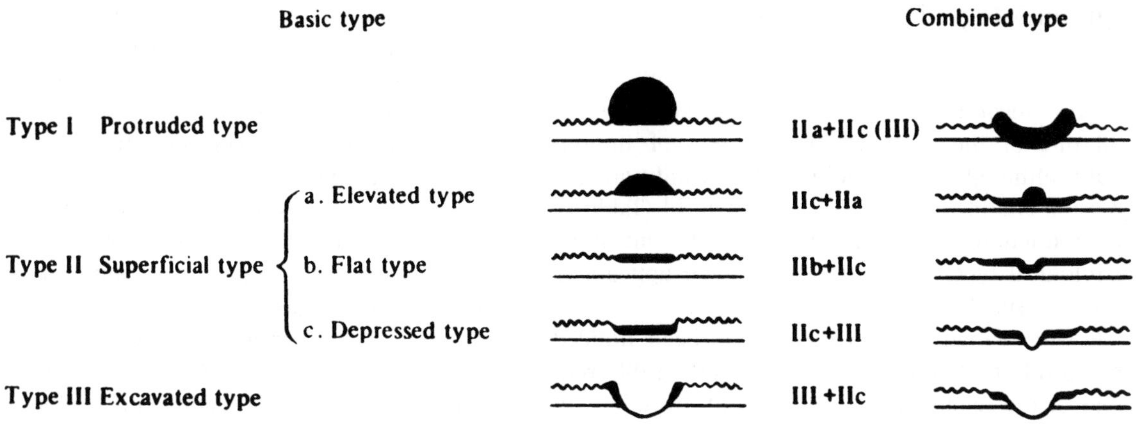

Fig. 1. Early gastric cancer: basic and combined types (Sakita and Oguro 1974). In an analysis of 17212 lesions (Fukutomi and Sakita 1984), the EGC depressed group (II c and III) accounted for 73.9%, the elevated group (I and II a) for 15.8%, the intermediate group (II a + II c) for 7.5% and the flat type (II b) for 1.0%

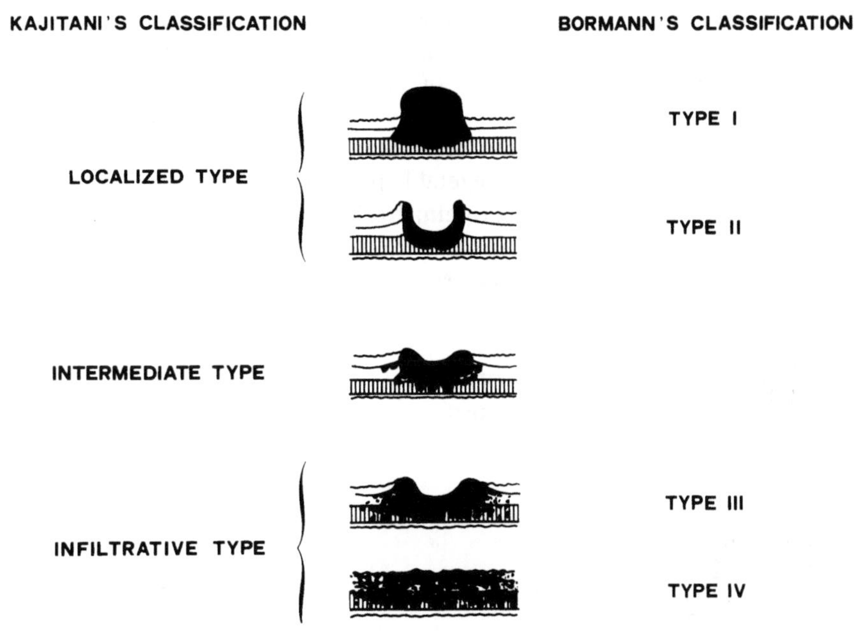

Fig. 2. Classification of advanced gastric cancer based on gross findings, according to Kajitani (1950) and Bormann (1926)

an expression of generalized involvement. Mesenchymal tumours, mainly leiomyosarcomas, account for 1%–2.5% of total gastric malignancies.

The term "early gastric cancer" (EGC) is used to describe an adenocarcinoma limited to mucosa or submucosa independent of size and lymph node invasion. Macroscopically, EGC can be divided into three main types – type I, protruded; type II, superficial (II a, elevated; II b, flat; II c, depressed); type III, excavated – with several combinations (Fig. 1).

"Advanced gastric cancer" (AGC) denotes a tumour infiltrating gastric wall beyond the submucosa. Five types were described by Bormann (1926): I, polypoid or fungating; II, ulcerating; III, ulcerating and infiltrating; IV, diffusely infiltrating; V, unclassifiable.

A simpler descriptive classification is generally adopted in the USA. Most lesions are described as ulcerative, approximately 10% can be classified as polypoid, and another 10% as scirrhous. In the USA, as in Europe, the superficial type (EGC) is uncommon.

After fixation, specimens may be classified into four types (Kajitani 1950): superficial (EGC), localized (Bormann's types I and II), infiltrative (Bormann's types III and IV) and intermediate (Fig. 2).

"Linitis plastica" denotes extensive neoplastic involvement of stomach with infiltration of the walls.

Epidemiology: Risk Factors

Gastric cancer is, considering the two sexes together, still one of the most common causes of tumour death, although its morbidity and mortality are decreasing sharply almost all over the world (Table 1). This reduction is especially evident for the intestinal histological type, while the diffuse type appears to be rather steady.

A wide variation in incidence has been noticed among different countries and even among different areas of the same country. The present attitude is to consider exogenous factors (dietary, environmental, economic, occupational) as leading causes of cancer of the stomach. A preeminent causative role is attributed to dietary habits. Countries where the incidence is high, generally vary quite widely in diet, so that it is very difficult to find a single guilty foodstuff. Notwithstanding, we can list some items associated with an increased incidence of gastric cancer:

High intake: salt; salted, pickled or smoked foods; complex carbohydrates; nitrates; vegetable proteins

Low intake: animal fat and protein; fresh green leafy vegetables; fresh citrus and other fruits; milk; vitamins A, E, C and other antioxidants

Interestingly, in a lot of countries gastric cancer mortality and stroke mortality are correlated (Fig. 3). Salt consumption has been identified as a common factor: where a programme of salt restriction was instituted, parallel reduction of mortality was observed. Salt seems not to be a carcinogen itself, but, because of its osmotic power, it causes mucosal lesions and slows gastric emptying, facilitating and prolonging contact with carcinogens.

A high salt intake, malnutrition or incorrect nutrition can cause atrophic lesions and achlorydria that may, according to Correa et al. (1975), be the first step in a sequence of events (atrophic gastritis, gastric atrophy, intestinal metaplasia, dysplasia) leading to cancer. These lesions may also be iatrogenic [gastric secretory inhibitors(?), gastric surgery] or genetic in origin. The occurrence of cancer, particularly of the diffuse type, in twins strongly suggests the existence of a genetic factor. However, this is difficult to evaluate, since members of the same family tend to be exposed to the same environmental factors. In any case, a genetic susceptibility to external and particularly to dietary factors may be supposed.

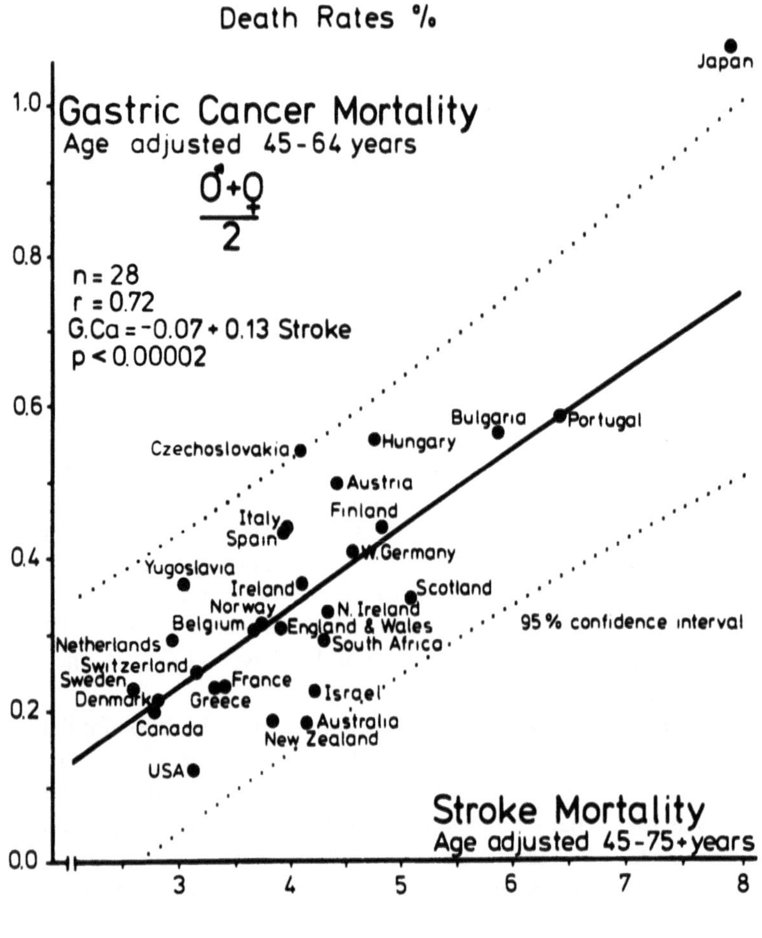

Fig. 3. Geographical relationship between stroke and gastric cancer mortalities, 1965–1970 (average of both sexes) (Joossens and Geboers 1983)

Histopathology

Early Gastric Cancer

According to Fukutomi and Sakita (1984), there are very neat correlations among macroscopic type, size and differentiation (Table 2). Age and histology are also related: differentiated adenocarcinomas are more frequent among the aged, while undifferentiated ones are more often observed among the young.

With regard to depth of invasion, slight invasion is predominant in types II b [mucosa (m) 87.3%] and II a (m 68.1%), while deep invasion is conspicuous in combined II a + II c [submucosa (sm) 69.2%], so that lymph node metastases are more common in II a + II c (18.4%) and less frequent in II b (7.0%) and II a (8.7%). On the whole, lymph node metastases occur in about 4% of cases of intramucosal invasion and about 20% of cases of submucosal invasion. For this purpose it is useful to divide submucosal EGC into two subtypes, sm I and sm II (Yamada et al. 1980). In the latter, submucosal invasion is massive and very deep so that it is not possible to exclude absolutely the invasion of muscularis propria. As a matter of fact, these tumours can be considered invasive in their initial stages as far as lymph node metastases and long-term survival are concerned.

On average, about 8%–12% of cancers of the stomach are multiple. Most multiple cancers are type II b, with type II a the next most frequent.

Table 3 shows the relationship between histological type, cancerous invasion and lymph node metastases.

In terms of growth patterns reflecting the biological behaviour (invasiveness, tendency towards metastases and prognosis), EGC can be classified into

Table 1. Significant (at least $P < 0.05$) changes in gastric cancer mortality over two 10-year periods (%)

Country	1955–1965	1968–1975/1979
Iceland	−133	n.s.
Finland	− 57	−54
Switzerland	− 52	−45
Australia	− 49	−33
Denmark	− 47	−29
Sweden	− 45	−26
Norway	− 44	−44
USA	− 44	−30
Canada	− 43	−39
Northern Ireland	− 36	n.s.
Netherlands	− 35	−34
Scotland	− 31	−22
France	− 30	−30
West Germany	− 27	−34
Belgium	− 25	−46
Hungary	− 24	−23
England and Wales	− 22	−32
Austria	− 21	−38
Czechoslovakia	− 20	−32
Italy	− 16	−30
Japan	− 12	−38
Ireland	n.s.	−35
New Zealand	n.s.	−32
Spain	n.s.	−29
Greece	n.s.	−16
Poland	n.s.	−31
Portugal	+ 10	−17

Modified from Joossens and Geboers (1983)

Table 2. EGC: macroscopic and histologic correlations

Lesions	*n*	Differentiated (%)	Undifferentiated (%)
Elevated (I, II a)	2 795	91.9	8.1
Intermediate (II a + II c)	1 253	80.0	20.0
Flat (II b)	312	74.1	25.9
Depressed (II c, III)	12 304	54.5	45.5
≤0.5 cm	474	80.4	19.6
0.6–1.0	1 369	75.5	24.5
1.1–2.0	4 056	67.7	32.3
2.1–4.0	6 414	63.5	36.5
>4.1	4 192	51.7	48.3

Modified from Fukutomi and Sakita (1984)

Table 3. EGC: histology, invasion and lymph node metastases

Histology	Invasion		Lymph node metastases	
	Mucosa	Submucosa	+	−
Papillary	688 (48.6%)	729 (51.4%)	177 (14.1%)	1082 (85.9%)
Tubular	4932 (53.1%)	4353 (46.9%)	864 (10.4%)	7433 (89.6%)
Poorly differentiated	1168 (42.1%)	1607 (57.9%)	386 (14.8%)	2214 (85.2%)
Signet-ring cell	1738 (59.5%)	1181 (40.5%)	272 (10.0%)	2440 (90.0%)
Others	238 (43.0%)	316 (57.0%)	57 (11.1%)	458 (88.9%)

Modified from Fukutomi and Sakita (1984)

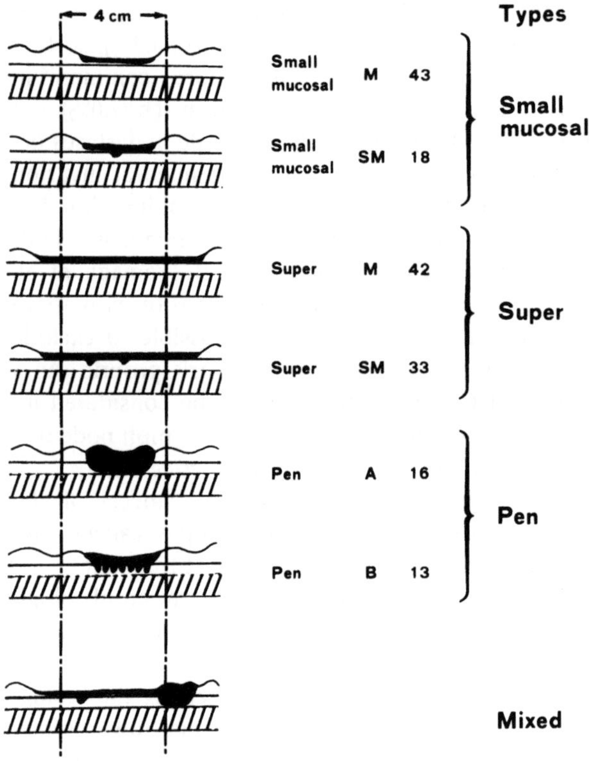

Fig. 4. Growth patterns of early gastric cancer and numbers of cases (Kodama et al. 1983)

the "small mucosal" type, the superficially spreading "super" type and the penetrating growth "pen" type, further subdivided into pen A, growing expansively, and pen B, deepening infiltratively (Fig. 4). The small mucosal, super and pen B types (especially depressed lesions), are characterized by a low incidence of vessel invasion and lymph node metastases and by a good prognosis after surgery (about 90% 10-year survival). In contrast, the pen A type (especially elevated lesions) is characterized by a relatively high incidence of vessel invasion and lymph node metastases and by a poor prognosis after surgery (64.8% 5-year survival) due to early recurrence in the form of liver involvement (Kodama et al. 1983).

Histological Classifications of Gastric Cancer

In the classification proposed by the WHO (Oota 1977) adenocarcinomas are divided into papillary, tubular, mucinous and signet-ring cell types, and graded as well, moderately or poorly differentiated. Undifferentiated and unclassified carcinomas are two separate groups.

The Japanese Research Society committee on histological classification of gastric cancer (1981 b) has proposed a similar classification, dividing gastric cancer into the specific and the common types. While the specific types are adenosquamous, squamous cell, carcinoid tumour, undifferentiated carcinoma and miscellaneous, the common types may be papillary, tubular (well or moderately differentiated), poorly differentiated, mucinous and signet-ring cell. As far as the amount of interstitial tissue is concerned, the following terms are used: medullary if it is scanty, scirrhous if it is abundant, and intermediate.

Laurén's classification (1965) has also been widely used for epidemiological purposes. The intestinal type (more frequent and mostly polypoid or fungating) looks like intestinal mucosa from a histological point of view and is associated with intestinal metaplasia (Fig. 5). Diffuse carcinoma (mostly infiltrating) is characterized by wider spreading in the mucosa and it often infiltrates the gastric wall extensively (Fig. 6). The intestinal type, predominant among populations at high risk for gastric cancer ("epidemic" type), is more frequent in men (2:1) and in older patients, has a better prognosis and is preceded by a prolonged precancerous process. The diffuse type, similar in frequency in most populations ("endemic" type), is more common in women and in younger patients, has a poorer prognosis and is not preceded by known precancerous changes.

The classification proposed by Ming (1977) is similar to that of Laurén in practice, but has the advantage that it can be applied also to those cases which remain unclassified by Laurén's system. This classification divides tumours into an expanding type (more frequent and mostly fungating) and an infiltrative type (mostly diffuse). Histogenesis, clinical and epidemiological correlations of the expanding and infiltrative types are similar to those of the intestinal and diffuse types in Laurén's classification.

Finally, in the classification of Mulligan and Rember (1954), gastric carcinomas are divided into three groups: mucous cell carcinoma, pylorocardial gland cell carcinoma and intestinal carcinoma. In some cases it is not possible to classify the tumour. This classification is interesting from a histogenetic point of view, but has not been widely used in practice.

Staging and Prognosis

The new TNM classification of gastric cancer (proposed at the Joint Meeting of the UICC, the AJC and the JJC in 1984 and approved by the UICC and the AJC in 1985 and by the JJC in 1986) was published

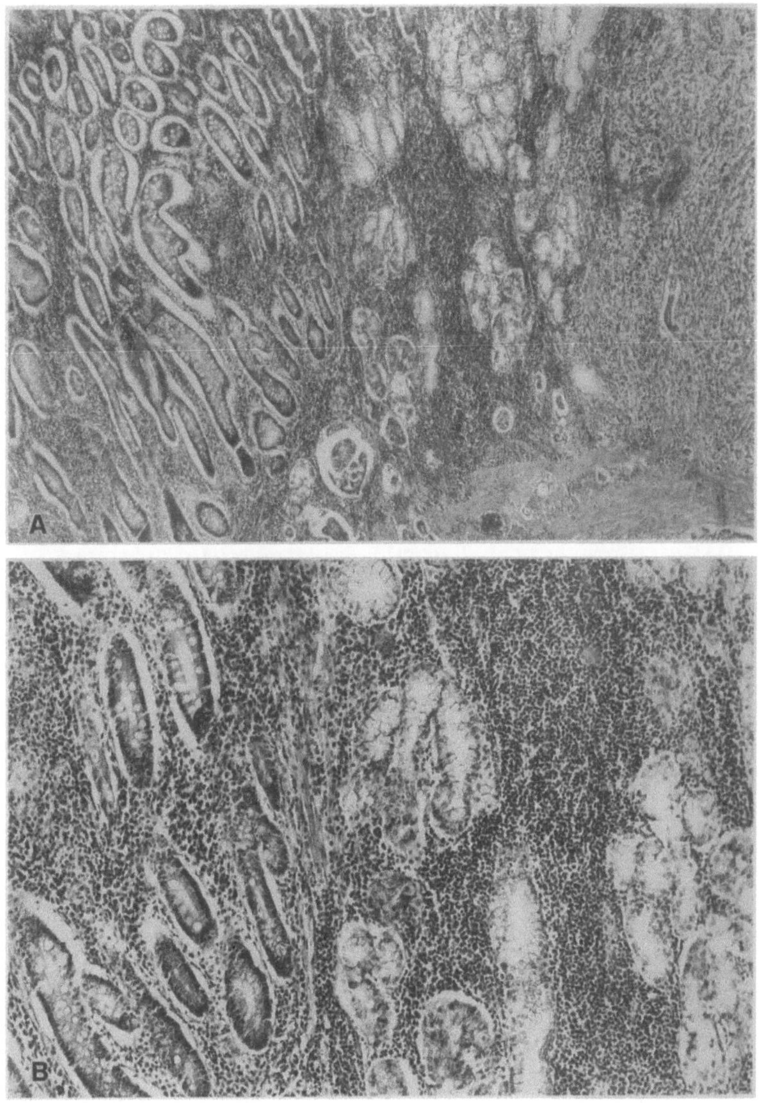

Fig. 5 A, B. Intestinal type adenocarcinoma. **A** *Right*, the neoplasia, partly differentiated in glandular structures; *left*, the gastric glands show complete intestinal metaplasia. HE, × 150. **B** Both in the lamina propria of metaplastic mucosa and in the interstitium of neoplasia we can see dense inflammatory infiltrate. HE, x 250. (Courtesy of Prof. G. Pettinato, Associate of Pathology, II Medical School, University of Naples)

in 1987 in the 4th edition of the TNM manual (Hermanek and Sobin 1987). The important improvements are as follows: (1) "Size of tumour" has been removed from the T category, first because it has no significant role in prognosis (K. Maruyama 1986, 1987) and secondly because, thanks to the new and more sophisticated diagnostic methods (X-ray: double-contrast method, CT, etc.; endoscopy and endoscopic biopsy; ultrasound: surface and endoscopic) the criterion of superficial extension may be substituted by the criterion of infiltration, so that clinical and pathological TNM almost completely coincide. (2) T and N are now given equal weight in the staging, because depth of invasion and lymph node metastasis have almost the same significance for prognosis (K. Maruyama 1986, 1987). (3) The category of N 3 has been completely abolished, as on the basis of several observations [2% and 3.8% 5-year survival rates in the experience of Miwa (1984) and Maruyama (1987) respectively] it is considered to represent distant metastasis. (4) As for all the organs of digestive tract, the old category G 3 (low degree of differentiation or undifferentiated) splits into G 3 (poorly differentiated) and G 4 (undifferentiated) (Table 4).

On the whole, the prognosis of gastric cancer depends on various factors:

- Distant metastases (including peritoneal dissemination and distant lymph node metastases) constitute the most important and definite variable in univariate analysis (5-year survival rate of 62.7% in M 0 and 2.9% in M 1, K. Maruyama 1986).
- Depth of invasion and/or invasion of contiguous structures. In the multivariate analysis (nine vari-

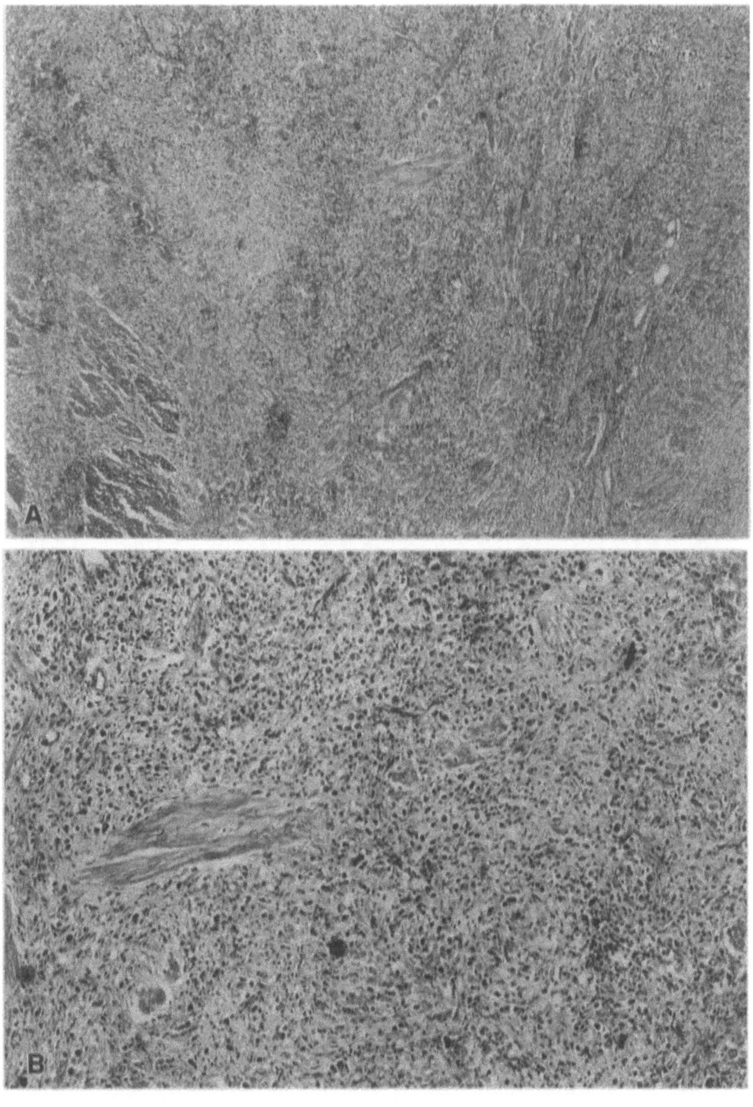

Fig. 6 A, B. Undifferentiated diffuse adenocarcinoma. **A** The neoplasia is formed by a sheet of non-cohesive pleomorphic cells infiltrating the whole thickness of the wall. Absence of glandular differentiation. HE, × 150. **B** Neoplastic cells show marked polymorphism and nuclear hyperchromasia. Parts of muscular layer can be seen HE, × 250. (Courtesy of Prof. G. Pettinato, Associate of Pathology, II Medical School, University of Naples)

ables) published by Cunningham et al. (1987), the best predictor of survival after curative resection was the presence or absence of serosal involvement ($P = 0.0004$). In the multivariate analysis (25 variables) published by K. Maruyama (1986, 1987) the most important prognostic factor (ratio of risk 4.69) was the depth of invasion: 5-year survival rate in m 94.2%, in sm 85%, in the proper muscular layer (pm) 80.9%, in invasion of subserosa (ss) 59.3%, in slight invasion of serosa (s 1) 44.4%, in severe invasion of serosa (s 2) 27.4% and in invasion of neighbouring organs (s 3) 10.2%.

- Involvement of locoregional lymph nodes. This represents the second best prognostic factor in Maruyama's multivariate analysis (ratio of risk 4.04): 5-year survival rate in N 0 81.5%, in N 1 49,7%, in N 2 24.2%, in N 3 5.9%, in N 4 1.9%.
- Number of lymph node metastases. As reported by Kim and Jung (1987), patients who had three or less positive lymph nodes had a better prognosis (5-year survival rate 44.9%) than those who had more than four positive lymph nodes (5-year survival rate 24.1%).
- Macroscopic characteristics. The rate of lymph node metastases increases and the 5-year survival rate decreases from Bormann's type I to type IV: 48.7%, 42.4%, 37.4%, 9,3% (K. Maruyama 1987). In Maruyama's multivariate analysis the type of cancer was the third most important prognostic factor (ratio of ris 1.76).
- Location of tumour. This represents the fourth most important factor in Maruyama's multivariate analysis (ratio of risk 1.50). Five-year survival rates: upper third 33.5%, middle third 59.8%, lower third 55.4%.

Table 4. New clinical TNM[a] categories, staging, and 5-year survival rates[b]

T – Primary tumour

TX	Primary tumour cannot be assessed
TO	No evidence of primary tumour
Tis	Carcinoma in situ: intraepithelial tumour without invasion of the lamina propria
T1	Tumour invades lamina propria or submucosa (98%, $n=2961$)
T2	Tumour invades muscularis propria or subserosa[1] (70%, $n=2481$)
T3	Tumour penetrates the serosa (visceral peritoneum) without invasion of adjacent structures[2, 3] (34%, $n=4943$)
T4	Tumour invades adjacent structures[2, 3] (16%, $n=1160$)

Notes:

[1] A tumour may penetrate muscularis propria with extension into the gastrocolic or gastrohepatic ligaments or the greater or lesser omentum without perforation of the visceral peritoneum covering these structures. In this case, the tumour is classified T2. If there is perforation of the visceral peritoneum covering the gastric ligaments or omenta, the tumour is classified T3.

[2] The adjacent structures of the stomach are the spleen, transverse colon, liver, diaphragm, pancreas, abdominal wall, adrenal gland, kidney, small intestine and retroperitoneum.

[3] Intramural extension to the duodenum or oesophagus is classified by the depth of greatest invasion in any of these sites including stomach.

N – Regional lymph nodes

NX	Regional lymph nodes cannot be assessed
NO	No regional lymph node metastasis (87%, $n=4817$)
N1	Metastasis in perigastric lymph node(s) within 3 cm of the edge of the primary tumour (45%, $n=3010$)
N2	Metastasis in perigastric lymph node(s) more than 3 cm from the edge of the primary tumour or in lymph nodes along the left gastric, common hepatic, splenic or coeliac arteries (24%, $n=2847$)

Note: involvement of other intra-abdominal lymph nodes is regarded as distant metastasis (2%, $n=151$)

M – Distant Metastasis

MX	Presence of distant metastasis cannot be assessed
MO	No distant metastasis (63%, $n=10131$)
M1	Distant metastasis (6%, $n=4314$)

Stage 0	Tis	N0	M0
Stage IA	T1	N0	M0 (99%, $n=2392$)
Stage IB	T1	N1	M0 (90%, $n=225$)
	T2	N0	M0 (88%, $n=1027$)
Stage II	T1	N2	M0 (79%, $n=68$)
	T2	N1	M0 (71%, $n=635$)
	T3	N0	M0 (69%, $n=870$)
Stage IIIA	T2	N2	M0 (52%, $n=404$)
	T3	N1	M0 (46%, $n=1143$)
	T4	N0	M0 (52%, $n=89$)
Stage IIIB	T3	N2	M0 (23%, $n=1290$)
	T4	N1	M0 (26%, $n=172$)
Stage IV	T4	N2	M0 (16%, $n=247$)
	Any T	Any N	M1 (10%, $n=2247$)

From Hermanek and Sobin (1987).

[a] The pT, pN and pM categories correspond to the T, N and M categories.

[b] The 5-year survival rates were calculated using the data of 11 845 resected cases collected by the Japan Research Society for Gastric Cancer.

- Grade of differentiation. This represents the fifth most important prognostic factor in Maruyama's multivariate analysis (ratio of risk 1.16), with 74.6% 5-year survival rate in well-differentiated, 61.2% in moderately differentiated, 46.9% in poorly differentiated and in signet-ring cell and 39.9% in mucinous carcinomas.
- Histological type. As reported by Hermanek (1987), while the prognosis for EGC is the same for both intestinal and diffuse types, that for AGC is decisively affected by histological type, with the following 5-year survival rates: pT2 64% and 45%, pT3–4 42% and 17%, pN+ 40% and 18% in intestinal and diffuse types respectively.
- Size of tumour. Since this is correlated with depth of invasion and lymph node metastases, it has no prognostic value in multivariate analysis when adjusted for other variables (K. Maruyama 1986).
- Host defence. Patients with evidence of host response (lymphoid infiltration of the primary tumour, sinus histocytosis and follicular hyperplasia in lymph nodes draining gastric tumours) have better survival (Giles 1986).
- Age and sex. As multivariate evaluation shows worse 5-year survival in male and younger patients (Bozzetti et al. 1986).

In the multivariate analysis of K. Maruyama (1986, 1987), the factors related to treatment (type of resection, surgical margin, combined resection, lymph node dissection, adjuvant chemotherapy, adjuvant immunotherapy, date of operation and surgeon) did not play a major role in the prognosis of gastric cancer.

Finally, all above-mentioned and previous reports indicate that the prognosis of gastric cancer patients depends mainly on three variables: depth of invasion, lymph node metastases and distant metastases.

Tumoral infiltration of the wall and/or contiguous structures and involvement of lymph nodes are closely interconnected: with the increase of depth of invasion there is a proportional increase not only of

Table 5. Correlation among depth of invasion of gastric wall, lymphnode metastases and long-term survival

Depth of invasion	Lymphnode metastases (%)				
	N0	N1	N2	N3	N4
Mucosa	92	6	0	2	0
Submucosa	84	10	3	2	0
Muscularis	53	20	18	9	0
Serosa	31	22	37	8	1
Adjacent structures	13	21	49	15	3
5-year survival rate (%)	81	60	31	21	0

Modified from Kodama (1981).

lymph node metastases, but also of positivity at a distance (N 2, N 3 and N 4) (Table 5).

Cytological and structural characteristics may also influence biological behaviour [presence of pepsinogen II-immunoreactive cells; mucinous character (Fiocca et al. 1988); production of epidermal growth factor (Tahara et al. 1986); higher levels of collagenases and a greater number of free laminin specific receptors, as reported in a cooperative study by Bucci et al. (1987)].

Natural History

While for the diffuse type of gastric cancer no precursor lesions have been identified, the intestinal type is preceded or at least accompanied, by atrophic, metaplastic and dysplastic changes.

Generally, a precancerous condition is a clinical situation in which there is a higher risk for the development of cancer. In the stomach such conditions may be: pernicious anemia (risk 4–6 times greater than that of the general population); polyps (rarely precursors of cancer but possibly sentinel markers, if hyperplastic), especially adenomatous polyps [relative risk variously reported; possible coexistence of gastric cancer; malignant changes through progressive stages (Kamiya et al. 1982)]; peptic ulcer (the sequence ulcer→cancer is very rare, probably accounting for no more than 1% of gastric carcinomas; there is a possibility of about 2% of misinterpreting benign ulcer and ulcerated cancer); Ménétrier's disease (degree of risk variously reported); stomach operations (some considerations suggest that the operation itself is not the only factor involved, and probably not even the decisive factor, but merely a co-factor) (Fig. 7).

Only histological examination is able to recognize the precancerous lesions: chronic atrophic gastritis (CAG), intestinal metaplasia (IM) and dysplasia (mild, moderate and severe).

Follow-up after CAG has shown an 8%–13% incidence of gastric cancer after 10–20 years, with a risk about 10 times greater than in a comparable healthy population. The risk is higher when the atrophy is more severe (above all in the antrum), in male subjects and in the aged (Sipponen et al. 1985) (Fig. 8).

The most important form of IM may be the incomplete colonic type II B (Jass 1980; Segura and Montero 1983). The presence of sulfomucins, however, might only indicate a more advanced stage of IM and thus might not be useful as a selective marker of a greater and more concrete risk. In the end, only an indefinable proportion of gastric carcinomas originate from areas of IM.

Dysplasia has a very low incidence (Nagayo 1983; Zampi et al. 1988) (Table 6) in endoscopic biopsies and surgical specimens. Hattori (1986), investigating the histogenesis of gastric adenocarcinomas, showed that IM, dysplasia and adenocarcinoma arise at the same time. This implies, according to him, that none of them has a precursor. On the basis of the above-mentioned observations (low incidence; association with gastric cancer in progress; tendency towards stability or regression, if isolated; slow and moderate neoplastic evolution) gastric dysplasia looks more like a paracancerous than a precancerous lesion.

Finally, Nagayo (1983) proposes that the sequences dysplasia →cancer and adenoma →cancer may be valid and operating only in some cases; frequently, cancer starts directly on gastric atrophic mucosa, the sequence being atrophy →cancer.

Probably, especially for the intestinal type of gastric cancer, the evolution of gastric mucosa from normal to atrophic, metaplastic, dysplastic and neoplastic takes a long time, not less than 20 years. This particularly slow evolution is widely confirmed by studies on growth curves of EGC (Concetti et al. 1981; Tsukuma et al. 1983).

The routes of spread for gastric carcinoma are similar to those for other intestinal tumours. They include direct extension (lesser and greater omentum, liver, diaphragm, pancreas, spleen, biliary tract, transverse colon), nodal metastases (local and distant), vascular metastases (liver, lungs, bone, brain, etc.) and peritoneal metastases (transperitoneal dissemination to surface of liver, visceral and parietal studding or seeding, pelvic metastasis – Krukenberg's ovary tumour and Blumer's rectal shelf). Direct extension to adjacent organs (e.g. oesophagus) may also be due to diffusion via the submucosal and subserosal lymphatics.

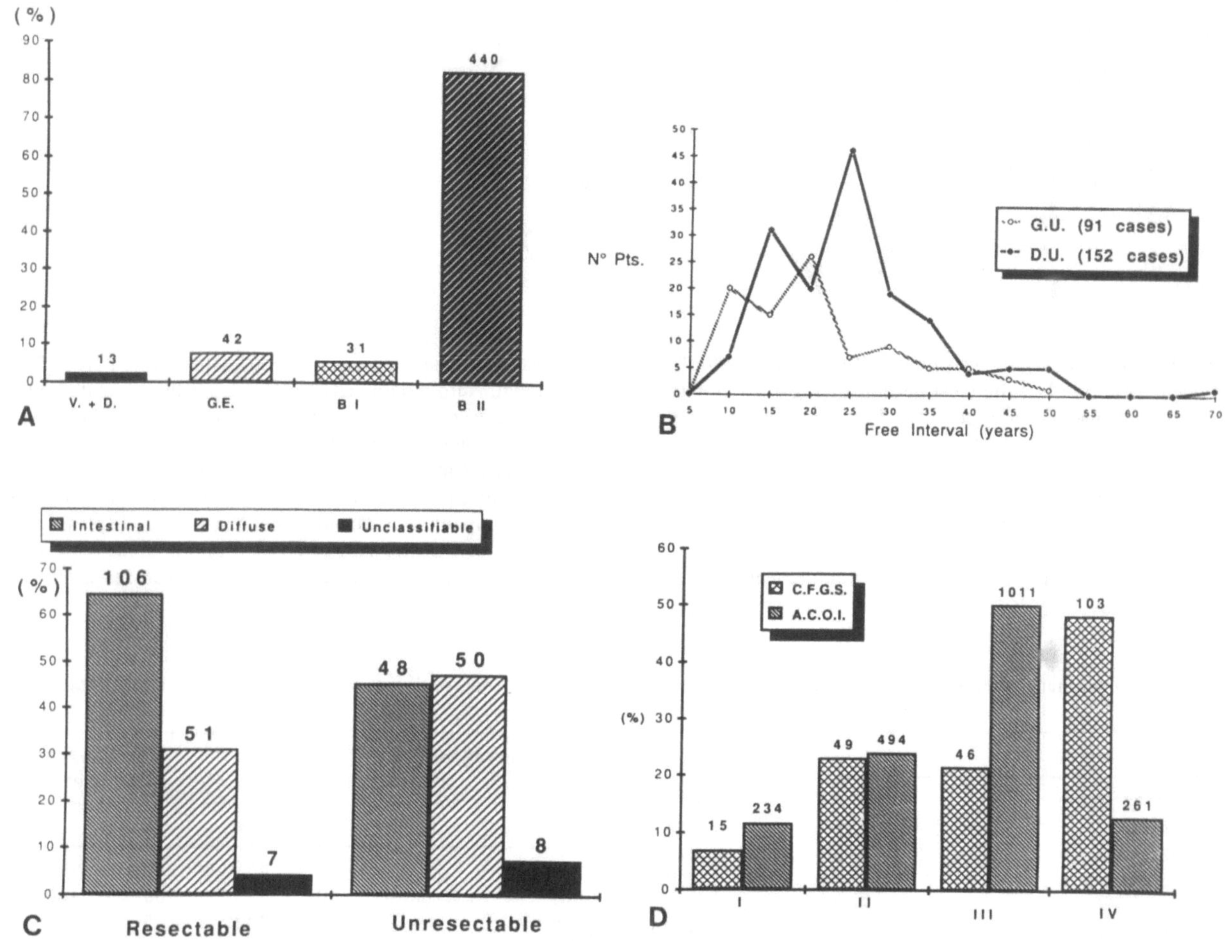

Fig. 7 A–D. Carcinoma following gastric surgery (CFGS): own national survey. **A** The differences in incidence of gastric cancer following operation using different techniques are not statistically significant. **B** Gastric ulcer (GU) is more frequently ($P \leq 0.01$) related to CFGS as the cause of the previous operation. The average free interval is about 22.3 years in patients operated on for GU and about 18.3 years in patients operated on for duodenal ulcer (DU). This difference has to be explained, considering that DU are usually operated on at a younger age than GU (ca. 40.4 and 46 years respectively in our survey). Comparing the distribution of free intervals (arranged in 5-year classes) between the previous operation and the development of CFGS, we obtain similar curves except for an anticipation of about 5 years in the case of GU. **C** Data we collected on distribution of different histological types of primary gastric carcinoma showed no statistically significant difference from the original data of Laurén. Among unresectable CFGS, however, there is a statistically significant ($P \leq 0.05$) prevalence of diffuse type carcinomas, which confirms the greater "aggressivity" of this type. **D** CFGS is diagnosed very late; 48.3% of patients are in stage IV. The difference from primary gastric cancer (2000 cases collected by the ACOI) is statistically very significant ($P \leq 0.001$)

Table 6. Hyperplasia and dysplasia of gastric mucosa (146 cases, 1293 endoscopic biopsies): associated lesions

	Simple hyperplasia		Severe hyperplasia		Mild dysplasia		Severe dysplasia	
	n	%	*n*	%	*n*	%	*n*	%
Superficial gastritis	10	6.8	1	0.7	–	–	–	–
Atrophic gastritis	27	18.5	2	1.4	2	1.4	–	–
Erosion	1	0.7	4	2.7	–	–	–	–
Ulcer	46	31.6	9	6.2	6	4.1	1	0.7
Polyp	25	17.1	4	2.7	1	0.7	–	–
Others	6	4.1	–	–	–	–	1	0.7

From Zampi (1988).

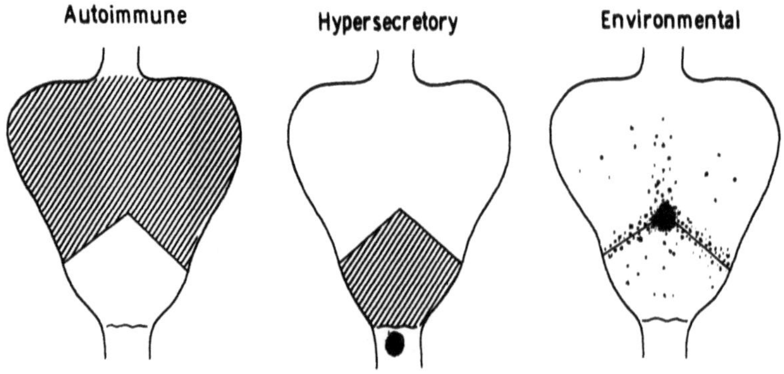

Fig. 8. The topographic distribution of the three types of chronic gastritis (CG). The *lines* and *dots* represent affected areas. The typical location of peptic ulcer accompanying each type of gastritis is shown. Autoimmune CG *(left)* is typically associated with pernicious anaemia, and, because of the presence of atrophy, metaplasia and dysplasia, it must be considered a real morphological precursor of cancer. However, since the incidence of pernicious anaemia among people over 65 years old is generally about 1%, the problem of the interrelation between pernicious anaemia and gastric cancer is, in numerical terms, minimal. Since in hypersecretory CG *(middle)* atrophy, metaplasia and dysplasia are rare, it should not be considered a real morphological precursor of cancer. Environmental CG *(right)*, on the other hand, is usually accompanied by atrophy, metaplasia and dysplasia and therefore must be considered a morphological precursor of cancer. This type of CG may very often be found in areas with high incidence of gastric cancer and, from a numerical point of view, it is the most important precancerous lesion (Correa 1980)

Table 7. Lymphatic metastases in gastric cancer (autopsy, 128 cases)

Metastatic region	*n*	%
Retroperitoneum	62	48.4
Mesentery	54	42.2
Perigastric	50	39.1
Head of pancreas	46	35.9
Neck	35	27.3
Hilum of liver	21	16.4
Paratracheal	20	15.6
Hilum of lung	18	14.1
Para-aortic	11	8.6
Mediastinum	10	7.8
Others	15	11.7

Modified from Yamada (1980).

Table 8. Metastatic involvement in gastric cancer (autopsy, 128 cases)

Metastatic organs[a]	Total metastases		Haematogenous metastases	
	n	%	*n*	%
Liver	60	46.9	60	100.0
Lung	50	39.1	50	100.0
Pancreas	50	39.1	5	10.0
Adrenal	37	28.9	21	56.7
Intestine	33	25.6	0	–
Spleen	31	24.2	8	25.8
Omentum	24	18.8	0	–
Ovary	22	17.2	10	45.4
Gallbladder and common bile duct	21	16.4	0	–
Bladder	18	14.1	2	11.1
Bones	15	11.7	15	100.0
Uterus	15	11.7	5	33.3
Kidney	11	8.6	3	27.3
Pleura	11	8.6	2	18.2
Diaphragm	11	8.6	1	9.1
Others	27	21.1	15	55.5

Modified from Yamada (1980).
[a] Contiguous metastases not considered.

On the whole, especially in Western countries, gastric cancer is detected late and thus treated at an advanced stage characterized by a high rate of lymph node, hepatic and peritoneal metastases. As reported by Yamada et al. (1980), in terminal stages of the disease (autopsy findings) the involvement of remaining and distant lymph nodes is very frequent, indeed almost ubiquitous (Table 7). As to vascular metastases, in all studies the liver is the organ most frequently involved. The most commonly involved distant organ is the lung, followed by the adrenals (Table 8). While the involvement of peritoneum, omentum, liver (by direct extension) and pancreas is very often observed, the involvement of spleen is relatively uncommon, especially if the neoplasm is not in the middle and upper part or on the back wall of the stomach.

K. Maruyama (1987), who followed up 98.8% of 4734 resected cases, reported that by the end of the 5th postoperative year, 2026 patients (42.8%) had died: 78 (3.8%) of postoperative complications, 1422 (70.2%) of recurrence of the primary cancer, 195

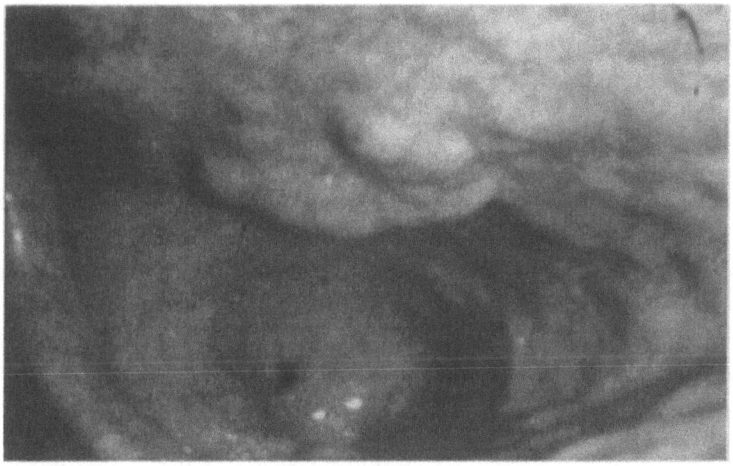

Fig. 9. Gastrocamera image: in the antrum a protruded lesion (EGC type II a) is evident

(9.6%) of other disease and 331 (16.3%) of unknown causes.

From an analysis of autopsy or reoperative findings we can get useful information about common patterns of tumor spread: in some cases there are especially liver metastases, in others we have lymph node metastases with distant involvement but only a few hepatic lesions. Peritoneal carcinosis is almost always associated with lymphatic involvement, while distant and/or liver metastases are relatively rare. Moreover, when Krukenberg's tumours are present, only few intraperitoneal metastases may be found. The knowledge of these patterns and their influence on prognosis allows us to choose the best surgical and/or combined therapies.

Screening of Asymptomatic Disease

Although we have recently seen an essential increase in rates of operability and resectability, results at a distance, in terms of global survival, are still extremely discouraging, especially in European and American countries. This is due to the very late detection of gastric cancer, and the only possible solution to the problem is to improve diagnosis. To achieve this, we should carry out mass screenings of asymptomatic people or selected groups (inhabitants of countries at high risk, particular occupations, family history of neoplasia, subjects more than 40 years old with dyspeptic symptoms, patients with well-known precancerous conditions or lesions). While the rate of EGC is very high in mass screenings, it is quite low in the follow-up of symptomatic patients.

One great restriction on mass screening is the absence of a preliminary test which is repeatable, cheap, selective, sensitive, specific, acceptable and with a good predictive value. For this reason, we should follow Japanese recommendations for annual indirect radiography or examination by gastrocamera (Fig. 9), followed by endoscopy with cytology and biopsy in suspect cases. Such an approach, however, contradicts some fundamental requisites of mass screening: the procedures utilized, even if reliable, are invasive, not easily acceptable, especially for Western people, and thus not always repeatable. Moreover, the absence of a simple and cheap method of preliminary selection and the need, from the outset, for optimal organization, expensive diagnostic techniques and highly trained medical and paramedical staff, the costs of such a programme are very high in relation to the benefits and unsustainable for most countries with a medium to low incidence of gastric cancer. Additionally, the incidence of gastric cancer has been shown to be on the decrease.

Even in Japan, Hirayama (1981), looking at the cost/benefit ratio in the context of a critical review of mass screening programmes for gastric cancer, says: "In order to make the current screening programme more effective, it is of utmost importance to delineate gastric cancer high risk groups as precisely as possible and concentrate screening to such groups".

An interesting alternative screening study, based on determination of fetal sulfaglycoprotein antigen in gastric juice and endoscopy in secretion-positive individuals, was reported by Hakkinen (1981). In view of the very high false-positive rate, however, this screening programme would also appear economically infeasible in the USA and Europe.

Of the other techniques used to select the population for conventional diagnostic methods (juice factors: acid output, beta-glucuronidase, lactic dehydrogenase, CEA and alpha-fetoprotein (AFP); serum tests: tetracycline, CEA and alpha-fetoprotein; urine test: diagnex blue), some are inappropriate but others are not worth further study.

Possible serological screening tests are pepsinogen I (PG I) pepsinogen II (PG II) and gastrin. Pernicious anemia, CAG type A, IM and the intestinal type of gastric cancer are characterized by serum PG I levels below 20–25 ng/ml. When this is associated with a high serum gastrin (>100 pg/ml) a prediction of antral sparing can be made. The contemporaneous dosage of PG I and PG II and the evaluation of their ratio seems to constitute the most reliable subclinical marker of atrophic gastritis of the corpus-fundum and/or antrum (Barbara et al. 1988). But these screening possibilities also require further study.

At present, it is clear that mass screening may not be used for gastric cancer. However, we must aim at the selection and follow-up of high-risk patients, and it is our contention that persistent dyspeptic symptoms, though vague, must be evaluated and studied vigorously.

Table 9. Incidence of symptoms (%) in 90 patients with EGC according to type

Symptoms	Type I	Type II	Type III	All
Epigastric pain	5.6	37.5	40.5	28.9
Vomiting	11.1	18.8	33.3	23.3
Other (weakness etc.)	22.2	6.3	11.9	23.3
Abdominal pain	16.7	31.3	9.5	18.9
Weight loss	16.7	18.8	11.9	18.9
Anorexia	11.1	12.5	11.9	14.4
Indigestion	5.6	18.8	14.3	12.2
Haematemesis and melaena	22.2	–	–	6.6
Dysphagia	–	–	–	1.1
Not known	5.6	–	7.1	4.4

Modified from Fielding et al. (1980).

Diagnosis of Symptomatic Disease

The symptoms of gastric cancer are initially vague, various and transient, encouraging procrastination. Several remedies relieve the symptoms, and nondiagnostic X-rays (often not double-contrast) may increase the delay. Finally, if the physician does not consider the possibility of cancer, the patient may be empirically treated for peptic disease or not treated at all, letting him think that there are no serious problems.

Even in large institutions or in international trials, a negative anamnesis is recorded in only a very small percentage of cases. Evident symptoms usually date back more than 6 months, and the average interval between the onset of symptoms and diagnosis is generally about 7 months. Finally, even today, we often find a palpable mass at the time of admission (Meyers et al. 1987). There is significant difference between AGC and EGC in the symptoms and their duration.

Table 9 shows the incidence of symptoms in EGC. Although symptoms are almost always present, they are by no means specific.

In AGC, pain, prevalent as first symptom, and weight loss, prevalent at the time of admission, are the most common findings. Other symptoms include nausea and vomiting, combined or alone, anorexia, dysphagia, weakness and eructation. Massive upper gastrointestinal bleeding is uncommon (Table 10).

Unfortunately, symptoms often begin to occur when the disease is at least moderately advanced,

Table 10. Gastric carcinoma symptoms: literature review and own series (%)

Author(s) (year)	La Due (1950)	Clarke (1961)	Kelsey (1967)	Goldsmith (1970)	Lundh et al. (1974)	Adashek et al. (1979)	Weed et al. (1981)	Own Series (1986)	Meyers et al. (1987)
No. of patients	1112	250	245	270	901	501	265	427	255
Symptom									
Weight loss	85	68	56	58	78	24	50	67	72
Pain	69	67	56	48	67	38	66	57	51
Vomiting (and nausea)	43	47	38	21	48	24	32	32	40
Anorexia	30			21	45	4	25	41	35
Dysphagia	20		9	17	29	13	23	11	22
Haematemesis	6	18		13		16	23	9	11
No symptoms	0.4	5	6					4	

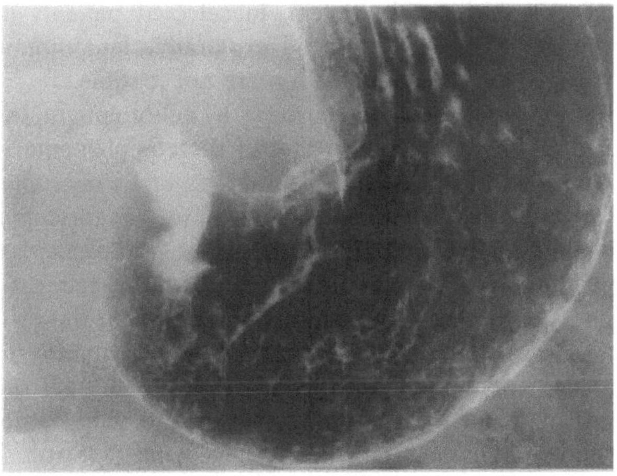

Fig. 10. Double-contrast radiography of the stomach: depressed area at level of angulus with clear interruption of plicae and areolae. On the lesser curvature a "plus" image can easily be seen. Histology: EGC type III. (Courtesy of L. Cirillo, I Department of Radiology, II Medical School, University of Naples)

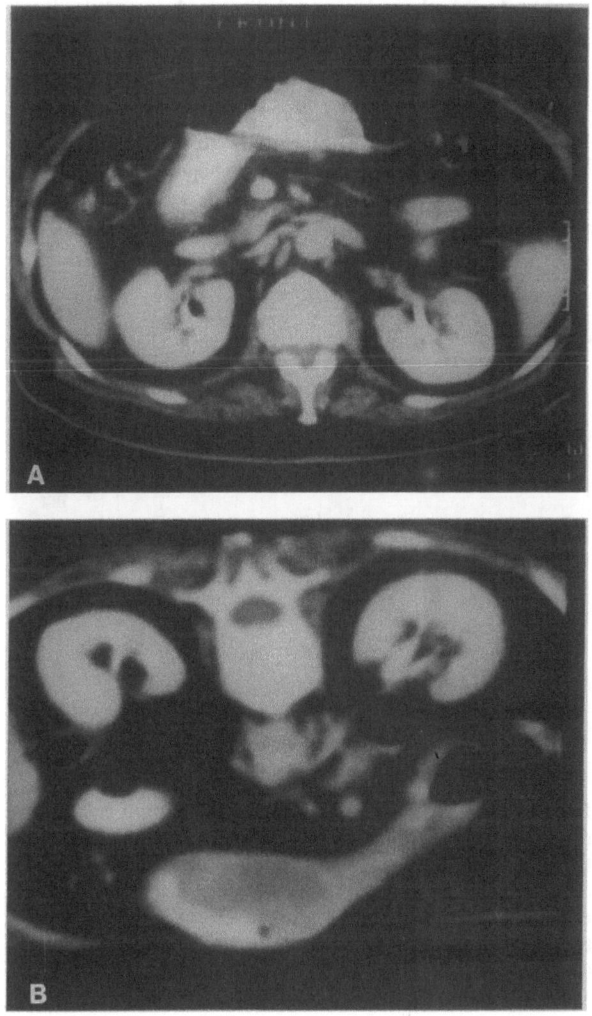

Fig. 11 A, B. CT scans of upper abdomen with Gastrografin and gaseous contrast. A rough, expansive, vegetating formation localized on the back wall of gastric antrum can easily be seen. The intraluminal outline of the neoplasm is well marked by gas in the supine position **(A)** and by gastrografin in the prone position **(B).** The fatty cellular tissue near the rear wall of the stomach shows no sign of infiltrative lesions; moreover, there are no signs of lumbo-aortic or mesenteric lymphadenopathies. (Courtesy of I. Marano, I Department of Radiology, II Medical School, University of Naples)

and signs such as palpable mass, ascites and jaundice frequently first become evident when the patients are already incurable.

About 10% of symptomatic carcinomas are missed in barium studies. The accuracy of barium roentgenography may be improved, 88% up to 95% by the use of a double-contrast technique, mostly in the detection of small or early lesions (Fig. 10).

Endoscopy is certainly the best diagnostic technique (98%), especially when associated with multiple biopsies and exfoliative cytology. When suspicious areas are detected, at least seven biopsy specimens (Graham et al. 1982) should be taken to obtain high diagnostic accuracy. However, the first biopsy should be done as carefully as possible, as bleeding in the target area may prevent the taking of multiple direct biopsy specimens (Iishi et al. 1985). The dye-spray method helps to select the biopsy sites. To improve the rate of diagnosis of EGC, it is of utmost importance to train endoscopists in the technique of biopsy. Gastroscopy with multiple target biopsy or cytology remains the most suitable technique for screening patients at risk for malignancy. Very strict follow-up, with frequency related to the current precancerous condition and to the precancerous lesion found, should be carried out. Endoscopy, in experienced hands, may also be useful in the evaluation of resectability (distensibility, peristaltic waves, pyloric function, wall involvement, size of tumour, proximal and distal extension).

CEA serum monitoring is not useful for diagnosis of primary gastric cancer. Gastric juice CEA levels, even if not diagnostic, are promising in the detection of patients at risk (Nitti et al. 1983). As far as tissue CEA is concerned, data are not yet evaluable.

In staging the disease (and in following up patients operated on or submitted to medical therapy), echotomography and computerized tomography (CT) are very important methods. They can be used to guide biopsy, cytology or needle aspiration, and to yield further information about extragastric extension of neoplasia, liver and lymph node metastases and peritoneal or pelvic spread. CT has high diagnostic accuracy with regard to the extent of intra-abdominal growth and resectability, and correlates well with the findings of surgery. Gastric carcinoma can be separated into four groups: I: gastric wall thickening absent or less than 1 cm; II: thickening of gastric wall more than 1 cm (Fig. 11); III: direct extension of tumour into adjacent organs, local or regional lymph node involvement (Fig. 12); IV: distant metastases (Fig. 13). Using this system, in selected patients it should be possible to avoid explorative laparotomy when resection and palliation are not feasible.

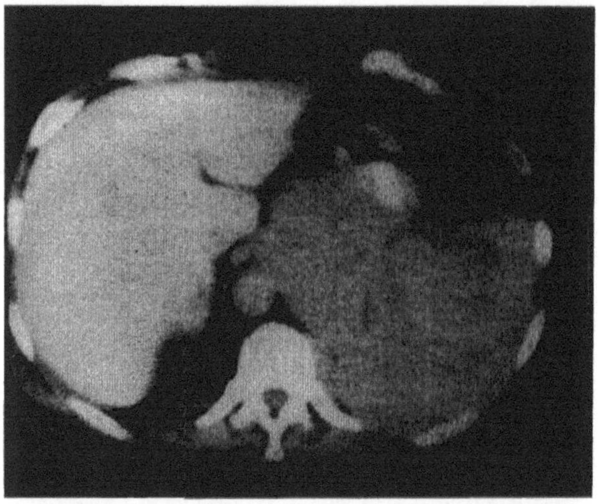

Fig. 12. CT scan of upper abdomen with barium swallow. A rough, expansive formation can be seen which, starting from the fundal and cardiac regions, widely infiltrates the surrounding fatty cellular tissue with signs of infiltrative involvement of the left diaphragmatic muscle; moreover, the lesion extends to the back of the left hypochondrium surrounding the spleen. (Courtesy of I. Marano, M. D., I Department of Radiology, II Medical School, University of Naples)

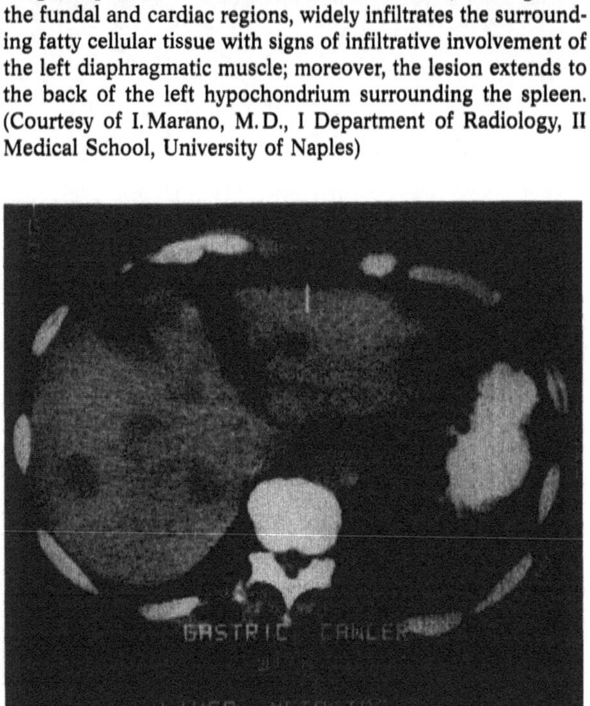

Fig. 13. CT scan of upper abdomen with Gastrografin. A rough thickening of the lesser gastric curvature and of part of the fundus can be seen. The presence of numerous hepatic metastatic lesions (CT-guided fine-needle aspiration biopsy) is a contraindication to surgery. (Courtesy of I. Marano, I Department of Radiology, II Medical School, University of Naples)

In view of the progress made by echotomography and CT in gastric cancer and of the complementary nature of the two methods, there is often no room for any other technique (scintigraphy, laparoscopy, lymphography, etc.) except for some very particular indications. A very new technique is gastroechography, i. e. the use of an echographic probe at the distal end of the endoscope. The irregular structure of malignant tumours with infiltration into the gastric wall and into neighbouring tissues and paragastric lymph node metastases can be visualized (Strohm and Classen 1987). However, this method is still too new to draw valid conclusions, and it is too expensive to be used routinely.

Surgical Treatment

Surgical Treatment of EGC

The choice of surgical treatment for EGC (laser therapy, local resection, partial or total gastrectomy, lymph node dissection, etc.) depends on a number of factors: age and general condition of the patient; site, size, type and possible multiplicity of the tumour; accompanying benign and/or precancerous lesions.

In Japan, R2 gastric resection (gastrectomy, omentectomy, complete removal of group 1 and 2 lymph nodes) has achieved general acceptance as the procedure of choice in the treatment of EGC.

Patients with m EGC have a 100% 5-year survival rate regardless of the kind of gastrectomy in both the single and multiple cancer groups (Kitaoka et al. 1984). The 5-year survival rate for patients with sm EGC who received R2 resection is significantly higher than that for patients with multiple EGC who received R1 resection (96.6% and 64.2% respectively) but not higher than in those with a single EGC and R1 resection[1]. In addition, 125 patients with m polypoid single EGC showed no lymph node metastases and had a 100% 20-year survival rate. Therefore, a new surgical treatment for EGC could be recommended: R1 resection is preferred for intramucosal carcinoma and single sm EGC, while R2 resection for multiple submucosal carcinoma. Laser therapy,

[1] For explanation of resection parameter R, see subsection "Lymphadenectomy" below.

local resection of the tumour or R0 resection may also be sufficient for an intramucosal single polypoid carcinoma less than 2.0 cm in diameter.

As described above, the pen A type of EGC is characterized by a poor prognosis after surgery (Kodama et al. 1983): radical surgery including extensive lymph node dissection and adequate chemotherapy may be warranted.

In inoperable cases of EGC (respiratory or cardiac disease, patient too old etc.), curative laser therapy may be performed. Takemoto (1986) described the state of laser therapy in Japan, collecting 785 treated cases of EGC. Recurrence was observed in only 80 of the 427 patients followed up for 1 year. In the other cases the observation period after laser treatment was too short to evaluate the therapeutic effect. Laser therapy was more effective in lesions smaller than 2 cm in diameter, in elevated lesions and in differentiated and mucosal cancers. The conclusion to be drawn from this review is that laser therapy of EGC should be considered particularly in inoperable cases because of the low incidence of recurrence. It is more accurate and effective in conjunction with ultrasonic endoscopy, a sensitive procedure for clarifying the depth of invasion. However, we need more experience before we can assess the value of laser therapy as a curative substitute for surgical treatment. Further studies are also required to evaluate the efficacy of local resection as definitive treatment for EGC in selected cases.

Surgical Treatment of AGC: General Considerations

Surgery is still, notwithstanding its limitations, the primary and principal treatment of AGC.

In Western countries, during the last 40 years we have observed a considerable increase in the rates of both operability (improved preoperative, anaesthesiological and intensive care techniques) and resectability (above all, an increase in the proportion of palliative resections), whereas the global long-term survival index has varied only slightly (ReMine 1964; Cady et al. 1977; Adashek et al. 1979; Moore 1986; Meyers et al. 1987).

Currently, in Western countries, the 5-year cure rates following resections for gastric adenocarcinoma are about 20%–30%, while Japanese reports indicate that the potential for cure is closer to 50%. In no other cancer do the results of treatment vary so much between one country and the rest of the world. Possible explanations include the very much higher rate of EGC (about 40% or more) and the significantly lower operative mortality (about 2%) recorded in Japan (de Aretxabala et al. 1987; Rohde et al. 1987b). According to Sasaki and Akai (1985), 30% of the decrease in gastric cancer mortality in Japan should be attributed to patients with EGC, 16% to improved diagnostic and therapeutic techniques and the remaining 54% to a lower incidence of gastric cancer.

There remain a lot of unresolved questions concerning the surgical therapy of AGC.

In almost all tumours of the upper or middle third of the stomach in order to obtain a 6-cm tumor-free margin of gastric wall it is necessary to carry out a total gastrectomy, extended to a varying degree, together with splenectomy, omentectomy and the required extent of lymph node removal. If cancer penetrates the gastric serosa on the back wall, the parietal peritoneum of the lesser sac over the pancreas should be removed too, as there may be microscopic disease. If cancer is adherent to the pancreas, caudal pancreatectomy should be performed en bloc. Pancreatic resection, however, is considered a serious risk factor by a lot of authors, as it increases postoperative morbidity and mortality. In the light of the extremely severe prognosis of cases in which cancer infiltrates the whole thickness of the stomach and contiguous organs, we have to ask ourselves whether it is worthwhile carrying out such procedures. The very low survival rates for patients with involvement of the serosa and adjacent organs seem to indicate that the use of extensive resection must be restricted in situations where it would significantly add to operative mortality. On the other hand, some published results suggest the superiority of extended surgical procedures, but the therapeutic role of such extensive surgery has yet to be validated by prospective randomized trials (Shiu and Decosse 1987).

Splenectomy may not be required when the tumour is located in distal stomach, antrum and lesser curvature/anterior wall, as in these cases metastasis to splenic lymph nodes is negligible (Table 11). Patients who have not been submitted to splenectomy have a more favourable prognosis, particularly regarding postoperative complications and long-term survival. Some undefined role of the spleen in immunocompetence may also be relevant.

Greater and lesser omentectomy and dissection of lymph nodes along the hepatic artery to the hilum of the liver and along the left gastric artery to the coeliac axis must be performed. Lymph nodes along the superior border of the pancreas, along the splenic artery and around the superior mesenteric artery should also be removed. Adherence to or invasion of the liver requires its wedge removal. A 3-cm margin

Table 11. Lymph node involvement in tumours located in distal (A), middle (M) and proximal (C) stomach

Lymph node group	Metastatic involvement (%)		
	A	M	C
1. Right paracardial	6.0	8.8	29.6
2. Left paracardial		13.7	21.0
3. Lesser curvature	26.3	27.2	42.2
4. Greater curvature	32.4	21.7	18.6
5. Suprapyloric	20.0	13.3	
6. Infrapyloric	13.3	9.9	1.7
7. Left gastric artery	13.3	9.5	19.6
8. Common hepatic artery	13.0	2.1	5.6
9. Coeliac artery	5.5	4.3	5.2
10. Splenic hilus		10.3	9.2
11. Splenic artery		10.2	24.0
12. Hepatic hilus	2.7		
13. Retropancreatic	1.8		
14. Mesenteric root	2.3		
15. Middle colic artery			
16. Para-aortic			

Modified from de Aretxabala et al. (1987).

of normal duodenum and a 6-cm margin of normal stomach should be included. If distal subtotal gastrectomy is required a gastrojejunostomy should be performed, as local recurrence may obstruct a gastroduodenostomy.

For tumours in which it is theoretically possible to carry out an oncologically correct subtotal distal resection, there is still heated discussion between the supporters of such a procedure and those who prefer, even in these conditions, to perform total gastrectomy (total gastrectomy *de principe*). No objective comparison between subtotal distal resection and total gastrectomy in terms of morbidity, mortality and long-term survival can be made. Until a few years ago, the indications for these two procedures were usually different, if not contrary. Total gastrectomy was usually reserved for patients with advanced lesions: in such cases, the results (more complications, higher mortality and lower long-term survival) relate only to the nature of the lesion and the condition of the host, not to the operation itself. In fact, in the series of those authors who carry out elective total gastrectomy (McNeer et al. 1974; Lortat-Jacob et al. 1975; Mazzeo and Forestieri 1979; Shiu et al. 1980), postoperative complications and mortality are about the same as for those who perform distal resections, while long-term survival is significantly higher. In our own experience the mortality for elective and required distal resections and for elective and required total gastrectomies is 2.4%, 9.2%, 4.4% and 11.1% respectively, while the 5-year survival rates are 23.5%, 12.0%, 39.2% and 13.8% respectively. The use of elective total gastrectomy even for lesions that might in theory be treated with subtotal distal resection obviously does not imply that total gastrectomy has to be carried out always and at any cost. The patient's age is often decisive. In our experience, total gastrectomy must be avoided in elderly patients (>68 years), because of the substantial increase in mortality (13% vs 4.6%).

As for the natural history of the disease, 30%–50% of resected patients will have recurrences limited to the gastric stump or bed. Two cautious conclusions can be advanced concerning the potential for improvement (Craven 1986): (1) The use of total gastrectomy would avoid gastric stump recurrence, the primary or single cause of failure in 10%–20% of cases. (2) Gastric bed recurrence could be reduced by more radical lymphadenectomy and/or by more effective adjuvant therapies (radiotherapy + chemotherapy, intraperitoneal chemotherapy, intraoperative radiotherapy).

Resection Margins

A proximal free margin of 6 cm seems to provide a sufficient warranty of local radicality.

Hornig et al. (1987) suggest a proximal margin of clearance of at least 5 cm (measured on a fresh and unstretched specimen, corresponding to 10 cm in situ) for resection of diffuse type gastric carcinoma. In fact, the prognosis is influenced by the extent of proximal margins of clearance (<5 cm or >5 cm) only in advanced diffuse type carcinoma (29.4% and 59.7% respectively), not in early diffuse type carcinoma (90% and 95% respectively) or advanced intestinal type carcinoma (50.8% and 62% respectively).

Bozzetti et al. (1982), on the contrary, claim that with the exception of depth of infiltration of the gastric wall, none of the evaluated parameters (tumour location, site, size, gross appearance, histological type, lymph node status) was significantly related to a higher rate of infiltration or could provide a clinicopathological guide to extension of the resection. The risk of proximal infiltration is significantly higher when the tumour infiltrates the serosa or spreads beyond it. Therefore the resection could be performed with a margin of 3 cm when the tumour does not infiltrate the serosa and 6 cm when there is serosal involvement or infiltration cannot be precisely assessed.

Palpation and gross inspection are unreliable methods for judging the adequacy of resection, and a frozen section is recommended. However, even with this technique a rate of 9%–21% false negatives has been reported (Schrock and Lawrence 1978; Papachristou et al. 1980). Cytology by scraping the edges of transection is also not considered fully reliable. A negative line of resection is an important, but not an absolute, requisite for 5-year survival (positive margins were present in 15% of 5-year survivors; White et al. 1975), and does not guarantee the absence of local recurrence (Serlin et al. 1977; Soga et al. 1985).

Lymphadenectomy

Apart from gastric lymphatic peculiarities, which can lead to various patterns of lymph node involvement, one must remember that location of neoplasia and depth of invasion are of fundamental importance. For this reason, to achieve a real increase of survival, it may be useful to determine patterns of lymphatic drainage, or sites of metastasis which must be resected, case by case (Table 11).

Among the proposed classifications, the best is that from the Japanese Research Society for Gastric Cancer (1981 a), which also gives some useful practical information about surgical technique (Figs. 14, 15). In this classification, alongside the established parameter N, the new concept R is introduced: R 0 = gastric resection + incomplete removal of lymph nodes of group 1; R 1 = gastric resection + complete removal of group 1 lymph nodes; R 2 = gastric resection + complete removal of group 1 and 2 lymph nodes; R 3 = gastric resection + complete removal of group 1, 2 and 3 lymph nodes.

With the aim of long-term survival, we must evaluate the real utility of an elective extended lymph

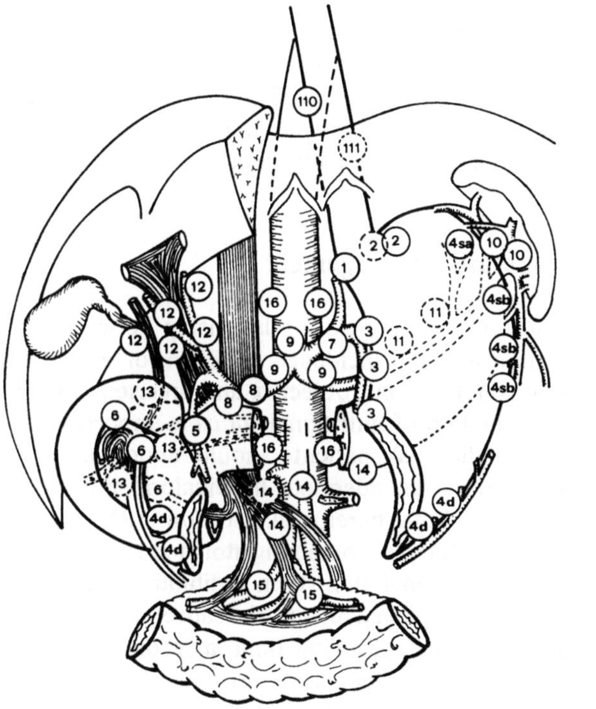

Fig. 14. Lymph node designations used by the Japan Research Society for Gastric Cancer. *1* right cardiac; *2* left cardiac; *3* along lesser curvature; *4* along greater curvature (*4 a* left group: *a* along short gastric arteries, *b* along left gastroepiploic artery; *4 d* right group: along right gastroepiploic artery); *5* suprapyloric; *6* infrapyloric; *7* along left gastric artery; *8* along common hepatic artery; *9* around coeliac artery; *10* at splenic hilus; *11* along splenic artery; *12* in hepatoduodenal ligament; *13* at posterior aspect of pancreas; *14* at root of mesentery; *15* around middle colic artery; *16* around abdominal aorta; *110* lower thoracic paraesophageal; *111* diaphragmatic

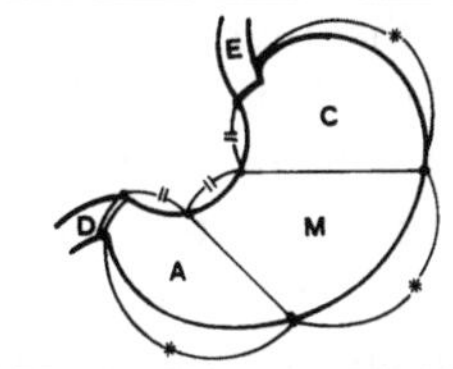

	AMC MAC MCA CMA	A AM	MA M MC	C CM
Group 1 (N_1)	1 2 3 4 5 6	3 4 5 6	3 4 5 6 1	1 2 3 4 s
Group 2 (N_2)	7 8 9 10 11	7 8 9 1	2** 7 8 9 10** 11	4 d 7 8 9 10 11 5* 6*
Group 3 (N_3)	12 13 14 110* 111*	2* 10* 11 12 13 14	12 13 14	12 13 14 110* 111*

Fig. 15. Groups and lymph node designations used by the Japan Research Society for Gastric Cancer according to tumor location. * Resection or non-resection of these lymph nodes does not affect the R number; ** these lymph nodes should be excised if the primary tumour site is MC, but excision is optimal if the primary tumour site is MA or M. In distal gastrectomy cases, resection or non-resection of 4sa lymph nodes does not affect the R number

node dissection. From first data it seems that such dissection is useless in stage I, may be effective in stages II and III when lymph node metastases are present, but in stage IV is not just useless, but harmful as far as postoperative morbidity and mortality are concerned.

In the retrospective study (8133 cases) published by Nishi et al. (1986) the prognosis of N 0 cases was excellent regardless of the extent of lymphadenectomy. In N 1 cases, the survival rates decreased together with R number (R 3 58.8%, R 2 45.3%, R 1 39.8%, R 0 5.9%). In the prognosis of N 2 cases no difference in the survival rates according to R number was apparent. Finally, in N 3 and N 4 cases there was no obvious difference in survival depending upon the extent of lymphadenectomy. Caution must still be exercised in drawing conclusions on the effect of lymph node dissection on survival from retrospective studies, and prospective studies are mandatory.

De Aretxabala et al. (1987) focused not on the efficacy of node dissection in relation to the survival rate, but rather on the interrelationships between number of nodes dissected, degree of node involvement and proportion of patients with node involvement. Routine lymph node dissection, at least R 2, allows excision of a greater number of metastatic nodes and the detection of more patients with such metastases. Furthermore, in this study the procedure was performed without affecting postoperative mortality.

In most Western countries it is not possible to draw any conclusions about the validity and utility of extended lymph node dissection, as it is less uniformly performed, pathologists may study only a few nodes, the proportion of positive nodes among those examined is rarely reported, and various groups of nodes are not likely to be identified unless specifically tagged by the surgeon.

Our opinion in this respect is that extended lymph node dissection, perhaps accompanied by resection of adjacent organs, may cause an increase of complications and mortality without a real improvement in survival, expecially in more advanced cases. There are probably clinically occult liver metastases and distant lymphatic or peritoneal foci of disease in most of these patients which are already beyond the scope of even the most extensive procedure at the time of surgery. Massive serosal involvement, which halves 5-year survival, would seem to be a contraindication to very extensive lymphatic removal. Most of these patients die because of diffuse metastasis, especially peritoneal and hepatic, independent of the surgical technique used. Moreover, the excision of additional organs to achieve complete lymph node removal is rarely indicated. On the whole, we think that the most useful approach is resection of perigastric and functionally contiguous lymph nodes, according to the location of neoplasia (usually an R 2 resection), without extension to anatomically and biologically distant lymph node groups. The increase of operative risk with extended lymph node dissection would be excessive in the case of prophylactic interventions (N −) and disadvantageous with curative ones (N +), since if the N 3 or N 4 nodes are involved and operation is at best palliative (5-year survival about 0%).

Palpation and gross inspection are unreliable methods for assessment of lymph node metastasis. In a prospective study (Rohde et al. 1987 a) of the difference between surgical and pathological stagings, the former was found to be less accurate (more false negatives) in the definition of depth of invasion and lymph node involvement. Therefore, histology-oriented frozen section of tumour, lymph nodes and resection margin seem mandatory. However, frozen section of lymph nodes is often not feasible because of their inaccessibility and it may add an unjustifiable degree of risk to patients with curable tumours owing to the possible spilling of tumour cells (Papachristou and Shiu 1981). Lymphatic staging by peroperative imprint cytology (Keighley et al. 1984) may be a rapid, reliable and relatively simple method of identifying lymphatic metastases.

Preoperative Management

Because of the very close relationship between malnutrition and the incidence of severe or even fatal septic complications, objective and precise preoperative evaluation of nutritional status is important. Selected higher risk patients should undergo, for at least 10 days, an adequate hypercaloric nutritional programme (total parenteral nutrition; TPN). As the flora of the tumour-containing stomach is varied and abundant, rational short-term antibiotic prophylaxis should be employed in gastric cancer surgery. Depending on the prevailing flora, a second- or third-generation, beta-lactamase resistant cephalosporin or penicillin + aminoglycosides, or monobactams (aztreonam) + metronidazole is indicated. Where it is necessary to extend the operation to a colic resection, such prophylaxis offers good protection against sepsis.

Finally, it is advisable to carry out functional respiratory evaluation. Patients should do respiratory physiokinesitherapy in the days before the operation, perhaps even being trained on the machines to be used after operation.

Surgical Technique

For gastric cancer, not including cardiac tumours, laparotomy alone is, in most cases, sufficient to give optimal exposure. The incision is median, extended for about four fingerbreadths under the navel; the ensiform apophysis may be resected.

The first step is, obviously, careful clinical and pathological staging of the abdominal cavity, obtaining all possible information about the neoplasia and its extravisceral extension. Then one must evaluate operability and the feasibility of carrying out the operation by laparotomy alone. The best exposure is obtained by section of the triangular ligament of the left hepatic lobe, which is displaced to the right, incision of the pre-oesophageal peritoneum and the blunt dissection of the oesophageal hiatus. These manoeuvres yield essential information about the upward extension of the neoplasia. To evaluate the mobility of the mass on deep strata, one must accurately explore the coeliac axis, the back gastric wall and the pancreas, by means of section of the lesser omentum and access to the epiploic retrocavity after coloepiploic detachment, which is carried out in the usual way, very close to the colon and in an almost avascular area, or, even better, by means of wide dissection of the two layers of mesocolon (Fig. 16).

The technique we shall describe is radical total en bloc resection by means of a standard systematic procedure, which may, however, be varied according to the specific case and to the surgeon's own preferences.

When we are convinced of operability, going rightwards we complete the coloepiploic detachment with section of the gastroepiploic vein at its confluence with the middle colic vein, and ligation of the right gastroepiploic artery at its origin. This dissection allows the lowering of the right colic corner and, after Kocher's manoeuvre, the mobilization of the duodenal C loop and of the head of the pancreas. In this way we gain access to the (lower) pancreaticoduodenal, subpyloric and retroduodenal pancreatic lymph nodes. Increasing duodenal mobilization (on the right) and resectioning Treitz's ligament and freeing the duodenojejunal flessure (on the left), we can reach, if this is necessary, the periaortic and pericaval areas and the lymph nodes of the upper mesenteric vein and artery (in the supraduodenal tract). It may even be possible to complete retropancreatic dissection in this way, behind the neck of the gland up to the splenomesenteric confluence.

Having thus completed the dissection of pancreaticoduodenal lymph nodes upwards, after complete section of the lesser omentum we proceed downwards and remove the periportal (lateral-posterior), periarterial and supra- and retropyloric lymph nodes (section of pyloric artery and gastroduodenal artery) (Fig. 17).

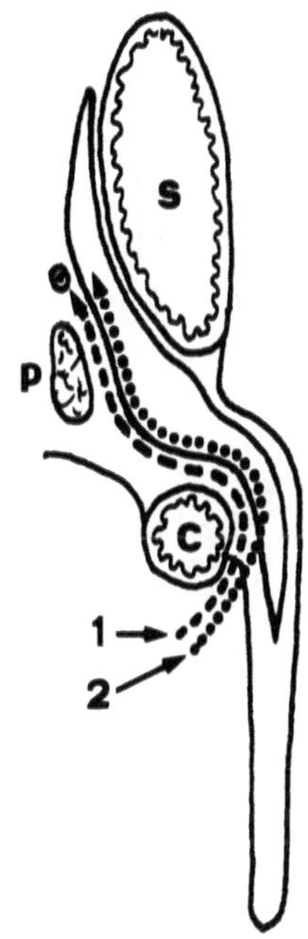

Fig. 16. Access to the omental retrocavity may be made by means of *1* wide dissection of the two layers of mesocolon or *2* classic coloepiploic detachment. *s*, stomach; *p*, pancreas, *c*, colon

Thus duodenal section (usually performed by means of linear or bilinear stapler, if we do not recover duodenal continuity) allows complete removal of the pancreaticoduodenal and retropyloric lymph nodes. Then, going upwards along the hepatic artery, after resecting the gastrohepatic ligament and the posterior peritoneum we complete the lymphadenectomy in the area of the hepatic artery and reach the coeliac axis (possibility of ligating the left gastric and splenic arteries at their origins).

Displacing the stomach upwards and leftwards, we apply tension to the gastric coronary vein and left gastric artery, which must be ligated and resected at their origins. When ligating left gastric artery it is necessary to take care to spare the large-diameter left hepatic artery. The dissection is completed along the higher part of the lesser curvature, following the pericardial tract up to the right pilaster of the diaphragm.

After left coloepiploic detachment, we resect the gastrosplenic omentum. We complete the cardiac resection on the left and at the back by resecting the gastrophrenic ligament. Finally, we resect the oesophagus.

Left lymphadenectomy, complete and extended, is typical of extensive total gastrectomy. We have already discussed the possibility of resecting the splenic artery. In this case, instead of resecting the gastrosplenic ligament, we incise the posterior perito-

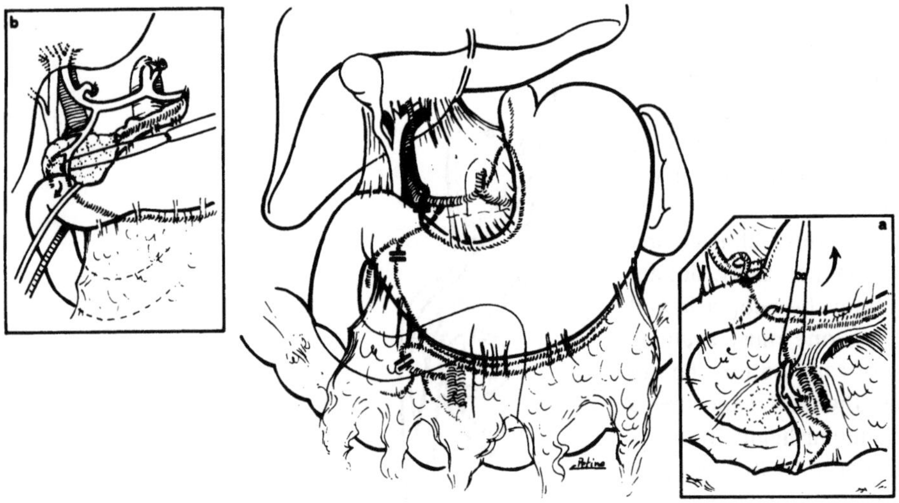

Fig. 17. Section of the gastroepiploic vein at its confluence with the middle colic vein (inset *a*) and of the right gastroepiploic, pyloric and left gastric arteries (inset *b*)

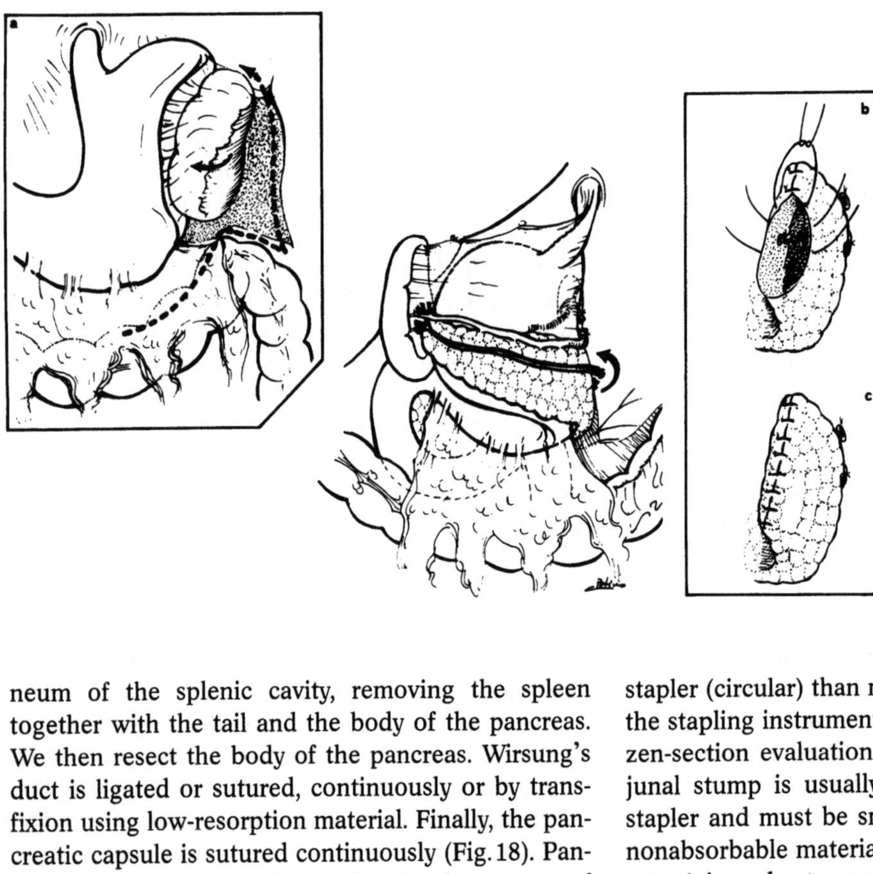

Fig. 18. Splenectomy combined with resection of body and tail of pancreas. *Inset a*, incision of the posterior peritoneum of the splenic cavity. *Inset b*, resection of the body of the pancreas – Wirsung's duct is ligated or sutured. *Inset c*, the pancreatic capsule is sutured continuously

neum of the splenic cavity, removing the spleen together with the tail and the body of the pancreas. We then resect the body of the pancreas. Wirsung's duct is ligated or sutured, continuously or by transfixion using low-resorption material. Finally, the pancreatic capsule is sutured continuously (Fig. 18). Pancreatic resection may be made also by means of mechanical sutures.

Resection of the body and tail of the pancreas will allow better peri-aortic toilet, together with the possibility of completely removing the suprapancreatic, subpancreatic and splenic hilar lymph nodes.

End-to-end or end-to-side oesophagojejunal anastomosis can be carried out when using a Roux-en-Y or an interposed ansa. The oesophagojejunal anastomosis is performed more frequently by means of a stapler (circular) than manually. The tissue "rings" in the stapling instrument may provide material for frozen-section evaluation of resection margins. The jejunal stump is usually closed by linear or bilinear stapler and must be small (possibly connected, with nonabsorbable material, to the diaphragmatic peritoneum) in order to avoid stasis. In interposition of a jejunal ansa, the jejunoduodenal anastomosis may be performed manually or by circular stapler.

Reconstructive Techniques After Total Gastrectomy

From a practical and operative point of view, we believe that the first duty of the surgeon is to carry out a reconstruction which causes the minimum oesophageal reflux. Accordingly, whatever the individual surgeon's preferences, we are sure that the best methods for reconstruction are jejunal interposition or Roux-en-Y with a sufficiently long ansa.

Roux-en-Y is easier and quicker than jejunal interposition, but the advantage of the latter is the recovery of duodenal transit. In order to choose between the two methods, we have to consider whether it is necessary to save this transit. From our clinical practice we realised, little by little, that patients with Roux-en-Y had a nutritional status no worse than that of patients with jejunal interposition; comparative trials confirmed these clinical doubts (Bradley 1979).

Recently, in order to evaluate the real utility of restoring duodenal transit to improve nutritional status, we assembled a homogeneous group of 28 patients who had undergone elective total gastrectomy from 1 to 5 years before without recurrences. We submitted this group to a series of diagnostic surveys and compared the data with those from 20 healthy people similar as far as age and sex were concerned. Eighteen of the 28 patients had received an oesophagojejunoduodenostomy, 10 a Roux-en-Y oesophagojejunostomy. Analysis of weight changes, H2 breath-test transit time evaluation, absorption of glucides (xylose test) and triglycerides and monitoring of serum bile acids (both total and primary) after standard meal stimulus, showed no significant statistical difference between the two groups (Fig. 19).

Weight loss is the most evident consequence of total gastrectomy. However, from our survey it is evident that changes in intestinal absorption deriving from ablation of the stomach are not sufficient to account for this loss of weight. An anamnestic review of our totally gastrectomized patients shows that for various reasons (disinformation, anxiety, lack of appetite, external conditioning etc.) they eat less than they should do. This, rather than malabsorption, is the problem. All the patients regained weight with a diet of 2600 kcal/day during the stay in hospital included in the survey.

We therefore now believe that the choice of reconstructive method has to take into account the age and general condition of the patient (i.e. surgical and anesthesiological risk), the urgency of the operation, the stage of neoplasia, its curability and, on the whole, life expectation. In other words, we should use omega oesophagojejunostomy in urgent cases, in anaesthesiological and surgical high-risk patients or when life expectation is quite low. In the vast majority of patients we prefer a Roux-en-Y ansa of at least 50 cm. Finally, in ideally suited patients it may well be better to use, even speculatively, an interposed jejunal ansa of at least 25 cm, useful in preventing reflux yet not so long as to create problems of emptying in the event of malposition.

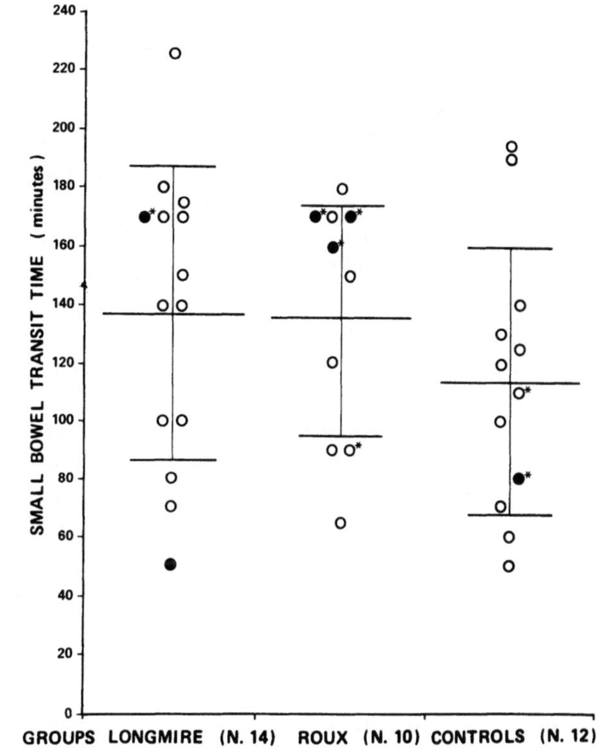

Fig. 19. Measurement of bowel transit time by means of lactulose H2 breath-test in totally gastrectomized patients and healthy controls. *Filled circles* indicate subjects with diarrhoea, *asterisks* those with premature H2 breath-test positivities, both due to bacterial overgrowth. On administration of metronidazole H2 breath-test values are brought back to normal and diarrhoea disappears. Irregularities of bile acids levels may also be due to bacterial overgrowth

Extended Operations

We must not forget that a deep lesion with considerable lymph node involvement and invasion of contiguous structures has an extremely unfavourable prognosis by itself (average survival 8 months; 5-year survival rate less than 10%). In these cases, extended operations do not raise the cure rate but they definitely increase immediate complications, mortality and morbidity and, very often, reduce the quality of life. In such conditions it will be better to do whatever is necessary to obtain the best cytoreduction, limiting morbidity and mortality, to carry out prophylaxis or therapy in the case of urgency and to assure the patient the best attainable quality of life.

Extension to the abdominal wall is simple and must always be carried out if the invasion is limited;

it would become dangerous if large enough to necessitate the use of a prosthesis, because of the risk of infection.

We have already said a lot about the spleen and the body and tail of the pancreas. Generally, in lesser involvement, splenectomy plus removal of the pancreatic capsule may be sufficient: the operation is easier and more complete with only a slight increase in morbidity and mortality. When there is greater involvement, splenectomy plus peripancreatic lymphadenectomy is advised so as to avoid the resection of the body and tail of the pancreas, and the associated high morbidity and mortality, if at all possible.

As far as gastric cancer with synchronous hepatic metastases is concerned, palliative resection of neoplasia and hepatectomy are fully justified in selected cases. As reported by Koga (1980), the postoperative mean survival time of H1 (liver metastases limited to one lobe) and H2 (a few scattered metastases 1 to 2 both lobes) patients was significantly longer in those treated by non-curative gastrectomy than in those receiving laparotomy alone (20.6 and 12.4 months vs 4.1 and 4.1 months). However, this improvement was observed only in patients without peritoneal metastases or direct invasion of other organs. There was no significant difference between the two operations in H3 (numerous scattered metastases to both lobes) patients. In cases of gastric cancer with liver metastases but without peritoneal dissemination, Okuyama et al. (1985) found the most favourable results with the best prognosis in the group receiving gastrectomy + hepatectomy + chemotherapy, using continuous intra-arterial infusion for the treatment of residual metastatic lesions in the liver.

A hepatic metastasis may be removed at a later stage if there are no signs of growth and/or host immune reactivity has improved or local chemotherapy has been successful. In recent years, whenever we have found hepatic metastases, whether resectable or not, we have inserted a totally implantable system (e.g. Port-a-cath) in subcutaneous tissue with a catheter in the gastroduodenal artery for local chemotherapy (Fig. 20).

Resection must always be extended to the small bowel and colon in operations carried out for purposes of prophylaxis or the treatment of emergencies (occlusion); preoperative barium enema may be very useful in this respect.

In the case of Krukenberg's tumour, ovariectomy must always be performed as it is simple and involves no increase in morbidity and mortality.

Extension to the left suprarenal gland should be carried out only if necessary; invasion of this gland excludes curative surgical management.

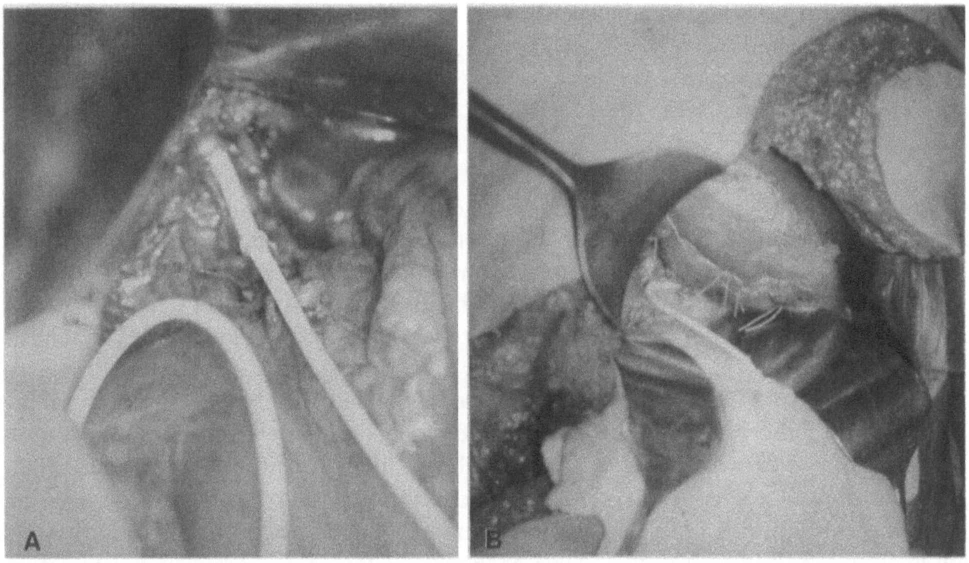

Fig. 20. A Catheter of Port-a-Cath, inserted via subcutaneous tissue into the gastroduodenal artery for local chemotherapy in a patient with bilobar liver metastases of gastric cancer. **B** Catheter of Infusaid 400 pump inserted via subcutaneous tissue into left branch of hepatic artery after right hepatectomy in a patient with multiple unilobar metastases of gastric cancer

Other Adjuvant and Palliative Treatment Forms

As regards adjuvant and palliative treatments, gastric cancers can be classified as follows:
- Local disease: the primary treatment is surgical, but radiotherapy, chemotherapy and immunotherapy have been and are being evaluated as adjuvant treatments.
- Disseminated disease: the treatment is principally palliative and symptomatic.
- Locally advanced, nonresectable or locally recurrent disease: chemotherapy and/or radiotherapy can improve survival in some patients.

Table 12. Activity of principal single-agent and combination therapies in advanced gastric cancer: literature review

	No. of patients	Partial + complete response (%)
5-FU	392	21
Mitomycin C	309	25
Doxorubicin	68	25
BCNU	56	18
Cis-platinum	37	24
FAM	198	42
MeCCNU + 5-FU	175	22
FAMe	90	30
FAP	52	37
FAB	35	52
BCNU + 5-FU	34	41
4-epi-DX + 5-FU	32	41
MTX + FA	30	63

Local Disease

A large number of controlled trials of various regimens of postsurgical adjuvant chemotherapy carried out in the USA, Europe and Japan have revealed very little advantage in terms of survival. Combination chemotherapy is usually considered more effective than single-agent chemotherapy in terms of response rate, duration of response and survival (Table 12).

In a controlled surgical adjuvant study from the Gastrointestinal Tumor Study Group (1982a), following curative resection for gastric adenocarcinoma 142 patients were randomized to receive adjuvant chemotherapy (MeCCNU and 5-FU) or to be followed up closely without it. The chemotherapy group was characterized by longer survival, longer disease-free intervals and reduction of liver metastases. Unfortunately, these results were not confirmed by similar studies published by the Veterans Administration Surgical Oncology Group (Higgins et al. 1983) (no statistically significant improvements in survival or reductions in risk of recurrence) and by the Eastern Cooperative Oncology Group (Engstrom et al. 1985) (sites of recurrence similar for both groups; clinically important haematological toxicity, two deaths among treated patients).

Furthermore, Cullinan et al. (1985) maintain that chemotherapy may be criticized because of the subjectivity in evaluating response rate and because of the better initial performance and nutritional status of responders than nonresponders, and state that the shorter survival of nonresponders is probably due simply to the deleterious effects of chemotherapy.

In Japan (Yoshida et al. 1984) adjuvant chemotherapy is usually administered almost immediately after surgery, whereas in Western countries it is not started until 3–6 weeks postoperatively.

In view of the very poor results of adjuvant systemic chemotherapy, we initiated, in patients with serosal invasion, a programme of adjuvant treatment by means of endoperitoneal chemotherapy with two catheters: one in the gastric bed, the other in the pouch of Douglas. (First cycle between 4th and 8th week: on days 1, 2, 3, 4 and 5, 1000 mg 5-FU + 100 mg Lederfolin + 2000 U heparin + 50 mEq sodium bicarbonate is administered in 2 l saline solution 0.9%. Second cycle between 12th and 16th week: repeat as in first cycle.)

Disseminated Disease

The only currently available treatment for disseminated forms of gastric cancer is chemotherapy. It is more successful in patients with a good performance status who are minimally symptomatic and whose disease is confined to the abdomen than in those with either widely disseminated metastatic disease or a poor performance status. Moreover, it is even possible that a chemotherapy programme does not result in prolongation of survival, but that we simply have the best response from those who would have survived the longest if not treated. Thus, response to chemotherapy may merely be another indicator of good prognosis, just like other factors (MacDonald et al. 1985).

Locally Unresectable or Partially Resectable Disease, Local Recurrence

Patients with locally unresectable, partially resectable or locally recurrent gastric cancers have been considered candidates for radiotherapy.

Current techniques permit the delivery of 40–52 Gy in 4–6 weeks, with acceptable complication rates. According to autopsy and reoperative series, most locoregional failures fall within the volume of a shaped gastric radiation portal. Patient tolerance of this therapy is improved by daily doses of 1.7–1.8 Gy. However, the presence of radiation-sensitive organs in the upper abdomen prevents us from administering doses (60–66 Gy) necessary to achieve a more permanent control.

On the other hand, when intraoperative radiotherapy is used a strong dose may be safely delivered to the unresectable remnants, as healthy contiguous organs can be shifted out of the field. However, the irradiated area is restricted and cannot include all foci of microscopic disease. Early results (Abe 1984; Timothy 1986) indicate that tumour control is possible and that major improvement in survival may be obtained in patients with advanced local disease without distant metastases.

The best therapeutic results would be obtained by means of surgical removal of all gross neoplasia and lymph nodes together with radiation + chemotherapy to control microscopic or subclinical residual disease. However, cumulative toxicity may reduce the benefits of such a combined therapy.

It must be said that at present no combined modality regimen is really successful. Further studies of radiotherapy + chemotherapy or intraoperative radiotherapy are mandatory, possibly in combination with other methods able to improve the efficacy of radiotherapy (i.e. hyperthermia and radiosensitizers). Finally, the use of neutron beams from modern cyclotrons in combination with surgery must be assessed (Catterall 1986).

Palliative Surgical Treatment

The role of surgery in patients with locally advanced or disseminated gastric cancer represents one of the biggest problems that surgeons have to face.

As surgery is the main treatment for gastric carcinoma, all tumours should be considered operable and potentially resectable until proven otherwise. Subjective judgements should be avoided, and decisions on operability should be based on operative and histological evidence only. The neoplasia should always be resected to avoid associated complications and to increase the potential benefit of adjuvant therapy, unless the removal of the stomach and adjacent structures would endanger the patient's survival.

The results of surgery (even if palliative) + radiotherapy + chemotherapy are better in terms of response and survival rates than those obtained without surgical treatment.

Experience has fully documented the failure of various bypass procedures. These do not always succeed in relieving obstruction, do not reduce morbidity, mortality and duration of hospital stay and provide no real relief (Adson 1964; Ekbom and Gleysteen 1980).

Palliative resection, when feasible, is very reasonable and may even be preferable to bypass procedures. Palliative total gastrectomy, however, is generally unacceptable because of its very high mortality and morbidity in such advanced cases, unless it is the only way to treat a complication.

Palliative resection of a gastric cancer should be carried out only if prognostic factors suggest survival of no more than a few months and if there is no increase in operative risk. For instance, it is of no use in the event of involvement of the peritoneum, adjacent organs and the liver.

Many surgeons wrongly consider even a few liver metastases to be much more important than multiple peritoneal metastases. In fact, while in cases of hepatic metastases survival of some months can be achieved, peritoneal carcinosis may cause intestinal occlusion within a few weeks. As mentioned above, Koga (1980a) and Okuyama (1985) confirmed that non-curative gastrectomy for gastric cancer with liver metastases is useful only if peritoneal involvement is absent. Moreover, as reported by Adson (1964), Nakajima (1978) and many others, the prognosis is very bad in patients with positive cytology of ascitic fluid. Finally, we must remember that, while we have effective complementary therapies to control hepatic metastases, no comparable treatment is available for peritoneal carcinosis. For this reason, palliative resection in patients with uncontrollable ascites and massive peritoneal involvement must be critically reviewed. In some patients with cytologically positive ascites we gave, with good results, six to eight weekly cycles of endoperitoneal chemotherapy, followed in some cases by palliative surgery.

Follow-up

Curative surgery for gastric cancer requires very frequent follow-up. The goal is, above all, the diagnosis of metastases or recurrence by means of anamnesis, physical findings, routine laboratory evaluation, tu-

Table 13. Postoperative follow-up programme in gastric cancer patients

	Months													
	3	6	9	12	15	18	21	24	30	36	42	48	54	60
Symptom review and physical examination	X	X	X	X	X	X	X	X	X	X	X	X	X	X
Routine laboratory tests and tumor markers	X	X	X	X	X	X	X	X	X	X	X	X	X	X
Echography	X	(X)	X	X	X	(X)	X	X	X	(X)	X	X	X	(X)
Barium swallow	X			X				X		X		X		X
Endoscopy		X		(X)		X			X		X		X	
Chest X-ray				X				X		X		X		X
CT		X				X				X				X

Laparoscopy, bone scan, monoclonal antibodies, immunoscan etc. are required in the event of specific findings ( ) optional.

mour markers, aspiration cytology, barium swallow, CT, echography and endoscopy (Table 13).

In the specific case of gastric cancer, even particularly strict follow-up will not yield valuable results in terms of further curative potential except in the case of isolated local recurrence (gastric stump or anastomosis). Notwithstanding this, follow-up may be useful in improving knowledge of the natural history of the disease and in evaluating the effectiveness of the therapy employed.

Patients should be followed up at least every 3 months during the first 2 years and at 6-months intervals thereafter. Careful symptom review, physical examination, routine laboratory tests, monitoring of tumour markers and abdominal echography should be done 3, 6, 9, 12, 15, 18, 21, 24, 30, 36, 42, 48, 54 and 60 months after surgery.

Serum CEA monitoring may be used to detect a recurrence of gastric cancer (Tamada et al. 1985), although some findings (Janssen and Oriasaeter 1986) strongly reduce the clinical value of serial CEA monitoring in the follow-up of treated patients. Similar discordances are found for other markers. With regard to AFP (Ishiguro et al. 1985), it seems that different patterns of AFP subfractions may facilitate differential diagnosis of primary hepatoma from hepatic metastases of gastric cancer.

Barium swallow should be carried out shortly after surgery and repeated yearly. Endoscopy is recommended at 6-month intervals during the first 18 months and yearly thereafter. It is also necessary (together with cytology and biopsy) in the case of symptoms and/or radiological findings suggestive of local relapse. Annual chest X-ray is recommended. CT scanning can be done 6, 18, 36 and 60 months after surgery. If a CT scan is made, echography may be omitted.

If patients are on adjuvant therapy their progress may be evaluated more specifically. In intraperitoneal chemotherapy, for instance, we perform CT peritoneography or a ^{99}Tc peritoneal scan (Fig. 21). Other studies (bone scan, monoclonal antibodies, immunoscan, laparoscopy, etc.) are required only to evaluate new or changing symptomatology or in the presence of specific findings.

Peritoneal and pleural effusions, if present, are tapped for cytology. Any enlarged superficial nodes are aspirated. The presence of recurrences may be confirmed, but not excluded, by means of percutaneous fine-needle aspiration of parietal or intra-abdominal masses (guided by CT or echography).

Finally, the possibility (about 10% of cases) of a second primary neoplasm, even in EGC, must be considered.

Recurrence and Treatment of Recurrence

Recurrence of EGC is very rare (2.8%; Kitaoka et al. 1984). The recurrence is mainly haematogenous (liver), ranging from 41.2% (Kitaoka et al. 1984) to 66.7% (Yamada et al. 1980). The rate of recurrence in multiple EGC is higher than that in single EGC (7.2% and 2.4% respectively; Kitaoka et al. 1984).

On the other hand, recurrence, often more than one type simultaneously, is the rule in AGC. Although autopsy findings show widespread disease in about three-quarters of patients, locoregional relapse should not be underestimated (McNeer et al. 1951;

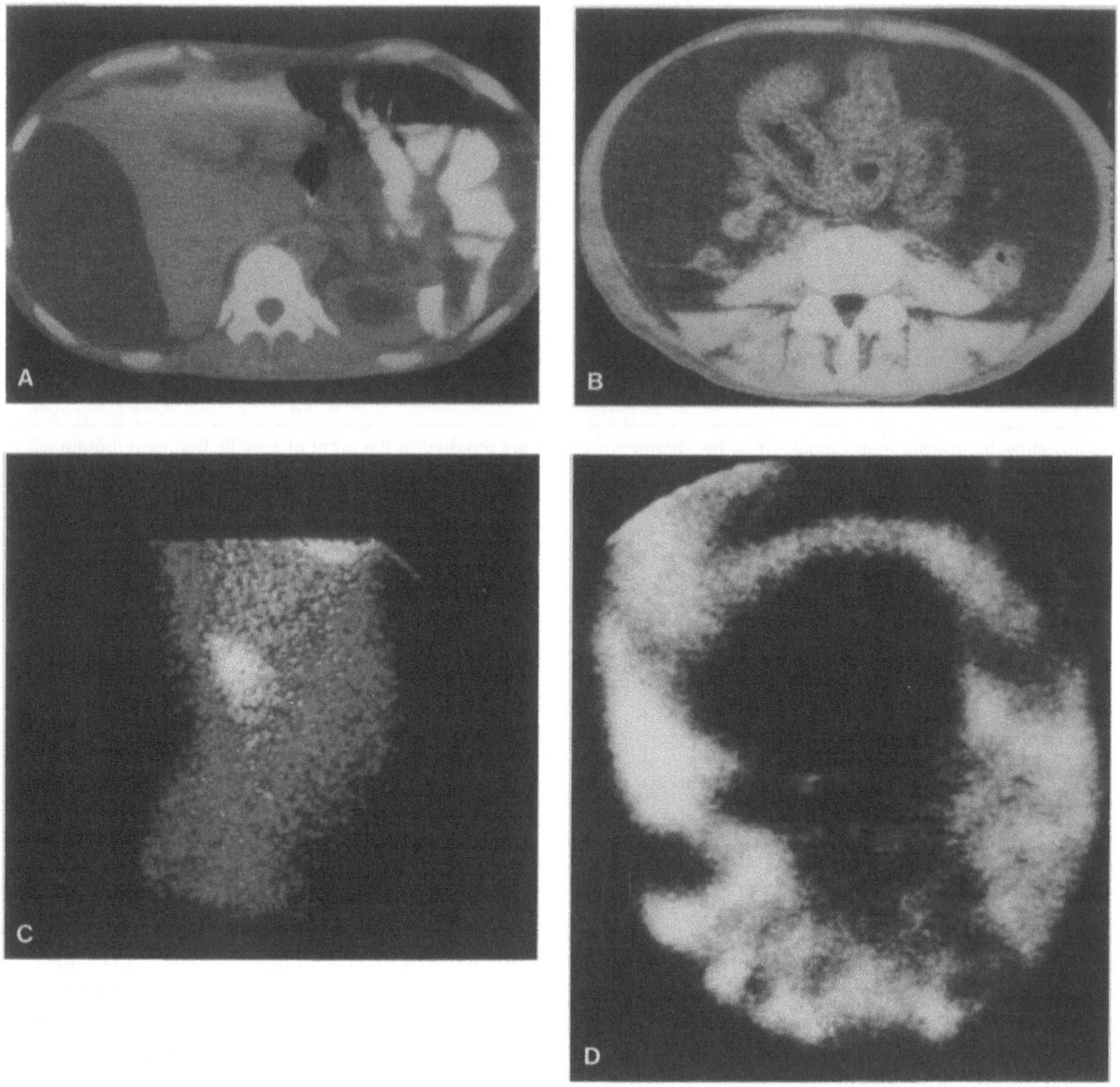

Fig. 21 A–D. F.V., male, 44 years old, submitted to total gastrectomy (October 1984) for gastric cancer (undifferentiated diffuse carcinoma, pT4 pN2 M0). Eighteen months after surgery, presence of ascites and bowel subocclusion. **A, B** Abdominal CT: medial dislocation of healthy liver by conspicuous ascites intestinal loops are displaced into left hypochondrium, free because of splenectomy. Small nodular lesions are evident on the surface of these loops, suggesting peritoneal carcinosis. (Courtesy of Prof. E. Porta, I Department of Radiology, II Medical School, University of Naples). **C** Monoclonal antibodies immunoscan of the abdomen [F (ab') 2 anti-CEA 131-I]. This lateral view after 48 h shows hyperaccumulation in the gastric bed, suggesting local recurrence. (Courtesy of Prof. M. Salvatore, Department of Nuclear Medicine, II Medical School, University of Naples). **D** Peritoneal scan with 99 Tc injected through a Port-a-Cath catheter positioned for intraperitoneal chemotherapy: regular distribution through viscera up to the diaphragm. (Courtesy of Prof. M. Salvatore and L. Celentano, Department of Nuclear Medicine, and W. Craus, Department of Surgical Semeiology, II Medical School, University of Naples)

Thomson and Robbins 1952; Serlin et al. 1977; Iwanaga et al. 1978; Koga et al. 1978; Yamada et al. 1980; Pichlmayr and Meyer 1981; Gunderson and Sosin 1982; Soga et al. 1985; Meyer and Pichlmayr 1987). In our own experience, the pattern of recurrence (isolated or multiple) is as follows: 28% gastric remnant (and/or gastric bed, 39% peritoneum, 18% liver, 15% abdominal lymph nodes (Table 14).

Generally, early or intermediate recurrence is characteristic of infiltrative, poorly differentiated adenocarcinoma with serosal invasion and peritoneal metastases, while late recurrence is characteristic of

Table 14. Patterns of recurrent gastric cancer: literature review and own experience (%)

Authors	No. rec.	Local	Peritoneum	Liver	Lymph-nodes
Iwanaga et al. (1978)	255	30	33	17	20
Koga et al. (1978)	105	20	49	16	14
Yamada et al. (1980)	281	26	48	21	5
Gunderson and Sosin (1982)	181	39	24	13	24
Soga et al. (1985)	120	42	42	4	12
Engstrom et al. (1985)	99	51	16	32	22
Own findings (1986)	67	28	39	18	15

No. rec., number of recurrences; local, mainly gastric remnant and/or gastric bed; peritoneum, localized or diffuse peritoneal seeding; liver, haematogenous metastases; lymph nodes, abdominal. N.B. These series include recurrences with one or more components. If more than one component has been detected, the recurrences are classified according to the most prominent site.

localized, differentiated adenocarcinoma without serosal invasion and with haematogenous (liver) metastases. It is most interesting that very late recurrences are more frequently local and are peculiar to primary lesions excised early (usual treatment: elective subtotal resection), whereas patients suffering from advanced tumours usually die prematurely because of liver metastases and/or peritoneal carcinosis. In these patients total gastrectomy is often of no use in terms of curative intent and local radicality and is also associated with an increase in complication and mortality. From this point of view it would be better to use total gastrectomy (elective or *de principe*) when curative resection is feasible, and subtotal resection (required or *de necessitè*) when it is not.

Local recurrences should not necessarily be considered as treatment failures. One in seven of such recurrences may be cured (Inberg et al. 1981). For instance, local recurrences in the gastric or oesophageal wall or at the anastomosis may still be resectable if detected early (19%; Papachristou and Fortner 1981). For the others, the average survival may be about 16 months. Of the 120 patients in the series of Soga et al. (1985), repeat resection could be carried out in 25 patients (20.8%), all with local recurrence. The 5-year survival rate was 21.4%. Resection of a local recurrence, even if palliative, should be carried out only if distant metastases are absent and the patient is able to tolerate further surgery with minimal risk.

In several studies on gastric cancer, systemic therapy has failed to reduce the recurrence rate (Engstrom et al. 1985). According to Gunderson (1983), however, about one-third of patients could potentially profit from effective local therapy, either alone or as an adjuvant to surgery.

As far as new ways of reducing recurrences or improving curability are concerned, we must look at more effective chemotherapeutic associations (to be administered even earlier), at the best combined radiotherapy-chemotherapy regimens, at intraoperative radiotherapy and at intraperitoneal or intrarterial chemotherapy. Present and future studies will provide more information.

Rehabilitation

Weight loss is often attributed to malabsorption alone, but insufficient intake may play a more important role. In fact, malabsorption of lipids and of proteins has been shown not to be the main cause of weight loss in most patients submitted to total gastrectomy; surprisingly inadequate feeding emerges as the cause of malnutrition and weight loss.

A moderate anaemia may be due to deficiency of iron and/or vitamin B 12 and/or folic acid. Iron malabsorption usually appears within the first year postoperatively. For this reason, parenteral administration of iron may be useful during the adaptation period, to be replaced after 1 year by the oral route. The lack of vitamin B 12 because of malabsorption may be corrected by parenteral administration (1000 μg every 2 months i.m.). Exogenous administration of folic acid may also be useful.

Dumping syndrome can be rectified by particular dietetic measures. In very rare untreatable cases surgery may be used (antiperistaltic interposition).

Reflux oesophagitis and oesophagitis following stenosis with dysphagia are a severe problem, as they can interfere with feeding. In most cases, conservative medical therapy with perendoscopic dilatation is suggested in the presence of anastomotic stricture. In very severe and untreatable cases, surgery in the form of a Roux-en-Y loop must be used. Obviously, in all these cases the nature of the problem should be identified clearly to avoid the concrete possibility of local recurrence. Other measures may include exogenous administration of pancreatic extracts, and of metronidazole when bacterial overgrowth is certain.

Cases in which only feeding jejunostomy is possible are fortunately very rare; in these circumstances the jejunostomy can be used at home with only minimal patient training. The same applies to cases in which protracted parenteral feeding is required.

Acknowledgements. The authors are very grateful to their colleagues Ciro Falasconi, Cesare Formisano and Eugenio Meucci for their contribution to this work.

Future developments

As we have already said, notwithstanding the increase in rates of operability and resectability, the survival of patients with gastric carcinoma is still discouraging and not much better than some years ago. In Japan, thanks especially to the mass screenings which have increased the EGC/AGC ratio, there have been considerable advances in curability. In most Western countries, however, in view of the constant decrease of frequency of gastric cancer, such mass screening cannot be justified, especially in terms of the cost/benefit ratio. Part of the problem is the absence of a selective, cheap, repeatable, sensitive and specific preliminary test. Currently in Western countries, it is only possible to carefully evaluate symptomatic patients and strictly follow up those with well-known precancerous lesions or conditions, increasing radiological and endoscopic definition.

As far as surgical therapy is concerned, only very slight improvements are possible. All data necessary for correct staging should be obtained preoperatively so as to enable optimal therapeutic planning. Apart from better definition through the improvement of traditional methods (endoscopy, radiology, CT, NMR, cytohistology), it may be useful, for instance, to obtain preoperative (gastroechography) or intraoperative (with a 7.5-MHz transducer; Machi et al. 1986) information about peritoneal involvement, because of its negative prognostic value. Preoperative or intraoperative information about some lymph node groups should also be useful. Perendoscopic lymphography is not very helpful in this sense; perendoscopic lymphoscintigraphy is very difficult, while gastroechography with target biopsies has to be developed. Finally, diagnosis by intraoperative cytohistology must become more accurate and more reliable.

As far as the diagnostic and therapeutic use of monoclonal antibodies is concerned, we cannot yet draw any conclusions.

Future research should concentrate on the discovery of new, more active drugs and new pharmacological associations (optimization of dosage) and on the codification of intraoperative radiotherapy and/or combined therapy.

References

Abe M (1984) Intraoperative radiation therapy for gastrointestinal malignancy. In: DeCosse JJ, Sherlock P (eds) Clinical management of gastrointestinal cancer. Nijhoff, Boston, pp 327–349

Adashek K, Sanger J, Longmire WP Jr (1979) Cancer of the stomach. Review of consecutive ten year intervals. Ann Surg 189: 6–10

Adson MA (1964) Palliative operations for gastric cancer. In: ReMine WH, Priestley JT, Berkson J (eds) Cancer of the stomach. Saunders, Philadelphia, pp 141–157

Barbara L, Biasco G, Brillanti S, Miglioli M (1988) Carcinoma gastrico: aspetti clinici. In: Mazzeo F, Forestieri P (eds) I tumori dello stomaco. SES, Naples (in press)

Bormann R (1926) Geschwülste des Magens und Duodenums. In: Henke F, Lubarsch O (eds) Handbuch der speziellen pathologischen Anatomie und Histologie, vol. 4. Springer, Berlin, p 865

Bozzetti F, Bonfanti G, Bufalino R, Menotti V, Persano S, Andreola S, Doci R, Gennari L (1982) Adequacy of margins of resection in gastrectomy for cancer. Ann Surg 196: 685–690

Bozzetti F, Bonfanti G, Morabito A, Bufalino R, Menotti V, Andreola S, Doci R, Gennari L (1986) A multifactorial approach for the prognosis of patients with carcinoma of the stomach after curative resection. Surg Gynecol Obstet 162: 229–234

Bradley E III (1979) Total gastrectomy. Clin Gastroenterol 8: 354–371

Bralow SP (1982) Diagnosis and staging of esophageal and gastric cancer. Cancer 50: 2566–2570

Bresalier RS, Boland CR, Itzkowitz SH, Kim YS (1984) Basic gastrointestinal oncology. Gastric cancer. In: Kern F Jr, Blum AL (eds) The gastroenterology annual vol 2. Elsevier, Amsterdam, pp 298–303

Bucci L, Gentile M, Grigioni W, Salvatore M, Lastoria S, Mazzeo F (1987) New trends in prestaging of colorectal cancer and early detection of local recurrence. In: Montori A, de Anna L, Piccione M, Masoni L (eds) Proceedings of the 4th International Symposium of Digestive Surgery and Endoscopy, Roma, 1986. Monduzzi, Bologna, pp 251–256

Cady B, Ramsden D, Stein A, Haggitt R (1977) Gastric cancer: contemporary aspects. Am J Surg 133: 423–430

Catterall M (1986) Fast neutron radiotherapy in advanced gastric cancer. In: Preece PE, Cuschieri A, Wellwood JM (eds) Cancer of the stomach. Grune and Stratton, London, pp 261–273

Cheli R, Giacosa A (1983) Atrophic gastritis. In: Sherlock P, Morson BC, Barbara L, Veronesi U (eds) Precancerous lesions of the gastrointestinal tract. Raven, New York, pp 155–169

Clarke JS, Cruze K, El Farra S, Longmire WP Jr (1961) The natural history and results of surgical therapy for carcinoma of the stomach. An analysis of 250 cases. Am J Surg 102: 143

Concetti HF, Kato Y, Sugano H, Kitagawa T (1981) Natural history of gastric carcinoma with special reference to the early cancer stage: a mitotic index study on original and recurrent carcinoma. Gan 72: 665–672

Correa P (1980) The epidemiology and pathogenesis of chronic gastritis: three etiologic entities. Front Gastroenterol Res 6: 98–108

Correa P (1985) Clinical implications of recent developments in gastric cancer pathology and epidemiology. Semin Oncol 12: 2–10

Correa P, Haenszel W, Cuello C, Tannenbaum S, Archer M (1975) A model for gastric cancer epidemiology. Lancet 2: 58–60

Craven JL (1986) Radical surgery for gastric cancer. In: Preece PE, Cuschieri A, Wellwood JM (eds) Cancer of the stomach. Grune and Stratton, London, pp 165–187

Cullinan SA, Moertel CG, Fleming TR, Rubin JR, Krook JE, Everson LK, Windschitl HE, et al. (1985) A comparison of three chemotherapeutic regimens in the treatment of advanced pancreatic and gastric carcinoma. Fluorouracil vs fluorouracil and doxorubicin vs fluorouracil, doxorubicin and mitomycin. JAMA 253: 2061–2067

Cunningham D, Coombes RD (1986) Current approaches to the chemotherapy of gastric cancer. In: Preece PE, Cuschieri A, Wellwood JM (eds) Cancer of the stomach. Grune and Stratton, London, pp 243–247

Cunningham D, Hole D, Taggart DJ, Soukop M, Carter DC, McArdle CS (1987) Evaluation of the prognostic factors in gastric cancer: the effect of chemotherapy on survival. Br J Surg 74: 715–720

Cuschieri A (1986) Reconstruction after gastric resection for cancer. In: Preece PE, Cuschieri A, Wellwood JM (eds) Cancer of the stomach. Grune and Stratton, London, pp 209–229

De Aretxabala X, Konishi K, Yonemura Y, Ueno K, Yagi M, Noguchi M, Miwa K, Miyazaki I (1987) Node dissection in gastric cancer. Br J Surg 74: 770–773

Douglass HO Jr, Nava HR (1985) Gastric adenocarcinoma – management of the primary disease. Semin Oncol 12: 32–45

Dupont JB Jr, Lee JR, Burton GR, Cohn I Jr (1978) Adenocarcinoma of the stomach: review of 1497 cases. Cancer 41: 941–947

Egawa S, Tsukiyama I, Yanagawa S, Akine Y, Watai K, Kawada Y, Ishioka K (1984) Treatment of metastatic gastric cancer by combined radiation and hyperthermia (report of two cases). Radiat Med 2: 270–272

Ekbom GA, Gleysteen JJ (1980) Gastric malignancy: resection for palliation. Surgery 88: 476–481

Engstrom PF, Lavin PT, Douglass HO Jr, Brunner KW (1985) Postoperative adjuvant 5-fluorouracil plus methyl-CCNU therapy for gastric cancer patients (EST 3275). Cancer 55: 1868–1873

Fielding JWL, Ellis DJ, Jones BG, Paterson J, Powell DJ, Waterhouse JAH, Brookes VS (1980) Natural history of "early" gastric cancer: results of a 10-year regional survey. Br Med J 281: 965–967

Fielding JWL, Newman CE, Ford CHJ, Jones BG (eds) (1981) Gastric cancer. Pergamon, Oxford

Fiocca R, Villani L, Tenti P, Solcia E, Cornaggia M, Riva C, Finzi G, Capella C (1988) Caratterizzazione istologica e linee cellulari differenziative del carcinoma gastrico in fase iniziale ed avanzata. In: Mazzeo F, Forestieri P (eds) I tumori dello stomaco. SES, Naples, (in press)

Forestieri P (1986) La strategia terapeutica nelle precancerosi gastriche. In: Bazan P (ed) Proceedings of the 10th National Congress of the Italian Society of Surgical Oncology (S.I.C.O.). Moduzzi, Bologna, pp 1497–1509

Forestieri P, Formisano C, Bucci L, Mazzeo F (1984) Gastrite atrofica e cancro dello stomaco. In: Marrano D, Campione O (eds) Proceedings of the 8th National Congress of the Italian Society of Surgical Oncology (S.I.C.O.). Monduzzi, Bologna, pp 813–821

Forestieri P, Formisano C, Mazzeo F (1987 a) The carcinoma following gastric surgery. Preliminary results of a national survey. In: Scientific Committee of First International Symposium (eds) Epidemiology, prevention and early detection of gastric cancer. CIC, Rome, pp 265–277

Forestieri P, Formisano C, Meucci E, Iovine L (1987 b) Studio retrospettivo sul "carcinoma dello stomaco operato" per l'individuazione di una popolazione a rischio. In: Bachi V, Badellino F (eds) Proceedings of the 9th National Congress of the Italian Society of Surgical Oncology (S.I.C.O.). Monduzzi, Bologna, pp 437–453

Forestieri P, Formisano C, Mazzeo F (in press) Chirurgia dello stomaco e del duodeno. In: Bazan P (ed) Le suturatrici meccaniche in chirurgia. Piccin, Padova (Progressi in chirurgia)

Fukutomi H, Sakita T (1984) Analysis of early gastric cancer collected from major hospitals and institutes in Japan. Jpn J Clin Oncol 14: 169–179

Gall FP, Hermanek P (1985) New aspects in the surgical treatment of gastric carcinoma – a comparative study of 1,636 patients operated on between 1969 and 1982. Eur J Surg Oncol 11: 219–225

Gastrointestinal Tumor Study Group (1982 a) Controlled trial of adjuvant chemotherapy following curative resection for gastric cancer. Cancer 49: 1116–1122

Gastrointestinal Tumor Study Group (1982 b) A comparison of combination chemotherapy and combined modality therapy for locally advanced gastric carcinoma. Cancer 49: 1771–1777

Gilbertsen U (1969) Results of treatment of stomach cancer. An appraisal and efforts for more extensive surgery and a report of 1,983 cases. Cancer 23: 1305–1308

Giles GR (1986) Staging and prognostic determinations of gastric cancer. In: Preece PE, Cuschieri A, Wellwood JM (eds) Cancer of the stomach. Grune and Stratton, London, pp 89–105

Giuli R (1978) Le traitement chirurgical des cancers de l'estomac. Ann Chir 32: 673–677

Goldsmith HS, Ghosh BC (1970) Carcinoma of the stomach. Am J Surg 120: 317

Graem N, Fischer AB, Beck H (1984) Dysplasia and carcinoma in the Billroth II resected stomach 27–35 years post-operatively. Acta Pathol Microbiol Immunol Scand [A] 92: 185–188

Graham DY, Schwartz JT, Cain GD, Gyorkey F (1982) Prospective evaluation of biopsy number in the diagnosis of esophageal and gastric carcinoma. Gastroenterology 82: 228–231

Grigioni WF, Bucci L, d'Errico A, Forestieri P, Milani M, Villanacci V, Mazzeo F (1984) Validità e limiti dell'esame istologico estemporaneo nell'apparato gastroenterico. In: Marrano D, Campione O (eds) Proceedings of the 8th National Congress of the Italian Society of Surgical Oncology (S.I.C.O). Monduzzi, Bologna, pp 21–25

Gunderson LL, Sosin H (1982) Adenocarcinoma of the stomach – areas of failure in a reoperation series (second or symptomatic looks). Clinicopathologic correlation and implications for adjuvant therapy. Int J Radiat Oncol Biol Phys 8: 1–11

Gunderson, LL, Hoskins B, Cohen AM, Kaufman S, Wood WC, Carey RW (1983) Combined modality treatment of gastric cancer. Int J Radiat Oncol Biol Phys 9: 965–975

Hakkinen I (1981) Application of serum and gastric juice tumour markers to early diagnosis and screening of gastric cancer. In: Fielding JWL, Newman CE, Ford CHJ, Jones BG (eds) Gastric cancer. Pergamon, Oxford, pp 85–94
Hallissey MT, Fielding JWL (1986) Screening for gastric cancer and premalignant lesions. In: Preece PE, Cuschieri A, Wellwood JM (eds) Cancer of the stomach. Grune and Stratton, London, pp 33–45
Hattori T (1986) Development of adenocarcinomas in the stomach. Cancer 57: 1528–1534
Hautefeuille P, Valleur P, Castaing D, Piel JL, Gerum A, Houdart R, Villet R, Galian A (1982) Influence de l'extension ganglionnaire sur la survie après résection de cancers gastriques infiltrants. Gastroenterol Clin Biol 6: 849–856
Herfarth C, Schlag P (1979) Gastric cancer. Springer, Berlin Heidelberg New York
Hermanek P (1987) Clinical significance of histologic classification in accordance with Laurén as an addition to pTNM. Scand J Gastroenterol [Suppl 133] 22: 31–32
Hermanek P, Riemann JF (1982) The operated stomach – still a precancerous condition?. Endoscopy 14: 113–114
Hermanek P, Sobin LH (eds) (1987) TNM classification of malignant tumours. Springer, Berlin Heidelberg New York, pp 43–46
Higgins GA, Amadeo JH, Smith DE, Humphrey EW, Keehn RJ (1983) Efficacy of prolonged intermittent therapy with combined 5-FU and Methyl-CCNU following resection for gastric carcinoma (a VASOG report). Cancer 52: 1105–1112
Hill MJ (1983) Environmental and genetic factors in gastrointestinal cancer. In: Sherlock P, Morson BC, Barbara L, Veronesi U (eds) Precancerous lesions of the gastrointestinal tract. Raven, New York, pp 1–22
Hirayama T (1981) Methods and results (cost-effectiveness) of gastric cancer screening. In: Fielding JWL, Newman CE, Ford CHJ, Jones BG (eds) Gastric cancer. Pergamon, Oxford, pp 77–84
Hirayama T (1984) Epidemiology of stomach cancer in Japan with special reference to the strategy for the primary prevention. Jpn J Clin Oncol 14: 159–168
Hollender LF, Kauffmann JP, Bur F, Meyer C, Bahnini J, Keller D, Cordeiro F, Pigache P (1983) Etude rétrospective de 384 exérèses pour cancers gastriques. Chirurgie 109: 731–741
Holyoke ED, Douglass HO Jr (1984) Carcinoma of the stomach. In: Pilch YH (ed) Surgical oncology. McGraw-Hill, New York, pp 543–558
Hornig D, Hermanek P, Gall FP (1987) The significance of the extent of proximal margins of clearance in gastric cancer surgery. Scand J Gastroenterol [Suppl 133] 22: 69–71
Iishi H, Tatsuta M, Okuda S (1985) Endoscopic diagnosis of minute gastric cancer of less than 5 mm in diameter. Cancer 56: 655–659
Iishi H, Yamamoto R, Tatsuta M, Okuda S (1986) Evaluation of fine-needle aspiration biopsy under direct vision gastrofiberscopy in diagnosis of diffusely infiltrative carcinoma of the stomach. Cancer 57: 1365–1369
Inberg MV, Heinonen R, Lauren P, Rantakokko V, Viikari SJ (1981) Total and proximal gastrectomy in the treatment of gastric carcinoma: a series of 305 cases. World J Surg 5: 249–257
Ishiguro T, Sugitachi I, Sakaguchi H, Itani S (1985) Serum alpha-fetoprotein in patients with primary hepatoma or hepatic metastasis of gastric cancer. Cancer 55: 156–159
Iwanaga T, Koyama H, Furukawa H, Taniguchi H, Wada A, Tateishi R (1978) Mechanisms of late recurrence after radical surgery for gastric carcinoma. Am J Surg 135: 637–640
Janssen CW Jr, Oriasaeter H (1986) Carcinoembryonic antigen in patients with gastric carcinoma. Eur J Surg Oncol 12: 19–23
Japanese Research Society for Gastric Cancer (1981a) The general rules for the gastric cancer study in surgery and pathology. Part I. Clinical classification. Jpn J Surg 11: 127–139
Japanese Research Society for Gastric Cancer (1981b) The general rules for the gastric cancer study in surgery and pathology. Part II. Histological classification of gastric cancer. Jpn J Surg 11: 140–145
Jass JR (1980) Role of intestinal metaplasia in the histogenesis of gastric carcinoma. J Clin Pathol 33: 801–810
Joossens JV, Geboers J (1983) Epidemiology of gastric cancer: a clue to etiology. In: Sherlock P, Morson BC, Barbara L, Veronesi U (eds) Precancerous lesions of the gastrointestinal tract. Raven, New York, pp 97–113
Kaibara N, Okamoto T, Kimura O, Iitsuka Y, Takebayashi M, Yurugi E, Nishidoi H, et al. (1983) Possible role of lymph node dissection in the surgical treatment of gastric cancer with disseminating peritoneal metastasis. Jpn J Surg 13: 404–408
Kajitani T (1950) Clinical classification of gastric cancer and its significance. Gan 41: 76–78
Kamiya T, Morishita T, Asakura H, Miura S, Munakata Y, Tsuchiya M (1982) Long-term follow-up study on gastric adenoma and its relation to gastric protruded carcinoma. Cancer 50: 2496–2503
Kanayama H, Hamazoe R, Osaki Y, Shimizu N, Maeta M, Koga S (1985) Immunosoppressive factor from the spleen in gastric cancer patients. Cancer 56: 1963–1966
Keighley MRB, Morris DL, Moore J, Thompson H (1984) Preoperative imprint cytology: lymphatic staging of gastric carcinoma. Accuracy and survival. J Exp Clin Cancer Res 3: 483–485
Kelsey JR Jr (1967) Cancer of the stomach. A clinical guide for diagnosis and treatment. Thomas, Springfield
Kim JP, Jung SE (1987) Patients with gastric cancer and their prognosis in accordance with number of lymph node metastases. Scand J Gastroenterol [Suppl 133] 22: 33–35
Kirchner R, Henke W, Wittekind C, Farthmann EH (1987) The surgeon's estimation of radicality and results of pathologic examination at margins of resection in gastric cancer surgery. Scand J Gastroenterol [Suppl 133] 22: 72–75
Kishimoto H, Koga S (1979) Evaluation of gastrectomy combined with the resection of other organs in the treatment of gastric cancer. Jpn J Surg 9: 173–179
Kitaoka H, Yoshikawa K, Hirota T, Itabashi M (1984) Surgical treatment of early gastric cancer. Jpn J Clin Oncol 14: 283–293
Kodama Y, Sugimachi K, Soejima K, Matsusaka T, Inokuchi K (1981) Evaluation of extensive lymph node dissection for carcinoma of the stomach. World J Surg 5: 241–248
Kodama Y, Inokuchi K, Soejima K, Matsusaka T, Okamura T (1983) Growth patterns and prognosis in early gastric carcinoma. Superficially spreading and penetrating growth types. Cancer 51: 320–326
Koga S, Kishimoto H, Tanaka K, Kawaguchi H (1978) Clinical and pathological evaluation of patients with recurrence of gastric cancer more than five years postoperatively. Am J Surg 136: 317–321
Koga S, Kawaguchi H, Kishimoto H, Tanaka K, Miyano Y, Kimura O, Takeda R, Nishidoi H (1980a) Therapeutic significance of noncurative gastrectomy for gastric cancer with liver metastasis. Am J Surg 140: 356–359
Koga S, Kishimoto H, Tanaka K, Miyano Y, Kawaguchi H, Ta-

keda R, Nishidoi H, Kimura O (1980 b) Results of total gastrectomy for gastric cancer. Am J Surg 140: 636–638

Koga S, Kaibara N, Kimura O, Nishidoi H, Kishimoto H (1981) Prognostic significance of combined splenectomy or pancreatico-splenectomy in total and proximal gastrectomy for gastric cancer. Am J Surg 142: 546–550

Koga S, Maeta M, Shimizu N, Osaki Y, Hamazoe R, Oda M, Karino T, Yamane T (1985) Clinical effects of total-body hyperthermia combined with anticancer chemotherapy for far-advanced gastrointestinal cancer. Cancer 55: 1641–1647

Kolaric K, Potrebica V, Stanovnik M (1986) Controlled phase III clinical study of 4-epi-doxorubicin + 5-fluorouracil versus 5-fluorouracil alone in metastatic gastric and recto-sigmoid cancer. Oncology 43: 73–77

La Due JS, Murison PJ, McNeer G, Pack GT (1950) Symptomatology and diagnosis of gastric cancer. Arch Surg 60: 305

Lambert R (1983) Principles of screening adapted to precancerous conditions of the gastrointestinal tract. In: Sherlock P, Morson BC, Barbara L, Veronesi U (eds) Precancerous lesions of the gastrointestinal tract. Raven, New York, pp 293–303

Laufer I (1977) Double contrast radiology in the diagnosis of gastrointestinal cancer. In: Glass J (ed) Progress in gastroenterology. Grune and Stratton, New York, pp 643–669

Laurén P (1965) The two histological main types of gastric carcinoma: diffuse and so-called intestinal-type carcinoma. Acta Pathol Microbiol Scand 64: 31–49

Lavin PT, Bruckner HW, Plaxe SC (1982) Studies in prognostic factors relating to chemotherapy for advanced gastric cancer. Cancer 50: 2016–2023

Le Chevalier T, Smith FP, Harter WK, Schein PS (1985) Chemotherapy and combined modality therapy for locally advanced and metastatic gastric carcinoma. Semin Oncol 12: 46–53

Lehnert T, Erlandson RA, Decosse JJ (1985) Lymph and blood capillaries of the human gastric mucosa. A morphologic basis for metastasis in early gastric carcinoma. Gastroenterology 89: 939–950

Lehtola J (1978) Family study of gastric carcinoma with special reference to histological types. Scand J Gastroenterol [Suppl] 13: 1–54

Li DKB, Burhenne HJ (1983) Computed tomography of the stomach and duodenum: a review. Am J Gastroenterol 78: 36–41

Liotta LA, Rao CN, Barsky SH (1983) Tumor invasion and the extracellular matrix. Lab Invest 49: 636–648

Longmire WP Jr (1981) The place of radical surgery in gastric cancer. In: Fielding JWL, Newman CE, Ford CHJ, Jones BG (eds) Gastric cancer. Pergamon, Oxford, pp 203–216

Lortat-Jacob J, Giuli R, Estenne B, Clot P (1975) Intéret de la gastrectomie totale pour le traitement des cancers de l'estomac. Etude de 482 interventions radicales. Chirurgie 101: 59–67

Lundell L, Grip I, Olbe L (1986) Pancreatic resection additional to gastrectomy for gastric cancer. Effect on postoperative morbidity. Acta Chir Scand 152: 145–149

Lundh G, Burn JI, Kolig G, Richard CA, Thomson JWW, van Elk PJ, Oszachi J (1974) A co-operative international study of gastric cancer. Ann R Coll Surg Engl 54: 219–228

Lygidakis NJ (1984) Carcinoma of the stomach; the value of radical surgery and early diagnosis in the outcome of the disease. An analysis of 389 cases treated between 1964 and 1983. J Exp Clin Cancer Res 3: 53–62

MacDonald JS, Cohn I Jr, Gunderson LL (1985) Cancer of the stomach. In: Devita VT, Hellmann S, Rosenberg SA (eds) Cancer. Principles and practice of oncology. Lippincott, Philadelphia, pp 659–690

Machi J, Takeda J, Sigel B, Kakegawa T (1986) Normal stomach wall and gastric cancer: evaluation with high-resolution operative US. Radiology 159: 85–87

Maruyama K (1986) Results of surgery correlated with staging. In: Preece PE, Cuschieri A, Wellwood JM (eds) Cancer of the stomach. Grune and Stratton, London, pp 145–163

Maruyama K (1987) The most important prognostic factors for gastric cancer patients. A study using univariate and multivariate analyses. Scand J Gastroenterol [Suppl 133] 22: 63–68

Maruyama K, Miwa K (1987) Japanese staging system for gastric cancer. Evaluation and documentation of tumor extension. Scand J Gastroenterol [Suppl 133] 22: 22–26

Maruyama M (1986) Comparison of radiology and endoscopy in the diagnosis of gastric cancer. In: Preece PE, Cuschieri A, Wellwood JM (eds) Cancer of the stomach. Grune and Stratton, London, pp 123–144

Mazzeo F, Forestieri P (1979) Linfoadenectomia nei tumori dello stomaco. In: Proceedings of the 3rd National Congress of the Italian Society of Surgical Oncology (S.I.C.O.). Rivista di Oncologia, pp 32–48

Mazzeo F, Forestieri P (1981) Possibilita' e limiti degli interventi allargati in chirurgia oncologica: stomaco. Folia Oncol 4: 220–229

Mazzeo F, Forestieri P (1985) La gastrectomia totale. In: Fegiz G (ed) Proceedings of the 87th National Congress of Italian Society of Surgery (S.I.C.). Masson Italia, Milano, pp 685–722

Mazzeo F, Forestieri P (eds) (1988) I tumori dello stomaco. SES, Naples, (in press)

Mazzeo F, Santangelo ML, Agresti A (1970) Cura chirurgica del carcinoma gastrico. Gli interventi palliativi e i reinterventi per recidive. In: Fegiz G (ed) Proceedings of the 72th National Congress Italian Society of Surgery (S.I.C.). E.M.E.S., Rome, pp 397–419

Mazzeo F, Forestieri P, Formisano C (1983 a) La gastrectomia totale di elezione nella terapia chirurgica del cancro dello stomaco. In: Pagan V, Zotti EF (eds) Proceedings of the 6th National Congress of the Italian Society of Surgical Oncology (S.I.C.O.). La Garangola, Padova, pp 136–142

Mazzeo F, Mozzillo N, Formato A, Forestieri P (1983 b) Fisiopatologia della sindrome da agastria. G Chir 4: 681–684

McConnell RB (1983) Genetics of precancerous conditions of the gastrointestinal tract. In: Sherlock P, Morson BC, Barbara L, Veronesi U (eds) Precancerous lesions of the gastrointestinal tract. Raven, New York, pp 23–42

McNeer G, Vandenberg H, Donn FY, Bowden LA (1951) A critical evaluation of subtotal gastrectomy for the cure of cancer of the stomach. Ann Surg 134: 2–7

McNeer G, Bowden L, Booher R, McPeak C (1974) Elective total gastrectomy for cancer of the stomach. Ann Surg 180: 252–256

Meyer HJ, Pichlmayr R (1987) Patterns of recurrence in relation to therapeutic strategy in gastric cancer. Scand J Gastroenterol [Suppl 133] 22: 45–48

Meyers WC, Damiano RJ, Postlethwait RW, Rotolo FS (1987) Adenocarcinoma of the stomach. Changing patterns over the last 4 decades. Ann Surg 205: 1–8

Ming SC (1977) Gastric carcinoma. A pathobiological classification. Cancer 39: 2475–2485

Miwa K (1984) Evaluation of the TNM classification of stomach cancer and proposal for its rational stage-grouping. Jpn J Clin Oncol 14: 385–410

Moore JR (1986) Gastric carcinoma: 30-year review. Can J Surg 29: 25–28

Morson BC, Sobin LH, Grundmann E, Johansen A, Nagayo T, Serck-Hanssen A (1980) Precancerous conditions and epithelial dysplasia in the stomach. J Clin Pathol 33: 711–721

Mozzillo N, Formato A, Greco L, Forestieri P, Mazzeo F (1982) Evaluation of intestinal reconstruction after total gastrectomy: Longmire procedure versus Roux en Y in view of intestinal absorption (Abstr). 1st International Congress of the European Society of Surgical Oncology, Athens

Mulligan RM, Rember R (1954) Histogenesis and biologic behaviour of gastric carcinoma. Arch Pathol 58: 1–25

Myren J (1983) Markers of cancer risk and surveillance of the gastric stump. In: Sherlock P, Morson BC, Barbara L, Veronesi U (eds) Precancerous lesions of the gastrointestinal tract. Raven, New York, pp 195–203

Nagata T, Ikeda M, Nakayama F (1983) Changing state of gastric cancer in Japan. Histologic perspective of the past 76 years. Am J Surg 145: 226–233

Nagayo T (1983) Precancerous changes of the stomach from the aspect of dysplasia of the gastric mucosa – histological study. In: Sherlock P, Morson BC, Barbara L, Veronesi U (eds) Precancerous lesions of the gastrointestinal tract. Raven, New York, pp 115–126

Nakajima T, Harashima S, Hirata M, Kajitani T (1978) Prognostic and therapeutic value of peritoneal cytology in gastric cancer. Acta Cytol (Baltimore) 22: 225–229

Nishi M, Nakajima T, Kajitani T (1986) The Japanese Research Society for Gastric Cancer – The general rules for the gastric cancer study and an analysis of treatment results based on the rules. In: Preece PE, Cuschieri A, Wellwood JM (eds) Cancer of the stomach. Grune and Stratton, London, pp 107–121

Nitti D, Farini R, Grassi F, Cardin F, di Mario F, Piccoli A, Vianello F, et al. (1983) Carcinoembryonic antigen in gastric juice collected during endoscopy. Value in detecting high-risk patients and gastric cancer. Cancer 52: 2334–2337

Noguchi Y, Ohta H, Tagaki K, Ike H, Takahashi T, Ohashi I, Kuno K, et al. (1985) Synchronous multiple early gastric carcinoma: a study of 178 cases. World J Surg 9: 786–793

Nomura AMY, Stemmermann GN, Samloff IM (1980) Serum pepsinogen I as a predictor of stomach cancer. Ann Intern Med 93: 537–540

Ohman U, Emas S, Rubio C (1980) Relation between early and advanced gastric cancer. Am J Surg 140: 351–355

Okuyama K, Isono K, Juan JK, Onoda S, Ochiai T, Yamamoto Y, Koide Y, Satoh H (1985) Evaluation of treatment for gastric cancer with liver metastasis. Cancer 55: 2498–2505

Oota K (1977) Histological typing of gastric and oesophageal tumours. WHO, Geneva

Papachristou DN, Fortner JG (1981) Local recurrence of gastric adenocarcinomas after gastrectomy. J Surg Oncol 18: 47–53

Papachristou DN, Shiu M (1981) Management by en bloc multiple organ resection of carcinoma of the stomach invading adjacent organs. Surg Gynecol Obstet 152: 483–487

Papachristou DN, Agnanti N, d'Agostino H, Fortner JG (1980) Histologically positive esophageal margin in the surgical treatment of gastric cancer. Am J Surg 139: 711–714

Pichlmayr R, Meyer HJ (1981) Patterns of recurrence in relation to therapeutic strategy. In: Fielding JWL, Newman CE, Ford CHJ, Jones BG (eds) Gastric cancer. Pergamon, Oxford, pp 171–184

Preece PE, Cuschieri A, Wellwood JM (eds) (1986) Cancer of the stomach. Grune and Stratton, London

Priestman TJ (1986) Adjuvant chemotherapy. In: Preece PE, Cuschieri A, Wellwood JM (eds) Cancer of the stomach. Grune and Stratton, London, pp 231–242

ReMine WH (1981) Preoperative assessment and palliative surgery. In: Fielding JWL, Newmann CE, Ford CHJ, Jones BG (eds) Gastric cancer. Pergamon, Oxford, pp 123–137

ReMine WH, Priestley JT, Botson J (1964) Cancer of the stomach. Saunders, Philadelphia

Rohde H, Koster R, Gebbensleben B, Stutzer H, Rau E (1987 a) Errors of surgical staging in patients with cancer of the stomach. Scand J Gastroenterol [Suppl 133] 22: 27–30

Rohde H, Rau E, Gebbensleben B, Stutzer H, Koster R, Salzberger B, Ahrens P (1987 b) What causes in-hospital mortality of surgical patients with cancer of the stomach? Scand J Gastroenterol [Suppl 133] 22: 76–79

Sakita T, Oguro Y (1974) Endoscopic diagnosis of early gastric cancer. In: Berry LH (ed) Gastrointestinal pan-endoscopy. Thomas, Springfield, pp 278–294

Sasaki J, Akai S (1985) Role of diagnostic and therapeutic improvements in the decline of gastric cancer mortality rate in Japan. Jpn J Cancer Res 76: 149–153

Schein PS, Smith FP, Woolley PV, Ahlgren JD (1982) Current management of advanced and locally unresectable gastric carcinoma. Cancer 50: 2590–2596

Schrock TR, Lawrence WW (1978) Total gastrectomy. Am J Surg 135: 348–355

Segura DI, Montero C (1983) Histochemical characterization of different types of intestinal metaplasia in gastric mucosa. Cancer 52: 498–503

Serlin O, Keehn H, Higgins G, Harrower H, Mendeloff G (1977) Factors related to survival following resection for gastric carcinoma. Cancer 40: 1318–1329

Shiu MH, Decosse JJ (1987) The importance of the extent of resection for prognosis of stomach cancer patients. Scand J Gastroenterol [Suppl 133] 22: 54–57

Shiu M, Papachristou D, Kosloff C, Eliopoulos G (1980) Selection of operative procedure for adenocarcinoma of the midstomach. Ann Surg 192: 730–738

Sipponen P, Kekki M, Haapakoski J, Ihamaki T, Siurala M (1985) Gastric cancer risk in chronic atrophic gastritis: statistical calculations of cross-sectional data. Int J Cancer 35: 173–177

Sjostedt S, Pieper R (1986) Gastric cancer. Factors influencing long-term survival and postoperative mortality. Acta Chir Scand [Suppl] 530: 25–29

Soga J, Kobayashi K, Saito J, Fujimaki M, Muto T (1979) The role of lymphadenectomy in curative surgery for gastric cancer. World J Surg 3: 701–708

Soga J, Suzuki T, Miyashita K, Muto T (1985) An evaluation of recurrent gastric carcinoma. J Exp Clin Cancer Res 4: 181–186

Soreide O, Lillestol J, Viste A, Bierkeset T (1982) Factors influencing survival in patients with carcinoma of the stomach. Acta Chir Scand 148: 367–372

Srivastava A, Hughes LE (1986) Role of palliative surgery in gastric cancer. In: Preece PE, Cuschieri A, Wellwood JM (eds) Cancer of the stomach. Grune and Stratton, London, pp 189–207

Suehiro S, Nagasue N, Ogawa Y, Sasaki Y, Hirose S, Yukaya H (1984) The negative effect of splenectomy on the prognosis of gastric cancer. Am J Surg 148: 645–648

Sugimaki K, Inokuki K (1984) Critical evaluation of prophylactic splenectomy in total gastrectomy for stomach cancer. Gan No Rinsho 30: 1057–1060

Strohm WD, Classen M (1987) Staging of gastric and esophageal carcinoma by means of endoscopic ultrasonography. Scand J Gastroenterol [Suppl 133] 22: 17–21

Tahara H, Sumiyoshi H, Hata J, Yasui W, Taniyama K, Hayashi T, Nagae S, Sakamoto S (1986) Human epidermal growth factor in gastric carcinoma as a biologic marker of high malignancy. Jpn J Cancer Res 77: 145–152

Takemoto T (1986) Laser therapy of early gastric carcinoma. Endoscopy [Suppl 1] 18: 32–36

Tamada R, Hiramoto Y, Tsujitani S, Nozuka T, Okamura T, Masuda H, Sugimachi K, Inokuchi K (1985) Serum CEA levels facilitate detection of recurrences of cancer in patients after gastrectomy. Jpn J Surg 15: 23–29

Tatsuta M, Okuda S, Tamura H, Taniguchi H (1982) Endoscopic diagnosis of early gastric cancer by the endoscopic congo red – methylene blue test. Cancer 50: 2956–2960

Thomson FB, Robins RE (1952) Local recurrence following subtotal resection for gastric carcinoma. Surg Gynecol Obstet 95: 341–344

Timothy AR (1986) Radiotherapy in gastric cancer. In: Preece PE, Cuschieri A, Wellwood JM (eds) Cancer of the stomach. Grune and Stratton, London, pp 249–259

Tsukuma H, Mishima T, Oshima A (1983) Prospective study of early gastric carcinoma. Int J Cancer 31: 421–426

Tytgat GNJ, Mathus-Vliegen EMH, Offerhaus J (1983) Value of endoscopy in the surveillance of high-risk groups for gastrointestinal cancer. In: Sherlock P, Morson BC, Barbara L, Veronesi U (eds) Precancerous lesions of the gastrointestinal tract. Raven, New York, pp 305–318

Utsunomiya J (1983) Clinical aspects of benign and malignant tumors. Gastric cancer. In: Kern F Jr, Blum AL (eds) The gastroenterology annual vol. 1. Elsevier, Amsterdam, pp 328–334

Vallgren S, Hedenbro J, Gotberg S, Walther B (1985) Preoperative computed tomography for evaluation of tumour growth in patients with gastric cancer. Acta Chir Scand 151: 571–573

Veronesi U, Montorsi W, Gennari L, Spinelli P, Emanuelli H (eds) (1984) I tumori gastroenterici. Ambrosiana, Milano

Weed TE, Nussle W, Ochsner A (1981) Carcinoma of the stomach. Why are we failing to improve survival? Ann Surg 191: 407–413

Weisburger JH, Wynder EL, Horn CL (1982) Nutritional factors and etiologic mechanism in the causation of gastrointestinal cancers. Cancer 50: 2541–2549

White RR, Mackie JA, Fitts WT Jr (1975) An analysis of twenty years experience with operations for carcinoma of the stomach. Ann Surg 181: 611–615

Yamada E, Miyaishi S, Nakazato H, Kato K, Kito T, Takagi H, Yasue M, et al. (1980) The surgical treatment of cancer of the stomach. Int Surg 65: 387–399

Yap P, Pantangco E, Yap A, Yap R (1982) Surgical management of gastric carcinoma. Follow-up results in 465 consecutive cases. Am J Surg 143: 284–287

Yoshida K, Ikeuchi H, Kano K, Machida T, Takahashi M, Miura Y, Miura N (1984) Results of surgical treatment of gastric cancer – special reference to pathological findings. Tohoku J Exp Med 144: 57–62

Zampi G, Amorosi A, Bianchi S (1988) Le precancerosi gastriche: precursori morfologici e reale potenziale evolutivo. In: Mazzeo F, Forestieri P (eds) I tumori dello stomaco. SES, Naples, (in press)

Pancreatic and Periampullar Carcinoma

W. Hohenberger, H. Zirngibl, and F. P. Gall

Definitions

It is useful to differentiate malignant tumours of the exocrine pancreas from periampullar carcinomas, even though the lesions often cannot be classified until surgery and in 10% of cases, identification is possible only on examination of the surgical specimen (Longmire and Traverso 1981; Warren et al. 1975). The difference lies mainly in the prognosis. Periampullar carcinomas cause obstructive jaundice at an early stage and are frequently only a few millimetres in diameter at the time of diagnosis. Lymphogenous and hematogenous metastases are less common and, with adequate techniques, the tumours can thus be resected curatively in about 70%–90% of cases. The average 5-year survival rate is 30% (Cubilla and Fitzgerald 1984) (Table 1). The ratio of pancreatic to periampullar carcinoma is around 5:1 to 10:1 (Forrest and Longmire 1979; Hermanek and Wörner 1979; Malagelada 1979; Rückert and Kümmerle 1979;

Table 1. Differences between pancreatic and periampullar carcinoma: histological and prognostic classification (University Department of Surgery, Erlangen, 1961–1982)

	Ductal carcinomas	Other exocrine carcinomas[a]	Endocrine carcinomas[b]	Periampullar carcinoma
Number of patients	399	4	18	86
Distant metastases on diagnosis	207 (51.8%)	0	5 (28%)	5 (6%)
Resection rate	69 (17.3%)	4	13 (72%)	65 (76%)
Survival rates (%)[c]				
1 year	13.4 ± 3.5		56.6 ± 23.9	51.3 ± 11.1
2 years	6.4 ± 2.6		57.8 ± 24.4	40.7 ± 11.2
5 years	1.8 ± 1.8		52.4 ± 28.2	27.5 ± 11.4
Median survival time (months)	3.1		55.8	12.0
Number of patients resected	69	4	13	65
Median tumour diameter (cm)	3.10	6.00	6.00	2.20
Lymph node metastases				
No	18 (26%)	1	6 (46%)	35 (54%)
Yes	47 (68%)	3	4 (31%)	25 (38%)
No data	4 (6%)	–	3 (23%)	5 (8%)
Curative operation				
Yes	45 (65%)	3	11 (85%)	59 (91%)
No	20 (29%)	1	2 (15%)	4 (6%)
No data	4 (6%)	–	–	2 (3%)
Survival rates after curative resection (%)[c]				
1 year	39.7 ± 11.9		70.4 ± 26.0	58.0 ± 12.5
2 years	26.6 ± 11.3		71.4 ± 26.5	48.9 ± 13.0
5 years	11.8 ± 11.2		62.2 ± 34.0	35.2 ± 13.8
Median survival time (months)	8.4			18.9

Only histologically confirmed tumours are included.
[a] Acinar cell carcinoma, cystadenocarcinoma, low-grade papillary carcinoma.
[b] Including combined exocrine/endocrine carcinoma.
[c] Calculated according to the actuarial method, age-corrected, postoperative mortality not excluded, 95% confidence limits.

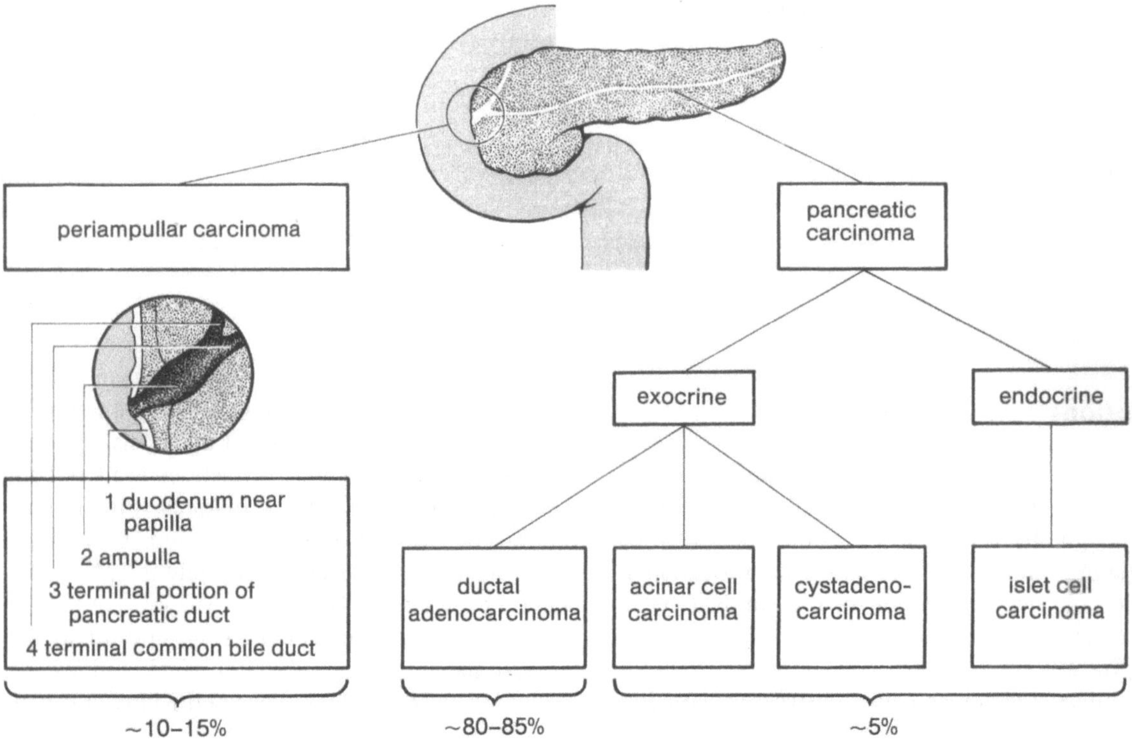

Fig. 1. Pancreatic carcinoma and periampullar carcinoma: classification. (From Hermanek 1984)

Trede 1982). Periampullar carcinomas are defined as tumours of the distal part of the common bile duct, the terminal part of the pancreatic duct, the ampulla of Vater and the area of the duodenum immediately adjacent to the papilla of Vater (Hermanek and Wörner 1979) (Fig. 1). The actual pancreatic carcinomas are divided into adenocarcinomas, acinar cell carcinomas and cystoadenocarcinomas; other rare types of tumour are also found. The most frequent malignant endocrine tumour of the pancreas is islet cell carcinoma.

Table 2. Increase in incidence of pancreatic carcinoma in Saarland, FRG

	Incidence per 100 000 population			
	Men		Women	
	Crude rate	World-standardized rate	Crude rate	World-standardized rate
1970–1972	7.2	5.9	4.7	2.5
1982–1984	10.6	7.4	9.6	3.9

Data from the Statistisches Amt des Saarlandes (1987).

Epidemiology

A rise in the incidence of pancreatic carcinoma, in some instances marked, has been reported worldwide. However, it is hard to tell whether this increase is genuine or attributable to improvements in diagnosis. All epidemiological investigations have the disadvantage that the diagnosis of pancreatic carcinoma is confirmed histologically in only 50%–70% of cases (Gudjonsson et al. 1978; Levin et al. 1981). The almost threefold increase in mortality in the USA between 1930 and 1980 must be seen against this background (Williams and Weissburger 1986). The increase in incidence in the Saarland is shown in Table 2 as an example for the Federal Republic of Germany. Table 3 illustrates the frequency of pancreatic carcinoma in various countries. Marked regional differences can be discerned, as well as variations among different ethnic groups in the same region. In general, pancreatic carcinoma is up to three times more common in men than in women. Overall it is one of the most frequently occurring malignancies.

Pancreatic carcinomas are very rare before 40 years, only about 1% being diagnosed in younger patients. The peak occurs between 60 and 80 years of age (Levin et al. 1981) (Fig. 2), with 80% of cases

Table 3. Standardized incidence of pancreatic carcinoma per 100 000 population in various countries

	Men		Women		Ratio men/women
	Frequency	Rank[a]	Frequency	Rank[a]	
Senegal, Dakar	1.0	15	1.0	16	1
Brazil, Sao Paulo	5.4	14	4.0	14	1.95
Canada, British Columbia	8.2	8	5.6	10	1.46
USA, San Francisco Bay Area					
Whites	9.3	7	6.4	10	1.45
Blacks	18.3	5	9.9	6	1.85
Chinese	6.4	9	5.7	10	1.12
Japanese	3.9	10	4.8	8	0.81
China, Shanghai	3.9	10	2.9	14	1.34
India, Bombay	2.0	15	0.9	23	2.22
Israel, all Jews	9.5	8	6.5	9	1.46
Japan, Nagasaki	8.7	7	6.4	9	1.36
Singapore					
Chinese	3.9	11	2.0	15	1.96
Malays	1.4	15	1.1	17	1.27
Indians	1.6	17	3.3	15	3.21
FRG, Hamburg	7.8	7	4.5	10	1.73
Finland	9.7	5	6.3	7	1.54
Italy, Varese	6.7	12	3.9	12	1.72
Switzerland, Geneva	8.8	11	5.0	12	1.76
GB, Birmingham	8.1	8	4.8	11	1.69
Poland, Cieszyn	2.5	17	0.9	24	2.78
Australia, New South Wales	8.1	8	8.7	10	0.93
New Zealand					
Maoris	14.8	4	10.2	8	1.45
Non-Maoris	8.6	8	5.0	10	1.72

From Waterhouse et al. (1982).

[a] Position in rank order of frequency: in Dakar, for example, pancreatic carcinoma is the 15th most common cancer among men and the 16th most common among women.

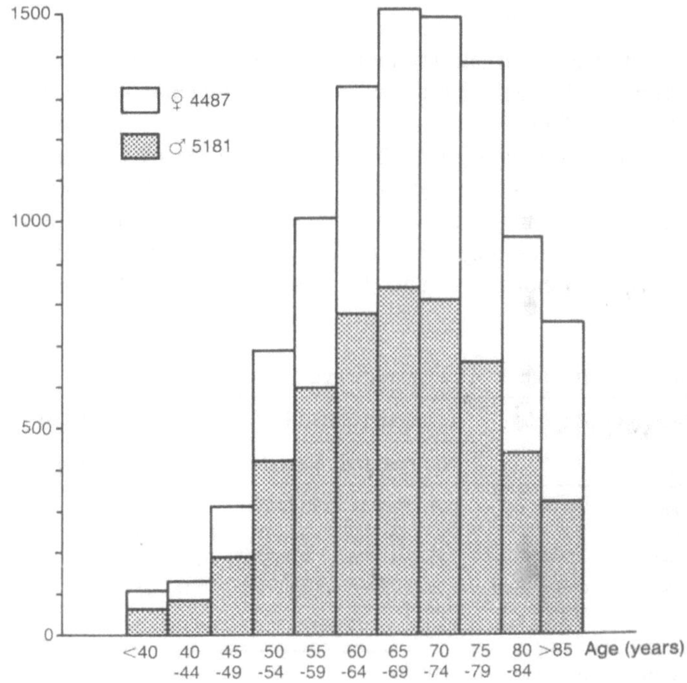

Fig. 2. Age and sex distribution of pancreatic carcinoma in the USA from 1973 to 1977 ($n = 9668$). (Modified from Levin et al. (1981)

involving patients from this age group (Gordis and Gold 1984). The prognosis is very poor, so that incidence and mortality do not differ to any great extent. In the FRG, with a total population of 61.6 million, 7448 people died of pancreatic carcinoma in 1983. This amounted to 4.9% of all cancer deaths (Statistisches Bundesamt 1984).

Nicotine abuse is viewed as the most important factor in the pathogenesis of pancreatic carcinoma, increasing the risk threefold. Opinions differ regarding coffee and alcohol, but their consumption has only a slight effect, if any. A diet rich in protein and fat has been proved to increase the risk significantly. Raw fruit and vegetables are thought to reduce the risk (Williams and Weissburger 1986).

The risk among diabetic women is 6 times greater than among non-diabetics. (Berg and Connolly 1979; Cohn and Hastings 1981; Fraumeni 1975; Moolgavkar and Stevens 1981; Sirinek and Aust 1986; Wynder 1975).

Chronic pancreatitis has repeatedly been suggested to be a risk factor, although there is no hard evidence for this proposition (Sarles and Sahel 1976). Only in the rare hereditary form of pancreatitis does the carcinoma rate seem to be higher.

Clinical Pathology

Pancreatic Carcinoma

Local Tumour Spread

As found both on surgery and on autopsy, the preferred site for pancreatic carcinoma is the head of the organ (Table 4).

Ductal carcinomas of the body and tail of the pancreas are, on the average, bigger, and have, in the overwhelming majority of cases, already penetrated into the surrounding tissue and, above all, already display lymphogenous and hematogenous distant metastases at the time of diagnosis (Baylor and Berg 1973; Cubilla et al. 1978b). A particular problem posed by pancreatic carcinomas, even in small tumours, is the early stage at which growth extends beyond the pancreas (Table 5). This is the case in 50%–86% of resected ductal pancreatic carcinomas (Hermanek 1984; Klöppel et al. 1979b).

Tumours of the head of the pancreas lead to stenosis of the intrapancreatic common bile duct. Despite this, obstructive jaundice is not an early symptom. Later, there is also duodenal stenosis. Neoplasms of the uncinate process may invade the root of the mesentery, or the area around the Treitz ligament on a broad front. Direct infiltration or extensive lymph node involvement at the superior margin of the pancreas leads to long stenoses of the common hepatic artery. Dorsal extension causes narrowing of the superior mesenteric artery. More common are alterations of the superior mesenteric vein, the splenic vein and/or the portal vein, initially demonstrated no more than angiographically. Back pain is generally caused by infiltration as a result of continuous tumour growth, or of extensive lymph node metastases into the retroperitoneum, or in the region of the coeliac trunk.

Although growth extending beyond the pancreas is very often encountered in pancreatic carcinoma and may entail local inoperability, this finding must, if necessary, be confirmed histologically, because one often finds peritumoral inflammation which may make it impossible even for the experienced surgeon to determine macroscopically, whether during exploration or on the basis of the operative specimen after surgery, precisely how far the tumour itself extends. This means, on the one hand, that inoperability (for example, apparent infiltration of the root of the mesentery) must be confirmed by means of intraoperative histological examination and, on the other hand, that the plane of resection, should resection be carried out, must be investigated for the possible presence of tumour tissue, especially if partial or even subtotal pancreatectomy has been per-

Table 4. Distribution of pancreatic carcinomas

Region of pancreas	Erlangen (1961–1981)		Becker et al. (1976)	Gudjonsson et al. (1978)	Klöppel et al. (1979b)
	Not resected	Resected	Autopsy material	Laparotomy ± resection	Autopsy material
Head	271 (79.2%)	52 (73%)	49 (53%)	51 (61%)	90 (69.8%)
Body	23 (6.7%)	5 (7%)	12 (13%)	7 (8%)	13 (10.1%)
Neck	11 (3.2%)	2 (3%)	16 (17%)	2 (2%)	17 (13.2%)
More than one region	37 (10.8%)	12 (17%)	16 (17%)	24 (29%)	9 (7.0%)
	342	71	93	84	129

Modified from Hermanek (1984).

Table 5. Tumour size and peripancreatic infiltration of ductal pancreatic carcinoma: histological findings after resection

Tumour diameter (mm)	Erlangen (1961–1981)		Klöppel et al. (1979 b)	
	n	Infiltration of peripancreatic tissue	*n*	Infiltration of peripancreatic tissue
11–20	6	2 (30%)	13	10 (77%)
21–30	18	11 (61%)	16	14 (88%)
31–40	10	4 (40%)	4	4 (100%)
41–50	12	6 (50%)	} 4	4 (100%)
>60	5	2 (40%)		

From Hermanek (1984).

formed. Residual tumour tissue is found later in 18%–45% of patients undergoing "radical" excision without intraoperative histology (Brooks and Culebras 1976; Castellanos et al. 1976; Collins et al. 1966; Forrest and Longmire 1979; Piorkowski et al. 1982; Warren et al. 1975).

Independently of the peritumoral inflammation, tumour-related stenosis of the pancreatic duct may lead not only to chronic pancreatitis in more peripheral parts of the organ, with all the morphological and histological consequences, but also to acute haemorrhagic-necrotizing pancreatitis.

The intracanalicular spread in the panreatic duct does not usually extend much more than 1–2 cm beyond the macroscopically visible border of the tumour, but has a bearing on the choice of the line of resection in partial subtotal duodenopancreatectomy.

Dispersal of tumour cells to the biopsy track after percutaneous needle biopsy (Smith et al. 1980), or to a percutaneous bile drainage tract (Kim et al. 1982) is an extremely rare occurence.

Histopathology

The classification of pancreatic carcinomas proposed by WHO (Gibson and Sobin 1978) is reproduced in Table 6. About 90% of all pancreatic carcinomas are of the ductal type.

In the section plane, ductal pancreatic carcinomas are moderately clearly delimited, compact, white nodules with no lobular structure. Diffusely infiltrating tumours may, however, include isolated normal lobules of parenchyma.

The histological variants of ductal carcinoma display differences in cytological architecture, in structural differentiation (tubulopapillary, tubular, solid, macradenous/micradenous), in mucous formation and in the nature of the stroma (dermoplastic or scirrhous carcinomas, carcinoma with osteoid formation).

For adenocarcinomas, the WHO classification provides for three grades of differentiation:

- Well differentiated: histologically and cytologically very similar to normal tissue
- Poorly differentiated: histological and cytological similarity to normal tissue discernible only with difficulty or not at all
- Moderately differentiated: tumours to which neither of the above descriptions applies

If different grades of differentiation are present, all must be taken into account and recorded.

The classification proposed by the American Joint Committee on Cancer (Beahrs and Myers 1983) also provides for three grades of malignancy, with the difference that only the least favourable grade present is recorded.

Multicentric growth

The reported frequency of multicentric growth in pancreatic carcinoma varies between 0% and 38% (Deixonne et al. 1986; Nagai et al. 1986). However, figures of over 15% include continuous tumour growth extending over several parts of the pancreas and non-invasive atypical proliferation of ductal epithelium, which can be referred to as dysplasia, or carcinoma in situ (Edis et al. 1980; Kozuka et al. 1979; Levin et al. 1978; Moossa 1982). Amongst our own patients, two of 69 resected ductal carcinomas (3%) turned out to be multicentric.

Lymphogenous Metastasis

Lymph channels lead from the pancreas to many lymph collecting stations, thus lymphogenous metastasis may be widespread. Two groups of *regional* lymph nodes must be distinguished: those near the pancreas (Fig. 3) and those somewhat further away. This second group includes the regional nodes along the superior mesenteric artery, the superior para-aortic nodes and the group of nodes at the coeliac trunk and at the porta hepatis (Fig. 4). The UICC classification of 1987 (Table 7) does not follow this subdivision (Hermanek and Sobin 1987).

Table 6. Classification of exocrine pancreatic carcinomas according to the WHO (Gibson and Sobin 1978), with frequencies among the patients of the University Department of Surgery, Erlangen (1961–1985)

Tumour type	Definition	Frequency (Erlangen)	
		All patients ($n = 524$)	Resected patients ($n = 113$)
Ductal pancreatic carcinoma			
Adenocarcinoma	Tumour forming glandular or papillary structures	457 (87.2%)	99 (87.6%)
Mucinous adenocarcinoma	Adenocarcinoma containing large amounts of extracellular mucus	19 (3.6%)	2 (1.8%)
Signet-ring cell carcinoma	Adenocarcinoma with prominent component of discrete cells distended with mucus	3 (0.6%)	–
Adenosquamous carcinoma	Adenocarcinoma containing unequivocal squamous carcinomatous elements, (keratin and/or intercellular bridges)	3 (0.6%)	1 (0.9%)
Squamous cell carcinoma	Tumour composed exclusively of cells showing squamous differentiation (intercellular bridges and/or keratin)	3 (0.6%)	–
Undifferentiated carcinoma	Epithelial tumour which is so poorly differentiated that it cannot be placed in any other category	29 (5.5%)	3 (2.7%)
Exocrine tumours with favorable prognosis			
Acinar cell carcinoma	Adenocarcinoma forming epithelial structures resembling pancreatic acinar tissue; identification requires absence of mucus and the positive demonstration of acinar cell characteristics	–	–
Cystadenocarcinoma	Cystic tumour, usually multilocular, lined by mucus-secreting epithelium, often with papillary infoldings	8 (1.5%)	6 (5.3%)
Low-grade papillary carcinoma	Not yet listed as separate category in WHO classification	2 (0.4%)	2 (1.8%)

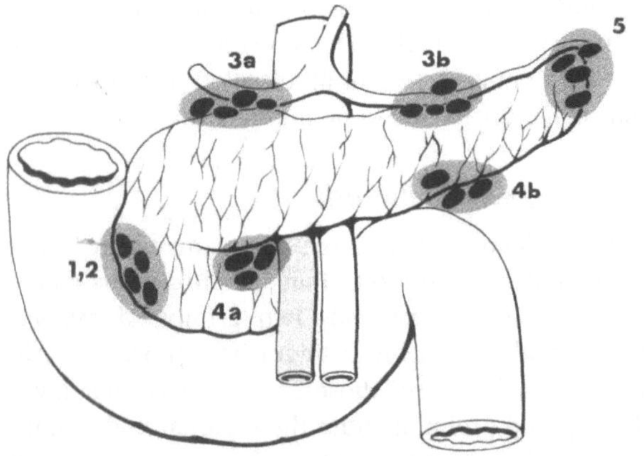

Fig. 3. Regional lymph nodes, first group. *1* Anterior duodenopancreatic; *2* posterior duodenopancreatic; *3* suprapancreatic: *a* head, *b* body/tail; *4* infrapancreatic: *a* head, *b* body/-tail; *5* splenic; *6* subpyloric or right gastroepiploic (not shown). (From Hermanek 1984)

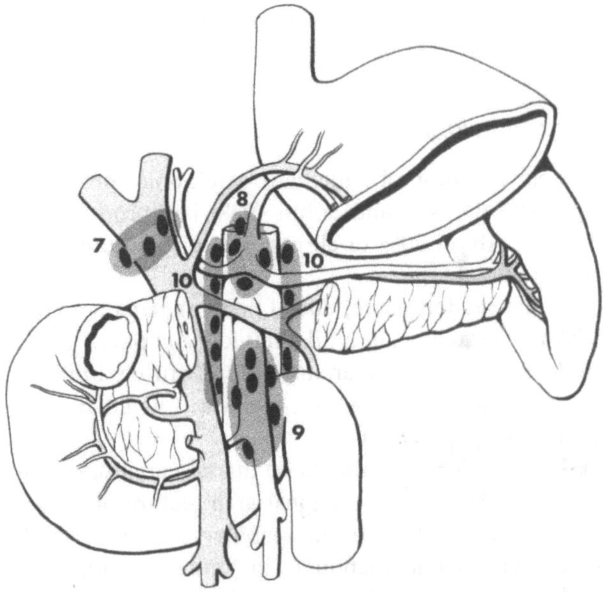

Fig. 4. Regional lymph nodes, second group. *7* At the porta hepatis; *8* celiac; *9* around the trunk of the superior mesenteric artery; *10* superior para-aortic. (From Hermanek 1984)

Table 7. TNM/pTNM classification and staging of pancreatic carcinoma

Rules for Classification

The classification applies only to carcinoma of the exocrine pancreas. There should be histological or cytological confirmation of the disease.

The following are the procedures for assessment of the T, N and M categories:

T categories Physical examination, imaging and/or surgical exploration
N categories Physical examination, imaging and/or surgical exploration
M categories Physical examination, imaging and/or surgical exploration

Anatomical Subsites

1. Head of pancreas[1]
2. Body of pancreas[2]
3. Tail of pancreas[3]
4. Entire pancreas

Notes: 1. Tumours of the head of the pancreas are those arising to the right of the left border of the superior mesenteric vein. The uncinate process is considered as part of the head.
2. Tumours of the body are those arising between the left border of the superior mesenteric vein and left border of the aorta.
3. Tumours of the tail are those arising between the left border of the aorta and the hilum of the spleen.

Regional Lymph Nodes

The regional lymph nodes are the peripancreatic nodes which may be subdivided as follows:

Superior Superior to head and body
Inferior Inferior to head and body
Anterior Anterior pancreaticoduodenal, pyloric and proximal mesenteric
Posterior Posterior pancreaticoduodenal, common bile duct and proximal mesenteric
Splenic Hilum of spleen and tail of pancreas

TNM Clinical Classification

T – Primary Tumour
TX Primary tumour cannot be assessed
T0 No evidence of primary tumour
T1 Tumour limited to the pancreas
T1a Tumour 2 cm or less in greatest dimension
T1b Tumour more than 2 cm in greatest dimension
T2 Tumour extends directly to any of the following: duodenum, bile duct, peripancreatic tissues
T3 Tumour extends directly to any of the following: stomach, spleen, colon, adjacent large vessels

N – Regional Lymph Nodes
NX Regional lymph nodes cannot be assessed
N0 No regional lymph node metastasis
N1 Regional lymph node metastasis

M – Distant Metastasis
MX Presence of distant metastasis cannot be assessed
M0 No distant metastasis
M1 Distant metastasis

pTNM Pathological Classification

The pT, pN and pM categories correspond to the T, N and M categories.

G Histopathological Grading

GX Grade of differentiation cannot be assessed
G1 Well differentiated
G2 Moderately differentiated
G3 Poorly differentiated
G4 Undifferentiated

Stage Grouping

Stage I	T1	N0	M0	(10 = 19%)[a]
	T2	N0	M0	
Stage II	T3	N0	M0	(2 = 4%)
Stage III	Any T	N1	M0	(38 = 72%)
Stage IV	Any T	Any N	M1	(2 = 4%)

From Hermanek and Sobin (1987).
[a] Frequency among ductal carcinomas resected in the University Department of Surgery, Erlangen, 1978–1982 (*n* = 53, unclassified 1 = 2%).

Ductal pancreatic carcinomas, even if small, are characterized by a high frequency of lymph node metastasis (Table 8). In tumours invading the peripancreatic tissue the rate reaches 80% or more, with involvement of the second group of regional nodes in about 30% (Gall et al. 1981; Hermanek and Giedl 1986). Even in small tumours, para-aortic nodes as far down as the trunk of the inferior mesenteric artery can be affected (Nagai et al. 1986).

One practical point of great significance is that we have hitherto observed no splenic lymph node metastases from carcinomas of the *head* of the pancreas.

It is essential that the surgeons remember the un-

Table 8. Ductal pancreatic carcinoma: lymphatic metastasis by tumour size and local infiltration (Erlangen 1961–1982)

	n	Lymph node metastases
Tumour size		
≤ 2.0 cm	7	4 (57%)
2.1–3.0 cm	25	16 (64%)
3.1–4.0 cm	10	9 (90%)
4.1–5.0 cm	6	5 (83%)
5.1–6.0 cm	7	6 (86%)
> 6 cm	11	8 (73%)
Confined to pancreas	9	4 (44%)
Peripancreatic infiltration	55	43 (78%)

Histological findings on tumour resection. Patients with insufficient data excluded.

Table 9. Correlation of local tumour infiltration with lymph node and distant metastasis in autopsy material

Extent of primary tumour	n	N0 M0	N+M0	N0 M1	N+M1
Confined to pancreas	2	1/2	-	1/2	-
Extending beyond pancreas	38	14%	14%	10%	62%
Infiltration of adjacent organs	79	3%	13%	3%	81%

From Klöppel et al. (1979 b).

reliability of macroscopic assessment of the regional lymph nodes: on histological examination Van Heerden et al. (1981) found metastases in about 50% of nodes which macroscopically appeared tumour-free.

Distant Metastases

The organ which is most frequently invaded by metastases of ductal pancreatic carcinoma is the liver. Circumscribed or diffuse lung involvement may also occasionally be the first manifestation of a pancreatic tumour (Rossman 1959).

In autopsy material, extrapancreatic tumour growth, lymph node and distant metastases are correlated (Klöppel et al. 1979 b) (Table 9). Amongst surgical patients, 31.3% display metastases in the liver, 1.8% to the lungs, 1.1% to the adrenals and 0.4% to the skin (Matsuno et al. 1986). Metastasis of regional lymph nodes, which according to the new UICC classification (Hermanek and Sobin 1987) also counts as distant metastasis, is present in 20.9%.

Diffuse peritoneal metastases are less frequent. Even in autopsy specimens they are found in only 22% of cases.

Characteristics of Exocrine Pancreatic Tumours with Favourable Prognosis

Acinar cell carcinoma and cystadenocarcinoma each accounts for only about 1% of pancreatic carcinomas.

Acinar cell carcinoma macroscopically resembles ductal pancreatic carcinoma. Histologically, the tumour cells are arranged in acini with a small central lumen. The tumour cells are large and polygonal, the cytoplasm is eosinophilically granulated and mucous formation is absent. Undifferentiated areas with small round cells may also be observed. The prognosis depends on the grade of differentiation. Well-differentiated acinar cell carcinomas may release lipolytic enzymes and cause tissue necrosis in the subcutis, the mesentery, the greater omentum and the fat marrow of the long tubular bones, as well as arthralgia. The tumours previously referred to as "metastasizing adenomas" belong to this type.

Cystadenocarcinoma is of ductal origin. The cysts are usually multilocular, but large unilocular cysts are occasionally formed. In multilocular tumours the cysts vary in size. Pancreatic cystadenocarcinomas are found mainly in the body and tail of the organ. Three times as many women as men are affected (Smithers et al. 1986).

In the case of single-cyst tumours, macroscopic differentiation from postpancreatic pseudocysts is almost impossible. For this reason, every cystic entity in the pancreas should be checked by means of intraoperative histological examination before fashioning a cystojejunostomy.

Two-thirds of all cystic mucigenous tumours of the pancreas are benign, the remaining one-third are malignant. Differentiation may be difficult and necessitates the preparation and analysis of a large number of tissue blocks, as atypias and infiltrations of the fibrous tissue can often be identified only on a few particular locations in the cyst. Cystadenocarcinomas probably arise from benign mucinous cystadenomas. Microcystic (glycogen-rich or serous) cystadenomas, on the other hand, do not tend to undergo malignant transformation.

A further malignant tumour of the exocrine pancreas is *low-grade papillary carcinoma* (synonyms: papillary cystic neoplasm, papillary epithelial neoplasm), which has been reported increasingly more often in recent years (Kaufman et al. 1986; Komorn et al. 1986; Rustin et al. 1986). This tumour occurs mainly in young women, displays predominantly local, infiltrating growth and seldom metastasizes. The prognosis is usually good.

The extremely rare pancreaticoblastoma in children should be considered a tumour of uncertain or multiple histogenesis, as should mixed-type acinar, ductal and/or endocrine carcinomas.

Other Malignancies of the Exocrine Pancreas

Non-epithelial pancreatic malignancies, such as fibrosarcoma, liposarcoma and angiosarcoma, neurogenic sarcomas and malignant fibrous histiocytomas are rare (Becker 1973; Cubilla and Fitzgerald 1980).

Periampullar Carcinoma

Tumour spread

Periampullar carcinomas spread exophytically in the ampulla and the duodenum, intracanalicularly in the common bile duct or the pancreatic duct, and also, especially in poorly differentiated tumours, by infiltration of the wall of the ampulla and the ducts, the neighbouring duodenal wall or the pancreatic tissue. The peripancreatic and periduodenal connective tissue is usually not reached until late in the development of the disease.

Cubilla and Fitzgerald (1984) describe a special form, namely intra-ampullar carcinoma, with a favorable prognosis as a result of early obstructive jaundice.

Periampullar tumours are considerably smaller than ductal carcinomas at the time of diagnosis. Of the 65 periampullar carcinomas resected in our own institution from 1961 to 1982, 9% were under 1 cm in diameter, 34% measured from 1.1 to 2 cm, 32% from 2.1 to 3 cm and only 17% were more than 3 cm (no exact measurements were made in the remaining 8%).

The first and almost the only lymphogenous metastasis is to the anterior and posterior duodenopancreatic nodes. Involvement of the nodes around the body or tail of the pancreas is almost unknown in operable patients. Similarly, intracanalicular spread towards the body of the pancreas, multicentricity and atypical hyerplasias of ductal epithelium in the body and tail need not be taken into consideration when planning surgery.

Histopathology

Periampullar carcinoma is classified according to the same criteria as ductal carcinoma (Table 6). Nevertheless, mucinous adenocarcinoma, adenosquamous carcinoma, signet-ring cell carcinoma and undifferentiated carcinoma rarely occur in the periampullar region. Tumours of this site are overwhelmingly adenocarcinomas, displaying tubular, papillary or tubopapillary structure. Polypoid ampullar carcinomas more often show a high grade of differentiation (Moossa 1982). They usually still contain residues of benign, generally villous, adenoma (Kozuka et al. 1981; Seifert 1982; Volkholz et al. 1981). Benign, usually villous, adenomas of the papillary region are very much rarer than carcinomas and are regarded as precancerous lesions. Papillary adenomas and papillary carcinomas are common in familial adenomatosis of the large intestine (Gardner's syndrome) (Bussey 1980). Definitive histological differentiation from periampullar carcinoma may be extremely difficult. Infiltrative growth is often demonstrated only after lengthy histological investigations of many sections. Endoscopic forceps biopsies which reveal only benign adenomatous structures by no means rule out carcinoma and for this reason a total biopsy is necessary, in the form of either snare biopsy or local surgical excision.

TNM/pTNM Classification and Staging

Pancreatic Carcinoma

The UICC introduced its first TNM/pTNM classification and staging system for pancreatic carcinoma in 1987 (Hermanek and Sobin 1987) (Table 7). Earlier classifications were published by Hermreck et al. (1974), the National Cancer Institute (Cubilla et al. 1978 a), Hollender and Meyer (1978), Gall et al. (1981) and Fortner (1981).

Tumours fulfilling the following conditions can be referred to as early carcinomas of the pancreas (Moossa and Levin 1981):

- Diameter under 2 cm
- No invasion of peripancreatic tissue
- No lymph node metastases
- No distant metastases (T1a, NO MO)

Early carcinomas are reported to comprise 0.4% of all diagnosed pancreatic carcinomas (Ichikawa 1986, personal communication). We found the same frequency (3/693) among our own patients from 1969 to 1984 (Gall and Kessler 1987). These three patients constituted 4% of our resected ductal pancreatic carcinomas.

Tsuchiya et al. (1986) state that 35.9% of pT1a pancreatic carcinomas already have lymph node metastases and thus can, by definition, no longer be referred to as early carcinomas.

Periampullar Carcinoma

The UICC also introduced a TNM/pTNM classification for periampullar carcinoma in 1987 (Hermanek and Sobin (1987) (Table 10).

Symptoms

Pancreatic Carcinoma

The most frequent symptoms of pancreatic carcinoma are weight loss, jaundice, upper abdominal pain and back pain (Table 11), all of which generally ap-

Table 10. TNM/pTNM classification and staging of carcinomas of the ampulla of Vater

Rules for Classification

The classification applies only to carcinoma. There should be histological confirmation of the disease.

The following are the procedures for assessment of the T, N and M categories:

T categories Physical examination, imaging and/or surgical exploration
N categories Physical examination, imaging and/or surgical exploration
M categories Physical examination, imaging and/or surgical exploration

Regional Lymph Nodes

The regional lymph nodes are:

Superior Superior to head and body of the pancreas
Inferior Inferior to head and body of the pancreas
Anterior Anterior pancreaticoduodenal, pyloric, and proximal mesenteric lymph nodes
Posterior Posterior pancreaticoduodenal, common bile duct, and proximal mesenteric

Note: The splenic lymph nodes and those at the tail of the pancreas are *not* regional; metastases of these lymph nodes are coded M1.

TNM Clinical Classification

T – Primary Tumour
TX Primary tumour cannot be assessed
T0 No evidence of primary tumour
Tis Carcinoma in situ

T1 Tumour limited to ampulla of Vater
T2 Tumour invades duodenal wall
T3 Tumour invades 2 cm or less into pancreas
T4 Tumour invades more than 2 cm into pancreas and/or into other adjacent organs

N – Regional Lymph Nodes
NX Regional lymph nodes cannot be assessed
N0 No regional lymph node metastasis
N1 Regional lymph node metastasis

M – Distant Metastasis
MX Presence of distant metastasis cannot be assessed
M0 No distant metastasis
M1 Distant metastasis

pTNM Pathological Classification

The pT, pN and pM categories correspond to the T, N and M categories.

G Histopathological Grading

GX Grade of differentiation cannot be assessed
G1 Well differentiated
G2 Moderately differentiated
G3 Poorly differentiated
G4 Undifferentiated

Stage Grouping

Stage 0	Tis	N0	M0
Stage I	T1	N0	M0
Stage II	T2	N0	M0
	T3	N0	M0
Stage III	T1	N1	M0
	T2	N1	M0
	T3	N1	M0
Stage IV	T4	Any N	M0
	Any T	Any N	M1

From Hermanek and Sobin (1987).

Table 11. Frequency of Symptoms before diagnosis of pancreatic carcinoma. (University Department of Medicine, Erlangen, 1971–1981; $n = 143$)

Symptom	%
Weight loss[a]	89
Upper abdominal pain	78
Lack of appetite	64
Jaundice	54
"Loss of energy"	39
Back pain	27
Vomiting	25
Diarrhea	24
Cholecystectomy	13

Modified from Lux and Lutz (1984).
[a] Mean weight loss 9.5 kg.

pear late in the course of the disease. With the exception of jaundice, which is 3 times as common in tumours of the head of the pancreas as in carcinomas of the body or tail of the organ, the symptoms do not vary with tumour location (Parker and Postlethwait 1985). Loss of appetite may occur early in the disease, with continuous, often marked, loss of weight. Fatty stools, denoting insufficiency of the exocrine pancreas, are observed only after destruction of two-thirds of the exocrine parenchyma. The pain is usually continuously progressive and epigastric or periumbilical in localization. At the time of diagnosis almost one-third of patients complain of severe, sometimes belt-like back pain and in the case of tumours of the head of the pancreas, pains radiating to the right shoulder-blade. Back pain is usually due to infiltration of the retroperitoneum and the solar plexus and then indicates inoperability.

With the exception of tumours in the immediate neighbourhood of the retropancreatic and intrapancreatic common bile duct, jaundice is also a late symptom. In most cases it develops without colics, but it is often associated with other kinds of pain. If the tumour has totally obstructed the bile duct the result is complete congestion with palpable enlargement of the gallbladder (Courvoisier's sign).

Psychic changes, including depression, sometimes occur months before clinical manifestation of the disease, as premonitory and prodromal signs. They probably represent a reaction to the unexplained upper abdominal symptoms. Thrombosis and thrombophlebitis are among the most frequent paraneoplastic phenomena in pancreatic carcinoma. Shivering, fever, haematemesis, melena and dermatomyositis are rare symptoms. Tryptic skin necrosis and joint pain occur only exceptionally, but are also observed in inflammatory conditions of the pancreas (Lux and Lutz 1984). A somewhat more frequent manifestation, particularly of small carcinomas close to the pancreatic duct, is a sometimes very severe haemorrhagic-necrotizing pancreatitis caused by obstruction of the duct. This possibility should be borne in mind in patients over 40 with acute pancreatitis of unexplained origin when ERCP, which we perform even during an attack of acute pancreatitis, reveals an interruption of the duct or a circumscribed narrowing of the main duct in an otherwise normal duct system.

Only 15% of patients consult a doctor within 1 month of the first symptoms, while 85% wait up to 6 months. Duration of symptoms for more than 2 years was observed in 13% of cases by Warren and Jefferson (1973). A delay in diagnosis on the part of the physician also seems to be fairly considerable. Moossa and Dawson (1981) report that 70% of patients in their study had undergone thorough examination, usually for biliary diseases, in the year preceding diagnosis. Another symptom which should give rise to suspicion of pancreatic carcinoma is the sudden onset of diabetes.

Periampullar Carcinoma

Jaundice in an otherwise symptom-free patient is the principal sign of periampullar carcinoma and occurs at an early stage of the disease. Upper abdominal pain and weight loss are each encountered in about 30% of cases. Manifest diabetes mellitus is found preoperatively in only about 7% of patients with periampullar carcinoma, as compared to 20%–30% of those with pancreatic carcinoma.

Gallstone disease is reported in 3 times as many patients with periampullar carcinoma as with ductal pancreatic carcinoma (20% vs 6%). Ten to eighteen per cent of patients with periampullar carcinoma have undergone biliary surgery between a few months and 4 years before definitive diagnosis (Moossa and Dawson 1981; Wise et al. 1976).

Screening for Asymptomatic Pancreatic Carcinoma

Pancreatic risk groups have hitherto been poorly defined, there are no established specific tumour markers, and even in the case of concrete suspicion, preoperative confirmation by ERCP and CT is successful in only 93% of cases (Moossa et al. 1980). For these reasons, specific screening for asymptomatic pancreatic carcinoma has not even been discussed hitherto.

In the context of general screening, sonography is the only fairly simple routine procedure which can be applied to the detection of pancreatic tumours. However, even sonographic evaluation is often hindered by air in the colon. The proportion of pancreatic carcinomas diagnosed in the asymptomatic stage as a result of screening, therefore, remains very small. Apart from this, even supplementary invasive diagnostic techniques often fail to differentiate pancreatic carcinoma from segmental pancreatitis with any certainty. Even after laparotomy with intraoperative punch biopsy, histological confirmation of a small pancreatic carcinoma is occasionally unsuccessful. We are convinced that the correct procedure in this situation (sonographic or CT suspicion of tumour, above all localized wall impression, or wall irregularity of the common bile duct, or the pancreatic duct, or displacement of these structures) is to resect the part of the pancreas affected. This is justified provided the surgeon can carry out the necessary surgery with an acceptable low risk of postoperative death. Our deviation from this practice in a few cases in recent years resulted in the deaths of two patients, about 1 year later, from pancreatic carcinomas that had not been confirmed initially. In contrast, there have been no postoperative deaths among patients who underwent resection for suspected carcinoma and turned out on histopathological analysis to have pancreatitis (Gall and Kessler 1987).

Diagnosis of Symptomatic Pancreatic and Periampullar Carcinoma

The information yielded by an investigation is usually discussed in terms of the specificity and sensitivity of the method. To assist interpretation of the data provided we wish to give a theoretical example: given a population of 100 000 containing 20 pancreatic carcinomas, in otherwise normal non-smokers, a marker substance with 90% sensitivity and 98% specificity will detect 18 of the 20 tumours, but will throw up about 2000 false positives, all of which will have to undergo the complete series of investigations (Holyoke et al. 1979).

Laboratory Investigations

Pancreatic carcinoma causes no specific changes in laboratory parameters. One indirect sign, an increase in gamma-GT and alkaline phosphatase, may precede the diagnosis of pancreatic carcinoma by a matter of months, even with alcohol abuse or in the absence of primary liver disease.

Only one substance, galactosyltransferase isoenzyme II (GT II), may, in future, be useful in detecting a high proportion of pancreatic carcinomas in combination with imaging techniques (Vilardell and Farré-Viladrich 1986). The sensitivity of GT II is 67.2% and the specificity 98.2%. However, it is also raised in the presence of other neoplasms.

The co-occurrence of diabetes and pancreatic carcinoma is well established. One-third of the patients with pancreatic carcinoma have manifest diabetes, a further third a diabetic metabolic state. In 69% of the patients reported by Moossa and Dawson (1981), the impairment had been present for less than 2 years.

Tumour Markers, Immunological and Chemical Investigation of the Pancreatic Secretion

Various tumour-associated antigens, such as CEA, AFP, Tennessee antigen and pancreatic oncofetal antigen (POA) may be increased in serum and in the pancreatic secretion in cases of pancreatic carcinoma. Their diagnostic value, however, is limited; they make no essential contribution to the differential diagnosis between carcinoma and chronic pancreatitis.

The highest predictive value among the tumour markers is currently displayed by the carbohydrate antigen 19-9 (CA 19-9) with sensitivity of 69–93% and specificity of 85% (Del Favero et al. 1986; Safi et al. 1986). The specificity, or rate of diagnosis, can be increased in combination with CEA, imaging techniques or fine-needle aspiration (Iishi et al. 1986; Tatsuta et al. 1985). However, CA 19-9 is much less informative in small tumours.

Another very promising tumour marker is the glycoprotein DU-PAN-2, which is raised in 94% of patients with pancreatic adenocarcinoma and returns to normal values after curative resection. DU-PAN-2 levels are increased in only 1% of normal healthy individuals (Makve et al. 1985).

Further promising markers are the leukocyte adherence inhibition test and POA, each with a sensitivity of up to 47.5% and a specificity of up to 89.9% (Moossa et al. 1980; Podolsky 1984).

Sonography

Pancreatic tumours of 2 cm or more in diameter are generally detected on sonography. Figures of 73%–94% are reported for sensitivity (Feinberg et al. 1977; Lutz 1987; Pollock and Taylor 1981; Rettenmeier 1976; Weill 1982) and 83%–96% for specificity.

The typical sonographic image in pancreatic carcinoma shows a localized enlargement of the pancreas with the fairly evenly echo-poor lesion standing out against the denser normal pancreatic tissue and surrounding structures. Smaller tumours have rounded contours, while larger tumours are irregular in form and sometimes display protrusions. Big tumours may show central zones of necrosis. A further sonographic sign which may indicate a pancreatic tumour is dilatation of the biliary tract. Obstruction of the pancreatic duct can also be demonstrated indirectly by distension of the duct to 3 mm or more. Finally, the generally echo-poor hepatic metastases indicate malignancy of a pancreatic lesion.

Differentiation between localized inflammatory processes and carcinoma of the pancreas is not possible by means of sonography alone, since in the absence of calcifications caused by inflammation the pictures are largely similar. Moreover, pancreatic carcinoma is known to occur simultaneously with pseudocysts and inflammation of the surrounding structures resulting from retention pancreatitis. It may also be difficult to differentiate pancreatic carcinoma from other tumours in the immediate neighbourhood, for instance bile duct carcinoma, lymph node metastases or infiltration from gastric carcinoma or carcinoma of the colon. Sonography does not yield reliable information on operability of pancreatic carcinomas: extensive peritumoral inflammation may simulate tumour infiltration of large vessels. Initial reports of endoscopic ultrasound have been optimistic: detection even of smaller lesions in the head of the pancreas seems to be improved (Strohm et al. 1984; Yasuda et al. 1984).

Conventional Radiography

With the recent advances in diagnosis, intravenous cholangiography has become obsolete in pancreatic carcinoma. Distension of the duodenal C-loop on conventional imaging of the gastroduodenal tract with contrast medium may point to a tumour of the head of the pancreas. Relevant functional pyloric or duodenal stenoses can be visualized by this method.

Mesentericography

Some investigators report the diagnostic accuracy of selective pancreatic angiography as 90% (Rosch and Keller 1981). Currently, the most significant contribution of this procedure is probably to the localization of endocrine pancreatic tumours.

The angiographic signs of a pancreatic tumour are pathological tumour vessels, displacement of arteries and infiltration, with stenosis, of long sections of arteries or of the splenic vein, the superior mesenteric vein or the portal vein. While constriction of the portal vein does not in itself represent a contra-indication to resection, infiltration of long sections of the common hepatic artery, the superior mesenteric artery, or the superior mesenteric vein is a sign of inoperability. In our experience, curative resection is possible in 70% of patients with a normal angiogram (Urakawa 1987).

Selective pancreatic angiography may make an important contribution to diagnosis when ERCP is not possible for anatomical reasons, or when the tumour is in the tail of the pancreas (Watanabe and Nishimura 1977).

According to Kümmerle et al. (1976), pancreatic carcinomas that can be visualized angiographically are rarely operable. Many surgeons demand a selective pancreatic angiogram before performing resection, in order to have a picture of any anomalies in the visceral arteries preoperatively, but in our experience this is not absolutely necessary.

Computed Tomography

Computed tomography (CT) is the second most important non-invasive diagnostic procedure after sonography, and is the principal imaging technique when the presence of a tumour in the body or the tail of the pancreas is uncertain. Ninety-five per cent of tumours with a diameter of 2 cm or more can be visualized (Ward et al. 1983). Smaller pancreatic tumours can generally be demonstrated only when they have caused a change in the shape of the organ, obstruction of the pancreatic duct or have infiltrated or displaced neighbouring organs and vessels (Bruch et al. 1987; Rosenberger et al. 1987). More than half of all pancreatic tumours are isodense without vascular enhancement.

Computed tomography is superior to sonography principally in the detection of hepatic metastases and the assessment of retroperitoneal or vascular infiltration and of enlarged lymph nodes (87% sensitivity and 90% specificity vs 69% and 82% respectively for sonography). In addition, sonography is technically unsatisfactory in 16% of cases (Hessel et al. 1982). One very important application is CT guidance of fine-needle aspiration in suspected pancreatic tumours (Wittenberg et al. 1984). The local operability of a pancreatic tumour cannot usually be determined on the basis of the CT scan alone.

Nuclear Magnetic Resonance

Nuclear magnetic resonance is still not universally available and its value in the diagnosis of pancreatic tumours is not yet clear (Ihse and Isaksson 1984).

Endoscopic Retrograde Cholangiopancreaticography

Endoscopic retrograde cholangiopancreaticography (ERCP) is always indicated when pancreatic carcinoma is suspected, but has not been demonstrated clearly by endoscopy, sonography or CT. With experience the imaging of pancreatic duct is successful in 92% of cases (Lux and Lutz 1984). In the remaining cases the endoscopic demonstration of tumour infiltration of the duodenum is sufficient to confirm the diagnosis.

In combination with ERCP, samples of pancreatic secretion can be collected for cytological examination. Furthermore, in the case of cholestasis, nasobiliary drains or endoprostheses can be inserted for drainage of the biliary tract.

The pancreaticographic findings (Fig. 5) may be the same in pancreatitis as in a pancreatic tumour, so the clinical findings must be borne in mind when interpreting the images. Solitary stenoses with irregular contours are a reliable sign of a carcinoma, as is

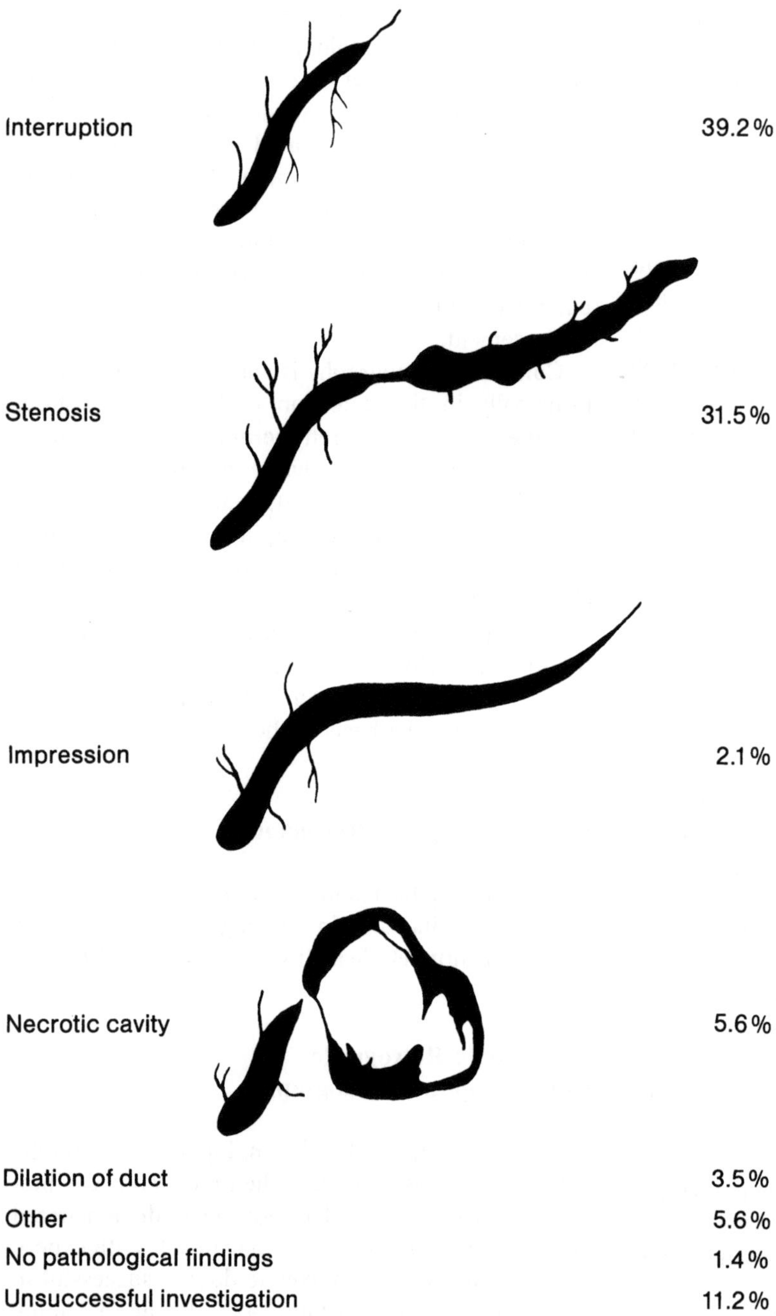

Fig. 5. Schematic diagrams and frequency of the various pathological findings in the pancreatic duct in 143 cases of pancreatic carcinoma. (From Lux and Lutz 1984)

the absence of post-stenotic changes, particularly in the side-branches (Anacker et al. 1975; Stadelmann et al. 1974). However, cyst formation and isolated stenoses are also found in 10% of cases of chronic pancreatitis (Classen et al. 1974).

In this context, circumscribed stenoses of the biliary tract are an additional sign of the presence of a pancreatic carcinoma, since, in most cases of chronic pancreatitis, there are long tubular stenoses of the distal common bile duct. The sensitivity of ERCP is reported as 80%–95%, the specificity as 90%–98% (Sirinek and Aust 1986).

The results of ERCP are distinctly better in tumours over 3 cm in diameter, than in smaller tumours (Yasuda et al. 1984). Combined with aspiration cytology, ERCP yields the correct diagnosis in about 90% of cases of pancreatic carcinoma.

Laparoscopy, Pancreatic Scintigraphy, Percutaneous Transhepatic Cholangiography

Laparoscopy, pancreatic scintigraphy and percutaneous transhepatic cholangiography have no current practical application in the diagnosis of pancreatic carcinoma.

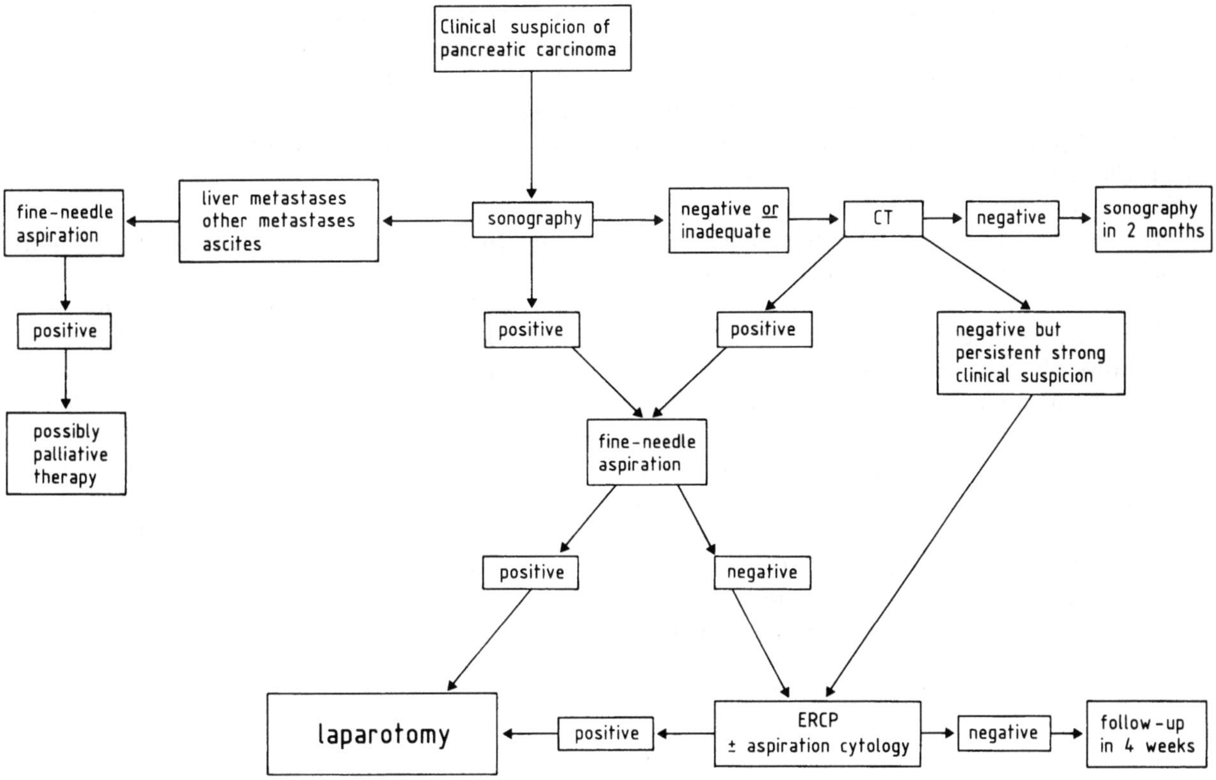

Fig. 6. Diagnostic strategy in the case of suspected pancreatic carcinoma

Micromorphological Diagnosis

Preoperative diagnosis of periampullar carcinomas usually ensues from examination of biopsy specimens obtained during gastroduodenoscopy. Forceps biopsy is useful only with obviously malignant findings: if the specimen contains only adenoma, snare biopsy or local excision is necessary for a definitive diagnosis.

In pancreatic carcinoma, forceps biopsy will be successful in confirmig the diagnosis preoperatively only in those cases where the tumour has broken through into the stomach or the duodenum. Laparoscopic biopsy seldom yields positive findings.

The choice of cytological investigations includes percutaneous ultrasound-guided or CT-guided fine-needle biopsy, endoscopic fine-needle biopsy and examination of the pancreatic juice and a brush smear from the pancreatic duct. The value of these techniques is limited by the 20%–30% false negative rate. The experience of the investigator is a crucial factor, especially with regard to cytological findings. False positives should not occur with experienced personnel (Gudjonsson et al. 1978; Malagelada 1979; Moossa and Dawson 1981; Seifert and Klöppel 1979).

Diagnostic Strategy if Carcinoma Is Suspected

The Erlangen strategy in the case of suspected pancreatic carcinoma is shown in Fig. 6. In order to diagnose pancreatic carcinoma at an early stage more frequently than has been the case hitherto, it seems particularly important to start paying closer attention to the previous history of the patient and to consistently take all appropriate diagnostic steps.

Surgical Therapy

Since chemotherapy and radiotherapy of pancreatic and periampullar carcinomas are largely ineffective as palliative measures, the only potentially curative means of treatment is surgical intervention. Even today, however, the operative mortality of pancreatic resection is 5%–15%. Since, in addition, the great majority of the patients are over 60 years of age, tumour resection should be performed only with curative intent. This was, in fact, possible in only about 30% of the patients with pancreatic carcinoma referred to our hospital for treatment. Hepatic metastases, juxtaregional lymph node metastases, large-scale invasion of the retroperitoneum or the root of the mesentery and ascites are all contraindications to pancreatic resection.

Confirmation of the criteria of local inoperability should be attempted by means of fine-needle biopsy. If this is not possible, exploratory laparotomy is indicated. The sonographic or CT demonstration of infiltration of neighbouring organs or the retroperitoneum is not sufficient to prove inoperability, as the accompanying peritumoral inflammation may simulate infiltration.

Obstructive jaundice is especially significant for preoperative planning. As a result of the often considerable delay in diagnosis, patients with this complication develop severe impairments of liver function, clotting and kidney function, distinctly increasing the risk associated with immediate radical surgery. However, preliminary biliary tract decompression by means of biliodigestive anastomoses or T drainage often renders a subsequent radical operation much more difficult by virtue of the sometimes considerable adhesions that ensue.

However valuable such operative bile draining techniques for normalization of liver function and coagulation may seem in the individual case, no clear benefit as regards mortality associated with the subsequent radical intervention has emerged from retrospective studies of operations with and without drainage (Kümmerle et al. 1976). Non-surgical means of preoperative bile drainage (endoscopic transpapillary insertion of bilioduodenal catheters, nasobiliary probe, percutaneous transhepatic drainage) should be preferred.

Percutaneous transhepatic bile drainage has the disadvantage of a complication rate of 10.1% and mortality of 1.6% (Hagenmüller and Classen 1982). Haemorrhages and bacterial infections are the principal complications. Endoscopic implantation of bilioduodenal endoprostheses fares somewhat better with a complication rate of 3.8%, though the mortality (1.7%) is similar (Hagenmüller and Soehendra 1983).

One particularly vociferous advocate of preliminary non-operative biliary drainage is Wiechel (1985), who observed no postoperative deaths among 74 patients undergoing subsequent radical resection of periampullar carcinomas. Opinions differ, however, in the literature. In prospective studies (Gundry et al. 1983; Hatfield et al. 1982), lowering of operative mortality by preoperative biliary decompression could not be conclusively demonstrated. The consensus is that jaundice of more than 4 weeks' duration with bilirubin concentrations over 20 mg% and consecutive liver insufficiency with serious impairment of blood clotting necessitates biliary drainage.

If cholestasis is of recent onset, associated disturbances of liver function and coagulation are usually only slight, so that in these cases there is no need to undertake drainage of the bile ducts, even endoscopically, before radical intervention.

Indications for the Various Curative Operations

The selection of the appropriate method for resection of carcinomas of the pancreas and the periampullar region is determined above all by the site of the tumour. The choice is between the following procedures:

- Right resection: partial or subtotal duodenopancreatectomy
- Total extirpation: conventional total duodenopancreatectomy or regional total duodenopancreatectomy
- Left resection: usually subtotal four-fifths resection for reasons of radicality
- Papillary excision

Partial Duodenopancreatectomy

The unilateral partial duodenopancreatectomy developed by Whipple (Whipple et al. 1935) is the classical radical operation for periampullar carcinoms. Since these tumours infiltrate the head of the pancreas only slightly, or not at all, a sufficiently large margin of clearance is guaranteed by partial duodenopancreatectomy, with division of the pancreas through the isthmus to the left of the portal vein. To ensure radicality, the uncinate process is removed completely – in contrast to the procedure in chronic pancreatitis – as this is the only way to allow systemic dissection of the regional lymph nodes of the first and second groups (see p. 583) along the mesenteric artery. Ductal carcinoma of the head of the pancreas is a definite contraindication to partial duodenopancreatectomy, as local recurrence rates of over 30% have been observed, due to the insufficient margin of clearance at the left border of resection (Brooks and Culebras 1976; Hicks and Brooks 1971; Ihse et al. 1977; Knight et al. 1978; Levin et al. 1978; Mongé et al. 1964a; ReMine et al. 1970).

Total Duodenopancreatectomy

Partial duodenopancreatectomy for ductal carcinoma of the head of the pancreas often leaves remnants of tumour which are detectable only microscopically at the lateral margin of resection (see above). For this reason, the long-term results of this operation proved unsatisfactory and total duodenopancreatectomy was very soon recommended for such tumours. Removal of the entire pancreas plainly obviates local recurrence at the margin of resection and avoids any chance of dissemination of the accumulated pancreatic juice from the pancreatic duct. A further argument for total extirpation is the occurrence of mulicentric pancreatic carcinoma, but the reported frequency of this varies. We have observed multicentric invasive growth in only 3% (2/69) of our pancreatic carcinoma patients.

Ductal pancreatic carcinoma can metastasize to many different groups of regional lymph nodes. Adequate dissection en bloc of all regional nodes is made much easier by total duodenopancreatectomy.

Another advantage of total extirpation of the organ is that pancreaticojejunal anastomosis is then not necessary because the pancreatic tissue is often friable; the fashioning of an anastomosis can easily lead to necrosis of the nearby pancreatic remnant and thus to insufficiency of the suturing, with a danger of peritonitis and pancreatic fistulae.

However, all these oncologically desirable advantages are gained at the price of considerable problems in the management of diabetes. In pancreoprivic diabetes there is no counter-regulation of the insulin level by glucagon, so fluctuations in blood sugar, which can lead to possibly fatal hypoglycemia shock, occur more frequently. In our view total duodenopancreatectomy is indicated in the following circumstances:

- Large ductal adenocarcinoma of the head of the pancreas infiltrating far into the body of the organ
- Carcinoma of the body of the pancreas extending into both the head and the tail
- Involvement of the whole organ.

Subtotal Duodenopancreatectomy

Total duodenopancreatectomy, despite its advantages, is burdened with a greater postoperative risk and a higher frequency of postoperative complications (Van Heerden et al. 1981; Herter et al. 1982; Kümmerle et al. 1984; Rückert and Kümmerle 1986) and for this reason we no longer employ it for ductal pancreatic carcinoma. Instead, we remove these tumours by means of subtotal duodenopancreatectomy, retaining a small remnant of pancreas on the left. This procedure should, however, be reserved for carcinomas of the head of the pancreas which extend only to, or slightly beyond, the isthmus and for tumours of the uncinate processus. Dividing the pancreas at the junction of the body and tail provides a 4.5 cm margin of clearance from the left border of the tumour, sufficient to ensure there will be no microscopic tumour residues at the line of resection. The preservation of the tail of the pancreas and the spleen does not violate the principle of radicality: Cubilla et al. (1978b) and Hermanek and Giedl (1987) found no involvement of the groups of lymph nodes at the hilus of the spleen in the cases of pancreatic carcinoma they studied. Subtotal pancreatic resection is also justified by the infrequency of multifocal tumours and the extremely low rate of second carcinoma in the pancreatic remnant.

The preservation of a distal remnant of pancreas has the advantage of averting diabetes in about two-thirds of the patients with normal carbohydrate metabolism before surgery. Our management of the retained stump of pancreas depends on the consistency of the pancreatic parenchyma. If there is distinct fibrosis as a result of retention pancreatitis, a pancreaticojejunal anastomosis is fashioned following occlusion of the pancreatic duct with an opacifying prolamine solution (Ethibloc). If the parenchyma is normal or friable in consistency, however, we forgo the creation of an anastomosis, choosing instead to occlude the duct system with prolamine and close the fishmouth-shaped plane of resection with interrupted sutures. This kind of closure of the pancreatic stump led, in 10% of cases, to a temporary pancreatic fistula, via the functional drain, which closed spontaneously some days later.

With subtotal duodenopancreatectomy, we have been able to achieve a decisive reduction in operative mortality, as compared to total extirpation, without sacrificing radicality. In our experience the postoperative course is also much less complicated than following total duodenopancreatectomy, hardly differing from partial duodenopancreatectomy in this respect.

Left Resection

Only rarely is a pancreatic carcinoma in the body or the tail of the organ diagnosed so early that it can be excised curatively, by means of subtotal left resection.

Smaller cystadenocarcinomas or endocrine tumours of the body and tail may permit left resection. In subtotal left resection the pancreas is divided to the right of the portal vein, enabling removal of the body and the tail of the pancreas with the spleen and the associated supra- and infrapancreatic lymph nodes as far as the portal vein.

Papillary Excision

Small periampullar carcinomas of the duodenal or ampullar type in older patients can be removed by means of local (papillary) excision if partial duodenopancreatectomy is no longer feasible because of increased operative risk.

Intraoperative Diagnosis, Local Inoperability, Resectability

Histological and Cytological Confirmation of Diagnosis

With the assistance of an experienced tumour pathologist, intraoperative histological confirmation of a pancreatic tumour is nowadays possible in the great majority of patients. In our hospital the rate of accurate diagnosis is 94% (Hermanek 1986 a).

The former practice of taking wedge-shaped biopsies from the tumour area has now been discontinued, since pancreatic fistulae, pacreatitis and bleeding may frequently ensue if the excision site is not removed in a subsequent resection. Since these wedge biopsies often sample tissue only from the marginal areas, in the presence of retention pancreatitis a carcinoma may be missed. Only tumours which make the surface of the pancreas bulge distinctly can be successfully diagnosed histologically by means of direct biopsy with a tangential incision, which has the advantage of obviating largely pancreas-specific complications.

For diagnosis of tumours of the head of the pancreas, we employ transduodenal punch biopsy with a Tru-Cut needle. The head of the pancreas, with the tumour, is mobilized according to Kocher and held between thumb and finger, the needle transfixing the duodenum by the shortest possible route before entering the pancreas (Fig. 7). Multiple puncture for tissue sampling is possible without increasing the risk of pancreatic fistulae and pancreatitis. Occasionally, however, there is bleeding from the parenchyma into the organ and, in exceptional cases clinically relevant pancreatitis appears. Tumours of the body and tail of the pancreas are punctured directly, sparing the pancreatic duct, if possible. Negative findings can be explained by the surgeon missing small tumours. Contrary to the many warnings in the literature, the appropriate technique of punch biopsy of the pancreas has revealed itself to be largely safe with a low complication rate (George et al. 1975; Hermanek 1983, 1986 a; Isaacson et al. 1974; Moossa 1982; Rosai 1981). Some authors prefer fine-needle biopsy for cytological diagnosis, as the smaller calibre of the neddle means that serious complications are unlikely (Bodner 1981; Gudjonsson et al. 1978). Only with experience on the part of the investigator can results be achieved which exhibit the same degree of comparability as those of biopsy excision of blocks of tissue. A compilation of data from the literature (Hermanek 1984) revealed average sensitivity of 83.2% for cytological diagnosis and 94.1% for histological examination of biopsy specimens. The surgeon should confirm the carcinoma histologically or cytologically before embarking on partial or total duodenopancreatectomy. This is possible nowadays in the overwhelming majority of cases. In cases where repeated punch biopsies of the suspicious area have failed to reveal a tumour, but the suspicion of carcinoma persists, we go on to resect the pancreas, on the grounds that a negative biopsy finding does not necessarily rule out malignancy (Bowden et al. 1965; Forrest and Longmire 1979; Fortner 1981; Gambill 1970; Hines and Burns 1976; Moossa 1982; Porter 1958; Trede 1982; Warren et al. 1962). An absolute precondition, however, is the presence of a tumour in the head of the pancreas which has been visualized on CT scan, the site of which, on bimanual palpation, agrees with the preoperative findings or which has led to compression of the bile duct or the pancreatic duct that is clearly documented on ERCP.

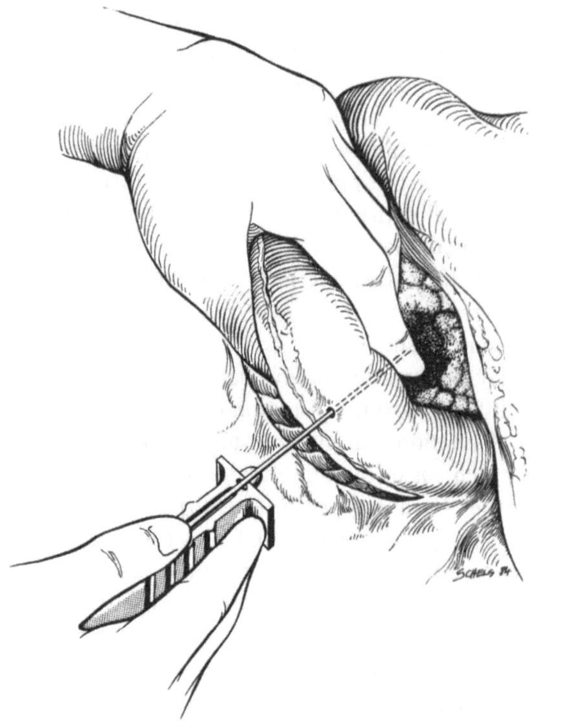

Fig. 7. Transduodenal punch biopsy of a pancreatic tumor using a Tru-cut needle. (From Gall and Zirngibl 1984)

We have followed up a few patients who did not undergo resection because their tumours were diagnosed histologically as benign, but who died 6 months to 1 year later of carcinoma of the pancreas.

A large tumorous process of the head of the pancreas, which seems, on the basis of the clinical symptoms, the preoperative diagnostic investigations and the intraoperative findings to have arisen against the background of chronic pancreatitis may indicate pancreatic resection in itself, without histological confirmation.

Intraoperative confirmation of the diagnosis is less difficult in periampullar carcinoma. The duodenal type is demonstrated by examination of a sufficiently large sample of the tumour excised locally after duodenotomy. Histological confirmation of the intra-ampullar type ensues by means of direct puncture of the bulging area of the papilla, also after duodenotomy. In the case of carcinoma of the distal common bile duct, the recommended procedure is either puncture following choledochotomy and intracanalicular needle advancement, or tissue sampling with biopsy forceps, or a sharp spoon.

Resectability, Local Inoperability

The criteria of resectability of pancreatic carcinoma are unmistakably influenced by the long-term results of surgical therapy, which remain very poor. The approaches to this problem vary all the way from extreme caution (Crile 1970) to ultraradical resection with removal of all pancreatic and juxtaregional lymph nodes from the diaphragm to the iliac bifurcation (Nagakawa et al. 1982) and additional resection of the retropancreatic segment of the portal vein and involved segments of artery (Fortner 1973). Despite differences of opinion, there are now generally recognized guidelines on the contraindications to radical surgery: proven distant metastases and tumour infiltration, whether diffuse or localized, into adjacent non curatively resectable extrapancreatic structures. It has been our experience that limited inflammatory processes close to a tumour can simulate tumour infiltration, so histological investigation of such local penetration is indispensable. Wide infiltration of the root of the mesentery along the superior mesenteric artery and vein, encirclement of the celiac trunk and an immobile carcinoma fixed in the retroperitoneum are all definitive criteria of inoperability. The same goes for diffuse permeation of the hepatoduodenal ligament with encircling of the proper hepatic artery, the portal vein and the common bile duct.

In the case of no more than circumscribed arterial infiltration, pancreatic resection, with resection of the involved arteries and implantation into the aorta, interposition of a vascular graft or anastomosis with the transposed splenic artery, has been carried out in selected cases (Fortner 1981). The effect of this extended operation on duration of survival cannot yet be assessed as there has been no large series, but one must be acquainted with these methods of vascular substitution in order to be able to complete the planned resection if arterial involvement is recognized too late to turn back.

In tumours of the head of the pancreas or the uncinate process, the retropancreatic segment of the portal vein can be infiltrated in a circumscribed fashion or obstructed with or without thrombosis. Many surgeons consider proof of such infiltration of the vessel wall to constitute inoperability, but in the context of total duodenopancreatectomy this complication can in fact be dealt with at no great risk, by transverse resection of the retropancreatic portion of the portal vein and end-to-end anastomosis without interposition of a synthetic graft.

The decision to extend the resection in the case of involvement of neighbouring organs (stomach, colon, adrenal) can be made only after histological classification of the tumour. Such extension is usually not justified in ductal carcinoma, with its generally unfavourable prognosis. If, on histology, the tumour turns out to be a less aggressive cystadenocarcinoma, acinar cell carcinoma or endocrine pancreatic carcinoma, extended resection en bloc, including the involved organs, is indicated.

The evaluation of regional lymph nodes no longer plays an important part in the assessment of resectability. The demonstration of a metastasized regional lymph node, previously sufficient for some surgeons to reject pancreatic resection, constitutes no contraindication provided the node concerned can be removed in the course of lymph node dissection. In the case of involvement of the juxtaregional lymph nodes, resection should not be performed unless indicated for other reasons. Hollender and Marrie (1981) carry out resection only when no more than three lymph nodes from four different defined groups are involved by carcinoma. Since the retropancreatic groups of lymph nodes are accessible only relatively late in the course of duodenopancreatectomy, we and others (Fortner 1981; Moossa 1982) omit biopsy of the regional lymph nodes, which are always removed systematically in the resection en bloc performed today.

Regional lymph node metastases which have grown together to form a conglomerate tumour including the vessels and fixed in the retroperitoneum obviously represent an absolute contraindication to resection.

Extended pancreatic resection is no longer indicated in the presence of histologically confirmed hepatic or peritoneal metastases. The removal of hepatic metastases, even if this were possible by means of local wedge excision or hemihepatectomy, does not prolong survival.

Resection Rates. A distinct improvement in the resection rate of periampullar carcinoma has been achieved during the past two decades. Jaundice is an early symptom of these tumours. The papillary region is easily accessible to diagnostic endoscopy and biopsy, so that advanced tumours are very seldom observed. Nowadays, 70%–85% of periampullar carcinomas can be curatively excised (Aston and Longmire 1973; Coutsoftides et al. 1977; Gall et al. 1981; Hollender and Marrie 1981; Nakase et al. 1977; Rückert and Kümmerle 1979; Van Heerden et al. 1981; Williams et al. 1979).

In ductal carcinoma, on the other hand, the situation has changed little despite new and more sophisticated diagnostic techniques and increasing surgical experience. The use of modern imaging procedures and ERCP has so far effected no great improvement in early diagnosis, so that the overwhelming majority of tumours are at a very advanced stage at the time of surgery. It is, therefore, not surprising that the resection rate for ductal pancreatic carcinoma, regardless of site, is only 15%–30% (Björck et al. 1981; Fortner 1984; Gall et al. 1981; Hollender and Marrie 1981; Kümmerle et al. 1984; Moossa 1982; Nakase et al. 1977; Shapiro 1975; Trede 1982).

Resection Techniques

Partial Duodenopancreatectomy

Partial duodenopancreatectomy is the preferred method for radical surgery of periampullar carcinomas. The distinguishing features as compared to the approach in benign processes (chronic pancreatitis) are the following:

- Histological confirmation and clarification of resectability
- Shifting of the line of resection of the left margin of the portal vein
- Complete excision of the uncinate process
- Right-side regional dissection of both groups of lymph nodes described above (see p. 583).

Resection of Head of Pancreas

The first step after laparotomy is painstaking inspection and palpation to exclude the presence of hepatic and peritoneal metastases. The head of the pancreas is exposed according to Kocher, so as to be able to check dorsal tumour penetration. The right flexure of the colon is then mobilized and the ileocolic vein identified. This vein serves as a guide for dissection up to its junction with the superior mesenteric vein. Incision of the omental bursa and upward retraction of the stomach then follows, facilitating the exposure of the portal vein at the inferior margin of the pancreas. Dissection along the colic vein also assist visualization of the portal vein. After ligation of the gastroepiploic vein, the anterior wall of the portal vein is exposed to view. The retroperitoneal freeing of the head of the pancreas must be accompanied by careful haemostasis, as icteric patients, in particular, tend to suffer widespread seeping haemorrhage with substantial loss of blood. The visualization of the retropancreatic segment of the portal vein represents the most important aspect of the exploration to determine resectability. Direct tumour contact with the wall of the vein is not often encountered in periampullar carcinoma. On elevating the inferior margin of the pancreas, this portion of the portal vein can largely be dissected free, under direct vision and using both blunt and sharp dissection, up to the surerior pancreatic margin. Attention must be paid to the inferior mesenteric vein and the splenic vein. Marked adhesions to the anterior wall of the vein should arouse suspicion of tumour infiltration. In this case blind, blunt dissection may easily result in laceration of the portal vein and the ensuing bleeding is hard to stem. Dorsal infiltration in tumours of the uncinate process is harder to evaluate than is ventral adhesion. After ligation of the veins which flow rightwards out of the uncinate processus and drain into the portal vein, however, the dorsal aspect of the portal vein can be exposed sufficiently to allow a clear demonstration of tumour invasion, if present. The last step is to check the hepatoduodenal ligament: tumour invasion from the superior pancreatic margin seldom reaches this far in periampullar carcinoma, but very frequently does so in carcinoma of the head of the pancreas.

Dissection of Regional Lymph Nodes

Since 1978, we have combined partial duodenopancreatectomy with systematic regional dissection of all groups of lymph nodes of both groups described

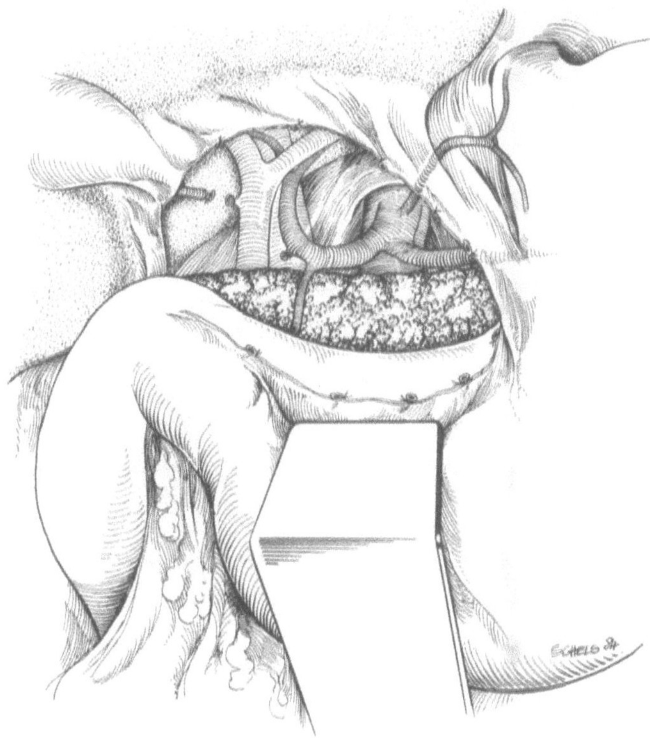

Fig. 8. Partial duodenopancreatectomy: situation after dissection of the hepatoduodenal ligament, the common hepatic artery and the celiac trunk. The right gastric artery has been divided and the gastroduodenal artery is exposed

above right of the aorta. The extra time this takes is minimal and we have not yet found any increase in surgical risk. Dissection in the subhepatic space is facilitated by two-thirds resection of the stomach and retraction of the inferior gastric stump caudally and to the right. After cholecystectomy and exposure of the common hepatic duct - taking care not to miss a possibly aberrant right hepatic artery dorsal and to the right of the common bile duct - lymph node dissection is commenced in the hepatoduodenal ligament at the porta hepatis. The common hepatic duct is divided cranial to the inflowing cystic duct and the chain of lymph nodes extending into the dorsal and ventral sides of the bile duct up to the porta hepatis is dissected away from the caudal direction. On the ventral side of the hepatoduodenal ligament dissection is continued along the right hepatic artery as far as the origins of the right gastric artery and the gastroduodenal artery, which are ligated and divided (Fig. 8). The lymph nodes at the left margin of the hepatoduodenal ligament are also freed from the portal vein, beginning at the porta hepatis and working distally. On exposing the common hepatic artery as far as the coeliac trunk these nodes are left in place on the surgical specimens in continuity with the upper pancreatic group of nodes. The dissection in this region is completed by ligation of the vena coronaria ventriculi and complete exposure of the ceoliac trunk, with removal of the lymph nodes along the right crus of the diaphragm.

The dorsal plane of dissection is represented by the anterior wall of the vena cava and the aorta (Fig. 9). Lymph node dissection caudal to the pancreas begins at the level of the origin of the inferior mesenteric artery with removal of the para-aortic and paracaval nodes en bloc with the surgical specimen as far as the level of the left renal vein. The superior mesenteric artery is reached 0.5–1 cm cranial to the left renal vein.

After raising the surgical specimen ventrally to the left, the dorsal aspect of the trunk of the superior mesenteric artery can be dissected away from the retroperitoneal connective tissue as far as the point where it enters the root of the mesentery without any danger of injuring lateral branches originating in this segment. This greatly facilitates the subsequent ventral exposure of the artery. The dorsal dissection is finished after the coeliac trunk is reached and exposed from the caudodorsal direction. Dissection of the uncinate processus may under some circumstances be facilitated by division, caudal to Treitz' ligament and skeletization, of the upper jejunum. Following this mobilization, the upper small intestine is drawn through under the root of the mesentery towards the right into the upper abdomen. The pancreas is divided after placement of sutures at the

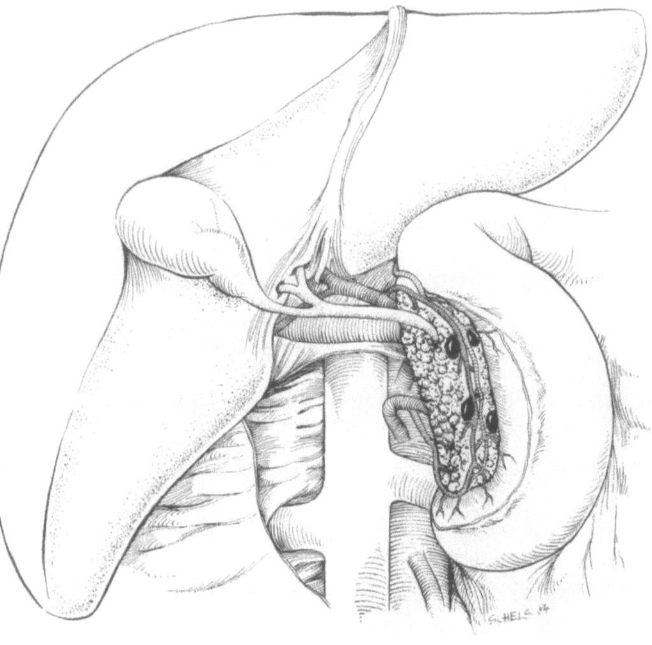

Fig. 9. Dorsal plane of dissection after clearance of the paracaval and para-aortic lymph nodes from the inferior mesenteric artery to behind the hepatoduodenal ligament

superior and inferior margins, left of the portal vein. Following careful displacement of the head of the pancreas to the right, the portal vein can be dissected away from the dorsal connective tissue and the uncinate processus. Veins draining into the portal vein from the dorsal must be identified and ligated. The surgical specimen then remains fixed in position only by its connective tissue adhesions to the superior mesenteric artery cranially and by the uncinate process hooking under the artery caudally (Fig. 10).

The trunk of the artery is located by means of palpation, and after the sharp division of the taut connective tissue at the anterior wall the artery is exposed from its point of origin from the aorta to the root of the mesentery. The surgical specimen is then tugged to the right and the last connections along the common hepatic artery as far as the coeliac trunk and along the superior mesenteric artery are dissected away stepwise, taking care not to damage the pancreaticoduodenal artery (usually two separate branches) where it originates from the right margin of the superior mesenteric artery. The final detachment of the uncinate process, which hooks under the mesenteric artery at this point, generally presents no problems after division of the pancreaticoduodenal branches.

Reconstruction of the Gastrointestinal Tract

The reconstruction of the gastrointestinal tract is carried out according to Child et al. (1978) with a retrocolically elevated loop of the upper small intestine. The weakest point of this reconstruction remains the pancreaticojejunal anastomosis. It can be fashioned without difficulty in chronic recurring pancreatitis because of the development of fibrous and connective tissue in the pancreas, but in resection of a carcinoma the normal soft, friable nature of the transverse section of the pancreas in the region of the line of resection, often only 1.5–2 cm in diameter, causes considerable problems of technique. However carefully the sutures are inserted there is a risk of segmental pancreatic necrosis resulting in postoperative suture insufficiency. The frequency of postoperative insufficiency and pancreatic fistulae is still reported as 10%–20% (Bodner 1981; Edis et al. 1980; Forrest and Longmire 1979). Because of the very good results achieved by means of occlusion of the pancreatic duct using prolamine (Ethibloc) in chronic pancreatitis, we have started occluding the duct of the pancreatic remnant in carcinoma surgery as well, in order to avoid such complications of the pancreaticojejunostomy. Despite this, we have experienced four cases of suture insufficiency in our patients in recent years: on surgical revision these failures were attributed to circumscribed pancreatic necrosis extending only slightly leftwards beyond the region of the anastomosis into the otherwise apparently normal remaining portion of the organ. This circumscribed necrosis is probably attributable to a local impairment of perfusion by one of the interrupted sutures. For this reason, we now omit pancreaticojejunostomy altogether in the case of a thin, friable pancreas, choosing instead blind closure of the pan-

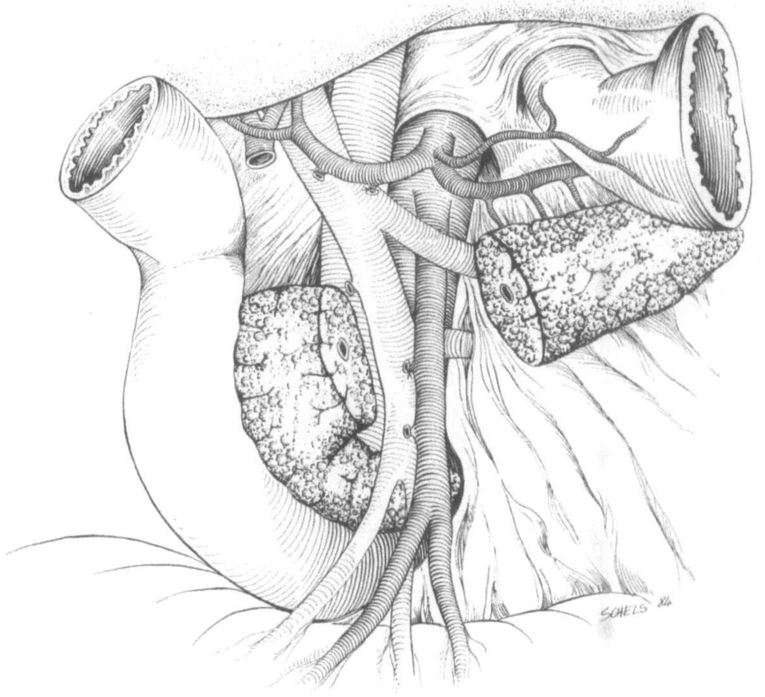

Fig. 10. Division of the pancreas left of the portal vein, complete detachment of the uncinate process after division of the pancreaticoduodenal branches

creatic stump with interrupted sutures after occlusion of the duct. Exocrine pancreatic insufficiency as a result of duct occlusion constitutes a relatively minor disadvantage, as lifelong substitution with preparations of pancreatic enzyme no longer presents problems. Most anastomoses of pancreas to small intestine probably become non-functional because of scar closure anyway, so that a loss of exocrine function in the long term must be assumed.

Subtotal Duodenopancreatectomy

Since 1980, we have been using subtotal instead of total duodenopancreatectomy to resect ductal carcinomas of the head of the pancreas which extend only slightly, if at all, to the region of the isthmus over the portal vein. Subtotal duodenopancreatectomy entails an extension of partial duodenopancreatectomy to the left. In our opinion, the subtotal operation may be employed when there is no tumour infiltration of the splenic vein. By contrast, Fortner (1984) performs subtotal duodenopancreatectomy with additional resection of the portal vein: in six out of eight patients it was necessary to remove the spleen because of venous congestion or a tear in the capsule.

The exposure and dissection of the head of the pancreas takes place as in partial duodenopancreatectomy, but for the subtotal resection the dissection is continued to the junction of the body and tail of the pancreas. On exposure of the splenic artery the suprapancreatic lymph nodes are left in place on the surgical specimen. When the lower margin of the pancreas is elevated, the visualization of the splenic vein and the ligation of the small lateral branches to the pancreas present no technical problems. This preparation can be facilitated by tunnelling the portal vein and then supporting the pancreas in a sling and pulling it in a ventral direction.

The lateral division of the organ ensues approximately halfway between the origin of the splenic artery and the hilus of the spleen, leaving a pancreatic stump 4–5 cm in length (Fig. 11).

After displacement of the pancreatic surgical specimen to the right, the splenic artery and splenic vein are elevated and the lymph nodes along the aorta are cleared. Our management of the pancreatic stump depends on the consistency of the parenchyma. If the pancreas is normal, i.e. somewhat friable, we do not fashion an anastomosis, but rather close the stump blind after occluding the pancreatic duct. This site is provided with a functional drain exiting to the left. Pancreatic fistulae have formed in only 10% of such cases and have always closed spontaneously within a short time.

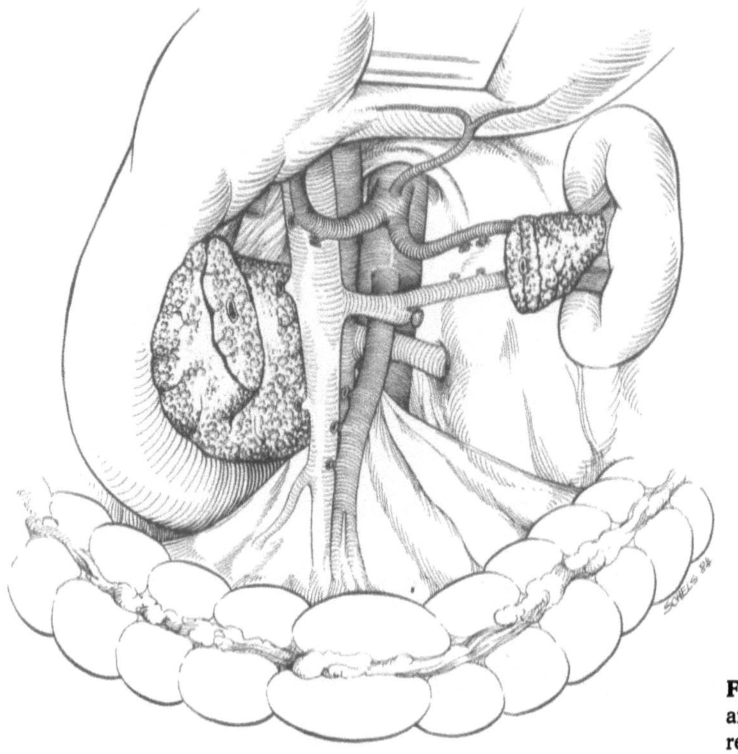

Fig. 11. Subtotal duodenopancreatectomy: situation after division of the pancreas and dissection of all regional lymph nodes

Total Duodenopancreatectomy

We combine total duodenopancreatectomy with regional lymph node dissection, the extent of which is portrayed in Fig. 12. The exposure of the head of the pancreas is as in partial duodenopancreatectomy, so only the left-sided pancreatic dissection will be described here.

After exposure of the coeliac trunk and ligation of the splenic artery at its origin, the gastric stump is retracted upwards and the left lateral lymph nodes from the limb of the diaphragm towards the hilus of the spleen are cleared, peeling the retroperitoneal tissue away from the aorta, the left crus of the diaphragm and the left adrenal capsule.

Mobilization of the left flexure of the colon facilitates access to the retroperitoneum. The spleen with the tail of the pancreas is now dissected away bit by bit from Gerota's fascia, exposing the left kidney, adrenal and renal vein. The supra- and infrapancreatic lymph nodes remain attached to the surgical specimen. Caution must be exercised in freeing the pancreas from the adrenal capsule, as laceration may well lead to diffuse haemorrhage, which in turn may necessitate excision of the adrenal.

When the dorsal dissection reaches the left margin of the aorta, dissection continues along the superior mesenteric artery, which has already been peeled away from the structures connected with it, working from right to left. Further detachment as far as the exposed portal vein now poses no great difficulty. After ligation of the splenic vein where it flows into the portal vein, the surgical specimen is displaced to the right, in order to be able to divide the structures connecting the head of the pancreas to the portal vein and the superior mesenteric artery and vein under direct vision.

In the case of tumour adhesion in the retropancreatic segment of the portal vein, after completion of left and right dissection the pancreas is connected only to the portal vein. In order to avoid portal haemorrhage due to passive hyperaemia in the intestinal region, the trunk of the superior mesenteric artery is clamped to reduce the blood flow to the area during resection of the portal vein. The portal vein is then clamped proximally and distally and divided at the superior and inferior margins of the pancreas and the surgical specimen is removed. On retracting the mesentery upward, an end-to-end anastomosis can be performed freely. In 22 duodenopancreatectomies with resection of the portal vein, we have not had to resort to inserting a prosthesis in one single case.

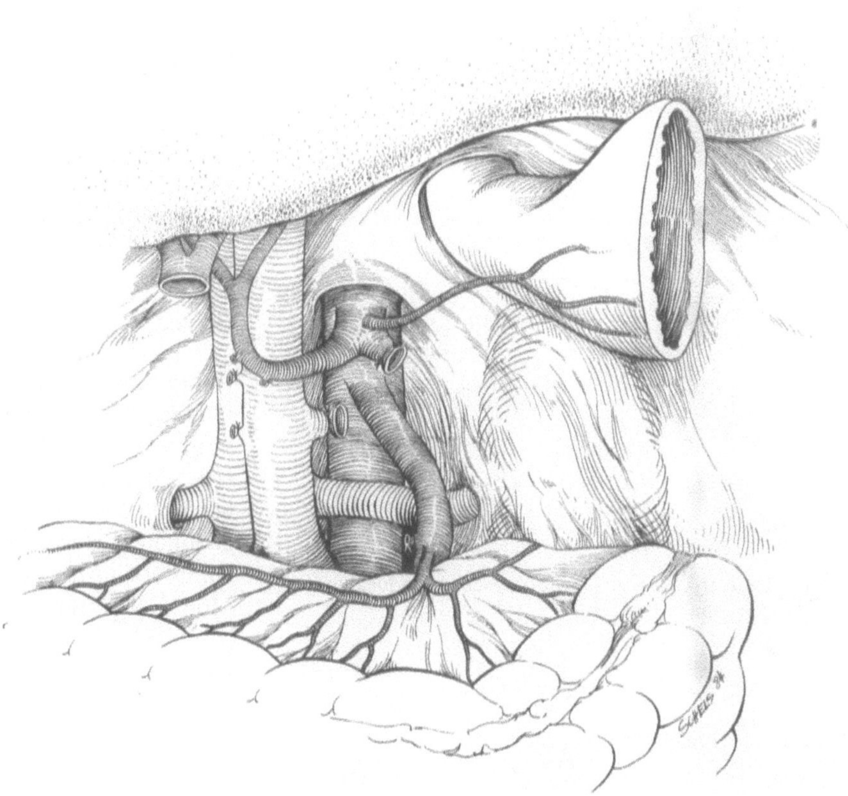

Fig. 12. Total duodenopancreatectomy: the limits of regional lymph node dissection

Left Resection

In tumours of the left side of the pancreas, for clarification of resectability, incision of the omental bursa and mobilization of the left flexure of the colon are followed by exposure of the full extent of the gland. Adenocarcinomas of the body and tail of the pancreas are rarely operable at the time of diagnosis: there is often already some degree of peripancreatic tumour infiltration cranially, caudally and dorsally into the retroperitoneum.

If operability is established, the first step comprises detachment of the greater omentum from the stomach along the greater curvature from the cardia to the pylorus, with ligation of the short gastric arteries and veins and the right gastroepiploic artery. There follows exposure of the common hepatic artery and identification of the celiac trunk with ligation of the trunk of the splenic artery. The retroperitoneum is then incised lateral to the spleen, the spleen is retracted upward, the tail of the pancreas is detached from the renal capsule, the splenic vein is ligated at its junction with the portal vein and the pancreas is divided to the right of the portal vein.

Extensive peritumoural callosities sometimes render left-to-right dissection extremely difficult. In this case it is better to divide the pancreas at the isthmus after exposure of the portal vein, in order to gain improved access for ligation of the splenic vein. The splenic artery is then exposed, ligated at its origin and the surgical specimen is scooped out from right to left.

The pancreatic duct of the remaining stump is sealed with a single purse-string ligature and the plane of the resection closed with interrupted sutures.

Papillary Excision

After mobilization according to Kocher, the duodenum is incised over the papillary region. The tumour is grasped with a clamp at its base and pulled ventrally to raise it from the posterior duodenal wall. The tumour is then excised in a circular fashion, using a diathermy knife, usually leaving a margin of clearance of no more than a few millimetres. Removal of the tumour leaves the congested common bile duct and pancreatic duct unattached; the lumina are sewn to the duodenal aperture, using interrupted sutures (Fig. 13).

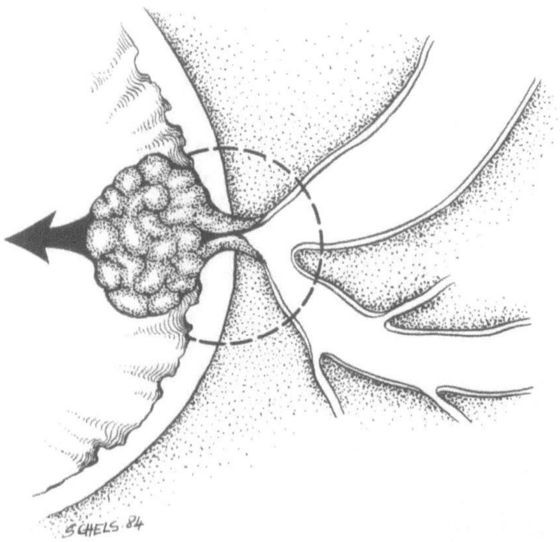

Fig. 13. Papillary excision: extent of resection in local excision of a papillary tumor

Non-resective Surgery

Because of the anatomical relationship of the head of the pancreas to the duodenum and the distal common bile duct, biliary and duodenal compression syndromes often develop when there are tumours of this region. Carcinomas of the head of the pancreas lead to obstructive jaundice in 65%–75% of cases. In addition, 40%–60% of such tumours display duodenal stenoses at the time of diagnosis (Moossa 1982) and in 5% the obstruction is complete (Sarr and Cameron 1982). Palliative diversions to deal with biliodigestive and gastroenteric obstruction are employed in cases of proven inoperability. Very occasionally, it is necessary to bypass stenoses of the transverse colon or small intestinal stenoses distal to Treitz' ligament by means of enteroenteric anastomoses. Cattell (1947) recommended palliative decompression of the post-stenotically dilatated pancreatic duct by means of pancreaticojejunostomy, claiming a pain-alleviating effect, but this technique has not been widely adopted.

Biliary Tract Drainage

Obstruction by the tumour leads to mechanical jaundice with unbearable itching, cholangitis, liver insufficiency and life-threatening bleeding due to coagulopathy (Moossa 1982). A large number of methods are available for surgical biliary decompression by means of anastomosis of the extrahepatic bile ducts with the stomach, duodenum or upper jejunum. One of these, cholecystogastrostomy, should no longer be employed because of the frequent reflux of food into the gallbladder with recurrent cholangitis. A factor which speaks against cholecystoduodenostomy, or choledochoduodenostomy, is the close proximity of the tumour to the anastomosis, which may then become prematurely non-functioning due to stenosis caused by tumour growth.

Cholecystojejunostomy

A prerequisite for cholecystojejunostomy is confirmation by preoperative or intraoperative cholangiography of a marked dilatation of the cystic duct. If this duct is narrow and tortuous, the drainage achieved by a gallbladder anastomosis is usually inadequate. Later dilatation of the cystic duct after decompression of the gallbladder cannot be expected. Moreover, ascending cholangitides may easily result in obliteration of a narrow cystic duct. Proven tumour invasion of the hepatoduodenal ligament is also a contraindication to cholecystojejunostomy, because progressing tumour infiltration blocks the lower part of the cystic duct at an early stage.

Hepaticojejunostomy

These has come to be a clear preference for hepaticojejunostomy, since the fashioning of a high anastomosis between the common hepatic duct, or its bifurcation, and a Roux-en-Y loop of small intestine is facilitated by the usually considerable dilatation of the proximal bile ducts. The high anastomosis also guarantees a large margin between the site of the operation and the upper border of the tumour, so that the anastomosis will remain patent even in the case of later infiltration of the hepatoduodenal ligament.

Gastrojejunostomy

Simultaneous creation of a gastrojejunostomy is always indicated in clinically manifest duodenal obstruction, or when tumour constriction is demonstrated intraoperatively. Opinions differ, however, regarding the advisability of gastrojejunostomy after every biliodigestive anastomosis for mechanical jaundice. In a compilation study by Sarr and Cameron (1982), repeat laparotomy for subsequent duodenal obstruction was necessary in 2%–50% (average 13%) of cases after biliary decompression. The simultaneous fashioning of a gastrojejunostomy had no effect on operative mortality (18% after biliary decompression alone, 17% with additional gastrotejunostomy). For this reason, simultaneous gastrojejunostomy is advisable, particularly in younger patients who may be expected to live longer (Diamond and Fisher 1975; Forrest and Longmire 1979; Herter et al. 1982; Moossa et al. 1979; Sarr and Cameron 1982). The risk of ulceration of the anastomosis in the course of the average survival of 8.5 months is reported as 3% (Sarr and Cameron 1982). The combination of gastroenterostomy with truncal vagotomy has often been advised, but we have never yet followed this recommendation.

Technique of Combined Biliodigestive and Gastrojenunal Diversion

The type of biliodigestive anastomosis we prefer in inoperable pancreatic carcinoma is hepatojejunostomy. After excision of the gallbladder, the common hepatic duct is divided as far proximally as possible. The distal bile duct stump is closed blind. The small intestine is divided sufficiently distal, about 50 cm from Treitz' ligament and the distal part is drawn retrocolically up to the porta hepatis. The anastomosis is carried out with thin resorbable sutures (4/0). The stitches pierce the whole wall of the bile duct, but only the serous and muscular layers of the intestine. This suture technique obviates strangulation and ischemia of the intestinal mucosa, which after the sutures are tied, prolapses into the bile duct and covers the anastomosis. The proximal loop of small intestine is then also drawn up retrocolically and anastomosed longitudinally with the posterior wall of the stomach. The end leading from the gastroenterostomy is then implanted in Y fashion in the distal loop of small intestine which has been anastomosed with the bile duct (Fig. 14).

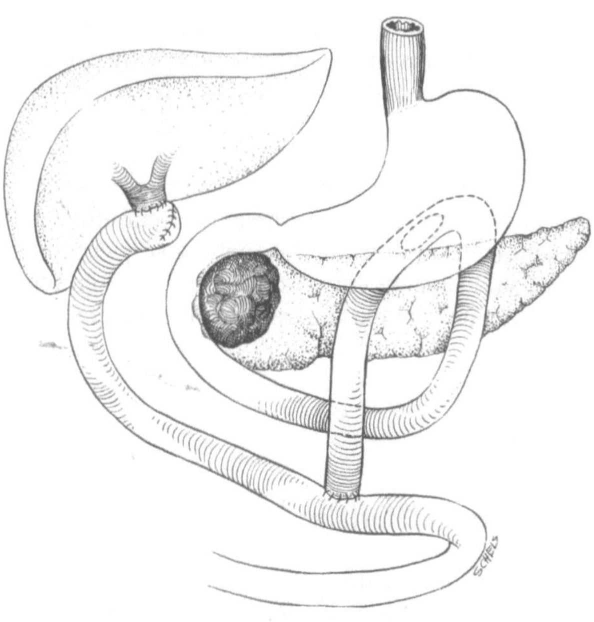

Fig. 14. Combined biliodigestive and gastrojejunal bypass operation

Endoscopic Bile Duct Decompression

Endoscopically placed nasobiliary drains, biliodudenal catheters (e.g. pigtail catheter) and endoscopic papillotomy have established themselves as alternatives to surgery for biliary decompression. They bear the advantage of low primary mortality, around 1.5%–2% (Hagenmüller and Classen 1982; Hagenmüller and Soehendra 1983; Riemann and Demling 1985), but suffer the disadvantage of frequent catheter changes as a result of occlusion and recurrent cholangitis.

These methods are nowadays part of the standard repertoire of any experienced gastroenterologist. They not only enable largely problem-free preoperative decompression of obstructive jaundice, but may also obviate laparotomy in some icteric patients whose tumours are definitely inoperable. The danger exists, however, that endoscopic procedures may be selected too often. We know from our own experience that internists sometimes postulate inoperability on grounds of age and insert a palliative endoprosthesis without even referring the patients to an experienced surgeon, thus throwing away the chance of curative radical surgery of tumours which are actually operable. In many cases, the possibility of radical surgery can be excluded only on laparotomy.

Surgery of Local Recurrences and Distant Metastases

With both ductal pancreatic carcinoma and periampullar carcinoma, local recurrences may occur in the pancreatic remnant, the root of the mesentery or in the position previously occupied by the pancreas. As a consequence of the broad infiltration of the retroperitoneum and of neighbouring organs, the prospects of being able to eliminate these recurrences are extremely remote. Because of the generally poor prognosis of ductal pancreatic carcinoma, operative excision of distant metastases in the liver or lung is inappropriate. Metastases of periampullar carcinoma can be dealt with according to the general rules for such surgery – solitary focus, exclusion of further distant metastases, limited intervention (e.g. wedge or partial liver resection, pulmonary wedge excision). The operative risk should be kept minimal, as the effect of such measures on the long-term prognosis cannot yet be evaluated.

Non-surgical Therapy

Carcinoma of the pancreas and the periampullar region can hitherto be cured only by surgery. The cure rate, however, remains low and for this reason adjuvant treatment following curative surgical resection has been investigated, with the main focus of interest being on intraoperative radiotherapy. This apparently prevents local recurrence in the radiation field, but the long-term survival rates are not affected (Hiraoka et al. 1984; Shipley et al. 1984 a).

Adjuvant external radiotherapy in combination with 5-fluorouracil (5-FU), on the other hand, seems to improve the cure rate significantly (Kalser and Ellenberg 1985). Greater experience is needed before this technique can be evaluated definitively.

Reduction of tumour-related pain and prolongation of survival time can apparently be achieved by intraoperative irradiation of non-resectable tumours (Nishimura et al. 1984; Shipley et al. 1984 b). The best results are obtained with the combination of local irradiation, implantation of ^{125}I seeds and chemotherapy (Dobelbower et al. 1986; Morrow et al. 1984; Wittington 1984). However, these methods need further investigation, as various studies have shown no discernable advantage in combination treatment (Gastrointestinal Tumour Study Group 1985), haemorrhage and obstruction have been observed in 50% of cases (Skibber et al. 1985), and local complications of the interstitial implantation of radioisotopes have resulted in perioperative mortality of up to 25% (Dobelbower and Milligan 1984).

High-frequency hyperthermia (Falk et al. 1986) and percutaneous intraluminal radionuclide therapy (Cutherell et al. 1986) are so far only experimental.

The value of chemotherapy remains unclear, but it has hitherto shown no promise as sole adjuvant treatment after macroscopically curative resection.

For palliative treatment, combinations of 5-FU + doxorubicin + mitomycin C (FAM) or streptozotocin + mitomycin C + 5-FU (SMF) seem superior to any of these drugs administered alone. Response rates of around 40% have been reported (review: Baumel and Deixonne 1986; Harvey and Schein 1984). However, a recent study of a larger patient population (Oster et al. 1986) did not confirm these results in advanced pancreatic carcinoma: the response rates were 14% with FAM and 4% with SMF.

Alleviation of pain is an important aspect of the treatment of patients with inoperable carcinoma infiltrating the hypogastric plexus. Beside intraoperative direct or later translumbar injection of the nerve plexus with about 20 ml 5% phenol or 80% alcohol, methods include neurosurgical interventions (e.g. unilateral or bilateral chordotomy), a peridural indwelling catheter and systemic administration of powerful analgesics.

Follow-up

Disturbances of carbohydrate metabolism and of digestion represent the main foci of attention in the postoperative care of patients with curatively resected pancreatic carcinoma. The carbohydrate metabolism must be regularly monitored, and if diabetes is observed it must be stabilized using the standard methods. Considerable problems may be encountered, particularly after total pancreatectomy.

Exocrine pancreatic insufficiency, whether immediate (after duct occlusion) or slowly developing (after obstruction of a pancreaticojejunal anastomosis) must be compensated by enzyme substitution.

Apart from clinical examination, the most important techniques for detection of local recurrences and distant metastases after curative surgery and for observation for progress during chemotherapy or radiotherapy are upper abdominal sonography and CT and lung X-ray. The tumour markers CA 19-9 and DU-PAN-2 seem to be useful for the early detection of recurrences and the evaluation of response to non-surgical treatment.

All programmes of follow-up after curative surgery usually consist of no more than checking for recurrences. Operative treatment of recurrences and distant metastases is possible only in very occasional cases, and chemotherapy or radiotherapy is currently indicated only within the framework of clinical trials.

Prognosis

Postoperative Mortality

In the past decade there has been a distinct decrease in postoperative mortality following resection of periampullar and ductal carcinoma. Through the concentration of patients in centres with more experience, postoperative complications which used to be frequent and often fatal, such as pancreatic fistulae, pancreatic necrosis and suture insufficiency, can be increasingly avoided.

Partial Duodenopancreatectomy

Earlier large compilation studies reported 20%–25% postoperative mortality after resection of the head of the pancreas (Fish and Cleveland 1964; Hermann 1979; Levin et al. 1978; Shapiro 1975), but from about the beginning of the 1970s the rate sank to around 15% (Tables 12, 13), and a further reduction to ca. 10% postoperative mortality after partial duodenopancreatectomy has been recorded recently (Kairahuoma et al. 1987; Matsuno and Sato 1986; Moossa et al. 1984; Tarazi et al. 1986). The outstanding results described by Van Heerden et al. (1984) and Trede (1985) – 4% and 1.1% respectively – represent the exception.

Table 12. Periampullar carcinoma: results of partial duodenopancreatectomy

Reference		*n*	Operative mortality (%)	Mean/median survival time (months)	Five-year survival rate excluding operative mortality (%)
Mongé et al. (1964 b)		120	18		24
Smith (1973)		180	4		30
Warren et al. (1975)		193	15		28
Sato et al. (1977)[a]		46	7		19
Forrest and Longmire (1979)[b]		30	13	44	21
Rückert and Kümmerle (1979)[c]		37	14		27
Sellner and Jellinek (1979)		25	20		30
Williams et al. (1979)[a]		27	11		27
Björck et al. (1981)		26	15		27
Cooperman et al. (1981)		56	14	30	25
Walsh et al. (1982)		44	16		16
Average[d]		784	13.4	–	24.9
Univ. Dept. Surgery,	1961–1977	18	22	30.1	42 ± 18%[e]
Erlangen	1978–1982	32	13		

[a] With one total duodenopancreatectomy.
[b] With four total duodenopancreatectomies.
[c] With six total duodenopancreatectomies.
[d] Calculated as arithmetic mean without weighting for patient numbers.
[e] 95% confidence limits.

Table 13. Ductal carcinoma of head of pancreas: results of partial duodenopancreatectomy

Reference		*n*	Operative mortality (%)	Mean/median survival time (months)	Five-year survival rate excluding operative mortality (%)
Aston and Longmire (1973)		39	10	15.4	6
Smith (1973)		44	21		6
Hermreck et al. (1974)		50	28	11.4	11
Shapiro (1975)		24	8	10.6	0
Coutsoftides et al. (1977)		23	12	15.0	0
Child et al. (1978)		26	19		
Forrest and Longmire (1979)		50	12	16.2	4
Edis et al. (1980)		124	16	10.0	5
Björck et al. (1981)		62	10		8
Cooperman et al. (1981)		27	11	15.0	11
van Heerden et al. (1981)		141	12		5
Cohen et al. (1982)		36	16	9.0	0
Average[a]		646	14.6	12.8	5.1
Univ. Dept. Surgery,	1961–1977	11	27	14.8	16 + 21%[b]
Erlangen	1978–1982	9	11		

[a] Calculated as arithmetic mean without weighting for patient numbers.
[b] 95% confidence limits.

Table 14. Ductal pancreatic carcinoma: results of total pancreatectomy

Reference		n	Operative mortality (%)	Mean/median survival time (months)	Five-year survival rate excluding operative mortality (%)
Pliam and Remine (1975)		33	21		14
Ihse et al. (1977)		58	23	20	4
Tryka and Brooks (1979)		25	12	24	18
Edis et al. (1980)		38	16	10	3
Cooperman et al. (1981)		43	28	15	6
van Heerden et al. (1981)		51	14	13	2
Moossa and Levin (1981)		45	9		
Fortner (1984)[a]		35	26	13	0
Average[b]		328	18.6	15.8	6.7
Univ. Dept. Surgery,	1961–1977	2	(50)	7.1	0
Erlangen	1978–1982	18	22		

[a] Regional duodenopancreatectomy: usually total, in a few cases subtotal.
[b] Calculated as arithmetic mean without weighting for patient numbers.

Total Duodenopancreatectomy

Total duodenopancreatectomy generally involves higher mortality than Whipple's operation, despite the fact that no pancreaticojejunal anastomosis is performed and therefore that the specific problems associated with this procedure do not arise (Table 14).

Extension of the operation to include regional lymph node dissection seems to have no unfavourable influence on operative risk, as Fortner (1984) reports 8% postoperative mortality since 1979 and other authors describe similar results (Matsuno and Sato 1986; Trede 1985; Van Heerden 1984).

Subtotal Duodenopancreatectomy

In the University Department of Surgery, Erlangen, subtotal duodenopancreatectomy has been performed in 37 patients (28 ductal carcinomas, nine large periampullar carcinomas with wide infiltration of the head of the pancreas) since 1980. There was only one postoperative death, caused by suture insufficiency of the pancreaticojejunostomy (Gall 1986). The postoperative mortality among our patients is thus 3%, much lower than our figure of 22% (4/18) for total pancreatectomy from 1978 to 1982. The literature contains only one other report of the mortality associated with subtotal duodenopancreatectomy: Fortner (1984) mentioned eight operations with no fatalities and shares our opinion that the subtotal procedure should be preferred to total pancreatectomy.

Left Resection

Left resection is the standard procedure for chronic pancreatitis of the tail of the pancreas and in this context displays an operative mortality of 5% (Gebhardt 1984), but it is seldom used as a therapeutic intervention in carcinomas of this region. The generally scanty reports in the literature indicate an average mortality of 25% (Coutsofides et al. 1977; Forrest and Longmire 1979; Herter et al. 1982; Knight et al. 1978; Longmire and Traverso 1981). However, the case numbers are low and the range of mortality wide. In Erlangen we lost none of the five patients who underwent left-sided four-fifths resection of a ductal carcinoma of the tail of the pancreas between 1961 and 1982.

Bypass Surgery

The operative mortality after bypass surgery of nonresectable tumours is 14% in our survey of the literature (Table 15) and 18% in a review by Sarr and Cameron (1984). The mean duration of survival worldwide is 6 months.

Exploratory Laparotomy

Purely exploratory laparotomy shows an average mortality of 32.5% (Table 16) – an expression of the advanced nature of the disease. Sarr and Cameron (1984) performed a survey and reported mortality of 27% with mean survival of 3.4 months.

Table 15. Ductal pancreatic carcinoma: results of bypass operation

Reference		n	Operative mortality (%)	Mean/median survival time (months)
Bowden et al. (1965)		114	5	5.0
Hermreck et al. (1974)		172	24	5.0
Hertzberg (1974)		148	13	6.8
Shapiro (1975)		24	4	8.1
Brooks and Culebras (1976)		35	14	5.6
Coutsoftides et al. (1977)		125	12	7.4
Trede et al. (1977)		43	32	1.5
Hoitsma et al. (1978)		35	14	9.5
Hollender (1978)		83	17	4.8
Knight et al. (1978)		153	22	6.7
Sato et al. (1978)		59	19	4.5
Forrest and Longmire (1979)		103	20	5.5
Jain et al. (1979)		92	22	7.0
Moossa et al. (1979)		31	7	6.0
Reed et al. (1979)		101	13	7.7
Schmid (1979)		33	9	4.8
Tryka and Brooks (1979)		35	14	5.6
van Heerden et al. (1981)		151	6	6.0
Ross and Jonas (1980)		55	13	6.7
Wangsuwanpor and Basse (1983)		68	12	8.0
Average[a]		1160	14.0	6.1
Univ. Dept. Surgery,	1961–1977	63	24	4.2
Erlangen	1978–1982	65	12	
	1-year survival rate		12 ± 6%[b]	
	2-year survival rate		2 ± 3%[b]	

Not a single patient survived for 5 years!
[a] Calculated as arithmetic mean without weighting for patient numbers.
[b] 95% confidence limits.

Table 16. Ductal pancreatic carcinoma: results after explorative laparotomy

Reference		n	Operative mortality (%)	Mean/median survival time (months)
Hermreck et al. (1974)		125	51	1.8
Hertzberg (1974)		21	43	1.6
Jones and Burns (1976)		22	40	3.0
Coutsoftides et al. (1977)		119	34	5.8
Knight et al. (1978)		133	25	3.5
Forrest and Longmire (1979)		67	44	3.6
Jain et al. (1979)		38	14	6.0
Moossa (1979)		74	8	2.5
Reed et al. (1979)		28	7	6.0
Average[a]		627	32.5	3.8
Univ. Dept. Surgery,	1961–1977	117	31	3.2
Erlangen	1978–1982	75	12	
	1-year survival rate		8 ± 5%[b]	
	2-year survival rate		4 ± 3%[b]	

Not a single patient survived for 5 years!
[a] Calculated as arithmetic mean without weighting for patient numbers.
[b] 95% confidence limits.

Long-term Prognosis, Overall Results

Numerous individual reports and compilation studies have been published on the late results of curative resection of periampullar and pancreatic carcinoma. According to a WHO study (Aoki and Ogawa 1987), despite all improvements in diagnostic and surgical techniques, the 5-year cure rate for pancreatic carcinoma is under 1%. Similarly poor results were found by Gudjonsson et al. (1978), who reported an absolute 5-year survival rate of only 0.4% for 15 000 pancreatic carcinomas compiled from the literature. The prognosis is so poor because 85%–90% of ductal pancreatic carcinomas have grown far beyond the border of the organs and have metastasized by the time of diagnosis (Cubilla et al. 1978 b; Hermanek 1984; Kümmerle et al. 1976; Lux et al. 1977; Trede et al. 1977). Since no risk groups have been defined and no suitable screening methods are available, and since the new imaging and endoscopic techniques have not increased the proportion of early carcinomas admitted for surgery, the prognosis of ductal pancreatic carcinoma will, at least for the next few years, remain extremely poor. A retrospective analysis of the 186 patients treated for exocrine pancreatic carcinoma at the University Department of Surgery, Erlangen, between 1964 and 1977 revealed that none survived 5 years (Hermanek and Wörner 1979). Our results have improved only slightly since then: the current 5-year survival rate for all patients with ductal pancreatic carcinoma is 1.8%, for curative resection 11.8% (Table 1).

Carcinomas of the periampullar region have a distinctly better prognosis. Jaundice is an early symptom and endoscopic biopsy techniques of diagnosis have been widely adopted, so carcinomas of the periampullar region are now usually referred for surgery at an early stage. This has led to an increase in resection rates to 70%–90% (Aston and Longmire 1973; Coutsoftides et al. 1977; Gall et al. 1981; Hollender and Marrie 1981; Nakase et al. 1977; Rückert and Kümmerle 1979; Van Heerden et al. 1981; Williams et al. 1979). The 5-year survival rates (including postoperative mortality) are 25% for all tumours, 35% for curative resection (Table 1).

Prognostic Influence of Tumour-associated Factors

The prognosis of ductal pancreatic carcinoma is so poor, even after curative resection (5-year survival rates of 5%–10%), that the influence of various possible prognostic factors is not at all clear.

Tumours sited in the body and tail of the pancreas exhibit a distinctly poorer prognosis than those in the head of the organ. In a survey compiling data from the literature (Gall and Zirngibl 1984), tumours that could be treated by left resection showed a 5-year survival rate of 0%, as against 5.1% for tumours of the head of the pancreas which could be treated by partial duodenopancreatectomy. The average duration of survival was 11.4 months and 13.7 months respectively.

Some authors (e.g. Edis et al. 1980; Herter et al. 1982) doubt whether early diagnosis can improve the poor prognosis of ductal pancreatic carcinoma, the reason for their scepticism being that they observed no difference in the duration of patient survival between tumours resected early and those which were already advanced. Our experience, however, is the opposite, that early treatment is clearly beneficial. Analysis of all curative resections of ductal carcinoma reveals a median duration of survival for patients staged pN0 of over 60 months. Metastatic involvement of one or two groups of regional lymph nodes reduces the median survival time to 9 months and 8 months respectively.

Moossa and Levin (1981) reported favourable results in early carcinoma: in a group of 17 patients the duration of survival ranged from 7 months to 9 years (average 28 months).

Tumour grade also seems to exert a certain influence on the prognosis (Klöppel et al. 1984).

Furthermore, tumour site is apparently of prognostic significance in periampullar carcinoma. Analysis of the data in the literature (Gall and Zirngibl 1984) reveals that the prognosis is better for carcinomas of the ampulla of Vater and of the periampullar duodenum (average survival 45.9 months and 41.3 months respectively) than for carcinomas of the distal common bile duct (28.5 months). This difference is reflected in the average 5-year survival rates (26.8%, 31.9% and 19% respectively). Similar results concerning the influence of tumour site on prognosis were reported in a compilation study by Hermann (1979).

Prognostic Influence of Therapy-associated Factors

Ductal Pancreatic Carcinoma

Partial vs Total Duodenopancreatectomy

Recent reports of late results still do not show clearly whether partial or total duodenopancreatectomy is more suitable for radical resection of ductal carcinomas of the head of the pancreas. Our survey of the literature reveals duration of survival of 12.8 months for partial duodenopancreatectomy (Table 13) and 15.8 months for total duodenopancreatectomy (Table 14). The 5-year survival rates are 5.1% and 6.7% respectively (Tables 13, 14). Other compilations report 5-year survival rates of 3%–5% for total duodenopancreatectomy (Björk et al. 1981; Gudjonsson et al. 1978; Hermann 1979; Nakase et al. 1977; Shapiro 1975). The long-term results in comparable tumours and the figures for operative mortality thus, similarly show no clear superiority of one procedure over the other.

Some authors, however, have reported serious difficulties in control of diabetes in 18%–25% of cases after total duodenopancreatectomy (Herter et al. 1982; Pliam and ReMine 1975).

Regional Duodenopancreatectomy

The effect of so-called regional total pancreatectomy on the duration of survival cannot yet be evaluated. Fortner (1984) attained a median survival time of 15 months using this method. Increasing the resection rate by performing ultraradical resection even in advanced tumours has not improved survival time. Ihse et al. (1977), in agreement with others (Björk et al. 1981; Brooks and Culebras 1976; Reed et al. 1979; Sato et al. 1977; Warren et al. 1975), demonstrated that the results of resection of stage III ductal pancreatic carcinoma (according to Hermreck et al. 1984) resembled those of palliative measures.

Subtotal Duodenopancreatectomy

We cannot yet report any late results for subtotal duodenopancreatectomy. However, the median duration of survival among our 35 patients – 12 months – does not differ from that following total duodenopancreatectomy. Thus we can conclude, at least provisionally, that subtotal duodenopancreatectomy is associated neither with lesser radicality nor with shorter survival.

Palliation or Resection?

The disappointingly low survival rates after resection have led some surgeons to employ only palliative measures in ductal pancreatic carcinoma. From the mid-1960s to the mid-1970s, several authors (Crile 1970; Feduska et al. 1971; Hertzberg 1974; Mongé et al. 1964; Shapiro 1975) reported that there was no difference in average survival between resection and palliative surgery without resection, and concluded that palliative measures should be preferred even for resectable ductal pancreatic carcinomas. The overwhelming majority of surgeons experienced in pancreatic surgery now reject this advice, however, since to follow it is to deny the opportunity of definitive cure, however slight, to patients with normal surgical risk and early-stage tumours. Our survey of the literature shows no great difference in operative mortality between palliative and resecting procedures (bypass surgery 14.0%, partial duodenopancreatectomy 14.6%, total duodenopancreatectomy 18.6%, resecting procedures overall 15.9%). The mean survival time for palliative bypass surgery is only 6.1 months, that for resecting interventions much higher: partial duodenopancreatectomy 12.8 months, total duodenopancreatectomy 15.8 months, overall 13.8 months (Tables 13–15).

A review by Moossa et al. (1979) of the results of 18 American authors revealed an average survival time of 4.3 months for bypass surgery, with no patients still alive after 5 years. Following curative surgery resection, the average duration of survival was 16.5 months and the 5-year survival rate 18%. Our own recent results confirm that curative tumour resection is now clearly superior to palliative surgery: the median survival time for ductal pancreatic carcinoma in the period 1978–1982 was 9.0 months in the 34 patients who underwent curative resection as opposed to only 3.6 months in the 64 patients undergoing bypass surgery. The age-corrected 2-year survival rates including postoperative mortality were $33\% \pm 17\%$ and $1\% \pm 3\%$ respectively. On the basis of these results resection has since been the favoured procedure in operable pancreatic carcinoma.

Periampullar Carcinoma

An average survival time of 7.4 months has been reported after palliative bypass surgery of inoperable periampullar carcinoma (Nakase et al. 1977). In contrast, survival times of 30–44 months are reported after partial duodenopancreatectomy (Table 12). Amongst our patients treated between 1960 and 1982, the median duration of survival was 6.7 months after bypass surgery ($n = 16$) but 30.1 months after partial duodenopancreatectomy ($n = 50$).

Malignant Tumours of the Endocrine Pancreas

Some malignant tumours of the endocrine pancreas are extremely rare. The current worldwide total of reported cases is just under 200 each for vipoma and glucagonoma and around 50 for somatostatinoma. The principal feature distinguishing endocrine from exocrine carcinomas is their more favourable prognosis. This is partially explained by the fact that the hormonal symptoms often result in early diagnosis of small tumours confined to the pancreas, but patients with distant metastases may also survive for surprisingly long periods, in some cases for several years. The median duration of survival in cases of proven malignancy is 4 years, and up to 19 years has been reported (Cubilla and Hajdu 1975).

Endocrine malignancies are not necessarily hormonally active. They are usually only 2–3 cm in diameter and unlike exocrine carcinomas show no preference for the head of the pancreas, but are distributed throughout the organ. Because of their rich vascularization, they are often strikingly dark red and soft and, therefore, difficult to detect by palpation when small. They are generally well delimited by a pseudocapsule. Depending on the tumour type, in up to 10% of cases the endocrine tumours are extrapancreatic, but produce hormones typical of the pancreas (glucagon, insulin, somatostatin, pancreatic polypeptide). Such tumours occur above all in the wall of the duodenum and the stomach (Stefanini et al. 1974), in the jejunum and the biliary tract in the case of somatostatinoma (Friesen 1987), and in the adrenal medulla and the neural tissue in the case of vipoma.

In endocrine neoplasms of the pancreas, as in other endocrine organs, it is particularly difficult to differentiate between benign and malignant tumours (Klöppel 1981). Frequently, neither biopsy nor examination of the excised tumour permits definitive diagnosis and the only proof of malignancy is provided by the demonstration of metastases. Histologically proven vascular invasion should be interpreted as a sign of malignancy (Cubilla and Hajdu 1975). The danger of metastasis increases with the size of the tumour. Every tumour over 2 cm in diameter, especially over 3 cm, is suspected of malignancy. The proportion of tumours comprised by malignancies varies according to type. Most enterochromaffin cell (EC) carcinoid tumours and somatostatinomas in the pancreas are malignant, glucagonomas are malignant in 60%–80% of cases, solitary gastrinomas in 60%, multicentric gastrinomas in over 90%, gastrinomas in the context of multiple endocrine neoplasia in just under 50%, vipomas in 40%, insulinomas in 40%, somatostatinomas and PPomas each in about 50% (Thompson and Eckhauser 1984).

Metastasis is usually to regional lymph nodes and the liver (Klöppel 1981). Recently, the immunohistological demonstration of HCG alpha-chains has been claimed to offer the possibility of diagnosing malignancy without proof of metastasis (Heitz et al. 1983).

Malignant endocrine pancreatic tumours are rare, comprising about 1%–3% of all malignant tumours of the pancreas and periampullar region. There is no sex preference, and the peak incidence is found in the fourth and fifth decades of life. The hereditary multiple endocrine neoplasia (adenomatosis) type I (MEN I, MEA I, Wermer's syndrome) is characterized by synchronous and metachronous development of hyperplasias, adenomas and malignant tumours of the parathyroid, the endocrine pancreas and the adenohypophysis (Heitz and Steiner 1981). Malignant endocrine pancreatic tumours, most frequently gastrinoma (about 20%) are also found in this context (Wermer 1974).

Classification

The endocrine system of the pancreas consists of the islets of Langerhans, the principal components of which are the glucagon-producing A cells and the insulin-producing B cells. Scattered hormone-producing cells of the diffuse endocrine system – clear-cell organ (Feyrter 1938), enteroendocrine cells – are found in the islets and in other parts of the pancreas, particularly the ducts. The islets and the diffuse endocrine system are now referred to together as the APUD cell system (APUD = amine precursor uptake and decarboxylation) (Pearse 1969).

Light microscopy yields limited information which is of assistance in classifying endocrine tumours. Together with clinical biochemical demonstration of hormones (radioimmunoassay in serum), the most important diagnostic technique is immunocytochemistry, which has greatly reduced the significance of electron microscopy (Heitz et al. 1982).

The WHO classification of endocrine pancreatic tumours is reproduced in Table 17 (Williams et al. 1980). Table 18 shows a classification based principally on immunocytochemistry. It must be borne in mind with such classifications that tumours are not infrequently immunohistologically multihormonal in structure, and in this event there is not always agreement between the histological and the clinical findings (Larsson et al. 1975), as the clinical symptoms seldom reflect the multihormonal nature of the process.

The most frequent malignant endocrine neoplasm is insulinoma, followed by gastrinoma. The other types of tumour are much rarer. Multiple lesions are found most commonly in malignant gastrinoma (25%), less often in insulinoma (10%).

Table 17. WHO classification of malignant endocrine pancreatic tumours

I. Islet cell carcinomas (tumours of cells occuring exclusively or almost exclusively in the islets of Langerhans)
1. A cell carcinoma (malignant glucagonoma)
2. B cell carcinoma (malignant insulinoma)

II. Malignant tumours of the diffuse endocrine system (malignant carcinoids) (tumours of diffuse endocrine cells occurring singly or in small groups mainly in the ducts)
1. Malignant G cell tumour (malignant gastrinoma, malignant G cell carcinoid)
2. Malignant EC cell carcinoid (malignant enterochromaffin cell carcinoid, malignant classical carcinoid, malignant argentaffinoma)
3. Other malignant carcinoids:
   a) malignant Verner-Morrison tumour (malignant vipoma, malignant D1 cell tumour)
   b) malignant D cell tumour (malignant somatostatino ma)

III. Poorly differentiated endocrine carcinoma (malignant epithelial tumour with little structural evidence of endocrine differentiation but frequently showing evidence of functional endocrine differentiation [production of multiple hormones including ectopic hormones]; histologically small cell carcinoma similar to oat cell carcinoma of the lung or a tumour made up of larger cells forming solid and ductular areas)

From Williams et al. (1980).

Table 18. Immunocytochemical classification of malignant endocrine tumours of the pancreas

Cell type	Hormone	Malignant tumour
A	Glucagon	Malignant Glucagonoma
B	Insulin	Malignant Insulinoma
D	Somatostatin	Malignant Somatostatinoma
D1	Vasoactive intestinal polypeptide	Malignant Vipoma
G	Gastrin	Malignant Gastrinoma
PP	Pancreatic polypeptide	Malignant PPoma
EC	Serotonin	Malignant Carcinoid
?	Ectopic ACTH	Malignant Ectopic ACTH tumor (corticotropinoma)

From Klöppel et al. (1979) b.
The light-microscopic structure of A and B cell tumours is of the islet cell tumour type, that of the other tumours is of the intestinal carcinoid type.

Diagnosis

The symptoms of hormonally active tumours are determined by the hormones produced. The appropriate diagnostic tests are listed in Table 19. Hormonally inactive tumours are discovered late – especially when not located in the head of the pancreas – and their symptoms resemble those of exocrine tumours.

For hormonely active and biochemically confirmed tumours, preoperative tumour localization is of crucial importance: it shortens operating time and lowers the number of blind resections, the frequency of postoperative complications and operative mortality.

The first attempts at localization of the tumour are made with sonograph and CT scan, but these methods detect only the larger tumours. In the case of tumours in the vicinity of the upper gastrointestinal tract or in the head of the pancreas, endoscopic ultrasound is more revealing, detecting tumours down to 5 mm in diameter. The most informative investigations as regards tumour site are angiography with selective visualization of the coeliac trunk and the superior mesenteric artery, and selective transhepatic catheterization of the pancreatic veins with blood sampling for hormone determination (Fig. 15).

The accuracy of angiography in insulinomas, which are relatively large, is reported as 65%–90% (Edis et al. 1976; Pistolesi et al. 1977; Stefanini et al. 1974). In gastrinomas, which are on average smaller, the corresponding figures are 40%–60% (Gray et al. 1970; Thompson et al. 1975). If angiography is unsuccessful, transhepatic catheterization of the pancreatic veins can be tried (Ingemansson et al. 1977). By way of a percutaneously, transhepatically placed catheter, blood samples are taken from various segments of the portal veins and the splenic vein for hormone determination. A distinctly increased concentration of hormone in one segment indicates the location of the tumour. The tumour site has been claimed to be detectable in about 70% of cases using this method (Günther et al. 1981). If all attempts at localization fail, the tumour may be extrapancreatic. This is the case in 1%–3% of insulinomas and glucagonomas, 30% of gastrinomas and 10%–20% of vipomas.

Treatment

Surgical Therapy

The therapy of choice in all malignant endocrine tumours is surgical excision. After median upper abdominal laparotomy, the basic surgical steps to achieve full exposure of the pancreas are incision of the omental bursa, Kocher mobilization of the duodenum as far as the abdominal aorta, incision of the retroperitoneum at the inferior margin of the pancreas and, in order to identify retropancreatic tu-

Table 19. Hormonal symptoms and diagnosis of malignant endocrine tumours of the pancreas

Tumour type	Symptoms	Diagnosis
Malignant Insulinoma	Hypoglycemia: transient neurological symptoms such as apathy, confusion and clouding of consciousness, transient neurological focal phenomena, psychic changes (irritability, abnormal behaviour or excitement states), permanent neurological deficit ("stroke") Gastrointestinal: hunger, nausea, vomiting	Hypoglycaemia High serum insulin Fasting test Insulin suppression test Insulin provocation tests (tolbutamide, glucagon, calcium-glucose infusion)
Malignant Glucagonoma	Mild diabetes mellitus Erythema necrolytica migrans (spots and popules at first, soon followed by vesicles, erosion, healing with hyperpigmented scar formation) Atrophic glossitis and stomatitis Normochromic anaemia Weight loss Ileus Thrombophlebitis	Serum glucagon
Malignant Gastrinoma	Recurring therapy-resistant gastric/duodenal ulcers, often with bleeding, perforation, pain as in ulcer disease Gastric hypersecretion, vomiting Watery diarrhoea Steatorrhoea	Analysis of gastric secretion with pentagastrin stimulation (high basal secretion, no or only slight increase in acid values after stimulation) Serum gastrin over 500 pg/ml (normal 20–50 pg/ml) Stimulation tests (secretin, calcium, glucacon)
Malignant Enterochromaffin cell carcinoid	Diarrhoea or possibly fully developed carcinoid syndrome (flush, colic, tachypnoea, cardiopathy, diarrhoea) Colicky abdominal pain	5-Hydroxyindoleacetic acid in urine serotonin in serum
Malignant Vipoma Malignant PPoma	WDHA syndrome (pancreatic cholera): watery diarrhoea, hypokalaemia, achlorhydria	Serum VIP Serum prostaglandin E, F Serum PP
Malignant Somatostatinoma	Diabetes mellitus Disturbances of digestion, e.g. steatorrhoea, hypohlorhydria Often cholelithiasis Anaemia	Serum somatostatin (ACTH, thyrocalcitonin)
Malignant Corticotropinoma	Cushing-like picture Hypokalaemic alkalosis Osteoporosis	Serum ACTH

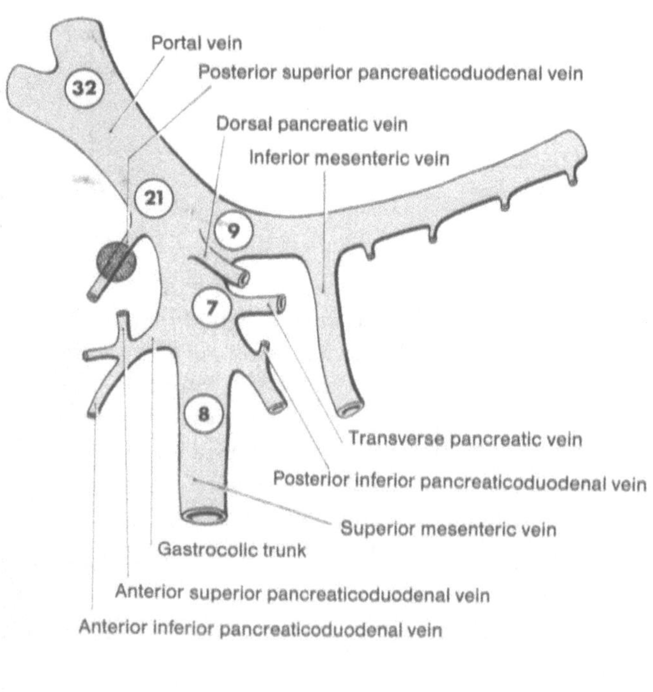

Fig. 15. Localization of an insulinoma in the upper dorsal quadrant of the head of the pancreas by means of selective blood sampling from the veins of the pancreas. Hatched circle: tumour; circled numbers: insulin level (μU/ml)

mours, mobilization of the tail of the pancreas from left-lateral to medial-ventral after the freeing and elevation of the spleen, together with the tail of the pancreas.

Particularly the regional lymph nodes, the liver and the duodenum must be painstakingly explored. All lesions which might be metastases are biopsied for intraoperative histological examination. Precise visualization and palpation of all segments of the pancreas is essential even after successful preoperative tumour localization, in view of the multifocal occurrence of gastrinoma, insulinoma and occasionally other tumours.

If no tumour can be seen or palpated, the newly developed method of intraoperative sonography can be employed to identify smaller processes in the pancreatic tissue. In addition, occult tumours can nowadays be localized by intraoperative hormone determination in selective blood samples from various segments of the portal vein and splenic vein (Turner 1978).

Smaller non-malignant tumours and non-curable tumours which already have distant metastases can be enucleated. This procedure, however, may well involve damage to the pancreatic duct, necessitating drainage of the defect into a Roux-en-Y loop. Failure to recognize such a ductal lesion intraoperatively may result in persisting pancreatic fistulae in over 10% of cases (Stefanini et al. 1974).

The rules of tumour surgery should be applied in all tumours over 2–3 cm in diameter, especially if malignancy is suspected and there are no distant metastases. Depending on tumour site, either left resection or partial duodenopancreatectomy with lymph node resection and prolamine occlusion of the remaining pancreas is carried out. In the case of local inoperability, reduction of tumour size is advisable in order to improve the hormonal symptoms and to increase the chances of successful medical therapy.

In malignant gastrinoma, complete excision of the primary tumour and any metastases present is impossible. Gastrectomy used to be the procedure of choice to avoid severe ulcerative complications, but nowadays ulcers can usually be prevented by using H_2-receptor antagonists.

The sometimes slow progression of endocrine pancreatic malignancies, even in the presence of hepatic metastases, seems to justify an aggressive approach, surgical resection of the primary tumour and regional lymph node metastases possibly being accompanied by local chemotherapy and/or embolization. However, no definitive recommendations have yet been formulated.

Medical Therapy

Details of medical therapy of malignant endocrine tumours are reported by Brennan and MacDonald (1982), Broder and Carter (1973 b), MacDonald et al. (1977) and Moertel et al. (1980).

Cytostatic therapy has been largely unsatisfactory so far. The drugs generally employed are streptozotocin, DTIC, adriblastin and 5-FU. Substances which inhibit the pathological hormone secretion or alleviate its effects are used in the case of inoperable tumours and distant metastases. In insulinomas, the agent of choice is diazoxide (300–500 mg/day), administered together with a mild saluretic to combat the simultaneous NaCl retention. Somatostatin can be given in an attempt to depress glucagon production in glucagonomas, and EC carcinoids can be treated with parachlorphenylalanine. Corticosteroids, or in the case of high prostaglandin E levels indomethacin, are used against vipomas. In gastrinomas, H_2-receptor antagonists (cimetidine, ranitidine), possibly in combination with anticholinergics, have proved their worth in combating ulcers.

Prognosis

In general, malignant endocrine tumours have a better prognosis than carcinomas of the exocrine pancreas. A mean postoperative duration of survival of about 3–4 years has been reported for malignant insulinoma (Broder and Carter 1973 a). Eighty per cent of patients with malignant glucagonoma survive for more than 2 years, 23% for more than 5 years (Binnick et al. 1977; Higgins et al. 1979). In the case of malignant gastrinoma with hepatic metastases, 42% of patients survive for 5 years and 30% for 10 years (Fox et al. 1974 a). Patients with metastastic vipoma have a life expectancy of about 12 months. It is very difficult to make statements concerning the prognosis of the other types of endocrine pancreatic tumours because of their rarity.

Prospects

Overall, the long-term results of treatment of pancreatic carcinoma remain disappointing. However, the improvements that have been achieved cannot be overlooked. Operative mortality of no more than 10% following tumour resection should now be the standard and a number of centres have mortality figures of less than 5% for resections of periampullar and pancreatic carcinoma. Further improvements cannot be expected, however, in the near future.

Clarification of the risk factors for pancreatic carcinoma has hitherto been no more than rudimentary and further epidemiological studies are necessary. Only in this way can any further high-risk groups be identified and specific screening programmes be initiated. However, the currently available investigation techniques are not capable of diagnosing early carcinomas accurately in sufficient numbers. Better tumour markers and endosonography may improve the situation in the future. The value of nuclear magnetic resonance has not yet been established, but, even assuming further positive experience, it will probably remain restricted to exceptional cases.

Radical surgery with extensive dissection of lymph nodes will remain the principal form of treatment, despite the fact that various surgeons are currently still (or again) omitting such lymph node dissection. The better long-term survival rates achieved in some centres cannot, however, be improved further by surgical therapy alone. Recent results seem to suggest that it might be possible to increase survival rates by means of local (perhaps intraoperative) radiotherapy in combination with systemic chemotherapy. We already know that not all patients benefit from chemotherapy; on the contrary, the side effects sometimes nullify the benefits achieved by other therapeutic procedures. A better definition of suitable patients is thus necessary.

Probably no essential improvement in the result of the treatment of pancreatic carcinoma is produced by any of the palliative measures.

References

Anacker H, Weiss HD, Kramann B (1975) Das Pankreaskarzinom im endoskopischen retrograden Pancreatico-Cholangiogramm. Fortschr Röntgenstr 122: 238–242

Aoki K, Ogawa H (1978) Cancer of the pancreas – international mortality trends. WHO Stat Rep 31: 2–27

Aston SJ, Longmire WP (1973) Pancreatico-duodenal resection. Arch Surg 106: 813–817

Baumel H, Deixonne B (1986) Therapeutic managements. In: Baumel H, Deixonne B (eds) Exocrine pancreatic cancer. Springer, Berlin Heidelberg New York, p 145

Baylor SM, Berg JW (1973) Cross classification and survival characteristics of 5000 cases of cancer of the pancreas. J Surg Oncol 5: 335–357

Beahrs OH, Myers MH – AJCC (1983) Manual for staging of cancer. Lippincott, Philadelphia

Becker V (1973) Bauchspeicheldrüse, Inselapparat ausgenommen. Springer, Berlin Heidelberg New York

Becker V, Kümmerle F, Schier J, Lenner V, Longdong W (1976) Tumoren des Pankreas. In: Forell MM (ed) Pankreas. Springer, Berlin Heidelberg New York (Handbuch der inneren Medizin, vol 3, part 6)

Berg JW, Connelly RR (1979) Updating the epidemiologic data on pancreatic cancer. Semin Oncol 6: 275–284

Binnick AN, Spencer SK, Dennison WL Jr, Horton ES (1977) Glucagonoma syndrome. Report of two cases and literature review. Arch Dermatol 113: 749–754

Björck S, Svensson JO, Macpherson S, Edlund Y (1981) Cancer of the head of the pancreas and choledochoduodenal junction: a clinical study of 88 Whipple resections. Acta Chir Scand 147: 353–359

Bodner E (1981) Chirurgie des Pankreas: Das Pankreaskarzinom. Acta Chir Austr 4: 94–100

Bowden L, McNeer G, Pack G (1965) Carcinoma of the head of the pancreas. Am J Surg 109: 578–582

Brennan MF, MacDonald JS (1982) Cancer of the endocrine system: The endocrine pancreas. In: de Vita VT Jr, Hellmann S, Rosenberg SA (eds) Cancer, principles and practice of oncology. Lippincott, Philadelphia

Broder LE, Carter SK (1973a) Pancreatic islet cell carcinoma. I. Clinical features of 52 patients. Ann Intern Med 79: 101–107

Broder LE, Carter SK (1973b) Pancreatic islet cell carcinoma. II. Results of therapy with streptozotocin in 52 patients. Ann Intern Med 79: 108–118

Brooks JR, Culebras JM (1976) Cancer of the pancreas. Am J Surg 131: 516–520

Bruch JM, Lopez FM, Lopez P, Narboni T, Raffael C (1987) Morphological examinations. In: Baumel H, Deixonne B (eds) Exocrine pancreatic cancer. Springer, Berlin Heidelberg New York, p 65

Bussey HJR (1980) Polyposis syndromes. In: Wright R (ed) Recent advances in gastrointestinal pathology. Saunders, Philadelphia

Castellanos J, Manifacio G, Lillehei RC, Shatney CH (1976) Total pancreatectomy for ductal carcinoma of the head of the pancreas: current status. Am J Surg 131: 595–598

Cattell RB (1947) Anastomosis of the duct of Wirsung: its use in palliative operations for cancer of the head of the pancreas. Surg Clin North Am 27: 636–643

Child CG III, Hinerman DL, Kauffman GL Jr (1978) Pancreaticoduodenectomy. Surg Gynecol Obstet 147: 529–533

Classen M, Koch H, Wurbs D, Demling L (1974) Diagnostic and therapeutic aspects of ERCP. In: Congr Intern Endosc Gastroint, Mexico

Cohen JR, Kuchta N, Geller N, Shires T, Dincen P (1982) Pancreaticoduodenectomy: a 40 year experience. Ann Surg 195: 608–617

Cohn I Jr, Hastings PR (eds) (1981) Pancreatic cancer. UICC Technical Report Series, vol 57. UICC, Geneva

Collins JJ Jr, Craighead JE, Brooks JR (1966) Rationale for total pancreatectomy for carcinoma of the pancreatic head. N Engl J Med 274: 599–602

Cooperman AM, Herter FP, Marboe CA, Helmreich ZU, Perzin KH (1981) Pancreatoduodenal resection and total pancreatectomy. An institutional review. Surgery 90: 707–712

Coutsoftides T, MacDonald J, Shibata HR (1977) Carcinoma of the pancreas and periampullary region: a 41 year experience. Ann Surg 186: 730–733

Crile G (1970) The advantages of bypass operations over radical pancreatoduodenectomy in the treatment of pancreatic carcinoma. Surg Gynecol Obstet 130: 1049–1053

Cubilla AL, Fitzgerald PJ (1976) Morphological lesions associated with human primary invasive nonendocrine pancreas cancer. Cancer Res 26: 2690–2698

Cubilla AL, Fitzgerald PJ (1980) Surgical pathology aspects of

cancer of the ampulla-head-of-pancreas region. In: Fitzgerald PJ, Morrison AB (eds) The pancreas. Williams and Wilkins, Baltimore
Cubilla AL, Fitzgerald PJ (1984) Tumors of the exocrine pancreas. Armed Forces Institute of Pathology, Washington DC, Sec Series, Fasc 19
Cubilla A, Hajdu SI (1975) Islet cell carcinoma of the pancreas. Arch Pathol 99: 204–207
Cubilla AL, Fitzgerald PJ, Fortner JG (1978 a) Pancreas cancer – duct cell adenocarcinoma: survival in relation to site, size, stage and type of therapy. J Surg Oncol 10: 465–482
Cubilla AL, Fortner J, Fitzgerald PJ (1978 b) Lymph node involvement in carcinoma of the head of the pancreas area. Cancer 41: 880–887
Cutherell L, Wanebo HJ, Tegtmeyer CU (1986) Catheter tract seeding after percutaneous biliary drainage for pancreatic cancer. Cancer 57: 2057
Deixonne B, Marty Double C, Pignodel C (1986) Pathological anatomy. In: Baumel H, Deixonne B (eds) Exocrine pancreatic cancer. Springer, Berlin Heidelberg New York, p 11
Del Favero G, Fabris C, Plebani M et al. (1986) CA 19-9 and carcinoembryonic antigen in pancreatic cancer diagnosis. Cancer 57: 1576
Diamond D, Fisher B (1975) Pancreatic cancer. Surg Clin North Am 55: 363–376
DiMagno EP, Malagelada JR, Taylor WF, Go VLW (1977) A prospective comparison of current diagnostic tests for pancreatic cancer. N Engl J Med 297: 737–742
Dobelbower RR Jr, Milligan AJ (1984) Treatment of pancreatic cancer by radiation therapy. World J Surg 8: 919
Dobelbower RR Jr, Merrick HW, Ahnja RK, Skeel RT (1986) 125 I interstitial implant, precision high-dose external beam therapy, and 5-FU for unresectable adenocarcinoma of pancreas and extrahepatic biliary tree. Cancer 58: 2185
Edis AJ, Mellrath DC, van Heerden JA, Fulton RE, Sheedy PF, John Service F, Dale AJD (1976) Insulinoma – current diagnosis and surgical management. Curr Probl Surg 13: 1–45
Edis AJ, Kiernan PD, Taylor WF (1980) Attempted curative resection of ductal carcinoma of the pancreas. Review of Mayo Clinic experience, 1951–1975. Mayo Clin Proc 55: 531–536
Falk RE, Moffat FL, Lawler M, Heine J, Makowka L, Fall JA (1986) Combination therapy for resectable and unresectable adenocarcinoma of the pancreas. Cancer 57: 685
Feduska NJ, Dent TL, Lindenauer SM (1971) Results of palliative operations for carcinoma of the pancreas. Arch Surg 103: 330–334
Feinberg SB, Schreiber DR, Goodale R (1977) Comparison of ultrasound pancreatic scanning and endoscopic retrograde cholangiopancreaticograms: a retrospective study. J Clin Ultrasound 5: 96–100
Feyrter F (1938) Über diffuse endokrine epitheliale Organe. Barth, Leipzig
Fish JC, Cleveland BR (1964) Pancreaticoduodenectomy for periampullary carcinoma. Ann Surg 159: 469–476
Forrest JF, Longmire WP Jr (1979) Carcinoma of the pancreas and periampullary region. Ann Surg 189: 129–138
Fortner JG (1973) Regional resection of cancer of the pancreas: a new surgical approach. Surgery 73: 307–320
Fortner JG (1981) Surgical principles for pancreatic cancer: regional total and subtotal pancreatectomy. Cancer 47: 1712–1718
Fortner JG (1984) Regional pancreatectomy for cancer of the pancreas ampulla, and other related sites. Tumor staging and results. Ann Surg 199: 418–425
Fox PS, Hofmann JW, DeCosse JJ, Wilson SD (1974 a) The influence of total gastrectomy on survival in malignant Zollinger-Ellison syndrome. Ann Surg 180: 558–565
Fox PS, Hofmann JW, Wilson SD, DeCosse JJ (1974 b) Surgical management of the Zollinger-Ellison syndrome. Surg Clin North Am 54: 395–407
Fraumeni JF Jr (1975) Cancer of the pancreas and biliary tract: epidemiological considerations. Cancer Res 35: 3437–3446
Friesen SR (1987) Update on the diagnosis and treatment of rare neuroendocrine tumors. Surg Clin North Am 67: 379
Gall FP (1986) Chirurgie des duktalen Karzinoms. In: Gall FP, Groitl H (eds) Fortschritte in der Pankreaschirurgie. Zuckschwerdt, München
Gall FP, Kessler H (1987) Das Frühkarzinom des exokrinen Pankreas: Diagnose und Prognose. Chirurg 58: 78
Gall FP, Zirngibl H (1984) Chirurgische Therapie der Pankreastumoren. In: Gebhardt C (ed) Chirurgie des exokrinen Pankreas. Thieme, Stuttgart
Gall FP, Hermanek P, Gebhardt C, Meier H (1981) Erweiterte Resektion der Pankreas- und periampullären Karzinome: Regionale, totale und partielle Duodenopankreatektomie. Leber Magen Darm 11: 179–184
Gambill EE (1970) Pancreatic and ampullary carcinoma: diagnosis and prognosis in relationship to symptoms, physical findings and relapse of time as observed in 255 patients. South Med J 63: 1119–1124
Gastrointestinal Tumor Study Group (1979) A multi-institutional comparative trial of radiation therapy alone and in combination with 5-fluorouracil for locally unresectable pancreatic carcinoma. Ann Surg 189: 205–208
Gebhardt C (1984) Chirurgische Therapie der chronischen Pankreatitis. In: Gebhardt C (ed) Chirurgie des exokrinen Pankreas. Thieme, Stuttgart
George P, Brown C, Gilchrist J (1975) Operative biopsy of the pancreas. Br J Surg 62: 280–283
Gibson JB, Sobin LH (1978) Histological typing of tumours of the liver, biliary tract and pancreas. International Histological Classification of Tumours, no 20. WHO, Geneva
Gordis L, Gold EB (1984) Epidemiology of pancreatic cancer. World J Surg 8: 808
Gray RK, Rosch J, Grollmann JH (1970) Arteriography in the diagnosis of islet cell tumors. Radiology 97: 39–44
Gudjonsson B, Spiro HM (1978) Biopsy techniques in the diagnosis of pancreatic cancer. Gastroenterology 75: 726–728
Gudjonsson B, Livstone EM, Spiro HM (1978) Cancer of the pancreas. Diagnostic accuracy and survival statistics. Cancer 42: 2494–2506
Gundry SR, Strodel WE, Knol JA, Eckhauser FE (1983) Efficacy of preoperative percutaneous biliary decompression in patients with obstructive jaundice. Gastroenterology 84: 1177 A
Günther R, Kümmerle F, Beyer J, Klose K, Kuhn FP, Rückert K (1981) Lokalisationsdiagnostik von Inselzelltumoren durch Sonographie, Computertomographie, Arteriographie und selective transhepatische Blutentnahme. Fortschr Geb Röntgenstr Nuklearmed Ergänzungsband 135: 657–662
Hagenmüller F, Classen M (1982) Therapeutic endoscopic and percutaneous procedures. In: Popper H, Schaffner F (eds) Progress in liver disease, vol 8. Grune and Stratton, New York
Hagenmüller F, Soehendra N (1983) Nonsurgical biliary drainage. In: Classen M, Schreiber HW (eds) Biliary tract disorders. Clinics in gastroenterology, vol 12. Saunders, Philadelphia
Harvey JH, Schein PS (1984) Chemotherapy of pancreatic carcinoma. World J Surg 8: 935
Hatfield ARW, Tobias R, Girdwood AH et al. (1982) Is preop-

erative biliary drainage necessary in obstructive jaundice surgery? Gut 23: A 449
Heitz PU, Steiner H (1981) Pluriglanduläre endokrine Regulationsstörungen. In: Doerr W, Seifert G (eds) Spezielle pathologische Anatomie, vol 14, part 2. Springer, Berlin Heidelberg New York
Heitz PU, Kasper M, Polak JM, Klöppel G (1982) Pancreatic endocrine tumors: immunocytochemical analysis of 125 tumors. Hum Pathol 13: 263–271
Heitz PU, Kasper M, Klöppel G, Polak JM, Vaitukaitis JL (1983) Glycoprotein-hormone alpha-chain production by pancreatic endocrine tumors: a specific marker for malignancy. Cancer 51: 277–282
Hermanek P (1983) Intraoperative Diagnostik des Pankreaskarzinoms. Langenbecks Arch Chir 359: 289–299
Hermanek P (1984) Pathologie der Pankreastumoren. In: Gebhardt C (ed) Chirurgie des exokrinen Pankreas. Thieme, Stuttgart
Hermanek P (1986) Intraoperative histologische Diagnostik. In: Beger HG, Bittner R (eds) Das Pankreaskarzinom. Frühdiagnostisches und therapeutisches Dilemma. Springer, Berlin Heidelberg New York Tokyo
Hermanek P, Giedl J (1986) Lymphogene Metastasierung des Pankreas- und periampullären Karzinoms. Häufigkeit, Topographie. In: Beger HG, Bittner R (eds) Das Pankreaskarzinom. Frühdiagnostisches und therapeutisches Dilemma. Springer, Berlin Heidelberg New York Tokyo
Hermanek P, Giedl J (1987) Pathologie des Pankreaskarzinoms. In: Gall FP, Gebhardt C, Groitl H (eds) Fortschritte in der Pankreaschirurgie. Zuckschwerdt, München, p 189
Hermanek P, Sobin LH (eds) (1987) TNM. Classification of malignant tumours. Springer, Berlin Heidelberg New York, p 65
Hermanek P, Wörner U (1979) Pathologie des Pankreaskarzinoms und des periampullären Karzinoms. In: Chirurgie der Bauchspeicheldrüse. Bericht über ein Symposium in Erlangen, vol 1. Braun-Dexon, Melsungen
Hermann RE (1979) Carcinoma of the pancreas and periampullary region. In: Egdahl RH (ed) Manual of surgery of the gallbladder, bile ducts, and exocrine pancreas. Springer, Berlin Heidelberg New York
Hermreck A, Thomas C, Friesen S (1974) Importance of pathologic staging in the surgical management of adenocarcinoma of the exocrine pancreas. Am J Surg 127: 653–657
Herter FP, Cooperman AM, Ahlborn TN, Antinori C (1982) Surgical experience with pancreatic and periampullary cancer. Ann Surg 195: 274–281
Hertzberg J (1974) Pancreatico-duodenal resection and bypass operation in patients with carcinoma of the head of the pancreas, ampulla, and distal end of the common duct. Acta Chir Scand 140: 523–527
Hessel SJ, Siegelman SS, McNeil BJ, Sanders R, Adams DF, Alderson PO, Friberg HJ, Abrams HL (1982) A prospective evaluation of computed tomography and ultrasound of the pancreas. Radiology 143: 129
Hicks RE, Brooks JR (1971) Total pancreatectomy for ductal carcinoma. Surg Gynecol Obstet 133: 16–20
Higgins GA, Recant L, Fischman AB (1979) The glucagonoma syndrome: surgically curable diabetes. Am J Surg 137: 142–148
Hines LH, Burns RP (1976) 10 years experience treating pancreatic and periampullary cancer. Am Surg 42: 441–447
Hiraoka T, Watanabe E, Mochinaga M, Tahiro S, Miyanichi Y, Nakamura J, Yokoyama J (1984) Intraoperative irradiation combined with radical resection for cancer of the head of the pancreas. World J Surg 8: 766
Hollender LF, Marrie A (1981) Pancreascarcinom und periampulläres Carcinom. In: Allgöwer M, Harder F, Hollender LF, Peiper HJ, Siewert JR (eds) Chirurgische Gastroenterologie, vol 2. Springer, Berlin Heidelberg New York
Hollender LF, Meyer C (1978) Operative Behandlung des Pankreaskarzinoms. Zentralbl Chir 103: 1256–1263
Holyoke ED, Douglas HO, Goldrosen MH, Ming Chu T (1979) Tumor markers in pancreatic cancer. Semin Oncol 6: 347
Ihse J, Isaksson G (1984) Preoperative and operative diagnosis of pancreatic cancer. World J Surg 8: 846
Ihse J, Lilja P, Arnesjö B, Bengmark S (1977) Total pancreatectomy for cancer. Ann Surg 186: 675–680
Iishi H, Yamamura H, Tatsuta M, Okuda S, Kitamura T (1986) Value of ultrasonographic examination combined with measurement of serum tumor markers in the diagnosis of pancreatic cancer of less than 3 cm in diameter. Cancer 57: 1947
Ingemansson S, Kuhl C, Larsson LI, Lunderquist A, Nobin A (1977) Islet cell hyperplasia localized by pancreatic vein catheterization and insulin radioimmunoassay. Am J Surg 133: 643–645
Isaacson R, Weiland LH, Mellrath DC (1974) Biopsy of the pancreas. Arch Surg 109: 227–230
Jain JM, Brief DK, Nozick J (1979) Carcinoma of the pancreas: fifteen years' experience. Am Surg 45: 15–20
Kairahuoma MJ, Kivinicuni H, Stahlberg M (1987) Pancreatic resection for carcinoma of the pancreas and the periampullary region in patients over 70 years of age. Br J Surg 74: 116
Kalser MH, Ellenberg SS (1985) Pancreatic cancer. Adjuvant combined radiation and chemotherapy following curative resection. Arch Surg 120: 899
Kaufman SL, Reddick RL, Stiegel M, Wild RE, Thomas PA-C, Thomas CG Jr (1986) Papillary cystic neoplasm of the pancreas: a curable pancreatic tumor. World J Surg 10: 851
Kim WS, Barth KH, Zinner M (1982) Seeding of pancreatic carcinoma along the transhepatic catheter tract. Radiology 143: 427–428
Klöppel G (1981) Endokrines Pankreas und Diabetes mellitus. In: Doerr W, Seifert G (eds) Pathologie der endokrinen Organe. Springer, Berlin Heidelberg New York (spezielle pathologische Anatomie, vol 14, part 1)
Klöppel G, Seifert G, Heitz PU (1979a) Endokrine Pankreastumoren. Morphologie und Syndrome. Dtsch Med Wochenschr 104: 1571–1577
Klöppel G, Sosnowski J, Eichfuss H-P, Rückert K, Klapdor R (1979b) Aktuelle Aspekte des Pankreaskarzinoms. Dtsch Med Wochenschr 104: 1801–1805
Klöppel G, Lingenthal G, Klapdor R, Kern HF, Rückert K, von Bülow M (1984) Morphologische Kriterien zum Wachstumsverhalten des Pankreaskarzinoms. Dtsch Med Wochenschr 109: 702–708
Knight RW, Scarborough JP, Goss JC (1978) Adenocarcinoma of the pancreas. A ten-year experience. Arch Surg 113: 1401–1404
Komorn HJ, Zirkin RM, Nathan LE (1986) Papillary cystic neoplasm of the pancreas: report of two cases of a surgically curable tumor. Surgery 99: 110
Kozuka S, Sassa R, Taki T et al. (1979) Relation of pancreatic duct hyperplasia to carcinoma. Cancer 43: 1418–1428
Kozuka S, Tsubone M, Yamaguchi A, Hachisuka K (1981) Adenomatous residue in cancerous papilla of Vater. Gut 22: 1031–1034
Kümmerle F, Kirschner P, Mangold G (1976) Zur Klinik und Chirurgie des Pankreaskarzinoms. Dtsch Med Wochenschr 101: 729–734

Kümmerle F, Trede M, Schwemmle K, Hollender LF (1984) Pankreaskopfcarcinom: Ist die totale Pankreatektomie noch das Verfahren der Wahl? Langenbecks Arch Chir 362: 71–74
Larsson LI, Grimelius L, Hakanson R, Rehfeld JF, Stadil F, Holst J, Angervall L, Sundler F (1975) Mixed endocrine pancreatic tumors producing several peptide hormones. Am J Pathol 79: 271–280
Levin B, ReMine WH, Hermann RE, Schein PS, Cohn I (1978) Panel: cancer of pancreas. Am J Surg 135: 185–191
Levin DL, Connelly RR, Devesa SS (1981) Demographic characteristics of cancer of the pancreas: mortality, incidence and survival. Cancer 47: 1456–1468
Liang V, Go W, Taylor WF, DiMagno EP (1981) Efforts at early diagnosis of pancreatic cancer. Cancer 47: 1698–1703
Longmire WP Jr, Traverso LW (1981) The Whipple procedure and other standard operative approaches to pancreatic cancer. Cancer 47: 1706–1711
Lutz H (1987) Diagnostischer Wert des Ultraschalls bei Pankreaserkrankungen. In: Gall FP, Gebhardt C, Groitl H (eds) Fortschritte in der Pankreaschirurgie. Zuckschwerdt, München, p 218
Lux G, Lutz H (1984) Diagnostik von Pankreastumoren. In: Gebhardt C (ed) Chirurgie des exokrinen Pankreas. Thieme, Stuttgart
Lux G, Schaffner O, Koch H, Rösch W, Stolte M (1977) Duodenoskopische Diagnose des Papillen- und Pankreaskarzinoms. Erfahrungen bei 100 Fällen. In: Lindner H (ed) Fortschritte der gastroenterologischen Endoskopie, vol 8. Witzstrock, Baden-Baden, pp 159–163
Macdonald JS, Widerlite L, Schein PS (1977) Biology, diagnosis and chemotherapeutic management of pancreatic malignancy. Adv Pharmacol Chemother 14: 107
Makve DM, Meyers WC, Bast RC, Seigler HF, Metzger RS (1985) Carcinoma of the pancreas. Therapeutic efficacy as defined by a serodiagnostic test utilizing a monoclonal antibody. Ann Surg 202: 440
Malagelada JR (1979) Pancreatic cancer. An overview of epidemiology, clinical presentation and diagnosis. Mayo Clin Proc 54: 459–467
Matsuno S, Sato T (1986) Surgical treatment for carcinoma of the pancreas. Experience in 272 patients. Am J Surg 152: 499
Matsuno S, Kato S, Kobari M, Sato T (1986) Clinicopathological study on hematogenous metastasis of pancreatic cancer. Jpn J Surg 16: 406
Moertel CG, Hanley JA, Johnson LA (1980) Streptozotocin alone compared with streptozotocin plus fluorouracil in the treatment of advanced islet-cell carcinoma. N Engl J Med 303: 1189–1194
Mongé JJ, Judd ES, Gage RP (1964a) Radical pancreatoduodenectomy: a 22 year-experience with the complications, mortality rate and survival rate. Ann Surg 160: 711–722
Mongé JJ, Dockerty MB, Wollaeger EE, Waugh JM, Priestley JT (1964b) Clinicopathologic observations on radical pancreatoduodenal resection for periampullary carcinoma. Surg Gynecol Obstet 118: 275–283
Moolgavkar SH, Stevens RG (1981) Smoking and cancers of bladder and pancreas: risks and temporal trends. J Natl Cancer Inst 67: 15–23
Moossa AR (1982) Pancreatic cancer. Approach to diagnosis, selection for surgery and choice of operation. Cancer 50: 2689–2698
Moossa AR, Dawson PJ (1981) The diagnosis of pancreatic cancer. Pathobiol Annu 11: 299–335
Moossa AR, Levin B (1981) The diagnosis of "early" pancreatic cancer. The University of Chicago experience. Cancer 47: 1688–1697
Moossa AR, Lewis MH, Mackie CR (1979) Surgical treatment of pancreatic cancer. Mayo Clin Proc 54: 468–474
Moossa AR, Mackie CR, Gelder FB, Dhorajiwala JM (1980) The value of tumor markers in the diagnosis and management of nonendocrine tumors of the pancreas. In: Moossa AR (ed) Tumors of the pancreas. Williams and Wilkins, Baltimore, p 397
Moossa AR, Scott MH, Lavelle-Jones M (1984) The place of total and extended total pancreatectomy in pancreatic cancer. World J Surg 8: 895
Morrow M, Hilario B, Brennan MF (1984) Comparison of conventional surgical resection, radioactive implantation, and bypass procedures for exocrine carcinoma of the pancreas 1975–1980. Ann Surg 199: 1
Nagakawa T, Kurachi M, Konishi K, Miyazaki I (1982) Translateral retroperitoneal approach in radical surgery for pancreatic carcinoma. Jpn J Surg 12: 229–233
Nagai H, Kuroda A, Morioka J (1986) Lymphatic and local spread of T 1 and T 2 pancreatic cancer. A study of autopsy material. Ann Surg 204: 65
Nakase A, Matsumoto Y, Uchida K, Honjo I (1977) Surgical treatment of cancer of the pancreas and the periampullary region. Ann Surg 185: 52–57
Nishimura A, Nakano M, Otsu H et al. (1984) Intraoperative radiotherapy for advanced carcinoma of the pancreas. Cancer 54: 2375
Oster MW, Gray R, Panasci L, Perry MC (1986) Chemotherapy for advanced pancreatic cancer. Cancer 57: 29
Parker GA, Postlethwait RW (1985) The continuing problem of carcinoma of the pancreas. J Surg Onc 28: 36
Pearse AGE (1969) The cytochemistry and ultrastructure of polypeptide hormone producing cells of the APUD series, and the embryologic, physiologic and pathologic implications of the concept. J Histochem Cytochem 17: 303–313
Piorkowski RJ, Blivernicht SW, Lawrence W Jr, Madarlaga J, Horsley JS, Neifeld JP, Terz JJ (1982) Pancreatic and periampullary carcinoma. Experience with 200 patients over a 12 year period. Am J Surg 143: 189–193
Pistolesi GF, Frasson F, Fugazolla C, Taddei GT, Caresano A (1977) Angiographic diagnosis of endocrine tumors of the pancreas. Radiol Clin 46: 401–421
Pliam MB, ReMine WH (1975) Further evaluation of total pancreatectomy. Arch Surg 110: 506–511
Podolsky DK (1984) Serologic markers in the diagnosis and management of pancreatic carcinoma. World J Surg 8: 822
Pollock D, Taylor KJW (1981) Ultrasound scanning in patients with clinical suspicion of pancreatic cancer. Cancer 47: 1662–1665
Porter MR (1958) Carcinoma of the pancreaticoduodenal area. Operability and choice of procedure. Ann Surg 148: 711–724
Reed K, Vose PC, Jarstfer BS (1979) Pancreatic cancer: 30 year review (1947–1977). Ann J Surg 138: 929–933
ReMine WH, Priestley JT, Judd ES, King JN (1970) Total pancreatectomy. Ann Surg 172: 595–604
Rettenmeier G (1976) Leistungsfähigkeit der Sonographie bei Erkrankungen der Bauchspeicheldrüse. In: Bartelheimer H, Classen M, Ossenberg FW (eds) Die Untersuchung der Bauchspeicheldrüse. Thieme, Stuttgart
Riemann JF, Demling L (eds) (1985) Endotherapie von Gallenwegserkrankungen. Thieme, Stuttgart
Rosai J (1981) Ackerman's surgical pathology, 6th edn. Mosby, St. Louis
Rosch J, Keller FS (1981) Pancreatic arteriography, transhepat-

ic pancreatic venography and pancreatic venous sampling in diagnosis of pancreatic cancer. Cancer 47: 1679–1684
Rosenberger J, Mödder U, Pichlmaier H, Friedmann G (1979) Die Computer-Tomographie des Pankreas. Münch Med Wochenschr 121: 1037–1040
Ross H, Jonas RA (1980) The results of surgery for carcinoma of the pancreas. Aust NZ J Surg 50: 454–458
Rossmann P (1959) Lungenmetastasen des Pankreaskrebses mit klinischem Bild des Alveolarkrebses. Zentralbl Allg Pathol 99: 301
Rückert K, Kümmerle F (1979) Das Papillenkarzinom. Chirurg 50: 308–312
Rückert K, Kümmerle F (1986) Ergebnisse der totalen Duodenopankreatektomie als Regeloperation beim Pankreaskarzinom. In: Beger HG, Bittner R (eds) Das Pankreaskarzinom. Frühdiagnostisches und therapeutisches Dilemma. Springer, Berlin Heidelberg New York
Rustin RB, Broughan TA, Hermann RE, Grundfest-Broniatowski SF, Petras RE, Hart WR (1986) Papillary cystic epithelial neoplasms of the pancreas. Arch Surg 121: 1073
Safi F, Beger HG, Bittner R, Büchler M, Krautzberger W (1986) CA 19-9 and pancreatic adenocarcinoma. Cancer 57: 779
Sarles H, Sahel J (1976) Die chronische Pankreatitis. In: Forell MM (ed) Pankreas. Springer, Berlin Heidelberg New York (Handbuch der inneren Medizin, vol 3, part 6)
Sarr MG, Cameron JL (1982) Surgical management of unresectable carcinoma of the pancreas. Surgery 91: 123–133
Sarr MG, Cameron JL (1984) Surgical palliation of unresectable carcinoma of the pancreas. World J Surg 8: 906
Sato T, Saitoh Y, Noto N, Matsuno S (1977) Follow-up studies of radical resection for pancreaticoduodenal cancer. Ann Surg 186: 581–588
Seifert E (1982) Diagnostik und endoskopische Therapie der Papillentumoren. Schweiz Rdsch Med Prax 71: 394–396
Seifert G, Klöppel G (1979) Diagnostic value of pancreatic biopsy. Pathol Res Pract 164: 357–384
Sellner F, Jelinek R (1979) Behandlungsergebnisse nach partieller Duodenopankreatektomie. Wien Med Wochenschr 23: 682–685
Shapiro TM (1975) Adenocarcinoma of the pancreas: a statistical analysis of biliary bypass vs. Whipple resection in good risk patients. Ann Surg 182: 715–721
Shipley WK, Tepper JE, Warshaw AL, Orlow EL (1984a) Intraoperative radiation therapy for patients with pancreatic carcinoma. World J Surg 8: 929
Shipley WK, Wood WC, Trepper JE, Warshaw AL, Orlow EL, Kaufmann SD, Battit GE, Nardi GL (1984b) Intraoperative electron beam irradiation for patients with unresectable pancreatic carcinoma. Ann Surg 200: 289
Sirinek KR, Aust JB (1986) Pancreatic cancer: continuing diagnostic and therapeutic dilemma. Surg Clin North Am 66: 757
Skibber JM, Weiss SM, Mohinddin M, Rosato FE (1985) Impact of radiotherapy in palliative gastroenterostomy in pancreatic cancer. Ann Surg 202: 725
Smith R (1973) Progress in the surgical treatment of pancreatic disease. Am J Surg 125: 143–153
Smith FP, Macdonald JS, Schein PS, Ornitz RD (1980) Cutaneous seeding of pancreatic cancer by skinny-needle aspiration biopsy. Arch Intern Med 140: 855
Smithers BM, Welch C, Goodall P (1986) Cystadenocarcinoma of the pancreas presenting in pregnancy. Br J Surg 73: 591
Stadelmann O, Safrany L, Löffler A et al. (1974) Endoscopic retrograde cholangiopancreaticography in the diagnosis of pancreatic cancer. Endoscopy 6: 84–93
Statistisches Amt des Saarlandes (1987) Morbidität und Mortalität an bösartigen Neubildungen im Saarland 1984. Statistisches Amt des Saarlandes, Saarbrücken
Statistisches Bundesamt Wiesbaden (1984) Gesundheitswesen, Fachserie 12, Reihe 4: Todesursachen. Kohlhammer, Stuttgart
Stefanini P, Carboni M, Patrassi N, Basoli A (1974) Beta-islet cell tumors of the pancreas: results of a study on 1067 cases. Surgery 75: 597–609
Strohm WD, Kurtz W, Hagenmüller F, Classen M (1984) Diagnostic efficacy of endoscopic ultrasound tomography in pancreatic cancer and cholestasis. Scand J Gastroenterol [Suppl 102] 19: 18–23
Tarazi RY, Hermann RE, Vogt DP, Hoerr SO, Esselstyn CB, Cooperman AM, Steiger E, Grundfest S (1986) Results of surgical treatment of periampullary tumors: a thirty-five-year experience. Surgery 100: 716
Tatsuta M, Yamamura H, Iishi H et al. (1985) Values of CA 19-9 in the serum, pure pancreatic juice, and aspirated pancreatic material in the diagnosis of malignant pancreatic tumor. Cancer 56: 2669
Thompson JC, Reeber DD, Villar HV, Fender HR (1975) Natural history and experience with diagnosis and treatment of the Zollinger-Ellison syndrome. Surg Gynecol Obstet 140: 721–739
Thompson NW, Eckhauser FE (1984) Malignant islet-cell tumors of the pancreas. World J Surgery 8: 940
Trede M (1982) Pankreaskarzinom. In: Encke A, Jungbluth KH, Röher HD, Trede M (eds) Aktuelle chirurgische Onkologie. Springer, Berlin Heidelberg New York
Trede M (1985) The surgical treatment of pancreatic carcinoma. Surgery 97: 28
Trede M, Kersting KM, Hottmeister A (1977) Das Pankreaskarzinom. Münch Med Wochenschr 119: 617–622
Tryka AF, Brooks JR (1979) Histopathology in the evaluation of total pancreatectomy for ductal carcinoma. Ann Surg 190: 373–379
Turner RC, Morris RJ, Lee ECG, Harris EA (1978) Localization of insulinomas. Lancet 1: 515–518
Tsuchiya R, Harada N, Miyamoto T, Trunoda T (1986) Importance of lymph node dissection in pancreatic cancer surgery. In: Gall FP, Gebhardt C, Groitl H (eds) Fortschritte in der Pankreaschirurgie. Zuckschwerdt, München, p 248
Urakawa Y (1987) Die Bedeutung der praeoperativen Angiographie für die Frage der Resektabilität von Karzinomen der pankreatoduodenalen Region. In: Gall FP, Gebhardt C, Groitl H (eds) Fortschritte in der Pankreaschirurgie. Zuckschwerdt, München, p 225
Van Heerden JA (1984) Pancreatic resection for carcinoma of the pancreas: Whipple versus total pancreatectomy – An institutional perspective. World J Surg 8: 880
Van Heerden JA, ReMine MH, Weiland LH, Mellrath DC, Ilstrup DM (1981) Total pancreatectomy for ductal adenocarcinoma of the pancreas. Mayo Clinic experience. Am J Surg 142: 308–311
Vilardell F, Farré-Viladrich A (1986) Tumor markers in cancer of the pancreas. Front Gastrointest Res 12: 137
Volkholz H, Stolte M, Klöppel G (1981) Das villöse Adenom der Papilla Vateri – Vorläufer des Pankreaskarzinoms? Verh Dtsch Ges Pathol 65: 375
Walsh DB, Eckhauser FE, Cronenwett JL, Turcotte JG, Lindenauer SM (1982) Adenocarcinoma of the ampulla of Vater. Diagnosis and treatment. Ann Surg 195: 152–157
Ward EM, Stephens DH, Sheedy PR II (1983) Computed tomographic characteristics of pancreatic carcinoma: an analysis of 100 cases. Radiographics 3: 547

Warren KW, Jefferson MF (1973) Carcinoma of the endocrine pancreas. In: Carey LC (ed) The pancreas. Mosby, St. Louis

Warren KW, Cattell RB, Blackburn JP, Nora PF (1962) A long-term appraisal of pancreaticoduodenal resection for periampullary carcinoma. Ann Surg 155: 653–662

Warren KW, Choe DS, Plaza J, Relihan M (1975) Results of radical resection for periampullary cancer. Ann Surg 181: 534–540

Watanabe M, Nishimura Y (1977) Recent advance in the diagnostic and therapy of cancer of the pancreas and the biliary tract, with special reference to the significance of combined use of endoscopic retrograde cholangiopancreatography and selective celiac arteriography. Gastroenterol Jpn 12: 88

Waterhouse J, Meier C, Shanmugaratnam K, Powell (eds) (1982) Cancer incidence in five continents. International Agency for Research on cancer, Sci Publ 42

Weill FS (1982) Ultraschalldiagnostik in der Gastroenterologie. Springer, Berlin Heidelberg New York

Wermer P (1974) Multiple endocrine adenomatosis: multiple hormone producing tumours, a familial syndrome. Clin Gastroenterol 3: 671–684

Whipple AO, Parsons WB, Mullins CR (1935) Treatment of carcinoma of the ampulla of Vater. Ann Surg 102: 763–776

Wiechel KL (1985) Perkutane transhepatische Drainage bei malignem Verschlußikterus. In: Riemann JF, Demling L (eds) Endotherapie von Gallenwegserkrankungen. Thieme, Stuttgart

Williams ED, Siebenmann RE, Sobin LH (1980) Histological typing of endocrine tumours. International histological classification of tumours, no 23. World Health Organization, Geneva

Williams GM, Weissburger JH (1986) Food and cancer: cause and effect? Surg Clin North Am 66: 873

Williams JA, Cubilla A, Maclean BJ, Fortner JG (1979) Twenty-two year experience with periampullary carcinoma at Memorial Sloan-Kettering Cancer Center. Am J Surg 138: 662–665

Wise L, Pizzinboro C, Dehner LP (1976) Periampullary cancer – a clinicopathological study of 62 patients. Am J Surg 131: 141–148

Wittenberg J, Ferrucci J, Warshaw AL (1984) Contribution of computed tomography to patients with pancreatic adenocarcinoma. World J Surg 8: 831

Wittington R, Sohin L, Mohinddin M, Cantor RJ, Rosato FE, Biermann WA, Weiss SM, Pajak TF (1984) Multimodality therapy of localized unresectable pancreatic adenocarcinoma. Cancer 54: 1991

Wynder EL (1975) An epidemiological evaluation of the causes of cancer of the pancreas. Cancer Res 35: 2228–2233

Yasuda K, Tanaka Y, Fujimoto S, Nakajima M, Kawai K (1984) Use of endoscopic ultrasonography in small pancreatic cancer. Scand J Gastroenterol [Suppl 102] 19: 9–17

Cancer of the Liver

O. J. Garden and H. Bismuth

Introduction

The prognosis for the patient with liver cancer remains poor, despite advances in our understanding of the pathogenesis, in detection and in treatment. Nonetheless, there has been a reappraisal of the management of both primary and secondary liver cancer in recent years. This chapter contains only limited description of the treatment of the rarer primary liver cancers, since this is based on that of hepatocellular carcinoma. Discussion of hepatic metastases will be limited to their management by surgical and radiological intervention in order to avoid unnecessary duplication of other chapters in this volume.

Hepatocellular Carcinoma

Hepatic parenchyma can give rise to benign and malignant tumours which possess different characteristics in children. For this reason, the more precise term "hepatocellular carcinoma" (HCC) is preferable to "hepatoma", "primary liver cancer" and "hepatocarcinoma".

There is great variation in the incidence of HCC worldwide (Table 1). The annual incidence in North America and Northern Europe represents approximately 2% of all cancers, whereas the incidence in some areas of Southern Africa and the Far East reaches 40 per 100 000 males, thus representing approximatively 40% of all cases (Lefkowitch 1981). This variation is ethnic as well as geographical. In all populations studied the incidence of HCC rises with age, but in areas with a high incidence the peak is

Table 1. Incidence of HCC in males by continent

Continent	Country	Rate/100 000/year
Africa	Mozambique	164.6
	Nigeria	10.2
	South Africa	
	black	12.3
	white	0.6
	Uganda	6.5
America	Chile	1.1
	Colombia	0.7
	USA	
	black	1.0
	white	0.2
Asia	Singapore (Chinese)	4.1
	Japan	0.4
	India	0.1
Europe	Scotland	0.4
	Denmark	0.4
	Austria	0.1
Oceania	Australia	0.2

After Doll (1969).

reached at about 40–50 years, whereas low-incidence areas, such as Northern Europe, have the peak at about 70 years.

In some areas there has been a definite increase in the incidence of HCC. Okuda (1986) has recently reported a rise in the incidence of primary liver cancer in the Osaka area from 16.3 per 100 000 male population in 1966–1968 to 34.2 per 100 000 in 1981–1982. It was the third most common cancer in that area, but will probably overtake lung cancer to become the second most common behind gastric cancer.

Aetiology

The varied distribution of HCC is related to two main aetiological factors: hepatitis B virus and cirrhosis.

The important link between hepatitis B virus and HCC has been demonstrated by several investigators (Blumberg and London 1981; Beasley and Hwang 1984). Not only is there an increased incidence of HCC in populations with a high carrier rate of hepatitis B surface antigen (HBsAg), but in some areas, such as Taiwan, where the carrier rate of HBsAg in the normal population is about 10%, 80% of patients with HCC are HBsAg positive (Tong et al. 1971). The annual incidence of HCC for HBsAg-negative patients is 3 per 100 000, compared to 528 per 100 000 in HBsAg-positive subjects (Beasley and Hwang 1984). This association still holds in areas with low carrier rates of hepatitis B virus (Bassendine et al. 1979).

In HBsAg-positive patients, the presence of cirrhosis greatly increases the risk of developing HCC, from an annual incidence of 201 per 100 000 men without cirrhosis to 2419 per 100 000 men with cirrhosis (Beasley and Hwang 1984). It should be noted that in certain cases HBsAg is no longer present in the serum but evidence of chronic infection by hepatitis B is provided by the presence of the virus DNA in the liver (Brechot et al. 1985). Harvey et al. (1984) showed that several members of the same family who had become infected by hepatitis B virus at birth subsequently developed HCC between the ages of 20 and 40 years. This suggests a familial disposition for HCC and that other members of the family should be screened.

Up to 84% of patients with HCC have an associated cirrhosis (Ihde et al. 1974; Bismuth et al. 1983; Okuda et al. 1986). Furthermore, the discovery rate of HCC in a survey in China was 15–38 per 100 000 in the general population whereas in the same provinces it was 330–985 per 100 000 of those with liver disease (Tang and Yang 1985). HCC develops more commonly in macronodular cirrhosis and arises frequently in haemochromatosis, where there is a 30% risk of developing a tumour if fibrosis or cirrhosis persists after treatment of the iron excess (Bomford and Williams 1976). The incidence of HCC in alcohol cirrhotics is between 5% and 25% (Powell et al. 1971; Johnson et al. 1978 b), in cryptogenic cirrhosis 10% (Powell et al. 1971). Tumours have developed infrequently in patients with primary biliary cirrhosis (Krasner et al. 1979) and secondary biliary cirrhosis (Jakobovitz et al. 1984). The development of HCC has been described in other liver diseases, but the association is tenuous. Other factors have been implicated in the development of HCC. Extensive epidemiological studies in China have shown an association between the source of drinking water and aflatoxin contamination of food and the risk of developing HCC. A fourfold increase in detection of aflatoxin food contamination was accompanied by a rise in liver cancer mortality from 8.3 to 25.6 per 100 000 population (Yu 1985). In general, however, the risk of developing HCC is maximal in HbsAg-positive subjects if they develop cirrhosis, are male and over 60 years of age.

Pathology

Although the distribution of the different types of HCC appears to vary from one part of the world to another (Okuda et al. 1984), they can be classified in terms of their macroscopic appearance. The invasive type has no defined edge and invades normal liver parenchyma and adjacent vessels. The multifocal type involves large areas of liver, and since it invariably arises in cirrhotic liver a multicentric origin seems likely. The expanding type has a definite edge which appears to push back normal liver and vessels but, at an advanced stage, this tumour is surrounded by small satellite lesions. The expanding type of HCC can be subdivided into three subtypes: nodular tumours arising in cirrhotic liver; pseudoadenomatous tumours which are homogeneous lesions resembling benign hepatocellular adenomas with necrotic and haemorrhagic areas and arise from normal liver; and sclerosing tumours, characterised by a diffuse fibrous reaction and normally found in non-cirrhotic liver. Fibrolamellar tumours belong to this last-named group.

All HCC have a rich arterial blood supply, and this accounts for the frequent episodes of intraperitoneal and intratumoral bleeding. Necrosis of the tumour can give rise to arteriovenous fistula. Direct local invasion of these tumours can occur in three ways. In 60% of cases there is spread via the branches of the portal veins (Carella et al. 1981; Makuuchi 1985). The tumour can progress to involve the portal vein itself or the superior mesenteric and splenic veins. This method of spread is important when deciding on the appropriate surgical treatment of these tumours. In about 20% of cases, the hepatic veins are involved by tumour invasion which can extend into the superior vena cava and right atrium. The third and least common method of spread is by invasion of the intrahepatic bile ducts, which may give rise to haemobilia or jaundice if major ducts are involved (Carella et al. 1981). Secondary spread of the tumour is frequent but limited. The commonest sites are the regional lymphatics, lymph nodes, lungs and bone.

The microscopic appearance of these tumours is variable, ranging from a more common trabeculated pattern, similar to the normal liver architecture, to a ductular or papillary pattern. Some clear cell and anaplastic forms occur. It is not uncommon to find a tumour possessing zones with differing degrees of differentiation. The histological features may give a guide to prognosis. Although Takashi et al. (1984) have suggested that the presence of a capsule indicates a good prognosis, this has not been confirmed in our experience (Zillhardt et al. 1985). We have noted that recurrence rates and long-term mortality are worse when the tumour has a less substantial reticulum framework on microscopy (Table 2). The fibrolamellar type of HCC belongs to the group with an even and abundant distribution of reticulum. This tumour variant, which is also known as eosinophil HCC, has received much attention in recent years because of its more favourable prognosis, but it comprises only about 0.2% of all HCC (Okuda et al. 1984). This type of tumour primarily affects a younger age group and represents 40% of primary liver cancers under 35 years of age (Farhi et al. 1983). These lesions usually arise in normal liver tissue and there is no apparent link between their development and hepatitis B virus infection. They are more commonly found in the left lobe of the liver and microscopically have abundant fibrous tissue and polygonal cells with granular cytoplasm (eosinophilic). This appearance may be homogeneous but recurrence of a fibrolamellar tumour has been described following previous resection of a mixed lesion (Zillhardt et al. 1985). Because of their similarity to benign hepatic adenomas and focal nodular hyperplasia, it has been suggested that fibrolamellar tumours may arise from these benign lesions (Vecchio et al. 1984).

Table 2. Value of reticulum framework as an indicator of prognosis in HCC

Reticulum framework	Number of patients	Tumour recurrence	Deaths
Even distribution	11	4	1
Uneven distribution	7	5	6
Sparse or absent	4	3	4

From Zillhardt et al. (1985).

Investigation

Hepatocellular carcinomas often present at an advanced stage because they have developed in an already diseased liver. A high degree of clinical awareness should therefore be maintained in order to detect any change in symptomatology or worsening of liver failure in the patient with established cirrhosis. Liver function tests are invariably abnormal on presentation and tend to show a cholestatic pattern (Ihde et al. 1974). Other biochemical tests may be abnormal but will not help to differentiate between HCC and other liver diseases. High serum vitamin B_{12} binding capacity has been observed in three-quarters of cases of fibrolamellar carcinomas (Paradinas et al. 1982; Denis et al. 1984) but it remains to be seen whether this tumour marker will be of value in diagnosis or prognosis. It may be of value along with other tumour markers, such as neurotensin (Collier et al. 1984), in monitoring treatment of this particular group of patients.

Table 3. Incidence of abnormal AFP levels in patients with and without liver disease

	Number of patients	Number with AFP >10 IU/l
Normal control	50	0
Cirrhosis	100	1
Cirrhosis and HCC	30	29
Normal liver and HCC	20	11
Secondary liver cancer	50	3

From Johnson et al. (1978 a).

Although serum carcinoembryonic antigen (CEA) may be elevated in some cases of HCC, serum alphafetoprotein (AFP) concentrations are more specific in diagnosis. Radioimmunoassay has improved the sensitivity of AFP measurement in the detection of HCC in areas with a low prevalence (Johnson et al. 1978 a). It is of particular value in detecting and excluding HCC in cirrhosis, but less useful in distinguishing between HCC and secondary hepatic deposits in patients without cirrhosis (Table 3). When AFP measurements have been used to monitor HBsAg-positive patients, tumours have not usually been detected until they have attained a diameter of about 2 cm (Yun-Fan et al. 1986; Okuda et al. 1975). Measurement of AFP has been used in mass screening for early detection of HCC. Tang and Yang (1985) undertook such a survey in over 2 million individuals in Shanghai and detected 351 subclinical cases of HCC (discovery rate 16 per 100 000). The asymptomatic patients tended to have small tumours which were amenable to surgical resection, resulting in higher survival rates than for clinically symptomatic patients. Regular measurement of AFP levels appears to be the only feasible means of detecting HCC in at-risk patients before the lesion presents clinically and at a time when surgical excision may still be possible. Unfortunately, the fibrolamellar variant of HCC which carries a favourable prognosis does not appear to be associated with high levels of AFP. All 10 of the patients studied by Paradinas et al. (1982) had normal AFP levels, although others have reported variable elevation of levels (Collier et al. 1984; Craig et al. 1980). AFP levels can also be used to measure response to therapy (Yamada et al. 1983).

In experienced hands, ultrasonography has proved valuable in the detection and management of hepatic tumours (Sheu et al. 1985; Okuda 1986). Tumours as small as 2 cm can be detected and are generally seen as hypoechogenic areas. Displacement of intrahepatic or hepatic veins may be seen with larger tumours, and invasion of intrahepatic or extrahepatic portal veins or hepatic branches draining into the inferior vena cava may be demonstrated. Interpretation of scans may be made difficult by the presence of cirrhosis, but the hypoechogenicity of HCC should allow differentiation from surrounding hyperechogenic fibrotic areas. Portal hypertension may be inferred from an increase in the diameter of the portal vein and its branches or from detection of splenomegaly and a collateral circulation. In a study where real-time ultrasound was prospectively undertaken in 528 high-risk subjects, Sheu et al. (1985) detected 24 cases of subclinical HCC in 42% of which AFP levels were normal. Prospective AFP measurement and ultrasonography in 432 patients with chronic type B hepatitis detected eight asymptomatic patients (six by AFP, seven by ultrasound) with HCC (Liaw et al. 1986). The combination of AFP measurement and liver ultrasonography offers the best prospect of identifying HCC at an early stage and at a time when surgical treatment is possible (Okuda 1986; Liaw et al. 1986; Tang and Yang 1985).

HCC have a characteristic angiographic appearance. The normal intrahepatic arteries are displaced around the tumour, which is supplied by large abnormal vessels. There is an extensive tumour blush, and arteriovenous malformations may be present. In the portal venous phase of the angiogram it may be possible to identify tumour thrombus, which is diagnostic of HCC. Distortion of the hepatic vascular tree may be less marked with small HCC. These features may be of value in differentiating metastatic from primary tumours, but angiography is of most value in determining the feasibility of surgery or in alerting the surgeon to vascular anomalies. Although it has been suggested that a combination of hepatic arteriography, portal venography and inferior venacavography may be necessary to decide on resectability (Williamson et al. 1980), it is our practice to rely on arteriography with portal venous phase radiology and ultrasonography preoperatively with ultrasound at the time of surgery.

Radionuclide imaging is a relatively obsolete investigation in the diagnosis of HCC, and computed tomography (CT) should be undertaken when ultrasound examination is completed. Lesions are generally of low density but are easily obscured by adjacent cirrhotic liver. Injection of contrast medium may assist in augmenting the image of the lesion, which is generally well defined due to its high vascularity but can be irregular when there are areas of haemorrhagic necrosis. Detection of small lesions is reported to have improved with intra-arterial injection of Lipiodol, an oily contrast medium which is more selectively taken up by HCC and remains visible on CT for several weeks (Maki et al. 1985). CT may on occasion demonstrate vascular invasion but is of greater value in detecting extrahepatic spread of tumour to lymphatics.

There is some debate as to whether biopsy of a suspected HCC should be undertaken before surgery (Ballet and Poupon 1985). Where preliminary investigations have demonstrated a lesion which is not amenable to surgical intervention, histology may be helpful in planning subsequent treatment. However, biopsy may compromise a potentially curative surgical resection, seeding of tumour has been noted even when fine-needle biopsy is employed (Ferruci et al. 1979). Biopsy under ultrasound guidance can give positive cytology in about 90% of cases (Montali et al. 1982; Grant et al. 1983; Cornud et al. 1985). However, most studies have been undertaken in patients with both primary and secondary tumours such that, although positive cytology is obtained, a definitive statement on the type of tumour can be given in only 77% of cases (Cornud et al. 1985). Furthermore, when the liver is cirrhotic, it is possible to identify the tumour type in less than half the cases (Messner et al. 1985). The debate regarding biopsy is further confused in a recent review by Okuda (1986) who states that a lesion which is clearly identified by ultrasound, CT or angiography and appears benign on histological examination is most likely premalignant. Invasion of surrounding parenchyma by normal-appearing hepatocytes from an adenomatous hyperplastic nodule has been seen, and small nodules of overt malignant cells have been demonstrated in several adenomatous hyperplastic nodules.

Peroperative ultrasonography has further improved the chances of detecting small lesions, allows assessment of the tumour and has increased the therapeutic possibilities (Makuuchi et al. 1981; Bismuth and Castaing 1985; Castaing et al. 1986a). It has advantages over conventional preoperative scanning: the liver can be scanned over its entire surface, so that the limits of the tumour and its relationship to vessels can be defined; the absence of a costal margin and abdominal wall and bowel gas improves the quality of the image, with better definition of structures. Intraoperative ultrasonography greatly facilitates the study of hepatic vessels, and using a segmental classification of the liver (Couinaud 1957; Bismuth et al. 1982) resectability of the tumour can be assessed or the extent of resection planned (Bismuth and Castaing 1985; Castaing et al. 1986b). Previously unrecognised invasion of a hepatic vein by tumour may change the surgical approach. For example, in the case of a tumour apparently confined to the posterolateral segment of the right hepatic lobe, scanning will determine whether multiple or contralateral metastases exist (inoperable tumour), localise the lesion exactly in the two lateral segments of the right hepatic lobe (segmentectomy VII or bisegmentectomy VII and VIII) and relate the tumour to the middle hepatic vein in order to determine whether a right hepatectomy with segmentectomy IV (extended right hepatectomy) is required. The sensitivity of this investigation has been demonstrated by Castaing et al. (1986a); 13 out of 40 histologically proven HCC less than 3 cm in diameter were not diagnosed by preoperative ultrasonography or angiography but where detected by peroperative scan.

Ultrasonography can be further used to guide biopsy of suspected lesions. It is of particular value in the cirrhotic liver where a limited resection is required in order to preserve function. It can be used to facilitate the passage of a needle into the segmental branch of the portal vein, to inject methylene blue, or of a small balloon catheter, in similar fashion, to occlude the segmental vessel. Accurate excision is facilitated by the injection of dye into this vessel (Makuuchi 1985; Castaing et al. 1986b).

Treatment

The prognosis for patients with HCC is generally dismal, with 66% of untreated sufferers dying within 6 months of presentation (Ihde et al. 1974) and less than 22% surviving the first year (Okuda 1986). However, the increasing early detection of HCC in asymptomatic patients has improved duration of survival (Table 4). Comparison of asymptomatic HCC found on screening with clinically apparent HCC has shown a fivefold increase in resection rates and a tenfold increase in 5-year survival rates (Tang 1985). Resection of the tumour offers the only hope of long-term survival (Okuda 1986). Unfortunately, surgical resection is possible in only a small proportion of HCC patients due to the extent of tumour spread on presentation and the severity of the associated

Table 4. Effect of screening for subclinical HCC on resectability and 5-year survival rates on patients in Shanghai

	n	Resected	Operative mortality	Five-year survival	
				Overall	Resection
HCC	466	24.7%	6.1%	4.2%	16.1%
Subclinical HCC	100	60%	1.7%	43.9%	72.9%

From Tang (1985).

cirrhosis (Okuda et al. 1984; Bismuth et al. 1986b). These lesions are often multifocal, and extrahepatic spread to lymph nodes, peritoneum, portal vein, lung and bone are often present at the time of presentation.

HCC tends to present in two patient types and this gives rise to differing approaches in management.

Cirrhosis

Many cirrhotic HCC patients have some degree of liver dysfunction, either because the tumour has arisen at an advanced stage in the cirrhotic process or because an exacerbation of liver disease has led to an incidental diagnosis of HCC. There is a significant risk of haemorrhage in these patients due to pre-existing coagulopathy or portal hypertension, and there is a danger of precipitating liver failure with the resection of functioning hepatic tissue. The risk of the patient developing hepatic insufficiency in the postoperative period is difficult to assess preoperatively, although attempts have been made to do so by estimating the percentage of functional parenchyma remaining after surgery (Bismuth et al. 1983; Okamoto et al. 1984). The decision on suitability for resection should be based on evaluation of the tumour by ultrasonography, selective coeliac and superior mesenteric angiography and CT of the liver and lungs. Evaluation of liver function has been assessed in our institution by using the simple classification presented in Table 5 (Bismuth et al. 1983). Estimates of the feasibility of resection have been undertaken using a previously described formula (Bismuth et al. 1983):

$$\frac{\text{Quantity of functional liver removed} \times \text{degree of liver insufficiency}}{\text{Total quantity of functional liver}}$$

Quantitive measurements of the total liver volume and the volume removed are based on ultrasound, CT and angiography. The degree of liver insufficiency is 1 for group A patients, 2 for group B and 3 for group C (see Table 5). It has been our policy, therefore, to resect no more than 50% of functional tissue in group A, 24% in group B and 17.5% in group C patients.

If postoperative morbidity and mortality are to be kept to a minimum, techniques have to be developed to minimise the resection of functioning liver tissue. The surgeon must make every attempt at the time of operation to obtain histological confirmation of the tumour and to exclude extrahepatic metastatic spread. He must achieve control of the arterial and portal venous inflow of the segment to be resected at an early stage, and dissection should be performed in such a way as to minimise blood loss. It is our policy to transect liver parenchyma using a Kelly dissector and Cavitron, ligating vessels and bile ducts as they come into view. Following resection, absence of biliary leakage is confirmed by injecting methylene blue through the cystic duct (Bismuth et al. 1982). Intraoperative ultrasonography has proved invaluable in localising the tumour with accuracy in cirrhotic liver and allows careful examination of related vessels (Makuuchi et al. 1981; Sheu et al. 1985; Castaing et al. 1986b). Methylene blue can be injected under ultrasound control into a proximally clamped branch of the portal vein, facilitating excision of a minimal amount of functioning tissue with the tumour (Makuuchi 1985). Ultrasonography has also been used to place a balloon catheter in the portal branch of the liver segment containing the HCC in order to selectively occlude the area to be resected (Shima; Bismuth et al. 1986b). The introduction of these methods has undoubtedly improved the surgeon's ability to remove the tumour safely, and this is reflected in the increasing number of resections undertaken in our own institution in the last 14 years. Nonetheless, the morbidity and mortality associated with resection in this high-risk group is considerable. In our own series of 270 patients with HCC, only 35 resections were feasible. No patient died at operation, but there were five postoperative deaths and 50% of the survivors developed significant postoperative complications (Bismuth et al. 1986b). The postoperative mortality and major complications are shown in Table 6. In only one

Table 5. Criteria used to assess relative risk of patients undergoing liver resection

Criteria	Value	Score
Serum albumin	< 3 g/100 ml	1
Serum bilirubin	> 30 mmol/l	1
Encephalopathy	disorientation in time/space and/or asterixis present	
Ascites (clinical)		1
Coagulation factors		
$\frac{\text{Prothrombin} + \text{factor II}}{2}$	60%–40%	1
	< 40%	2
Assessment		
Group A: total score 0		
Group B: total score 1–2		
Group C: total score ⩾ 3		

From Bismuth et al. (1983).

Table 6. Postoperative risk related to severity of liver disease in 35 patients undergoing liver resection for HCC

Group	Number of patients	Postoperative deaths	Postoperative liver failure
A	25	0	6
B	8	4	3
C	2	1	1

From Bismuth et al. (1986b).

patient (in group B) was the extent of the resection close to the 24% acceptable limit previously described. The risk of complications or death was related to the severity of hepatic insufficiency. Nineteen of the 30 patients discharged from hospital have since died, 17 of them from recurrent disease.

The proportion of smaller HCC which are being resected has increased due to ultrasonography and AFP screening of at-risk patients (Bismuth et al. 1986b). Tang (1985) has shown an increased resectability rate on earlier detection of these small lesions, with an overall 5-year survival rate of 43.9%, but a recent natural history study of HCC measuring less than 3 cm in diameter has shown a 3-year survival rate of only 13% in this group (Ebera et al. 1986). It has yet to be seen whether a similar aggressive approach to small HCC will produce favourable long-term survival rates elsewhere, since it appears that there may be important differences between the Far East and Western countries with regard to the behavioural pattern of the tumour and the underlying cirrhosis.

Non-cirrhotic Disease

The risks following resection in the non-cirrhotic patient are about 15%–20% lower than in the cirrhotic patient. The non-cirrhotic patient, however, tends first to present with symptoms when the tumour has reached a considerable size, whereas the lesion involving cirrhotic liver is identified more often on routine screening. Although tumours in non-cirrhotic liver disseminate in the same way as in cirrhotic liver, we have found that 55% of these lesions are amenable to resection (Bismuth et al. 1984). There is less risk of liver failure, since the remaining liver parenchyma is normal and, on occasion, the normal unaffected lobe has hypertrophied (Bismuth et al. 1983). Extended right hepatectomy (right liver + segment IV or segment IV + I) can be undertaken for tumours arising in the right lobe and extending to the left. Excision may not be possible where such large tumours penetrate posteriorly and prejudice the venous drainage of the left lobe by invasion of the left hepatic vein. Peroperative ultrasonography is of value in assessing resectability by demonstrating invasion and involvement of the hepatic veins (Bismuth et al. 1984). If the tumour abuts onto the inferior vena cava, it may be advantageous to use a vascular isolation technique (Heaney et al. 1966; Huguet et al. 1976; Bismuth et al. 1984), dividing all the ligamentous attachments of the liver and freeing the entire inferior vena cava behind the liver. The liver is completely isolated by clamping the inferior vena cava above and below along with the vessels at the porta hepatis. Resection of the tumour can then be performed safely under optimal haemostasis within an hour.

The outcome for non-cirrhotic patients undergoing resection of HCC is considerably better than for these with cirrhosis (Bismuth et al. 1983; Okuda 1986). Of the last 42 non-cirrhotic patients to undergo curative resection in our institution, 24 were still alive at the time of writing and six of these had survived beyond 5 years (Bismuth et al. 1983). The fibrolamellar variant of HCC carries a more favourable prognosis, with 5-year survival of 63% (Craig et al. 1980). Every attempt should be made to excise fibrolamellar tumours, even if this involves extensive resection. If the tumour is too extensive to allow safe curative resection, there may be an indication for liver transplantation. To date, the long-term results of transplantation for HCC have not been encouraging, with a 60% incidence of recurrence in the grafted liver or at extrahepatic sites (Calne et al. 1981; Iwatsuki et al. 1985). In an analysis of liver transplantation data from 540 patients, Scharschmidt (1985) reviewed the records of 140 patients who had undergone transplantation for neoplastic disease. One- and 3-year survival was 26% and 12% respectively and was similar for patients transplanted before and after January 1980, despite improvements in surgical technique, supportive care and immunosuppressive therapy. Tumour recurrence may be due to the presence of extrahepatic deposits, which are common with these large tumours but which are not identified by preoperative investigation. For this reason, it is our practice when considering such patients for transplantation to undertake an exploratory operation to identify extrahepatic metastases. Despite normal preoperative investigations, we have found on exploration that 50% of cases have extrahepatic spread, usually confined to lymph nodes (Bismuth et al. 1986b). The debate as to whether resection or transplantation should be undertaken will continue, but the need for trial dissections should be obviated by adequate preoperative investigation and peroperative ultrasonography.

The outlook for patients who are unsuitable for resection is poor, with an average duration of survival of 2–6 months (Ihde et al. 1974; Okuda 1986). The results of chemotherapy have been generally disappointing. Some success, however, has been reported with doxorubicin when given systemically (Falkson et al. 1978; Ballet et al. 1982) and by intra-arterial hepatic infusion (Bern et al. 1978). The most encouraging results have followed the administration of doxorubicin in cycles using a dose of 60 mg/m^3 at 3-weekly intervals (Johnson et al. 1978b). Among patients unsuitable for surgical intervention, some form of regression, as demonstrated by imaging and AFP levels, was seen in 25% of cases. Less than 10% of patients achieved complete remission of symptoms, but median survival was 2 years. Despite these encouraging results, further large studies have shown little evidence to suggest that the duration of survival is improved by chemotherapy (Okuda 1986).

Both cryosurgery and high-power YAG laser beam vaporisation have been shown to be effective in small numbers of patients with superficial lesions (Tang 1985). Where surgical excision was not possible due to the situation of the tumour or due to coexisting cirrhosis, 1- and 2-year survival rates of 60% and 20% respectively were obtained with cryosurgery. Transarterial embolisation has the obvious advantage, over surgical ligation, of avoiding laparotomy, but it also delays collateral resupply of the tumour by obliterating the hepatic artery and the branches feeding the tumour (Blumgart and Allison 1982). Embolisation does produce pain and fever as a result of the liver cell necrosis, but this is usually short-lived. Of 120 patients with unresectable hepatoma so treated, 96% demonstrated a substantial fall in AFP along with a selective disappearance of tumour vessels and an isolated decrease in tumour density on CT scanning (Yamada et al. 1983). Seventy-five per cent of tumours showed a 50% reduction in size. Embolisation can be combined with selective chemotherapy (Maki et al. 1985), and we have been encouraged by our early results using this particular technique, which is employed as palliation for those patients who present with large irresectable HCC. Both chemotherapy and embolisation may be considered for patients in whom there is doubt regarding the feasibility of resection of the HCC. A favourable response to therapy may be achieved, with reduction in tumour size sufficient to allow safe resection. Patients with such lesions should thus be carefully monitored.

Hepatoblastoma

Hepatoblastoma is the most common liver tumour of childhood and invariably presents before the age of 3 years, at a time when HCC is rare (Ishak and Glunz 1967; Weinberg and Finegold 1983). It is more common in boys than in girls, but does not appear to be associated with chronic hepatitis B infection and is found in non-cirrhotic liver.

Hepatoblastoma generally presents as a large lesion with abdominal pain, weight loss and abdominal distension. It is lobulated and may contain areas of necrosis and haemorrhage. Microscopically, epithelial and mixed types of tumour have been identified (Ishak and Glunz 1967). The former type comprises either foetal or embryonic hepatocytes, whilst the latter has both these primitive hepatocytes with a proliferation of collagen. In some mixed hepatoblastomas areas of osteoid tissue and cartilage may be present. Irrespective of the type, there is generally invasion of the portal vein branches and/or hepatic veins.

On clinical examination the liver is generally palpable. The levels of AFP are almost always elevated (Okuda et al. 1980), and several cases of precocious puberty have been reported, with production of gonadotrophin (Beach et al. 1984). Ultrasonography and CT will invariably detect these tumours because of their size on presentation, though arteriography will be necessary to delineate the vascular supply of the tumour. The diagnosis is confirmed by needle or surgical biopsy.

Treatment

The treatment of choice for hepatoblastoma is total excision, and this can be undertaken in about 70%–75% of cases (Okuda et al. 1980; Weinberg and Finegold 1983). The principles of excision are the same as for HCC. Local recurrence of metastatic spread following resection usually ensues within 3 years but may occur later. Transplantation of the liver has been undertaken in children, but where primary liver malignancy was the main indication there have been no 5-year survivors. However, one transplanted patient who was found incidentally to have a liver malignancy survived beyond 6 years (Iwatsuki et al. 1985).

Some success has been reported by Weinberg and Finegold (1983) in the treatment of unresectable lesions with doxorubicin, vincristine, cyclophosphamide, 5-fluorouracil and cisplatinum. It has been

proposed that preoperative chemotherapy may allow excision of a previously unresectable tumour in a few patients (Forouhar et al. 1984), and others have suggested that systemic chemotherapy following resection has improved long-term survival (Weinberg and Finegold 1983).
The prognosis for patients with hepatoblastoma will depend on whether the lesion is resectable and on the type of malignant hepatocytes. Recurrence and metastases are more frequent in the embryonic type than in the tumour containing foetal cells. The 5-year survival rate following surgical resection is 62% compared with only 45% overall (Okuda et al. 1980).

Cholangiocarcinoma

Cholangiocarcinomas arise from the epithelial cells of the bile ducts; only those arising from the intrahepatic ducts are considered as liver tumours. Such tumours are less frequent than those arising in the extrahepatic biliary tree and are about 15 times less common than HCC (Okuda et al. 1980).

Cholangiocarcinoma affects the 50–80 age group and has a male predominance which is somewhat less pronounced than that of HCC. Like hepatoblastoma, it tends to arise in normal liver tissue with no history of infection. There is debate whether it may be caused by biliary stasis (Kawarada and Mizumoto 1984), and an association between cholangiocarcinoma and Caroli's syndrome (Dayton et al. 1983) has been suggested.

Cholangiocarcinoma usually presents with abdominal pain, jaundice or an abdominal mass (Okuda et al. 1980; Kawarada and Mizumoto 1984). Both gamma-glutamyl transpeptidase and alkaline phosphatase tend to be elevated on presentation, but AFP is not often elevated. Ultrasonography usually shows a solid large tumour, but the lesions are generally hypovascular on angiography. The diagnosis can be confirmed by biopsy. Tumour spread is to the peritoneal cavity, diaphragm and lungs.

The outlook for patients with cholangiocarcinoma is poorer than for those with HCC. Less than 10% of tumours are amenable to resection, and even in these cases survival beyond 3–4 years is uncommon (Okuda et al. 1980; Kawarada and Mizumoto 1984). Both radiotherapy and chemotherapy have been used, but their value is debatable (Kawarada and Mizumoto 1983).

Cystadenocarcinoma

Cystadenocarcinoma always arises from cystadenoma, an extremely rare tumour affecting females over 40 years of age (Ishak and Glunz 1977). The diagnosis is established by ultrasonography and CT scanning, which show a multiloculated fluid-filled lesion. This feature differentiates cystadenoma/cystadenocarcinoma from the unilocular benign cyst. Where investigation demonstrates a benign cystadenoma, this should be resected before malignant transformation occurs. A benign cyst should be deroofed when symptoms arise, but this is not often required. In case of doubt as to the diagnosis, surgical exploration is indicated. Transformation to cystadenocarcinoma should be strongly suspected when ultrasonography demonstrates a number of papillary projections into the lumen (Stanley et al. 1983). Percutaneous biopsy under ultrasonography guidance can be performed to confirm the diagnosis, but surgical exploration is advisable to enable peroperative ultrasonography and definitive biopsy.

Angiosarcoma

Angiosarcoma (synonyms: haemangioendothelioma, haemangioendotheliosarcoma, haemangioblastoma) develops from the endothelial cells lining the hepatic sinusoids. It is extremely rare, although it is the most common of the liver sarcomas (annual incidence 0.25 per million), and normally affects the 50–70 age group (Locker et al. 1979). In a number of cases it may be possible to identify a causal relationship, e. g. exposure to thorotrast, radiation, arsenic, vinyl chloride or ingestion of steroids (Popper et al. 1978; Locker et al. 1979).

Characteristically, angiosarcomas are ill-defined and multiloculated with areas of necrosis and haemorrhage. Adjacent liver may be fibrotic or cirrhotic when a precipitating factor has been demonstrated. The presentation of this rare tumour does not distinguish it from other primary malignancies and there is invariably an elevation of gamma-glutamyl transpeptidase and alkaline phosphatase. AFP and CEA are normal. On occasion, there is an associated thrombocytopenia, evidence of haemolysis or a disseminated intravascular coagulation due to the destruction of blood cells and consumption of coagulation factors by this vascular lesion. Ultrasonography and CT show a solid tumour, but angiography may be diagnostic by showing a peripheral hypervascular zone with pooling of contrast and a central avascular area (Locker et al. 1979).

The diagnosis can only be confirmed by histology, but percutaneous biopsy should be avoided because of the risk of causing haemoperitoneum. Biopsy should therefore be undertaken via the transjugular route or at surgery. Angiosarcoma carries a poor prognosis, with median survival of 6 months. The tumour extends to peritoneum, diaphragm and pleura, with distant metastases to lung and bone. Excision is not always possible, and other treatment modalities have not been well assessed with this rare lesion (Locker et al. 1979).

Other Sarcomas

Although other primary sarcomas of the liver have been described, they are extremely rare. Undifferentiated embryonic sarcoma is usually found in children less than 10 years of age and consists of well-defined, rapidly growing cystic lesions (Stocker and Ishak 1978). Differentiated lesions include fibrosarcoma, leiomyosarcoma and malignant epithelioid haemangioendothelioma. The last-named lesion, only recently recognised and reviewed by Ishak et al. (1984), pursues a much less aggressive course than hepatic angiosarcoma. It infiltrates and obliterates hepatic and portal venous channels and may lead to extensive hepatic fibrosis. Immunohistochemical staining for factor VIII-related antigen is present to a variable extent in all of these tumours. Because of their relative rarity, the most effective treatment for these lesions is not known. Hepatic resection may not be possible because of the diffuse hepatic involvement and liver transplantation should be considered if disease is localised to the liver. Nonetheless, survival beyond 5 years has been described in patients who received no treatment (Ishak et al. 1984).

Secondary Hepatic Tumours

Secondary tumours are the most common type of liver malignancy in Western countries and may originate from any part of the body. According to Willis (1973), one-third of patients with malignant disease have hepatic metastases at autopsy (Table 7). Clinicians have tended to focus their attention on the management of liver metastases from colorectal carcinoma since other tumours tend to have a poor prognosis irrespective of evidence of hepatic involvement (Bengmark et al. 1972). Colorectal tumours tend to spread predominantly to the liver, where their growth is generally slow. Since the primary carcinoma can be controlled by wide resection, there is an increasing trend to offer patients intervention for their secondary lesion. Treatment of hepatic metastases from other primaries will not be discussed here, but the indications for surgical intervention are similar to those in colorectal metastasis.

Table 7. Frequency of hepatic metastases at autopsy

Primary site	Frequency of hepatic metastases (%)	
	Literature survey	Willis
Oesophagus	27	41
Stomach	33	46
Pancreas	60	73
Large bowel	33	53

From Willis (1973).

Liver secondaries are present in 15%–25% of patients with colorectal cancer at the time of their initial presentation. Of 550 patients undergoing radical resection of a primary colorectal cancer, 186 developed recurrence and in 74 (40%) this involved the liver. In only 41 patients (22%), however, was the liver the sole site of secondary spread (Russel et al. 1984). The authors indicated that treatment aimed only at the liver is unlikely to improve survival in disseminated disease and is likely to benefit only a small number of patients. Hepatic metastases may go unnoticed at the time of surgery for the primary colorectal lesion, it has been noted that some of these patients with "occult" hepatic metastases succumb to the malignancy without evidence of dissemination to other sites (Finlay and McArdle 1986). Further evidence to support the treatment of colorectal metastases has come from a natural history study of 466 patients (Wagner et al. 1984). Of the 214 patients considered in retrospect to be suitable for resection, 39 had a single metastasis, with a 3-year survival rate of 21%. Few properly controlled trials of treatment have been undertaken, but the evidence for surgical resection and hepatic dearterialisation or embolisation will be discussed below. The use of cytotoxic agents in the management of disseminated colorectal cancer is discussed by B. Arnesjø et al. in this volume.

Resection

In a review of 141 patients who had undergone resection of hepatic metastases for colorectal cancer over a 35-year period, Adson (1986) noted 3- and

5-year survival of 40% and 25% respectively. A comparison of this treated group with an untreated control group managed in the same institution (Wagner et al. 1984) showed a significant difference in 3-year survival (40% vs 21%). Some authors have found that Dukes' classification of the primary tumour at the time of apparently curative resection is useful in identifying those patients who would benefit from hepatic resection (Adson 1986; Fortner et al. 1984), but this has not been confirmed by others (Ekberg et al. 1986). The size of the lesion only appears to influence operative mortality (Ekberg et al. 1986), and survival does not appear to be influenced by the presence of multiple resectable secondary lesions (Adson 1986); this latter author, however, included all cases where there was more than one tumour deposit as multiple lesions. Ekberg et al. (1986) showed in a smaller study that 41% of patients with less than four metastases survived 3 years, whereas there were no 3-year survivors among those who underwent resection of four or more metastatic deposits. The removal of synchronous or metachronous lesions does not appear to influence survival, but most authors agree that spread of tumour beyond the liver carries an unfavourable prognosis (Ekberg et al. 1986; Adson 1986; Iwatsuki et al. 1983; Fortner et al. 1984). The extent of the resection does influence operative mortality (Adson 1986), and inadequate resection is associated with poor long-term survival (Ekberg et al. 1986).

Selection of patients for hepatic resection of colorectal metastases should be based on these criteria, and careful consideration must be given to the extent of resection. We have had no operative or postoperative mortality in our own experience of 54 resections (Bismuth et al. 1986a) and the figure is below 6% in most large series (Adson 1986; Ekberg et al. 1986). Although there appears to be no significant difference in survival rates between patients undergoing resection of synchronous or metachronous hepatic tumours, it is our policy not to remove both primary and secondary lesions at the same time, in order to enable evaluation of tumour evolution and of response to chemotherapy. Screening patients for the development of liver metastases is time-consuming and expensive but is at present the only way of detecting recurrent disease at a potentially curable stage. Elevation of serum CEA concentration occurs late in recurrent colorectal cancer (Finlay and McArdle 1983), so this investigation must be supplemented by ultrasound and CT if liver metastases are to be detected. It is our policy to vigorously exclude metastatic spread to other sites when patients are referred for consideration of liver resection. This includes colonoscopy to detect local recurrence, CT of the thorax, abdomen and pelvis, and bone scanning. Even when these investigations fail to identify extrahepatic spread, metastatic deposits to lymphatics and lymph nodes may be detected at laparotomy (Ekberg et al. 1986). Assessment of resectability will be based on coeliac and superior mesenteric angiography, ultrasonography and CT.

The principles of surgical resection are identical to those for HCC, although the presence of normal liver tissue will allow larger resections with less risk of precipitating hepatocellular failure. Peroperative ultrasonography is invaluable in assessing suitability for resection and in deciding the extent of resection. We have found that it provides additional information, changing the planned surgical procedure, in 36% of cases undergoing resection of hepatic metastases (Castaing et al. 1986a). The type of resection undertaken for these tumours has changed with experience. We have been disappointed by the results of localised tumour excision, and feel that extensive resections (hemihepatectomy) are inappropriate for small lesions. It is our practice to base excision on the tumour size and we are prepared to excise six segments to achieve this (e.g. right hepatectomy + segments I and IV). When the tumour is small and localised a segmentectomy may be undertaken, ensuring a 2-cm margin of clearance around the tumour. These segmentectomies are facilitated by the use of peroperative ultrasonography, which localises associated vessels and can be used to locate balloon catheters in portal vessels so as to reduce blood loss (see above). It is necessary to control the arterial branch supplying the hepatic lobe in advance of attempted resection.

The 5-year survival rates of up to 40% in patients undergoing resection of hepatic metastases from colorectal carcinoma will encourage surgeons to consider intervention in these patients (Iwatsuki et al. 1983; Adson 1986). But it remains to be seen whether surgical resection will play a part in the management of patients with liver metastases from other primary sites.

Hepatic Dearterialisation and Embolisation

When the hepatic metastasis is so situated that safe surgical excision is not possible, hepatic dearterialisation may be considered. There is, however, a lack of data suggesting clinical benefit. Response to treatment is difficult to assess, but may be judged by diminution in tumour size on CT, a fall in CEA levels or tumour devascularisation on angiography.

Surgical devascularisation can be achieved by simple ligation of the hepatic artery or by radical dissection and division of vessels in the lesser omentum, conserving only the portal vein and common bile duct. The former approach is associated with a large fall in liver blood flow but a drop of less than 10% in tumour blood flow (Taylor et al. 1979). Furthermore, collateral blood flow to the tumour has been demonstrated within a short period of time following ligation of the hepatic artery. A series of 97 patients with colorectal liver metastases treated in this way had a median survival of only 9.5 months (Petrelli et al. 1984). More extensive surgical dearterialisation may reduce the collateral circulation that may persist with ligation of the hepatic artery alone, but the associated high morbidity and mortality has prevented its general use.

A less invasive means of achieving tumour devascularisation is hepatic arterial embolisation. The materials most commonly used for embolisation have been Gelfoam and Ivalon. Both ethanol and Lipiodol have been added to emboli to occlude tumour vessels more effectively. Liver failure is a relative contraindication to embolisation, but if portal vein occlusion exists, massive liver necrosis may ensue. All patients will demonstrate a rise in serum lactic dehydrogenase, transaminases and alkaline phosphatase. We prefer to administer prophylactic antibiotics to reduce the risk of sepsis and abscess formation. Few studies have looked exclusively at the management of hepatic metastases of colorectal carcinoma, but favourable responses have been described (Chuang et al. 1982). Similar responses have recently been reported with combined embolisation and intra-arterial infusion of cytotoxic agents.

Summary

There is uncontrolled evidence to suggest that survival can be prolonged for many patients with either primary or secondary liver tumours by means of the various therapeutic options described. Most patients with malignant hepatic tumours have extrahepatic spread that precludes any benefit from surgical intervention, and those patients who appear to have lesions amenable to resection require careful preoperative assessment. The advent of peroperative ultrasonography has improved patient selection and limits the risk of precipitating liver failure by minimising the size of resection. Patients with apparently irresectable lesions should be closely monitored, since both chemotherapy and embolisation may reduce tumour bulk sufficiently to allow surgical excision. The improvement in therapeutic techniques and the low operative mortality among our own patients has allowed us to pursue an aggressive treatment programme. Should there be a suspicion of recurrent HCC on follow-up we have no hesitation in undertaking second-look laparotomy to consider further resection, although this approach is still being evaluated in hepatic metastases. In the long term, survival rates will improve only if patients are referred for treatment at an earlier stage. This will require screening of those at "high risk" of developing HCC and of patients having undergone apparently curative resection of a primary tumour of the gastrointestinal tract.

References

Adson MA (1986) Liver resection in primary and secondary liver cancer. In: Bengmark S, Blumgart LH (eds) Liver surgery. Livingstone, Edinburgh, pp 63–80

Ballet F, Poupon R (1985) Stratégie diagnostique dans les tumeurs de foie. Gastroenterol Clin Biol 9: 39–41

Ballet F, Barbare JC, Petit J, et al. (1982) Faut-il traiter par l'adriamycine par voie générale le carcinome hépatocellulaire sur cirrhosis non operable? Gastroenterol Clin Biol 6: 267–271

Bassendine MF, Chadwick RG, Lysolotis T, et al. (1979) Primary liver cell cancer in Britain – a viral aetiology? Br Med J 1: 166

Beach R, Betts P, Radford M, Millward-Sadler H (1984) Production of human chorionic gonadotrophin by a hepatoblastoma resulting in precocious puberty. J Clin Pathol 37: 734–737

Beasley RP, Hwang LY (1984) Epidemiology of hepatocellular carcinoma. In: Kyas GN, Dienstag JL, Hoofnagle JN (eds) Viral hepatitis and liver disease. Grune and Stratton, Orlando, pp 209–224

Bengmark S, Hafstrom L, Olsson A (1972) The natural history of primary and secondary liver tumours. V. The prognosis for conventionally treated patients with liver metastases from breast cancer. Digestion 6: 321

Bern MM, MacDermott W, Cady B, et al. (1978) Intraarterial hepatic infusion and intravenous adriamycin for treatment of hepatocellular carcinoma. Cancer 42: 399–405

Bismuth H, Castaing D (1985) Echographie per-operatoire du foie et des voies biliaires. Flammarion, Paris

Bismuth H, Houssin D, Castaing D (1982) Major and minor segmentectomies "réglées" in liver surgery. World J Surg 6: 10–24

Bismuth H, Houssin D, Mazmanian G (1983) Postoperative liver insufficiency: prevention and management. World J Surg 7: 505–510

Bismuth H, Houssin D, Michel P (1984) Chirurgie des carcinomes hépatocellulaires: une nouvelle approche. Chirurgie 11: 509–516

Bismuth H, Castaing D, Arrisueno Gomez de la Torre C (1986a) Chirurgie d'exérèse des métastases hépatiques des cancers colo-rectaux. Chirurgie 112: 45–49

Bismuth H, Houssin D, Ornowski J, Meriggi F (1986b) Liver

resections in cirrhotic patients: a western experience. World J Surg 10: 311–317

Blumberg BS, London WT (1981) Hepatitis B virus and the prevention of primary hepatocellular carcinoma. N Engl J Med 304: 782

Blumgart LH, Allison DJ (1982) Resection and embolisation in the management of secondary hepatic tumours. World J Surg 6: 32–45

Bomford A, Williams R (1976) Long term results of venesection therapy in idiopatic haemochromatosis. Q Med J 45: 611–613

Brechot C, Degos F, Lugassy C, et al. (1985) Hepatitis B virus DNA in patients with chronic liver disease and negative tests for hepatitis B surface antigen. N Engl J Med 312: 270–276

Calne RY, Williams R, Lindop M, et al. (1981) Improved survival after orthotopic liver grafting. Br Med J 283: 115–118

Carella G, Degott C, Benhamou JP (1981) Invasion of the lumen of the bile duct by hepatocellular carcinoma. Liver 1: 251–254

Castaing D, Emond J, Kunstlinger F, Bismuth H (1986a) Utility of operative ultrasound in the surgery of liver tumours. Ann Surg 204: 600–605

Castaing D, Kunstlinger F, Bismuth H (1986b) Ultrasonographie per-opératoire en chirurgie hepatique. J Belge Radiol 69: 1–8

Chuang VP, Wallace S, Soo CS, et al. (1982) Therapeutic Ivalon embolization of hepatic tumours. AJR 138: 289–294

Collier NA, Weinbren K, Bloom SR, et al. (1984) Neurotensin secretion by fibrolamellar carcinoma of the liver. Lancet 1: 538–540

Cornud F, Vissuzaine C, Sibert A, et al. (1985) Sensibilité de la ponction biopsie à l'aiguille fine dans le diagnostic histologique de tumeurs malignes hépatiques et pancréatiques. Gastroenterol Clin Biol 9: 47–50

Couinaud C (1957) Le foie. Etudes anatomiques et chirurgicales. Masson, Paris

Craig JR, Peters RL, Edmundson HA, Omata M (1980) Fibrolamellar carcinoma of the liver: a tumour of adolescents and young adults with distinctive clinico-pathologic features. Cancer 46: 372–379

Dayton MT, Longmire WP, Tompkins RK (1983) Caroli's disease: a premalignant condition? Am J Surg 112: 82–84

Denis J, Grippon P, Legendre C, Tubiana JM, Levy VG (1984) Carcinome fibrolamellaire: un carcinome hépatobiliaire de pronostic favorable. Gastroenterol Clin Biol 8: 920–924

Doll R (1969) The geographical distribution of cancer. Br J Cancer 23: 1–8

Ebera M, Ohto M, Shinagawa T, et al. (1986) Natural history of minute hepatocellular carcinoma smaller than three centimetres complicating cirrhosis: a study in 22 patients. Gastroenterology 90: 289–298

Ekberg H, Tranberg KG, Andersson R, et al. (1986) Determinants of survival in liver resection for colorectal secondaries. Br J Surg 73: 727–731

Falkson G, Moertel CG, Lavin PH, et al. (1978) Chemotherapy studies in primary liver cancer. Cancer 42: 2149–2156

Farhi DC, Shikes RH, Murari PJ, Silverberg SG (1983) Hepatocellular carcinoma in young people. Cancer 52: 1516–1525

Ferrucci JT, Wittemberg J, Margulies MN (1979) Malignant seeding of the tract after thin-needle aspiration biopsy. Radiology 130: 345–346

Finlay IG, McArdle CS (1983) Role of carcinoembryonic antigen in detection of asymptomatic disseminated disease in colorectal carcinoma. Br Med J 286: 1242–1244

Finlay IG, McArdle CS (1986) Occult hepatic metastases in colorectal cancer. Br J Surg 73: 732–735

Forouhar FA, Quinn JJ, Cooke R, Foster JH (1984) The effect of chemotherapy on hepatoblastoma. Arch Pathol Lab Med 108: 311–315

Fortner JG, Silva JS, Golbey RB, et al. (1984) Multivariate analysis of a personal series of 247 consecutive patients with liver metastases from colorectal cancer. Treatment by hepatic resection. Ann Surg 199: 306–316

Grant E, Richardson J, Smirniotopoulus J, Jacobs N (1983) Fine needle biopsy directed by real-time sonography. AJR 141: 29–32

Harvey VJ, Woodfield DG, Probert JC (1984) Maternal transmission of hepatocellular cancer. Cancer 54: 1360–1363

Heaney JP, Stanton WK, Halbert DS, et al. (1966) An improved technique for vascular isolation of liver: Experimental study and case reports. Ann Surg 163: 237–241

Huguet C, Gallot D, Offenstradt G, Coldigner M (1976) Exclusion vasculaire totale du foie dans la chirurgie d'exérèse large. Nouv Presse Med 5: 1189–1193

Ihde DC, Sherlock P, Winnawer SJ, Fortner JG (1974) Clinical manifestations of hepatoma: a review of six years experience at a cancer hospital. Am J Med 56: 83

Ishak KG, Glunz PR (1967) Hepatoblastoma and hepatocarcinoma in infancy and childhood. Report of 47 cases. Cancer 20: 396–422

Ishak KG, Sestechenn IA, Zachary M, et al. (1984) Epithelioid hemangioendothelioma of the liver: a clinicopathologic and follow-up study of 32 cases. Hum Pathol 15: 839–852

Iwatsuki S, Shaw BW, Starzl TE (1983) Experience with 150 liver resections. Ann Surg 197: 247–259

Iwatsuki S, Shaw BW, Starzl TE (1985) Five year survival after liver transplantation. Transplant Proc 17: 259–263

Jakobovitz A, Dubley FJ, Allen P (1984) Primary liver cell carcinoma complicating secondary biliary cirrhosis. Br Med J 289: 227

Johnson PJ, Portmann B, Williams R (1978a) Alpha-fetoprotein concentrations measured by radioimmunoassay in diagnosing and excluding hepatocellular carcinoma. Br Med J 2: 661–663

Johnson PJ, Williams R, Thomas H, et al. (1978b) Induction of remission in hepatocellular carcinoma with doxorubicin. Lancet 1: 1006–1009

Kawarada Y, Mizumoto R (1984) Cholangiocellular carcinoma of the liver. Am J Surg 147: 352–359

Krasner N, Johnson PJ, Portmann B, Watkinson G, MacSween RNM, Wiliams R (1979) Hepatocellular carcinoma in primary biliary cirrhosis: report of four cases. Gut 20: 255–258

Lefkowitch JH (1981) The epidemiology and morphology of primary malignant liver tumours. Surg Clin North Am 61: 169

Liaw YF, Tai DI, Chu CM, et al. (1986) Early detection of hepatocellular carcinoma in patients with chronic type B hepatitis. Gastroenterology 90: 263–267

Locker GY, Doroshaw JH, Zwelling LA, Chabner BA (1979) The clinical features of hepatic angiosarcoma: a report of four cases and a review of the English literature. Medicine (Baltimore) 58: 48–64

Maki S, Komo T, Maeda H (1985) Image enhancement in computed tomography for sensitive diagnosis of liver cancer and semiquantitation of tumour selective drug targeting with oily contrast medium. Cancer 56: 751–757

Makuuchi M (1985) Interventional ultrasound during liver surgery. In: Watanabe H, Makuuchi M (eds) Interventional real-time ultrasound. Igakushoin, Tokyo, pp 122–140

Makuuchi M, Hasegawa A, Yamazaki S (1981) Intraoperative ultrasonic examination for hepatectomy. Jpn J Clin Oncol 11: 367–369

Messner M, Deugnier Y, Bernard-Griffiths L, et al. (1985) Valeur de la cytoponction écho-guidée dans le diagnostic des tumeurs sur cirrhose. Etude de 29 cas. Gastroenterol Clin Biol 9: 42–46

Montali G, Solbiato L, Crole F, Ierace T, Ravetto C (1982) Fine needle aspiration biopsy of liver focal lesions ultrasonically guided with a real-time probe. Report of 126 cases. B J Radiol 55: 717–723

Okamato E, Kyo A, Yamaniaki N, Tanaka N, Kuwata K (1984) Prediction of the safe limits of hepatectomy by combined volumetric and functional measurements in patients with impaired liver function. Surgery 95: 586

Okuda K (1986) Primary liver cancer. Quadrennial review lecture. Dig Dis Sci 31: 133S–146S

Okuda K, Korada K, Obata H, et al. (1975) Clinical observation during a relatively early stage of hepatocellular carcinoma with special reference to serum fetoproteins levels. Gastroenterology 69: 226–234

Okuda K, and the liver cancer study of Japan (1980) Primary liver cancers in Japan. Cancer 45: 2663–2669

Okuda K, Obata H, Nakajima Y, et al. (1984) Prognosis of primary hepatocellular carcinoma. Hepatology 4: 3S–6S

Okuda K, Peters SL, Simson IW (1986) Gross anatomic features of hepatocellular carcinoma from three disparate geographic areas. Proposal of new classification. Cancer 54: 2165–2173

Paradinas FJ, Melia WM, Wilkinson ML, et al. (1982) High serum vitamin B12 binding capacity as a marker of the fibrolamellar variant of hepatocellular carcinoma. Br Med J 285: 840–842

Petrelli NJ, Barcewitz PA, Evans JT, et al. (1984) Hepatic artery ligation for liver metastases in colorectal carcinoma. Cancer 53: 1347–1353

Popper H, Thomas LB, Telles NC, et al. (1978) Development of hepatic angiosarcoma in man induced by vinyl chloride, thorotrast, and arsenic. Comparison with cases of unknown aetiology. Am J Pathol 92: 349–369

Powell LW, Mortimer R, Harris OD (1971) Cirrhosis of the liver: a comparative study of the four major aetiological groups. Med J Aust 1: 941

Russel AH, Tong D, Dawson LE, Wisbeck W (1984) Adenocarcinoma of the proximal colon. Sites of initial dissemination and patterns of recurrence following surgery alone. Cancer 53: 360–367

Scharschmidt BF (1985) Human liver transplantation: analysis of data on 540 patients from four centers. In: Gips CH, Krom RAF (eds) Progress in liver transplantation. Nijhoff, Dordecht, pp 249–266

Sheu JC, Sung JL, Chen DS, et al. (1985) Early detection of hepatocellular carcinoma by real-time ultrasonography. Cancer 56: 660–666

Stanley J, Vujic I, Gobien RP, Reines HD (1983) Evaluation of biliary cystadenoma and cystadenocarcinoma. Gastrointest Radiol 8: 245–248

Stocker JT, Ishak KG (1978) Undifferentiated (embryonal) sarcoma of the liver. Report of 31 cases. Cancer 42: 336–348

Takashi K, Kenpi T, Takashi M, Toshya F, Keiso S, Kiyoshi I (1984) Limited hepatic resection effective for selective cirrhotic patients with primary liver cancer. Ann Surg 199: 51–54

Tang Z (1985) Surgical treatment of subclinical hepatocellular carcinoma. In: Tang Z (ed) Subclinical hepatocellular carcinoma. Springer, Berlin Heidelberg New York, pp 63–75

Taylor I, Bennett R, Sherriff S (1979) The blood supply of colorectal metastases. Br J Cancer 39: 749–756

Tang Z, Yang B (1985) Early detection of subclinical hepatocellular carcinoma. In: Tang Z (ed) Subclinical hepatocellular carcinoma. Springer, Berlin Heidelberg New York, pp 12–21

Tong MJ, Sun S, Schaefter BT, et al. (1971) Hepatitis-associated antigen and hepatocellular carcinoma in Taiwan. Ann Intern Med 75: 687–691

Vecchio FM, Fabiano A, Ghirlanda G, Manna R, Massi G (1984) Fibrolamellar carcinoma of the liver: the malignant counterpart of focal nodular hyperplasia with oncotic change. Am J Clin Pathol 81: 521–526

Wagner JS, Adson MA, van Heerden JA, et al. (1984) The natural history of hepatic metastases from colorectal cancer. A comparison with resective treatment. Ann Surg 199: 502–507

Weinberg AG, Finegold MJ (1983) Primary hepatic tumors of childhood. Hum Pathol 14: 512–537

Williamson BWA, Blumgart LH, McKellar NJ (1980) Management of tumours of the liver. Am J Surg 139: 210–215

Willis RA (1973) Secondary tumours of the liver. In: Willis RA (ed) The spread of tumours in the human body, 3rd edn. Butterworth, London, p 175

Yamada R, Sato M, Kawabata M, et al. (1983) Hepatic artery embolisation in 120 patients with unresectable hepatoma. Radiology 148: 397–401

Yu S (1985) Epidemiology of liver cancer. In: Tang Z (ed) Subclinical hepatocellular carcinoma. Springer, Berlin Heidelberg New York, pp 189–211

Yun-Fan L, Dar In T, Chia-Ming C, et al. (1986) Early detection of hepatocellular carcinoma in patients with chronic type B virus: a prospective study. Gastroenterology 90: 263–267

Zillhardt P, Szekely AM, Houssin D, Santelli G, Lemaigre G, Bismuth H (1985) Carcinome hépatocellulaire sur foie non scirrhotique. Ann Pathol 5: 239–247

Cancer of the Biliary Tract

O. SØREIDE and L. H. BLUMGART

Introduction

Cancer of the bile duct system may arise in any part of the biliary tract – from the intrahepatic biliary radicles to the inflow into the duodenum. Cholangiocarcinoma – the tumour derived from bile duct epithelium – originating from the intrahepatic ductal system may be symptomatically and clinically indistinguishable from other solid liver lesions, whereas tumours located in the pancreatic and ampullary region represent a heterogeneous group which may originate from the true periampullary tissues, the pancreas, the duodenal mucosa or the common bile duct. Thus, this chapter will deal with primary malignant tumours of the left and right hepatic ducts and their confluence, the common hepatic and bile ducts above the pancreas, and with tumours originating in the gallbladder and cystic duct.

Cancer of the bile ducts is rare and carries a poor prognosis. Although uncommon, the wider application of new investigative techniques such as percutaneous transhepatic cholangiography (PTC), endoscopic retrograde cholangiography (ERC), ultrasound (US) and computed tomography (CT) has led to important progress in the morphological diagnosis of jaundice and subsequently to an increasing interest in ascertaining optimal treatment strategies.

A major problem when reviewing the literature on biliary tract tumours is that the reports often encompass decades during which changes in diagnostic and treatment options were made. Similarly, randomized trials – although admittedly difficult to perform – are rarely found, making comparison between treatment approaches difficult. However, improvements in imaging can help select those patients most suitable for surgical intervention, and this chapter suggests that resectional surgery offers the best palliation and the only chance of survival.

Incidence and Epidemiology

A major problem in the study of biliary tract cancer has been the failure of the International Classification of Diseases (ICD) to distinguish between cancers of the liver and biliary system until 1958 (seventh revision). A subsite specification was introduced with the eighth revision, but many national statistics, many cancer registries and even clinical studies group all bile duct tumours together despite major differences in incidence and epidemiology of gallbladder and other bile duct cancers.

The frequency of biliary tract tumours in autopsy series was found to be 0.43% for gallbladder cancer in a review of 206 098 autopsies (Arminsky 1949), and 0.12% for other extrahepatic bile duct cancers in a review of 129 571 autopsies (Sako et al. 1957). However, the incidence of this disease at autopsy varies considerably, and estimates of the frequency of the disease based on autopsy studies are inaccurate, probably due to selection of certain patient groups in the hospitals in which autopsy studies are performed.

The rarity of the disease is further underlined by looking at the proportion of these tumours in relation to other malignant diseases. Based on national cancer registry data, cancer of the gallbladder and extrahepatic bile ducts comprises 0.8% of all malignant tumours registered (1968–1975) and 2.8% of all gastrointestinal malignancies (Cancer Registry of Norway 1980).

The descriptive epidemiology of bile duct cancer reveals an international variation in incidence rates from approximately 2 per 100 000 inhabitants per year in low risk countries (United Kingdom, Norway, United States), to approximately 4–6 per 100 000 in medium risk areas (Canada, Japan, Hawaii, Israel, France). The highest rates (8–10 cases per 100 000 inhabitants) are reported for Rhodesian Africans, Colombians and El Paso Latins (Fraumeni 1975; Diehl 1980).

Gallbladder cancer is more common than other bile duct cancers, the proportions being approximately 75% and 25%, respectively (Krain 1972; Shani et al. 1974, Maram et al. 1979). Tumours of the gallbladder and bile duct show epidemiological distinctions. Gallbladder cancer is twice as common in women than men, while bile duct malignancies have a 60% male predominance (Fraumeni 1975). In both categories the risk increases steadily with age, with a consistent preponderence of females with gallbladder cancer and males with bile duct cancer.

Due to the deficiences in coding practice alluded to above, it is difficult to determine secular trends (Diehl 1980).

Etiology

Usually no clear causative factor can be identified, but the geographical variations suggest a possible role for environmental factors. There exist some coincidental relationships of other conditions with cholangiocarcinoma. Several observations demonstrate the central importance of cholelithiasis as a risk factor for gallbladder cancer, and the frequencies of gallstones and gallbladder cancer run in parallel from one population to another (Hart et al. 1971; Diehl 1980). The frequency of cancer in gallbladders with intramural calcification (porcelain gallbladder) is reported to be exceptionally high (10%–20%; Cornell and Clarke 1959; Etala 1962). Although suggested, a similar relationship is hard to document for other biliary tract cancer.

The association to inflammatory bowel disease, in particular chronic ulcerative colitis, was first reported by Parker and Kendall (1954). It has been estimated that the risk of biliary tract tumours is 10–30 times greater than in the general population (Ritchie et al. 1974; Christophi and Hughes 1985; Mir-Madljessi et al. 1987). The prevalence of bile duct cancer in patients with colitis is in the order of 0.5%–1% and tumours appear 2–3 decades earlier than usual (Akwari et al. 1975; Mir-Madjlessi et al. 1987). Prior proctocolectomy does not prevent the occurrence of cancer (Ritchie et al. 1974).

Recent literature also suggests a clear relationship between primary sclerosing cholangitis (PSC) and bile duct malignancy with cancer occurring in 2%–9% of patients with PSC (Wee et al. 1985; Aadland et al. 1987; Mir-Madjlessi et al. 1987). As nearly all patients with PSC also have inflammatory bowel disease, it is difficult at this time to establish the sequential relationship between colitis, PSC and cancer although Wee et al. (1985) have provided evidence that patients with colitis and bile duct cancer seem to have PSC prior to the development of the malignancy.

Congenital cystic dilatation of any part of the biliary tract is associated to cholangiocarcinoma (Kagawa et al. 1978; Rossi et al. 1987; Todani et al. 1987).

The incidence of carcinoma arising in choledochal cysts varies with age at the initial appearance of symptoms, from 0.7% in cysts that appear before 10 years of age, to 6.8% in the second decade, and 14.3% for older patients (Voyles et al. 1983a). Early excision of the cyst is recommended, in particular in view of recent findings from Japan showing that approximately 20% of cancers related to choledochal cysts occur in patients who had undergone various internal drainage procedures in the past (Todani et al. 1987). Komi et al. (1986) have – in a histological study of excised cysts – also been able to correlate age of the patients with increasing epithelial metaplasia.

Some studies suggest a relationship between infection with *Clonorchis sinensis* and bile duct cancer (Belamaric 1973). This and other liver flukes may potentiate the carcinogenic action of certain chemicals on the biliary epithelium (Flavell and Lucas 1983). Typhoid carriers have been shown to have a mortality from "hepatobiliary cancers" six times that of controls, which was consistent with the postulated conversion of bile to carcinogens of the infectious agent (Welton et al. 1979).

Other reported positive associations with biliary carcinoma include congenital biliary atresia, ileal disease, obesity, diabetes and use of oral contraceptives or postmenopausal estrogens although none has been formally examined (Fraumeni 1975; Diehl 1980).

The relationship between benign tumours of the biliary tract, especially the gallbladder, and later development of frank malignancies is not clearly established, although malignant transformation is thought to occur, especially when papillomatosis is present (Sawyer 1970; Arbab and Brasfield 1976; Gouma et al. 1984; Kozuka et al. 1984). Many surgeons advocate cholecystectomy in any patient in whom a polyp-like lesion is found in the gallbladder. However, several studies have shown that the size of the lesion is a vital indicator of malignancy as cancer is – nearly without exception – only seen in polyps exceeding 10 mm in diameter (Piehler and Crichlow 1978; Kozuka et al. 1982; Koga et al. 1988). Consequently a more expectant approach to the patients with a small polyp may be justified.

A new concept of the etiology of biliary tract cancer has recently been proposed (Suda et al. 1983; Kimura et al. 1985; Nagata et al. 1985; Sameshima et al. 1987), based on the demonstration of the existence of an anomalous ductal junction between the common bile duct and the pancreatic duct. This anomaly permits reflux of pancreatic juice into the bile duct. Such anomaly is frequently seen in patients with choledochal cyst, but cancer may occur even in the absence of cystic dilatation of the bile ducts (Yamauchi et al. 1987). Carcinoma may be considered to arise as a consequence of inflammatory degeneration of the bile duct wall produced by bile stasis and reflux of pancreatic juice.

Pathology

Localization of Tumour

Extrahepatic bile duct tumours are unevenly distributed along the duct. Figure 1 gives the location of lesions based on Longmire's classification (Longmire et al. 1973), and the frequency distribution based on some major series (Tompkins et al. 1981; Kinami and Miyazaki 1982; Evander et al. 1982; Langer et al. 1985). This classification has importance for diagnosis, treatment and prognosis.

Gallbladder cancer tends to occur most commonly in the fundus and neck. However, a major problem is the fact that most cancers (80%–90%) present at an advanced stage (Morrow et al. 1983).

Macroscopic Appearance

Bile duct carcinomas have been recently described as sclerosing, nodular or papillary (Weinbren and Mutum 1983). The sclerosing lesion extends along the duct, thickening the ductal wall and proceeding to extraductal extension producing a fibrous mass.

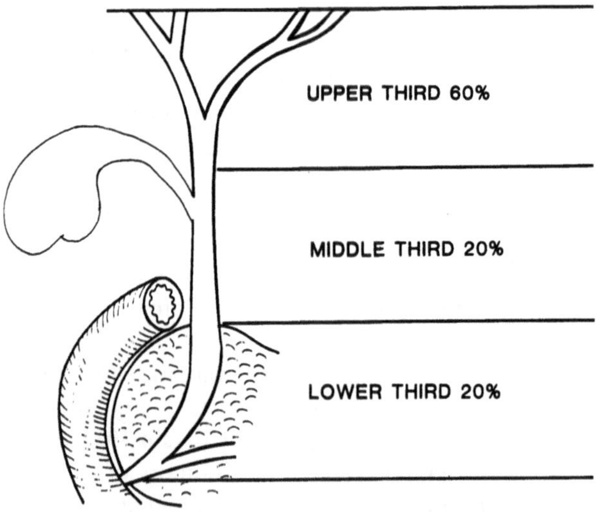

Fig. 1. Anatomical distribution of extrahepatic bile duct tumours

Encasement and compression of the hepatic artery and portal vein are frequently seen. A nodular cholangiocarcinoma has a base which is continuous with the duct wall and projects into the duct lumen. Papillary tumours present as a friable mass, usually with extension into surrounding structures and with accompanying sclerosis of the ductal wall. The sclerotic type is most commonly seen in the proximal duct(s), whereas the nodular and papillary types are encountered in the distal duct. The macroscopic appearance might have prognostic implications, with the best survival for the papillary type and the worst for sclerosing tumours (Todoroki et al. 1980; Nichols et al. 1983; Kozuka et al. 1984).

Gallbladder cancer can be almost imperceptible and may be identified in an in situ phase as microscopic plaques on normal-appearing mucosa (Rosen 1978). In localized gallbladder cancer, small growths – sessile or pedunculated – are seen. More commonly, an obvious, advanced infiltrating malignant tumour is encountered (Piehler and Crichlow 1978; Rosen 1978).

Histological Findings

Carcinomas of the gallbladder and extrahepatic biliary ducts are generally morphologically similar, with approximately 90% being adenocarcinomas (Arminsky 1949; Sako et al. 1957; Shani et al. 1974; Piehler and Crichlow 1978). Squamous cell, mixed adenosquamous and undifferentiated carcinomas also occur. Metastatic lesions – especially to the gallbladder – have been described (Beaver et al. 1986).

The microscopic characteristics of adenocarcinomas have recently been outlined (Weinbren and Mutum 1983). Special features of cholangiocarcinomas include mucin secretion, either free in stroma or intracellularly. There may be cells of differing character within the same acinar formation, and invasive characteristics with perineural, neural and lymphatic involvement are common. Of particular importance to the surgeon is the infiltrating spread of cancer cells below a tumour-free epithelial surface (Weinbren and Mutum 1983; Kozuka et al. 1984). Lymphatic metastases may occur in up to 50% of patients (Kuwayti et al. 1957). Tumours of the gallbladder with a high mucopolysaccharide content may permit longer survival (Johnson et al. 1986).

The staging system for gallbladder cancer – based on the microscopic findings – developed by Nevin et al. (1976) correlates with the clinical course and has important consequences for the management of patients. There are five stages of the disease:

Stage I: mucosal involvement only
Stage II: Involvement of mucosa and muscularis
Stage III: mucosal, muscularis and subserosal involvement
Stage IV: involvement of all three layers and the cystic duct lymph node
Stage V: involvement of the liver by direct extension or metastasis to distant organs

No similar staging system has been developed for other bile duct tumours.

Clinical Features

The literature is abundant with descriptions of patient symptoms and signs. As a general rule, however, detailed analysis of these is of limited value due to the poor sensitivity of each symptom. Experienced clinicians will, however, correctly identify 90% of the patients in whom the symptoms are actually due to mechanical obstruction (Wheeler et al. 1979; O'Connor et al. 1983).

The single most important symptom for extrahepatic bile duct cancer is jaundice, which is found in 90%–98% of cases (Andersson et al. 1977; Alexander et al. 1984; Langer et al. 1985). Jaundice is most often progressive, but fluctuations have been registered in up to 11% of the patients (Andersson et al. 1977). Similarly, it should be noted that incomplete obstruction and obstruction affecting only part of the biliary tract – for instance, a single right or left hepatic duct – frequently fail to cause jaundice and hyperbilirubinaemia and are first suspected because of an unexplained increase in alkaline phosphatase activity in patients investigated due to upper abdominal pain and discomfort (Zeman et al. 1980).

All other symptoms recorded are either unspecific and related to the jaundice (itching, dark urine, pale stools), or common both in benign and malignant biliary diseases (upper abdominal pain, seen in 50%–60% of patients with extrahepatic bile duct cancer). Other nonspecific complaints relate to the malignancy (anorexia, weight loss). Cholangitis is a feature of the disease, but is an unusual presenting complaint, as is haemobilia.

The symptom patterns in gallbladder cancer are somewhat different. Three groups can be identified, each representing about a third of the patients:

Group I: manifestations of biliary lithiasis with acute or chronic "cholecystitis"; the diagnosis is usually unsuspected and may be made at the time of cholecyst-

ectomy or later as an incidental pathological finding in gallbladders removed for presumed benign biliary disease.
Group II: the features of obstructive jaundice.
Group III: symptoms of a nonspecific advanced malignancy.

It is important to realize that in only 8.6% or less of the patients is gallbladder cancer accurately diagnosed before operation (Piehler and Crichlow 1978), although recently the newer diagnostic imaging modalities have resulted in better preoperative definition of the disease (Collier et al. 1984; Ouchi et al. 1987).

Investigations, Diagnostic Strategy and Assessment of Resectability

Most patients evaluated are those with obstructive jaundice, the overriding objective being to identify potentially treatable causes without subjecting the patient to needless risk, discomfort or expense. In this respect, it is important to realize that approximately 50% of jaundiced patients will have a primary extrahepatic malignancy or metastatic cancer as the cause (Croker 1985).

Until recently, the diagnosis of cholangiocarcinoma was, with few exceptions, made either at laparotomy or at autopsy (Klatskin 1965; Longmire et al. 1973). The recognition that jaundice can be investigated and the cause even treated without recourse to major abdominal surgery has led to an important change in the attitude towards these patients. However, the fact that in a recent series 61% (57/94) of patients with cholangiocarcinoma at the confluence of hepatic ducts had undergone previous surgery (Blumgart et al. 1984a) indicates that many clinicians and surgeons are unaware of the fact that an ordered use of radiological tests should be successful in imaging the obstructive lesion in nearly all cases, and help select appropriate therapy.

The tests performed should answer the following questions:

1. What is the cause of the obstruction?
2. If organic stenosis, is the cause benign or malignant?
3. Is the stenosis or suspected tumour resectable?
4. If not resectable, can the radiological tests help select the best palliative treatment?

Several studies have described diagnostic strategies in jaundice and the usefulness of various tests (Thomas et al. 1982; Lindberg et al. 1983; Scharschmidt et al. 1983; Saint-Marc Girardin et al. 1985). Most studies have, however, addressed only the first two questions, while it is the last two which are of paramount importance to the surgeon.

Table 1 gives the radiological tests which the authors have found useful in the evaluation of suspected biliary tract tumours, and the information which each test may give. It is now widely accepted that US should be the first imaging procedure in patients with jaundice – indeed, in any patient with suspected biliary tract disease. As indicated in Table 1, US not only demonstrates bile duct dilatation, but may give additional information regarding tumour extension and resectability (Gibson et al. 1986; Okuda et al. 1988).

Direct cholangiography – PTC or ERC – provides the most useful and accurate information. The choice between the two often depends on local circumstances, and they may be regarded as complementary. However, for the majority of patients the preoperative determination of proximal extension of the tumour into the liver has important therapeutic implications, and this is the main reason for advocating PTC in most cases of suspected high malignant

Table 1. Diagnostic tests in evaluation of jaundiced patients and the specific information obtained from each test in patients with biliary tract tumours

Test	Information obtained
Ultrasound	Obstruction +/– Level of obstruction Cause of obstruction Vascular involvement Metastases Liver atrophy
Percutaneous transhepatic cholangiography	Level of obstruction Liver atrophy Cause of obstruction Resectability (proximal extent of lesion) Infection (bile culture) Treatment options
Endoscopic retrograde cholangiography	Level of obstruction Cause of obstruction (Treatment options)
Cytology	Tissue confirmation
Angiography	Resectability (vascular involvement) Road map Liver atrophy
Computed tomography	Obstruction +/– Level of obstruction Liver atrophy Resectability (caudate or caval vein involvement) Metastases

biliary tract obstruction. ERC seems unable to provide sufficient information as to the proximal duct anatomy and extent of the lesion (Tanaka et al. 1988). It is important not to accept a single cholangiographic diagnosis but to pursue the examination until the entire intrahepatic biliary tree has been outlined (Fig. 2; Voyles et al. 1983b). A clear demonstration of the cholangiographic anatomy of the left hepatic duct is particularly important in selecting patients for a possible palliative biliary-enteric anastomosis. Diagnostic difficulties may arise in the case of multifocal or diffuse sclerosing carcinomas, where the cholangiographic findings may mimic sclerosing cholangitis. This situation may be found in up to 10% of bile duct tumours (Nichols et al. 1983).

Cholangiographic features of the neoplastic obstruction itself have generally been of little help in determining resectability or prognosis (Liquory and Canard 1983), although a recent study from Japan suggests that the cholangiographic changes – dividing the type of obstruction into protuberant, papillary, sclerosing or constricted – are related to resectability (Okuda et al. 1988). The highest resection rate was found for papillary type obstruction, while only 10% of the sclerosed type could be surgically removed. The classification (or typing) system for hilar cholangiocarcinoma based on the proximal extent of the lesion proposed by Bismuth and Corlette (1975) will help select patients suitable for resective surgery (Fig. 3; see below) and the usefulness of this classification system in selecting treatment has now been well demonstrated (Pichlmayr et al. 1988; Bengmark et al. 1988; Bismuth et al. 1988). Similarly, intrahepatic ductal changes consisting of stricturing, distortion or non-filling of the main duct (or

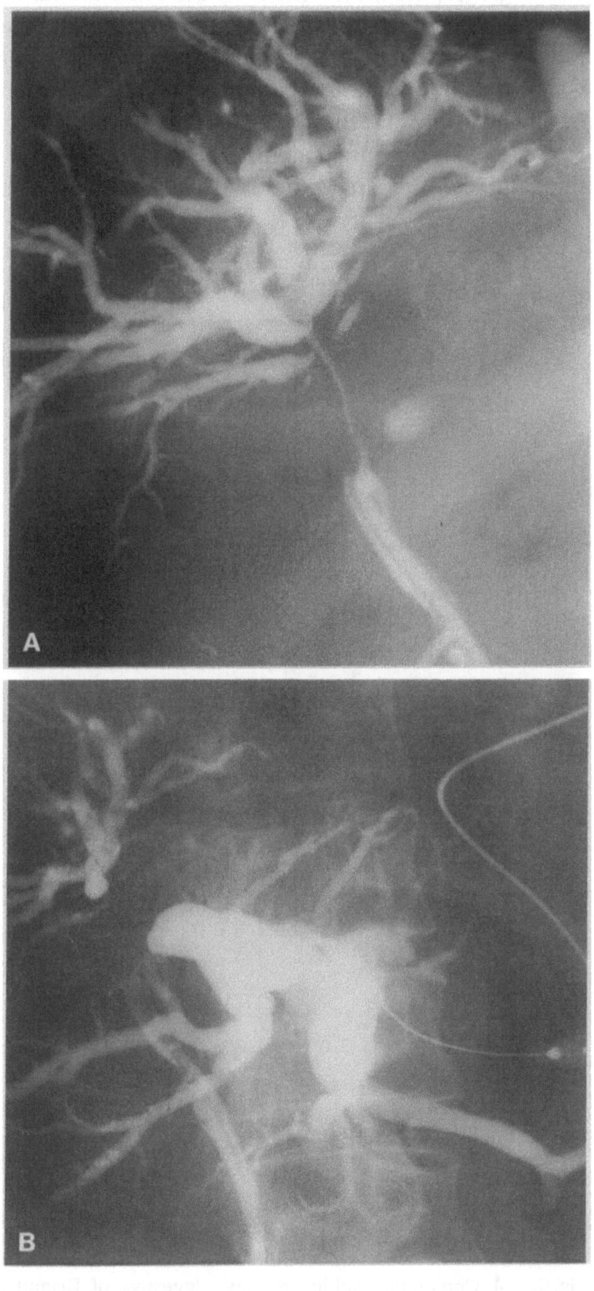

Fig. 2. **A** Preoperative percutaneous cholangiography demonstrating filling of the right hepatic ducts only. **B** A separate puncture on the left side demonstrates a hypertrophic left lobe. These pictures illustrate the need for complete visualization of all intrahepatic biliary ducts

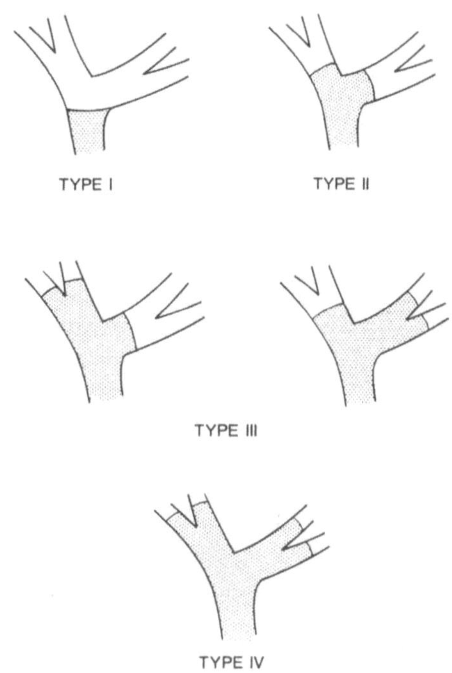

Fig. 3. Typing system for hilar cholangiocarcinoma based on proximal extent of tumour

its branches) draining the segment V area (Couinaud 1957) of the right lobe of the liver strongly suggest carcinoma of the gallbladder (Collier et al. 1984).

Partial liver atrophy is a feature which has received little attention in the past and may be demonstrated at cholangiography (Fig. 4). It may follow unilateral bile duct and/or portal vein obstruction (Ham 1979; Blumgart 1985). The radiological signs of atrophy include crowding and irregularity of the bile ducts within the affected area. US and CT may confirm the diagnosis of atrophy (Gibson et al. 1986; Carr et al. 1985). Drainage of dilated ducts within an atrophic segment may not be effective in relieving obstruction, and resection of liver, leaving an atrophic remnant, is dangerous and associated with liver failure in the postoperative period. Unilobar atrophy is often associated with hypertrophy of the contralateral lobe; this may cause diagnostic difficulties since the large, palpable liver is not a tumour mass (Tsuzuko et al. 1973).

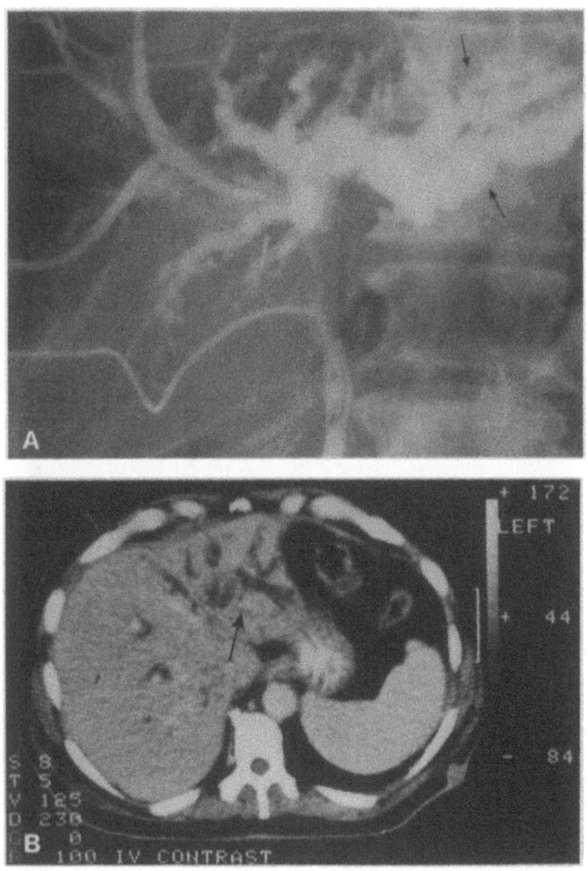

Fig. 4. **A** Cholangiographic signs of liver atrophy. Note crowding and irregularity of bile ducts of the left liver *(arrows)*. **B** CT scan confirms left liver atrophy. Note small left lobe and dilated crowded ducts *(arrow)*

Previous studies have demonstrated the value of arteriography and portography in assessing the resectability of biliary malignancies (Williamson et al. 1980). Currently, involvement of the main trunk of the portal vein [with very few exceptions (Sakaguchi et al. 1986)], involvement of both branches of the portal vein, bilateral involvement of hepatic artery and portal vein, or a combination of vascular involvement to one side of the liver with extensive cholangiographic involvement on the other are taken as signs of irresectability (Blumgart 1985; Fig. 5). The radiographic evidence of involvement of major veins usually signifies compression rather than frank invasion by tumour (Beazley et al. 1984). However, the fibrous reaction adjacent to the abutting and compressing tumour usually involves the

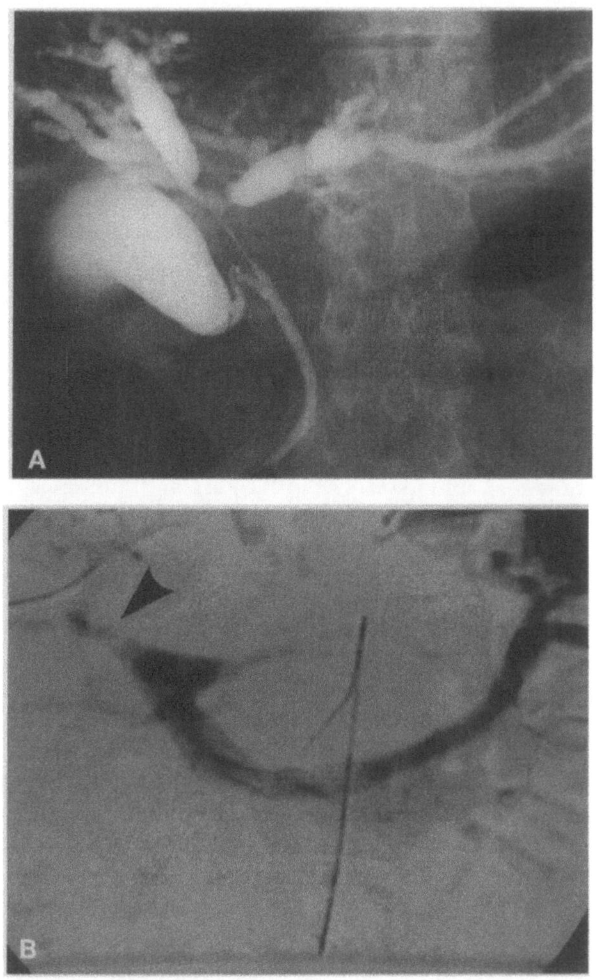

Fig. 5. **A** Cholangiographic findings suggestive of Bismuth type III hilar cholangiocarcinoma (second order duct involvement on the right side, first order on the left). **B** Angiography demonstrates involvement of the right portal vein *(arrowhead)*. The preoperative radiological findings suggest that right hepatectomy (or lobectomy) must be performed

vein to such an extent as to make removal of the tumour impossible, although localized lesions in which the sole barrier to excision is venous involvement may be excised, including a segment of portal vein with subsequent porta-portal anastomosis (Blumgart et al. 1984a).

It is important to realize that, in the presence of a localized bile duct stricture and in the absence of angiographic vascular involvement, it is impossible to make a definitive diagnosis. Although most isolated bile strictures are neoplastic, a significant proportion (10%) will have a benign lesion (Hadjis et al. 1985). Thus, it is important that claims of successful long-term results for the management of cholangiocarcinoma should be accompanied by tissue confirmation of the malignant nature of the lesion. Preoperative aspiration cytology will confirm the malignancy in 50%–90% of cases (Benjamin et al. 1987; Okuda 1988; Søreide 1988). Transpapillary biopsies and brush cytology from the common bile duct may be equally effective (Aabakken et al. 1986). Cytological examination of bile obtained following percutaneous catheter drainage may yield positive results in approximately a third of the patients (Harell et al. 1981; Muro et al. 1983).

The value of CT scanning in the preoperative evaluation of bile duct and gallbladder cancer is not established. As a general rule, CT does *not* demonstrate the bile duct tumour but may show metastases or liver atrophy (Carr et al. 1985; Okuda et al. 1988). The limitations of cholangiography and angiography in the assessment of bile duct tumours include a failure to demonstrate involvement of the caudate lobe (segment I) or of the inferior vena cava. CT scanning may improve assessment in the future. Magnetic resonance imaging is similar to CT and its value in these cases is limited at the moment (Okuda et al. 1988).

Itai et al. (1980) claim that gallbladder cancer can be diagnosed by CT in 74% of cases. It is evident that CT – or any other diagnostic modality – is accurate when an extensive lesion is present and incorrect preoperative diagnosis is still the rule rather than the exception (Ouchi et al. 1987). Currently, US is probably the best diagnostic test for early gallbladder cancer although difficulties in interpretation are frequently encountered as gallstones are also present in 60%–90% of cases, and localized benign lesions, tumour-like lesions (cholesterol or hyperplastic, inflammatory polyps) and chronic cholecystitis with thickening and/or irregularity of the gallbladder wall may mimic cancer.

In summary, the ordered use of imaging procedures outlined above, and the exclusion of patients unfit for major surgery, will identify the 60%–90% of patients with bile duct tumours located in the middle third that will come to laparotomy. For hilar lesions, Fig. 6 shows – based on extensive experience (Voyles et al. 1983b; Blumgart et al. 1984) – that approximately 40% of the patients will be identified as irresectable on the basis of PTC findings and general fitness, and a further 20% will be excluded after the angiographic studies. Thus, only 40% of the patients with a hilar lesion will come to laparotomy, and the proportion who are actually suited for resection is in the order of 15%–20%.

Currently, no information is available as to the proportion of gallbladder cancers that are accurately diagnosed preoperatively and thought to be resectable. An extensive review (Piehler and Crichlow

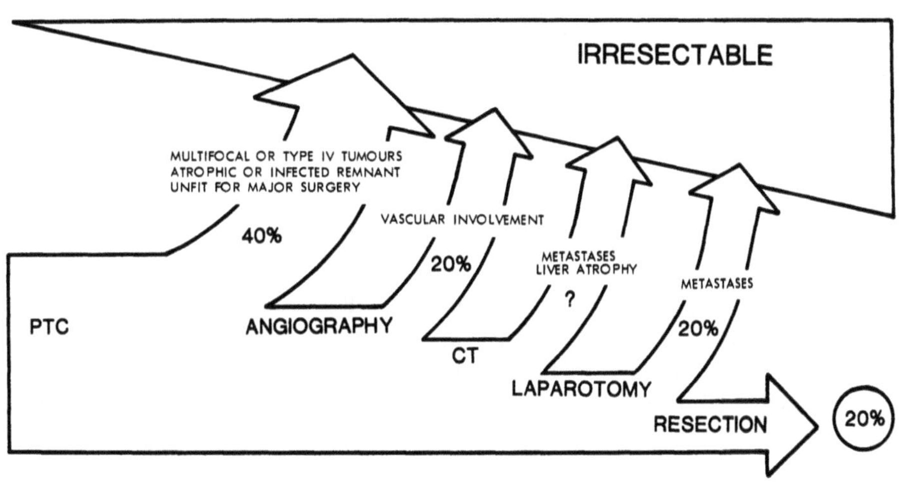

Fig. 6. Preoperative investigative strategy in patients with hilar cholangiocarcinoma. Each step will identify further patients unsuitable for resection

Table 2. Overview of treatment options for biliary tract cancer

Potentially curative surgery
Pancreaticoduodenectomy (Whipple's operation)
Local resection of extrahepatic biliary tract
Liver resection with biliointestinal reconstruction
Liver transplantation
Palliative Treatment
Palliative surgery
- Biliointestinal bypass
- Surgically placed catheters
Percutaneous intubational techniques
- External drainage ("PTD")
- Exteriorized stents
- Endoprosthesis
Endoscopic intubational techniques
- Endoprosthesis
Radiotherapy
- Internal
- External

1978) clearly indicates that preoperative diagnosis will be accurate in less than 10% of the patients. Unfortunately, recent data suggest that improvements in imaging have so far not improved the prognosis for patients with gallbladder cancer (Klamer and Max 1983; Morrow et al. 1983).

Treatment Options and Complications

Table 2 gives an overview of treatment options for patients with biliary tract cancer. In this context, palliative treatment usually means treatment of jaundice and pruritus. It should, however, be noted that since all palliative treatment modalities carry a significant complication rate and risk, jaundice alone is not an absolute indication for biliary decompression – especially in the asymptomatic, old and frail patient.

A major controversy surrounding surgery for obstructive jaundice has been the claim that preoperative percutaneous biliary drainage will significantly diminish postoperative morbidity and reduce operative mortality. Early studies of the value of preoperative drainage used historical controls to reach this conclusion. However, recent prospective, controlled studies have neither confirmed the beneficial effect of preoperative drainage (Hatfield et al. 1982; McPherson et al. 1984; Pitt et al. 1985) nor shown a reduced surgical morbidity in the drained patients. Indeed, any benefit is at least cancelled out by a significant complication rate related to the drainage procedure itself (Smith et al. 1985). Thus, routine preoperative drainage is not indicated except in the septic patient with cholangitis.

Extrahepatic Bile Duct Cancer: Potentially Curative Surgery

Middle Third Tumours

As already mentioned, 60%–90% of patients with middle third tumours will come to laparotomy (Tompkins et al. 1981; Kinami and Miyazaki 1982; Langer et al. 1985; Nakayama et al. 1988), but the actual resectability rate varies from 13% (Evander et al. 1980) to 82% (Kinami and Miyazaki 1982). Occasionally, local resection with reconstruction by means of a Roux-en-Y loop is sufficient, similar to the treatment of type I hilar lesion (Fig. 3). However, many lesions, if resectable, require wide excision, including the head of the pancreas (Whipple's procedure).

The overall hospital mortality following resection of middle duct tumours ranges from zero (Tompkins et al. 1981) to 35% (Andersson et al. 1977). However, recent data suggest that even for the difficult operation of pancreaticoduodenectomy, mortality of less than 5% can be anticipated in experienced hands (Rossi et al. 1985).

Upper Third Tumours ("Hilar Cholangiocarcinoma")

As outlined in Fig. 6, the resectability rate for hilar cholangiocarcinoma is 15%–20% of all patients evaluated and in whom tissue confirmation of the diagnosis is obtained (Blumgart et al. 1984; Langer et al. 1985; Bismuth et al. 1988). Higher resectability rates (up to 75%) can be found in the literature (Mizumoto et al. 1986), but it is not always evident whether the rate is based on those actually explored, or on the total number of patients evaluated.

As mentioned above, we have shown that preoperative investigations can help select the patients most suitable for resection. The type of resection chosen is determined partly by the fact that dissection of the biliary tree past secondary bifurcations cannot generally be accomplished without hepatic parenchymal resection. In addition, vascular involvement, especially portal venous encasement, dictates partial hepatectomy. Thus, it is possible to give recommendations as to the type of resection needed for hilar lesions (Table 3).

The technique of local resection includes a complete clearance of all lymph nodes in the hepatoduodenal ligament en bloc with the bile duct and gallbladder (Blumgart 1988). Hepatic resection may be required as indicated by intrahepatic ductal or vascular involvement (Table 3; Blumgart et al. 1984;

Table 3. Selection of treatment based on preoperative radiological studies for patients with high bile duct tumours. The tumour type corresponds to the Bismuth classification shown in Fig. 3. The primary surgical option for each tumour type is modified based on the angiographic findings

Tumour type based on PTC	Primary surgical option	Vascular involvement		
		MPV ± MHA	RPV ± RHA	LPV ± LHA
Type I	Local resection	Irresectable	Right hepatectomy[a]	Left hepatectomy[a]
Type II	Local resection	Irresectable	Right hepatectomy[a]	Left hepatectomy[a]
Type III (left)	Left hepatectomy	Irresectable	Irresectable	Left hepatectomy[a]
(right)	Right hepatectomy	Irresectable	Right hepatectomy[a]	Irresectable

[a] Liver resection is contraindicated if the liver remnant is atrophic.
MPV, main portal vein; MHA, main hepatic artery; RPV/LPV, right and left portal veins; RHA/LHA, right and left hepatic arteries.

Bengmark et al. 1988; Bismuth et al. 1988; Pinson and Rossi 1988). Although extensive vascular involvement is considered a contraindication to resection (Table 3), some of these tumours can be removed by concomitant excision of segments of the portal vein followed by portal reconstruction (Tsuzuki et al. 1983; Boerma et al. 1985; Sakaguchi and Nakamura 1986; Blumgart 1988). Central hepatic resection (Hart and White 1980; White 1988) or partial resection of segment IV (Launois et al. 1979) has been used to facilitate exposure of the hilar area. Biliary-enteric continuity, either to one or more hepatic ducts, is re-established with Roux-en-Y hepaticojejunostomy. Cameron et al. (1982) and others stent the anastomosis with transhepatic or transjejunal silicone tubes; but, employing our preferred technique of biliointestinal anastomosis (Blumgart and Kelley 1984) stents can be safely omitted in the majority of patients.

A major problem in resection of bile duct tumours is related to the submucosal spread of cholangiocarcinoma and the reactive fibrosis that accompanies the tumours, sources of considerable difficulty in determining the point for tumour-free surgical transection of involved ducts. A fairly high proportion of patients undergoing extensive resection have had involved resection margins (Evander et al. 1980; Alexander et al. 1984; Beazley et al. 1984; Bengmark et al. 1988). However, a few surgeons have pursued a policy of radical excision of hilar cholangiocarcinoma, and results may improve with increasing experience.

Resection of hilar tumours carries high morbidity, with figures up to 50% reported (Tsuzuki et al. 1983). A major problem seems to be anastomotic complications with bile leaks. A recent study suggests, however, that biliary fistula – admittedly a significant clinical problem – will close spontaneously in these patients (A. Czerniak, J. H. Thompson, I. S. Benjamin, O. Søriede, L. H. Blumgart, to be published). The hospital mortality following resection is around 10% (Ottow et al. 1985), with figures ranging from 3% (Langer et al. 1985) to 25% (Skoog and Thoren 1982; Kinami and Miyazaki 1982). The mortality differs between the two types of resection, close to zero for local resection (Blumgart et al. 1984). Major hepatic resection carries mortality rates ranging from 4% to 27% (Pinson and Rossi 1988; Bengmark et al. 1988).

Gallbladder Cancer: Potentially Curative Surgery

Reference must be made to the staging system for gallbladder cancer developed by Nevin et al. (1976; see "Histological Findings" above) and to the clinical presentation of the disease.

For the very few patients in whom the diagnosis is established preoperatively and where localized disease is found at operation (Stages II–IV), the minimal operation should include cholecystectomy and excision of the pericholedochal nodes as lymphatic spread is found in a high proportion of cases (Fahim et al. 1962; Vaittinen 1970). A complete dissection is best performed by excision of the extrahepatic bile duct, and lymph node clearance by skeletization of the vessels in the hepatoduodenal ligament as in the operation for type I hilar cholangiocarcinoma. Whether wedge resection of the gallbladder liver bed should be added to the procedure is far from established, although some data suggest marginally better 5-year survival by inclusion of limited liver resection (Vaittinen 1970; Morrow et al. 1983; Ouchi et al. 1987). If at operation more advanced locoregional disease is found (stage V), a formal partial hepatectomy (segments IV, V and VI) or lobectomy may be added, although reports of long-term survival are only anecdotal (Adson 1973; Piehler and Crichlow 1977; Ouchi et al. 1988).

No optimal treatment strategy has been established for the group of patients in whom the diagnosis is established by histological examination of a gallbladder removed for gallstone disease. As pointed out by Piehler and Crichlow (1977), the majority of successes in treatment have come after simple cholecystectomy, which suggests that the stage of the disease rather than extent of operation is the decisive factor. In the absence of hard data, our opinion is that for patients where the incidental cancer is of stages I–III, no further surgical therapy is usually indicated. However, we are fully aware that the practice of several experienced surgeons is to reoperate with lymphadenectomy and resection of the adjacent liver. Adjunctive radiotherapy may increase survival in these patients (Treadwell and Hardin 1976).

It should be noted, however, that if surgeons were to adopt the habit of routinely inspecting the gallbladder directly after removal, intraoperative diagnosis of the early lesion, providing an immediate opportunity to extend the procedure as necessary, would increase.

Liver Transplantation

Patients with tumours found to be irresectable (Table 3), but without evidence of distant metastases, may theoretically be treated by liver replacement. Indeed, liver grafting has been tried by leading transplant centres, but disappointing results – caused by early tumour recurrence and death – led to the opinion that patients with bile duct cancer should perhaps not undergo transplantation (Starzl et al. 1985; Calne et al. 1986). In the Cambridge experience, the median survival for 26 patients with cholangiocarcinoma treated with liver grafting was less than 6 months, with only one patient surviving beyond 5 years (O'Grady et al. 1988). Recently, however, Pichlmayr et al. (1988), in Hanover, have provided evidence that improved selection of patients – in particular, avoiding liver grafting in patients with lymph node metastases – may improve results. A cautious approach to the problem of liver transplantation for irresectable bile duct cancer seems justified.

Palliative Treatment

Most patients with biliary cancer will need some form of biliary decompression as a palliative measure. Assessment of the results of the various palliative methods is no less difficult than for resection, one of the main problems being selection of patients. For instance, patients submitted to intubation who might have been suitable for resection constitute a relatively low-risk group, whereas others are possibly too ill to tolerate any form of treatment at all. Another important problem is that histological confirmation of the nature of the stricture has not been available in many series.

The Bismuth classification of hilar lesions (Fig. 3) with the identification of patients in whom the left and right hepatic ducts (or segmental ducts) are separated by tumour (types III–IV), highlights the question of whether drainage of only part of the liver suffices to relieve jaundice and pruritus. There is, however, abundant evidence that partial drainage is adequate unless the undrained remnant is infected or the drained liver atrophic (Bismuth and Corlette 1975; Longmire and Tompkins 1975; Blumgart 1985).

Palliative Surgery

Several surgical bypass possibilities have been described (Blumgart and Kelley 1984; Ottow et al. 1985). The two most popular are the retrograde intrahepatic cholangiojejunostomy proposed by Longmire and Sanford (1948), where retrograde drainage is established through the intrahepatic portion of the dilated biliary tree within the left liver (and modifications thereof), and anastomosis to the left ducts approached through the umbilical fissure (segment III-bypass), developed by Soupault and Couinaud (1957) and popularized by Bismuth and Corlette (1975). The Longmire operation is difficult to perform, is associated with significant morbidity, and may give only partially satisfactory results (Longmire et al. 1973; Ragins et al. 1973). We and others (Traynor et al. 1987) have used the segment III approach increasingly, achieving satisfactory results with few problems related to the procedure itself. Complete preoperative cholangiographic visualization of the bile duct anatomy allows selection of candidates for this operation.

According to a recent review (Ottow et al. 1985), the 30-day mortality associated with these procedures is approximately 20% although significantly lower (Bismuth et al. 1988) and higher (Lai et al. 1987) figures are found.

Some authors argue strongly that palliative bypass surgery is superior to other non-surgical procedures as survival and quality of life are improved (Deveraux and Greco 1986; Bismuth et al. 1988; Miyazaki et al. 1988). However, the UCLA experience does not support these enthusiastic reports, indeed, the worst results were found in the palliative surgery group (Lai et al. 1987). Andreani et al. (1986) also conclude – based on an excellent review – that endoprostheses are preferable to surgical bypass if irresectability is obvious. Case selection may underline these differences in opinion, but, in general, surgical bypass seems to offer advantage in patients who will tolerate operation and in whom the ductal anatomy is favourable.

The technique of drainage via a surgically placed catheter was popularized by Terblanche et al. (1972). Modifications of the U-tube technique using T-tubes, Y-tubes, or straight transhepatic tubes have been described by several authors (Ottow et al. 1985). In a modification of this technique the proximal end of a transtumour tube is buried beneath the skin where it can be recovered at a later time for irrigation or drainage (exoendoprosthesis; Blumgart et al. 1981). More recently, a subcutaneous reservoir which allows bile sampling, irrigation and transtubal radiology has been developed (Voyles 1985). Operative mortality with these types of intervention averages 15% (Ottow et al. 1985). However, advances in preoperative evaluation as well as in radiological and endoscopic intubation techniques seem to have considerably reduced the need for these procedures.

Non-Surgical Biliary Drainage

Non-surgical biliary drainage may be accomplished by any of several intubation techniques (Table 2). External drains are placed percutaneously. They may lead to metabolic derangements, may create a portal of entry for bacteria, and the tubes need daily care, but the advantage is easy exchange in the case of blockage.

Tubes that stent a tumour and are brought out through the skin may be referred to as "exteriorized stents". This technique may permit internal radiotherapy, but the complications of infection and the inconvenience to the patient are significant.

Endoprostheses are tubes that stent the tumour. They are internal and can be introduced using radiological percutaneous or endoscopic techniques. The quality of life seems to be superior to that with external tubes, but exchange is less easy, especially if the percutaneous technique has been employed.

Although some authors claim that a particular technique is superior to others, several uncontrolled studies and reviews on the topic (Burchart 1982; Hagenmüller and Soehendra 1983; Leung et al. 1983; Classen et al. 1984; Cotton 1984; Huibregtse and Tytgat 1984; Malangoni et al. 1985; Ottow et al. 1985; Pogany et al. 1985; Andreani et al. 1986; Lammer et al. 1986) seem to permit the following conclusions in relation to the use of drainage for biliary decompression:

1. The technical success rate of biliary drainage is about the same for the endoscopic and the percutaneous transhepatic routes.
2. The two techniques are equally effective in relieving jaundice.
3. Endoscopically and percutaneously placed endoprosthesis are equally successful.
4. Perihilar tumours are more difficult to traverse with the endoscopic technique.
5. For periampullary lesions (not discussed here) the endoscopic approach seems preferable.
6. The mortality and morbidity are similar for all types of intubation with complication rates of 10%–30% and 30-day mortality of 20%–30%. Whether the deaths were a result of the procedure rather than a natural outcome of advanced disease is not always clear.
7. Endoscopically inserted prostheses are easier to replace in case of occlusion.
8. Readmissions for local complications are frequent.

Randomized trials should provide the most scientifically persuasive information as to the comparison of the two methods for endoprostheses insertion. Such a study – including both hilar and low bile duct lesions – has recently been published (Speer et al. 1987), and the conclusion was that the endoscopic method had a significantly higher success rate for relief of jaundice (81% versus 61%) and significantly lower 30-day mortality (15% versus 33%). The higher mortality after percutaneous stents was due to complications related to liver puncture (haemorrhage and bile leaks). We will argue that local expertise should primarily dictate treatment alternatives. Furthermore, percutaneous and endoscopic techniques can be usefully combined if there is difficulty in negotiating a stricture endoscopically (Robertson et al. 1987).

Radiotherapy

Studies of the use of radiotherapy for cancer of the bile duct have not been carried out in a systematic way. A number of investigators have used internal (Levitt et al. 1988) and/or external radiation in conjunction with intubation (Iwasaki et al. 1977; Pilepich and Lambert 1978; Chitwood et al. 1982; Fletcher et al. 1983; Mornex et al. 1984; Meyers and Jones 1987). Claims of benefit are clouded by the small numbers and the heterogeneity of the patients and the problem that histological or cytological proof of the disease has not been obtained in many long-term survivors. Complications related to the irradiation itself, which are additional to those related to the intubation, are not infrequent, including duodenitis or ulceration with associated gastrointestinal bleeding, as well as duodenal stenosis and fibrotic changes in the normal biliary tract (Sindelar et al. 1982).

The position of adjuvant radiotherapy - perhaps consequent to incomplete resection - has yet to be explored. A new concept in the treatment of bile duct cancer is the combination of intraoperative radiation therapy with surgery (Iwasaki et al. 1988). The authors conclude that this expensive and cumbersome technique, eventually combined with postoperative external radiation, would improve the prognosis of the patient with advanced bile duct cancer. However, the number of patients treated is small, and data are not easily interpreted. Results from prospective, controlled studies are awaited.

Chemotherapy

The role of cytostatic drug therapy - given either as adjuvant treatment to patients undergoing resection or to those with advanced disease - is at present a confusing subject. A substantial number of studies - especially from the United States and Japan - claim improved survival. However, we do not at present recommend such treatment as the lack of hard scientific data supporting such a practice is striking. In recent years, cytostatic drugs have also been given by hepatic artery infusion. It appears that partial response rates are higher than in systemic therapy, but serious biliary toxicity in nearly half the patients is a problem (Oberfield and Rossi 1988).

Survival

The prognosis for patients with biliary tract tumours is dismal. In bile duct cancer, overall survival at 5 years may approach 8% in recent series (Tompkins et al. 1981; Langer et al. 1985), whereas 1-year and 5-year survival for patients with gallbladder cancer was 11.8% and 4.1%, respectively, in a collected series of 5836 patients (Piehler and Crichlow 1978).

Survival for bile duct cancer appears to be related to resectability of the tumour, its location and pathological type. The mean (or median) survival for patients resected for attempted cure ranges from 11 to 33 months (Ottow et al. 1985), with 5-year survival rates of 20%-40% in recent series (Alexander et al. 1984; Langer et al. 1985; Pinson and Rossi 1988). Direct comparison with palliative treatment modalities is difficult, but reviews (Ottow et al. 1985) and comparative studies (Alexander et al. 1984) clearly suggest that resection is superior to palliative measures.

Some authors have had favourable experience with resection in which residual disease is left behind, reporting median survival of up to 16 months (Evander et al. 1980; Alexander et al. 1984; Pinson and Rossi 1988). As the quality of life for resected patients may be superior to that for patients treated by palliation (Blumgart et al. 1984), despite residual tumour in the resection margin in some cases (Beazley et al. 1984; Bengmark et al. 1988), this finding may indicate that an aggressive surgical approach in these patients is justified. It is in this situation that postoperative radiotherapy may have a place, as suggested by Cameron et al. (1982).

Most authors also find that patients with distal tumours fare much better than those with proximal and mid-duct tumours (Tompkins et al. 1981; Alexander et al. 1984; Nakayama et al. 1988), with a difference in median survival between high- and low-duct tumours of approximately 12 months. However, such differences may be more apparent than real and may be related to the later presentation of hilar lesions and the fact that treatment modalities for hilar tumours need further refinement. Survival is approximately twice as long in patients with papillary lesions as in those with infiltrating tumours (Tompkins et al. 1981; Nichols et al. 1983; Kozuka et al. 1984; Langer et al. 1985), but the effect of tumour differentiation is more controversial and seems not to be clearly established.

For patients with gallbladder cancer, the main prognostic determinants are tumour stage according to the system developed by Nevin et al. (1976) and to the clinical presentation, i.e. whether the tumour was an unexpected finding after cholecystectomy for presumed benign disease (Piehler and Crichlow 1978). These two variables are of course interrelated, as the majority of tumours found incidentally will be in a favourable stage.

Nevin et al. (1976) concluded that 76% of his patients with tumours invading mucosa or muscularis (stages I and II) were cured, and that all patients in similar stages surviving the operation itself (reported in the literature up to that time) survived 5 years. Morrow et al. (1983) found cumulative 5-year survival of 41% for patients with stages I-III tumours. No patient with stage IV-V tumours lived beyond 18 months.

The effect of clinical presentation on survival was

clearly documented in the review by Piehler and Crichlow (1978). Five-year survival was 15% in patients in whom the tumour was found following elective cholecystectomy for benign disease, 3% in patients in whom tumours were identified by the surgeon and thought to be resected, and 0.4% in patients undergoing palliative procedures for unresectable disease.

Future Perspectives

When reviewing the extensive literature, the need for a clinical staging system enabling comparison of results in similar patients undergoing varying forms of treatment becomes apparent. Tissue verification of the malignancy is imperative regardless of treatment approach (Blumgart et al. 1984). The role of aggressive surgical therapy with curative intent, based on well-defined preoperative imaging criteria, seems to be firmly established but may need verification, especially regarding the role of non-curative resections, the possible effect of adjuvant radiotherapy and the effect on the quality of life. All palliative treatment modalities carry a significant risk of complications and death. Further trials comparing the different palliative treatment strategies are clearly needed so as to allow evaluation of complications, mortality, survival and, most important, patient comfort.

References

Aabakken L, Kåresen R, Serck-Hanssen A, Osnes M (1986) Transpapillary biopsies and brush cytology from the common bile duct. Endoscopy 18: 49–51

Aadland E, Schrumph E, Fausa O, Elgjo K, Heilo A, Aakhus T, Gjone E (1987) Primary sclerosing cholangitis: a long-term follow-up study. Scand J Gastroenterol 22: 655–664

Adson MA (1973) Carcinoma of the gallbladder. Surg Clin N Am 53: 1203–1216

Akwari OE, van Heerden JA, Foulk WT, Baggenstoss AH (1975) Cancer of the bile ducts associated with ulcerative colitis. Ann Surg 181: 303–309

Alexander F, Rossi RL, O'Bryan M, Khettry U, Braasch JW, Watkins E (1984) Biliary carcinoma. A review of 109 cases. Am J Surg 147: 503–509

Andersson Å, Bergdahl L, van der Linden W (1977) Malignant tumours of the extrahepatic bile ducts. Surgery 81: 198–202

Andréani T, Buffet C, Etienne JP (1986) Non-surgical management of malignant obstructive jaundice. Gastroenterol Clin Biol 4: 308–318

Arbab AA, Brasfield R (1976) Benign tumors of the gallbladder. Surgery 61: 535–540

Arminsky TC (1949) Primary carcinoma of the gallbladder. A collective review with the addition of twenty-five cases from the Grace Hospital, Detroit, Michigan. Cancer 2: 379–398

Beaver BL, Denning DA, Minton JP (1986) Metastatic breast carcinoma of the gallbladder. J Surg Oncol 31: 240–242

Beazley RM, Hadjis N, Benjamin IS, Blumgart LH (1984) Clinicopathological aspects of high bile duct cancer. Experience with resection and bypass surgical treatments. Ann Surg 199: 623–635

Belamaric J (1973) Intrahepatic bile duct carcinoma and *C. sinensis* infection in Hong Kong. Cancer 31: 468–473

Bengmark S, Ekberg H, Evander A, Klofver-Stahl B, Tranberg K-G (1988) Major liver resection for hilar cholangiocarcinoma. Ann Surg 207: 120–125

Benjamin IS, Krausz T, Domizio P, Lazzara S, Blumgart LH (1987) Cytological diagnosis of hepatobiliary and pancreatic malignancy. Gut 28: A 1401

Bismuth H, Corlette MB (1975) Intrahepatic cholangioenteric anastomosis in carcinoma of the hilus of the liver. Surg Gynecol Obstet 140: 170–178

Bismuth H, Castaing D, Traynor O (1988) Resection or palliation: priority of surgery in the treatment of hilar cancer. World J Surg 12: 39–47

Blumgart LH (1985) Bile duct strictures. In: Fromm D (ed) Gastrointestinal surgery, vol 2. Livingstone, New York, pp 755–811

Blumgart LH (1988) Cancer of the bile ducts. In: Blumgart LH (ed) Surgery of the liver and biliary tract. Churchill Livingstone, London.

Blumgart LH, Kelley CJ (1984) Hepaticojejunostomy in benign and malignant high bile duct strictures: approaches to the left hepatic ducts. Br J Surg 71: 257–261

Blumgart LH, Voyles CR, Smadja C (1981) Exo-endoprosthesis for relief of obstructive jaundice. Lancet 2: 306–307

Blumgart LH, Benjamin IS, Hadjis NS, Beazley RT (1984) Surgical approaches to cholangiocarcinoma at confluence of hepatic ducts. Lancet I: 66–70

Boerma EJ, Bronkhorst FB, van Haelst UJGM, de Boer HHM (1985) An anatomic investigation of radical resection of tumour in the hepatic duct influence. Surg Gynecol Obstet 161: 223–228

Burcharth F (1982) Nonsurgical drainage of the biliary tract. Semin Liver Dis 2: 75–86

Calne RY, Williams R, Rolles K (1986) Liver transplantation in the adult. World J Surg 10: 422–431

Cameron JL, Broe P, Zuidema GD (1982) Proximal bile duct tumours. Surgical management with silastic transhepatic biliary stents. Ann Surg 196: 412–417

Cancer Registry of Norway (1980) Survival of cancer patients. Cases diagnosed in Norway 1968–1975. Norwegian Cancer Registry, Oslo

Carr D, Hadjis NS, Banks LM, Hemingway AP, Blumgart LH (1985) Computed tomography of hilar cholangiocarcinoma. A new sign. AJR 145: 53–56

Chitwood WR, Meyers WC, Heaston DK, Herskovic AM, McLeod ME, Jones RS (1982) Diagnosis and treatment of primary extrahepatic bile duct tumors. Am J Surg 143: 99–105

Christophi C, Hughes ER (1985) Hepatobiliary disorders in inflammatory bowel disease. Surg Gynecol Obstet 160: 187–192

Classen M, Kawai K, Geenen J (eds) (1984) Non-operative biliary drainage. Springer, Berlin Heidelberg New York

Collier NA, Carr D, Hemingway A, Blumgart LH (1984) Preoperative diagnosis and its effect on the treatment of carcinoma of the gallbladder. Surg Gynecol Obstet 159: 465–470

Cornell CM, Clarke R (1959) Vicarious calcification involving the gallbladder. Ann Surg 149: 267–272
Cotton PB (1984) Endoscopic methods for relief of malignant obstructive jaundice. World J Surg 8: 854–861
Couinaud C (1957) Le foie. Etudes anatomiques et chirurgicales. Masson, Paris
Croker JR (1985) Biliary tract disease in the elderly. Clin Gastroenterol 14: 773–809
Devereux DF, Greco RS (1986) Biliary enteric bypass for malignant obstruction. Cancer 58: 981–984
Diehl AK (1980) Epidemiology of gallbladder cancer: a synthesis of recent data. JNCI 65: 1209–1214
Etala E (1962) Cancer de la vesicula biliar. Prensa Med Argent 49: 2283–2299
Evander A, Fredlund P, Hoevels J, Ihse I, Bengmark S (1980) Evaluation of aggressive surgery for carcinoma of the extrahepatic bile ducts. Ann Surg 191: 23–29
Fahim RB, McDonald JR, Richards JC, Ferris DO (1962) Carcinoma of the gallbladder: a study of its mode of spread. Ann Surg 156: 114–124
Flavell DJ, Lucas SB (1983) Promotion of *N*-nitrosodimethylamineinitiated bile duct carcinogenesis in the hamster by the human liver fluke, *Opisthorchis viverrini*. Carcinogenesis 4: 927–930
Fletcher MS, Brinkley D, Dawson JL, Nunnerberg H, Williams R (1983) Treatment of hilar cholangiocarcinoma by bile drainage combined with internal radiotherapy using ^{192}iridium wire. Br J Surg 70: 733–735
Fraumeni JF Jr (1975) Cancers of the pancreas and biliary tract: epidemiological considerations. Cancer Res 35: 3437–3446
Gibson RN, Yeung I, Thompson JN, Carr DH, Hemingway AP, Bradpiece HA, Benjamin IS, Blumgart LH, Allison DJ (1986) Bile duct obstruction: radiologic evaluation of level, cause and tumor resectability. Radiology 160: 543–547
Gouma DJ, Singh Mutum S, Benjamin IS, Blumgart LH (1984) Intrahepatic biliary papillomatosis. Br J Surg 71: 72–74
Hadjis NS, Collier NA, Blumgart LH (1985) Malignant masquerade at the hilum of the liver. Br J Surg 72: 659–661
Hagenmüller F, Soehendra N (1983) Non-surgical biliary drainage. Clin Gastroenterol 12: 297–316
Ham J (1979) Partial and complete atrophy affecting hepatic segments and lobes. Br J Surg 66: 333–337
Harell GS, Anderson MF, Berry PF (1981) Cytologic bile examination in the diagnosis of biliary duct neoplastic strictures. AJR 137: 1123–1126
Hart J, Modan B, Shani M (1971) Cholelithiasis in the aetiology of gallbladder neoplasms. Lancet 1: 1151–1153
Hart MJ, White TT (1980) Central hepatic resection and anastomosis for stricture or carcinoma at the hepatic bifurcation. Ann Surg 192: 299–305
Hatfield ARW, Tobias R, Terblanche J, Girdwood AH, Fataar S, Harries-Jones R, Kernoff L, Marks IN (1982) Preoperative external biliary drainage in obstructive jaundice: a prospective controlled clinical trial. Lancet 2: 896–899
Huibregtse K, Tytgat GNT (1984) Endoscopic placement of biliary prostheses. In: Salmon P (ed) Advances in gastrointestinal endoscopy, vol 1. Chapman and Hall, London, pp 219–231
Itai Y, Araki T, Yoshikawa K, Furui S, Yashiro N, Tasaka A (1980) Computed tomography of gallbladder carcinoma. Radiology 137: 713–718
Iwasaki Y, Ohto M, Todoroki T et al. (1977) Treatment of carcinoma of the biliary system. Surg Gynecol Obstet 144: 219–224
Iwasaki Y, Todoroki T, Fukao K, Ohara K, Okamura T, Nishimura A (1988) The role of intraoperative radiation therapy in the treatment of bile duct cancer. World J Surg 12: 91–98
Johnson LA, Lavin PT, Dayal YY, Geller SA, Doos WG, Cooper HS, Gresber JE, Masse ST, Weiland LH, Moertel CG, Engstrøm PF (1986) Gallbladder adenocarcinoma: prognostic significance of tumour acid mucopolysaccharide content. J Surg Oncol 33: 243–245
Kagawa Y, Kashihara S, Kuramoto S, Maetani S (1978) Carcinoma arising in a congenitally dilated biliary tract. Report of a case and review of the literature. Gastroenterology 74: 1286–1294
Kimura K, Ohto M, Saisho H et al. (1985) Association of gallbladder carcinoma and anomalous pancreaticobiliary ductal union. Gastroenterology 89: 1258–1265
Kinami Y, Miyazaki I (1982) Operative results of extrahepatic bile duct carcinoma. Jpn J Surg 12: 171–177
Klamer TW, Max MH (1983) Carcinoma of the gallbladder. Surg Gynecol Obstet 156: 641–645
Klatskin G (1965) Adenocarcinoma of the hepatic ducts at its bifurcation within the porta hepatis. An unusual tumour with distinctive clinical and pathological features. Am J Med 38: 241–256
Koga A, Watanabe K, Fukuyama T, Takiguchi S, Nakayama F (1988) Diagnosis and operative indications for polypoid lesions of the gallbladder. Arch Surg 123: 26–29
Komi N, Tamura T, Tsuge S, Miyoshi Y, Udaka H, Takehara H (1986) Relation of patient age to premalignant alterations in choledochal cyst epithelium: histochemical and immunohistochemical studies. J Pediatr. Surg 21: 430–433
Kozuka S (1982) Relation of adenoma to carcinoma in the gallbladder. Cancer 50: 2226–2234
Kozuka S, Tsubone M, Hachisuka K (1984) Evolution of carcinoma in the extrahepatic bile ducts. Cancer 54: 65–72
Krain LS (1972) Gallbladder and extrahepatic bile duct carcinoma. Analysis of 1808 cases. Geriatrics 27: 111–117
Kuwayti K, Baggenstoss AH, Stauffer MH, Priestley JT (1957) Carcinoma of the major intrahepatic and the extrahepatic bile ducts exclusive of the papilla of Vater. Surg Gynecol Obstet 104: 357–366
Lai ECS, Tompkins RK, Roslyn JJ, Mann LL (1987) Proximal bile duct cancer. Quality of survival. Ann Surg 205: 111–118
Lammer J, Neumayer K (1986) Biliary drainage endoprostheses: experience with 201 placements. Radiology 159: 625–629
Langer JC, Langer B, Taylor BR, Zeldin R, Cummings B (1985) Carcinoma of the extrahepatic bile ducts: results of an aggressive surgical approach. Surgery 98: 752–758
Launois B, Campion J-P, Brissot P, Gosselin M (1979) Carcinoma of the hepatic hilus. Surgical management and the case for resection. Ann Surg 190: 151–157
Leung JWC, Emery R, Cotton PB, Russell RCG, Vallon AG, Mason RR (1983) Management of malignant obstructive jaundice at the Middlesex Hospital. Br J Surg 70: 584–586
Levitt MD, Laurence BH, Cameron F, Klemp PFB (1988) Transpapillary iridium-192 wire in the treatment of malignant bile duct obstruction. Gut 29: 149–152
Lindberg G, Björkman A, Helmers C (1983) A description of diagnostic strategies in jaundice. Scand J Gastroenterol 18: 257–265
Liquory C, Canard JM (1983) Tumours of the biliary system. Clin Gastroenterol 12: 269–295
Longmire WP Jr, Sanford MC (1948) Intrahepatic cholangiojejunostomy with partial hepatectomy for biliary obstruction. Surgery 24: 264–276

Longmire WP Jr, McArthur MS, Bastounis EA, Hiatt J (1973) Carcinoma of the extrahepatic biliary tract. Ann Surg 178: 333–343

Longmire WP Jr, Tompkins RK (1975) Lesions of the segmental and lobar hepatic ducts. Ann Surg 182: 478–495

Malangoni MA, McCoy DM, Richardson JD, Flint LM (1985) Effective palliation of malignant biliary duct obstruction. Ann Surg 201: 554–559

Maram ES, Ludwig J, Kurland LT, Brian DD (1979) Carcinoma of the gallbladder and extrahepatic biliary ducts in Rochester, Minnesota, 1935–1971. Am J Epidemiol 109: 152–157

McPherson GAD, Benjamin IS, Hodgson HJF, Bowley NB, Allison DJ, Blumgart LH (1984) Preoperative percutaneous transhepatic biliary drainage: the result of a controlled trial. Br J Surg 71: 371–375

Meyers WC, Jones RS (1988) Internal radiation for bile duct cancer. World J Surg 12: 99–104

Mir-Madjlessi SH, Fasmer RG, Swik MV (1987) Bile duct carcinoma in patients with ulcerative colitis. Relationship to sclerosing cholangitis: report of six cases and review of the literature. Dig Dis Sci 32: 145–154

Miyazaki K, Nagafuchi K, Nakayama F (1988) Bypass procedure for bile duct cancer. World J Surg 12: 64–67

Mizumoto R, Kawarada Y, Suzuki H (1986) Surgical treatment of hilar carcinoma of the bile duct. Surg Gynecol Obstet 162: 153–158

Mornex F, Ardiet JM, Bret P, Gerard JP (1984) Radiotherapy of high bile duct carcinoma using intracatheter iridium-192 wire. Cancer 54: 2069–2073

Morrow CE, Sutherland DER, Florack G, Eisenberg MM, Grage TB (1983) Primary gallbladder carcinoma: significance of subserosal lesions and results of aggressive surgical treatment and adjuvant chemotherapy. Surgery 94: 709–713

Muro A, Mueller PR, Ferrucci JT, Taft PD (1983) Bile cytology: a routine addition to percutaneous biliary drainage. Radiology 149: 846–847

Nagata E, Sakai K, Kinoshita H, Kobayashi Y (1985) The relation between carcinoma of the gallbladder and an anomalous connection between the choledochus and the pancreatic duct. Ann Surg 202: 182–190

Nakayama F, Mingazaki K, Nagafuchi K (1988) Radical surgery for middle and distal thirds bile duct cancer. World J Surg 12: 60–63

Nevin JE, Moran TJ, Kay S, King R (1976) Carcinoma of the gallbladder – staging, treatment and prognosis. Cancer 37: 141–148

Nichols DA, MacCarty RL, Gratley TA (1983) Cholangiographic evaluation of bile duct carcinoma. AJR 141: 1291–1294

Oberfield RA, Rossi RL (1988) The role of chemotherapy in the treatment of bile duct cancer. World J Surg 12: 105–108

O'Connor KW, Snodgrass PJ, Swonder JF et al. (1983) A blinded prospective study comparing four current non-invasive approaches in the differential diagnosis of medical versus surgical jaundice. Gastroenterology 84: 1498–1504

O'Grady JG, Polson RJ, Rolles K, Calne RY, Williams R (1988) Liver transplantation for malignant disease. Results in 93 consecutive patients. Ann Surg 207: 373–379

Okuda K, Ohto M, Tsuchiya Y (1988) The role of ultrasound, percutaneous transhepatic cholangiography, computed tomographic scanning and magnetic resonançe imaging in the preoperative assessment of bile duct cancer. World J Surg 12: 18–26

Ottow RT, August DA, Sugarbaker PH (1985) Treatment of proximal biliary tract carcinoma: an overview of techniques and results. Surgery 97: 251–262

Ouchi K, Owada Y, Matsuno S, Sato T (1987) Prognostic factors in the surgical treatment of gallbladder carcinoma. Surgery 101: 731–737

Parker RG, Kendall EJ (1954) The liver in ulcerative colitis. Br Med J 2: 1030–1032

Pichlmayr R, Ringe B, Lauchart W, Bechstein WO, Gubernatis G, Wagner I (1988) Radical resection and liver grafting as the two main components of surgical strategy in the treatment of proximal bile duct cancer. World J Surg 12: 68–77

Piehler JM, Crichlow RW (1977) Primary carcinoma of the gallbladder. Arch Surg 112: 26–30

Piehler JM, Crichlow RW (1978) Primary carcinoma of the gallbladder: collective reviews. Surg Gynecol Obstet 147: 929–942

Pilepich MV, Lambert PM (1978) Radiotherapy of carcinomas of the extrahepatic biliary system. Radiology 127: 767–770

Pinson CW, Rossi RL (1988) Extended right hepatic lobectomy, left hepatic lobectomy, and sceletonization resection for proximal bile duct cancer. World J Surg 12: 52–59

Pitt HA, Gomes AS, Lois JF, Mann LL, Deutsch LS, Longmire WP Jr (1985) Does preoperative percutaneous biliary drainage reduce operative risk or increase hospital cost? Ann Surg 201: 545–552

Pogany AC, Kerlan RK Jr, Ring EJ (1985) Percutaneous biliary drainage. Clin Gastroenterol 14: 387–402

Ragins H, Diamond A, Meng C-H (1973) Intrahepatic cholangiojejunostomy in the management of malignant biliary obstruction. Surg Gynecol Obstet 136: 27–32

Ritchie JK, Allan RN, Macartney J, Thompson H, Hawley PR, Cooke WT (1974) Biliary tract carcinoma associated with ulcerative colitis. Q J Med 43: 263–279

Robertson DAF, Ayres R, Hacking CN, Shepherd H, Birch S, Wright R (1987) Experience with a combined percutaneous and endoscopic approach to stent insertion in malignant obstructive jaundice. Lancet 2: 1449–1452

Rosen VJ (1978) The gallbladder and extrahepatic biliary tracts. In: Coulson WF (ed) Surgical pathology, vol 1. Lippincott, Philadelphia, pp 260–274

Rossi RL, Heiss FW, Beckmann CF, Braasch JW (1985) Management of cancer of the bile duct. Surg Clin N Am 65: 59–78

Rossi RL, Silverman ML, Braasch JW, Monson JL, Relline SG (1987) Carcinomas arising in cystic conditions of the bile ducts. A clinical and pathologic study. Ann Surg 205: 377–384

Saint-Marc Girardin M-F, le Minor M, Alperovitch A, Roudot-Thoroval F, Metreau J-M, Dhumeaux D (1985) Computer-aided selection of diagnostic tests in jaundiced patients. Gut 26: 961–967

Sakaguchi S, Nakamura S (1986) Surgery of the portal vein in resection of cancer of the hepatic hilus. Surgery 99: 344–349

Sako K, Seitzinger GL, Garside E (1957) Carcinoma of the extrahepatic bile ducts; review of the literature and report of six cases. Surgery 42: 416–437

Sameshima Y, Uchimura M, Muto Y, Maeda J, Tsuchiyama H (1987) Coexistent carcinoma in congenital dilatation of the bile duct and anomalous arrangement of the pancreatico-bile duct. Carcinogenesis of coexistent gall bladder carcinoma. Cancer 60: 1883–1890

Sawyer KC (1970) The unrecognized significance of papillomas, polyps and adenomas of the gallbladder. Am J Surg 120: 570–578

Scharschmidt BF, Goldberg HF, Schmid R (1983) Approach to the patient with cholestatic jaundice. N Engl J Med 308: 1515–1519

Shani M, Hart J, Modan B (1974) Cancer of the biliary system: a study of 445 cases. Br J Surg 61: 98–100

Sindelar WF, Tepper J, Travis EL (1982) Tolerance of bile duct to intraoperative irradiation. Surgery 92: 533–540

Skoog V, Thorén L (1982) Carcinoma of the junction of the main hepatic ducts. Acta Chir Scand 148: 411–415

Smith RC, Pooley M, George CRP, Faithful GR (1985) Preoperative percutaneous transhepatic internal drainage in obstructive jaundice: a randomized, controlled trial examining renal function. Surgery 97: 641–647

Soupault R, Couinaud CL (1957) Sur un procéde nouveau de derivation biliaire intrahepatique. Les cholangio-jejunostomies gauches sans sacrifice hépatique. Presse Med 65: 1157–1159

Speer AG, Cotton PB, Russel RCG, Mason RR, Hatfield ARW, Leung JWC, MacRae KD, Hooghton J, Lennon CA (1987) Randomized trial of endoscopic versus percutaneous stent insertion in malignant obstructive jaundice. Lancet 2: 57–62

Starzl TE, Iwatsuki S, Shaw BN Jr, Gordon RD (1985) Orthotopic liver transplantation in 1984. Transplant Proc 17: 250–254

Suda K, Miyano T, Koruma I, Matsumoto M (1983) An abnormal pancreatico-choledocho-ductal junction in cases of biliary tract carcinoma. Cancer 52: 2086–2088

Søreide O (1988) Percutaneous aspiration cytology. In: Blumgart LH (ed) Surgery of the liver and biliary tract. Churchill Livingstone, London, pp 327–335

Tanaka M, Ogawa T, Matsumoto S, Nakayama F (1988) The role of endoscopic retrograde cholangiopancreatography in preoperative assessment of bile duct cancer. World J Surg 12: 27–32

Terblanche J, Saunders SJ, Loow JH (1972) Prolonged palliation in carcinoma of the main hepatic duct junction. Surgery 71: 720–731

Thomas MJ, Pellegrini CA, Way LW (1982) Usefulness of diagnostic tests for biliary obstruction. Am J Surg 144: 102–108.

Todani T, Watanabe Y, Toki A, Uroshihara N (1987) Carcinoma related to choledochal cysts with internal drainage operations. Surg Gynecol Obstet 164: 61–64

Todoroki T, Okamura T, Fukao K, Nishimura Y, Otsu H, Sato H, Iwasaki Y (1980) Gross appearance of carcinoma of the main hepatic duct and its prognosis. Surg Gynecol Obstet 150: 33–38

Tompkins RK, Thomas D, While A, Longmire WP Jr (1981) Prognostic factors in bile duct carcinoma. Analysis of 96 cases. Ann Surg 194: 447–456

Traynor O, Castaing D, Bismuth H (1987) Left intrahepatic cholangioenteric anastomosis (round ligament approach): an effective palliative treatment for hilar cancers. Br J Surg 74: 952–954

Treadwell TA, Hardin WJ (1976) Primary carcinoma of the gallbladder. The role of adjunctive therapy in its treatment. Am J Surg 132: 703–706

Tsuzuki T, Hoshimo Y, Uchiyama T et al. (1973) Compensatory hypertrophy of the lateral quadrant of the left hepatic lobe due to atrophy of the rest of the liver appearing as a mass in the left upper quadrant of the abdomen. Ann Surg 177: 406–410

Tsuzuki T, Ogata Y, Iida S, Nakanishi I, Takenaka Y, Yoshii H (1983) Carcinoma of the bifurcation of the hepatic ducts. Arch Surg 118: 1147–1151

Vaittinen E (1970) Carcinoma of the gallbladder. A study of three hundred and ninety cases diagnosed in Finland, 1953–1967. Ann Chir Gynaecol suppl 168, Fenn 59

Voyles CR, Smadja C, Shands WC, Blumgart LH (1983 a) Carcinoma in choledochal cysts. Age-related incidence. Arch Surg 118: 986–988

Voyles CR, Bowley NJ, Allison DJ, Benjamin IS, Blumgart LH (1983 b) Carcinoma of the proximal extrahepatic biliary tree. Radiologic assessment and therapeutic alternatives. Ann Surg 197: 188–194

Voyles CR (1985) The exo-endoprosthesis in proximal biliary-enteric anastomosis. Am J Surg 149: 80–83

Wee A, Ludwig J, Coffey RJ, LaRusso NF, Wiesner RH (1985) Hepatobiliary carcinoma associated with primary sclerosing cholangitis and chronic ulcerative colitis. Hum Path 16: 719–726

Weinbren K, Mutum SS (1983) Pathological aspects of cholangiocarcinoma. J Pathol 139: 217–238

Welton JC, Marr JS, Friedman SM (1979) Association between hepatobiliary cancer and typhoid carrier state. Lancet 1: 793–794

Wheeler PG, Theodossi A, Pickford R, Laws J, Knill-Jones RP, Williams R (1979) Non-invasive techniques in the diagnosis of jaundice – ultrasound and computer. Gut 20: 196–199

White T (1988) Skeletization resection and central hepatic resection in the treatment of bile duct cancer. World J Surg 12: 48–51

Williamson BW, Blumgart LH, McKellar NJ (1980) Management of tumours of the liver. Combined use of arteriography and venography in the assessment of resectability especially in hilar tumours. Am J Surg 139: 210–215

Yamauchi S, Koga A, Matsumoto S, Tanaka M, Nakayama F (1987) Anomatous punction of pancreaticobiliary duct without congenital choledochal cyst: a possible risk factor for gallbladder cancer. Am J Gastroenterol 82: 20–24

Zeman R, Taylor KJW, Burrell MI, Gold J (1980) Ultrasound demonstration of anicteric dilatation of the biliary tree. Radiology 134: 689–692

Small Bowel Cancer

U. Metzger

Introduction

Although the surface area of the small bowel is estimated at 4500 m^2, tumors are a clinical rarity. Only 0.5–1% of all malignant neoplasms are located in the small intestine. In autopsy series, however, the rate is much higher (4%–5% of malignant neoplasms), indicating low detection rates during the patients' lifetime (Schippers et al. 1982; Mason 1986). The average annual incidence is estimated at 0.7 and 0.6 per 100 000 for males and females respectively (Barclay and Schapira 1983; American Cancer Society, 1986). The rarity of these tumors means that no single institution or physician has extensive experience. Table 1 shows the type, location and frequency of both benign and malignant tumors of small bowel from 11 large series (Mason 1986). In the experience of many centers, the most common malignant tumor of the small bowel is actually metastatic lesions – most frequently from primary neoplasms of the ovary, stomach, colon and pancreas, as well as malignant melanoma. Most benign tumors of the small bowel are undiagnosed in the lifetime of the patient and are discovered if at all, as incidental findings at autopsy. The carcinoid tumors belong to the endocrine malignancies of the gut and are described by Stadil and Kohlet, this volume. Adenocarcinomas are most often located in the periampullar region of the duodenum and in the proximal jejunum. Lymphomas occur most often in the distal part of the small intestine and are usually of the non-Hodgkin's type. Sarcomas comprise leiomyosarcomas, hemangioendotheliomas and others.

Table 1. Tumors of the small intestine

	Duodenum	Jejunum	Ileum	Total
Malignant				
Adenocarcinoma	97	99	34	230
Lymphoma	6	64	85	155
Sarcoma	15	29	37	81
Miscellaneous	1	4	4	9
	119	196	160	475
Carcinoid	15	19	229	263
Benign				
Leiomyoma	31	84	61	176
Adenoma	42	42	41	125
Lipoma	25	17	48	90
Miscellaneous	33	18	24	75
Hemangioma	3	39	23	65
Neurofibroma	4	7	3	14
Lymphangioma	0	2	4	6
Fibroma	0	6	4	10
Fibromyoma	0	1	0	1
	138	216	208	562
				1300

From Mason (1986).

Both carcinoids and adenocarcinomatous tumors of the small intestine are associated with a high incidence of primary malignant neoplasms at other sites (17.0% and 20.3% respectively; Barclay and Schapira 1983). Alexander and Altemeier (1968) reported 83 of 112 patients with primary neoplasms of the small intestine as having another independent neoplasm at death. Of those with benign intestinal neoplasms, 57% had another benign neoplasm elsewhere and 23% had a primary malignancy at another location.

The etiology of small bowel carcinoma is unclear. Williamson et al. (1983) analyzed 171 patients with malignant small bowel tumors and found for the 68 adenocarcinomas an 80% preponderance of localization in the duodenum and proximal jejunum. A similar distribution in the upper small bowel in carcinomas induced in rats by the colonic carcinogen azoxymethane suggests defense mechanisms within ileal mucosa, as well as etiologic links between colorectal carcinoma and proximal small bowel cancer. Although the etiology of small bowel carcinoma is unknown, there are several clinical entities with clearly increased risks of small bowel malignancy. Greenstein et al. (1981) found a significant increase in the incidence of small bowel cancers in Crohn's disease, especially in defunctioned ileal loops. Familial polyposis of the colon and Gardner's syndrome are autosomal dominant forms of colonic polyposis; however, generalized polyposis has been recorded with associated small bowel carcinoma (Ross and Mara 1974). Isolated polyps are most commonly adenomatous and in the adult may have a relationship to malignancy. Adenomatous polyps may originate at the ampulla of Vater and cause obstructive symptoms. In general these polyps are benign; however, if villous adenomas arise in the duodenum or proximal small intestine, they are frequently malignant (one-third of cases) (Cooperman et al. 1978; Everett et al. 1981). Juvenile polyposis is most commonly found in the colon and rectum. Isolated examples of generalized gastrointestinal polyposis are reported with and without family history; these polyps have no apparent relationship to malignancy. Other syndromes associated with small intestinal neoplasms, like Peutz-Jegher's syndrome and von Recklinghausen's disease, bear no apparent risk of development of cancer. Jejunal cancer was also found as a complication of celiac disease (nontropical sprue), with a latent interval of 9 to 10 years. In each case the underlying condition had been treated by withdrawal of gluten from the diet and prolonged corticosteroids (Williamson et al. 1983).

It has sometimes been said that the lower the location of the cancer in the small intestinal tract, the better the prognosis. If one considers all cancers this may be true because carcinoids, with their better prognosis, are twice as common in the ileum as are adenocarcinomas. However, if one considers a single histologic type, the results are equally good in jejunum and ileum for carcinoids and equally bad for adenocarcinomas.

There is no standardized staging procedure for small bowel tumors, but in the case of adenocarcinoma, the UICC TNM classification as used for colorectal carcinoma is recommended.

Diagnosis and Treatment

The number and variety of small bowel tumors found at autopsy suggest that many such tumors are asymptomatic. When symptoms do arise, they are usually related to either obstructive phenomena or bleeding. Because the content of the small intestine is largely liquid, the degree of obstruction must be almost complete before symptoms are noted. Obstruction is the most common complication (50%) of benign tumors, and intussusception is the most common presentation. Bleeding is associated with angiomatous lesions and also with benign myomas, fibromas, and metastatic tumors. The rate of bleeding may be quite variable, from occult blood loss causing marginal anemia to exsanguinating hemorrhage. In a collective review of 373 malignant tumors, Schippers et al. (1982) found pain in 65%, weight loss in 49%, nausea and vomiting in 31%, bleeding in 29%, palpable tumor mass in 25% and perforation in 6.4% of cases. Early symptoms include uncharacteristic diffuse abdominal pain, anemia and weight loss. Due to the nonspecific nature of these symptoms, a fatal diagnostic delay of 10–12 months is encountered in almost all reported series.

The specific diagnosis of small intestinal neoplasms is now theoretically possible by direct visualization and biopsy through various fiberoptic endoscopes capable of traversing the entire small bowel from either end. Radiologic contrast studies utilizing various forms of barium are thought to represent the best technique for demonstration of lesions in the middle stretch of the small intestine. Sonography and computerized tomography are useful for large and palpable masses. Lesions that are bleeding at the time of investigation may be identified by arteriography if the bleeding rate is greater than 2 ml/min. However, the diagnostic sensitivity of all these measures is relatively poor and about half of the small bowel tumors are found only at laparotomy. Clearly, lack of visibility is one problem. Lack of symptoms of a specific nature may be another, difficulty in diagnosis a third. Perhaps most important, in view of the autopsy series, is a low index of suspicion on the part of the attending physician. It may be helpful to recall that around 5% of gastrointestinal malignancies and 25% of benign gastrointestinal lesions are to be found in the small intestine. Explorative laparotomy is therefore indicated whenever clinical suspicion of a small bowel tumor persists. The search for occult fecal blood is the only screening method available for selected high-risk patients, but the efficacy and the true value of such screening is not known at present.

The treatment of both benign and malignant lesions of the small bowel is primarily surgical. Segmental resection is sufficient for benign lesions, and extended segmental resection including the regional lymph nodes is used for malignant lesions. Very frequently, particularly in metastatic disease, there will be extension of the malignant process beyound the scope of total excision. Palliative surgery should be performed, however, to lessen the chance of obstruction, perforation and hemorrhage. In malignant tumors of the duodenum, radical pancreaticoduodenectomy may be necessary. When malignant tumors of the terminal ileum are encountered, right colectomy is usually part of the operative procedure along with ileotransverse colostomy. If malignant lymphoma is encountered, staging procedures to determine the extent of intra-abdominal spread must be performed. This includes sampling of intra-abdominal and periaortic nodes, liver biopsy and often splenectomy. In addition, the focal disease in the small bowel is usually resected with healthy margins, and the patient is given proper systemic therapy. The surgical therapy of carcinoid tumours is discussed by Stadil and Kohlet, this volume. Radiotherapy is limited by morbidity of the small intestine. No significant responses have been reported in the treatment of adenocarcinomas. Radiotherapy may be indicated in conjunction with systemic therapy for bulky lymphoma.

Systemic chemotherapy is indicated for Hodgkin's as well as for non-Hodgkin's lymphoma with or without residual disease following surgery. There is no indication for adjuvant treatment in adenocarcinomas and sarcomas. Depending on histologic grading, doxorubicin-containing chemotherapy might be useful for disseminated sarcomas. Very little has been published on the role of chemotherapy in the treatment of advanced adenocarcinoma of the small bowel, which has been considered resistant to this modality. At the M.D. Anderson Hospital, only one partial and two minor responses were seen in a total of 21 single-agent and multidrug chemotherapy treatments containing fluoropyrimidines (Jigyasu et al. 1984). As a working approach to this problem, one can suggest that the same palliative chemotherapy be used for this disease as for colorectal carcinoma.

Results and Follow-up

Some 55%–68% of patients have resectable disease at the time of laparotomy (Schippers et al. 1982; Williamson et al. 1983). Except for lymphomas and carcinoid tumors, there are no long-term survivors with unresectable lesions. Among 150 primary gastrointestinal lymphomas collected from 1974 to 1982 at the University of Vienna School of Medicine, the 28 cases of intestinal lymphomas localized in the small and large bowel without any site prevalence presented with Ann Arbor stage I in 14%, stage II in 82%, and stage III in 4%. Tumor resection was performed in 90% of all cases and was followed by multiagent chemotherapy in 53%. Radical tumor resection was obtained in only 28.6% of the intestinal lymphomas and was closely related to tumor stage. Survival analyses demonstrated a significant influence of the presenting tumor stage on prognosis as expressed by the overall 2-year survival rate of 70% for stage I vs 39% for stage II. Radical tumor resection was a major determinant of survival and cure of disease, as exhibited by the disease-free 2-year survival rate of 57% after radical resection vs 8% after nonradical resection of malignant lymphomas. Diffuse tumor growth and tumor penetration through the wall beyond the serosa decreased the survival rate (Dragosics et al. 1985). In the Stanford experience of diffuse histiocytic lymphoma (48 patients: 27 stomach, 12 small intestine, 9 others), the probability of cure was approximately 75% for stage IE patients. If the patient had regional lymph node involvement or pathologic stage IIE disease, combination chemotherapy was combined with radiotherapy in a sequence determined on an individual basis and resulted in a cure rate of approximately 40% (Gray et al. 1982).

In a review of 2837 carcinoid tumors, Godwin (1975) found 5-year survival rates of 58%–71%. The prognosis is much poorer for adenocarcinoma and sarcoma. In a collective of 309 patients, Schippers et al. (1982) found 21% 5-year survival, very similar to the 22.5% reported by Williamson et al. (1983) from the Massachusetts General Hospital among 40 curatively resected carcinomas. The Mayo Clinic reported 5-year survival of 22% for adenocarcinoma and 52% for carcinoid (Pagtalunan et al. 1964). The Roswell Park Memorial Institute found 5-year survival of 16% for adenocarcinoma and 56% for carcinoid (Goel et al. 1976).

Follow-up examinations should be performed in all patients with or without curative resection. Early detection of recurrent tumor is difficult, but endoscopy and/or radiologic contrast studies may be useful. No reports of curative reintervention or experience of the value of tumor markers are available in the literature. More important than early detection of recurrence is monitoring of primary treatment side effects, e.g. malabsorption and inadequate nutrition following extensive resection, late toxicities of radiotherapy and chemotherapy. Follow-up of carcinoid tumors is described by Stadil and Kohlet, this volume. The prognosis of small bowel cancer can only be improved by earlier diagnosis, i.e. by a higher index of suspicion on the part of the attending physician. Sophisticated combined modality approaches will further increase the survival of patients with malignant lymphoma. For sarcomas and adenocarcinomas, efficient cytotoxic drugs are needed for palliative treatment of disseminated disease as well as for adjuvant therapy.

References

Alexander JW, Altemeier WA (1968) Association of primary neoplasms of the small intestine with other neoplastic growths. Ann Surg 167: 958–962

American Cancer Society (1986) Cancer statistics. CA 36: 1, 9–25

Barclay THC, Schapira V (1983) Malignant tumors of the small intestine. Cancer 51: 878–881

Cooperman M, Clausen KP, Hecht C, Lucas JG, Keith LM (1978) Villous adenomas of the duodenum. Gastroenterology 74: 1295–1299

Dragosics B, Bauer P, Radaszkiewicz T (1985) Primary gastrointestinal non-Hodgkin's lymphomas. Cancer 55: 1060–1073

Everett GD, Shirazi SS, Mitros FA (1981) Villous tumours of the duodenum. Am J Gastroenterol 75: 376–380

Godwin DJ (1975) Carcinoid tumors – an analysis of 2837 cases. Cancer 36: 560–566

Goel IP, Didolkar MS, Elias EG (1976) Primary malignant tumors of the small intestine. Surg Gynecol Obstet 143: 717

Gray GM, Rosenberg SA, Cooper AD, Gregory PB, Stein DT, Herzenberg H (1982) Lymphomas involving the gastrointestinal tract. Gastroenterology 82: 143–152

Greenstein AJ, Sachar DB, Smith H, Janowitz HD, Aufses AH (1981) A comparison of cancer risk in Crohn's disease and ulcerative colitis. Cancer 48: 2742–2745

Jigyasu D, Bedikian Y, Stroehlein JR (1984) Chemotherapy for primary adenocarcinoma of the small bowel. Cancer 53: 23–25

Mason GR (1986) Tumours of the duodenum and small intestine. In: Sabiston DC Jr (ed) Davis-Christopher textbook of surgery. Saunders, Philadelphia

Pagtalunan RJG, Mayo CW, Dockerty MB (1964) Primary malignant tumors of the small intestine. Am J Surg 108: 13

Ross JRE, Mara JE (1974) Small bowel polyps and carcinoma in multiple intestinal polyposis. Arch Surg 108: 736–739

Schippers E, Langer S, Flosdorff W, Hilber U (1982) Das primäre Dünndarmmalignom. Chirurg 53: 364–369

Williamson RCN, Welch CE, Malt RA (1983) Adenocarcinoma and lymphoma of the small intestine. Ann Surg 197: 172–178

Cancer of the Colon and Rectum

B. ARNESJØ, J. F. HALVORSEN, and A. O. MYKING

Definition

The synonymous terms "colorectal cancer", "cancer of the large intestine" and "cancer of the large bowel" will in this chapter be used to denote malignant tumours coded according to the Eighth Revision of the International Classification of Diseases (ICD) as 153 (cancer of the colon, excluding rectum) and 154 (cancer of the rectum and rectosigmoid junction) considered in an aggregate. Other malignant diseases such as cancer of the appendix and anal cancer will be considered elsewhere in this volume.

More than 98% of all malignant tumours of the large intestine are adenocarcinomas – 5%–10% of the mucinous type. Tumours of nonepithelial origin, such as carcinoids, malignant melanomas, lymphosarcomas or other forms of malignant haematological tumours and sarcomas, are seldom encountered. Some of these rare tumour forms will be mentioned elsewhere in this volume and others are similar in clinical presentation and surgical treatment to adenocarcinomas.

Epidemiology

The incidence of colonic and rectal cancer is increasing in an almost parallel fashion in all age groups in nearly all European countries (for references see Ziegler et al. 1985; Hill 1987; Adami 1988). There is a slow shift from a predominantly rectal primary localization to predominance in the colon. Within the colon there is an increase of proximally localized tumours. The sex ratios of colonic and rectal cancer differ, with rectal cancer being distinctly more common among males in most countries. Colonic cancer affects both sexes at rather similar rates.

In areas where the incidence of both cancers is comparatively low, the proportion of the total formed by rectal cancers is high. The proportion of colon cancer is highest in high-incidence areas.

The incidence varies among countries and regions in Europe (Correa and Haenszel 1978; Schottenfield and Winawer 1984; Silverberg 1984). The highest incidence (>35 annually diagnosed cases per 100 000 inhabitants) is found in some areas of Britain and Scandinavia and in Switzerland. Central European countries have intermediate, the Mediterranean countries and Finland low incidence (<25 per 100 000). Intermediate or low rates have been reported from Eastern European countries.

Subsequent to moving from an area with low to one with high incidence, even the first generation of immigrants commences a continuous adaptation to the higher incidence of the new country. Observed racial differences seem mainly related to socioeconomic factors, since the rates for different ethnic groups living in the same area tend to converge over time. This is in contrast to stomach cancer and may reflect the relatively low influence of constitutional factors in the development of colorectal cancer. There is also a marked variation within countries. Densely populated areas with a high average income and a high educational level tend to have a higher incidence.

Age-specific incidence rates of both colonic and rectal cancer rise from the age of 10–15 years up to 80–84 years. Most reports indicate a significant risk for colorectal cancer above the age of 40 years, after which it is almost doubled each decade. About 10% of the paediatric and young adult patients have a known predisposing disease, such as familial polyposis, ulcerative colitis or Crohn's disease, and others belong to "cancer-disposed families". Between 30% and 50% of the paediatric cases and around 15% of those diagnosed at an age below 30 years have mucinous carcinomas, compared to 5% of older adults. Since colloid or mucinous cancers have more aggressive growth characteristics they contribute to the relatively poor prognosis in young cases.

Etiology

Inflammatory bowel diseases, hereditary abnormalities and dietary factors have been ascribed etiological roles in colorectal cancer (for references see Lipkin and Good 1978; Levin and Riddell 1984; Ziegler et al. 1985; Thompson 1986; Hill 1987; Williams and Northover 1987).

Severe, extended and long-lasting ulcerative colitis increases the likelihood of developing colorectal carcinoma to about 40% after 25 years, irrespective of the age of onset. The cancer risk in this disease is correlated to the number of symptomatic attacks and to the extent of the disease. Multifocal carcinomas may develop in these cases.

Patients with Crohn's disease of the colon carry a 20 times higher risk of developing colorectal cancer than an age-matched control population.

Familial polyposis of the colon and Gardner's syndrome are hereditary disorders associated with adenomatous polyps of the colon and rectum which have a dominant mode of inheritance. In familial polyposis 80% of the sufferers will develop colorectal carcinoma, usually at an early age and often at multiple sites. Gardner's syndrome occurs about half as often as familial polyposis and is characterized by colorectal polyposis and soft tissue or bone abnormalities – features often not coexisting in a single patient, but recognizable on a family basis. The cancer risk is probably similar to that of familial polyposis. In Turcot's syndrome, colorectal adenomatous polyposis is combined with central nervous system tumours. Recent investigations have indicated genetic defects localized to the mucosa of intestinal polyps in familial polyposis syndromes. Bodmer et al. (1987) localized the gene for familial adenomatous polyposis to chromosome 5, and Solomon et al. (1987) suggested that becoming recessive for this gene may be a critical step in the progression of a relatively high proportion of colorectal cancers. Screening investigations are now performed for the identification of relatives who are at risk of developing polyposis and patients with de novo polyposis.

Other hereditary polyposis syndromes, such as Peutz-Jeghers syndrome and generalized juvenile polyposis, although exhibiting a somewhat higher risk of malignant degeneration, are usually not associated with colorectal adenocarcinomas. The intestinal polyps are hamartomatous and not adenomatous in these conditions.

Families exist in which adenocarcinomas occur at a high rate at an early age and, at times, at multiple primary sites. Such family members may develop colorectal carcinomas or may have concomitant malignant neoplasms such as endometrial and breast carcinomas. The hereditary pattern in such families is not known.

Relatives of patients with "sporadic" colorectal cancer have an increased risk for colorectal cancer. Whether this reflects true genetic influence or environmental factors cannot be answered at present. A mixing with patients with manifest or de novo familial polyposis cannot be excluded.

A previous history of colorectal polyps of the adenomatous type or colorectal cancer represents an increased risk for a new primary colorectal cancer (Brahme et al. 1974; Morson and Bussey 1985). Several studies have indicated a two- to threefold increase in incidence in this population in comparison with an age-matched control population. Also, since endoscopic or surgical excision of benign colorectal adenomas reduces the risk of manifest cancer, several investigators advocate control programmes for such patients. It is now generally accepted that benign polyps may develop into manifest cancer with time. Such transition is supported by the fact that cancer is found in 1% of adenomas up to 1 cm in size, in 10% of adenomas between 1 cm and 2 cm and in 30%–50% of adenomas above 2 cm. There is also a higher cancer rate in adenomas that have a villous component microscopically. In addition, patients with multiple adenomas have a greater chance of developing malignancy than those with solitary adenomas. When one adenoma is detected there is a 40%–50% chance of additional adenomas elsewhere in the large bowel and a 30% chance of new adenomas developing.

Alimentary factors assumed to play a role in the development of colorectal cancer are meat, fat and dietary fibre. The action of intestinal bacteria – mainly anaerobic – on bile acids and fatty acids with the formation of carcinogenic substances has also been discussed (for references see Greenwald and Lanza 1986).

A correlation between the incidence of colorectal cancer and the GNP (gross national product) per capita has been demonstrated in epidemiological studies. High meat and low cereal consumption is characteristic of countries with high incidence rates. An increased intake of meat, fat of animal origin and refined carbohydrates at the expense of food of vegetable origin – with its high content of dietary fibre – occurs in countries with a high GNP per capita. The relative food fibre deficiency in "rich" countries causes better growth conditions for the intestinal bacterial flora, slower transit of intestinal contents and smaller fecal volumes. These effects may cause an intestinal environment with enhanced conversion of animal fats and bile acids by bacterial enzymes. Two studies – one performed in Copenhagen and Finland and one in Israel – have demonstrated low fibre intake in areas with high colorectal cancer incidence. Detailed comparisons revealed no differences in intestinal transit time but a markedly lower meat intake, a higher fibre intake, a reduced anaerobe/aerobe bacterial faecal excretion ratio and a higher faecal excretion of lactobacilli in the low-incidence populations. There were no differences in the excretion of faecal bile acids and neutral sterols.

Several hydrocarbons have been shown to induce experimental adenomatous polyps or manifest colorectal cancer. Antioxidant compounds such as selenium, α-tocoferol and phenolic antioxidants are capable of inhibiting this carcinogenic action. Extensive research is now going on in this field.

Histopathology

Adenocarcinoma is the most frequently occurring malignancy of the large bowel. Of 628 colonic and 494 rectal malignancies registered in 1982–1986 in our department of pathology there were only five epidermoid carcinomas, six undifferentiated carcinomas and four carcinoid tumours. Sarcomas or malignant lymphomas were not seen at all. This pattern is common in Europe.

Carcinoma

Most colorectal cancers are fungating or ulcerating tumours, the latter often with elevated edges projecting into the lumen. Simultaneously there is a mainly cross-sectional infiltrative growth in the bowel wall. This infiltration may cause constriction and stenosis and a considerable part of the tumour mass may project into the lumen.

Colorectal cancers may be subdivided into different grades of malignancy. Unfortunately, criteria for such histological grading are often arbitrary and depend on the traditions of different laboratories. In the last WHO proposal (Morson and Sobin 1976) a division into adenocarcinomas, mucinous carcinomas, signet-ring cell carcinomas, undifferentiated carcinomas and unclassified carcinomas was suggested. These carcinomas should also be subdivided into three differentiation classes – well, moderately well and poorly differentiated. In practice, it may seem difficult to classify other tumours than adenocarcinomas according to their differentiation.

Others have adopted Broders' scale for the estimation of malignancy grade. The anaplastic changes are described in four grades (I–IV) (Dukes 1940; Zamcheck et al. 1975). Microscopically, colorectal tumours – almost without exception – are characterized by a more or less uniform glandular structure and the presence of small amounts of mucus (Fig. 1). The ability to form glandular structures decreases in parallel with increasing cellular pleomorphism and nuclear atypia. With an excessive mucus content, these tumours are classified as signet-ring cell, colloid or mucoid carcinomas. Borderline findings are common, making classification difficult. As previously mentioned, mucoid carcinomas constitute about 5%–10% of all colorectal carcinomas in adults.

Typical colorectal adenocarcinomas have a macroscopic extent corresponding well with the microscopic growth. The border between normal mucosa and tumour is fairly abrupt. A transitional zone may exist, with hyperplasia, stretching, branching and elongation of the glands and with inconsistent atypia of epithelial cells (Saffos and Rhatigan 1977). The good correspondence between the macro- and microscopic tumour borders makes the assessment of the tumour area easy. A systematic study of the resection margins of surgical specimens from patients with colorectal cancer was carried out by Haugen and Svaar in 1982 (personal communication). Only two of a total of 214 resected specimens had tumour infiltration in one of the resection margins. These two cases had additional metastases to the peritoneum and liver or infiltration of the vaginal wall at the time of surgery. The average distance from the primary tumour to the nearest resection border was 5.2 ± 3.8 cm (means $\pm$ SD). From these results, it seems unnecessary to examine the resection margins histologically provided that the resection has been performed at least 5 cm from the tumour.

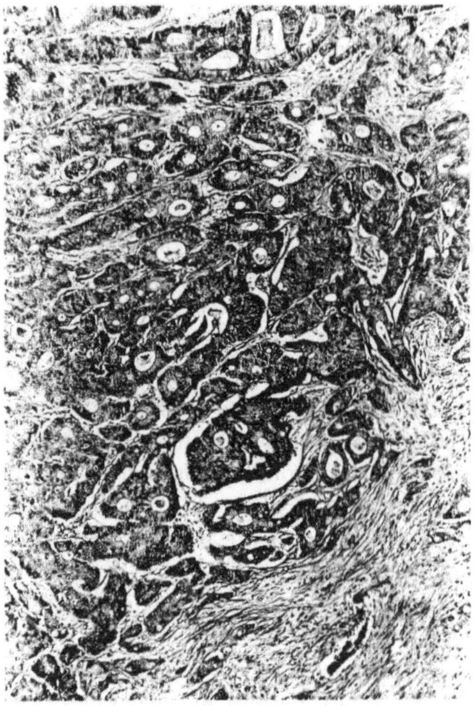

Fig. 1. Microphotograph illustrating an infiltrating part of a moderately well-differentiated adenocarcinoma of the colon. There are small amounts of mucus within the glandular spaces. This is the usual or "classical" type of colorectal carcinoma

Linitis plastica is extremely rare in colorectal cancer. Until 1982, only 52 such cases had been reported in the Anglo-Saxon literature (Ojeda et al. 1982). It is a matter of definition whether these tumours should be designed adenocarcinoma. Their diffuse infiltration can cause a rigid, diffusely thickened bowel wall with indistinct tumour margins, making peroperative histology necessary.

Carcinoids

Colorectal carcinoid tumours are rare. They are located mainly in the proximal colon and to a lesser extent in the rectum. They constitute 0.3% of all colorectal malignancies (for review see Horn 1949). Macroscopically they present with a yellowish cut surface. Small tumours are usually found in the submucosal layer and have the appearance of rounded nodules on the mucosal surface. Large tumours may ulcerate (Peskin and Orloff 1959). Colorectal carcinoids are usually neither argentaffin nor argyrophil in nature (Morson and Sobin 1976). Apart from that, the histological picture does not differ from the classical one. Some mucus production may be seen and does not exclude the diagnosis of a carcinoid tumour. Until 1959 there were no reports of carcinoid syndromes developed on the basis of rectal carcinoids (Peskin and Orloff 1959).

There are considerable difficulties in predicting the future behaviour of carcinoid tumours on the basis of their histological appearance. Nuclear pleomorphism and high mitotic activity should, however, arouse suspicion of malignancy. Caecal carcinoids metastasize more often than those elsewhere in the colon (Pearson and Fitzgerald 1949). Peskin and Orloff (1959) reported that rectal carcinoids bigger than 2 cm were malignant in nine out of 10 cases, whereas only one of 15 carcinoids smaller than 2 cm exhibited malignant behaviour.

Leiomyosarcomas

Colorectal leiomyosarcomas constitute less than 0.1% of all malignant colorectal tumours (MacKenzie et al. 1954). Small intestinal leiomyosarcomas are found 8 times and gastric leiomyosarcomas 20 times more often than colorectal ones. They arise 5 times more often in the colon than in the rectum. The tumours are well demarcated but have no capsule. Their size may vary considerably and lesions bigger than 15 cm may be found. There are four main types: intracolic (submucosal), extracolic (subserosal), combined (dumbbell) and constrictive (intramural). They are often rounded in shape with intact mucosa. Ulcerations and cystic degeneration may occur late but do not necessarily indicate malignancy. They may occur in infancy and in the late senium as well (Posen and Bar-Moar 1983; Rao et al. 1980).

Criteria for malignancy in gastrointestinal and retroperitoneal leiomyomas have been analysed by Ranchod and Kempson (1977). All tumours having more than five mitoses per 10 high-power fields behaved aggressively and merited the designation leiomyosarcoma. Forty per cent of the leiomyosarcomas had fewer mitoses. Tumour necrosis indicated malignancy despite infrequent mitoses.

Leiomyoblastomas and clear cell or epitheloid cell leiomyosarcomas are rare tumours with similar malignancy criteria (Ranchod and Kempson 1977). The pathologist must always report on malignancy with reservation, although the mitotic activity may be a good indicator.

Histopathological Prediction of Prognosis

Histological Grading

There is an inverse relationship between tumour malignancy grade and survival (Newland et al. 1981). Assessment, however, is difficult, since other prognostic factors such as depth of penetration, venous invasion and lymphatic spread are also important. Therefore, grading is difficult to analyze as a single and independent variable. Mucinous carcinomas generally have a worse prognosis than other carcinomas.

Recently, flow cytometric analyses of the DNA distribution in malignant and paraneoplastic cells from the colon and rectum have contributed considerably to our understanding of the relationship between cellular anaplasia and prognosis (for references see Lærum and Weiz 1987). Such analyses have the obvious advantage over histological interpretation of malignant cells that they give measurable and highly reproducible results. Further research seems to be necessary in order to include flow cytometric analyses in the routine evaluation of colorectal cancer patients. With the rapidly expanding knowledge within this field it would seem adviseable not to wait too long.

Site

Proximal colon carcinomas seem less infiltrative and may have a smaller potential for lymph node and liver metastases than rectosigmoid carcinomas (Halvorsen and Seim 1987). Pulmonary metastases are also more common in distal tumours – a fact that might be dependent on direct venous drainage into the systemic circulation.

Tumour Size and Local Extension

The prognosis is excellent in patients having a small focal cancer within a polyp. Metastases are rare in these cases (Scarborough et al. 1965; Palacios and Wellman 1966; Morson et al. 1984). The lack of lymphatic vessels in the lamina propria of the large bowel makes tumour penetration into the submucosal layer a prerequisite for lymphatic metastases (Fenoglio et al. 1973). By contrast, intramucosal stomach carcinomas may occasionally give rise to lymph node metastasis, probably due to a different lymphatic arrangement (Morson and Dawson 1979).

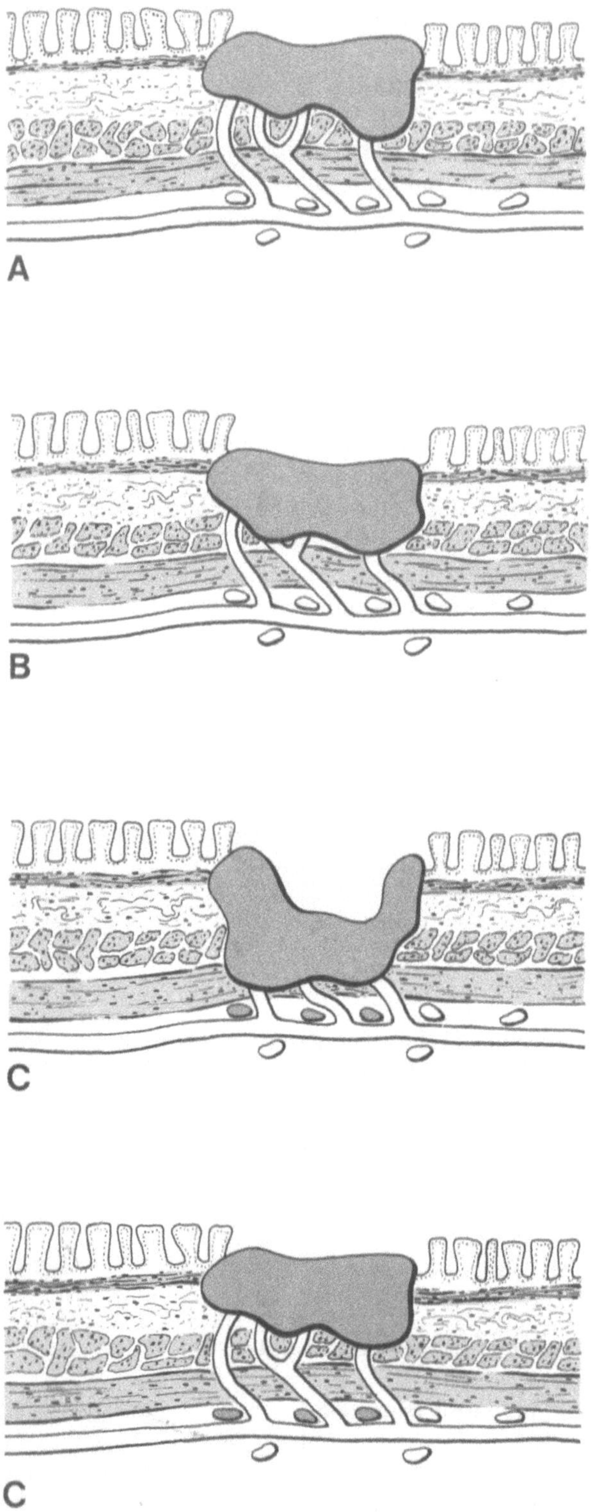

Fig. 2. Illustration of Dukes' stages A, B and C. *A* denotes cases where tumour growth has penetrated into the muscle layers, but not beyond. There is no lymph node involvement. *B* denotes cases where tumour growth has penetrated through the muscle layers into the pericolic or perirectal tissue without lymphatic involvement. *C* denotes cases where lymph node spread has occurred, regardless of local tumour penetration (Modified from WHO 1976)

A standardized system for the estimation of the depth of tumour penetration was proposed by Dukes in 1940. This system was originally developed for rectal carcinomas but was later adapted for colorectal carcinomas in general (Fig. 2). It gained general acceptance and is still the preferred system. In stage A tumour growth is confined to the bowel wall, in stage B there is extension into the perirectal or pericolic tissues but no lymph nodes are involved and in stage C there is lymph node involvement.

In 1979 Morson and Dawson reviewed this subject and claimed that patients with Dukes' A cancer almost invariably can be surgically cured. The 5-year survival rate drops to about 70% in Dukes' B cancer, whereas in Dukes' C cancer only one-third of the patients survive for 5 years. The prognosis in Dukes' C varies with the number of nodes involved; for three or less 5-year survival was 45% but with more than three it was only 15%. Growth into intramural veins has little effect on the prognosis, whereas extramural venous spread reduces overall survival to 25%.

These figures were somewhat modified in a prospective study reported by Newland et al. in 1981. In their series of 503 patients the figures were corrected for the mortality of an age-matched normal population. The 5-year survival was 79.7%, 74.8% and 49.4% for Dukes' stages A, B and C respectively.

Tumour size has been found to correlate positively with depth of penetration but has no relation to the presence or absence of lymph node metastases. The predictive value of tumour size and depth of penetration of the tumour has, therefore, been questioned. The prognostic discriminant value of these parameters, as used in the TNM system, has also been doubted (Wolmark et al. 1984).

The markedly lower 5-year survival rate in Dukes' stage C emphasizes the superiority of lymph node metastases over local tumour size and penetration as a predictor of outcome.

An elaborate scoring system based on a comprehensive set of discrete histopathological parameters has been suggested and is claimed to yield prognostic information superior to that obtained with other classifications (Jass et al. 1987).

Relationship Between Histological Grade and Extent of Local, Venous and Lymphatic Spread

In Dukes' original report of 985 rectal carcinomas (Dukes 1940), there was a positive correlation between histological malignancy grade (Broders grading) and the extent of local tumour growth. Of 14 patients with grade IV cancers, none belonged to

Dukes' stage A, one to stage B and 13 to stage C. Similar findings were reported by Zamchek et al. in 1975 and Newland et al. in 1981. The latter authors also demonstrated a positive correlation between the histological grade of malignancy and the venous and lymphatic spread. The correlations between prognostic parameters such as the level of serum carcinoembryonic antigen (CEA), tumour histopathology including stroma reaction, lymphatic and venous spread and Dukes' stage were strong, and even stronger and more reliable when combined.

Responses of Regional Lymph Nodes and Tumour-Adjacent Stroma

The presence of mononuclear cells (lymphocytes, plasma cells and macrophages) within or in the vicinity of the primary tumour indicates a favourable prognosis (Svennevig et al. 1984). A similar influence seems to exist in the presence of enlarged regional lymph nodes with a prominent paracortical response, particularly when combined with sinus histiocytosis (Patt et al. 1974). A prominent local lymphoid and regional lymph node response may be observed to a greater degree in Dukes' stage B than in Dukes' stage C (Pihl et al. 1980). This has been taken as evidence for a favourable host vs tumour relationship and has been suggested as a prognostic predictor within Dukes' stage B (Svennevig et al. 1984). Similar observations have been made in several other types of human malignancies (Patt et al. 1974; Berlinger et al. 1976; Kodama et al. 1976; Muldon and Brady 1976; Syrjänen and Hjelt 1977).

Natural History

Previously unrecognized colorectal cancer may be found in a considerable proportion of carefully performed postmortem examinations. In highly reliable reports from the General Hospital of Malmö (Sweden) where there is only one hospital, 26% of the colonic cancers and 11% of the rectal cancers had not been recognized before death (Berge et al. 1973; Ekelund 1974). Thus, the true incidence of colorectal cancer was 56.8 new cases per 100 000 inhabitants per year, after correction for a necropsy rate of 80%. The frequency of carcinoma of the colon and rectum not diagnosed before necropsy was 1.65%. The incidence of clinically diagnosed colorectal carcinomas during the same period was 40.2 per 100 000. At the time of clinical cancer diagnosis 22.2% of patients had coexisting polyps – solitary in 52% of cases. Altogether 29.1% had polyps prior to or after cancer diagnosis. In 2.4% of patients the carcinomas were multiple and in 75% of these cases there were multiple polyps. Nearly all polyps were adenomatous and generally located close to the carcinoma, particularly in rectal cancer patients. The polyps had a distribution similar to the carcinomas.

The distribution of the clinically diagnosed primary cancer lesions in Malmö was as follows: rectum 38%, sigmoid colon 29%, descending colon 4.5%, transverse colon 11%, ascending colon 18%. The colonic tumour distribution was the same in both sexes but rectal cancer was more common in men. 17% of the tumours were classified to Dukes' stage A, 38% to Dukes' stage B, 24% to Dukes' stage C and 21% had distant metastases. The proportion of patients with localized tumour was somewhat higher in proximal cancers. Recent stage distribution data in clinically detected colorectal cancers reveal exactly the same staging, but only if the stages Dukes' A and B are taken together. Thus it might seem that there has been a shift towards less advanced cancers since the early 1970s. Whether this reflects a true "downstaging", changes in pathologists' attitudes or other factors cannot be established at present.

The material from Malmö is interesting since it reflects the total colorectal cancer situation in a defined and well-controlled population, including those tumours undetected before death. However, the stage and behaviour of undetected tumours if allowed to grow cannot be established. A more active diagnostic attitude, with screening of asymptomatic populations, may disclose a greater proportion of such "undetected" tumours, which, in turn, may change the overall results of treatment. Screening of an asymptomatic population with repeated rectosigmoidoscopies and removal of all detected adenomas in the rectum resulted in a cancer incidence 85% lower than expected (Gilbertsen and Nelms 1978). Those cancers that developed after the first examination were all in an "early" stage.

Clinically detected colorectal cancers have a growth rate corresponding to an average "tumour doubling time" of about 625 days as measured by double-contrast barium enema (Welin et al. 1963). Lung metastases from the same tumour types grow 5 times faster. Exfoliation of faster-growing tumour tissue from the primary tumour might explain this difference, but seems implausible as the sole reason. However, this phenomenon provides support for the clinical impression that metastases – once present – may markedly enhance patient deterioration.

There are several ways in which colorectal cancer can spread: local, lymphatic and haematogenous spread and implantation. Local spread can occur by perineural infiltration and by direct infiltration of adjacent organs and structures. A prerequisite for lymphatic and haematogenous spread is tumour growth into the submucosal intestinal layer. Haematogenous spread takes place via three main venous routes – portal to the liver, caval to the lungs and lumbar to the spine.

Almost half of all colorectal cancer patients have metastases at operation (Sugarbaker et al. 1982). Above one-fifth of these have distant metastases, nearly all with deposits in the liver. About 50% of those with liver metastases also have extrahepatic manifestations. In half of the remaining 50% the liver manifestations are confined to one lobe. Some of these patients have solitary lesions. The fact that a few patients macroscopically have a resectable primary colorectal cancer and concomitant unilobar secondary hepatic spread with no signs of extrahepatic spread has attracted considerable interest recently. By radical removal of the primary tumour and liver resection the 5-year survival rate in these relatively rare patients has been improved from zero to about 25% – a result far better than in several other surgically treated forms of cancer. Better primary selection and better detection of those developing metachronous liver metastases after primary surgical treatment have been achieved with modern imaging techniques – also used intraoperatively.

Between 60% and 70% of the clinically detected primary colorectal cancers can be treated surgically with curative intention. Palliative surgical procedures can be performed in about 20%. Five to ten per cent are beyond surgery. About 75% of palliative operations consist of resection – bypass procedures or colostomies form the remainder. Abdominoperineal resection is performed in 50% of patients with rectal cancer, low anterior resection in 25% and palliative procedures such as colostomy in the remainder (Murphy 1979; Vana et al. 1979a, b; Arnesjø et al. 1984).

The postoperative mortality varies between 2% and 10% in most reports, with the highest figures after emergency operations. Postoperative complications have been reported at rates of up to 50%. Wound dehiscence, infection, urinary tract infection and cardiopulmonary complications are the most common.

The prognosis may vary in relation to the clinical features. Diagnosis in asymptomatic patients, long duration of symptoms, age higher than 70 years, low preoperative CEA, haemorrhage as presenting symptom and a polypoid configuration of the primary tumour are indicators of a relatively good prognosis. Low age at diagnosis, high preoperative CEA, intestinal obstruction, perforation or abscess formation, circumferential bowel lumen involvement, involvement of adjacent organs, tumour ulceration or distal intestinal location of the primary lesion may be predictors of relatively short survival. However, these signs should not be used as criteria for prognostic evaluation. Although not perfect, histopathological findings such as tumour size, differentiation, stage and spread are much better parameters for predicting prognosis in the individual patient.

The overall survival in both colonic and rectal cancer is improving in most countries (Sugarbaker et al. 1982). The reason for this cannot be firmly established. Better diagnostic facilities, particularly colonoscopy, better results of surgery and a more active surgical treatment of elderly patients may contribute. Until now no beneficial effects on survival of oncological therapy other than surgery have been demonstrated.

In colonic cancer the death rate is highest during the 1st year after diagnosis. Almost 50% of the deaths occur during this year. During the next 2–5 years the death rate still exceeds the expected, but at the end of this period there is only a slight excess, indicating that survivors at 5 years enjoy practically the same life expectancy as the general population. The 5-year survival rate is approximately 40% in both sexes. The death rate correlates with age and stage of disease at treatment.

In rectal cancer the overall 5-year survival rate is rather similar to that of colonic cancer, i.e. 30%–40%. However, the shape of the survival curves differs for the two sites. For cancer of the rectum the slope of the curve is steeper than expected at the end of the 5-year period, particularly among males. Thus, survival 5 years after radical treatment for rectal cancer does not mean a regained normal life expectancy. Sex, age and stage of disease at radical treatment correlate with survival. The prognosis is best in young women with localized rectal cancer.

Screening of Asymptomatic Disease

Surveillance of faecal occult blood is a method of screening for colorectal cancer which has been tried extensively in recent years (Adamsen and Kronborg 1984; Simon 1985; Winawer et al. 1985; Carlsson et al. 1986; Hardcastle et al. 1986; Klaaborg et al. 1986;

Williams and Northover 1987). An increasing prevalence of benign and malignant colorectal tumours, longer patient survival in "earlier" stages of disease, and the possibility of avoiding cancer development by detection and removal of premalignant polyps all speak in favour of such screening provided that it is cheap and simple to perform. Arguments against such screening are the relatively low sensitivity and specificity of the available tests and the low compliance of the population. This leads to complex examination programmes following false-positive tests and a false sense of security in false-negative individuals. In addition, faecal blood screening has not yet been demonstrated to have any beneficial effect on survival in colorectal cancer. Thus, there is insufficient support for general screening programmes involving tests for occult faecal blood. At the meeting of the International Workgroup on Colorectal Cancer in Geneva (1980) the following recommendations were made:

1. Persons at risk for colorectal cancer should be encouraged to contact the health care system.
2. The relative risk should be assessed by family and personal history questionnaires.
3. Once patients are in the system, screening should be added to other aspects of medical evaluation.
4. Screening should include proctosigmoidoscopy once every 3–5 years, beginning between the ages of 40 and 50 years. Rigid sigmoidoscopy should be used if this is the only available instrumentation, but flexible sigmoidoscopy, either the 60-cm scope used by a trained endoscopist or a 35-cm scope used by a general practitioner, is preferred.
5. Screening should include faecal occult blood testing annually, beginning between 40 and 50 years of age.
6. Diagnostic work-up of patients with a positive screening test should include colonoscopy.

Other screening programmes have been suggested but cannot be generally recommended at present. Among these, immunological tests, estimation of circulating tumour markers, detection of deficient deoxyribonucleic acid repair in circulating lymphocytes, cytological lavage examinations and histological examination of mucosal biopsies have been proposed to have diagnostic value. Despite being indicative of the presence of cancer, the sensitivity and specificity of these tests are too low to justify their use in the screening of symptomatic as well as asymptomatic risk groups. Furthermore, the efficacy of several of these different methods, solitarily or in combination, has not yet been fully evaluated. Endoscopic mucosal biopsies and some of the immunological tests, however, have a definite role in the follow-up of patients with inflammatory bowel disease and in those previously treated for colorectal cancer. Direct colonoscopy in symptomatic patients and high-risk groups has the highest diagnostic value.

Diagnosis of Symptomatic Disease

Cancer of the colon and rectum may present in three main ways: as non-urgent cases with insiduously developing chronic symptoms affecting bowel function or general health (75%); as emergencies with acute bowel obstruction (18%); or as emergencies with perforation of the colon and peritonitis (7%) (Goligher and Smiddy 1957).

In non-urgent cases the main symptoms are alteration of the bowel habits (constipation, diarrhoea or both), passage of blood and mucus, abdominal pain, flatulent distension, borborygmi, a palpable mass and impairment of general health. The presentation of symptoms is somewhat dependent upon the site and type of growth.

With growths in the right colon bowel symptoms may be completely absent, the main symptom being impairment of general health with loss of weight and anaemia. In many cases a vague constant pain is present in the right side of the abdomen.

With cancers of the left colon disturbances of bowel habits are frequent, the more so the further distally the lesion is situated. Blood and mucus may be recognized by the patient in the motion, the more so the closer the growth is to the rectum. Obstructive symptoms with flatulent distension, colicky pains and borborygmi, relieved by the passage of flatus, may be experienced.

With carcinomas of the distal sigmoid colon and the rectum bleeding is the main symptom, frequently accompanied by disturbance of bowel habit. The patient often has a sense of incomplete evacuation, and may have to visit the toilet a number of times during the early hours of the day ("morning diarrhoea"). Pain in the rectum is a sign of advanced disease, except with growths in the lower part of the rectum invading the skin-lined anal canal.

Colorectal cancer should be borne in mind in any patient above the age of 40 with symptoms as described above, particularly if they persist for more than 2–3 weeks.

The abdomen may be distended due to chronic intestinal obstruction or ascites. A mass may be felt, usually in the right side. The liver should be examined for enlargement, firmness and nodularity. Digital palpation of the rectum is essential, though only tumours within 10 cm of the anus may be felt. Occult blood in the stool may be demonstrated by chemical tests in the majority of cases.

Rigid sigmoidoscopy will identify carcinomas of the rectum and in many instances also of the lower 5–10 cm of the sigmoid. In order to examine the rest of the large bowel, barium enema, preferably a double-contrast barium examination, or colonoscopy will have to be performed. About 5% of the carcinomas are missed on air-contrast barium enema, in particular those situated in the sigmoid colon, where diverticular disease or overlapping of barium-filled loops of bowel may obscure them. In such cases colonoscopy offers a better chance of detection. Double-contrast barium enema or colonoscopy should be done preoperatively to detect synchronous carcinoma or adenoma, unless bowel obstruction makes this impossible. At endoscopy, biopsies for tissue diagnosis are taken and polyps removed whenever possible.

Until recently the preoperative assessment of rectal cancer was made by digital examination and endoscopy. Although digital examination provides fairly accurate information in the staging of rectal tumours (Nicholls et al. 1982), its use is limited to lesions located within 10 cm of the anal verge. Hildebrandt and Feifel (1985) reported that intrarectal ultrasonography for tumours in the lower two-thirds of the rectum provides a more sensitive method of assessing the local extent of rectal cancer. Computerized tomography (CT) has been reported to be a sensitive method of assessing tumours with a significant degree of extraluminal extension, but its value for correct staging of tumours confined to the rectal wall has been questioned (Nicholls et al. 1982).

Dissemination may be obvious from the presence of liver enlargement, ascites and abdominal masses away from the primary tumour. Digital examination of the rectum may reveal involvement of the pelvic peritoneum or the ovaries. Metastases may be found on chest X-ray or on ultrasound or CT scans of the liver.

Acute obstruction of the colon is more commonly seen with cancers of the left than with those of the right colon. The obstruction is often insiduous in onset, and the patient may have gone for days without passage of gas or stools. A plain X-ray of the abdomen will show widening of the colonic gas shadow proximal to the lesion. With obstructing growths in the caecal region there will be gas shadows and fluid levels in the small intestine, whereas the colon may be empty. An emergency barium or Gastrografin enema examination will show the site of the obstructing lesion.

Perforation of the colon in patients with colorectal cancer may take place through the tumour itself or through the bowel wall proximal to the tumour, most often through a stercoraleous ulcer in the caecum or sometimes elsewhere in the colon, both in the presence of distal obstruction. The perforation may occur into the free peritoneal cavity, in which case the patient presents with signs of generalized peritonitis, or it may be localized with the formation of an abscess. In the former situation a plain abdominal X-ray may show pneumoperitoneum, and in the latter ultrasonography or CT may reveal an abscess cavity.

Surgical Treatment

The aim of surgery is to remove the tumour-bearing segment of the bowel and the regional lymphatic vessels and nodes accompanying the blood vessels supplying the segment.

Right hemicolectomy is performed for growths of the right colon (caecum, ascending colon and hepatic flexure), extended right hemicolectomy for growths of the right transverse colon. Growths of the middle third of the transverse colon are removed by transverse colectomy with anastomosis of the two flexures. In the left colon (left third of transverse colon, splenic flexure, descending and sigmoid colon) some modification of left hemicolectomy is performed. With a growth in a long sigmoid loop on an ample mesosigmoid, sigmoid resection will suffice. More limited resections are made in poor-risk patients and patients with inoperable metastases.

Carcinomas in the upper third of the rectum are dealt with by anterior resection, growths in the middle third by low anterior resection and tumours in the lower third by abdominoperineal resection. In selected cases local excision of low rectal carcinomas may be performed. Other modalities for the surgical treatment of low-lying rectal cancers are transsacral resection (Localio et al. 1983), transsphincteric resection (Mason 1972) and abdominoanal resection (Parks and Percy 1982).

In addition to the above-mentioned bowel resections it may sometimes be necessary to resect part of a neighbouring viscus such as the stomach, a loop of small intestine, the uterus or adnexae, the urinary bladder, the posterior vaginal wall or a portion of the abdominal wall.

Preoperative Bowel Preparation

A number of regimens are in use to empty the large bowel prior to surgery. In our department, 2 days of fluid diet and X-Prep with a saline enema on the evening before surgery results in a fairly clean bowel, except in cases of severe obstruction. In such cases an attempt is made to empty the colon from below with repeated saline enemas. If this is unsuccessful, a preliminary transverse loop colostomy with washout of the distal colon followed by definitive surgery 1–2 weeks later may be contemplated.

Prophylaxis Against Infection and Thromboembolism

A variety of antibiotics in various combinations is used for the purpose of infection prophylaxis. The scheme should include agents effective against both aerobes and anaerobes, and in our department doxycycline 400 mg and metronidazole 1500 mg or tinidazole 1600 mg given as a continuous peroperative infusion results in an infection rate of about 4% (Norwegian Study Group for Colorectal Surgery 1985).

Postoperative thrombosis represents a substantial risk which cannot be completely avoided. Several prophylactic regimens have been suggested. In our department we use pre-, per- and postoperative s.c. heparin according to a Scandinavian protocol (Bergquist and Lindblad 1988).

Surgical Technique

The abdomen is opened through a midline incision which gives excellent access to all parts of the large bowel and the upper rectum, as well as the whole of the peritoneal cavity.

The liver is examined for the presence of metastases. The colon is palpated for the detection of synchronous carcinoma and adenoma, although this is preferably done preoperatively by colonoscopy or double-contrast barium enema. The regional lymph nodes, the ovaries and the peritoneum, especially the pelvic peritoneum, are examined for the presence of secondary deposits.

The "no-touch", or rather the "minimal-touch" technique is practised whenever possible. Since recent observations seem to indicate that blood transfusion influences the prognosis adversely (Burrows and Tartter 1982), care is now being taken to achieve immediate haemostasis and avoid transfusion. The bowel lumen on both sides of the tumour is tied off with tapes to prevent intraluminal spread of viable cancer cells. The supplying vessel (the ileocolic, middle colic, inferior mesenteric or superior haemorrhoidal artery) is ligated centrally, followed by ligation of the corresponding vein. Then the bowel segment to be removed is mobilized together with its mesentery. The bowel is divided between soft clamps, and an end-to-end anastomosis is effected using a one- or two-layer interrupted Vicryl or Dexon suture 3–0. The mesenteric defect is closed with a continuous Vicryl or Dexon suture 3–0.

For resectable growths of the upper third of the rectum, anterior resection with an end-to-end anastomosis between the upper sigmoid and the rectal stump using a single-layer row of inverting, interrupted Vicryl or Dexon sutures 3–0 is practised. For growths of the middle third of the rectum low anterior resection using the same suture technique is performed whenever possible. We have grown disenchanted with the EEA stapler as we have seen too many anastomotic strictures (five of 45 stapled low anterior resections). With growths in the lower third and advanced tumours in the middle third of the rectum an abdominoperineal resection is performed. Local excision by the peranal approach in low-lying rectal cancers (<6–7 cm from the anal verge) may be done in selected well-differentiated, small carcinomas of Dukes' A stage, or as a compromise operation in patients too frail for a major surgical procedure.

At the end of the operation the peritoneal and pelvic cavities are rinsed with 5–7 litres of normal saline to remove blood and detritus. Drains are not used, except in low anterior or abdominoperineal resection, in which case a suprapubic closed suction drain is placed through an extraperitoneal tunnel into the depth of the pelvis to avoid haematoma formation. The drain is removed when drainage falls to below 50 ml/day, usually 1–2 days postoperatively. In operations for rectal carcinoma the pelvic peritoneum is not closed, loops of small bowel being allowed to fill the pelvic cavity. In abdominoperineal resection the muscular pelvic floor and the skin are closed separately. The abdominal incision is closed in layers with continuous sutures.

In abdominoperineal resection a sigmoid colostomy is made in the left iliac region. The defect between the cut edge of the mesosigmoid and the anterolateral abdominal wall may or may not be closed. We do not close it, but leave it wide open to accommodate any loops of small bowel which might find their way into it. No case of intestinal obstruction due to incarceration of small intestine in this region has been observed in 15 years of following this practice.

The nasogastric tube is removed as soon as the patient is awake and any nausea has subsided, usually within 12 h of the operation. In low anterior or abdominoperineal resection the bladder catheter is retained for a week.

Malignant Colorectal Polyp

The malignant colorectal polyp removed at endoscopy represents a special problem. If removal is complete and the carcinoma well or moderately well differentiated, no further surgical treatment is required (Morson et al. 1984).

Acute Colorectal Obstruction

With growths of the right colon a right hemicolectomy or extended right hemicolectomy with an end-to-end anastomosis is usually possible, as the anastomosis is between the terminal ileum, which may or may not be dilated, and the transverse colon distal to the obstruction, which is usually empty.

When the obstruction is due to a carcinoma of the left colon, and the colon proximal to the growth is only moderately dilated, a primary left hemicolectomy may be contemplated. The contents of the bowel proximal to the growth may be milked into the segment to be removed or washed into a suitable receptacle by perfusion of the colon through a catheter placed in the caecum (Dudley et al. 1980). When the proximal colon is more than moderately dilated it is safer to perform a staged operation. A temporary transverse loop colostomy is made, followed by definitive surgery 2 weeks later. The colostomy is usually closed simultaneously.

With obstructing lesions of the rectum a temporary loop sigmoidostomy is made, which may then be resected together with the bowel at the definitive operation 2 weeks later.

Colorectal Carcinoma with Perforation

If the perforation has taken place at or close to a growth of the left colon, sigmoid colon or rectosigmoid junction, radical resection of the tumour-bearing bowel segment with a colostomy and closure of the distal bowel is performed (Hartmann's method). The bowel ends may then be reunited at a later date when the peritonitis has subsided.

If the perforation is elsewhere in the colon in a case of distal obstruction, the site of the perforation is exteriorized as a tube colostomy and an additional transverse loop colostomy is made to give adequate decompression of the large bowel. Radical operation of the distal obstructing lesion may then be performed when the peritonitis has subsided.

The peritoneal cavity is irrigated peroperatively with large amounts of warm saline. Systemic administration of broad-spectrum antibiotics effective against both aerobes and anaerobes is instituted as soon as peritonitis due to perforation of a carcinoma has been diagnosed, usually preoperatively, and continued postoperatively for as long as necessary.

Patients with localized peritonitis due to perforation of a carcinoma, usually of the caecum or ascending colon, are treated more or less along the same lines as the elective cases. Radical resection of the tumour-bearing bowel segment with primary anastomosis is performed, and broad-spectrum antibiotic treatment is given per- and postoperatively for about a week, unless septic complications necessitating longer treatment occur.

Adjuvant Chemotherapy and Immunotherapy

The handling of growths at operation probably releases malignant cells into the venous circulation. Therefore, the practice of infusing cytostatics into the portal vein and also into the systemic circulation during curative resection of a colorectal cancer, in the hope of minimizing the incidence of distant metastases, has been suggested (Cruz et al. 1956). A number of drugs have been used for this purpose, both single and in combination, most of them to no avail. Taylor et al. (1979; Taylor 1978) perfused the liver through the portal circulation with a daily dose of 1000 mg 5-fluorouracil for the first 7 postoperative days. Favourable long-term results were reported, but confirmation is needed before such adjuvant therapy can be recommended (Taylor et al. 1985).

The Gastrointestinal Tumor Study Group (1984) gave systemic adjuvant chemotherapy with 5-fluorouracil and semustine, immunotherapy with BCG, combination therapy with 5-fluorouracil, semustine and BCG, and no adjuvant treatment to four groups of patients who had had curative surgical resection for modified Dukes' stage B_2, C_1, or C_2 colon carcinoma. No difference was found between the three treatment arms and the control group of the study.

Buyse et al. (1986) studied the effect of chemotherapy in colorectal cancer by combining the results of all controlled randomized trials which had tested such treatment alone or in combination with other treatment forms versus no treatment. There was no overall benefit, but in trials only testing 5-fluorouracil alone or in combinations, the odds of death were 14% lower and the 5-year survival 4.3% higher in treated patients than in control patients.

Adjuvant Preoperative and Postoperative Radiotherapy in Curative Resection of Rectal Cancer

A number of studies have been reported in which preoperative adjuvant radiotherapy was given in doses ranging from 5 to 20 Gy in patients undergoing ostensibly curative resection for rectal cancer. Most of these studies have shown no advantage of radiotherapy as regards survival (Duncan 1985; Cummings 1986; Påhlman and Glimelius 1988). The Gastrointestinal Tumor Study Group (1985) gave 40–48 Gy postoperatively and postoperative chemotherapy (5-fluorouracil and MeCCNU), separately and combined, to patients with Dukes' B and C lesions, and reported a lower incidence of local and distant recurrences in the three treatment arms, especially with combined radio- and chemotherapy, than in the control arm. The MRC Working Party is currently evaluating the timing of adjuvant radiotherapy in relation to definitive surgery based on the pretreatment assessment of the mobility of the cancer. If it is tethered the probability of curative resection is low and preoperative radiotherapy may be of substantial benefit. If the cancer is mobile, the patient should proceed immediately to definitive surgery. Patients with Dukes' B and C growths should then be considered for postoperative radiotherapy in a dose of 40 Gy in 20 fractions over 4 weeks (Duncan 1985).

The use of radiotherapy as adjuvant to surgery in Dukes' B and C rectal cancers has been studied in several series. Pre- or postoperative radiotherapy at the primary treatment or at local relapse after curative surgery, respectively, has caused a "downstaging" after surgical resection and increased the resectability rate (Lise et al. 1987; Buyse et al. 1986). Several other trials are now in progress using different radiation dosages in rectal or rectosigmoid cancer, but there is as yet no evidence that this therapy has any beneficial effect upon survival or mortality. In some series the local recurrence rate has been reduced. After reviewing all recent randomized controlled trials published up to 1986, Buyse et al. (1986) summarized the effect of radiotherapy or radiotherapy combined with other forms of treatment as adjuvant to surgical excision of rectal cancer. Using two statistical methods and two endpoints (mortality odds ratio and 5-year survival benefit) they could demonstrate that the odds of death are 16% lower and of 5-year survival 4.2% higher in the treated group than in untreated control patients. There were 30% lower odds of death and 7.2% improvement in 5-year survival in curatively resected patients, which, however, might be ascribed to bias since resectability was not known prior to entry in the trials.

Buyse et al. (1986) concluded that adjuvant 5-fluorouracil or radiotherapy in colorectal cancer may improve the survival rate marginally, but that this improvement might be biased, since it is based only on published trials, which might have better results than unpublished ones.

Disseminated Disease

At the time of operation 40%–50% of patients with colorectal cancer will have distant metastases, about half of which will be clinically evident. The presence of distant metastases is not normally a contraindication to palliative excision of the primary growth, unless there is widespread affection of the liver or the peritoneal cavity.

A solitary liver deposit or a small cluster of nodules close to the edge of a liver lobe may be managed by a wedge resection at the primary operation. More centrally placed hepatic metastases necessitating formal lobectomy are best left for a second intervention 2–3 months later. In the interval between the operations the liver is examined with ultrasonography, CT and hepatic angiography to chart the pattern of metastases. In patients with solitary or localized clusters of metastases hepatic resection may be performed. Ridge and Daly's collective review (1985) recorded a 20% 5-year survival in such patients.

Attempts have been made to dearterialize widespread hepatic metastases by ligation of the hepatic artery. Hepatic artery ligation may be supplemented by infusion of a cytotoxic agent through the artery or the portal vein (Taylor 1978; Ekberg 1986). However, the mortality is high and the benefit is marginal.

The presence of widespread peritoneal deposits invariably signifies that the duration of survival will be short, and is thus a contraindication to even a palliative excision, unless there is acute bowel obstruction, in which case a bypass procedure or a loop colostomy may be performed.

In female patients with colorectal cancer coming to laparotomy 5%–6% will have ovarian deposits, one-third of which will be occult (Goligher 1984). This has prompted the policy of removing the ovaries routinely in women over the age of 40 without obvious deposits elsewhere. Though the benefit is quantitatively small, the addition of such a simple measure to the bowel resection may be justified.

In cases of extensive nodal involvement beyond the reach of curative resection a palliative resection of the bowel lesion is performed.

Pulmonary metastases occur in 5%–15% of patients who have undergone potentially curative resections. They are usually multiple and are often associated with recurrence elsewhere. In the case of a solitary deposit, pulmonary resection, lobectomy or even pulmonectomy may be performed, resulting in 5-year survival rates of 20%–40% (Mühe et al. 1981).

In cases with widespread metastases which are not amenable to surgery, the choice is between palliative radiotherapy, chemotherapy or both. The literature on chemotherapeutic regimens is vast, and although a 20%–40% response rate is claimed for some of these schedules, there is no significant prolongation of the patients' lives (Ridge and Daly 1985; Buyse et al. 1986).

Radiotherapy for advanced colorectal cancer has been restricted to palliation of pain, bleeding and tenesmus, with objective regression being achieved in 80% of the cases. Survival, however, has not been prolonged.

Follow-up

The purpose of follow-up is to detect metachronous cancers and adenomas, local recurrence and metastatic disease in the hope of their being amenable to surgical treatment. For the detection of metachronous cancers, adenomas and anastomotic recurrences, colonoscopy at regular intervals is recommended. The interval between these examinations is a matter of debate as they put a strain on colonoscopic resources. A "clean colon" having been established by colonoscopy prior to or immediately following surgery, 2-yearly check examination has been suggested (Williams 1985).

Regular monitoring of CEA offers a fairly reliable indicator of recurrent disease or distant metastases (Northover 1985). A rise in CEA was the first indication of recurrence in 60% of cases in two large British series (Tate 1982; Hine and Dykes 1984).

In our department, patients who have undergone an ostensibly curative resection for colorectal cancer are monitored with measurements of CEA at 3-monthly intervals. Clinical examination is performed every 6 months for the first 2 years, and then once a year for the next 3 years. If there is a rise in CEA, a vigorous search for the cause is conducted, including chest X-ray, colonoscopy, ultrasonography of the liver and CT of the abdominal and pelvic cavities. In patients operated upon with low anterior resection for rectal cancer, intrarectal ultrasonography is as accurate as CT in identifying local recurrence, with the added advantage of simplicity and low cost (Romano et al. 1985).

Routine second-look operation for the purpose of removing residual disease, as suggested by Gilbertsen and Wangensteen (1962), has not received universal acceptance. Whether a policy of second-look operation based on serial CEA determinations has any merit remains to be seen. Martin et al. (1980) reported that about 60% of their CEA-detected recurrences were resectable. Schiessel et al. (1986) estimated that 42% of their operations for local recurrence were radical, with 3-year survival of 30%.

Survival and Recurrence: A Review of the Main Clinical Trials

The literature on survival and recurrence after surgery for colorectal cancer is vast, and readers are referred to the excellent review of the trials prior to 1982 given by Goligher (1984). The main points emerging from these reports are as follows: There has been a steady increase in the resectability rate, and an impressive decline in operative mortality over the past three to four decades. The 5-year survival in these series is variously reported as crude survival, corrected survival and absolute survival rate, making comparison somewhat difficult.

The five-year survival rate in rectal cancer is related to the Dukes' stage of the tumour, the corrected survival rate being approximately 95% for Dukes' A, 80% for Dukes' B and 30% for Dukes' C cases (Dukes 1957). A similar correlation of Dukes' stage and prognosis also exists in cancer of the colon.

When there is invasion of a neighbouring viscus or the abdominal wall, the 5-year survival rate is approximately the same as in Dukes' C cases (Bonfanti et al. 1982). From the studies by Bussey (1963) it appears that the majority of patients who are going to die from recurrence of rectal carcinoma do so during the first 5 years and only relatively few between 5 and 10 years. After 10 years there are very few recurrences.

The pattern of recurrence following "curative" colorectal surgery is disseminated disease in 73% and local disease in 27% (Gilbert et al. 1984). Ekberg (1986) reviewed the pattern of recurrence after curative resection of colorectal cancer in 562 patients reported in seven recent publications. Seventy-nine per cent had intra-abdominal, 46% hepatic (16% hepatic only), 26% peritoneal and 56% resection site recurrences. A maximum of 10% of the patients survived for 5 years after evidence of recurrence had been demonstrated. The relapse pattern and rate varied in relation to the site and stage of the primary tumour. Enker et al. (1979) reported on relapse-free 5-year survival in 216 patients: Dukes' A 100%; B_1 74%; B_2 65%; C_1 68%; C_2 57%; metastatic cancer 4%.

The incidence of local recurrence is dependent upon the Dukes' stage of the growth, the tumour differentiation, whether or not obstruction or perforation have been present, and the mobility of the tumour (Phillips et al. 1984a). In patients operated upon for rectal and rectosigmoid cancer, recurrence rates were significantly higher after anterior resection than after abdominoperineal resection (Phillips et al. 1984b). Quirke et al. (1986) concluded that inadequate lateral clearance was the main cause of local recurrence in rectal cancer.

High ligation of the inferior mesenteric vessels during surgery for rectal cancer does not seem to improve the prognosis (Pezim and Nicholls 1984). The role of iliac node dissection is debatable, with some reports showing no effect (Glass et al. 1985) and others claiming improvement in the 5-year survival rate for patients with Dukes' B and C lesions (Enker et al. 1979).

Isolated or multiple liver metastases situated in one hepatic lobe constitute an important clinical problem. The 5-year survival after resection of such synchronous or metachronous metastases ranges between 20% and 42% (Burcharth et al. 1986; Ekberg 1986). Although not tested in controlled trials, these results have been claimed to be much better than in matched historical control groups.

Lobar resections or segmentectomies of tumour-involved areas of the liver have gained popularity in several centres, whereas results of simple metastasectomies have not been reported. This problem is now being studied in several institutions, as are the detection and selection of those patients that might benefit from such advanced surgical treatment. The presence of extrahepatic tumour manifestations contraindicates liver surgery, which, according to most authors, should not be performed simultaneously with the colorectal surgery.

Future Developments

The prognosis in colorectal carcinoma has not changed appreciably over the last three to four decades, and the little improvement that has occurred is due mainly to decreased operative mortality. At presentation many patients are already beyond surgical cure. As the prognosis is clearly related to the Dukes' stage of the growth, early detection would improve the results. Screening the general population for faecal occult blood has been suggested, but the logistics of such a programme are staggering (Ekelund et al. 1985; Carlsson et al. 1986). As probably the majority of colorectal cancers develop from adenomas, colonoscopy and polyp removal may reduce the incidence of colorectal cancer in the future, but again there will be considerable strain on endoscopic resources, as these patients and those who have been operated on for colorectal carcinoma will have to be followed for many years.

Improvement in survival following surgery for rectal cancer is only likely with the use of adjuvant therapy. Since not all patients require such treatment, and since the associated morbidity might be considerable, only high-risk groups should be treated in this manner. The wide range of operative techniques now available necessitates tailoring of the surgical treatment to the individual patient. An extended staging system based on CT of the liver and the pelvis, ultrasonography of the liver, measurement of CEA and acute-phase reactant protein and multiple superficial and deep biopsies to determine the histological grade of the tumour and its DNA cellular content has been suggested to select patients more accurately for the correct treatment (Williams et al. 1985).

In the follow-up of patients operated on for colorectal cancer, monoclonal antibodies may prove a useful tool in the detection of occult metastases and in the targeting of antitumour agents (Armitage et al. 1985).

Recently reported randomized clinical trials demonstrated that there may be a small but statistically significant effect of radiotherapy in rectal cancer and of chemotherapy regimens containing 5-fluorouracil in colorectal cancer. In order to prove such effects there is a need for trials with larger series of patients than has been the case so far, since the treatment benefits that may be expected are of small magnitude.

References

Adami HO (1988) Aspects of descriptive epidemiology and survival in colorectal cancer. Scand J Gastroenterol 23, Suppl 149: 6–20

Adamsen S, Kronborg O (1984) Acceptability and compliance in screening for colorectal cancer with fecal occult bloodtest. Scand J Gastroenterol 19: 531–534

Amorn J, Knight WA (1978) Primary linitis plastica of the colon. Report of two cases and review of the literature. Cancer 41: 2420–2425

Angerås U, Jönsson N, Jönsson P-E (1983) Primary anorectal malignant melanoma. J Surg Oncol 22: 261–264

Armitage NC, Perkins AC, Pimm MV, Farrands PA, Baldwin RW, Hardcastle JD (1985) The localization of an antitumour monoclonal antibody (791/36) in gastrointestinal tumours. Br J Surg 71: 407–412

Arnesjø B, Høst H, Høie J, Solheim K, Ylvisaker Ø (1984) Surgical oncology in Norway. Norges Offentlige Utredninger 1982: 29

Berge T, Ekelund G, Mellner C (1973) Carcinoma of the colon and rectum in a defined population. Acta Chir Scand 438: 11–86

Bergquist D, Lindblad B (1988) Thromboembolic problems in colorectal cancer surgery. Scand J Gastroenterol 23, Suppl 149: 74–81

Berlinger NT, Tsakraklides V, Pollak K, Adams GL, Yang M, Good RA (1976) Immunological assessment of regional lymph node histology in relation to survival in head and neck carcinoma. Cancer 37: 697–705

Bodmer WF, Bailey CF, Bodmer J, Bussey HJR, Ellis A, Gorman P, Lucibello FC et al. (1987) Localization of the gene for familial adenomatous polyposis on chromosome 5. Nature 328: 614–616

Bonfanti G, Bozzetti F, Doci R, Baticci F, Marolda R, Bignami P, Gennari L (1982) Results of extended surgery for cancer of the rectum and sigmoid. Br J Surg 69: 305–307

Brahme F, Ekelund G, Norden JG, Wenckert A (1974) Metachronous colo-rectal polyps; comparison of development of colo-rectal polyps and carinomas in persons with and without histories of polyps. Dis Colon Rectum 17: 166–171

Burcharth F, Höckerstedt K, Lempinen M, Søreide O (1986) Liver cancer. Ann Surg Gynaecol [Suppl] 200: 96

Burrows L, Tartter P (1982) Effect of blood transfusions on colonic malignancy recurrence rate. Lancet 2: 662

Bussey HJR (1963) The long term results of surgical treatment of cancer of the rectum. Proc R Soc Med 56: 494–496

Buyse M, Zeleniuch-Jaquotte A, Chalmers TC (1986) Adjuvant therapy of colorectal cancer: a meta-analysis of published clinical trials. N Engl J Med (in press)

Carlsson U, Ekelund G, Eriksson R, Fork T, Janzon L, Leandoer L, Lindström C, Trell E (1986) Evaluation of possibilities for mass screening for colorectal cancer with Hemoccult fecal blood test. Dis Colon Rectum 29: 553–557

Correa P, Haenszel W (1978) The epidemiology of large-bowel cancer. Adv Cancer Res 26: 1–141

Cruz EP, McDonald GO, Cole WH (1956) Prophylactic treatment of cancer: the use of chemotherapeutic agents to prevent tumour metastasis. Surgery 40: 291–296

Cummings BJ (1986) A critical review of adjuvant preoperative radiation therapy for adenocarcinoma of the rectum. Br J Surg 73: 332–338

Dudley HAF, Radcliff AG, McGeehan D (1980) Intraoperative irrigation of the colon to permit primary anastomosis. Br J Surg 67: 80–81

Dukes CE (1937) Histologic grading of rectal carcinoma. Proc R Soc Med 30: 371–376

Dukes CE (1940) Cancer of the rectum: an analysis of 1000 cases. J Pathol 50: 527–537

Dukes CE (1957) Discussion of major surgery in carcinoma of the rectum with and without colostomy, excluding the anal canal and the rectosigmoid. Proc R Soc Med 50: 1031–1035

Duncan W (1985) Adjuvant radiotherapy in rectal cancer: the MRC trials. Br J Surg [Suppl] 72: 59–66

Ekberg H (1986) Colorectal liver cancer; resection and regional chemotherapy. Dissertation, University of Lund Department of Surgery Bull 61

Ekelund G (1974) On colorectal polyps and carcinoma with special references to their interrelationship. Dissertation, Studentlitteratur, Lund

Ekelund G, Carlsson U, Janzon L (1985) The feasibility of large scale population screening. Br J Surg [Suppl] 72: 71–72

Enker WE, Laffer UT, Block GE (1979) Enhanced survival of patients with colon and rectal cancer is based upon wide anastomotic resection. Ann Surg 190: 350–360

Fenoglio CM, Gordon IK, Lane N (1973) Distribution of human colonic lymphatics in normal, hyperplastic, and adenomatous tissue. Gastroenterology 64: 51–66

Gastrointestinal Tumor Study Group (1984) Adjuvant therapy of colon cancer – results of a prospectively randomized trial. N Engl J Med 310: 737–743

Gastrointestinal Tumor Study Group (1985) Prolongation of disease-free interval in surgically treated rectal carcinoma. N Engl J Med 312: 737–743

Gilbert JM, Jeffrey I, Evans M, Kark AE (1984) Sites of recurrent tumour after "curative" colorectal surgery: Implications for adjuvant therapy. Br J Surg 71: 203–205

Gilbertsen VA, Nelms JM (1978) The prevention of invasive cancer of the rectum. Cancer 41: 1137–1139

Gilbertsen VA, Wangensteen OH (1962) A summary of thirteen years' experience with the "second look program". Surg Gynecol Obstet 114: 438–422

Glass RE, Ritchie JK, Thompson HP, Mann CV (1985) The results of surgical treatment of cancer of the rectum by radical resection and extended abdomino-iliac lymphadenectomy. Br J Surg 72: 599–601

Goligher JG (1984) Surgery of the anus, rectum and colon, 5th ed. Bailliere Tindall, London

Goligher JC, Smiddy FG (1957) The treatment of acute obstruction or perforation with carcinoma of the colon and rectum. Br J Surg 45: 270–274

Greenwald P, Lanza E (1986) Role of dietary fiber in the prevention of cancer. In: de Vita VT, Hellman S, Rosenberg SA (eds) Important advances in oncology 1986. Lippincott, Philadelphia

Halvorsen TB, Seim E (1987) Tumour site: a prognostic factor in colorectal cancer? A multivariate analysis. Scand J Gastroenterol 22: 124–128

Hardcastle JD, Armitage NC, Chamberlain J, Amar SS, James PD, Balfour TW (1986) Fecal occult blood screening for colorectal cancer in the general population. Results of a controlled trial. Cancer 58: 397–403

Hildebrandt U, Feifel G (1985) Preoperative staging of rectal cancer by intrarectal ultrasound. Dis Colon Rectum 28: 42–46

Hill M (1987) Neoplasms: epidemiology. Curr Opin Gastroenterol 3: 4–8

Hine KR, Dykes N (1984) Serum CEA testing in the postoperative surveillance of colorectal carcinoma. Cancer 49: 689–693

Horn RC (1949) Carcinoid tumors of the colon and rectum. Cancer 2: 819–836
Jass JR, Love SB, Northover JMA (1987) A new prognostic classification of rectal cancer. Lancet 1: 1303–1306
Klaaborg K, Stahl Madsen M, Söndergaard O, Kronborg O (1986) Participation in mass screening for colorectal cancer with fecal occult blood test. Scand J Gastroenterol 21: 1180–1184
KodamaY, Soejima K, Inokuchi K (1976) Reactive hyperplasia of paracortex and germinal centers of the regional lymph nodes in gastric carcinoma cases as a favourable prognostic indicator. Jpn J Surg 6: 9–18
Laerum OD, Weiz H (1987) Übersicht Zytometrie prämaligner Zustände. Arch Geschwulstforsch 57 (2): 151–171
Levin B, Riddell HR (1984) Frontiers in gastrointestinal cancer. Elsevier, New York
Lise M, Gerard A, Nitti D, Zane D, Buyse M, Arnaud JP, Metzger U (1987) Adjuvant therapy for colorectal cancer: the EORTC experience and a review of the literature. Dis Colon Rectum 30: 847–854
Lipkin M, Good RA (1978) Gastrointestinal tract cancer. Plenum, New York
Localio SA, Eng K, Gouge TH, Ranson JHC (1983) Abdominosacral resection for carcinoma of the midrectum: 10 years' experience. Ann Surg 188: 475–480
MacKenzie DA, Donald JR, Waugh JM (1954) Leiomyoma and leiomyosarcoma of the colon. Ann Surg 139: 67–75
Martin EW, Cooperman M, Carey LC, Minton JP (1980) Sixty second look procedures indicated primarily by rise in serial carcinoembryonic antigen. J Surg Res 28: 389–394
Mason AY (1972) Trans-sphincteric exposure of the rectum. Ann R Coll Surg Engl 51: 320–321
Morson BC, Bussey HJR (1985) Magnitude of risk for cancer in patients with colorectal adenomas. Br J Surg [Suppl] 72: 23–28
Morson BC, Dawson IMP (1979) Gastrointestinal pathology. Blackwell, Oxford, pp 173, 651
Morson BC, Sobin LH (1976) Histological typing of intestinal tumours. World Health Organization, Geneva (International histological classification of tumours no 15)
Morson BC, Whiteway JE, Jones EA, Macrae FA, Williams CB (1984) Histopathology and prognosis of malignant colorectal polyps treated by endoscopic polypectomy. Gut 25: 437–444
Muldoon CJ, Brady MP (1976) Regional lymph nodes in cancer. Ir J Med Sci 1945: 84–85
Mühe E, Gall FP, Angermann B (1981) Surgical treatment of metastases to the lung and liver. Surg Gynecol Obstet 152: 211–214
Murphy GP (1979) Commission on cancer. Long-term patient care evaluation study of cancer of the colon. American College of Surgeons, 55 East Erie Street, Chicago, IL 60611, USA
Newland RC, Chapuis PH, Pheils MT, Chir M, Pherson JG (1981) The relationship of survival to staging and grading of colorectal carcinoma. Cancer 47: 1424–1429
Nicholls RJ, Mason AY, Morson BC, Dixon AK, Kelsey-Fry I (1982) The clinical staging of rectal cancer. Br J Surg 69: 404–409
Northover JMA (1985) Carcinoembryonic antigen and recurrent colorectal cancer. Br J Surg [Suppl] 72: 44–46
Norwegian Study Group for Colorectal Surgery (1985) Should antimicrobial prophylaxis in colorectal surgery include agents effective against both anaerobic and aerobic microorganisms? A double-blind, multicenter study. Surgery 97: 402–407
Ojeda VJ, Mitchell KM, Walters NJ, Gibson MJ (1982) Primary colo-rectal linitis plastica type carcinoma: report of two cases and review of literature. Pathology 14: 181–189
Påhlman L, Glimelius B (1988) Perioperative radiotherapy in rectal carcinoma. Scand J Gastroenterol 23, Suppl 149: 82–89
Palacios R, Wellman K (1966) Adenomatous polyps of colonic carcinoma and pulmonary metastases. Gastroenterology 51: 82–86
Parks AG, Percy JP (1982) Resection and sutured colo-anal anastomosis for rectal carcinoma. Br J Surg 69: 301–304
Patt JW, Brynes RK, Vardiman JW, Coppleson LW (1974) Mesocolic lymph node histology is important prognostic indicator for patients with carcinoma of the sigmoid colon: an immunomorphologic study. Cancer 35: 1388–1397
Pearson CM, Fitzgerald PJ (1949) Carcinoid tumors – a reemphasis of their malignant nature. Cancer (Nov): 1005–1026
Peskin GW, Orloff MJ (1959) A clinical study of 25 patients with carcinoid tumors of the rectum. Surg Gynecol Obstet (Dec): 673–682
Pezim ME, Nicholls RJ (1984) Survival after high or low ligation of the inferior mesenteric artery during curative surgery for rectal cancer. Ann Surg 200: 729–733
Phillips RKS, Hittinger R, Blesovsky L, Fry JS, Fielding LP (1984 a) Local recurrence following "curative" surgery for large bowel cancer. I. The overall picture. Br J Surg 71: 12–16
Phillips RKS, Hittinger R, Blesovsky L, Fry JS, Fielding LP (1984 b) Local recurrence following "curative" surgery for large bowel cancer. II. The rectum and sigmoid. Br J Surg 71: 17–20
Pihl E, Nairn RC, Milne BJ, Cuthbertson AM, Hughes ESR, Rollo A (1980) Lymphoid hyperplasia. A major prognostic feature in 519 cases of colorectal carcinoma. Am J Pathol 100: 469–481
Posen JA, Bar-Moar JA (1983) Leiomyosarcoma of the colon in an infant. Cancer 52: 1458–1461
Quirke P, Dixon MF, Durdey P, Williams NS (1986) Local recurrence of rectal adenocarcinoma due to inadequate surgical resection. Histopathological study of lateral tumour spread and surgical excision. Lancet 2: 996–999
Ranchod M, Kempson RL (1977) Smooth muscle tumors of the gastrointestinal tract and retroperitoneum. A pathologic analysis of 100 cases. Cancer 39: 255–262
Rao BK, Kapur MM, Roy S (1980) Leiomyosarcoma of the colon: a case report and review of literature. Dis Colon Rectum 23: 184–190
Ridge JA, Daly JM (1985) Treatment of colorectal hepatic metastases. Surg Gynecol Obstet 161: 597–607
Romano G, de Rosa P, Vallone G, Rotondo A, Grassi R, Santangelo ML (1985) Intrarectal ultrasound and computed tomography in the pre- and postoperative assessment of patients with rectal cancer. Br J Surg [Suppl] 72: 117–119
Saffos RO, Rhatigan RM (1977) Benign (nonpolypoid) mucosal changes adjacent to carcinomas of the colon. A light microscopy study of 20 cases. Hum Pathol 8: 441–449
Scarborough R, Dockerty M, Gershon-Cohen G, et al. (1965) Adenomatous polyps of the rectum and the colon. Dis Colon Rectum 8: 85–96
Schiessel R, Wunderlich M, Herbst F (1986) Local recurrence of colorectal cancer: effect of early detection and aggressive surgery. Br J Surg 73: 342–344
Schottenfield D, Winawer SJ (1984) Large intestine. In: Schottenfield D, Fraumeni JF (eds) Cancer epidemiology and prevention. Saunders, Philadelphia
Silverberg E (1984) Cancer statistics, 1984. CA 34: 7–23

Simon JB (1985) Occult blood screening for colorectal carcinoma: a critical review. Gastroenterology 88: 820–837

Solomon E, Voss R, Hall V, Bodmer WF, Jass JR, Jeffreys AJ, Lucibello FC, et al. (1987) Chromosome 5 allele loss in human colorectal carcinomas. Nature 328: 616–619

Sugarbaker PH, Macdonald JS, Gundersen LL (1982) Colorectal cancer. In: de Vita VT, Hellman S, Rosenberg SA (eds) Cancer – principles and practice of oncology. Lippincott, Philadelphia

Svennevig JL, Lunde OC, Holter J, Bjørgsvik D (1984) Lymphoid infiltration and prognosis in colorectal carcinoma. Br J Cancer 49: 375–377

Syrjänen KJ, Hjelt LH (1977) Paracortical activity of the regional lymph nodes as a prognostic determinant in gastric carcinoma. Scand J Gastroenterol 12: 897–902

Tate H (1982) Plasma CEA in the post-surgical monitoring of colorectal carcinoma. Br J Cancer 46: 323–330

Taylor I (1978) Cytotoxic perfusion for colorectal liver metastases. Br J Surg 65: 109–114

Taylor I, Rowling J, West C (1979) Adjuvant cytotoxic liver perfusion for colorectal cancer. Br J Surg 66: 833–837

Taylor I, Machin D, Mullee M, Trotter G, Cooke T, West C (1985) A randomized controlled trial of adjuvant portal vein cytotoxic perfusion in colorectal cancer. Br J Surg 72: 359–363

Thompson H (1986) Pathology of inflammatory bowel disease. Curr Opin Gastroenterol 2: 397–404

Vana J, Mittleman AI, Schmitz RL, Baker HW, Smart CR, Murphy GP (1979a) Long-term patient care evaluation study for carcinoma of the rectum. American College of Surgeons, 55 East Erie Street, Chicago, IL 60611, USA

Vana J, Bedwani RN, Holyoke ED, Schmitz RL, Lawrence W Jr, Smart CR, Murphy GP (1979b) Short-term patient care evaluation study for carcinoma of the rectum. American College of Surgeons, 55 East Erie Street, Chicago, IL 60611, USA

Welin S, Jouker J, Spratt JS, et al. (1963) The rates and patterns of growth of 375 tumors of the large intestine and rectum observed serially by double contrast enema study. AJR 90: 673–687

WHO (1976) Histological typing of intestinal tumours. International histological classification of tumours, no 15. WHO, Geneva

Williams CB (1985) Polyp follow-up: how, who and how often? Br J Surg [Suppl] 72: 25–25

Williams CB, Northover JMA (1987) Colorectal cancer – screening of high-risk groups. GI Rep 2: 1–7

Williams NS, Durdey P, Quirke P, Robinson PJ, Dyson JED, Dixon MF, Bird CC (1985) Preoperative staging of rectal neoplasm and its impact on clinical management. Br J Surg 72: 868–874

Winawer S, Schottenfield D, Sherlock P (1985) Screening for colorectal cancer: the issues. Gastroenterology 88: 841–844

Wolmark N, Fisher ER, Wie HS, Fisher B, et al. (1984) The relationship of depth of penetration and tumor size to the number of positive nodes in Dukes' C colorectal cancer. Cancer 53: 2707–2712

Zamcheck N, Doos WG, Prudente R, Lurie B, Gottlieb LS (1975) Prognostic factors in colon carcinoma. Hum Pathol 6: 31–45

Ziegler RG, Devesa SS, Fraumeni JF (1985) Epidemiologic patterns of colorectal cancer. In: de Vita VT, Hellman S, Rosenberg SA (eds) Important advances in oncology 1986. Lippincott, Philadelphia

Tumours of the Anal Region

J. M. A. NORTHOVER and J. P. S. THOMSON

Introduction

Tumours of the anal region may be benign or malignant and may arise from the epithelium or other nearby tissues. This chapter will concentrate mainly on malignant tumours arising from squamous epithelium, not only because this is the commonest form of anal malignancy but also because it is attracting considerable attention by reason of its possible viral aetiology and also because of the introduction of possible non-operative therapeutic measures.

Definition

The anal canal is an area of embryological fusion where the entodermal hindgut fuses with the ectodermal proctodeum. It is now generally agreed that the fusion occurs over an area of about 2 cm between the lower rectum and the line of the anal valves. This zone is sometimes referred to as the transitional zone, as it has a mixture of different types of epithelium – columnar, cuboidal and stratified squamous. Figure 1 shows the location of this zone and the epithelia which are found in this region.

Tumours are classified into those arising from the epithelium distal to the transitional zone ('anal margin tumours') and those arising from the transitional zone itself ('anal canal tumours').

In general terms tumours arising from the anal margin tend to be similar to tumours found in the skin and carry a better prognosis than those arising from the anal canal. It is, however, important to state that on occasions the distinction between anal margin and anal canal tumours may be difficult. Further-

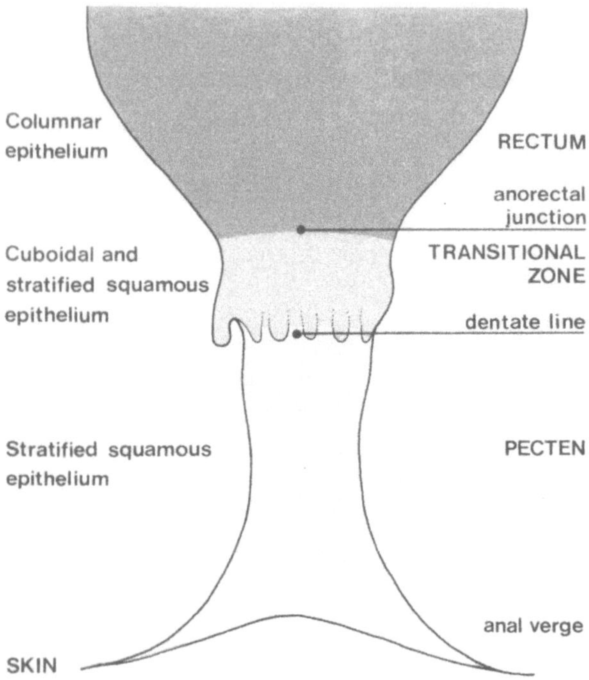

Fig. 1. A diagram of a coronal section through the anal canal to show the different epithelia

Table 1. Rare anal and perianal tumours

Tissue	Type(s) of tumour
Internal sphincter (smooth muscle)	Smooth muscle tumours (leiomyoma and leiomyosarcoma)
Striated muscle	Rhabdomyosarcoma
Ischiorectal fossa (adipose tissue)	Fibrosarcoma, liposarcoma
Lymphoid tissue	Leukaemia, lymphoma

more, some tumours apparently arising in the anal canal actually represent downward spread of tumours in the lower rectum. Non-epithelial tumours arise from surrounding lymphoid tissue, muscle or fat. All these tumours are exceedingly rare but should be noted (Table 1).

Epidemiology

Anal cancer is a rare disease in Western countries, though in some parts of the world, such as north east Brazil and some parts of India, it is a much more common condition. Apart from poor living conditions in the affected regions, no major factors have been suggested to account for this geographical difference.

Lately strong evidence has emerged in the USA to associate anal cancer with sexual activity. Several studies from the western USA have demonstrated a correlation between the incidence of anal cancer and indicators of male homosexuality (Daling et al. 1982; Austin 1982). Daling et al. (1982) examined the Washington State syphilis and cancer registries and reported an increased incidence of anal cancer in single men and in men with positive syphilis serology. Austin (1982) compared the incidence of anal cancer in the city of San Francisco, which has proportionately the largest male homosexual community in the world, with the incidence in adjacent urban communities and demonstrated a higher incidence of anal cancer in single men than in all other marital, sexual and geographical groups. Peters and Mack (1983) examined the incidence of anal cancer in both sexes in Los Angeles County and demonstrated that single men had a 6 times greater incidence of anal cancer than married men. Married women and women who had never married showed no difference in anal cancer incidence, but separated and divorced persons of both sexes had a higher incidence than married persons. In another study, Peters et al. (1984) found parallels between the descriptive epidemiology of squamous cell carcinoma of the cervix, vulva, penis and anus. No similar epidemiological studies have been performed in Europe. More recently, Daling et al. (1987) have reported the results of a case control study in which receptive anal intercourse carries a relative risk of 33:1 in males, though in females the ratio was reported as only 3:1. A history of sexually transmitted diseases, especially genital warts in homosexual men, and current smoking were other substantial risk factors.

This circumstantial evidence for a sexual association in this disease may gain firmer corroboration in the finding of human papilloma virus (HPV) in anal cancers. The occasional progression from condylomata acuminata to invasive malignancy is well known. Recently there have been isolated reports of a few cancers in which DNA hybridisation techniques have allowed demonstration of HPV DNA within the genome (Hill and Coghill 1986; Beckman et al. 1984; Wells et al. 1987).

A recent study using Southern blot analysis found HPV16 DNA in 60% of anal squamous cell cancers (Palmer et al. 1987). In situ hybridisation has since shown that HPV DNA is located in the malignant cells of the tumour rather than the stroma, adding further weight to the aetiological role for HPV in this disease (Scholefield et al., 1988).

Table 2. WHO classification of anal tumours

	Anal canal	Anal margin
I. Epithelial tumours	A. Benign B. Malignant 1. Squamous cell carcinoma 2. Basaloid carcinoma 3. Mucoepidermoid carcinoma 4. Adenocarcinoma 5. Undifferentiated carcinoma 6. Unclassified carcinoma	A. Benign 1. Squamous cell papilloma 2. Others B. Malignant 1. Squamous cell carcinoma 2. Basal cell carcinoma 3. Others C. Bowen's disease D. Paget's disease
II. Non-epithelial tumours		
III. Malignant melanoma		
IV. Unclassified tumours		
V. Secondary tumours		
VI. Tumour-like lesions		A. condylomata acuminata B. Giant condyloma C. Pseudoepitheliomatous hyperplasia D. Fibrous polyp E. Others

Histopathology

With so many different types of tumour a classification is essential. That suggested by the World Health Organisation (Morson 1976) is set out in Table 2.

Squamous Cell Carcinoma

Squamous cell carcinomas arising from the anal margin behave in very much the same way as squamous cell carcinomas arising from the skin at other sites in the body. They tend to be well differentiated with good keratin production. On the other hand, anal canal tumours are less well differentiated and therefore carry a poorer prognosis. Anal canal squamous cell carcinoma is 3 times more common than carcinoma of the anal margin, and whilst the age incidence is the same, anal canal carcinoma occurs more commonly in women (3:2) and anal margin carcinoma more frequently in men (4:1) (Morson and Dawson 1979).

Basaloid (or cloacogenic) carcinoma is a common variant of squamous cell carcinoma and is so called because of the resemblance on histological examination to basal cell carcinoma. However, its behaviour is quite unlike that tumour, with the potential to metastasize.

Bowen's disease (squamous cell carcinoma in situ) only rarely affects the perianal skin. Strauss and Fazio (1979) reported 12 cases from the Cleveland Clinic seen over a period of 25 years. Only a small proportion (5%–20%) will develop invasive carcinoma. Nevertheless, it is usually advisable to excise the area. Alternatively, the condition can be treated chemotherapeutically with 5-fluourouracil ointment (Efudix). This treatment, though, produces considerable soreness and requires very careful supervision.

The rare mucoepidermoid carcinoma of the anal canal is characterised by areas of neoplastic columnar epithelium with some mucus production in the better differentiated tumours.

Adenocarcinoma

Adenocarcinoma may appear in the upper anal canal, as previously stated as the result of downward spread of a rectal adenocarcinoma. The pathology and management of this tumour is therefore that of a lower-third rectal tumour. Two rarer forms of adenocarcinoma are that arising in the anal glands or their ducts and that complicating long-standing anal sepsis.

Secondary adenocarcinoma may occur in the anal canal with a separate primary tumour in the more proximal rectum. This spread may occur as the result of exfoliation and intraluminal spread into a wound at the anal margin, for example a fissure in ano or a post-haemorrhoidectomy wound (implantation metastases). Alternatively, there may be venous spread into the haemorrhoidal venous plexus, giving rise to metastases which are covered by squamous epithelium (non-implantation metastases). Secondary tumours in the anal canal or at the anal margin are very unusual.

Malignant Melanoma

Malignant melanoma is a tumour which arises in the transitional zone of the anal canal, and approximately one malignant melanoma is seen for every 250 rectal adenocarcinomas (Morson and Dawson 1979). Macroscopically, this rare tumour may not always exhibit obvious pigmentation and may also spread in the submucosal plane upwards into the rectum. This may cause confusion in the diagnosis. Treatment is unrewarding in that most patients die from metastases in a very short time after any operative procedure, which is usually excision of the rectum. Occasionally, though, a patient may survive and this justifies the attempt at treatment. Wanebo et al. (1981 b) report an 8% 5-year survival rate in a series of 51 patients. It was thought that the patients who survived had tumours with little depth of invasion. Ward et al. (1986) report no long-term survivors in a series of 21 patients treated at St Mark's Hospital. Furthermore, there was no difference between those treated by excision of the rectum and those treated by local excision.

Basal Cell Carcinoma

Basal cell carcinoma (rodent ulcer) occasionally occurs in the perianal skin. Why this should be so is obscure, as this area is not usually exposed to sunlight! However, whilst some such tumours have followed the use of radiotherapy for the treatment of benign disease, e.g. intractable pruritus, most are of unknown aetiology. Local excision is usually all that is required for successful management, and should local recurrence occur, this operation may be repeated.

Extramammary Paget's Disease

Paget's disease is a rare disorder which affects apocrine sweat glands. Probably as many as 80% of such tumours in the perianal region are associated with malignancy at some stage in the natural history of the disease.

Experience in the management of this condition is inevitably limited, but most surgeons consider wide local excision to be the first stage of management. If the distal anal canal is involved or malignancy is present, then excision of the rectum may be required. Inguinal lymph node involvement may occur and is best managed by block dissection. Conventional radiotherapy seems to be of little value in this condition, and despite radical local treatment the mortality from this form of Paget's disease is high (Lock et al. 1977).

Staging

Malignant tumours of the anal region spread in the usual ways – direct spread, lymphatic spread and vascular spread. The fundamental difference between anal tumours and rectal tumours is that the lymphatic spread of the former may be not only to the perirectal, para-aortic lymph nodes and the iliac lymph nodes, but also to the inguinal lymph nodes of either side. This precludes the use of the Dukes' classification of staging these lesions. The TNM classification may be applied but as Papillon (1982) has indicated, it is difficult to distinguish tumours limited to the internal sphincter (T1) from those that involve the external sphincter (T2). Furthermore, extension of the tumour into the rectum or perianal skin (T3) does not necessarily mean a worse prognosis. Modifications of this system based on tumour size, the extent of local lymph node involvement and metastatic spread have been described, but no classification has been widely used (Greenall et al. 1985 a).

Screening

Hitherto patients have not been screened for anal cancer. With the interest in the possible viral aetiology for this tumour and the knowledge that homosexuals and those with a history of anal condylomata acuminata are among the high-risk groups, however, screening programmes may well be developed (cf. screening for cervical carcinoma).

Diagnosis

Anorectal bleeding, anal pain, a change in bowel habit and pruritus ani are the usual symptoms associated with a squamous cell carcinoma of the anal region. It is important to remember, though, that this disorder may present with inguinal lymph node enlargement or with distant metastases. Greenall et al. (1985 a) have drawn our attention to the importance of benign conditions such as condylomata acuminata, chronic fistulae and leukoplakia, and of previous irradiation, as features common in patients with anal margin tumours but rare in patients with anal canal tumours.

On examination, the essential physical sign of malignancy is the presence of induration, and this will distinguish a malignant ulcer from other forms of ulceration such as occurs with a fissure in ano,

Crohn's disease and primary chancre. It may be difficult to examine the lesion adequately because of discomfort, and in this instance examination under anaesthesia can be very valuable: a more accurate idea of the degree of spread may be obtained, and the involvement of perirectal and iliac lymph nodes may be determined more accurately. Biopsy is an essential investigation and may be done at the same time. Biopsying anal tumours without anaesthesia may cause the patient a lot of unnecessary discomfort on account of the somatic innervation of the distal part of the anal canal.

Clinical examination is still the principal method of assessment, but the various imaging techniques – ultrasound, computerised tomography, magnetic resonance – may find a place in the evaluation of these patients.

Treatment

Development of Surgical Approach

Although uncommon, anal carcinoma has provoked an abundant literature regarding its treatment over the past half century. Gabriel advocated implantation of radium for low-grade tumours in his presidential address to the Proctology Section of the Royal Society of Medicine in 1940, but felt that radical perineal excision was required if cure was to be attempted in other cases. By 1960, however, he felt that local excision produced better results than local irradiation for early margin lesions, and that abdominoperineal excision was superior to the perineal approach in those cases requiring radical surgery. Excision of the inguinal nodes was not performed prophylactically. Others agreed with this policy. In the past 20 years radical surgery has been the mainstay of treatment in most parts of the world. The prognosis improved in the postwar period; while only 28% of patients survived for 5 years in the interwar years, by the 1960s this figure had risen to 46%, partly, it was suggested, due to the more radical surgical approach. Anal margin lesions carried a more favourable prognosis, despite the predominant use of conservative surgery in two-thirds of cases: 60% of patients at St Mark's survived for 5 years following local excision.

Several authors in the past 20 years have, due to paucity of cases, described series extending back for half a century in which results have been variable. Surgical treatment of anal margin lesions has led to 40%–88% 5-year survival, while patients with anal canal lesions fared worse, only 20%–65% surviving for this period (Wolfe and Bussey 1968; Cortese 1975; Singh et al. 1981; Madden et al. 1981; Pyper and Parks 1985).

Radiotherapy

Although most reports have stressed the central role of surgery in the curative treatment of anal cancer, several groups have advocated radiotherapy as the primary modality. Their central argument is that the evolution of modern radiotherapeutic methods has allowed many patients to undergo successful radical treatment without the inevitable sacrifice of anal function. Methods available include external beam, interstitial therapy, and combinations of either or both of these with subsequent surgery (Franklin 1980; Cummings 1982; Papillon et al. 1983; James et al. 1985; Harnett et al. 1985). One important problem with radiotherapy in this region in the past was the fine line between underdosage (treatment failure) and overdosage (radionecrosis), but modern techniques have made major morbidity a relatively minor problem. Papillon (1982) has perhaps been the strongest and most consistent advocate of a radiation-based approach to this disease. He has used radiation alone, split into two periods, for the management of the 80% of cases in which there is no deep infiltration of surrounding tissues. In more advanced lesions he has used initial radiation followed 2 months later by radical excision. Of those patients cured, 75% have retained anal function.

Despite the apparent advantages of radiation compared to ablative surgery, it was not until the development of the multimodality approach in the 1970s that surgeons began tentatively to release their hold on anal cancer as a 'surgical' disease.

Multimodality Approach

Over the past decade there has been an increasing body of evidence that the combination of chemotherapy and irradiation offers patients the prospect of a cure rate at least equal to that produced by surgery but with retention of anal function. The first report from Nigro's group appeared in 1974, when they recorded encouraging results achieved using preoperative chemoradiotherapy in three patients suffering from anal canal cancer. Arguing that such lesions are surgically unfavourable due to profuse blood supply, diffuse lymphatic drainage (both facilitating early spread) and anatomical difficulties, they suggested the use of combined preoperative chemotherapy and irradiation. They gave 30 Gy in 15 2-Gy doses over a 3-week period. 5-Fluorouracil, 25 mg/kg body weight daily, was given by infusion for 5 days at the beginning of the radiation course. In addition a bolus of mitomycin C, 0.5 mg/kg body weight, was given on the 1st day. Six weeks later the patients were offered abdominoperineal excision of the rectum, using a "wide perineal phase" and excising the rectovaginal septum. Groin dissection was not employed. In all cases the lesion had disappeared clinically following chemoirradiation; one patient refused surgery, while in the other two there was no histological sign of cancer in the operative specimen.

Three years later the same group reported on ten patients, including the original three (Buroker et al. 1977). The dose of chemotherapeutic agents was now related to body surface area, but otherwise there was no change in management. In six the tumour had clinically resolved and showed no tumour in the operative specimens; in all of these the lesion had been less than 4 cm in diameter prior to treatment. All patients remained well and disease-free up to 53 months postoperatively. With these spectacular early results, Nigro et al. (1974) questioned the need for abdominoperineal excision as a routine following chemoirradiation. They indicated that they were now performing "excisional biopsy" if the lesion had disappeared and not proceeding further if the histology was negative.

By 1983 the Wayne State series comprised 28 patients (Nigro et al. 1983). The initial course of 5-flourouracil was now being repeated on days 29 to 32. Twelve patients had undergone rectal excision, and 14 who were clinically clear after chemoirradiation had had biopsy which showed no evidence of residual tumour. Two others who were clinically free of disease after chemoirradiation were not biopsied and did not undergo further surgery. Twenty-two patients remained disease-free up to 8 years postoperatively. Five had died of cancer, four of these having had primary tumours larger than 7 cm and no tumour in the operative specimen. The authors emphasised the need for careful biopsy, taking deep tissue, under general anaesthesia in those in whom the tumour could no longer be seen macroscopically after initial therapy. They were now convinced of the efficacy of this regimen in those without evidence of dissemination, and suggested its routine adoption. They argued that the chemotherapy element was necessary, as it potentiated the irradiation and dealt with extrapelvic disease. They felt that those patients with primary tumours larger than 6 cm, who appeared to be the group at greatest risk of recurrent disease, might benefit from a further course of chemotherapy after anorectal excision if this had been necessary.

By the next year, 1984, Nigro was able to report on 104 cases, 44 treated at his institution and a further 60 treated elsewhere by the same regimen. Patients with known distant metastases were excluded, and only four had palpable inguinal deposits. Ninety-seven patients had no clinically apparent residual tumour after chemoradiation. Thirty-one patients had undergone anorectal excision, regardless of macroscopic appearance; 22 were found to have no cancer in the specimen. Sixty-two underwent excision biopsy of the area, only one showing microscopic evidence of tumour residue. Eleven patients had apparent resolution of disease after chemoradiation and were not biopsied. Local recurrence occurred in seven patients up to 1 year after negative local excision; anorectal excision was performed in these cases. Systemic toxicity due to chemoradiation was reported as mild or moderate in 99 patients. Eighty-two patients were alive and apparently disease free up to 11 years following treatment. Nigro concluded that this regimen was as effective as abdominoperineal excision in terms of cure. Whether chemotherapy improved on the results achieved with radiation alone was unclear, and could only be clarified by means of a randomised trial.

The Memorial Hospital group entered the field in 1976, from a different direction. Newman and Quan (1976) reported three patients with surgically incurable epidermoid anal cancer who were subjected to combination therapy. The first died following perforation of a duodenal ulcer during therapy, but the second patient was clinically "cured" by chemoradiation alone, despite late presentation, and in the third the anorectal excision specimen following chemoradiation was tumour-free. The regimen used in these cases differed from the Wayne State protocol in minor details. The second patient received repeated doses of mitomycin C and required further irradiation after 10 months for a scrotal recurrence which then resolved. Two years later the group reported on ten patients with tumours at various stages on initial treatment; this showed several further cases of apparent complete resolution (Quan et al. 1978). It thus seemed that this therapeutic approach might be effective, at least achieving good palliation, in patients previously beyond salvage. By 1983 the same group had collected 37 patients; 19 (53%) had no tumour in the operative specimen, while overall 35 (94%) had shown a "major clinical response" to pretreatment (Michaelson et al. 1983). With a median follow-up of 28 months, recurrence had been observed in 3/18

(17%) who had undergone anorectal excision and 4/17 (24%) in whom local excision had been carried out. Clearly it was too early to comment on cure rate, but the combined approach had been shown by a second group to have considerable promise (Greenall et al. 1985 a, b).

Cummings and colleagues in Toronto were the first group to offer 5-year survival figures for the combined approach and to attempt comparison of this regimen with radical radiotherapy (Cummings et al. 1984). They compared a series of 51 patients treated by radical radiotherapy (RT) between 1958 and 1978 with 30 patients who received combined therapy (FUMIR) between 1978 and 1982. The RT group was cut to 25 by excluding those patients who had not received radiotherapy that was comparable with that used in the later FUMIR group. The combined therapy regimen was very similar to that used by Nigro and the Memorial Hospital group, the main difference being that the radiation dose was 50 Gy rather than 30 Gy. Moreover, the radiation was delivered in two steps; in the first, 25 Gy/10 fractions/ 2 weeks was delivered to a large volume, including the pelvic and inguinal nodes, while in the second period, following straight on, radiation was delivered to the anal region only. The toxicity of this regimen was sufficient to lead to a change in approach after the first 16 patients. There was now a 4-week break between the two 25-Gy courses and the chemotherapy regimen was repeated at the beginning of the second course. No biopsies were performed routinely, the only indication being apparent residual tumour. Primary control was recorded at 6 months post treatment in 60% of RT patients and 94% of FUMIR patients. Surgical excision of residual disease was possible in six of the ten patients not initially controlled in the RT group and in one of the two in the FUMIR group. Acute haematological and intestinal toxicity occurred in many patients in the FUMIR group, although this decreased when the split regimen was adopted. Surgery for radiation complications was necessary in 3/25 (12%) of the RT group and 5/30 (17%) of the FUMIR group. Colostomy was never required for failure of primary tumour control in the FUMIR patients, though four needed this for radiation complications; in contrast, 7/25 (28%) RT patients needed colostomy for failed primary control and one for radiation damage. There was no difference in survival figures between the RT and FUMIR groups at the time of reporting. This study, although open to the criticism that the comparison was sequential rather than randomised, strongly suggested that combined (FUMIR) therapy had advantages in terms of quality of life (through anal conservation) without any sacrifice of survival prospects. The relatively high toxicity, both acute and late, compared infavourably with the lower radiation dose regimens reported by others. Other groups have reported noncontrolled series supporting the chemoradiation approach (Flam et al. 1983; Sischy et al. 1982; Wanebo et al. 1981 a; Boman et al. 1984).

Amid the steadily growing body of reports on the superiority of chemoradiation over surgery, there has been one eloquent argument to the contrary. The Mayo Clinic group, led by Moertel, updated their experience in a report on 118 patients treated predominantly by abdominoperineal excision; 71% survived for 5 years (Boman et al. 1984). The authors argued that local excision is the appropriate treatment for the smallest lesions, with radical radiotherapy and surgical salvage for large lesions. As 50% of the rest are cured by surgery, preoperative chemoradiation would be unnecessary. Thus a policy of uniform chemoradiation, they suggested, does not help the majority. The Mayo group felt that preoperative chemoradiation should be confined to lesions of 3 cm or more in diameter (size correlates well with degree of spread). They suggested that a trial to examine the efficacy of systemic adjuvant therapy would show no difference, and that a trial of surgery alone against surgery and postoperative radiotherapy would be the most appropriate study.

Summary

Carcinoma of the anus is a rare disease in Western countries, but epidemiological evidence suggests that it may be increasing in certain groups. The trend away from radical surgery in the primary treatment of this condition has reached a stage at which controlled evidence to support this approach is probably not necessary. The relative role of radiation alone and chemoradiation, and the different regimens within these approaches, leaves much room for future research, though the small numbers of cases at individual centres will make large comparative trials difficult to mount.

References

Austin DF (1982) Etiologic clues from descriptive epidemiology: squamous cancer of the anus. NCI Monogr 62: 69–90

Beckman AM, Daling JR, McDougall JK (1984) Human papillomavirus DNA in anogenital carcinomas. J Cell Biochem [Suppl] 9C: 68

Boman BM, Moertel CM, O'Connell MJ, Scott M, Weiland LH, Beart RW, Gunderson LL, Spencer RJ (1984) Carcinoma of the anal canal. A clinical and pathologic study of 188 cases. Cancer 54: 114–125

Buroker TR, Nigro N, Bradley G, Pelok L, Chomchai C, Considine B, Vaitkevicius VK (1977) Combined therapy for cancer of the anal canal: a follow-up report. Dis Colon Rectum 20: 677–678

Cortese AF (1975) Surgical approach for treatment of epidermoid anal carcinoma. Cancer 36: 1869–1875

Cummings BJ (1982) The place of radiation therapy in the treatment of carcinoma of the anal canal. Cancer Treat Rev 9: 125–147

Cummings B, Keane T, Thomas G, Harwood A, Rider W (1984) Results and toxicity of the treatment of anal canal carcinoma by radiation therapy or radiation therapy and chemotherapy. Cancer 54: 2062–2068

Daling JR, Weiss NS, Klopfenstein LL, Cochran LE, Chow WH, Daifuku R (1982) Correlates of homosexual behaviour and the incidence of anal cancer. JAMA 247: 1988–1990

Daling JR, Weiss NS, Hislop TG et al (1987) Sexual practices, sexually transmitted diseases, and the incidence of anal cancer. N Engl J Med 317: 973–977

Flam MS, John M, Lovalvo LJ, Mills RJ, Ramalho LD, Prather C, Mowry PA, Morgan DR, Lau BP (1983) Definitive nonsurgical therapy of epithelial malignancies of the anal canal. Cancer 51: 1378–1387

Franklin A (1980) Anal cancer treated by fast neutron radiation. Br J Surg 67: 469–472

Gabriel WB (1940) Squamous cell carcinoma of the anus and anal canal: an analysis of 55 cases. Proc R Soc Med 34: 139–160

Gabriel WB (1960) Discussion on squamous cell carcinoma of the anus and anal canal. Proc R Soc Med 53: 403–420

Greenall MJ, Quan SHQ, DeCosse JJ (1985a) Epidermoid cancer of the anus. Br J Surg [Suppl] 72: 97–103

Greenall MJ, Quan SHQ, Urmacher C, DeCosse JJ (1985b) Treatment of epidermoid carcinoma of the anal canal. Surg Gynecol Obstet 161: 509–517

Harnett AN, Doughty D, Plowman PN (1985) A simple brachytherapy technique for early anal carcinoma. Br J Radiol 58: 258–261

Hill SA, Coghill SB (1986) Human papillomavirus in squamous carcinoma of the anus (Letter). Lancet 2: 1333

James RD, Pointon RS, Martin S (1985) Local radiotherapy in the management of squamous carcinoma of the anus. Br J Surg 72: 282–285

Lock MR, Katz DR, Parks AG, Thomson JPS (1977) Perianal Paget's disease. Postgrad Med J 53: 768–772

Madden MV, Elliot MS, Botha JBC, Louw JH (1981) The management of anal carcinoma. Br J Surg 68: 287–289

Michaelson RA, Magill GB, Quan SHQ, Leaming RH, Nikrui M, Stearns MW (1983) Preoperative chemotherapy and radiation therapy in the management of anal epidermoid carcinoma. Cancer 51: 390–395

Morson BC (1976) Histological typing of intestinal tumours. World Health Organisation, Geneva

Morson BC, Dawson IMP (1979) Gastro-intestinal pathology. Blackwell, Oxford, pp 735–756

Newman HK, Quan SHQ (1976) Multi-modality therapy for epidermoid carcinoma of the anus. Cancer 37: 12–19

Nigro ND (1984) An evaluation of combined therapy for squamous cell cancer of the anal canal. Dis Colon Rectum 27: 763–766

Nigro ND, Vaitkevicius VK, Considine B (1974) Combined therapy for cancer of the anal canal: a preliminary report. Dis Colon Rectum 17: 354–356

Nigro ND, Seydel HG, Considine B, Vaitkevicius VK, Leichman L, Kinzie JJ (1983) Combined preoperative radiation and chemotherapy for squamous cell carcinoma of the anal canal. Cancer 51: 1826–1829

Palmer JG, Shepherd NA, Jass JR, Crawford LV, Northover JMA (1987) Human papilloma virus type 16 in anal squamous cell carcinoma. Lancet 2: 42

Papillon J (1982) Rectal and anal cancers. Springer, Berlin Heidelberg New York

Papillon J, Mayer M, Montbarbon JF, Gerard JP, Chassard JL, Bailly C (1983) A new approach to the management of epidermoid carcinoma of the anal canal. Cancer 51: 1830–1837

Peters RK, Mack TM (1983) Patterns of anal carcinoma by gender and marital status in Los Angeles County. Br J Cancer 48: 629–636

Peters RK, Mack TM, Bernstein L (1984) Parallels in the epidemiology of selected anogenital carcinomas. INCI 72: 609–615

Pyper PC, Parks TG (1985) The results of surgery for epidermoid carcinoma of the anus. Br J Surg 72: 712–714

Quan SHQ, Magill GB, Leaming RH, Hajdu SI (1978) Multidisciplinary preoperative approach to the management of epidermoid carcinoma of the anus and anorectum. Dis Colon Rectum 21: 89–91

Scholefield JH, Coates TJ, Palmer JG, Shepherd NA, Northover JMA (1988) The use of in-situ hybridization to demonstrate the intra-nuclear and morphological distribution of HPV 16 DNA in anal cancer. Brit J Surg vol: 75 p 1248

Singh R, Nime F, Mittelman A (1981) Malignant epithelial tumors of the anal canal. Cancer 48: 411–415

Sischy B, Remington JH, Hinson EJ, Sobel SH, Woll JE (1982) Definitive treatment of anal-canal carcinoma by means of radiation therapy and chemotherapy. Dis Colon Rectum 25: 685–688

Strauss RJ, Fazio VW (1979) Bowen's disease of the anal and perianal area: a report and analysis of twelve cases. Am J Surg 137: 231–234

Wanebo HJ, Futrell W, Constable W (1981a) Multimodality approach to surgical management of locally advanced epidermoid carcinoma of the anorectum. Cancer 47: 2817–2826

Wanebo HJ, Woodruff JM, Farr GH, Quan SH (1981b) Anorectal melanoma. Cancer 47: 1891–1900

Ward MN, Romano G, Nicholls RJ (1986) Anorectal malignant melanoma. Br J Surg 73: 68–69

Wells M, Griffiths S, Lewis F, Dixon MF, Bird CC (1987) Identification of human papillomavirus in paraffin sections of anal condylomas and squamous carcinomas by in situ DNA hybridisation. J Pathol (in press)

Wolfe HRI, Bussey HJR (1968) Squamous cell carcinoma of the anus. Br J Surg 55: 295–301

Cancer of the Kidneys

W. Vahlensieck and N. Jaeger

Definitions

Kidney tumours may originate in the renal parenchyma or in the urothelium of the cavity system (carcinoma of the renal pelvis). The two types of tumour present essential differences with regard to incidence, the preoperative diagnostic procedures needed, treatment and prognosis (Vahlensieck and van der Weyer 1960).

The commonest parenchymatous tumour of the kidney is the renal cell carcinoma (Grawitz tumour). Such tumours are often termed 'renal adenocarcinomas' in the Anglo-American literature, but in Germany we have differentiated for a considerable time between the rarer adenocarcinoma and the more common hypernephroma or hypernephroid renal carcinoma. Clinically, however, there is no difference: diagnosis, treatment and prognosis are the same. As a result, and especially in accordance with the report by Mostofi (1967), the term 'renal cell carcinoma' is used to include both varieties (Hermanek et al. 1976).

Much rarer are malignant mesenchymal growths such as fibrosarcomas, liposarcomas, myosarcomas, angioendotheliomas, haemangiopericytomas and osteogenic sarcomas. The embryonic adenosarcoma (Brich-Hirschfeld-Wilms tumour) is in a category of its own with regard to treatment and prognosis and is the commonest tumour in childhood (Schmiedt et al. 1982; Vahlensieck and Gödde 1965).

Renal Cell Carcinomas

Epidemiology and Risk Factors

According to figures published by the Federal Statistical Office (1982), in the year 1981 there were 3798 deaths as a result of malignant changes of the renal parenchyma in the German Federal Republic; this amounts to 2.4% of all cancer deaths. Kidney cell carcinomas amount to 80%–85% of parenchymatous tumours and so form the largest proportion of such growths (Flamm and Wöber 1981; Schmiedt et al. 1981). In 2% of cases the tumours are bilateral, though it remains uncertain whether the lesion on one side represents a metastasis from the other (Schmiedt et al. 1982).

The average age at first diagnosis is between 53 and 61 years (Table 1) (Egger et al. 1979; Robson 1963). Men are affected twice as often as women (Table 1).

Renal cell carcinomas are diagnosed most commonly in North America and North Europe, less frequently in Africa, Asia and South America. Grouping within a family is observed only rarely (Steinberg et al. 1972; Brühl and Vahlensieck 1976), but is the predominant presentation of Hippel-Lindau disease (polycystic kidneys, cerebral and retinal angiomas), in which more than 60% of patients develop renal cell carcinomas, often bilaterally, at an average age which is about 15 years lower than for the sporadically occurring variety.

Exposure to radioactivity may be among the aetiological factors. Twenty-one per cent of proved Thorotrast-induced tumours were found to be renal cell carcinomas (Wenz 1967; Swarm 1967). In animal experiments it was possible to produce renal carcinomas with chemical carcinogens such as diethylstilboestrol. The fact that it is possible to influence the progression of a renal cell carcinoma by changes in the hormone metabolism (progesterone etc.) and in the immune system makes it probable that these factors, too, play a part in causation (Bloom 1973b). Both epidemiological studies and animal experiments have demonstrated a significant connection between nicotine abuse and the development of renal cell carcinomas, nitrosamine being considered the most important carcinogen. Weir and Dunn (1970) found that the risk for smokers was 2.46 times that of non-smokers. It also seems that obesity, especially in women, and excessive intake of animal fats favour the development of renal cell carcinomas (Sufrin 1982).

Table 1. Average age, age range and sex ratio of patients with renal cell carcinoma

Reference	*n*	Average age (years)	Age distribution (years)	Sex ratio (M:F)
Boxer et al. (1979)	106	55.7	–	2.2:1
Cox et al. (1970)	143	–	–	2.0:1
Egger et al. (1979)	283	60.9	–	–
Engelmann et al. (1983)	132	59.9	–	1.2:1
Jonitz and Hallwachs (1982)	136	–	–	1.1:1
McNichols et al. (1981)	506	55.3	27–79	1.8:1
Middelton and Presto (1973)	61	53.4	20–76	–
Patel and Lavengood (1978)	166	–	24–85	1.6:1
Robson et al. (1969)	88	53.0	19–81	–
Swanson and Borges (1983)	193	57.9	30–81	2.39:1
Thompson et al. (1975)	150	–	15–84	–
Waters and Richie (1979)	130	56.5	30–80	–

Histopathology

Parenchymatous renal tumours are subdivided into adenocarcinomas and hypernephroid carcinomas in the German literature (Brühl and Vahlensieck 1976; Zollinger 1966). Hermanek et al. (1976), on the other hand, do not believe that any useful purpose is served by making such a distinction, as only about 5% of the tumours are of non-hypernephroma type. In agreement with the relevant Anglo-American literature (Mostofi 1967; Javadpour 1984) they combined adenocarcinoma and hypernephroid carcinoma under the collective term of 'renal cell carcinoma'.

The so-called renal cortical adenoma (< 3 cm) is nowadays thought to be indistinguishable from renal cell carcinoma. Even such small tumours may grow, infiltrate and metastasize, and so must always be considered as small adenocarcinomas in an early stage (Kline and Valensi 1976). Renal cell carcinomas originate in the proximal tubules; they may be divided into clear cell and granular cell types. The cells may be arranged in solid, cystic, trabecular, tubular or papillary groups. The occasional (1.8%) cases in which sarcomatous changes are encountered have a particularly bad prognosis (Bennington 1973). If the tumour consists entirely of clear cells (cells rich in cytoplasm and optically empty with small nuclei without any striking atypical appearance), arranged in small nests or strands, then one is dealing with a grade I renal carcinoma according to the classification by Hermanek et al. (1976). A kidney carcinoma may, however, show glandular-papillary structures, acidophil cells and sarcoma-like components. Such features indicate that the tumour is not in grade I of the Hermanek classification. Tumours consisting exclusively of glandular or glandular-papillary architecture or entirely of granular cells in a microscope field at magnification × 64, or showing areas of sarcomatous change, are classed as grade III tumours. Those tumours which cannot be allocated to either grade I or III are considered to belong to group II (Hermanek et al. 1976; see 'Classification' below).

This classification is clearly of great prognostic significance. Schmiedt et al. (1981) were able to demonstrate a correlation between histological grade and 3-year survival rate. Other pathological features also have a prognostic significance: Brühl and Vahlensieck (1976) point out that cases with histologically proved tumour cells within the small veins have an appreciably reduced chance of cure. In view of the close anatomical relationship between the thin-walled capillaries and the tubular epithelial or tumour structures, destruction of the separating layer (endothelial cells) is easily brought about (Mostofi 1967), particularly in the presence of a rise of blood pressure or a lack of oxygen. As a consequence, tumour cells may spread into the pulmonary circulation and tumour emboli may arise.

It is not surprising, therefore, that metastases are disseminated most commonly through the renal veins. Histological examination (Middleton 1967; Mims et al. 1966) has shown that malignant infiltration or thrombus formation in the intrarenal veins occurs in 30% of cases. This results in an early spread of the tumour cells by the following routes (Bennington and Beckwith 1975):

1. Inferior vena cava→right side of heart→pulmonary circulation
2. Secondarily from the pulmonary circulation through the pulmonary artery into the systemic circulation and the corresponding parenchymatous organs
3. In a retrograde direction via the left testicular or ovarian vein into the pelvis
4. Into the spine through Batson's plexus and the paravertebral veins

In addition, lymphatic spread may occur to the regional and juxtaregional lymph nodes via the perinephric lymph vessel plexus (Brühl and Vahlensieck 1976). At the time of diagnosis, distant metastasis may have occurred to the following organs (Stähler et al. 1981): lungs (9.5%), bones (5.5%), liver (2.9%), brain (1.2%), adrenals (1.2%), contralateral kidney (0.3%).

Natural History

The pathology of renal cell carcinoma is multiple. Electron microscopy has shown a similarity between the cells of the proximal tubule and those of the carcinoma, as a result of which the proximal convoluted tubule is considered to be the site of origin. It is, however, uncertain whether this malignant growth passes through a stage in which it appears to be a cortical adenoma (Sun et al. 1977; Cooper and Waysman 1971; Pinals and Krane 1962).

Symptomatology

In cases where the tumour is diagnosed accidently, half of all patients with renal cell carcinoma have no subjective complaints (Chisholm 1974; Glenn 1964). As all relevant signs depend on local extension of the tumour or on dissemination of the growth, symptoms differ in the early and late stages of the disease.

Early Stages

There are no genuine early symptoms (Rattenhuber et al. 1981). Many tumours are discovered by chance during routine investigations – usually as a result of an ultrasound study of the upper abdomen (Jaeger and Vahlensieck 1985). As a result of a review of 204 patients with renal cell carcinomas, Vahlensieck and Gödde (1968) stress that early signs such as fever, gastrointestinal complaints, a rise of diastolic blood pressure and microscopic haematuria must always be carefully investigated so as to detect a kidney tumour as early as possible and thus be able to proceed to surgery at a favourable time.

Between 13% and 43% of all patients with a renal cell carcinoma are hypertensive (König et al. 1975; Andreew et al. 1971), a pathological rise in diastolic pressure being of special significance (Vahlensieck and Gödde 1968; Gütgemann and Vahlensieck 1964). A causative connection between the hypertension and the kidney tumour may be expected in about 10%–15% of patients (Rattenhuber et al. 1981). In such cases, the blood pressure frequently reverts to normal after removal of the tumour by nephrectomy (Mast et al. 1978). The following are pathogenetic causes of the hypertension (Sutter and Simma 1978):

- Arteriovenous shunts in the tumour
- Compression of the renal artery by the tumour
- Increased formation of vasopressor substances
- Polycythaemia

It is debatable whether an increase in plasma renin, produced autonomously by the tumour, is responsible for the rise in blood pressure (Sufrin et al. 1977; Mast et al. 1978).

Late Stages

Varying and specific symptoms such as a fall in general performance, lack of appetite, tiredness and loss of weight may all be signs that the disease has reached an advanced stage (Chisholm and Roy 1971; Cox et al. 1970; Flamm and Wöber 1981; Ruedi et al. 1975). Such complaints tend in general to appear rather earlier than the 'classical triad' of symptoms – haematuria, palpable tumour, pain in the lumbar region – indicating that the tumour has reached a very late stage (Vahlensieck and Gödde 1965) (Table 2).

Macroscopic haematuria as a result of infiltration of the tumour into the renal cavity system is the commonest first symptom, and occurs in 35%–70% of patients (Glenn 1964; McLaughlin 1979; Cox et al. 1970; Flamm and Wöber 1981). The haematuria is usually painless and is intermittent in over 60% of cases (Holland 1973). Palpable masses in the flank are encountered only if the tumour is growing at the lower pole of the kidney and has reached a considerable size (Rattenhuber et al. 1981; Schmiedt et al. 1981); the frequency of this is given in the literature as 15%–39% (Table 3). Pain in the flank as an initial symptom may be dull, stabbing or colicky. Its causes may be stretching of the capsule, local extension of the tumour, strain on the vascular pedicle or urinary obstruction (Altwein 1979; Schmiedt et al. 1981).

A varicocele appearing for the first time after the age of 30 years and not disappearing if the patient lies down must make one consider a renal tumour as its cause. A tumour of appropriate size and site or a metastasis in a lymph node may compress or infiltrate the spermatic vein and produce congestion of

Table 2. Frequency of the "classical triad" of symptoms in patients with renal cell carcinoma

Reference	*n*	Frequency (%)
Altwein (1979)	–	11.0
Boxer et al. (1979)	106	6.7
Hajdu and Thomas (1967)	100	15.0
König et al. (1975)	219	13.7
Patel and Lavengood (1978)	166	5.0
Ruedi et al. (1975)	156	20.0
Schmiedt et al. (1981)	–	13.0
Skinner et al. (1972b)	309	9.0
Waters and Richie (1979)	130	4.0

Table 3. Frequency of haematuria, lumbar pain and palpable abnormality in patients with renal cell carcinoma

Reference	Haematuria		Lumbar pain		Palpable abnormality		Total no. of cases
	%	*n*	%	*n*	%	*n*	
Altwein (1979)	40.0	–	48.0	–	39.0	–	–
Boxer et al. (1979)	35.0	37	32.0	34	35.0	37	106
Cox et al. (1970)	47.0	67	55.0	79	15.0	21	143
Hallwachs et al. (1969)	73.8	31	71.5	30	33.0	14	42
Jonitz and Hallwachs (1982)	48.5	66	39.7	54	24.3	33	136
Oliver et al. (1979)	53.0	94	24.0	43	19.0	34	178
Patel and Lavengood (1978)	35.0	58	34.0	56	30.0	50	166
Petkovic (1970)	76.0	114	75.0	112	–	–	150
Rüedi et al. (1975)	63.0	98	49.0	76	46.0	72	156
Schmiedt et al. (1981)	65.0	–	34.0	–	19.0	–	–
Waters and Richie (1979)	52.0	68	38.0	49	21.0	27	130

the intrascrotal venous plexus. According to Schmiedt et al. (1981), this is found in nearly 6% of cases. Wagle and Murphy (1971), on the other hand, observed a symptomatic varicocele in only 1.7% of their cases. It is not uncommon for patients to first consult their doctor when signs of distant metastases occur, local signs of the primary tumour being entirely absent; 5.4%–9.3% of renal cancers are found only when a primary growth is searched for once metastases have been identified (Cherrie et al. 1982; Pauer et al. 1981).

Laboratory Findings

In laboratory results, too, one may distinguish between early and late changes.

Early Signs

Microscopic haematuria is the earliest and most important laboratory abnormality. The finding of erythrocytes in the urinary sediment on even a single occasion demands establishment of the cause (Bauer and Rattenhuber 1981). A review of the literature by Vahlensieck and Gödde (1968) revealed that this abnormality is found in 80%–100% of cases; they themselves encountered it in 87% of 204 patients. They believe it to be caused by venous stasis due to compression of the parenchyma as a result of expansion of the tumour.

Late Signs

Anaemia is a common sign in advanced cases of renal cell carcinoma (Hallwachs et al. 1969; Schmitz 1967; Skinner et al. 1972b; Waters and Richie 1979), caused by the haematuria or by a deficiency of erythropoietin as a result of the destruction of functioning renal parenchyma. On the other hand, polycythaemia is encountered in 1.5% of cases (Chisholm and Roy 1971) due to the excessive production of erythropoietin by the tumour. The polycythaemia frequently disappears after excision of the tumour and kidney if no metastases are present.

In addition to an increase in the production of renin and erythropoietin, other endocrine paraneoplastic conditions are also encountered. These include the formation of prostaglandin A and E and the ectopic production of parathormone (hypercalcaemia), gonadotrophins, prolactin and ACTH (Chisholm 1980). A frequently mentioned (though rare) complex of laboratory findings is the Stauffer syndrome, which is not specific for renal cell carcinoma but is important in the diagnosis of the presence of a tumour. Holland (1973) and Ruedi et al. (1975) obtained relevant results in only 15% of their patients. This paraneoplastic syndrome consists of a reversible liver dysfunction of unknown aetiology (Stauffer 1961). It presents with hepato- or splenomegaly and the following changes in laboratory parameters:

- Rise in alkaline phosphatase
- Prolongation of prothrombin time
- Increase in Bromsulphalein retention
- Changes in electrophoresis (reduction in albumin fraction, rise in alpha-2-globulin)

Growth and Behaviour of Tumour

If the growth has not been excised the disease often takes an unexpected course. There may be fulminating progression and early death, the tumour or a metastasis may remain static for many years, there may be spontaneous regression of metastases after excision of the tumour and kidney, distant metastases may first appear after several years and there may be an improvement in survival rate after the excision of solitary distant metastases (Bartley and Hultquist 1950; Everson and Cole 1966; Garfield and Kennedy 1972; Rafla 1970). The rare spontaneous remissions of metastases must be caused by endocrine and immunological factors. In 1982 Katz and Schapira reported 89 well-documented cases of spontaneous remission of metastases of renal cell carcinoma, mostly in the lungs, the favourable outcome based in all probability on endocrinological and immunological factors. Sternsward et al. (1970) discovered tumour-specific antigens which stimulated the formation of lymphocytes and so produced a cellular immune response. This, however, does not justify inactive management once such a tumour has been diagnosed. Riches (1964) found that the 5-year survival rate was less than 5% in patients whose tumour was not treated surgically.

Classification

Grading

As suggested by the UICC, the pathohistological findings with regard to this tumour are divided into three grades. Classification of the cell changes into various categories is an important factor for the assessment of the prognosis (Altwein 1979; Rauschmeier et al. 1984). Various methods have been used for such grading, depending on nuclear morphology, arrangement of the cells in the tumour or cell types themselves. Skinner et al. (1972b) placed the main emphasis on the morphology of the cell nuclei and largely disregarded the way the cells were arranged. The scheme proposed by Hermanek et al. (1976) is based both on the cell type and on the histological form of organisation:

Grade I: the tumour is entirely solid and all the cells are of the 'clear' type.

Grade II: criteria for neither grade I nor grade II applicable.

Grade III: the structure of the tumour is entirely glandular or papillary-glandular; only granular cells are present in at least one microscopic field of vision with magnification × 64; a tumour with areas of sarcoma-like changes.

Staging

Staging of renal tumour is at the present time carried out according to two different systems (Holland 1973; Robson et al. 1969; Harmer 1978). While in the USA the established method is that proposed by Robson, in Europe the TNM system suggested by the UICC is preferred. In this system the extension of the primary tumour is designated by the symbols T0–T4 and involvement of the regional or juxtaregional glands with N0–N3 (Table 4). Distant metastases are designated M1, and involvement of veins, typical of renal cell carcinomas, is designated V1 or V2 (Table 4).

The preoperative TNM classification may be compared with the postoperative histological findings, where individual categories are preceded with a lower-case 'p'. That the preoperative assessment often over- or underestimates the true situation as established pathologically and histologically after operation may be seen from Table 5, which also shows the percentage of agreement with the diagnostic methods used, such as angiography and computerised tomography (CT).

The value of pre- and postoperative staging, as suggested by the UICC, lies in the help it gives in the precise planning of treatment, the exact evaluation of the results of comparable treatment and the indications it supplies as to prognosis (Stähler et al. 1981). It also has the advantage that it can be transcribed into the Robson classification, whereas the reverse is not the case.

The classification advocated by Robson consists of a modification of the proposal by Flocks and Kadesky (1958), who divided tumours of the renal parenchyma into four groups. Robson et al. (1969) also divided such tumours into four categories, regardless of metastases:

Table 4 a. Pretreatment clinical TNM classification as proposed by the UICC

Primary tumour

T0 No evidence of the existence of a primary tumour

T1 Small tumour without enlargement of the kidney with minimal distortion or deformity of calyces and limited vascular changes, surrounded by renal parenchyma

T2 Larger tumour with deformity and/or enlargement of the kidney or involvement of the calyces or the renal pelvis. Continuity of cortex maintained according to angiographic appearance

T3 Spread into the perirenal fat or into the fatty tissue surrounding the renal pelvis or into the vessels of the renal hilum

T4 Involvement of neighbouring organs or abdominal wall

Regional lymph nodes

N0 No evidence of regional lymph node involvement

N1 A single node on the same side involved

N2 A node on opposite side affected, or bilateral nodes, or several regional lymph nodes involved

N3 Fixed regional lymph nodes (this can only be established at operation)

Distant metastases

M0 No distant metastases

M1 Proved distant metastases

Table 4 b. Postoperative pathological and histological classification as proposed by the UICC

Primary tumour

The pT categories correspond to the T categories

Regional lymph nodes

The pN categories correspond to the N categories

Invasion of veins

V0 Veins do not contain any tumour

V1 Renal vein contains tumour

V2 Tumour within vena cava

Table 5. Accuracy (%) of angiography and CT during staging of renal cell carcinoma (agreement between preoperative tumour staging T and pathological and histological findings pT)

Reference	Angiography (%)	CT (%)	Cases (*n*)
Bracken and Jonsson (1979)	36	–	–
Cronan et al. (1982)	61	91	23
Egger et al. (1979)	63–83	–	268
Engelmann et al. (1983)	–	64	86
Futter et al. (1979)	45	–	54
Levine et al. (1979)	–	88	17
Schoenenberger and Probst (1982)	–	84	38
Weymann et al. (1980)	68	83	40/54

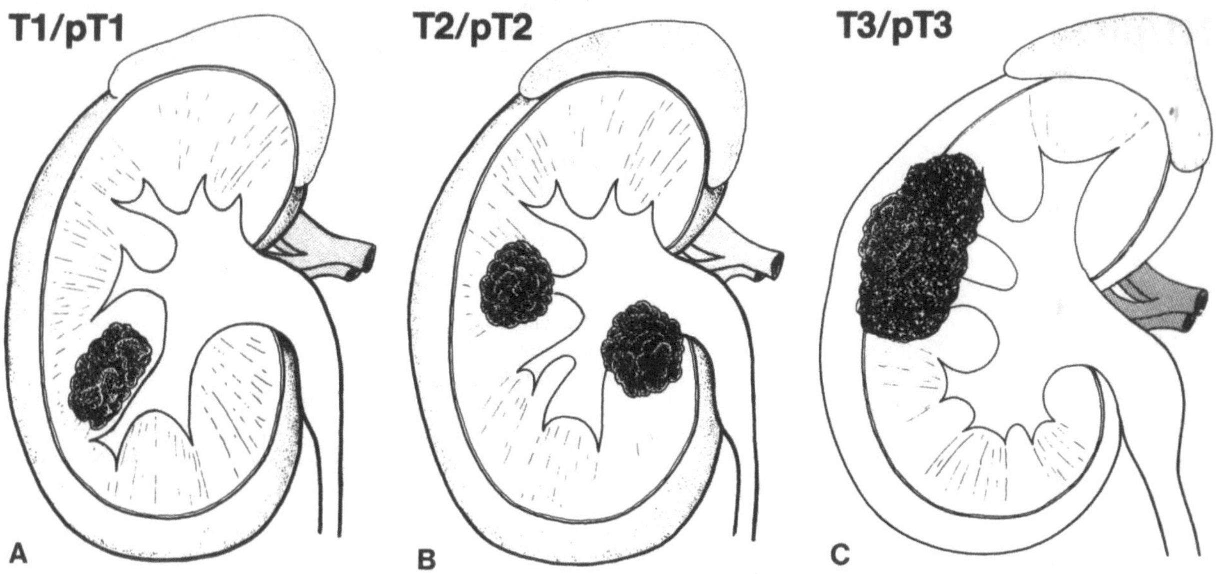

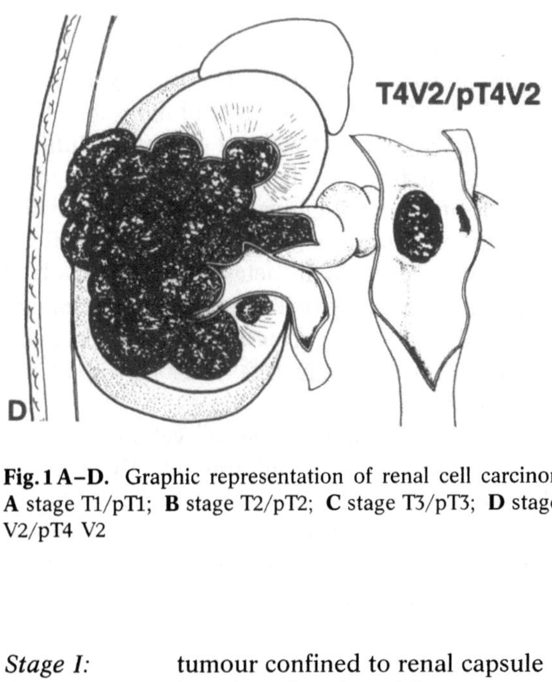

Fig. 1 A–D. Graphic representation of renal cell carcinoma: **A** stage T1/pT1; **B** stage T2/pT2; **C** stage T3/pT3; **D** stage T4 V2/pT4 V2

Stage I:	tumour confined to renal capsule
Stage II:	invasion of perirenal fat
Stage III A:	entry into renal vein or inferior vena cava
Stage III B:	involvement of regional lymph nodes
Stage III C:	veins and lymph nodes involved
Stage IV A:	invasion of neighbouring organs
Stage IV B:	distant metastases

This staging refers entirely to the postoperative pathological and histological findings, whereas the TNM system of the UICC distinguishes between the preoperative and the postoperative state (see above). The deciding criteria for the preoperative assessment are the clinical examination, routine urography, ultrasound, angiography, lymphography and, if possible, CT (Harmer 1978) (Figs. 1, 2).

Prognostic Factors

The essential factors affecting the progression of a renal cell carcinoma are, in addition to the patient's sex, the time interval between the first symptom and the establishment of the diagnosis (Brühl et al. 1976), the extent of the tumour at the time of treatment (staging), the histologically verified degree of malignancy (grading) (Hermanek et al. 1976) and the surgical procedure or other treatment employed (Robson 1963).

Age and Sex

Böhminghaus et al. (1982) found that the age of the patient has no bearing on the prognosis, but they were able to show that the outlook does depend on the patient's sex; 57% of the female patients but only 47% of the males survived for 5 years after operation.

Staging and Grading

Disregarding all other factors, the extent of the tumour at the time of treatment is an important prognostic indicator. This applies not only to its absolute size but also to its spread within the kidney and its extension into the venous vascular system. With regard to the absolute size of the tumour, Petkovic (1970) believes that only a diameter in excess of

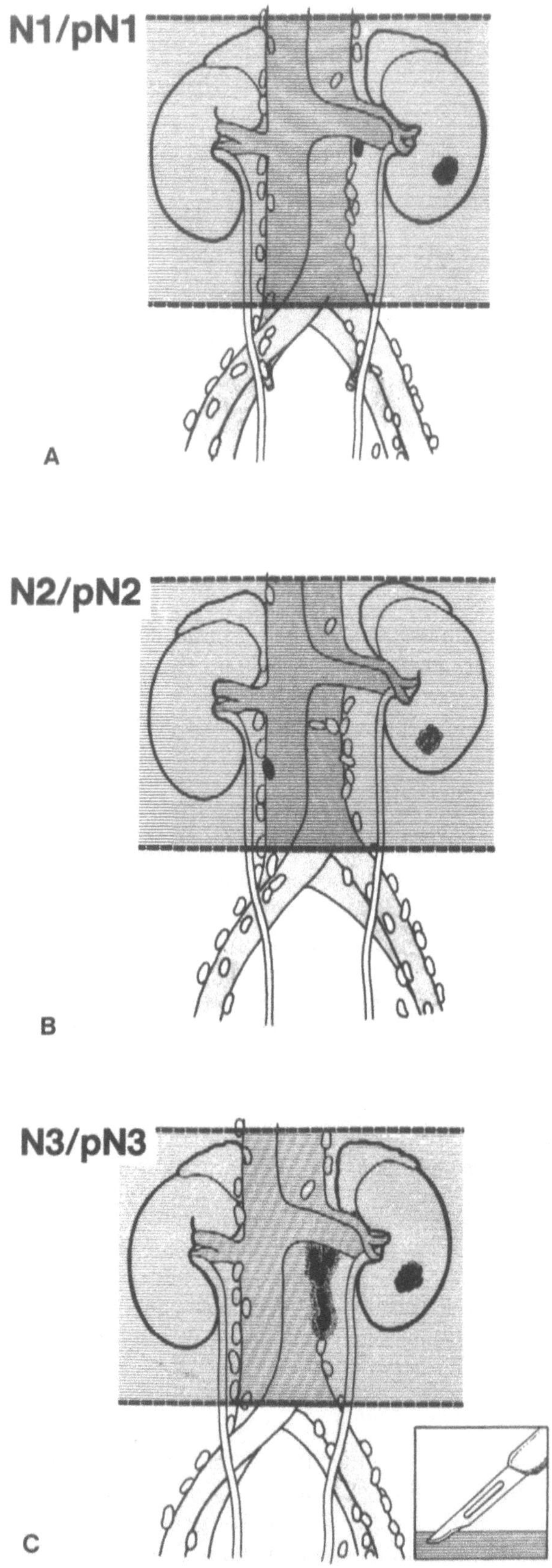

Fig. 2 A–C. Graphic representation of renal cell carcinoma with lymph node metastases: **A** stage N1/pN1; **B** stage N2/pN2; **C** stage N3/pN3

Table 6. Five-year survival rates in patients with renal cell carcinoma according to UICC tumour stage

Reference	pT1		pT2		pT3		pT4	
	(*n*)	(%)	(*n*)	(%)	(*n*)	(%)	(*n*)	(%)
König et al. (1975)	62	62	–	–	78	30	–	–
Rost and Brosig (1977)	15	67	4	75	15	27	–	–
Egger et al. (1979)	–	63	–	40	–	29	–	15
Altwein (1979)	–	66	–	66	–	25	–	10
Van der Werf-Messing et al. (1981)	61	64	38	60	67	33	7	0
Flamm (1982)	–	–	26	65	25	49	–	–
Own patients (1972–1982)	7	100	57	60	66	35	14	0

10 cm worsens the prognosis significantly. The TNM system takes less heed of the size of the tumour but pays more attention to its spread and effect in the surrounding tissues. In stage T1, as may be seen from Table 6, a 5-year survival rate of more than 50% is to be expected almost without exception. Infiltration into the perinephric fat, however, or spread to the vessels of the renal hilum (stage T3), reduces the chances of cure appreciably. The prognosis is affected even more adversely if metastases have involved the regional or juxtaregional lymph nodes. Schmiedt and Rattenhuber (1981) recorded a 5-year post-surgery survival rate of only 10% once spread to the lymph nodes had occurred.

The prognostic significance of venous involvement has been variously interpreted. There is no doubt that the technique of removing tumour thrombi, especially from the vena cava, has made a considerable impact (Molitor and Weißbach 1981). Skinner et al. (1972 b) and Petkovic (1975) were unable to establish any appreciable reduction in the chance of cure, but McNichols et al. (1981) and Oliver et al. (1979) noted that a tumour thrombus in the renal vein or vena cava worsened the prognosis by 10%. Schmiedt and Rattenhuber (1981) observed that only a quarter of patients in stage V1/2 survived for more than 5 years. Leyendecker (1985) evaluated 184 patients and found the following:

1. The proportion of patients with a tumour thrombus in the renal vein or inferior vena cava amounted to 13%.
2. Renal carcinoma with tumour thrombi in the renal vein could be of any grade of malignancy.
3. Renal carcinomas with tumour thrombi in the renal vein did not metastasise more frequently than

a comparable group of lesions without such thrombi. If, however, such thrombi were found in the vena cava, there was a 15% higher chance of metastasis.

In morphological investigations Leyendecker was also able to show that the free surface of tumour thrombi was covered by endothelium and a layer of subendothelial connective tissue of varying thickness; she assumed, therefore, that the endothelium prevented the dissemination of tumour cells from the thrombus into the circulation.

The chances of curative treatment in the presence of distant metastases are very poor. Egger et al. (1979) found a 53% 5-year survival rate in patients without metastases, but in the presence of haematogenous spread the expectation of living this long was reduced by 40%. None of the patients in whom metastases had reached multiple organs survived for more than 5 years.

Surgical Procedures

Regarding various surgical procedures, Sigel et al. (1981) were able to demonstrate that an abdomino-transperitoneal approach gave a 58% 5-year cure rate, while a lumbar approach produced a rate of only 48%. Routine lymph node dissection in the area of the local lymphatic drainage is recommended (Vahlensieck 1976). Only in this way is it possible to obtain exact evidence of the presence of regional metastases, which had occurred in 16.7% of our patients ($n = 170$). This technique also enables the surgeon to ligate the renal vessels before the tumour is even touched, so avoiding any extensive mobilisation and dissemination of tumour cells into the pulmonary and systemic circulation with a consequent appreciable impairment of the prognosis.

Screening for Asymptomatic Disease

Half the patients with a renal tumour do not have any subjective complaints (Chisholm 1974; Glenn 1964). There are no true early symptoms. Disability and gross clinical signs only make their appearance late in the course of the illness. The symptoms of a renal cell carcinoma are an expression of advanced tumour growth and have changed little in the past 30 years despite improvements in investigations and diagnosis (Rattenhuber et al. 1981). Many months frequently elapse between the appearance of early and often unspecific symptoms and the establishment of the diagnosis. According to Flamm and Wöber (1981) most patients present a history covering between 3 and 6 months, this delay being caused, in the opinion of Paul (1967), by the following factors:

- An early phase with few symptoms
- Haematuria considered trivial by patient and doctor, or overlooked
- Incomplete investigation if symptoms are unspecific or unusual
- Misjudgement in the presence of other urological conditions (prostatic adenoma, renal stones, urinary infections etc.).

The length of the history is an unimportant prognostic factor (Brühl et al. 1976). Patients with a 1-month history and a 5-year survival rate of 62% may be compared to others whose history goes back over 6 months and who have a 5-year survival rate of only 30% (Böhminghaus et al. 1982). In many cases (4%–30%) renal tumours are encountered by chance during routine investigations (Patel and Larengood 1978); it is to be expected that this rate will rise as a result of the more frequent use of upper abdominal ultrasound examination, particularly within the framework of preventive care.

In order to attain the best chances of cure it is essential to recognise and attack a renal tumour at an early stage. How large the number of 'chance' diagnoses can be, i.e. how often symptomless renal tumours may be detected by modern, noninvasive techniques, is illustrated in a study by Rattenhuber et al. (1981): 25% of their cases of renal carcinoma, which were completely asymptomatic and had not extended beyond the kidney, were picked up incidentally during transabdominal ultrasound investigations. Sigel et al. (1981) therefore advocate that abdominal sonography has to be included in the annual preventive checks for men and women. We, too, would plead that preventive examinations of all patients over the age of 40 should include upper abdominal sonography and examination of the urine with special reference to the presence of red blood cells. Only in this way will it be possible to treat these tumours during their initial stages and so to improve appreciably the chances of cure by means of radical surgery.

Diagnosis of Symptomatic Cases

In the event of relevant signs or abnormal laboratory results indicating a malignant process affecting the kidneys, specific investigation is essential. A number of investigative techniques are available to identify the primary tumour and metastases, if present. In the past, intravenous urography took pride of place, but nowadays upper abdominal sonography is increasingly used as the first line of attack in the search for such tumours (Gebauer and Ribka 1981).

Sonography

Conventional imaging procedures cannot easily distinguish between cystic and solid space-occupying lesions of the kidney. An ultrasound scan, on the other hand, may give precise information about the nature of the appropriate material examined (Gebauer and Ribka 1981; Thurn and Bücheler 1982). Jonitz and Hallwachs (1982) and Kolle (1981 b) found that in 90% of cases it is possible to distinguish between a cyst and a solid structure by means of sonography. Difficulties are encountered only if the tumour originates in the upper pole of the kidney (Gebauer and Ribka 1981), the demonstration of which may be made difficult by the bony thorax, the posterior pleural reflection or intestinal gas formation. Examination of the kidneys should be followed by liver sonography, as this procedure is more accurate than liver scintigraphy, which will only detect metastases of a diameter greater than 2 cm (Schmiedt et al. 1981). Opinions differ about the value of sonography. Whereas Kolle (1981 b) always uses angiography for the definition of tumours found by sonography and CT, and Petri et al. (1978) consider ultrasound as a merely ancillary investigation, Cronan et al. (1982) believe it to be a low-risk alternative to angiography, the latter procedure being reserved for selected cases. Jonitz and Hallwachs (1982) employ angiography only for technical reasons relevant to their surgical requirements if the presence of a tumour has been established by sonography and CT.

Intravenous Urography

Very subtle interpretation of the urogram may have great influence on subsequent procedures in the treatment of a renal tumour. Even the slightest pathological change in the collecting system or the smallest alterations in shape, contour, or position of the kidney demand explanation, even if noted on the opposite side. A prerequisite to radical surgery of a renal tumour is the demonstration of an unremarkable pyelogram on the contralateral side with a correct time relationship in the excretion of the contrast material.

Space-occupying lesions may, however, commence at the periphery and so produce slight and easily overlooked change, or no change at all, in the calyceal pattern. Sigel (1965) described such malignancies as "masked renal tumours" though with the aid of tomography such lesions, too, can be recognized. The diagnosis or suspicion of tumour formation can be settled in 96%–97% of cases by means of urography (Cox et al. 1970; Hallwachs et al. 1969; König et al. 1975).

Computerised Tomography

Since the introduction of CT in the 1970s a completely new chapter has been opened with regard to the diagnosis of renal tumours. This technique of investigation is not only able to distinguish simple renal changes from solid space-occupying lesions (Jonitz and Hallwachs 1982) but also provides exact information about local and regional extensions of the tumour and its limits (Cronan et al. 1982; Levine et al. 1979; Marshal et al. 1979; Schoenenberger and Probst 1982; Weyman et al. 1980) (Table 5). Kidney tumours with a diameter of as little as 1 cm are picked up with certainty by CT (Gebauer and Ribka 1981). Levine et al. (1979) noted that malignant tumours which could not be demonstrated urographically or by ultrasound could be seen on CT. Differences in density in the retroperitoneal space enable CT to provide evidence of, among other things, perinephric extensions of the tumour (Jonitz and Hallwachs 1982; Levine et al. 1979; Schoenenberger and Probst 1982). Even the presence and extent of regional lymph node metastases can be established (Kessler et al. 1981; Levine et al. 1979; Weyman et al. 1980). The available literature gives no clear indication whether CT is able to define tumour emboli in the renal veins or inferior vena cava: Levine et al. (1979) and Schoenenberger and Probst (1982) show on the basis of 17 and 38 cases respectively that involvement of the veins cannot always be exactly documented by means of CT; in 50% and 26% of cases respectively the intraoperative and pathological findings were not in agreement with the CT assessment. Engelmann et al. (1983), on the other hand, found a specificity of 97% for this technique in 86 evaluated CT scans for stages V1 and V2.

Angiography

Angiography of the renal artery is a precise and informative method for the demonstration or exclusion of a renal tumour (Table 5). In addition to size and location of the tumour, evidence may be obtained about the vascular morphology of the tumour and the organ which contains it (Lang 1973). This is particularly necessary when the evidence obtained from sonography, intravenous urography and CT is inadequate for precise preoperative definition of the tumour or if it is proposed to proceed to embolisation of the renal artery after diagnosis. The general angiography preceding a selective procedure may provide information concerning the existence of accessory renal arteries. In addition, lumbar and intercostal arteries may communicate with the tumour (Schmiedt and Rattenhuber 1981) if the tumour has penetrated the capsule. To avoid any intraoperative dissemination of the tumour it is necessary to ligate these vessels in addition to the main renal artery as a preliminary procedure (Jonitz and Hallwachs 1982). Two methods are available to demonstrate the vessels: conventional catheter angiography and digital subtraction angiography (DSA).

For conventional angiography, puncture of the femoral artery is required with direct demonstration of the arterial tree after the injection of the contrast medium (Kolle 1981b), carried out over three consecutive phases (Hallwachs et al. 1969): At the start of the procedure, during the arterial phase, the destruction of the normal vascular architecture may be demonstrated in addition to the tumour's own vessels and any arteriovenous anastomoses (Lang 1973). There follows a parenchymatous phase during which the size of the kidney or any extension may be seen. A blurred outline of the space-occupying lesion within the parenchyma provides evidence of a malignant process (Altwein 1979). Finally, in the venous phase, there may be a more rapid demonstration of the renal vein due to arteriovenous shunts (Hallwachs 1969). Occasionally tumour thrombi may be observed growing from the tumour into the renal veins or even into the inferior vena cava (Lang 1973; Schefft et al. 1978).

DSA is a new, less invasive method for the visualisation of arteries (Fischer and Schultz 1983) which is increasingly replacing conventional arteriography (Lackner et al. 1984a). The technique is based on computer subtraction of a blank picture – the so-called mask – from a filled one of the area under investigation (Arlat 1985). The contrast material is injected intravenously (Lackner et al. 1983). The advantage of intravenous DSA is that it reduces the risks of the investigation and the stress on the patient to a minimum (Arlat 1985; Bargon 1985). Arterial puncture may be unavoidable in the search for tumour-specific vessels (Arlat 1985), but even so the complication rate is less with this procedure than with conventional angiography, as there is a reduction in the amount of contrast medium required and the quantity of iodine administered (Grabbe et al. 1984; Lackner et al. 1984b).

Cavography

If involvement of the veins is suspected, the issue may often be settled by means of cavography, particularly in right-sided tumours (Kolle 1981a; Staehler et al. 1981) (Fig. 3). In the presence of appropriate findings this method of investigation often has a decisive bearing on the planning of the operation (Siminovitch et al. 1982a).

Diagnosis of Metastases

The following investigations are suggested to ascertain the presence or absence of dissemination (lymph node or distant metastases), with its adverse effect on prognosis:

- Pedal lymphography
- Chest X-ray
- Scintigraphy of skeleton
- CT of head

Opinions differ about the indications for preoperative lymphography: whereas Kessler et al. (1981) insist on the routine X-ray demonstration of the retroperitoneal lymph nodes once the presence of a renal tumour has been confirmed, Rübben and Lutzeyer (1981) avoid this procedure, as complete demonstration of the regional lymph node filter sites is impossible. According to Rübben and Lutzeyer (1981) the accuracy of this method of investigation lies between 40% and 60%. Kolle (1981b) is also doubtful about this procedure, as there is a high rate of false-positive and false-negative results. Furthermore, omission of pedal lymphography may be justified by the fact that lymphadenectomy is carried out in any case as part of a radical excision of the tumour and kidney (Kolle 1981b; Schmiedt et al. 1981; Schoenenberger and Probst 1982). X-raying the thorax in two planes helps to provide information concerning pulmonary metastases of a renal cell carcinoma, the incidence of which has been stated as 30%–56% (Brühl and Vahlensieck 1976). In the presence of suspicious small round foci, the plain chest X-ray should be followed by tomography (Bischoff and Sommerkamp 1977; Schmiedt et al. 1981). The most conclusive procedure for the exclusion of small metastatic round foci is a CT scan of the lungs (Schmiedt et al. 1981; Staehler et al. 1981).

Scintigraphy of the skeleton is used for the diagnosis of bony metastases (Bischoff and Sommerkamp 1977; Veyhl et al. 1981). CT of the head is employed if there is any clinical suspicion of cerebral metastases. This method is more sensitive than any

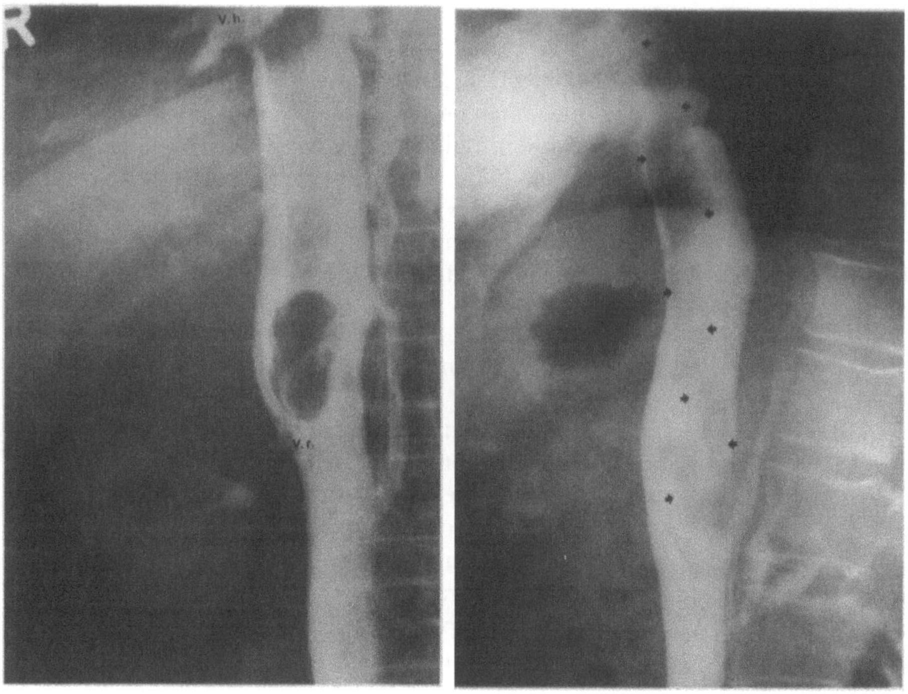

Fig. 3. Transfemoral cavography demonstrating a tumour thrombus *(arrows)* in the vena cava of a right-sided renal cell carcinoma. *V. h.*, vena hepatica; *V. r.*, vena renalis

other diagnostic procedure to date, including cerebral angiography and brain scintigraphy (Lanksch and Ringel 1981).

Surgical and Combined Treatment of Local and Regional Disease

The only treatment that promises any hope of success in the case of primary unilateral kidney tumour which has not disseminated consists of the radical removal of the growth (Angervall and Wahlquist 1978; Flamm et al. 1981; Fuselier et al. 1983; Marshall 1982; Oliver et al. 1979; Robson et al. 1969; Schmiedt et al. 1981; Skinner et al. 1972b; Vahlensieck 1973; Waters and Richie 1979). The limits of operability are set by any infiltration into neighbouring organs (stage T4) or impairment or absence of the contralateral kidney (Flamm and Wöber 1981; Pauer et al. 1981; Tolia and Whitmore 1975). If the general condition of the patient is good, then neither advanced age nor a large tumour is a contraindication to surgery (Bischoff and Sommerkamp 1977).

As early as 1976 Vahlensieck called for transperitoneal removal of the tumour and the kidney combined with retroperitoneal clearance of lymph nodes so as to put the prognosis on a firmer footing and to aim at cure despite the presence of lymph node metastases. Then as now, the following conditions must be fulfilled if surgery of the renal tumour is to have any hope of success (Graham and Glenn 1979; Nagel et al. 1969; Sigel and Held 1963; Vahlensieck 1976):

- Sufficiently radical surgery
- Good preservation of the vessels
- Avoidance of rough handling of the tumour-bearing organ before ligation of the renal artery and vein
- Prevention of dissemination of tumour cells during the operation

Basically, the surgeon may choose one of three main approaches: the intercostal-lumbar, the abdomino-transperitoneal and the thoracoabdominal.

The lumbar incision was rejected by Schmiedt (1973), who claimed that this approach was only justified after preoperative embolisation of the renal artery or if the patient's ability to withstand anaesthesia was limited. En bloc resection, i.e. extrafascial removal of the kidney containing the tumour with the pericapsular fatty tissue and the adrenal, is impossible with an incision in the flank (Sigel and Held 1963). Because of the narrow approach the para-aortic or paracaval lymph nodes are not reliably accessible. Before the renal pedicle is divided the kidney must be mobilised and displaced (Klosterhalfen 1968). This may lead to massive haemorrhage from the capsular veins and the haematogenous dissemination of tumour cells into the venous drainage area [the renal vein and renal capsular veins, which anastomose with the vertebral venous plexus, the adrenal-lumbar veins, the phrenic vein and the azygos vein (Schmiedt 1973)]. This anatomical situation makes it necessary to avoid all manipulation of the tumour until the kidney has been fully devascularised, to prevent any tumour dispersal. Klosterhalfen (1975) therefore believed that the lumbar approach is only suitable for palliative procedures. The advantages of the abdominotransperitoneal or thoracoabdominal route may be summarised as follows (Brosig and Buchberger 1962; Klosterhalfen 1975):

a) Manipulation and displacement of the kidney containing the tumour is largely unnecessary before ligation of the vessels, as they are directly exposed.
b) Primary ligation of the artery and vein is possible, avoiding tumour dissemination. The field for lymph gland dissection (which should precede searching for the renal artery and vein) is clear. A tumour thrombus in the vena cava can easily be isolated (Fig. 3).

In view of its high complication rate, the indications for preoperative embolisation are limited to the treatment of bulky cancers which are likely to present difficulties during surgery (De Kernion 1980; Flamm et al. 1981). Bischoff (1978) does not use this method at all because of its very serious side effects. Sigel et al. (1981) and Teasdale et al. (1982) do not believe that this procedure offers any advantage over others in the surgical treatment of an operable renal tumour provided a suitable approach is used. Kaisary et al. (1984) were unable to find any effect on the immune system in their 55 patients, while Kurth et al. (1984) observed extended (36 months) complete remission in 25 patients, thought to be due to an effect on the body's own defence mechanism. The decision whether the approach to a renal tumour should be transperitoneal or thoracoabdominal will depend in the first instance on the findings before treatment. Not only the size but also the site of the growth must be taken into consideration. Mayor (1975) and Oliver et al. (1979) advocate the abdominoperitoneal technique if the tumour arises mainly in the lower pole and the thoracoabdominal route for growths of the upper pole. In the view of Klosterhalfen (1975), opening of the thorax provides greater safety and better room for manoeuvre for the isolation of a tumour embolus of the inferior vena cava than does a purely abdominal approach. The disadvantage of such a two-cavity route is the large number of complications that may arise, such as haemothorax, serous effusions, pneumothorax or empyema of the pleurae. As a result this route should not be routine in the surgery of renal tumours but should be reserved for those that cannot be dealt with abdominally (Hienzsch 1972). Various incisions are used in the abdominotransperitoneal method. While in earlier years the *Rippenbogenrand* (costal margin) incision was advocated (Sigel and Held 1963) median upper and lower laparotomy has been preferred more recently (Swanson and Borges 1983). A further possibility is the extended transverse incision (Schmiedt et al. 1981). All the incisions aim to reach and deal with renal vessels. According to Hienzsch (1972) no incision should be employed routinely; rather the approach should be varied as the situation demands in the light of the pretreatment investigations (CT, angiography).

Lymph node excision may precede or follow the nephrectomy. No standardised criteria are available to define its extent (Herrlinger et al. 1983; Siminovitch 1982b). The so-called facultative dissection is limited to the removal of suspect nodes. It may contain nodes removed by chance for staging purposes (Herrlinger et al. 1983; McNichols et al. 1981). 'Regionally limited lymphadenectomy' encompasses a circumscribed area along the hilum of the affected side (De Kernion 1980; Middleton and Presto 1973; Siminovitch 1982). 'Extended systematic dissection' covers the whole area of lymphatic drainage, starting at the aortic bifurcation and reaching upwards to the diaphragm, and includes the para-aortic, paracaval and interaortocaval glands (Angervall and Wahlquist 1978; Herrlinger et al. 1983; Robson et al. 1969; Veyhl et al. 1981). Various retrospective investigations have shown that the demonstration of histologically verifiable lymph node involvement is dependent on the surgical technique employed: Chlepas et al. (1977) found, in 195 patients with renal tumours, that using the lumbar approach ($n = 33$) it was only possible to discover lymph node invasion in 6%; those operated on transperitoneally ($n = 132$) had an incidence of 17% of such involvement if the lymphadenectomy was carried out facultatively. Extended systematic dissection ($n = 30$) brought lymphatic metastases to light in 37% of cases. To operate in cases of hypernephroid carcinoma without systematic dissection means, in the opinion of Chlepas et al. (1977), that unrecognized lymph node metastases will be left behind in the field of operation, and these authors consider systematic lymphadenectomy to be the method of choice.

Herrlinger et al. (1983) make the following points:

- Radical surgery is the only curative procedure at present.
- In 44% of cases in which lymph node metastases are proved, these are micrometastases invisible to the surgeon.

- During facultative dissection over 30% of affected nodes are missed.

They were able to improve the 5-year survival rate for all patients operated on with the intention of cure from 50% ± 9% with facultative dissection to 63% ± 12% if systematic dissection was used. A renal cell carcinoma in a functionally or anatomically single kidney is best treated by the surgical removal of the tumour while sparing and retaining the remaining healthy renal parenchyma (Graham and Glenn 1979; Malek et al. 1976; Palmer and Swanson 1978; Jaeger et al. 1985). Account must be taken of the size of the tumour, the topography of its vascular supply and the exclusion of multiple distant metastases (Orestano et al. 1975). Although partial nephrectomy and tumour enucleation do not meet the requirements of radical tumour excision, these procedures may nevertheless be successful. Wickham (1975) collected 48 cases of a tumour in a solitary kidney, 28 of which were subjected to partial nephrectomy; after an average of 2.5 years 70% of these were still alive. Only isolated cases are amenable to extracorporeal dissection ('bench surgery') or to cooling by intra-arterial perfusion. As we have seen vascular complications after balloon occlusion, we prefer simple surface hypothermia with ice (Jaeger et al. 1985).

Adjuvant Treatment

No form of adjuvant treatment has established itself as standard therapy be it as an additional measure after the surgical removal of an advanced primary tumour (stage T4) or as prophylaxis against possible recurrence after removal of the kidney containing the tumour.

Radiotherapy

The value of pre- and postoperative irradiation with regard to prognosis is disputed (Angervall and Wahlquist 1978; Brühl et al. 1976; Cox et al. 1970; Waters and Richie 1979). Van der Werf-Messing et al. (1981) investigated the effect of preoperative irradiation in a prospective study ($n = 126$), but were unable to find a statistically significant difference in 5-year survival rate between the patients irradiated preoperatively and those who were only treated surgically. In another prospective study, Juusela et al. (1977) even found a poorer prognosis for preoperatively irradiated patients: 47% 5-year survival in patients whose operation was preceded by radiotherapy compared with 63% in those who only had surgery. As a result, considerable doubt has been cast on radiotherapy as a preoperative measure.

Irradiation at a later stage has been tested in numerous studies. Some authors obtained better results with postoperative radiotherapy than with tumour excision and nephrectomy alone, whereas others believe that the prognosis is worsened (Bloom 1973a). Vahlensieck (1973) considered postoperative radiotherapy to be without value, as it apparently blocks the defence system and so hastens the progression of micrometastases already present at the time of operation or causes a flare-up of circulating tumour cells.

Chemotherapy

The adjuvant use of cytostatics after tumour removal and nephrectomy may be regarded with considerable scepticism, if not rejected completely, in light of the many unsuccessful trials and the occurrence of a variety of complications. Vahlensieck (1973) observed 157 patients whose tumour and kidney had been removed and came to the conclusion that the 5-year and 10-year survival rates were more favourable in patients who had had only surgery than in those who had had cytostatic treatment after their operation. It must be assumed that this procedure, like radiotherapy, weakens the body's own defence system; this, of course, also applies to adjuvant combination chemotherapy and irradiation, which, according to investigations in our clinic, produces even less favourable results (Vahlensieck 1973). We therefore do not use intra- or postoperative cytostatics as long as we consider the radical operation to have been successful and thus expect a high 5-year survival rate. Other adjuvant treatments – hormones (progesterone or anti-oestrogene), interferon or other prophylactic immunotherapeutic measures – are not justified either (Pontes and Huben 1984). Instead, we place great emphasis on improving the patient's health in general during the postoperative phase by measures such as convalescence in a sanatorium and hope thereby to stimulate the body's own defence system.

Treatment of Disseminated Disease

About one-third of patients with renal cell carcinoma have clinical signs of metastases at the time of diagnosis. The occasional observation of spontaneous regression of lung metastases, in particular, after excision of the primary renal cell carcinoma (Garfield and Kennedy 1972) has prompted many urologists to subject such advanced cases to radical excision of the tumor-bearing kidney. In a retrospective study Osterhage and Frohmüller (1983) found that the survival time of these patients depended on whether one or more organs were affected by metastases and which organ it was that contained the secondary growth. The prognosis was best if there was a solitary metastasis in a regional lymph node or in the skeleton.

The expectation of life for patients with disseminated hypernephroid carcinoma is hardly better after removal of kidney and tumour plus adjuvant chemotherapy than after removal of the tumour and kidney alone (Heising and Engelking 1983). In an extensive review of 200 cases in the literature, Talley (1973) was able to show that nearly 90% of all renal cell carcinomas were primarily resistant to cytostatics, and even combination therapy was no more successful (Behrendt 1979; Klippel and Altwein 1981). The only substances which provide a glimmer of hope are vinblastine and ifosfamide, with a combination of which Weissmüller et al. (1983) obtained a response rate of 35%. Because of the serious side effects, and especially as a result of complications due to immunosuppression, Brühl et al. (1976) were very reluctant to use cytostatic drugs.

An alternative to cytostatic treatment of disseminated renal cell carcinoma is the use of hormones or antihormones. The justification for such treatment lies in the fact that in animal experiments, kidney malignancies have been induced by oestrogens and inhibited by the administration of progesterones or testosterone (Possinger et al. 1981; Rattenhuber et al. 1981; Weissmüller et al. 1983). The results of treatment are disappointing even if, before treatment, the types of steroid receptors present are established in a tumour preparation and the hormones used appear to be correctly selected. Among 20 patients with tumour dissemination only a single one had a partial response of the secondary deposit (Weissmüller et al. 1983). Even with the combined use of chemotherapy (vinblastine) and the antihormone tamoxifen, Wagner et al. (1983) obtained a response rate of only 18%.

A form of treatment that has gained in importance in recent years is immunotherapy (Schärfe et al. 1983). The theoretical advantage is that tumour cells should be destroyed selectively without any damaging effect on the body's own healthy cells (Klippel and Altwein 1981). An essential requirement is the surgical removal of the primary growth or reduction of the bulk of tumour cells present by extensive excision of metastases (Klippel et al. 1981). Tykkae et al. (1974) were able to confirm the effectiveness of immunotherapy: after 5½ years 23.6% of the 31 patients who received immunotherapy were still alive, whereas every one of 23 patients in a control group had died.

Follow-up

Continued care of patients who have had their tumours removed by nephrectomy presents problems, because in cases of recurrent disease – particularly with multiple metastases – we have only very limited forms of treatment at our disposal. On average, secondary growths are discovered after a 14-month disease-free interval; rapid progression and survival of only 7–13 months can then be expected. Metastases may, however, make their appearance as late as 10–20 years after primary treatment (Rathert 1982).

As a general guide, patients should be followed up 3-monthly in the 1st year, 6-monthly in the 2nd year and annually thereafter. The laboratory tests required at the 3-monthly visits are erythrocyte sedimentation rate (ESR), red cell count, Quick's test, gamma-glutamyl transpeptidase, alkaline phosphatase, creatinine and urinalysis. Possible pulmonary metastases or retroperitoneal recurrences should be sought by radiological examination of the thorax (after 3–6 months) or by CT of the thorax and abdomen (after 6–12 months). At yearly intervals the examination should include an excretion urography and bone scintigraphy. At each examination an ultrasound scan is carried out of the original site of the tumour and of the contralateral kidney.

Treatment of Recurrences

While the appearance of a recurrence in the area of a radical tumour excision indicates a poor prognosis in every case despite "second-look" intervention, the surgical removal of a solitary distant metastasis which has appeared at an interval after treatment of the primary tumour offers considerable hope of success, the outlook being the better the later after the original nephrectomy the metastasis has appeared. According to Swanson and Borges (1983) the 5-year survival rate is 45% for solitary metastases treated with the intention of cure which have appeared on average 15 months after nephrectomy. Secondary bone deposits, too, if recognized in time, can be resected en bloc, the defect stabilised osteosynthetically and healed with adjuvant gestagen therapy (Hubmer et al. 1983; Strube et al. 1983). The results of the treatment of recurrences with chemotherapy, hormones or antihormones and immunotherapy are no more encouraging than in the therapy of primary dissemination (see 'Treatment of Disseminated Disease' above) (Wagle and Murphy 1971; Weissmüller et al. 1983). The expectation of life after the occurrence of multiple distant metastases is only 5–11 months (Heising and Engelking 1983).

Disease-free Interval and Survival

The natural history of renal cell carcinomas is very variable. A few patients may display spontaneous regression or arrest of the growth of the tumour for many years, but such an exceptional outcome in a very small number of individuals must not deceive us about the generally high malignancy of this tumour; the 3-year survival rate of untreated patients amounts to only 4.4% (De Kernion 1980). The decisive factor determining survival is the presence or absence of metastases in lymph nodes and at distant sites. A more accurate prognosis can be expressed in the context of the disease stage the patient has reached only if he has had treatment, usually surgery. The average 5-year survival rate for all stages taken together is 50% according to Rathert (1982) and 45% in our own patients (1972–1982). If the prognosis is broken down according to the pathologically and histologically verifiable pT staging, then a deterioration of the prognosis is obvious above all if the tumour has spread to the perirenal or peripelvic fatty tissue (stage pT3) (Table 6). Even using Robson's classification, the results of treatment deteriorate if invasion of the perirenal fatty tissue has occurred (Table 7). Lymph node metastases worsen the prognosis appreciably; the 5-year survival rate is only 10% in such cases (Schmiedt and Rattenhuber 1981). Equally unpropitious are initial distant metastases, which, if multiple or in a number of organs, allow no hope of cure (Angervall and Wahlquist 1978; Patel and Lavengood 1978).

Contradictory opinions have been expressed about the prognosis of a tumour thrombus in the renal vein and/or the vena cava. While Angervall and Wahlquist (1978), Fuselier et al. (1983), Petkovic (1970) and Skinner et al. (1972 a) were unable to find any reduction in the chances of cure, McNichols et al. (1981) and Oliver et al. (1979) considered the prognosis to be worse.

Future Development

As the results of the treatment of renal cell carcinoma are at present unsatisfactory, we must seek ways and means to improve them. As with all malignant tumours, the chance of cure is the better the earlier the diagnosis is made, and the best hope lies in the early discovery of an asymptomatic renal carcinoma by sonography. Furthermore, if a renal cell carcinoma is borne in mind in the interpretation of the clinical signs and symptoms the interval before confirmation of the diagnosis, may be shortened. This applies in particular to the paraneoplastic syndrome and to a strongly raised ESR in the absence of infection. The inclusion of routine urinalysis in preventive or screening programmes is essential, as this should show up haematuria, the commonest symptom of these tumours.

Only surgical extirpation will at the present time allow cure of a renal cell carcinoma. Advances in

Table 7. Five-year survival rates in patients with renal cell carcinoma according to Robson's staging

Reference	Stage I		Stage II		Stage III		Stage IV	
	(*n*)	(%)	(*n*)	(%)	(*n*)	(%)	(*n*)	(%)
Robson et al. (1969)	32	66	14	64	24	42	12	11
Böttiger (1970)	31	76	12	65	16	35	32	5
Skinner et al. (1972 b)	102	65	22	47	108	51	77	8
Boxer et al. (1979)	18	56	5	100	10	50	26	10
Sigel et al. (1981)	107	73	33	54	136	35	38	15
McNichols et al. (1981)	177	67	57	51	209	34	56	14
Haschek (1981)	78	64	41	51	103	35	21	10
Schmiedt and Rattenhuber (1981)	164	80	23	55	27	10[a]	79	0
					53	25[b]		
Waters and Richie (1979)	36	51	54	59	8	12	32	0
Own patients (1972–1982)	58	65	37	57	17	19	32	11

[a] Stage III a: lymph node metastases only.
[b] Stage III b: vein invasion without lymph node metastases.

clinical and experimental research may be expected to improve supplemetary treatment of T1–4 N0 M0 tumours or to improve specific systemic therapy of TX NX M1 tumours; this may take the form of newly developed chemotherapeutic agents or improved means of targeting immunotherapy.

Carcinoma of the Renal Pelvis

Epidemiology and Aetiology

Tumours arising from the urothelium of the renal pelvis differ from renal cell carcinomas in location, histology and biological behaviour (Gödde and Vahlensieck 1968). They are rare, amounting to only 0.2% of all malignancies and 4.5%–9% of malignant renal tumours (Rathert 1982). Men are as a rule affected 2–3 times as often as women; the highest incidence lies between 50 and 60 years of age (Zingg 1982). In nearly 50% of patients a further urothelial tumour is or will be present at another site (Ammon et al. 1981).

Many tumour-inducing substances have been suggested to cause renal pelvic carcinomas: Thorotrast, not used in Germany since the Second World War, produced such tumours after a latency period of 15–40 years in 50% of cases in addition to radiation fibrosis (Rathert 1982). A carcinoma is found in 25% of cases after chronic irritation of the renal pelvis by stones and/or chronic inflammation (Bennington and Beckwith 1975). Petkovic (1975) reported a form of endemic nephritis in Yugoslavia which is often combined with a carcinoma of the renal pelvis. Phenacetin and nicotine are other possible causes (Rathert et al. 1975); there is a significant increase in incidence after phenacetin abuse or the use of other analgetics such as paracetamol, which may be converted by bacteria into oncogenic metabolites.

Pathological Anatomy

In 25% of cases renal pelvic carcinoma arises from multiple locations, which must be interpreted as primarily multifocal growth; spread by cellular seeding along the urinary passages is less likely. It is even more unlikely that tumour has extended along the lymphatics (Babaian and Johnson 1980). Bilateral incidence is rare, occurring in only 1%–2% of cases with the exception of tumours arising after endemic nephritis or abuse of nicotine or phenacetin (10%) (Zingg 1982). Some 80%–90% of renal pelvic tumours are papillary and in part solid transitional epithelial carcinomas, 5%–20% are squamous epithelial carcinomas (Zingg 1982). Adenocarcinomas are the exception.

Classification

As the UICC has not carried out any classification of renal pelvic carcinomas, the staging proposed by Bennington and Beckwith (1975), based on a comparison of patients from various centres, has been adopted:

Stage I: papillary carcinoma of mucous membrane without invasion
Stage II: infiltration of tumour into lamina propria
Stage III: extension of tumour into or beyond muscularis
Stage IV: infiltration of tumour into renal parenchyma

In addition to the tendency to infiltration, the degree of malignancy (grade) also has a decisive bearing on the prognosis. This classification is very similar to the one for tumours of the urinary bladder (Rathert 1982).

Symptoms

The dominant symptom of a carcinoma of the renal pelvis, and in 70%–80% of cases the initial symptom, is haematuria visible to the naked eye (Voss et al. 1977). Pain is the second most common symptom, occurring in 40%–60%, and microscopic haematuria is noted in 17%–30%. A urinary tract infection is present in 20%–30% of patients (Rathert 1982).

Diagnosis

Urothelial tumours of the renal pelvis may be identified by urography, retrograde pyelography or cytology. Angiography, lymphography and sonography are of secondary importance; CT is useful for the demonstration of lymph node metastases. In doubtful cases the diagnosis may be established by lavage cytology of the renal pelvis or by ureterorenoscopy (Papadopoulos et al. 1986).

Treatment

In view of the tendency of renal pelvic carcinomas to multilocular growth, the aim of surgery is to excise the kidney, the ureter, the ureteric ostium and a cuff of the bladder, a procedure which may be accomplished via lumbotomy and inguinal or suprapubic incision (Zingg 1982). If the intramural segment of the ureter is left behind, recurrence at that site, which carries mortality of more than 70% (Strong and Pearse 1976), may be expected in 22% of cases.

Methods in which parts of these structures are preserved, such as partial resection of the renal pelvis, transparenchymal electroresection or laser coagulation of the tumour, may be imployed as palliative procedures (Zingg 1982) in cases where the contralateral kidney is not present or not functioning.

Prognosis

The 5-year survival rate of renal pelvic carcinomas has been stated to be between 40% and 65% (Schabert and Nagel 1975; Voss et al. 1977) and is dependent on the degree of infiltration and the grade of histological differentiation. Non-infiltrating tumours in stages I and II have a 5-year survival rate of more than 80%, infiltrating tumours without penetration of all layers of the wall a rate of 40%–50%. Undifferentiated carcinomas with infiltration, on the other hand, show a poor prognosis, with a 5-year survival rate of 15%–20% (Rathert 1982).

References

Altwein JE (1979) Urologie. Enke, Stuttgart

Ammon J, Karsten JH, Rathert R (1981) Urologische Onkologie, 2nd edn. Springer, Berlin Heidelberg New York

Andreew A, Ranft A, Templin R (1971) Auswertung von 75 Patienten mit einem hypernephroiden Nierencarcinom. Zentralbl Chir 96: 1487–1494

Angervall L, Wahlquist L (1978) Follow-up and prognosis of renal carcinoma in a series operated by perifascial nephrectomy combined with adrenalectomy and retroperitoneal lymphadenectomy. Eur Urol 5: 13–17

Arlat IP (1985) Digitale Subtraktionsangiographie. Klinikarzt 14: 527–537

Babaian RJ, Johnson DJ (1980) Primary carcinoma of the ureter. J Urol 123: 357–359

Bargon G (1985) Die digitale Subtraktionsangiographie (DSA). Klinikarzt 14: 524–527

Bartley O, Hultquist GT (1950) Spontaneous regression of hypernephroma. Acta Pathol Microbiol Scand [A] 27: 448–451

Bauer HW, Rattenhuber U (1981) Labordiagnostik und paraneoplastische Syndrome. In: Rattenhuber U, Wieland W (ed) Diagnostik und Therapie des Nierenkarzinoms. Zuckschwerdt, München, pp 44–51

Behrendt H (1979) Retrospective and prospektive clinical aspects in hypernephroma. In: Löhr E (ed) Renal and adrenal tumours. Springer, Berlin Heidelberg New York, pp 200–211

Bennington JL (1973) Cancer of the kidney – etiology, epidemiology and pathology. Cancer 32: 1017–1029

Bennington JL, Beckwith JB (1975) Tumor of the kidney, renal pelvis, and ureter. In: Firminger HJ (ed) Atlas of tumor pathology, fasc. 12. AFIP, Washington, pp 93–110

Bischoff W (1978) Nierenembolisation. Akt Urol 9: 117–137

Bischoff W, Sommerkamp H (1977) Zur Problematik der operativen Therapie maligner Nierentumoren. Schweiz Med Wochenschr 107: 699–704

Bloom HJG (1973 a) Adjuvant therapy for adenocarcinoma of the kidney: present position and prospects. Br J Urol 45: 237–257

Bloom HJG (1973 b) Hormone-induced and spontaneous regression of metastatic renal cancer. Cancer 32: 1066–1071

Boehminghaus R, Greipel V, Schwartmann KP (1982) Analyse der Langzeitergebnisse nach Nephrektomie wegen Hypernephrom anhand von 442 Fällen. Urologe [A] 21: 201–204

Böttiger LE (1970) Prognosis in renal carcinoma. Cancer 26: 780–787

Boxer RJ, Wajsman J, Lieber MM, Mampaso FM, Skinner DG (1979) Renal carcinoma: computer analysis of 96 patients treated by nephrectomy. J Urol 122: 598–601

Bracken B, Jonsson K (1979) How accurate is angiographic staging of renal carcinoma? Urology 14: 96–99

Brosig W, Buchberger HG (1962) Transperitoneale Nephrektomie. Chirurg 33: 181–185

Brühl P, Vahlensieck W (1976) Zur Epidemiologie und Pathologie maligner Nierentumoren. Wien Med Wochenschr 126: 169–174

Brühl P, Scheef W, Albert H, Bücheler E (1976) Perspective nouvelles dans le traitement du carcinoma hypernephroide du rein. J Urol Nephrol 82: 417–427

Cherrie RJ, Goldman DG, Lindner A, De Kernion JB (1982) Prognostic implications of vena cava extension of renal cell carcinoma. J Urol 128: 910–912

Chisholm GD (1974) Malignant disease of the kidney: an appraisal of diagnosis and management. Ann R Coll Surg Engl 55: 21–27

Chisholm GD (1980) Clinical and biochemical markers in renal carcinoma. Renal cancer UICC-technical report series, vol 49, pp 182–198

Chisholm GD, Roy RR (1971) The systemic effects of malignant renal tumours. Br J Urol 43: 687–700

Chlepas S, Hermanek P, Sigel A (1977) Regionale Lymphknotenmetastasen beim Nierenparenchymkrebs. Urologe [A] 16: 208–212

Cooper PH, Waysman J (1971) Tubular differentation and basement membrane production in renal adenoma. J Pathol 109: 109–116

Cox CE, Lacy SS, Montgomery WG, Boyce WH (1970) Renal adenocarcinoma: 28-year review, with emphasis on rationale and feasibility of preoperative radiotherapy. J Urol 104: 53–61

Cronan JJ, Zeman RK, Rosenfield AT (1982) Comparison of computerized tomography, ultrasound and angiography in staging renal cell carcinoma. J Urol 127: 712–714

De Kernion JB (1980) Lymphadenectomy for renal carcinoma. Urol Clin North Am 7: 697–703

Egger B, Hartung R, Pollak E (1979) Staging und therapeutische Ergebnisse bei 288 hypernephroiden Nierenkarzinomen. Med Welt 30: 920–928

Engelmann U, Klose KJ, Bürger RA, Jacobi GH (1983) Die Treffsicherheit der Computertomographie in der therapeutischen Stadieneinteilung des Nierenzellkarzinoms. Akt Urol 14: 51–57

Everson TC, Cole WH (1966) Spontaneous regression of ade-

nocarcinoma of the kidney. In: Boyd W (ed) Spontaneous regression of cancer. Charles C Thomas, Springfield, pp 11-87
Federal Statistical Office (1982) Statistisches Bundesamt, Gruppe VII D. Sterbefälle 1981 nach Altersgruppen, Auszug aus Tabelle N 50
Fischer P, Schultz E (1983) Zum Auflösungsvermögen der digitalen Videosubtraktionsangiographie (DVSA). RoFo 138: 45-49
Flamm J (1982) Zur operativen Therapie maligner Nierentumoren. Wien Med Wochenschr 132: 49-53
Flamm J, Wöber L (1981) Der maligne Nierentumor. Wien Med Wochenschr 131: 579-585
Flamm J, Burkert S, Grof F (1981) Zur Problematik der transfemoralen Katheterembolisation von Nierentumoren. Akt Urol 12: 19-22
Flocks RH, Kadesky MC (1958) Malignant neoplasm of the kidney. An analysis of 353 patients followed five years or more. J Urol 79: 196-201
Fuselier HA, Guice SL, Brannan W, Ochsner MG, Sangisetty KV, Beckmann EN, Barnes CA (1983) Renal cell carcinoma: the Ochsner medical institution experience (1945-1978). J Urol 130: 445-448
Futter NG, Collins JP, Walsh WG (1979) Inaccuracies in angiographic staging of renal cell carcinoma. Urology 14: 629-630
Garfield DH, Kennedy BJ (1972) Regression of metastatic renal cell carcinoma following nephrectomy. Cancer 30: 190-194
Gebauer A, Ribka A (1981) Sonographie und Computertomographie in der Diagnostik des Nierenkarzinoms. In: Rattenhuber U, Wieland W (ed) Diagnostik und Therapie des Nierenkarzinoms. Zuckschwerdt, München, pp 84-91
Glenn JF (1964) Clinical and surgical considerations of renal malignancy. NC Med J 25: 367-374
Gödde St, Vahlensieck W (1968) Nierentumoren ohne Makrohämaturie. Langenbecks Arch Klin Chir 321: 74-85
Grabbe E, Witte G, Jend HH, Bücheler E (1984) Die angiographische Oberbauchdiagnostik mit Hilfe der DSA. RoFo 140: 3-9
Graham SD, Glenn JF (1979) Enucleative surgery for renal malignancy. J Urol 122: 546-549
Gütgemann A, Vahlensieck W (1964) Therapie und Prognose des einseitig renal bedingten Bluthochdrucks. Med Welt 48: 2557-2561
Hajdu SI, Thomas AG (1967) Renal cell carcinoma at autopsy. J Urol 97: 978-982
Hallwachs O, Beduhn D, Harbst H (1969) Die diagnostische Treffsicherheit der verschiedenen radiologischen Untersuchungsmethoden bei Nierentumoren. Urologe 8: 138-143
Harmer MH (1978) TNM-classification of malignant tumors, 3rd edn. UICC, Geneva, pp 109-112
Haschek H (1981) Zur operativen Therapie des Nierenkarzinoms. In: Rattenhuber U, Wieland W (ed) Diagnostik und Therapie des Nierenkarzinoms. Zuckschwerdt, München, pp 130-133
Heising J, Engelking R (1983) Prognose des hämatogen metastasierten Nierenzell-Karzinoms (pT_{1-4} N_X M_X) nach Tumornephrektomie plus Ifosfamid. In: Kaufmann J (ed) Verhandlungsbericht der Deutschen Gesellschaft für Urologie. Springer, Berlin Heidelberg New York, pp 75-77
Hermanek P, Sigel A, Chlepas S (1976) Histological grading of renal cell carcinoma. Eur Urol 2: 189-191
Herrlinger A, Sigel A, Schrott KM (1983) Die Bedeutung der lymphogenen Metastasierung des Nierencarcinoms für das Vorgehen bei der radikalen Tumor-Nephrektomie. In: Kaufmann J (ed) Verhandlungsbericht der Deutschen Gesellschaft für Urologie. Springer, Berlin Heidelberg New York, pp 104-106
Hienzsch E (1972) Operationen an den Nieren. In: Heise GW, Hienzsch E (eds) Urologische Operationslehre. Thieme, Leipzig, pp 23-59
Holland JM (1973) Cancer of the kidney - natural history and staging. Cancer 32: 1030-1042
Hubmer G, Gnad H, Vilits P (1983) Das Hypernephrom mit solitärer Fernmetastase: Ergebnisse der Tumornephrektomie und Metastasenchirurgie. In: Kaufmann J (ed) Verhandlungsbericht der Deutschen Gesellschaft für Urologie. Springer, Berlin Heidelberg New York, pp 47-49
Jaeger N, Vahlensieck W (1985) Prognose beim Nierencarcinom. Lebensversicherungsmedizin 37: 75-78
Jaeger N, Weissbach L, Vahlensieck W (1985) Value of enucleation of tumour in solitary kidneys. Eur Urol 11: 369-373
Javadpour N (1984) Cancer of the kidney. Thieme-Stratton, New York
Jonitz H, Hallwachs O (1982) Das Nierenkarzinom - ein häufig zu spät diagnostizierter Tumor. Diagnostik 15: 1204-1210
Juusela H, Malmio K, Alfthan O, Oravisto KJ (1977) Preoperative irradiation in the treatment of renal adenocarcinoma. J Urol Nephrol 11: 277-281
Kaisary AV, Williams G, Riddle PR (1984) The role of preoperative embolization in renal cell carcinoma. J Urol 131: 641-646
Katz SE, Schapira HE (1982) Spontaneous regression of genitourinary cancer - an update. J Urol 128: 1-4
Kessler N, Rath M, Bauer HW (1981) Wertigkeit der Lymphographie und Computertomographie bei der präoperativen Abklärung von Lymphknotenmetastasen des Nierenkarzinoms. In: Rattenhuber U, Wieland W (eds) Diagnostik und Therapie des Nierenkarzinoms. Zuckschwerdt, München, pp 75-83
Kline MJ, Valensi OJ (1976) Proximal tubular adenomas of kidney with so-called onkocystic features. Cancer 38: 906-912
Klippel KF, Jacobi GH, Schulte-Wissermann H (1981) Aktive Immuntherapie beim metastasierenden Hypernephrom. Akt Urol 12: 161-165
Klippel KF, Altwein JE (1981) Palliative Therapiemöglichkeiten beim metastasierten Hypernephrom. Dtsch Med Wochenschr 104: 28-31
Klosterhalfen A (1968) Thorako-abdominale Nephrektomie bei großen Nierentumoren. Urologe 7: 146-148
Klosterhalfen H (1975) Die Behandlung der Tumoren der Niere und der oberen Harnwege. In: Nagel R (ed) Verhandlungsbericht der Deutschen Gesellschaft für Urologie. Springer, Berlin Heidelberg New York, pp 85-91
König K, Schröder RH, Schwenn S (1975) Symptomatik und Überlebensdaten bei 219 Patienten mit Hypernephrom. In: Nagel R (ed) Verhandlungsbericht der Deutschen Gesellschaft für Urologie. Springer, Berlin Heidelberg New York, pp 169-173
Kolle P (1981 a) Die Rolle der Kavotomie bei der Radikaloperation des Nierenkarzinoms. Fortschr Med 99: 1626-1629
Kolle P (1981 b) Urologische Röntgendiagnostik einschließlich Renovasographie und Kavographie beim Nierenkarzinom. In: Rattenhuber U, Wieland W (ed) Diagnostik und Therapie des Nierenkarzinoms. Zuckschwerdt, München, pp 60-74
Kurth KH, Cinqualbre J, Oliver RTD, Schulmann CC (1984) Embolization and subsequent nephrectomy in metastatic renal cell carcinoma. World J Urol 2: 122-126

Lacker K, Janson R, Franken Th, Harder Th, Thurn P (1983) Digitale Subtraktionsangiographie (DSA). Dtsch Med Wochenschr 180: 350–355

Lackner K, Harder Th, Herter M (1984 a) Anatomische Auflösung der intraarteriellen digitalen Subtraktionsangiographie der Niere bei Verwendung unterschiedlicher Kontrastmittelkonzentrationen. RoFo 140: 695–698

Lackner K, Harder Th, Herter M, Leipner N (1984 b) Vergleich der intraarteriellen digitalen Subtraktionsangiographie mit der konventionellen Arteriographie. RoFo 141: 616–624

Lang EK (1973) Arteriography in the diagnosis and staging of hypernephromas. Cancer 32: 1043–1052

Lanksch W, Ringel K (1981) Zur Diagnostik und Therapie von zerebralen Nierenkarzinom-Metastasen. In: Rattenhuber U, Wieland W (eds) Diagnostik und Therapie des Nierenkarzinoms. Zuckschwerdt, München, pp 160–165

Levine E, Lee KR, Weigel J (1979) Preoperative determination of abdominal extent of renal cell carcinoma by computed tomography. Radiology 132: 395–398

Leyendecker R (1985) Nierenkarzinom. Inaugural dissertation University of Bonn

Malek RS, Utz DC, Culp OS (1976) Hypernephroma in the solitary kidney: experience with 20 cases and review of the literature. J Urol 116: 553–556

Marshal G, Baert A, Wilms G (1979) Value of computerized tomography and ultrasonography in the diagnosis of renal and adrenal space-occupying lesions. In: Löhr E (ed) Renal and adrenal tumours. Springer, Berlin Heidelberg New York, pp 98–122

Marshall FF (1982) Guest editorial; renal cell carcinoma. J Urol 128: 923

Mast GJ, Braedel HU, Ziegler M (1978) Hypertonie als Folge tumoröser und solitärer zystischer Nierenveränderungen. Akt Urol 9: 89–94

Mayor G (1975) Zur Frage der Zugangswege bei Nierentumoren. In: Nagel R (ed) Verhandlungsbericht der Deutschen Gesellschaft für Urologie. Springer, Berlin Heidelberg New York, pp 123–124

McLaughlin AP (1979) Tumor of the kidney. In: Early LE, Gottschalk CW (eds) Strauss and Welt's diseases of the kidney, vol 2, 3rd edn. Little Brown, Boston, pp 988–1005

McNichols DW, Segura JW, de Weerd JH (1981) Renal cell carcinoma: long-term survival and late recurrence. J Urol 126: 17–23

Middleton RG (1967) Surgery for metastatic renal cell carcinoma. J Urol 97: 973–977

Middleton RG, Presto AJ (1973) Radical thoraco-abdominal nephrectomy for renal cell carcinoma. J Urol 110: 36–37

Mims MM, Christensen B, Schulmberger FL, Goodwin WE (1966) A 10-year evaluation of nephrectomy for renal cell carcinoma. J Urol 95: 10–17

Molitor D, Weißbach L (1981) Operative Konzeption zur Beseitigung eines Tumorthrombus aus der unteren Hohlvene bei hypernephroidem Carcinom. Urologe [A] 20: 187–189

Mostofi FK (1967) Pathology and spread of renal cell carcinoma. In: King JS (ed) Renal neoplasia. Little Brown, Boston, pp 41–85

Nagel R, Baumgärtel H, Rilling J, Taenzer V, Haasner E (1969) Die Bedeutung der caudalen Venocavographie für die operative Behandlung maligner Nierentumoren. Urologe 8: 129–135

Oliver JA, Laplante MP, Reid EC, Schual RS (1979) Results of radical nephrectomy in 178 cases of renal cell adenocarcinoma. Can J Surg 22: 409–412

Orestano R, Urlesberger K, Marberger M, Georgi M, Rauchenwald W, Hohenfellner R (1975) Operative Behandlung maligner Tumoren in der Einzelniere. Akt Urol 6: 33–39

Osterhage HR, Frohmüller H (1983) Ergebnisse der Tumornephrektomie beim metastasierenden Nierencarcinom. In: Nagel R (ed) Verhandlungsbericht der Deutschen Gesellschaft für Urologie. Springer, Berlin Heidelberg New York, pp 50–51

Palmer JM, Swanson DA (1978) Conservative surgery in solitary and bilateral renal carcinoma: indications and technical considerations. J Urol 120: 113–117

Papadopoulos I, Figge M, Weißbach L (1986) Bioptische Sicherung von Urotheltumoren durch Ureterorenoskopie. In: Ackermann R (ed) Verhandlungsbericht der Deutschen Gesellschaft für Urologie. Springer, Berlin Heidelberg New York, pp 234–238

Patel NP, Lavengood RW (1978) Renal cell carcinoma: natural history and results of treatment. J Urol 119: 722–726

Pauer W, Mikuz G, Jakse G (1981) Ist die Nephrektomie beim metastasierenden Nierenkarzinom sinnvoll? Akt Urol 12: 146–149

Paul D (1967) Zur Prognose der bösartigen Nierengeschwülste unter besonderer Berücksichtigung der Anamnesedauer. Z Urol Nephrol 60: 459–464

Petković S (1970) Die Pathologie und Prognose der Nierenparenchymtumoren. Akt Urol 1: 178–183

Petković S (1975) The staging of renal parenchymal tumours. Br J Urol 47: 13–16

Petri E, Weitzel D, Halbauer U (1978) Nierensonographie – Fehlinterpretationen und Ursachen. Urologe [A] 17: 143–146

Pinals RA, Krane SM (1962) Medical aspects of renal carcinoma. Postgrad Med J 38: 507–514

Pontes EJ, Huben RP (1984) Immunotherapy of renal cell carcinoma. World J Urol 2: 142–145

Possinger K, Hartenstein R, Ehrhart H (1981) Chemotherapie des Adenokarzinoms der Niere. In: Rattenhuber U, Wieland W (eds) Diagnostik und Therapie des Nierenkarzinoms. Zuckschwerdt, München, pp 183–190

Rafla S (1970) Renal cell carcinoma: natural history and results of treatment. Cancer 25: 26–32

Rathert P (1982) Das Nierencarcinom: praktische Probleme der Diagnose und Therapie. GBK-Mitteilungsdienst 10: 11–15

Rathert P, Melchior H, Lutzeyer W (1975) Phenacetin: a carcinogen for the urinary tract? J Urol 113: 653–657

Rattenhuber UI, Bauer HW, Krebs E (1981) Symptomatologie des Nierenkarzinoms. In: Rattenhuber U, Wieland W (eds) Diagnostik und Therapie des Nierenkarzinoms. Zuckschwerdt, München, pp 38–43

Rauschmeier H, Hofstädter R, Jakse G (1984) Tumor grading: an important prognostic factor in renal cell carcinoma. World J Urol 2: 103–108

Riches EW (1964) The natural history of renal tumours. In: Riches EW (ed) Tumors of the kidney and ureter, vol 2. Williams and Wilkins, Baltimore; E and S Livingstone, Edinburgh, pp 124–136

Robson CJ (1963) Radical nephrectomy for renal cell carcinoma. J Urol 89: 37–42

Robson CJ, Churchill BM, Anderson W (1969) The results of radical nephrectomy for renal cell carcinoma. J Urol 101: 297–301

Rost A, Brosig W (1977) Preoperative irradiation of renal cell carcinoma. Urology 10: 414–417

Rübben H, Lutzeyer W (1981) Kritische Analyse der Indikation der TNM-orientierten urologischen Tumordiagnostik. Urologe [A] 20: 31–37

Rüedi P, Mayor G, Sulmoni A (1975) Klinische und therapeutische Erfahrungen an der Urologischen Universitätsklinik Zürich bei 156 Hypernephromfällen. Z Urol 68: 493–498

Schabert O, Nagel R (1975) Therapie und Prognose primärer Nierenbecken- und Harnleitertumoren. In: Nagel R (ed) Verhandlungsbericht der Deutschen Gesellschaft für Urologie. Springer, Berlin Heidelberg New York, pp 184-187

Schärfe T, Klippel KF, Hohenfellner R (1983) Pilotstudie Immuntherapie des metastasierenden Hypernephroms: Technik und Anwendung. In: Kaufmann J (ed) Verhandlungsbericht der Deutschen Gesellschaft für Urologie. Springer, Berlin Heidelberg New York, pp 78-80

Schefft P, Novick AC, Straffon RA, Stewart BH (1978) Surgery for renal cell carcinoma extending into the inferior vena cava. J Urol 120: 28-31

Schmiedt E (1973) Nierentumoren. Chirurg 44: 485-489

Schmiedt E, Rattenhuber U (1981) Operative Therapie des Nierenkarzinoms - Indikation, Methode, Ergebnisse und Prognose. In: Rattenhuber U, Wieland W (eds) Diagnostik und Therapie des Nierenkarzinoms. Zuckschwerdt, München, pp 134-139

Schmiedt E, Rattenhuber U, Tauber R, Wieland U (1981) Nierentumoren. In: Zenker R, Deucher F, Schink W (eds) Chirurgie der Gegenwart, vol 6. Urban and Schwarzenberg, München, pp 1-50

Schmiedt E, Rattenhuber U, Wieland W (1982) Parenchymatöse Nierentumoren. In: Hohenfellner R, Zingg EJ (eds) Urologie in Klinik und Praxis. Thieme, Stuttgart, pp 490-508

Schmitz W (1967) Zur Klinik und Therapie der Nierengeschwülste. Urologe 6: 139-145

Schoenenberger A, Probst P (1982) CT-Staging des hypernephroiden Karzinoms. Urologe [A] 21: 195-200

Sigel A (1965) Maskierte Nierentumoren. Urologe 4: 86-93

Sigel A, Held L (1963) Die Zugangswege der Nierenchirurgie. Urologe 2: 144-153

Sigel A, Chlepas S, Schrott KM, Hermanek P (1981) Die Operation des Nierentumors. Chirurg 52: 545-553

Siminovitch JP, Montie JE, Straffon RA (1982a) Inferior venacavography in the preoperative assessment of renal adenocarcinoma. J Urol 128: 908-909

Siminovitch JP, Montie JE, Straffon RA (1982b) Lymphadenectomy in renal adenocarcinoma. J Urol 127: 1090-1091

Skinner DG, Pfister RF, Colvin R (1972a) Extension of renal cell carcinoma into the vena cava: the rationale for aggressive surgical management. J Urol 107: 711-716

Skinner DG, Vermillion CD, Colvin R (1972b) The surgical management of renal cell carcinoma. J Urol 107: 705-710

Staehler G, Mellin HE, Rattenhuber U (1981) Staging des Nierenkarzinoms. In: Rattenhuber U, Wieland W (eds) Diagnostik und Therapie des Nierenkarzinoms. Zuckschwerdt, München, pp 52-59

Stauffer MH (1961) Nephrogenic hepatosplenomegaly. Gastroenterology 40: 694-696

Steinberg SM, Brodowski HS, Goep CE (1972) Renal carcinoma in mother and daughter. Cancer 29: 222-223

Sternswand J, Almgard IE, Frawzen S, von Schreeb T, Wedstrom LB (1970) Tumor distinctive cellular immunity to renal carcinoma. Clin Exp Immunol 6: 938-946

Strong DW, Pearse HD (1976) Recurrent urothelial tumors following surgery for transitional cell carcinoma of the upper urinary tract. Cancer 38: 2173-2179

Strube HD, Hohenfellner R, Ritter G, Schärfe T (1983) Besonderheiten und spezielle operative Behandlungsmöglichkeiten bei Skelettmetastasen des Hypernephroms. In: Kaufmann J (ed) Verhandlungsbericht der Deutschen Gesellschaft für Urologie. Springer, Berlin Heidelberg New York, pp 54-57

Sufrin G (1982) The challenges of renal adenocarcinoma. Surg Clin North 62: 1101-1118

Sufrin G, Mirland EA, Moore RH, Chu TM, Murphy GP (1977) Hormone beim Nierenkarzinom. Akt Urol 8: 17-24

Sun CN, Bissada NK, White HJ, Redman JF (1977) The spectrum of ultrastructural patterns of renal cell adenocarcinoma. Urology 9: 195-198

Sutter A, Simma W (1978) Hypernephrom als Ursache eines Hochdrucks. Urologe [A] 17: 76-78

Swanson DA, Borges PM (1983) Complications of transabdominal radical nephrectomy for renal cell carcinoma. J Urol 128: 704-707

Swarm RL (1967) Introduction experience with colloidal thorium dioxide. Ann NY Acad Sci 145: 806-819

Talley RW (1973) Chemotherapy of adenocarcinoma of the kidney. Cancer 132: 1062-1065

Taesdale C, Kirk D, Jeans WD, Penry JB, Tribe CT, Slade N (1982) Arterial embolization in renal carcinoma: a useful procedure? Br J Urol 54: 616-619

Thompson LM, Shannon H, Ross G, Montie J (1975) An analysis of factors affecting survival in 150 patients with renal carcinoma. J Urol 114: 694-696

Thurn P, Bücheler E (1982) Einführung in die Röntgendiagnostik. Thieme, Stuttgart

Tolia BM, Whitmore WF (1975) Solitary metastasis from renal cell carcinoma. J Urol 114: 836-838

Tykkae H, Kjelt L, Oravisto KJ, Turunen M, Tallberg Th (1974) Disappearance of lung metastases during immunotherapy in five patients suffering from renal cell carcinoma. Scand J Respir Dis [Suppl] 89: 123-128

Vahlensieck W (1973) Zytostatika in der Urologie. In: Nagel R (ed) Verhandlungsbericht der Deutschen Gesellschaft für Urologie. Springer, Berlin Heidelberg New York, pp 171-179

Vahlensieck W (1976) Lymphadenektomie bei Nierencarcinomen. Vortrag anläßlich des II. Kongresses der Europäischen Gesellschaft für Urologie, 24-26 Sept, Prague

Vahlensieck W, Gödde St (1965) Diagnostik, Therapie und Prognose von Wilms-Tumoren. Med Welt 33: 1850-1852

Vahlensieck W, Gödde St (1968) Importance of early diagnosis of renal tumors. Minn Med 51: 1545-1548

Vahlensieck W, van der Weyer KH (1960) Zur Differentialdiagnostik retroperitonealer Geschwülste. MMW 102: 783-792

Van der Werf-Messing B, van der Heul RO, Ledeboer RCh (1981) Renal cell carcinoma trial. In: Wannenmacher M, Schreiber HW, Gauwerky R, Ladner HA, Knüfermann H, Slanina J (eds) Kombinierte chirurgische radiologische Therapie maligner Tumoren. Urban and Schwarzenberg, München, pp 169-175

Veyhl H, Eisenberger F, Wanner K (1981) Therapieergebnisse beim Nierenkarzinom. Fortschr Med 99: 1623-1625

Voss T, Hermanek P, Chlepas S, Fischer M (1977) Klinische Pathologie und Therapie der Urotheltumoren des Nierenhohlsystems und Harnleiters. Urologe 16: 93-96

Wagle BG, Murphy GP (1971) Hormonal therapy in advanced renal cell carcinoma. Cancer 28: 318-321

Wagner H, Possinger K, Wilmanns W, Marx FJ, Wieland W (1983) Disseminated renal cell carcinoma combination chemotherapy with vinblastine/tamoxifen. Proceedings of Second European Conference on Clinical Oncology in Amsterdam, p 151

Waters WB, Richie JP (1979) Aggressive surgical approach to renal cell carcinoma: review of 130 cases. J Urol 122: 306-309

Weir JM, Dunn JE Jr (1970) Smoking and mortality: a prospective study. Cancer 25: 105-111

Weissmüller J, König HJ, Missmahl M (1983) Behandlungsergebnisse der zytostatischen Therapie beim metastasierten Nieren-Carcinom. In: Kaufmann J (ed) Verhandlungsbericht der Deutschen Gesellschaft für Urologie. Springer, Berlin Heidelberg New York, pp 69–71

Wenz W (1967) Tumors of the kidney following retrograde pyelography with colloidal thorium dioxide. Ann NY Acad Sci 145: 145–148

Weyman PJ, McClennan BL, Stanley RJ, Levitt RG, Sagel SS (1980) Comparison of computed tomography and angiography in the evaluation of renal cell carcinoma. Radiology 137: 417–424

Wickham JEA (1975) Conservative renal surgery for adenocarcinoma. The place of bench surgery. Br J Urol 47: 25–36

Zingg EJ (1982) Die Tumoren des Nierenhohlsystems und des Harnleiters. In: Hohenfellner R, Zingg EJ (eds) Urologie in Klinik und Praxis. Thieme, Stuttgart, pp 509–519

Zollinger HU (1966) Niere und ableitende Harnwege. In: Doerr W, Uehlinger W (eds) Spezielle pathologische Anatomie, vol 3. Springer, Berlin Heidelberg New York, pp 672–696

Cancers of the Urinary Bladder, Ureters and Urethra

L. DENIS, R. HALL and G. JAKSE

Definition

Transitional cell epithelium (urothelium) lines the urinary tract from the calyces of the kidney to the urethra, including the ducts of the prostate. Transitional cell cancer (TCC) accounts for 95% of all urothelial tumours. Almost all TCC originates in the bladder as ureteral and urethral cancers are relatively rare. Bladder cancer of this type will be the subject of this chapter.

Epidemiology – Risk Factors

Bladder cancers rank tenth in the World Health Organization prevalence statistics. TCC account for about 5% of all malignant tumours in males in Europe. The peak incidence is between 50 and 70 years, with a male to female ratio of 5 to 1. The rising incidence may be due to the aging of the European population in the first place, but unfortunately also due to probable carcinogenic exposure. One-third of all

TCC relates in some way to exogenous influences, such as lifestyle (tobacco), social organisation (cars, food preservatives), industrial exposure (aromatic derivatives) and even medical treatment (radiotherapy, cyclophosphamide) with drug abuse (phenacetin) in certain European regions. Aromatic amines have been identified in animal experiments as aetiological agents and clearly related to the development of human bladder cancer. Undoubtedly there are many other risk factors involved: smoking and industrial exposure seem to be most prominent. A latency time of many years compounds the problem of defining risk factors. Squamous cell cancer accounts for 3% of all bladder tumours in Europe but is heavily endemic in Egypt and other African or Asian countries. This endemic incidence is caused by parasitic disease (bilharziasis) and concomitant long-standing infection. Adenocarcinoma (30% of which arise in the urachus) accounts for 2% of all bladder cancers.

Histopathology

Transitional cell epithelium transforms into neoplastic epithelium by two main pathways. About two-thirds of all bladder cancers are initially papillary in configuration and develop from normal or hyperplastic epithelium without nuclear abnormalities, and only an increase in the number of cell layers is indicative of the diagnosis. Cytological examination of cells shed in the urine reveals only normal or, at most, atypical-looking cells. One-third of bladder cancers present as sessile lesions with nodular or ulcerative forms. The preneoplastic epithelial phase of medium- and high-grade tumours is not well defined but is thought to derive from a flat lesion where cellular anaplasia is present (Friedell 1976). The criteria for anaplasia include not only increased cellularity, but also nuclear abnormalities among other morphological features. This form of TCC in situ must, by definition, have enough cellular anaplasia to be recognised as cancer and by necessity will be at least grade 2 and usually grade 3. Cytological examination of the urine, if properly performed, will yield the diagnosis by detecting malignant cells in nearly 100% of these cases (Koss et al. 1985).

Carcinoma in situ can be *primary,* without any other bladder cancer, or *secondary* where it is either concomitant with visible neoplasm, persisting after removal of detectable tumour or developing after a tumour-free interval. The symptoms and prognosis of in situ disease are determined by the extent and the location of the bladder lesions.

In general, *papillary* tumours are of low grade with low invasive potential (10%) where the DNA patterns are largely diploid. In contrast, *sessile tumours* and the rare high-grade papillary tumours have a strong invasive potential (70%); their DNA patterns are largely aneuploid. Tumours and mucosal changes of different degrees of malignancy or malignant potential may coexist in different areas of the urothelium, which makes it imperative to evaluate the urothelium by random biopsy and cytology in every case of bladder cancer.

Spread of bladder cancer occurs by:

- Direct infiltration of the bladder wall where the basement membrane is the first subtle marker of invasive potential and invasion of muscle is particularly sinister.
- Lymphatic spread occurs first to the regional (obturator, external and internal iliac) nodes and then to para-aortic, mediastinal and supraclavicular nodes.
- Vascular dissemination – distant metastases affect the lungs, bone and liver most commonly.

In conclusion, we face a tumour of very heterogeneous nature, and all efforts should be made to establish the type and grade of the tumour, its depth of invasion, extent and location.

Natural History

The natural history of low-grade papillary tumours depends upon their size, multiplicity, breach of the basement membrane and the presence of dysplasia or atypia elsewhere in the urothelium. They usually appear in the lowest part of the bladder and are multiple in 50% of patients. In the latter case they express a transformation of the total urothelium, and it is no surprise that recurrences, or new occurrences, reappear in 60%–80% of patients. Being a urothelial disease, we find synchronous tumours of the upper urinary tract in up to 5% and recurrences in prostatic ducts and the prostatic and other parts of the urethra in another 5% of cases.

These tumours are superficial in relation to the bladder wall, but early invasion of the basement membrane (T1) leads to significant differences in prognosis and survival (Richards and Schröder 1985). Progression to invasive disease is usually late and associated with the deterioration in the grade of the tumour. Recurrent tumours may appear late in the natural history of the disease, and there is a smaller probability of tumour recurrence with increased length of tumour-free survival. Most patients die from unrelated disease.

Carcinoma in situ is, by definition, a superficial tumour, but its natural history is quite different. It may appear as a focal disease but is usually of a multifocal nature with involvement of the ureters or the urethra in 50% of cases. When associated with papillary tumours, it influences their natural history and leads to invasive disease in the majority of cases without adequate treatment (Jakse et al. 1980). Cancer invading the bladder wall muscle or beyond at the time of first diagnosis (T3, T4) occurs in approximately one-third of patients.

Multiplicity is frequent, as in papillary tumours, and once again concomitant carcinoma in situ influences the course of the disease and its treatment (Lutzeyer et al. 1982; Wolf et al. 1985). Regional lymph node involvement is much more common with invasive tumours and is related to the depth of invasion: 30% of T3 tumours have regional node metastases, and up to 10% show para-aortic involvement (Prout et al. 1979; Skinner 1980). This factor clearly limits local treatment of invasive disease, but even more unfortunate is the fact that 70% of these patients develop distant metastases within the 1st year after diagnosis indicating that we are facing a systemic disease (Prout and Kopp 1984).

There is a general consensus that even our sophisticated diagnostic methods cannot assess the correct nodal staging, and surgery is the only means to obtain reliable information of nodal metastases. Lymphangiography or computed tomography followed by fine needle aspiration may obviate the need for surgical diagnosis if positive. Chest X-ray, isotope scans of bone and ultrasound or CT scans of liver may identify distant metastases.

However, the greatest problem is the undetectable distant metastasis that is present at the time of diagnosis. It should be stressed that nodal status is an important clue to this development since few patients with negative nodes harbour distant metastases. An unsolved problem is, of course, the biological evaluation of the tumour and its potential for invasion. Blood group iso-antigens, ploidy and chromosomal markers are among the investigations that may provide additional information on tumour behaviour. Also unsolved, but well recognised, is the status of the host which is difficult to describe and is one of the important but underevaluated factors in most randomised trials.

The TNM classification of bladder cancer is illustrated in Table 1 and Fig. 1, and its pathological classification in Fig. 2.

Staging

The clinical staging of bladder cancer cannot always be accurate, but assessment of its extent and invasion is a great help in determining the likely prognosis and thus the best treatment for the vast majority of patients. Furthermore, if we want to compare treatment results, it is necessary to agree upon a universal staging system such as the TNM system which is accepted by the International Union Against Cancer and the American Joint Commission on Staging (Hermanek and Sobin 1987; Beahrs and Myers 1982). Adequate staging according to these rules should be an inseparable part of each diagnostic work-up of a patient with bladder cancer. For publication and randomised studies, exact description of the diagnostic methodology employed is imperative and randomised studies should involve a central pathology review.

Changes in the current criteria for bladder cancer staging are being studied. Among the many suggestions of importance are the documentation of:
- Multiplicity of tumours
- Search for carcinoma in situ
- Importance of the basement membrane
- Presence of muscle in the tumour biopsy specimen

Table 1. TNM categories in bladder cancer

T – Primary Tumour	
TX	Primary tumour cannot be assessed
T0	No evidence of primary tumour
Tis	Carcinoma in situ: "flat tumour"
	Ta Non-invasive papillary carcinoma
T1	Tumour invades subepithelial connective tissue
T2	Tumour invades muscle (inner half)
T3	Tumour invades deep muscle or perivesical fat
	T3a Tumour invades deep muscle (outer half)
	T3b Tumour invades perivesical fat
T4	Tumour invades any of the following: prostate, uterus, vagina, pelvic wall, abdominal wall
N – Regional Lymph Nodes	
NX	Regional lymph nodes cannot be assessed
N0	No regional node metastasis
N1	Metastasis in a single lymph node 2 cm or less in greatest dimension
N2	Metastasis in a single lymph node more than 2 cm but not more than 5 cm in greatest dimension, or multiple nodes, none more than, 5 cm in greatest dimension
N3	Metastasis in a lymph node more than 5 cm in greatest dimension
M – Distant Metastasis	
MX	Presence of distant metastasis cannot be assessed
M0	No distant metastasis
M1	Distant metastasis

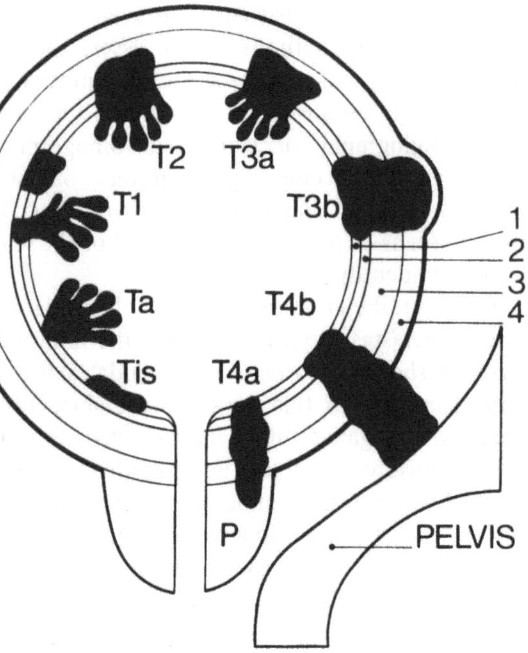

Fig. 1. T categories according to Hermanek and Sobin (1987). *1*, Urothelium; *2*, submucosa; *3*, muscle; *4*, serosa; *P*, prostate

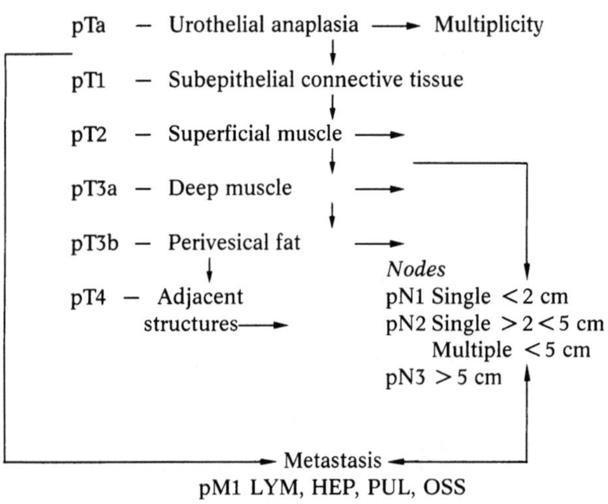

Fig. 2. Pathological *(p)* classification of bladder cancer. pTis may be concomitant to all T. Regional lymph node invasion pN1–3 and pM1 LYM (extraregional lymph nodes), HEP (lung), PUL (lung) and OSS (bone) should be evaluated as lethal disease

Prognosis – Prognostic Factors

As few patients die of primary superficial bladder cancer within 5 years of diagnosis most studies of prognostic factors have disease-free interval, recurrence rate or progression to higher stage rather than survival as end points of the study. T category and grade have withstood the test of time because they correlate with prognosis even in Ta, T1 and certainly T2 tumours (Cutler et al. 1982; Kurth 1984). Randomised studies have established the prognostic significance of recurrence rate before treatment and the total number of tumours and tumour size as important prognostic factors (Dalesio et al. 1983). Urothelial changes such as carcinoma in situ in normal-looking epithelium, positive cytology and no response to intravesical instillations of chemotherapeutic agents are also ominous signs of poor prognosis.

Stage and grade definitely correlate with survival in invasive bladder cancer where the additional factors of positive random mucosal biopsies, total tumour mass and even tumour morphology decrease the chance of a favourable outcome (Prout 1979; Slack and Prout 1980; Richards et al. 1986). In addition, the age and performance status of the patient, the length of the history, the presence of tumour markers and abnormal cell kinetics all influence the outcome of treatment. The downstaging of the primary tumour after preoperative radiotherapy is of prognostic value (Whitmore et al. 1977; van der Werf-Messing 1983).

Screening of Asymptomatic Disease

It is clear that haematuria, be it macroscopic or microscopic, will lead to suspicion of urothelial cancer until proven negative. Furthermore, properly conducted cytological examination of the urine is capable of detecting G2 and G3 bladder tumours, especially carcinoma in situ. However, the screening of populations for bladder cancer by these methods is not cost effective, and screening has to be restricted to high-risk patients (e.g. workers exposed to carcinogens) where urine analysis for haematuria and malignant cells is indicated.

Many patients with recurrent bladder tumours have no symptoms to suggest recurrence, and, for this reason, careful regular follow-up by urine cytology and cystoscopy is imperative for all patients with bladder cancer. The utilisation of new flexible fibre optic cystoscopes (Powell et al. 1984) and the use of transabdominal ultrasound may be helpful in this follow-up (Denis et al. 1984a).

Diagnosis of Symptomatic Disease

A consistent well-constructed work-up is essential to assess the invasive potential of the tumour according to prognostic factors (Fig. 3).

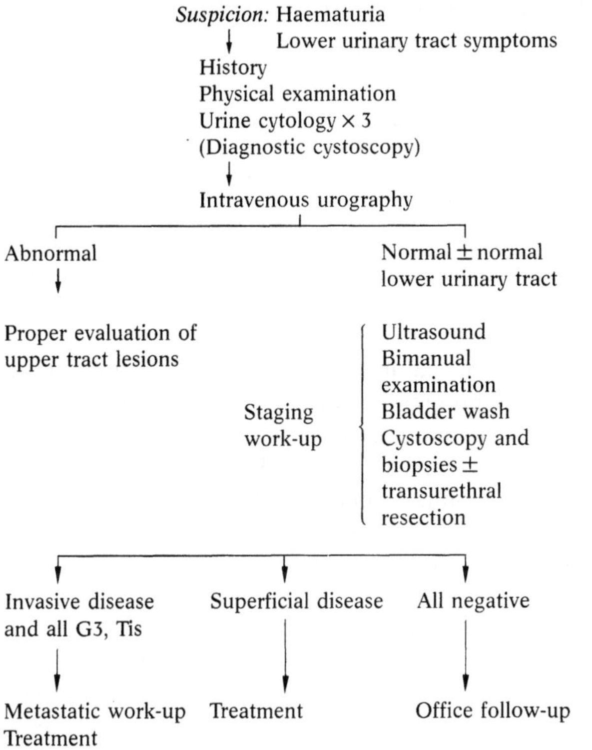

Fig. 3. Algorythm of diagnostic work-up of suspected bladder cancer. (From Niijima et al. 1986)

Painless haematuria is associated with bladder cancer in over one-half of the cases, and as soon as this symptom is observed, diagnostic investigation should start without delay. The complete history and physical examination will be followed by intravenous urography. These X-rays provide an overview of the entire urinary tract to exclude other possible causes of haematuria, and special attention is given to space-occupying lesions of the kidneys, radiolucent filling defects of the pelvi-calyceal systems and ureter, the possibility of low ureteric obstruction and intravesical lesions.

Transabdominal or transrectal ultrasound and a triple cytological examination of the urine may confirm the diagnosis, but a negative result from these examinations does not exclude urothelial cancer, and *a diagnostic cystourethroscopy is essential in all patients.*

Pain and dysuria are usually late symptoms in the development of bladder cancer when obstruction of the urinary tract, secondary infection and blood clots complicate primary disease. Suprapubic pain, severe frequency and dysuria, however, may be the first signal of carcinoma in situ, and the presence of these symptoms concomitant with "prostatism", without clear evidence of bladder outflow obstruction, is an indication for very careful cystoscopy and cytological examination of the urine.

After these preliminary investigations, *a staging cystoscopy* should be performed under general or spinal anaesthesia so that bimanual examination, mucosal biopsies and transurethral resection of the tumour may be performed. This will also be the definitive treatment for Ta and T1 tumours. This endoscopic assessment starts with a bimanual examination (of the empty bladder), one hand suprapubically and one finger in the rectum or vagina, to evaluate the size and mobility of palpable pelvic tumours. This examination should be repeated after the endoscopic resection. The cystoscopy proper evaluates bladder capacity, bladder wash cytology (which provides better cellular material for cytological examination and cytoflowmetry studies), a description of the growth pattern, size and location of the tumour(s). Also, field changes such as red patches of hyperaemia, mucosal oedema, cystitis cystica or ulceration will be noted. Endoscopic photography, if available, is especially useful in this respect. The next step is a cold cup biopsy of all suspicious areas of bladder mucosa, three to six biopsies of normal-looking mucosa next to the tumour and in opposed sites of the bladder and, finally, the complete resection of the tumour if possible. This resection biopsy will include the main tumour plus the base of the tumour together with some underlying muscle so that possible invasion may be assessed (Soloway et al. 1986). Very small papillary tumours may be coagulated but must be biopsied first to provide histological proof of malignancy.

The invasive process can be corroborated by intravesical ultrasound (Niijima and Nakamura 1982; Denis et al. 1984a). All this information should be recorded on a bladder diagram which forms an integral part of the patient's record. An example of such a diagram utilised in the studies of the EORTC GU Group is shown in Fig. 4.

All tumours with muscle invasion require investigation for possible metastases. Investigation can include chest X-ray, liver ultrasonography, bone scan, computed tomography of the pelvis and lymphangiography with fine needle aspiration of suspicious nodes. Nuclear magnetic resonance is at the stage of clinical evaluation. Some examples of medical imaging of the pelvis in bladder cancer patients are presented in Fig. 5.

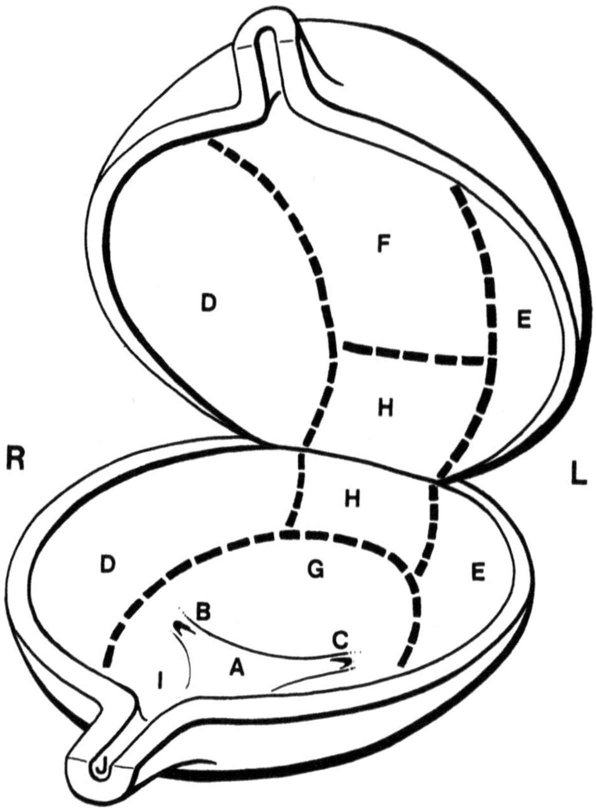

Fig. 4. Schematic representation of cystoscopical findings. Operating theatre diagram utilised in the EORTC GU Group prospective studies in bladder cancer. All biopsy sites are marked after a drawing of the tumour configuration. *A*, trigone; *B*, right ureteral orifice; *C*, left ureteral orifice; *D*, right wall; *E*, left wall; *F*, anterior wall; *G*, posterior wall; *H*, dome; *I*, neck; *J*, prostatic urethra; *K*, prostatic substance

Surgical and Combined Treatment of Loco-Regional Disease

Endoscopic resection is the preferred treatment for visible Tis, Ta, T1 and occasional papillary well-differentiated T2 tumours. This treatment is usually completed at the same time as the staging cystoscopy under anaesthesia. Resection by high-frequency current is primarily utilised, but where one is dealing with multiple lesions, simple coagulation after adequate resection biopsy of the largest tumours is acceptable. Laser coagulation is under clinical investigation. Partial cystectomy may occasionally be more suitable for single, large, superficial tumours at the dome or anterior wall of the bladder. Single, small papillary Ta tumours with negative cytology are of a good prognostic category and require no further treatment. T1 tumours of high grade have a definitely worse prognosis which justifies additional therapy in some patients.

Table 2. Chemoresection studies in superficial bladder cancer

Drug	CR/PR (%)	LT	ST
TTPA	50–70	++	+
ADM	66–78	++	− (negative)
MMC	47–81	++	− (negative)
BCG	65–81	++	+

CR/PR, complete remission/partial remission; LT, local toxicity; ST, systemic toxicity.

Since the natural history of most Ta tumours in terms of progression to invasion and survival is so slow, large randomised studies on superficial bladder cancer have to be conducted to determine the best form of treatment because long-term remission occurs in 60%–80% of cases. Intravesical treatment with cytotoxic chemotherapy is the treatment of choice in recurrent tumours with bad prognostic profiles. Chemoresection by intravesical instillation can be effective in about half the patients. The drugs of proven benefit for this purpose are thiotepa (TTPA), adriamycin (ADM), etoglucid and mitomycin C (MMC) and the immunomodulator bacille Calmette-Guerin (BCG) (Denis et al. 1984c). However, the cost effectiveness of intravesical therapy is poor in relation to simple endoscopic surgery which is the best primary treatment for the majority of Ta or T1 tumours. Chemotherapy, as an initial treatment, should generally be confined to patients with carcinoma in situ or phase II chemoresection trials.

Intravesical radium implantations have only been reported to be superior to transurethral resection in patients with T1 tumours (van der Werf-Messing et al. 1984). A randomised clinical trial is still needed to confirm this possibility.

The situation is very different in the presence of carcinoma in situ where we deal with a mucosal field change disease. Intravesical chemotherapy is the treatment of choice because it effects treatment of the total bladder mucosa. The aim of treatment is to destroy all visible lesions, obtain negative cytology and render patients symptom free. Effective therapy has been reported with ADM, MMC, TTPA and BCG (Jakse et al. 1980; Herr et al. 1987) (Table 2).

Careful follow-up, including biopsies of the prostatic urethra, is indicated since failure of this treatment necessitates cystectomy. The presence of Tis in the lower ureters, the prostatic fossa or the ducts of the prostate may be difficult to identify but requires aggressive treatment, usually cystourethrectomy.

Invasion of the bladder muscle is associated with poor prognosis. Invasion of muscle is, of course, only one aspect of tumour "aggression" where grade, tu-

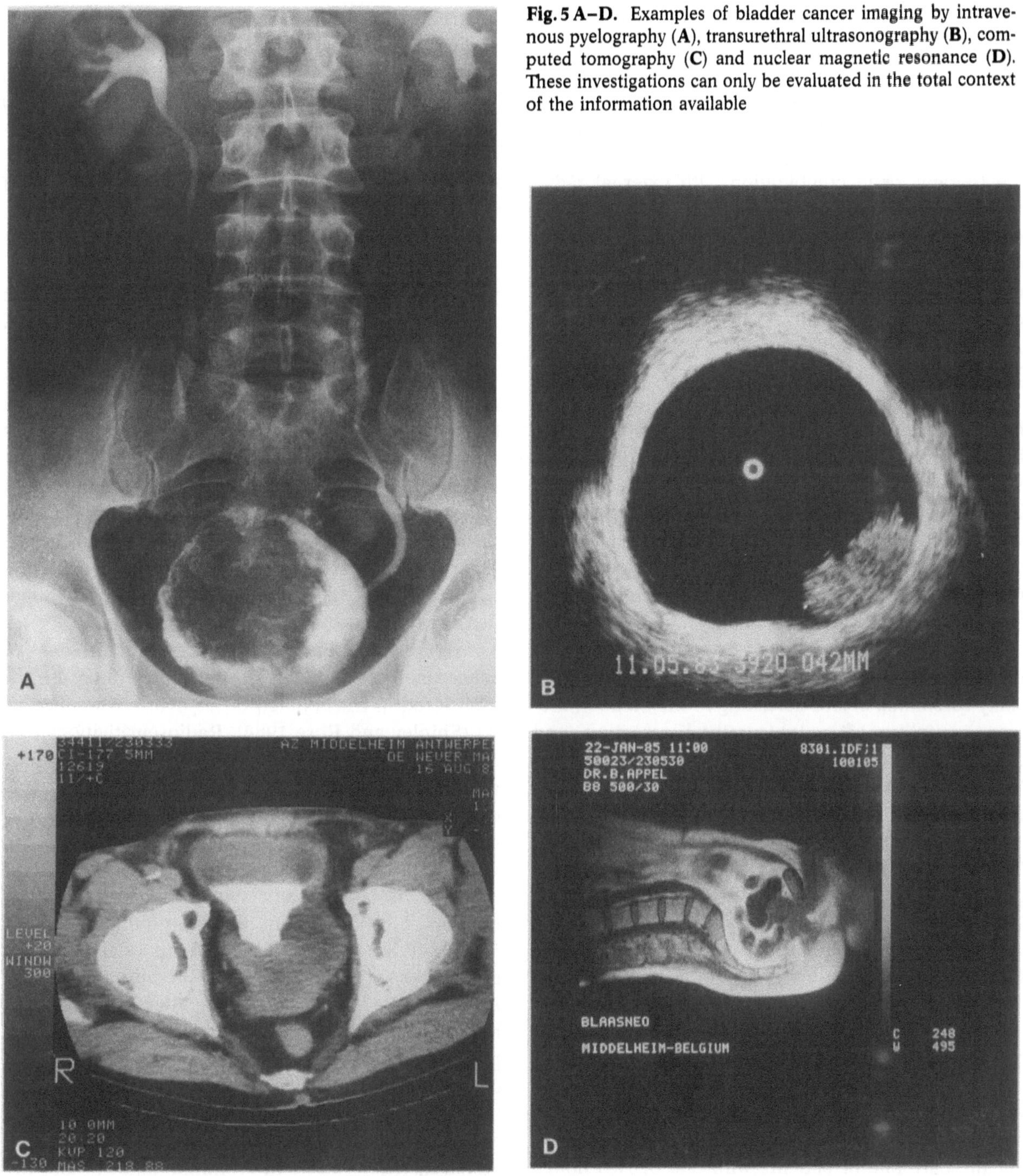

Fig. 5 A–D. Examples of bladder cancer imaging by intravenous pyelography (**A**), transurethral ultrasonography (**B**), computed tomography (**C**) and nuclear magnetic resonance (**D**). These investigations can only be evaluated in the total context of the information available

mour mass and biological behaviour determine the final outcome of disease. More than 80% of grade 3 tumours are associated with muscle invasion (Friedell 1976), and more than 70% of invasive cancers are associated with carcinoma in situ (Prout et al. 1979).

Treatment of a loco-regional nature yields results of less than 50% 5-year survival overall. The popular transurethral resection used alone is suitable for T2 tumours only if they are well differentiated and show papillary invasion on a broad but shallow front. In general, if T2 cases of G2 and G3 grade are included, transurethral resection alone allows progression in nearly 50% of cases in 3 years. The results in higher T categories are worse, and combination with radiotherapy does improve results in selected subsets of patients. Once again, the exception may be the combination of resection and interstitial radiation in selected solitary T3a tumours less than 5 cm in diameter where 5-year survival of 70% has been reported (van der Werf-Messing et al. 1984).

Partial cystectomy (segmental resection) as a single therapy, or in combination with external radiotherapy, is strictly limited to single tumours with negative random biopsies, limited involvement of one ureteric orifice, where resection includes a minimal zone of 2 cm of normal mucosa around the tumour. Despite this, recurrent disease occurs in up to 70% of cases, and overall 5-year survival is 30%–50%.

Cystectomy seems the logical choice for the treatment of invasive bladder cancer still restricted to the bladder. The term "radical cystectomy" is usually reserved for the extirpation of the regional nodes combined with the bladder and its perivesical tissue, with the inclusion of the prostate and seminal vesicles and the urethra in certain cases. Cystectomy as primary treatment is usually indicated for T2 G3, T3 and T4 tumours.

A second indication for cystectomy is limited to treatment failures in superficial bladder cancer, especially carcinoma in situ persisting in the bladder, ureter or urethra after transurethral resection and chemotherapy for accepted periods of time. The term "salvage cystectomy" is reserved for cystectomy after "curative" doses of external radiotherapy.

The mortality rate following cystectomy is 1%–3% in series published in 1982 (Denis et al. 1982). This is probably due to better patient preparation, meticulous operative technique and postoperative care, where minimal requirements involve bowel preparation, peroperative antibiotics and drainage and postoperative intravenous nutrition.

The technique involves a median laparotomy; the removal of the bladder with the prostate and seminal vesicles in males and with the uterus and anterior vaginal wall in females, plus a pelvic lymphadenectomy. The role of careful radical dissection in improving the cure rate in patients with one or two nodes positive is still in doubt: claims are made that radical lymph node removal may cure patients with limited nodal involvement (Skinner 1982). Most reports, however, indicate that positive lymph nodes are an indication of systemic disease. A nerve-sparing cystectomy may be attempted in selected cases. Urethrectomy is performed when the tumour invades the prostate or urethra or the operation is being performed for widespread carcinoma in situ.

The operative morbidity can be serious, especially after radiotherapy: wound infection, fistula, bowel obstruction and the usual complication of extensive surgery requires additional surgery in 10% of cases. Cystectomy by its very nature requires supravesical urinary diversion. A long list of procedures testify that we do not have the perfect diversion. Ureterostomy, transureterocutaneostomy, ileal and colon conduit, ureterosigmoidostomy and bladder replacement by ileum, caecum or rectum have been reported (Sonoda et al. 1986).

The curative results of cystectomy are usually reported as approximately 30% 5-year survival and the maximal results reach 50% (Hohenfellner and Jacobi 1984).

Most surgical research has focused on the continent ileal reservoir as advocated by Kock et al. (1982) popularised by the Mainz or Bern adaptations of the technique. The concept is sound in that a low-pressure, high-capacity reservoir with continent and nonrefluxing valves is produced, but complications resulting in up to 30% of reinterventions have been reported (Skinner et al. 1987). An attractive alternative is of course the internal replacement of the bladder as proposed by Camey and le Duc (1979).

External radiotherapy is also able to cure invasive cancer in about 30% of cases when 50–70 Gy are administered in fractionated doses over a 6-week period (Shipley and Rose 1984). Radiosensitivity can be recognised after 40 Gy by tumour reduction, and for these reasons combined therapy was instituted. Preoperative radiotherapy followed by cystectomy was introduced to reduce tumour burden, diminish the viability of tumour cells and hope for cure of microscopic metastases in adjacent lymph nodes. The reduction of local recurrent disease and the increase of 5-year survival to 50% of the patients established the credentials of this combined therapy (Slack and Prout 1980). However, it has been demonstrated by a randomised trial that cystectomy with and without preoperative irradiation is equally effective in terms of survival (Crawford et al. 1987). No matter what the explanation, the fact remains that both surgery and radiotherapy can only be effective in loco-regional disease (Jakse and Frommhold 1984), and the majority of patients develop distant metastases in the 1st year after diagnosis, which points to common but undetected micrometastases as the overriding cause of treatment failure.

Adjuvant Treatment

The promising results of chemotherapy in disseminated disease (Stoter 1985) have lead to adjuvant therapy with cytotoxic agents after cystectomy and radiotherapy. Early trials were disappointing: adjuvant 5-fluorouracil (5FU), ADM plus 5FU and a combination of methotrexate (MTX), ADM, 5FU and bleomycin have all proved to be ineffective in increasing survival after surgery and/or radiotherapy (Richards et al. 1983; Corder et al. 1984). By contrast, the addition of high-dose MTX after partial cystectomy has been reported to decrease the incidence of local recurrence and increase 3-year survival (Socquet 1981).

Practically all current studies utilise *cis*-platinum which is recognised as the most efficient single agent in the treatment of bladder cancer. The lack of measurable parameters, the toxicity of treatment and the physical condition of the treated patient obstruct proper randomisation which in consequence jeopardises the result of treatment (Prout and Kopp 1984).

To avoid these obstacles and to test the effect of chemotherapy against the untreated primary tumour, the treatment sequence has been reversed and chemotherapy is given before definitive surgery.

This treatment is called "neo-adjuvant" (a misnomer) or upfront chemotherapy. The term "neo-adjuvant" utilised in most publications is considered as primary chemotherapy followed by surgery (Fagg et al. 1984; Denis et al. 1984b, 1986a) or by radiotherapy (Raghavan et al. 1985; Shipley et al. 1987). These first preliminary results were followed by a vast number of phase II trials utilising a selection of combination chemotherapy followed by different types of locoregional treatment (Splinter et al. 1988). All combination chemotherapy includes *cis*-platinum (CDDR) with additional MTX or vinblastine (VBL), ADM or epirubicin treatment in a series of cycles (Denis et al. 1987; Sternberg et al. 1987; Shipley et al. 1987).

These studies have demonstrated that neo-adjuvant chemotherapy is able to downstage invasive bladder cancer to pT0. The pathological complete remission obtained is associated with long-term survival free of disease after initial treatment. The clinical complete response did differ from pathological response as expected. Unfortunately, no benefit of neo-adjuvant chemotherapy could be shown in the non-responding patients. This leaves us with a situation where a subset of patients with invasive bladder tumour might greatly benefit from this type of treatment. Randomised prospective trials are needed to answer questions as to what treatment combination could be most efficient. The obvious advantages of downstaging in up to 30% of the patients has to be balanced against the toxicity in all of the patients treated. A minimal course of chemotherapy to evaluate the response of the untreated primary tumour could be a temporary empirical solution to this complex problem in patients with invasive bladder cancer with poor prognostic factors and acceptable physical condition.

Treatment of Disseminated Disease

Cis-platinum (DDP), MTX, VBL and ADM have been shown to be the most active drugs against metastatic TCC. When used as single agents, they produce an overall remission rate of 20%–30% in phase II trials. However, very few long-lasting remissions have been seen and in real life the term "complete response" is a misnomer as other metastases inevitably appear sooner or later.

Recent combinations of DDP and MTX (Stoter et al. 1986) and MTX, VBL, ADM and *cis*-platinum (Sternberg et al. 1988) appear to be more effective and yield complete remissions of measurable disease in 20% and 30%, respectively. Both regimens are toxic.

Most patients with metastases from bladder cancer die within 6–12 months. Phase II trials usually show increased survival for those patients showing objective evidence of response. Occasionally, this increased survival may be beneficial to the patient and their family, but survival is prolonged by only a few months at best, and this advantage must be weighed up against the treatment toxicity. At the present time, systemic chemotherapy should not be recommended automatically for patients with metastases and should only be used in the context of prospective clinical trials.

Disseminated disease is often associated with very advanced cancer in the pelvis which may cause severe discomfort, haematuria with clot formation, frequency, dysuria and retention of urine. For such patients, local palliative treatment is required. Palliative transurethral resection, external radiotherapy and chemotherapy may each, separately, or in combination bring temporary relief to the patient. Local arterial embolisation or formalin instillations are sometimes effective in stopping bleeding. Urinary diversion is rarely indicated in these circumstances: cystectomy may palliate but usually complicates the last weeks or days of a patient's life by substituting the pain and anxiety of major surgery.

Follow-up

Suberficial Bladder Cancer

Papillary superficial bladder cancer has to be followed for recurrence and progression. A time-honoured schedule to control recurrent disease is a cystoscopy every 3 months during the 1st year, every 4 months during the 2nd year of a disease-free period and, thereafter, every 6–12 months for 5 years. This schedule has been questioned in the event of single papillary G1 tumours. The availability of expert urinary cytology and transabdominal ultrasound may permit less frequent cystoscopy, but, in general, regular cystoscopy is unavoidable.

A second examination is urography which, if normal at diagnosis, can be repeated every 3 years at discretion. It should be stressed that if cystoscopy is negative but cytology is positive, a new urogram should be obtained in every instance.

Carcinoma in situ must be followed meticulously. Urine cytology is essential and flow cytometry may be used if available. Endoscopy is best performed under general or regional anaesthesia since extra biopsies of suggestive lesions are essential, together with inclusion of lesions in the prostate and the urethra.

Invasive Bladder Cancer

All patients treated without cystectomy should undergo the same follow-up schedule as for superficial tumours, with the addition of laboratory studies (haematology, renal and liver function) and examinations for metastases. These tests, with physical examination, enquiry concerning quality of life and a chest X-ray, should be repeated every 3 months for 2 years and then every 6 months for 3 years. Liver ultrasound together with kidney ultrasound and bone scan may be performed less frequently. Abdominal computed tomography scan will be performed 6 and 12 months after surgery and then as indicated. Opportunities should be given on these occasions for the patient to voice his apprehensions and allow an objective evaluation of the psychosocial situation of the patient.

The above schedule is even more important in patients after cystectomy, when all kinds of problems, particularly related to urinary diversion, require the special control and attention of the physician responsible (Neal 1985).

Treatment of Recurrence

Superficial Bladder Cancer

All therapeutic efforts are directed against the well-documented recurrent nature of superficial bladder tumours. After the initial complete endoscopic destruction of all visible tumour, prophylactic instillation with cytotoxic drugs or immunostimulators needs to be carefully considered. A great variety of prognostic factors cause disparity in the results of published phase II trials organised to evaluate prophylactic therapy. An added problem is the definition of recurrence since it is established that surgical destruction is not always complete (Heney et al. 1983). A recurrence at the same place as the original tumour at the time of the first follow-up cystoscopy should be classified as residual disease. All other tumours can be considered as true recurrences or, preferably, new occurrences.

The time interval between the initial complete removal of tumour and the first recurrence is termed "disease-free interval". This parameter, however, only considers the first recurrence and ignores all future recurrences. For this reason results should be presented by utilising the "recurrence rate", which is the total number of occasions when recurrences are found in a group of patients divided by the sum of months of follow-up. The frequently employed "percentage of patients with recurrence" should not be used since it ignores the duration of follow-up which is variable for each series and for each individual patient (Sylvester 1985).

No superiority has been established for any one of the four most commonly used drugs, namely ADM, MMC, TTPA, and epodyl (Denis et al. 1986). Nor has any particular sequence of intravesical treatment been shown as best. Initial weekly therapy followed by monthly instillations are probably necessary as instillation of TTPA only at the time of control cystoscopies has proved to be ineffective (Medical Research Council 1985). The EORTC Genito-Urinary Tract Cooperative (GU) Group has conducted two randomised studies to compare the benefit of early or late instillations and seek to demonstrate if treatment should continue for longer than 6 months. The negative results favour a limited treatment period (Bouffieux et al. 1988).

Because the recurrence of G1 and G2 Ta tumours is low, and the chance of progression appears very small, prophylactic chemotherapy is probably not necessary. By contrast, these risks in G3 T1 tumours are so high that some form of additional treatment is certainly indicated. Good results have been reported for BCG (Morales 1984; Herr et al. 1987), which can be considered an alternative to chemotherapy.

Recurrent disease after intravesical instillation may be treated by instillations with a second drug since tumour ablation, and diminished recurrence rates have been reported by switching TTPA and MMC following failed therapy (Prout et al. 1983).

Invasive Bladder Cancer

Recurrent disease usually spells doom and all efforts should be made to provide optimal therapy at the time of first diagnosis. Tumour recurring after transurethral resection or inadequate partial cystectomy for invasive bladder cancer usually progresses rapidly and definitive treatment with radiation or cystectomy is needed urgently. If radiotherapy, given with curative intent, proves ineffective and invasive disease persists or recurs, "salvage" cystectomy may be effective in a few patients (Blandy et al. 1980). However, the chance of cure is small because metastases are usually developing, and for most patients salvage cystectomy is a palliative procedure. It should be remembered that some patients treated with radiotherapy develop noninvasive recurrences. For this reason regular cystoscopy is worthwhile after radiation and transurethral resection performed when tumours arise. Salvage chemotherapy is seldom beneficial in this situation and remains experimental.

Recurrent disease in the pelvis after cystectomy cannot be excised, and radiotherapy is only palliative. Chemotherapy may be tried, but results after previous surgery are much worse than in untreated patients.

Results of Therapy in Randomised Trials

Superficial Bladder Cancer

The EORTC GU Group has performed a series of randomised trials to evaluate the prophylactic benefit of intravesical chemotherapy after complete removal of the tumour. The studied drugs included TTPA (30 mg), teniposide (VM)-26 (50 mg), ADM (50 mg), epodyl (1.3 g) versus no treatment in two studies. Endpoints of each study focused mainly on the rate of tumour recurrence. Prophylactic treatment was clearly better than no treatment, but no clear superiority could be established for any of the active drugs. The knowledge acquired on prognostic factors permits the identification of subgroups of patients at different risk levels, and new agents such as MMC and BCG, are now being evaluated in randomisations in time and duration of treatment (Denis et al. 1986 b; Herr et al. 1987).

Invasive Bladder Cancer

Radiotherapy can be delivered in different fractionation techniques and combined with subsequent surgery. Attempts at randomised trials have failed to confirm a benefit for preoperative radiotherapy (Bloom et al. 1982; Hall and Heath 1981). No significant difference in survival could be demonstrated in a series of 475 patients, but patients with tumours downstaged by radiotherapy alone survived longer (Slack et al. 1977). While there is no discussion on the benefit of radiotherapy in a subset of patients, the question remains as to whether we may be dealing with a less aggressive tumour biology. Adjuvant therapy has proved even more difficult to analyse in these patients, and no clear advantage has been demonstrated so far in a prospective study. Preoperative chemotherapy awaits evaluation in a prospective fashion after analysis of the ongoing phase II studies (Sylvester et al. 1988).

Rehabilitation

Treatment of bladder cancer has considerable impact on the functional, psychological, social and economic life of the patient. Proper rehabilitation starts with the evaluation of personal values, sexual orientation and subjective assessment of the patient before treatment. All clinical studies should make efforts to evaluate quality of life and consider disease symptoms, side effects of treatment, functional status, psychological distress, sexuality, social interaction and satisfaction with medical treatment. At the time of regular follow-up examinations, symptoms are always recorded, but systematic recording of sexual and social problems is seldom performed. Self-administered questionnaires specifically designed for an older population could provide important information for the final evaluation of therapy. Hospital attendance for intravesical manipulations interrupt lifestyle, often disturb micturition and cause other side effects. Radiotherapy in the short term gives rise to fatigue, malaise, frequent micturition, diarrhoea and rectal irritation plus late side effects which can include contracted bladder, haemorrhagic telangiectasia and gastrointestinal problems.

Systemic chemotherapy causes nausea and vomiting which cannot always be suppressed by supplementary medication. Hair loss is very distressing, and the disturbance of renal and haematopoietic function may prove very toxic. Each drug or combination carries specific side effects. Loss of bladder function, and the need for urinary diversion following total cystectomy requires a particularly well-organised rehabilitation programme including counselling for the almost invariable loss of sexual function. The urinary stoma requires adequate prosthetic devices and specialised care. Most countries have stoma care self-help groups with the backing of stoma care nurses, but psychological adaptation and acquaintance with urinary devices starts with visits to the patient before surgery. Uretero- and transureterocutaneostomy are the least demanding procedures for the patient but require meticulous surgical technique. This type of diversion is usually temporary to save critical operating time but may also be permanent with dilated ureters. Their main disadvantage is stenosis of the ureter at the site of implantation in the skin.

Ureterosigmoidostomy is a time-tested procedure which is reserved for normal ureters and upper tracts and is contraindicated after irradiation to the pelvis and with diverticulosis. Preoperative testing is required, as is special follow-up for electrolyte imbalance by reabsorption and colonoscopy for colonic tumour formation.

Because ureterosigmoidostomy has a high incidence of late complications, the most popular diversion for the last three decades has been the ileal conduit. A segment of ileum, jejunum or colon is isolated and the ureters implanted. The ileal conduit is an adequate diversion if the myriad of minor problems with stoma care are solved for the patient in a satisfactory way. Unfortunately, the many reports of late complications of the upper tract in 30%–60% of the patients stress the importance of a constant follow-up and remind us that no diversion is as good as the patient's bladder. Bladder replacements require the cystectomy to stop at the external sphincter.

Tumours of the Ureter

The aetiological factors and natural history of ureteral tumours are similar to those of bladder cancer. More than 95% of the tumours arise from the urothelium as TCC. About two-thirds are located in the distal portion of the ureter. Multiple tumours can be found in up to 25% of cases. A history of a prior bladder cancer is given in more than 20% of the patients. Urography is the main diagnostic tool giving radiographic changes in up to 80% of cases. Retrograde ureterogram complemented by saline barbotage of the respective ureter yielding a high percentage of malignant cells will be diagnostic in most of the patients. Cystoscopy, mandatory in all patients, will confirm or disclose synchronous bladder cancer. Ureteroscopy, if possible, is becoming the standard diagnostic test in suspected ureteral tumours. Other diagnostic tests such as antegrade pyelography via percutaneous puncture of the renal calyceal system, computed tomography or ultrasound are indicated on rare occasions. Metastatic work-up is obligatory.

Radical surgery, including complete removal of kidney, ureter, bladder cuff and periorganic adipose tissue (perifascial nephroureterectomy), as well as regional lymphadenectomy, is considered the surgical therapy of choice in multiple or high-stage tumours. The overall 5-year survival rate is about 60%. Conservative surgery has been reported with increasing frequency. Distal ureteric tumours (pelvic portion) can be resected by removing a bladder cuff. The resulting defect is bridged by means of psoas hitch or Boari technique. This approach is feasible in tumours of all stages of the distal ureter, whereas conservative management, i.e. ureteral resection and end-to-end anastomosis, should only be considered in a small solitary low-grade tumour in other sections of the ureter. Ureteral tumours arising in a single kidney should be treated as a special problem, and several operative procedures, such as intestinal interposition, renal autotransplantation, prosthesis, etc., depend on the patient's age and general condition and the surgeon's preference and experience. Bilateral tumours are rare and should also be treated in a very individualised manner.

Follow-up investigations should include cystoscopy, urine cytology, sonography of the tumour bed and metastatic work-up. Urography and ureteroscopy in selected cases should be done once a year to detect asymptomatic tumours of the residual renal unit (Jakse and Marberger 1985).

Tumours of the Urethra

Primary malignant tumours of the urethra are rare. However, in patients with transitional cell carcinoma undergoing cystectomy the incidence of urethral tumours is about 4%–12%. Carcinoma in situ or atypical urothelium are found in as many as 18% of the autopsy cases. This percentage increases in those patients who died of multifocal bladder cancer.

In the case of a patient undergoing radical cystectomy without urethrectomy, regular follow-up examination with urethral washings and/or urethroscopy are necessary.

Papillary growths of the prostatic urethra can be managed effectively by transurethral resection. Although these lesions do not occur often, a careful endoscopy of the total urethra is mandatory in all patients followed for bladder cancer.

Future Development

The recognition that TCC can degenerate into two different pathways of tumour formation is a turning point in the treatment and research of bladder cancer. It underlines the fact that all aspects of a newly diagnosed bladder cancer should be properly evaluated and organised to lead to treatment decisions based upon hard clinical data. This evaluation should be sought in consensus opinion, especially with regard to the histo- and cytopathology of the tumour, and its clinical work-up, which should enable the medical community to compare the clinical results of treatment (Denis 1986 c).

Clinical research is to be seen as prospective. Randomised trials will focus primarily on new concepts derived from the complete work-up before treatment of preneoplastic lesions, grading methodology, tumour markers and therapeutic approaches to cure. Chemotherapy given in a systemic fashion will be most important in the treatment of invasive tumours. Basic research will focus on the nature of normal and cancerous urothelial cells with emphasis on the basic mechanisms of markers to define the biological potential of the tumour. This programme should be completed by the evaluation of animal and in vitro models both for superficial and invasive bladder cancer.

References

Beahrs OH, Myers MH (1983) Manual for staging of cancer. American Joint Committee on Cancer. Lippincott, Philadelphia

Blandy JP, England HR, Evans SJW, Hope-Stone HF, Mair GMM, Mantell BS, Oliver RTD, Paris AMI, Risdon RA (1980) T3 bladder cancer – the case for salvage cystectomy. Br J Urol 52: 506–510

Bloom HGH, Hendry WF, Wallace DM, Skeet RG (1982) Treatment of T3 bladder cancer: controlled trial of preoperative radiotherapy and radical cystectomy versus radical radiotherapy. Br J Urol 54: 136–151

Bouffieux C, Denis L, Kurth KH, de Paine M, Sylvester R et le groupe genitourinaire de l'EORTC (1988) Quel chimiotherapie intravesicale pour quelle tumeur de vessie. J Urol (Paris) (in print)

Camey M, le Duc A (1979) L'enterocystoplastie après cystectomie totale pour cancer de la vessie. Ann Urol (Paris) II: 642–658

Corder MP, McFadden DB, Stump DC (1984) Chemotherapy of advanced transitional cell carcinoma of the bladder. In: Smith PH, Prout GR Jr (eds) Bladder cancer – urology I. Butterworths International Medical Reviews, London, pp 240–276

Crawford ED, Das S, Smith JA (1987) Preoperative radiation therapy in the treatment of bladder cancer. Urol Clin North Am 14: 781–787

Cutler SJ, Heney NM, Friedell GH (1982) Longitudinal study of patients with bladder cancer: factors associated with disease recurrence and progression. In: Bonney WW (ed) AUA monographs, vol I: Bladder cancer. Williams and Wilkins, Baltimore, pp 35–46

Dalesio O, Schulman CC, Sylvester R, de Pauw M, Robinson M, Denis L, Smith P, Viggiano G, members of the EORTC Genito-Urinary Tract Cooperative Group (1983) Prognostic factors in superficial bladder tumors. A study of the European Organization for Research on Treatment of Cancer Genito-Urinary Tract Cooperative Group. J Urol 129: 730–733

Denis L (1987) Deeply invasive transitional cell carcinoma. In: Resnick MI, Kursh E (eds) Current therapy in genito-urinary surgery. Decker, Toronto, pp 63–69

Denis L, Smith P, Pavone-Macaluso M (1982) Clinical bladder cancer. Plenum, New York

Denis L, Braeckman J, Keuppens F (1984 a) Ultrasonography and computed tomography in the staging of bladder and prostate cancer. In: Kurth K, Debruyne F, Schröder F, Splinter T, Wagener T (eds) Progress and controversies in oncological urology. Liss, New York, pp 3–21

Denis L, Hendrickx G, Braeckman J, Debruyne R (1984 b) Interest of preoperative chemotherapy in the treatment of infiltrative bladder cancer. Acta Urol Belg 52: 579–582

Denis L, Murphy G, Prout G, Schröder F (1984 c) Controlled clinical trials in urologic oncology. Raven, New York

Denis L, Dalesio O, van Oosterom AT (1986 b) Bladder cancer. In: Slevin ML, Staquet MJ (eds) Randomized trials in cancer: a critical review by sites. Raven, New York, pp 645–660

Denis L, Niijima T, Prout GR, Schröder F (eds) (1986 b) Developments in bladder cancer. Liss, New York

Denis L, Calais de Silva F, Hendrickx G (1988) Preoperative chemotherapy in T3 T4 NX M0 bladder cancer with cisplatin and methotrexate. In: Smith PH, Pavone-Macaluso M (eds) Management of advanced cancer of the prostate and bladder. Liss, New York, pp 571–577

Fagg SL, Dawson-Edwards P, Hughes MA, Latief TN, Rolfe EB, Fielding JWL (1984) Cisplatinum (DDP) as initial treatment of invasive bladder cancer. Br J Urol 56: 296

Friedell GH (1976) Carcinoma, carcinoma in situ and "early lesions" of the uterine and the urinary bladder: introduction and definitions. Cancer Res 36: 2482–2484

Hall RR, Heath AB (1981) Radiotherapy and cystectomy for T3 bladder cancer. Br J Urol 53: 598–601

Hall RR, Newling DWW, Ramsden PD, Richards B, Robinson MRG, Smith PH (1984) Treatment of invasive bladder cancer by local resection and high dose methotrexate. Br J Urol 56: 668–672

Heney NM, Ahmed S, Flanagan MJ, Frable W, Corder MP, Haferman MD, Hawkings IR (1983) Superficial bladder cancer: progression and recurrence. J Urol 130: 1083–1086

Hermanek P, Sobin LH (1987) TNM classification of malignant tumours. Springer, Berlin Heidelberg New York

Herr H, Landone VP, Whitmore FW Jr (1987) An overview of intravesical chemotherapy for superficial bladder tumours. J Urol 138: 1363–1368

Hohenfellner RH, Jacobi GH (1984) Radical cystectomy without preoperative radiotherapy for invasive bladder carcinoma: a justified approach? In: Kurth KH, Debruyne FMJ, Schröder FH, Splinter TAW, Wagener TDJ (eds) Progress and controversies in oncological urology. Liss, New York, pp 313–342

Jakse G, Frommhold H (1984) Combined radiation and chemotherapy for locally advanced bladder cancer. In: Kurth KH, Debruyne F, Schröder F, Splinter T, Wagener T (eds) Progress and controversies in oncological urology. Liss, New York, pp 365–372

Jakse G, Marberger H (1985) Culp D, Loening S (eds) Tumours of the ureter in genito-urinary oncology. Lea and Fehger, Philadelphia, p 277

Jakse G, Hofstädter F, Leitner G (1980) Carcinoma in situ der Harnblase. Urologe [A] 19: 93–99

Kock NG (1971) Ileostomy without external appliances. Ann Surg 173: 545–566

Koss LG, Deitch D, Ramanathan R, Sherman A (1985) Diagnostic value of cytology of voided urine. Acta Cytol (Baltimore) 29: 810–816

Kurth KH (1984) Superficial TCC bladder cancer: the impact of tumor differentiation on recurrence, progression and survival. In: Küss R, Khoury S, Denis L, Murphy GP, Karr JP (eds) Bladder cancer. A. Pathology, diagnosis and surgery. Liss, New York, pp 307–318

Medical Research Council Working Party on Urological Cancer (1985) The effect of intravesical thiotepa on the recurrence rate of newly diagnosed superficial bladder cancer: an MRC study. Br J Urol 57: 680–685

Miyakawa M, Raghavan D, Riedl H, Robinson MRG, Worden JN (1986) Quality of life assessment in bladder cancer clinical trials: conceptual, methodological and practical issues. In: Denis L, Niijima T, Prout GR, Schröder F (eds) Consensus in bladder cancer. Liss, New York, pp 149–170

Morales A (1984) Long term results and complications of intracavitary bacillus Calmette-Guérin therapy for bladder cancer. J Urol 132: 452–457

Neal DE (1985) Complications of ileal conduit diversion in adults with cancer followed up for at least five years. Br Med J [Clin Res] 290: 1695–1697

Niijima T, Nakamura S (1982) Transurethral ultrasonography: bladder cancer staging and other clinical application. In: Denis L, Smith PH, Pavone-Macaluso M (eds) Clinical bladder cancer. Plenum, New York, pp 47–54

Powell PH, Manohar V, Ramsden PD, Hall RR (1984) A flexible cystoscope. Br J Urol 56: 622–624

Prout GR Jr, Kopp J (1984) Evaluation and management of patients with primary bladder carcinoma protocols of the NBCP Collaborative Group A. In: Denis L, Murphy G, Prout G, Schröder F (eds) Controlled clinical trials. Raven, New York, pp 221–240

Prout GR Jr, Griffin PP, Shipley WU (1979) Bladder carcinoma as a systemic disease. Cancer 43: 2532–2539

Prout GR Jr, Koontz WW Jr, Coombs LJ, Hawkings IR, Friedell GH for the National Bladder Collaborative Group A (1983) Long term fate of 90 patients with superficial bladder cancer randomly assigned to receive or not receive thiotepa. J Urol 130: 677–680

Raghavan D, Pearson B, Duval P, Rogers J, Meagher M, Wines R, Mameghan H, Boulas J, Green D (1985) Initial intravenous cisplatinum therapy: improved management for invasive high risk bladder cancer? J Urol 133: 399–402

Richards B, Schröder F (1983) Superficial bladder tumours. Liss, New York

Richards B, Bastable JR, Freedman L, Glashan RW, Harris G, Newling W, Robinson MR, Smith PH (1983) Adjuvant chemotherapy with doxorubicin (adriamycin) and 5-fluorouracil in T3 NX M0 bladder cancer treated with ratiotherapy. Br J Urol 55: 386–391

Richards B, Aso Y, Bollack C, Fossa S, Koontz W, Matsuda M, Matsumoto K, Prout G, van der Werf-Messing B, Wolf H (1986) Prognostic factors in infiltrating bladder cancer. In: Denis L, Niijima T, Prout GR, Schröder F (eds) Developments in bladder cancer. Liss, New York, pp 271–286

Shipley WV, Rose MA (1984) Bladder cancer. The selection of patients for full-dose irradiation. Cancer 55: 2278–2284

Shipley WV, Prout GR Jr, Einstein AB (1987) Treatment of invasive bladder cancer by cisplatin and irradiation in patients unsuited for surgery. JAMA 258: 931–937

Skinner DG (1982) Management of invasive bladder cancer: a meticulous pelvic node dissection can make a difference. J Urol 128: 34–36

Skinner D, Lieskorsky G, Boyd SD (1987) Continuing experience with the continent ileal reservoir (Kock pouch) as an alternative to cutaneous urinary diversion: an update after 250 cases. J Urol 137: 1140–1145

Slack NH, Prout GR (1980) The heterogeneity of invasive bladder carcinoma and different responses to treatment. J Urol 123: 644–652

Slack NH, Bross IDJ, Prout GR Jr (1977) Five year follow-up results of a collaborative study of therapies for carcinoma of the bladder. J Surg Oncol 9: 393–405

Socquet Y (1981) Combined surgery and adjuvant chemotherapy with high dose methotrexate and folinic acid rescue (HDMTX-CF) for infiltrating tumours of the bladder. Br J Urol 53: 439–443

Soloway M, Kurth KH, Herr H, Huland H, Denis L, Suzuki K, Blandy J, Hisazumi H, Koontz W, Tsugawa R (1986) Surgical techniques in the management of patients with superficial bladder cancer. In: Denis L, Niijima T, Prout GR, Schröder F (eds) Developments in bladder cancer. Liss, New York, pp 123–132

Sonoda T, Debruyne FMJ, Prout GR Jr, Matsuda M, Blandy JP, Hohenfellner R, Keuppens F, Matsumoto K, Ogata J, Whitmore WF Jr (1986) Surgical techniques in invasive bladder cancer. In: Denis L, Niijima T, Prout GR, Schröder F (eds) Developments in bladder cancer. Liss, New York, pp 138–148

Sternberg CN, Yagoda A, Scher HI, Watson RC, Herr HW, Sogoni PC, Morse MJ, Fair WR, Whitmore WF, Vaughan ED, Bander N, Weiselberg LR, Geller N, Hollander PS (1988) M-VAC for advanced transitional cell carcinoma of urothelium. J Urol 139: 461–469

Stoter G (1985) Chemotherapy for metastatic bladder carcinoma. World J Urol 3: 110–114

Stoter G, Child JA, Fossa SD, Boven E, Denis L, Splinter WG, van Oosterom AT, de Pauw M, Sylvester R for the EORTC Genito-Urinary Group (1987) Combination chemotherapy with cisplatin (CDDP) and methotrexate (MTX) in advanced transitional cell cancer of the bladder. J Urol 137: 663–667

Sylvester R (1985) The analysis of results in prophylactic superficial bladder cancer. In: Schröder FH, Richards B (eds) Superficial bladder tumours. Liss, New York, pp 3–11

Sylvester TAW, ten Kate FJW, Schröder FH, Denis L, Newling D, Jones WG, Jacquimin D, Becker-Kruger CGG, Sloter G, de Voegt HJ, de Paine M (1988) Neo-adjuvant chemotherapy in T3–4 N0-X M0 transitional cell carcinoma of the bladder. In: Khoury S, Murphy G, Chatelain C, Dews L (eds) Therapeutic progress in urological cancers. Liss, New York (in print)

Van der Werf-Messing B (1983) Radiation therapy of carcinoma of the urinary bladder in clinical bladder cancer. In: Denis L, Murphy G, Prout G, Schröder F (eds) Controlled clinical trials in urologic oncology. Raven, New York, pp 83–89

Van der Werf-Messing B, Menon RS, Hopp WC (1984) Interstitial radiotherapy of carcinoma of the bladder at the Rotterdam Radiotherapy Institute (RRTI). In: Küss R, Khoury S, Denis L, Murphy G, Karr JP (eds) Bladder cancer. Liss, New York, pp 71–85

Whitmore WF, Batata MA, Ghoneim MA, Grabstald H, Unal A (1977) Radical cystectomy with or without prior irradiation in the treatment of bladder cancer. J Urol 118: 184–187

Wolf H, Olsen PR, Højgaard K (1985) Urothelial dysplasia concomitant with bladder tumours as a determinant factor for future new occurrences in patients treated with full course radiotherapy. Lancet I: 1005

Carcinoma of the Prostate

F. H. SCHROEDER

Introduction

In most countries of the western world, prostatic carcinoma is the second most frequent cause of cancer death among males. In spite of great efforts throughout the world, the proportion of men dying from this, in many respects puzzling, disease has not changed very much in recent years. Management of prostatic carcinoma has remained controversial throughout the world for several reasons that will be explained in some detail. Prior to the great contributions of Huggins and Hodges (1941), which resulted in the introduction into clinical routine of endocrine management of prostatic carcinoma, the treatment of this tumor was purely symptomatic. In subsequent years, treatment of prostatic cancer patients by estrogens and/or castration became standard treatment. The evidence of the effectiveness of this treatment, resulting from mostly retrospective studies throughout the world, was considered so convincing that for the following 25 years no major clinical research impulses aimed at further objectivating the effect of this management.

Patients with prostatic carcinoma seemed to be in an exceptional position because, different from other human malignancies, there was something that could be done effectively about this tumor in the disseminated stage. It was generally believed that endocrine management, besides offering good palliation, would also lead to prolongation of life. The data published by the Veterans Administration Cooperative Urological Research Group (VACURG; 1967), which initially indicated that, in comparison to placebo treatment in a prospective randomized study, endocrine treatment would offer a delay of progression but no prolongation of life, therefore came as a great surprise. In addition to the timing, the optimal way of endocrinologically managing prostatic carcinoma is also still up for discussion. The controversy culminates in the question as to whether complete androgen withdrawal will produce better clinical results than castration only. Also, the role of estrogens in prostatic cancer tissue and their exploitation for therapeutic purposes is still entirely unclear.

There is an appreciable difference in the prognosis of patients with disseminated and locally confined prostatic carcinoma which seems to be independent of treatment. Still, there is no clear evidence that aggressive management of locally confined prostatic carcinoma results in a significant prolongation of life. The reasons for this discrepancy are not clearly understood at present. There is little doubt that there is a great variance in the aggressiveness of individual tumors. On the other hand, due to the age group involved, competing and unrelated causes of death play an important role.

Much of the controversy concerning the proper management of locally confined disease as well as of metastatic disease must be seen against the background of the fact that only 25%–50% of patients suffering from this disease will usually die *of* prostatic carcinoma. Unfortunately, the multifactorial problem of identifying those patients that are at risk and selecting them for more aggressive treatment has still not been solved. A solution is not foreseeable in the near future.

For these reasons it seems understandable that points of view that are often related to the quality of the patient's life and not to the risk presented by the tumor play a role in treatment decisions to be taken. It is only logical that such considerations will result in different answers.

Much clinically oriented basic research has been carried out in the field of prostatic cancer. This has mainly concentrated on pathological aspects, the development of proper prognostic factors and response criteria, the development of experimental models for this tumor, the mechanisms of endocrine dependence, and the mechanisms and changes that occur with hormone-independent growth of prostatic cancer. This research has greatly contributed to a better understanding and to a better classification of this disease. It has, however, not led to a prolongation of life. An important improvement of the prognosis of our patients can only result from a better understanding of the mechanisms that eventually lead to hormone-independent growth of prostatic cancer. Genetic instability and clonal selection have been pointed out as the major factors that seem to be involved. It seems that an important step forward in the management of this disease can only be made if either transition from the hormone-dependent to the hormone-independent state can be controlled in some way or if, in addition to the endocrine-dependent part of each individual tumor, also the hormone independent cell populations can be managed effectively by means of cytostatic drugs.

Epidemiology

Definitions

For proper understanding of many epidemiological and clinical aspects of prostatic carcinoma, it is important to understand and to use correctly some of the terms that describe the various stages at which the disease is commonly diagnosed during life or at postmortem examination. Much like other tumors, especially carcinoma of the breast, prostatic carcinoma is frequently encountered at autopsy, without ever having led to clinical symptoms. Such tumors are commonly called "latent" if they are locally confined to the prostate and "occult" if metastases are present. Prostatic carcinoma is named "focal carcinoma" if one or more small foci are encountered at routine examination of the organ at autopsy or after surgical removal of prostatic hyperplasia for obstruction. Various definitions of focal carcinoma are available in the literature. Usually, a microscopic carcinoma is considered focal if it does not exceed the size of one to three microscopic fields at a magnification of 200. The important issue is the differentiation of the focal tumor from the locally more extensive carcinoma. This becomes a crucial issue whenever a focal carcinoma is diagnosed clinically at the time of treatment of benign prostatic hyperplasia (BPH). In this case, one speaks of an "incidental carcinoma" whenever prostatic carcinoma is found histologically whereas a careful rectal examination revealed no abnormality. In this case, the delineation of the true focal tumor from the locally extensive incidental carcinoma is of great clinical importance. This issue will be discussed later on in this chapter. Prostatic carcinoma is termed "clinical" whenever the tumor can be detected by routine diagnostic measures such as rectal examination, determination of serum prostatic acid phosphatase, bone scan, etc.

Incidence and Mortality

In speaking about the incidence of prostatic cancer, one again has to differentiate clearly between the incidence of clinical carcinoma, the incidence of focal tumors, and the incidence of latent or occult carcinomas found at autopsy. The differences in the incidence of focal tumors found at autopsy or at clinical studies of BPH is of great epidemiological and clinical importance. On the one hand, the focal tumor must be considered the precursor of all clinical cancer; on the other hand, the incidence of focal tumors is so much higher that a different etiology for both lesions is very probable. For the pathogenesis of clinical carcinoma, the following simple scheme is generally agreed upon:

Focal carcinoma→promoting factors→clinical carcinoma, hormone dependent→promoting factors →clinical carcinoma, hormone independent.

The pathogenesis of hormone-independent prostatic carcinoma which ultimately leads to the death of our patients requires, according to this scheme, at least two mutational steps.

The factors promoting focal carcinoma to clinical carcinoma may vary geographically. This may explain the great differences that are encountered in the incidence of clinical carcinoma in various parts of the world. The lowest incidence rates are found in Asian countries like China, Japan, and Singapore, where in 1975 four to five males per 100 000 were found to have clinical carcinoma. Chinese and Japanese living in Hawaii at the same time had incidence rates of 26 and 36 per 100 000 male inhabitants. The increasing incidence of prostatic cancer in migrants from regions with a very low incidence to regions with a higher incidence was recognized by Haenszel and Kurihara (1968) and Akazaki and Stemmermann (1973). This observation indicates that the differences found in various regions are not only due to racial characteristics but also to environmental promoting factors.

Zaridze et al. (1984) described an increase in the incidence of prostatic carcinoma amounting to 2%–6% in most countries of the Western world for the years between 1960 and 1975. During the same period of time, prostatic cancer mortality has also been increasing in the same countries. There are a few exceptions, including Egypt and Barbados. Table 1 shows mortality rates in various countries of various regions of the world in decreasing order. The northern European countries are only surpassed by the Black population of the United States and of some Caribbean islands. It is evident that the lowest mortality rates are found in some Oriental countries.

Incidence and mortality of prostatic carcinoma also very strongly depend on age. Table 2 shows the incidence and mortality of prostatic cancer in the Netherlands in 1975–1976. Beside the clear increase with age, which has been shown to be exponential, it is evident that in the total population, mortality is almost one-third less than the incidence. If one considers the age groups from 55 to 79, in which about 75% of all tumors were diagnosed, the mortality rates amount to an average of 56% of the incidence. Of the total population of 2169 cases, 1560 or 71% died of prostatic carcinoma. The most relevant reason for this phenomenon lies in the fact that, inherent to the age groups involved, competing causes of death, especially from cardiovascular reasons, play an important role. Patients tend to die with their disease rather than from their disease.

On the whole, in most Western countries the incidence of prostatic carcinoma amounts to 10% of all malignancies in the male. This makes, in most cancer statistics, prostatic carcinoma the second most frequent male malignancy, which is only surpassed by carcinoma of the lung. Complete reviews of the epidemiology of cancer of the prostate have recently been published by Wynder et al. (1977) and Flanders (1984). The peculiar relationship between focal carcinoma, locally extensive latent carcinoma, and age has been subject to several studies among which the one by Breslow et al. (1977) and the one by Cohen et al. (1985) may be interesting for review.

Table 1. Age-standardized prostate cancer mortality rates per 100 000 inhabitants by country. (Data from American Cancer Society 1975)

Country	Mortality rate
Sweden	18
Netherlands	15
Federal Republic of Germany	14
United States	14
England	12
Italy	10
Chile	10
Israel	7
Greece	6
Hong Kong	4
Japan	4
Taiwan	1

Table 2. Incidence and mortality rate of malignant neoplasms of the prostate by age, 1975–1976. (Figures are given per 100 000 of the average Dutch male population.) (Data from Centraal Bureau voor de Statistiek 1979)

Age	Incidence (absolute)	Incidence	Mortality rate
40–44	2	0.5	–
45–49	7	1.9	0.5
50–54	33	9.2	2.8
55–59	69	22.5	8.8
60–64	175	63.0	24.8
65–69	345	149.0	74.9
70–74	475	269.1	156.0
75–79	508	440.7	294.4
80–84	354	533.0	521.0
85+	201	518.9	815.8
	2169	31.8	22.8

Risk Factors

It is obvious from the geographical differences observed throughout the world and the migrant studies cited above that risk factors play an important role in the promotion of prostatic carcinoma from the focal to the clinical state. The major epidemiological lead in explaining the differences between Oriental and Western countries may be diet. The total fat consumption in Oriental countries amounts to less than 20% of that of Western countries. A recent study in the United States has shown that overweight men had a significantly higher risk of fatal prostatic cancer. In the same study by Snowdon et al. (1984) the heavy use of milk, cheese, eggs, and meat produced suggestive positive associations toward fatal prostatic cancer.

In spite of suggestive differences (stature, hair growth, and hair distribution) between oriental and western races, no endocrinological differences have been found between such races that might contribute to the explanation of differences in incidence of prostatic carcinoma. It is, however, possible that this problem has not been studied sufficiently. Like prostatic hyperplasia, prostatic carcinoma seems to be extremely rare in males whose plasma testosterone is at castration level.

Some occupational hazards have been identified. These result mainly from industrial exposure to cadmium and other heavy metal ions. Sexual habits, socioeconomic status, sexual frustration, and a number of other possible risk factors are reviewed in the epidemiological literature cited above. A recent report by Kroes et al. (1986) indicates an experimental approach to the study of dietary risk factors in prostate carcinogenesis which may be helpful in the future and which may lead to a preventive approach in the management of this tumor.

Histopathology and Grade of Malignancy

Origin and Localization

Adenocarcinoma of the prostate originates from the prostatic epithelium, usually of the peripheral zone of the prostate. The peripheral zone, in the anatomical understanding of this organ by McNeal (1969), is located close to the fibrous capsule of the prostate. McNeal (1981) differentiates between two different pathways for the progressive evolution of lesions to prostatic carcinoma. The first type of atypical development consists of intraductal hyperplasia with progressive nuclear atypicality. The second form of premalignant change originates from repeated budding and branching of new acini without nuclear atypicality. BPH develops in the transition zone and the periurethral region in the system of McNeal. BPH and carcinoma of the prostate frequently occur in the same patient. A transition from BPH to prostatic carcinoma is, however, unlikely. The frequent coincidence of both lesions seems to be based on their frequency and similar age distribution.

Premalignant changes can be frequently seen in the prostate and can be easily confused with focal carcinoma. This was pointed out by Kastendieck et al. (1976). These authors characterized dysplasia carefully by morphological means and, much like McNeal (1981), relate dysplastic lesions to an immature metaplastic cell type often found in the prostate. The differentiation of dysplastic lesions from focal carcinoma is difficult and may lead to clinical confusion as has been pointed out by Brawn (1982).

Several studies are available in the literature that deal with the localization of the malignant lesion within the prostate. Two of these studies, both dealing with radical prostatectomy specimens, will be referred to in this context. Kastendieck et al. (1976) and Kastendieck (1980) report on a study of 50 total prostatectomy specimens. In this study 98% of the tumors were localized either in the peripheral zone of the prostate alone or in the peripheral and the central zone. Only one tumor (2%) was localized in the central part of the prostate only. Penetration of the capsule was seen in 80%, and infiltration of the seminal vesicles in 24% of the cases. In 60% of all cases, the tumor was multifocal within the gland.

Byar et al. (1972) reported on 208 radical prostatectomy specimens. In 85% of their cases, prostatic carcinoma was multifocal within the gland. Of all the tumors, 94% were detected in the outer subcapsular (peripheral) zone. A total of 109 tumors were located both centrally and peripherally. Only one tumor was located centrally. Capsular invasion was common and depended on the total tumor volume within the gland. Of all cases 84% showed perineural invasion. This was considered to be an early event in the development of invasive prostatic carcinoma which did not have prognostic impact in these patients.

Both groups used a step-sectioning technique of the whole organ. The fact that prostatic carcinoma originates exclusively close to the prostatic capsule in the peripheral zone leads to palpable changes of the dorsal surface of the prostate and makes the tumor detectable by rectal examination.

Grade of Malignancy

Prostatic carcinoma occurs in different histomorphological architecture which may be more or less closely related to the histology of the tissue of origin. Besides variation in architecture, there is also a variation in the size and shape of the cells, the nuclei, and the nucleoli (anaplasia). In most prostatic carcinomas, up to four different architectural patterns can be detected (pleomorphism). The pattern of growth and the histological or cytological appearance of the nucleus are related to the prognosis of the individual patient. Systematic attempts to correlate these variations in histomorphology to the prognosis of the individual patient are called "grading".

Various systems which are all based on either variations in the architecture and/or variations in the appearance of cells and nuclei have been created and reported in the literature. Probably most commonly used in clinical practice is the system by Gleason et al. (1974) which applies exclusively the architectural parameters of a maximum of two different patterns present in each tumor. This system, much like others, has been shown to correlate closely with prognosis, as has been impressively shown by Gleason et al. (1977). Other grading systems, like the one proposed by Mostofi (1975) and by Gaeta (1981) use architectural as well as cytological parameters for grading. It has been shown by Esposti (1971) and subsequently by many others that grading is also possible on the basis of purely cytological criteria on specimens obtained by means of fine needle aspiration biopsy.

The problem of all grading systems has been intra- and interobserver reproducibility. With most systems using three, four, or five different grades of malignancy, lack of reproduction of the original grading by the same pathologist or a different pathologist by one or even two steps in the various systems is not uncommon. Interobserver variability comparing different systems has recently been studied by Ten Kate et al. (1986). This study revealed large differences when five different grading systems were cross-examined by five experienced pathologists. The Gleason system in this study turned out to be the most reproducible way of grading.

In a recent study Schroeder et al. (1985) have examined in a multivariate analysis the various parameters that are commonly used in grading prostatic carcinoma. This study comes to the conclusion that only three parameters, architecture, nuclear anaplasia, and mitoses, are independent variables with prognostic impact. These authors also conclude that the fraction of any given tumor with the poorest differentiation determines the prognosis independently of its size. This casts some doubt on the Gleason system which neglects poorly differentiated tumor of small size in the presence of two larger fractions of better differentiation.

The problems around the reproducibility of histological grading on one side, and the certainty of the strong prognostic correlation of the grade of malignancy on the other have led to several attempts to automate the process of grading. Diamond et al. (1982) have applied morphometrical techniques to the evaluation of the nuclei of prostatic cancer cells. They found a correlation of a nuclear roundness factor, which is representative of nuclear anaplasia, with the prognosis of 17 patients after radical prostatectomy. This correlation was stronger than conventional grading. Benson and Walsh (1986) applied flow cytometry to biopsy and radical prostatectomy specimens. They found a very close correlation with a newly developed flow-cytometric grading index with local tumor extension. The future will have to show whether automated systems will lead to a more accurate and more reproducible way of determining the malignant potential of individual prostatic carcinomas.

Rarely, prostatic carcinomas occur that do not originate from the glandular epithelium of the peripheral zone. They all represent different but quite rare entities.

Prostatic adenocarcinomas of ductal origin (ductal carcinoma) have been the subject of several publications, including the one by Greene et al. (1979). The tumor arises from primary or secondary prostatic ducts and has distinct histological features. In many respects, including acid phosphatase production, the tumor corresponds to prostatic adenocarcinomas. Usually there is, however, no hormone responsiveness. The recommended treatment is radical excision.

Primary transitional cell carcinoma of the prostate originates from the transitional epithelium of the prostatic urethra. The simultaneous presence of carcinoma of the bladder infiltrating the prostate must be carefully excluded. These tumors do not respond to hormonal management, their prognosis is poor if radical excision fails. Radiotherapy did not reveal favorable results in a series by Kirk et al. (1979). Other entities are the leiomyosarcoma and the rhabdomyosarcoma of the prostate gland and the papillary and mucus-forming adenocarcinomas of the prostate.

Natural History

The natural history of a disease is best described by its natural course without any interference by treatment. The natural course of any disease will be determined by factors that characterize the prognosis of an individual tumor and host factors that may interfere. Much like the effect of treatment, the natural course can be defined by the rate of disease progression in time and by survival figures. In the case of prostatic carcinoma, where many other causes of death may interfere, survival figures that are corrected for intercurrent disease are particularly useful.

The effect of any management by means of surgical or conservative measures should in some way correct and improve the natural course of this disease. Treatment only makes sense if significant improvement can be achieved as far as the rate of progression, the rate of survival, and the comfort of the patient are concerned.

The classical article on the natural history of prostatic carcinoma was undoubtedly the one written by Whitmore (1973). For all practical purposes, he shows that it is wise to consider the incidentally found latent carcinoma, the locally confined tumor, and the metastatic tumor as separate disease entities. Because of their exceedingly high frequency, incidentally found latent carcinoma of the prostate (stage A) cannot be considered as usually progressing to the higher stages. On the other hand, the much lower incidence of locally confined carcinoma (stage B, 10%) and other clinical observations suggest that there is direct progression of some of the clinically occult tumors to locally progressive and even metastatic states. Locally invasive prostatic carcinoma with capsular penetration is diagnosed, according to Whitmore's large literature survey, in roughly 40% of the cases. About half of these patients will have lymph node metastases if investigated further. Roughly 50% of all cases documented in this survey show evidence of metastatic disease.

The more recent data of the surveys of the American College of Surgeons on prostatic cancer, published by Mettlin et al. (1982), show a tendency toward more frequent early diagnosis. In this report, incidental carcinoma (state A) amounted to 23%, locally confined palpable lesions (stage B) to 33.9%, locally extensive (stage C) disease to 19.5%, and metastatic tumors (stage D) to 23.6%. In this survey, which deals with almost 20000 patients, there is clearly a shift to more frequent early diagnosis of this disease in the United States.

Still, considering our lack of understanding of the way prostatic cancer progresses in morphology, its biological potential to metastasize, and its development from small to larger local lesions, it remains wise to consider separately the natural history by stages. In this chapter, the TNM classification will be introduced later but will already be used in this context. Unfortunately, there is little information in the literature on the course of untreated prostatic carcinoma by stages. The older information contained in Whitmore's paper will not be reviewed again, only recent information will be added.

Incidental Carcinoma

Incidentally found prostatic carcinoma is described in the TNM system as T0pT1–pT3. The tumor is not palpable on rectal examination and is found incidentally at the time of surgical intervention for BPH. Most of these tumors are small and well differentiated. From the large volume of literature on this subject, the study by Cantrell et al. (1981) is selected for review. In this study, 170 patients were followed for 2–15 years, with an average of 4 years, after they had been identified at the time of surgery for BPH to have incidental prostatic carcinoma. The size of the tumor, in this case the percentage of slide surface occupied by tumor, was the most important discriminating parameter between poor and good prognosis in a multivariate analysis. The grade of malignancy was the second most important parameter. Excepting prostatic surgery, no other treatment was used. During the observation period, no patient with a low-grade lesion and only one of 48 patients with a tumor size of less than 5% of the slide surface (2%) showed progression. The majority of all patients (60%) belonged to this favorable category. Of the remaining patients with more than 5% cancer tissue occupying their total slide surface, 32% showed progression. In a later oral communication with longer follow-up, the progression rate in those patients with less than 5% slide surface went up to 18%. In the so-called focal study by VACURG (1968), two of 30 patients (6.7%) showed progression within 6.8 years.

Locally Confined Carcinoma (Category T1–2N0M0)

Very little information is available in the recent literature on untreated patients with the locally confined nodule, which is commonly treated by radical prostatectomy or radiotherapy. The VACURG study of radical prostatectomy reported by Byar et al. (1981) contains a placebo-treated control arm of 20 patients. Seven of these (35%) showed progression within 7.7 years.

Locally Extensive and Metastatic Carcinoma

Virtually no information is available on the course of untreated locally extensive (T3NXM0) and metastatic (M+ and M1) prostatic carcinoma. It was shown by Kramer et al. (1981) that, independently of the extent of lymph node metastases in N+ disease, median time to progression amounts to 20 months. This is delayed to roughly 60 months by castration, as reported by van Aubel et al. (1985). With endocrine management in the European Organization for Research and Treatment of Cancer (EORTC) study 30761 reported by Pavone Macaluso et al. (1986), median time to progression was significantly different for locally extensive, nonmetastatic (T3NXM0) patients and patients with metastatic disease (M1). It amounted in the latter group to less than 1 year and in the first group to almost 2.5 years.

A complete description of the natural history of prostatic cancer is beyond the scope of this chapter. Only prospective clinical trials which include delayed control arms will be helpful in otaining further knowledge about the natural course of this disease.

Diagnosis and Staging

Diagnosis

Early prostatic carcinoma is usually asymptomatic. *Symptoms* that lead to the diagnosis of locally confined tumors are often due to acompanying BPH. Some degree of perineal and suprapubic discomfort, which is often reported by such patients, is identical to complaints caused by chronic or acute prostatitis. This symptom may, however, be due to prostatic carcinoma. The symptom tends to disappear with radical prostatectomy and to reoccur in patients with local recurrence.

As reported above, prostatic carcinoma usually originates close to the prostatic capsule and not in the region of the prostatic urethra. Therefore, it usually takes time until infiltration of the periurethral area and obstructive symptoms occur, which are more frequently related to locally extensive tumors. On the other hand, in some instances, rapidly developing urethral obstruction with residual urine is due to prostatic carcinoma which rapidly proliferates. Some patients will present with acute or chronic urinary retention as their initial symptom. This is usually an expression of a rapid rate of growth and a poor prognosis.

The lack of early symptoms of this tumor is probably the reason why most carcinomas are diagnosed in the metastatic or locally quite advanced stage. The obstructive symptoms encountered in patients with locally advanced tumors are identical to those caused by prostatic hyperplasia and consist of a slow urinary stream, frequency, hesitancy, urgency, and sometimes urge incontinence. In patients with metastases, the sites most frequently involved are regional and subregional lymph nodes. These metastases usually also remain asymptomatic. Bone metastases are the second most frequent and usually occur in the true pelvis or in the lumbar spine. In this case, bone pain, sciatic pain due to compression of lumbar roots, or, occasionally, spontaneous fractures will result. Such complaints are frequently the first presenting symptom of prostatic cancer. It may also happen that at the time of diagnosis the disease process is so advanced that anorexia, a decreased performance status, anemia, and other symptoms of a generalized disease process are present.

On *physical examination*, only very few specific findings are recognized. Most important are the findings on rectal examination. Rectal examination can be carried out with the patient standing and bent forward, in lithotomy position, and in knee-elbow position. Each one of the positions has its advantages and disadvantages. The standing position allows the finger to penetrate more deeply, but the pelvic floor is not relaxed. The lithotomy position and the knee-elbow position probably allow a better judgement on the consistency and delineation of the prostate. A full bladder can imitate a much larger prostate and make delineation of the basis impossible. Early prostatic cancer appears as a difference in consistency or a small nodule without (T1 category) or with (T2 category) deformation of the contour of the prostate. The lateral sulci and seminal vesicles should not be involved. A tumor of the category T3 is characterized as extending beyond the capsule of the prostate with or without involvement of the lateral sulci and/or the seminal vesicles. A tumor which is fixed to the surroundings or which is infiltrating neighboring structures such as the rectum, the bladder neck, the levator ani muscles, or the external sphincter belongs to the category T4. TX classification is used whenever the minimum requirements to assess the primary tumor cannot be met. A tumor which is not palpable at all but found as an incidental finding at the time of surgical treatment of prostatic obstruction is assigned the category T0. In this case, exceptionally, the tumor is assigned a pT category on the basis of the information available from the surgical specimen. This information on the T classification is based on the third revised edition of the TNM classification of malignant tumors of the International Union against Cancer (UICC) (Harmer 1982).

Recently, transrectal ultrasonography has been advocated as an adjuvant technique in diagnosing prostatic carcinoma and in determining its local extent. Prostatic carcinoma most frequently presents as an echopenic lesion (black area) in the ultrasonogram. Occasionally, the lesion may be hyperechoic and, rarely, isoechoic. Capsular deformation and interruption are other signs of prostatic carcinoma. These developments have been reviewed by Peeling and Griffiths (1984). The usually echopenic appearance of prostatic cancer is confirmed in recent articles by Dähnert et al. (1986) and Rifkin et al. (1986). Chodak et al. (1986) evaluated transrectal ultrasonography in a blind study of 260 men to evaluate the capability of the new technique in the detection of prostatic carcinoma. They found that the sensitivity of transrectal ultrasonography in this respect was 86%, but the specificity was only 41%. This correlated with positive and negative predictive values of transrectal ultrasonography of 36% and 89%, respectively. These authors concluded that transrectal ultrasonography is not as yet ready for use in screening programs.

Roughly half of the suspicious findings on rectal examination are confirmed by histological or cytological studies to consist of prostatic carcinoma. This was first clarified by Jewett (1956). Beside prostatic cancer, BPH, prostatic calculi, and chronic prostatitis are the most frequent causes of nodules, indurations, and irregularities of the dorsal surface of the prostate. It is evident that treatment decisions may not be based on the findings of rectal examinations alone. Prostatic biopsy can be carried out by means of a transperineal biopsy, under local or general anesthesia, using a needle that is suitable to produce a core of tissue for histological examination. The biopsy needle is guided by an index finger in the patient's rectum. The alternative technique is aspiration cytology which was established by Franzen et al. (1960). Both techniques, especially the aspiration biopsy, require a certain skill and routine. Both techniques allow the determination of the grade of malignancy of a given tumor. This was pointed out by Esposti (1971) and by Faul (1983) who studied a large number of patients comparing histological and cytological findings. With both techniques, false positive findings are rare. Negative findings with persistent suspicion on rectal examination should lead to repeating the biopsy.

Grading from biopsy specimens is possible but difficult because of the pleomorphic character of most prostatic carcinomas and of their multifocal origin. The possibility of missing the poorly differentiated fraction of a tumor by histological biopsy has serious implications if treatment decisions are to be based on grading. Undergrading has been reported to range from 20%–65% by Garnett et al. (1984), Kastendieck (1980), and Ackermann and Müller (1981).

Staging

In patients with prostatic carcinoma, the local extent of the tumor and the presence or absence of metastases are probably the most decisive prognostic factors. Locally confined prostatic carcinoma is amenable to potentially curative treatment, metastatic prostatic carcinoma can only be managed palliatively at this time.

In Europe, the TNM classification of prostatic carcinoma is generally accepted. A comparative evaluation of the various grading systems available has recently been published by Ten Kate (1986). For complete reference to the TNM system, the original publication of the UICC should be consulted. The usual T categories have already been described above. Lymph node metastases are described as categories NX, N0, and N1–N4. N1 applies to the involvement of a single homolateral regional lymph node. In N2 disease, unilateral or bilateral multiple regional lymph nodes are involved. N3 applies to fixed regional lymph nodes, and N4 to evidence of juxtaregional lymph node metastases.

Metastases are indicated by the M0, MX, and M1 categories. For postsurgical, histopathological classification, the pT categories are applied which roughly correspond to the T categories. pT1 prostatic carcinoma applies to focal (single or multiple) carcinoma. the grade of malignancy is indicated by the categories G1, G2, and G3. Biochemical evidence of metastases is not yet accepted for staging. Stage grouping has not yet been introduced. The general rules of the TNM system also apply to prostatic cancer. This information is based on the 1982 edition of the TNM system. A new edition has appeared (Hermanek and Sobin 1987) but is not generally accepted by the urological community.

Whenever localized prostatic carcinoma is diagnosed, and a curative approach is considered, staging efforts are more comprehensive than in situations where palliative treatment must be applied.

In staging the primary tumor, understaging is frequently seen and may occur as frequently as in 40%–50% of the cases, as reported by Schroeder (1980). In the same report, overstaging was seen in 15% of the cases. The contribution of transrectal ultrasonography to improving the accuracy of T classification is not yet clear but has been recently reviewed by Peeling (1984). Computer scanning has not contributed to a better T classification. The role of nuclear magnetic resonance is not yet entirely clear.

Cystoscopic examination and bimanual examination under anesthesia are considered useful to exclude bladder neck infiltration.

Grade and local tumor extension together are strong determinants for the presence of lymph node metastases. Relevant data related to this problem have recently been published by Grayhack and Assimos (1983), Smith et al. (1983), Catalona et al. (1982), Wilson et al. (1983), and Segalowsky et al. (1982). Roughly, the categories T1–2, T3, and T4 correlate with 25%, 50%, and 80% lymph node metastases, respectively. In grade 1 tumors, lymph node involvement is rarely seen, grade 2 and grade 3 carcinomata present with 25%–80% of lymph node metastases. The literature has been reviewed by Hoekstra and Schroeder (1981).

Unfortunately, there is no accurate means of lymph node staging, short of lymphadenectomy or open lymph node biopsy. Both CT scanning and lymphangiography offer an accuracy of roughly 75% in identifying pelvic nodal metastases. False negatives are more frequent than false positives, which amount to 35% versus 15%, respectively. Reviews are available from Hoekstra and Schroeder (1981) and Bosch and Schröder (1986). In general, even involvement of a single lymph node means that prostatic carcinoma has to be considered as a generalized disease, which is not within reach of local management.

Metastatic disease is suspected on the basis of biochemical parameters such as the determination of acid phosphatase, prostate-specific antigen, or other nonspecific parameters which are indicative of generalized metastatic disease. Bone metastases are detected with bone scans approximately 20% more frequently with conventional X-ray techniques. Changes on bone scans are, however not specific for prostate cancer metastases. Confirmation of abnormal findings on bone scans are therefore mandatory by X-ray, biochemical parameters, or bone biopsy.

Screening

Screening for prostatic cancer can be subdivided into screening for early disease and screening for metastatic disease. As long as no curative treatment is available for metastatic disease and as long as early treatment of metastatic disease is not definitely proven to be advantageous, it does not make much sense to engage in such programs.

The idea of screening for early disease sounds logical in the face of the very much poorer prognosis of patients suffering from metastases as compared to patients undergoing potentially curative treatment for locally confined prostatic carcinoma. The idea of screening for this entity appears to be very attractive at first sight because the lesion can be easily palpated on rectal examination in most instances. The low sensitivity of 69% determined by Guinan et al. (1980) can be much improved by combining rectal examination with biopsy techniques. The specificity, which means in this context the capability of rectal examination to exclude the presence of prostatic cancer, was found to be 89%. Prior to considering screening programs, the following critical considerations are, however, necessary:

- If one were to concentrate on the risk groups above the age of 50, the incidence of prostatic cancer per year would range between 50 and 100 per 100 000. Chodak and Schoenberg (1984) have shown that the yield in the age group between 51 and 80 years could be as high as 1.7%. About half of the patients he found were potentially curable.
- The cost of screening large numbers of potential patients by well-trained personnel is appreciable.
- It will become clear from the section on treatment (see Locoregional Tumor Extension – Potentially Curative Management) that the benefit to the patients treated for early detected local lesions, as far as survival goes, is probably marginal and lies in the range of 15% improvement of their corrected survival.
- It is doubtful whether the natural history of this disease warrants aggressive treatment.

Diagnosis of Metastatic Disease and Markers

Diagnosis of Metastases

In order of their frequency, lymph nodes, bones, and lungs are the most frequent sites of metastases from prostatic carcinoma. Other soft-tissue metastases like liver metastases and skin metastases are rare in this tumor.

The intensity of the search for metastases in each individual case will depend on factors like the age and condition of the patient, the local extension of the tumor, and the results of initial screening tests such as physical examination, the determination of serum markers, and bone scan study. If these studies are negative, and the patient is eligible for a potentially curative approach, the possibility of lymph node metastases being present becomes a very important issue. It has been estimated that in the presence of bone metastatic disease, the incidence of lymph node metastases may be as high as 80%. This is, however, not precisely known because lymph node staging is rarely, if ever, carried out in the presence of a prognostically overruling factor like bone metastases.

The incidence of lymph node metastases, in dependence on tumor grade and local extension (T category), has already been referred to in the section on staging of this chapter. The tools available for diagnosing lymph node metastases are: physical examination, computer scanning, lymphangiography, aspiration biopsy, open biopsy, and lymph node dissection. In the area of the true pelvis where the first regional metastases occur, ultrasound studies have proven not to be very useful. A report by Hoekstra and Schroeder (1981) gives an indication of the role of lymphangiography in diagnosing nodal metastases. This paper also gives a complete review of the literature on this subject and on the subject of correlation between T cateogry, G category, and the presence of lymph node metastases. When compared to the results of lymph node dissection, the overall accuracy of lymphangiography is roughly 75%, with a specificity of 79% and a sensitivity of 67%. Bosch and Schroeder (1986) recently compared the results of surgical staging to those of CT scanning and lymphangiography. They concluded that neither one of the radiological techniques is superior to the other, that grade and pT category allow prediction of the presence of lymph node metastases to a high degree and that the major benefit of radiological staging may be the identification of those cases that have advanced nodular disease. In these cases, lymph node dissection can be avoided. If, for any reason, the presence or absence of lymph node metastases becomes a crucial issue for further treatment decisions, surgical lymph node staging is the only accurate technique available at this moment.

In some cases, lymphadenectomy or open lymph node biopsy can be replaced by transperitoneal fine needle aspiration biopsy under X-ray or ultrasound control. There is a considerable volume of literature on this subject. One of the early systematic applications of the technique is reported by Pollen and Schmidt (1979). These authors studied 12 soft-tissue masses among which were six lymph nodes. All masses were identifiable by some means as being suspicious lesions. Göthlin and Höiem (1981) systematically punctured normal-appearing lymph nodes in 24 patients with low-grade prostatic carcinoma after lymphangiography. When six to ten apparently normal pelvic lymph nodes were punctured in each of these patients, lymph node metastases were identified in six of them (25%). Luciani and Piscidi (1983) reported on 24 patients with localized prostatic carcinoma who had undergone percutaneous aspiration biopsy and pelvic lymph node dissection. They found positive cytology in 11 patients, which was confirmed by lymphadenectomy in all cases. In one additional patient, lymphadenectomy revealed metastatic disease which had not been identified by aspiration biopsy. These results are encouraging and warrant further clinical investigation. The future will show what the role of routine biopsy in the management of this disease will be.

Bone metastases are best detected by bone scanning. This was clearly established in a series of classical articles by Chisholm et al. (1982). This group found that in 23% of their X-ray-negative cases, the bone scan was positive. This agrees with the observation of others. Hot spots seen on bone scans are not specific for prostatic carcinoma. Degenerative bone changes, old fractures, and metastases from other tumors will give the same appearance. Only about 10% of bone metastases coming from prostatic carcinoma are lytic and may not show up on bone scans, all other metastases are osteoblastic. If hot spots in ribs are the only lesions that seem to indicate metastatic disease, according to the authors' experience with many attempts to prove such lesions by biopsy, it is wise to assume that these are not caused by metastatic disease and to wait for further signs of progression. This is especially true if serum acid phosphatase or prostatic acid phosphatase show normal values.

Some authors, including Huben and Schellhammer (1982), question the routine use of bone scans for screening for metastases. If, in their series of 100 patients, an elevation of serum acid phosphatase in combination with bone pain had been used as an indication for bone scanning, no single patient with bone metastases would have been missed. The literature is reviewed by the two authors and seems to confirm their observation. The possible mechanisms of spread of prostatic cancer to bone, the incidence of metastases depending on stage, host factors, and the impact on calcium metabolism have been reviewed by Jacobs (1983). Future development in this field may be expected from the development of radioimmunoscanning utilizing labeled monoclonal antibodies against prostatic proteins. The increasing volume of literature in this field has been started off by the communication of Goldenberg et al. (1983).

Unusual soft-tissue metastases to liver, skin, or other organs are best detected with routine techniques such as ultrasound and CT scanning. These metastases are often suspected in the presence of positive serum markers with negative bone scans.

Markers

Human prostate contains large amounts of acid and alkaline phosphatase. This was stated by Gutman et al. (1936). Acid phosphatase has become a very commonly used tissue and serum marker for this disease. Determined enzymatically, acid phosphatase is a valuable marker for the presence of metastatic disease, with a high sensitivity and, unfortunately, a low specificity. Normal serum acid phosphatase does not exclude metastatic disease; some prostatic cancers do not produce large amounts of acid phosphatase.

In more recent years, polyclonal and monoclonal antibodies have become available against prostatic acid phosphatase. These have led to the now common radioimmuno- and enzymoimmunoassay for this enzyme. One of the original assays (Foti et al. 1977) seemed promising even for early detection of the primary tumor. Unfortunately, later observations have not confirmed the data. Vihko et al. (1985), who have contributed by developing several immunoassays for prostatic acid phosphatase, have shown that there is a strict correlation of prostatic acid phosphatase levels with the extent of disease. They found 38% elevated values in T0–T2M0 disease and 70% elevation in the presence of metastatic disease. With an increase of specificity of the assay methods to the prostatic antigen, acid phosphatase is more frequently elevated, but, unlike in the enzyme assay, elevations above normal are not indicative for metastatic disease. Higher cut-off values must be defined for prediction of metastatic disease. Such an attempt was recently made in a large series of observations by Oosterom et al. (1986) who found that elevations of prostatic acid phosphatase up to 8 μg per liter would predict metastases with an accuracy of just above 70%. The normal values in most assays range between 2 and 3 μg per liter. After prostatic massage, transient, moderate elevations of acid phosphatase may occur. This problem has been discussed by Pearson et al. (1983) and Bhat et al. (1981). BPH may lead to an elevation of serum acid phosphatase. A critical analysis of this phenomenon is found in the paper by Oosterom et al. (1986).

Prostatic acid phosphatase is also helpful as a tissue marker, especially in situations where the origin of metastatic deposits is unclear. Among other reports in the literature, Joebsis et al. (1978) have demonstrated these new technical possibilities.

Other markers for prostatic carcinoma include some that are ready for routine clinical use and others that are still investigational. Papsidero et al. (1980) identified prostate-specific androgen in 1980 and subsequently introduced the substance into clinical use as a serum and tissue marker. The evaluation of this new marker is still ongoing, but first results seem to indicate that prostate-specific antigen may be superior to prostatic acid phosphatase. Both markers together seem to greatly enhance the diagnostic and prognostic value of serum markers in prostatic carcinoma. Original data are presented by Kuriyama et al. (1982), Siddall et al. (1986). The clinical significance of both important markers, prostatic acid phosphatase and prostate-specific antigen, have recently been completely reviewed by Chu and Murphy (1986).

The significance of alkaline phosphatase for prostatic carcinoma has been reviewed by Wajsman et al. (1978). This enzyme was found to be elevated in 91% of patients with metastatic bone disease. Alkaline phosphatase may also be a prognostic indicator. Alkaline phosphatase is not tissue specific for prostate and is frequently elevated in liver disease. This may limit the importance of this marker for prostatic carcinoma, especially in the presence of specific markers, such as prostatic acid phosphatase and prostate-specific antigen.

Other prostatic markers which are still investigational include creatinine kinase BB (Silverman et al. 1981), estramustine-binding protein (Björk et al. 1982), aminopeptidase (Mattila 1969), acute phase reactant proteins (Milford Ward et al. 1977), urinary fibronectin (Webb and Lin 1980), carcinoembryonic antigen (Kane et al. 1976), neuraminic acid (Moss et al. 1979), placental lactogen (Schmidt et al. 1982), and an enzme index reported by Brendler et al. (1985).

Prognostic Factors and Response Criteria

"Prognostic factors" may be defined as parameters that closely correlate with the prognosis of the individual patient. Often, prognostic factors are obtained only on one occasion, for example, at the time of diagnosis of the primary or of the metastases. This is true for the local extension of the primary tumor, its grade of malignancy, the presence or absence of lymph node metastases, and the presence or absence of other distant metastases. Response criteria should closely correlate with response to treatment. Such parameters should be repeatedly evaluable and, if at all possible, bidimensionally measurable. Typical examples are palpable and measurable lymph node or skin metastases, lung metastases, liver metastases with ultrasound or CT imaging, the primary tumor evaluated by ultrasound, biochemical parameters such as acid phosphatase, prostate-specific antigen, or other useful markers. For biochemical markers, very high sensitivity and specificity are required for qualification as a response criterion. This is also the reason why, up to now, none of the serum markers for prostatic cancer have qualified as a response parameter in the sets of response criteria currently used. Response criteria may have to differ in the evaluation of hormone responsive and hormone unresponsive prostatic carcinoma. The phase II situation requires more stringent parameters than phase III trials.

Subjective response and quality of life are important aspects of cancer therapy. For this reason, beside evaluating objective response, valid subjective response criteria should be and are being developed by various research groups.

Prognostic factors and response criteria have been reviewed by Schroeder (1982) and Schroeder et al. (1984 b). WHO guidelines for evaluating response to cancer treatment were published in 1979. Response criteria commonly used in the United States have been reviewed by Murphy and Slack (1980). A critical analysis of response criteria in hormone unresponsive prostatic carcinoma patients has been presented by Yagoda et al. (1979).

The understanding of the various sets of response criteria used in clinical trials is of crucial importance for the correct interpretation of the treatment results. Important differences exist, especially between the trials of the EORTC Genitourinary (GU) Group and those American trials that were conducted by the National Prostatic Cancer Project (NPCP) or by using the criteria of this group. The main difference between these sets of criteria lies in the fact that frequently, in the United States, the "stable disease" (SD) category is classified as a response, whereas in Europe the corresponding "no change" (NC) category is not considered a response to treatment. The proportion of patients in this group usually amounts to 40%–50%. Internationally recognized response parameters are all bidimensionally measurable lesions. Unfortunately, for unknown reasons, the primary tumor shows a divergent behavior from distant metastases; its contribution to the evaluation of response is, therefore very limited. Only lytic bone metastases are measurable. Although the frequent blastic metastases are evaluable, they are not used in evaluating response. New lesions indicate progression. Nonspecific parameters, such as marker elevation, performance status, anemia, etc., are necessary to identify progression in case a patient deteriorates because of cancer but remains objectively stable.

A large number of prognostic factors and response criteria are presently under investigation. These include the volume of the primary tumor measured by ultrasound, receptor studies in prostatic tissue, serum markers, repeated fine needle aspiration biopsy, immunological demonstration of metastases, etc. For prognosticating localized disease, the prediction of lymph node metastases by evaluating grade and stage with more efficient techniques is of great importance.

Locoregional Tumor Extension – Potentially Curative Management

It has been stressed in the previous sections on the natural history and staging that, in dealing with localized prostatic carcinoma, there is a risk of overtreating nonaggressive lesions on the one hand, and of treatment failure by underestimation of the local extension, the grade of malignancy, and the lymph node status on the other. As has been summarized by Elder and Catalona (1984), there may be a slight chance for cure of an occasional patient with minimal lymph node involvement, otherwise the presence of lymph node metastases seem to be a sharp cut-off point for curability of this disease. Even in locally advanced disease, the rate of local recurrence is only about half of that of distant failure. In the large amount of material of Schroeder and Belt (1975) local recurrence occurred in 12.7% and distant metastases in 23% in 213 stage C cases. Because of a high rate of understaging by rectal examination of T2 tumors and a considerable rate of overstaging of T3 tumors, it is difficult to use the T1–2 group as a cut-off point for treatment with curative intent. On the other hand, the presence of a T4 tumor will usually make radical prostatectomy impossible. Radiotherapy may be applied to this lesion. Incidentally found prostatic carcinomas of the category T0pT1G1 are watched by most clinicians. This problem has been discussed above.

Three techniques are available for the mangement of locally confined disease: external beam radiotherapy, interstitial radiotherapy using ^{125}I or iridium, and radical prostatectomy.

Indications and Limitations of Locoregional Treatment

Whatever treatment is used in the management of T1–T2 prostatic carcinoma, the benefit in terms of statistically improved survival will be marginal with the background of the relatively low expected progression rate (35% per 7.7 years; Byar et al. 1981). Unfortunately, the risk of untreated T3 carcinoma with or without lymph node involvement is not known. Based on published results of various forms of treatment of this group of patients, it is safe to assume that the risk of progression of the untreated tumor is significantly higher than that of the T1 and T2 categories.

Not only the T1 category, but also the grade of the malignancy is an important prognostic determining factor in localized disease. This is shown in Table 3. The grade of malignancy in this series was determined by radical prostatectomy specimens. In spite of radical prostatectomy and, in a number of patients, adjuvant hormonal treatment, the rates of treatment failure clearly correlate more strongly with grade than with stage. If all information shown in this table were available preoperatively, one would be inclined to identify all G1 tumors as a low-risk group and all G3 tumors as a high-risk group and use this information for treatment decisions. Unfortunately, the determination of tumor grade and stage on the basis of rectal examination and biopsy is highy unreliable. In a recent study of 107 patients who were considered to be potential candidates for radical prostatectomy by Bosch and Schroeder (1986), understaging by rectal examination occurred in six of seven T1 patients and in 17 of 24 T2 patients

Table 3. Death from prostatic carcinoma correlated with T, pT, and G categories in patients with locally confined prostatic cancer treated by radical prostatectomy. (Adapted from Schroeder 1980)

T and P categories	Grade (nuclear pleomorphism)								
	Patients (*n*)	G1 Dead from carcinoma		Patients (*n*)	G2 Dead from carcinoma		Patients (*n*)	G3 Dead from carcinoma	
		(*n*)	(%)		(*n*)	(%)		(*n*)	(%)
T0	10	0	0	23	6	26.1	5	2	40.0
pT1	6	0	0	4	0	0	0	0	0
T1–2	33	3	9.1	125	18	14.4	31	10	32.3
pT2	28	2	7.1	72	7	9.7	14	2	14.3
T3	15	1	6.7	73	21	28.8	27	12	44.4
pT3	22	1	4.6	146	38	26.0	51	22	43.1

(71%). In patients who were judged as having grade 1 on the basis of a transperineal histological biopsy specimen, grade 2 or 3 was found in 10 out of 14 (71%); of 45 patients who were graded grade 2 on the basis of their biopsy, seven were found to have grade 3 tumors at the time of radical prostatectomy (20%). This amounted to a total undergrading of 17 out of 70 patients (24%). At least four other references in the literature are available which show undergrading in 39% to 66% of cases. At this moment, it is not known whether fine needle aspiration biopsy would allow a better sampling of the tumor and whether, in this way, undergrading could be reduced. For the time being, it seems to be impossible to use preoperative grading for treatment decisions. The dilemma remains. If grade 3 tumor is identified preoperatively, there is a high risk for the patient, but the results of treatment will be discouraging. Whenever a well-differentiated, confined tumor is identified preoperatively, there is a high risk of a hidden poorly differentiated tumor, and there is also the possibility that one is dealing with a "toothless lion," as the nonaggressive type of well-differentiated prostatic carcinoma was termed by Gittes and Chu (1976). The treating physician and patient remain confronted with the impossible task of weighing against each other an unknown, possibly high risk of their disease, a treatment of questionable effectiveness, and its associated complications. In this decision process, the age of the patient, considerations of quality of life, skills and preferences of urologists and radiotherapists, and other, quite subjective, factors will continue to play an important role.

The Role of Lymphadenectomy

The presence of lymph node metastases in this group of patients represents the most important prognostic factor. Independently of the number of lymph node metastases, the median time to progression in this group of patients amounts to about 20 months. The relevant literature was recently reviewed by Van Aubel et al. (1985). Unfortunately, none of the noninvasive imaging techniques, such as ultrasound studies, CT scanning, and lymphangiography, are sufficiently accurate to confirm or exclude the presence of lymphatic spread. The only safe and effective means of diagnosing lymph node metastases remains open surgical lymph node biopsy and dissection. There is a large volume of literature available on this subject, which has been reviewed by Hoekstra and Schroeder (1981) and Bosch and Schroeder (1986). Grade and T category are strong predictors of the presence or absence of lymph node metastases. This correlation has been reviewed by several authors, including Donohue et al. (1981), Zincke et al. (1982), and Freiha et al. (1979). Because of the limitations stemming from the inaccuracy of preoperative determination of stage and tumor extension, it is still felt at present that surgical lymph node evaluation cannot be omitted on the basis of these prognostic factors.

Technically, lymph node dissection can be limited to the area in between the bifurcation of the common iliac artery, the medial margin of the external iliac artery, the entry of the lacuna vasorum, and the deepest point of the obturator fossa. Since no curative intent is involved in carrying out nodal dissections, the finding of Whitmore (1984), that a dissection in this area is representative of the results of more extensive dissections, can be applied.

When a radical prostatectomy is planned, the author relies on frozen sections for the exclusion of nodal metastases. In a series of 107 cases, our false negative rate was 7% (Bosch and Schroeder 1986). The experience reported in the literature on this subject is quite variable and will always depend on the way the surgical material is sampled and reviewed.

Surgical complications of lymphadenectomy are not negligible. Large series of patients have been reviewed by Herr (1979a), Lieskowski et al. (1980), and Brendler et al. (1980). In these publications, postoperative complications occurred in 7%–16% of cases. Occasional deaths from myocardial infarction and pulmonary embolism are reported. Other complications are wound infections, deep vein thrombosis, lymphoceles, prolonged lymphatic drainage, and hematomas.

The optimal management of patients with regional lymph node metastases is not known. Van Aubel et al. (1985) and Bosch and Schroeder (1986) have reported prolonged survival with endocrine management, which amounts to a median time to progression of 61 months. It is, however, unclear at this moment, whether early hormonal treatment will prolong life in these patients.

Radical Prostatectomy

History

Since the beginning of this century, the possibility of radically removing the prostate and its surrounding tissues, including the prostate capsule and the seminal vesicles, has been considered an intriguing possibility for cure of locally confined prostatic cancer. Problems that have been associated with this approach have been the risk of incontinence resulting from the total disruption of the urethra and impotence which, as we know now, is due to the surgical damage of two peripheral nerves responsible for erection. Probably, the first planned radical prostatectomy was carried out by Billroth in 1867 in Vienna. He removed a prostatic tumor using a perineal midline incision. This approach was, however, not followed up in Europe. Young (1945) and his school at the Johns Hopkins Hospital deserve credit for having further developed the indications and the technique of radical prostatectomy. Belt et al. described a new perineal approach to the prostate in 1939. The most important recent technical contribution is the description of a potency-preserving approach by Walsh and Donker (1982).

Surgical Technique

Surgically, the prostate can be approached by the perineal and the retropubic routes. The perineal route is the traditional approach to radical prostatectomy favored by Young and Belt in the above-mentioned articles. More recently, the retropubic approach has become more common for two reasons: due to the high accuracy of lymph node staging by frozen section, lymphadenectomy and total prostatectomy are commonly carried out in one operation. The precise description of the nerve-sparing technique via the retropubic route by Walsh and Donker (1982) and the existing uncertainty about possible potency preservation using the perineal route plead for the retropubic approach. It is good practice to define a "total prostatectomy" as total removal of the prostate with its capsule, a manchet of bladder neck and the seminal vesicles, whereas the term "radical prostatectomy" is reserved for the combination of total prostatectomy with a pelvic lymph node dissection. Descriptions of the surgical technique are available in various urological text books. Walsh (1986) has described his approach in Campbell's Urology. Details of the nerve-sparing approach are reported by Lepor et al. (1985).

Results by T Category

In virtually all well-documented series of patients with locally confined prostatic carcinoma, statistically significant correlations between progression and survival rates on the one hand, and T categories, or the American staging systems, are found. The important point made by these findings is that local tumor burden is a very powerful prognostic factor. Recent studies by McNeal et al. (1986) and Stamey (personal communication, at the American Urology Association, 1986) correlate the volume of the primary tumor as determined by histopathological and ultrasound studies to the extent of the disease as determined by studying metastases at autopsy, prostate-specific antigen in patients, and the grade of malignancy in both the primary tumor and metastases. The investigators conclude that tumor volume is a highly critical determining factor of those studied. For example, bone metastases were never found below a local tumor volume of 4 ml. There is no doubt that primary tumor volume must be considered a prognostic factor on a "sliding scale." The ideal definition of T categories would be by primary tumor volume in cubic centimeters. Since this has been, up to now, impossible, staging systems arbitrarily define estimations of primary tumor volume. These produce, to a certain degree, comparable prognostic subgroups if handled strictly and, preferably, by the same investigator or group of investigators.

At the present time, a considerable number of staging systems are used that are not entirely comparable. This makes comparison from one series to another very difficult and questionable. The subject has been reviewed by Herr (1983). For this reason it is also impossible to compare, in a reliable fashion, the results of treatment in groups of patients that have not been defined in an identical fashion. Since reliable randomized studies are missing in this field, it is impossible to give a decisive opinion about the best treatment for the groups of patients involved.

Category T0pT1–3. The tumor described by this formula is the incidentally found prostatic carcinoma which would, in the American classification, be classified as an A1 or A2 tumor. Many of the aspects of this tumor have been dealt with above, essential references have already been given.

Category T0pT1G1–2. Radical prostatectomy is not considered to be indicated in T0pT1G1–2 tumors. This is especially true if a second-look transurethral resection has not revealed residual tumor. The chance of progression is small. Regular follow-up examinations, including a rectal examination, are indicated.

Category T0pT2–3G2–3. This category has a poor prognosis. In spite of radical prostatectomy, cancer mortality may amount to 40%–50% of these cases, as has been shown by Schroeder et al. (1984a). The only randomized study including patients in this category is the focal study of VACURG, reported by Byar et al. (1981). No difference in surival was found when 30 patients treated by placebo were compared to 31 patients treated by radical prostatectomy plus placebo, with a median follow-up of 6.8 years. This study has been rightly criticized for several good reasons, among others, by Walsh (1981). The study was not completed, bone scans were not performed for staging, no stratification into focal and nonfocal disease was applied, surgery was spread over many institutions which contributed, on average, one patient each.

Beside lymph node dissection and radical prostatectomy, radiotherapy is a frequently applied option. The proportion of patients who are at risk of dying of this disease is high if estimations are based on the numbers of those that escape treatment. Probably, a number of these patients could be cured by radical prostatectomy and maybe also by radiotherapy.

This view is shared by several authors whose series include this category of patients. Middleton et al. (1986) treated 40 stage A2 patients by means of radical prostatectomy. He found 91% to be free of tumor at the 5-year follow-up interval. The result was identical to that obtained in B1 patients. Usually, the results are identical or superior to the theoretical life expectancy of the age group involved.

Categories T1 and T2. The studies reporting on 15-year observations in patients with T1 and T2 tumors treated by radical prostatectomy clearly show that the proportion of patients dying from prostatic carcinoma per 5-year interval remains about the same throughout this long period of time (Herr 1983; Schroeder and Belt 1975). This stresses the necessity of long-term observations for the judgement on treatment success. Series with such long observation periods are available but they do not usually include lymph node dissections. An important prognostic factor remains unknown. Comparison of treatment results is difficult because of the variable staging systems used in various series. Gross survival over 5, 10, and 15 years was 75%–80%, 45%–50%, and 20%–30%, respectively, in such series. The theoretical life expectancy is usually slightly higher or identical to these results. Results obtained for stages T1 and T2 disease, which have in common the fact that the tumor is confined to the prostate, are significantly better than survival obtained for stage T3 disease. Subclassification into T1 and T2 roughly comparable to the B1 and B2 categories in the American systems (Jewett 1956; Whitmore 1980) allows the identification of subgroups with a different prognosis after radical prostatectomy. As shown by Elder et al. (1982), it is especially the B2 subcategory (involvement of at least one or more lobes of the prostate) in which clinical understaging of the primary is very common. Of his B2 patients, 66% were shown to have histological extention of tumor beyond the prostate capsule. Disease-free survival in this group over 5, 10, and 15 years amounts to roughly 73%, 50%, 25%, respectively. No patient who showed grade 3 prostatic carcinoma survived for 15 years disease-free, especially if the seminal vesicles were involved.

The large discrepancy between overall survival and disease-free survival observed in the Johns Hopkins series (Elder et al. 1982) may be, in part, due to the fact that lymph node staging had not been carried out in these patients. It is surprising that in a more recent, but also large series of 215 patients in whom lymph node dissection was used as a selection criterium, disease-free survival rates were almost identical to uncorrected survival (Gibbons et al. 1984). Also, as one would expect by applying this selection criterion, overall projected 15-year survival figures are in the range of 50% and considerably higher than in older series that do not apply an effective method of lymph node evaluation.

Local control rates are excellent. The overall rate of recurrence in the series of Jewett (1975) and Schroeder and Belt (1975) is almost identical and amounts to 6%–7%.

Category T3. In this group of locally advanced tumors with penetration of the capsule and/or palpable involvement of the seminal vesicles after lymph node staging, a subset of roughly 30% of patients can be identified who probably benefit from radical prostatectomy (Bosch et al. 1987). At this moment, no criteria are available to select this group of patients efficiently prior to radical prostatectomy. Long-term results of radical prostatectomy combined with lymphadenectomy resulting from series of patients not using adjuvant hormonal or other treatment are not available at this time. In the series reported by Bosch (1987), treatment failures in such a population of patients ranged between 20% and 50% at 2 years.

Long-term results of the management of locally extensive prostatic carcinoma (category T3, stage C3) by radical prostatectomy have been published, among others by Flocks (1973), Tomlinson et al. (1977), and Schroeder and Belt (1975). The series by Schroeder and Belt reports on 213 patients with histological stage C tumors with 5-, 10- and 15-year survival rates of 64%, 36%, and 20%, respectively. Local recurrences amounted to 12.7%.

Many other series include histologically extensive tumors because of the high probability of understaging stage T2 lesions. In the series of Schroeder and Belt, this probability amounted to more than 50%.

Adjuvant Treatment

In many older series, including the one by Belt and Schroeder (1972), adjuvant hormonal management was applied with variable indications. Results obtained in that particular series suggested that 5-year survival was greatly improved if patients received estrogens, but their 10- and 15-year survival rates were not influenced further by the effect of hormonal management. The improvement of early survival is also evident in the series of patients, reported by Zincke et al. (1986), with locally advanced and N+ disease managed by radical prostatectomy in combination with endocrine management at the Mayo Clinic. On the background of the results reported by Van Aubel et al. (1985) it appears questionable whether radical prostatectomy adds any benefit to the hormonal mangement of locally unresectable disease.

Complications of Radical Prostatectomy

Complications of radical prostatectomy using the retropubic and the perineal approaches have been reviewed by Ackermann and Frohmueller (1983). Surgical complications include the possibility of rectal injury, ureteral injury, and severe bleeding. Early postoperative complications may consist of impaired renal function, pulmonary embolus, myocardial infarction, wound infections, lymphocele formation, and hematoma. Late complications include incontinence which happens in 1%–12.5% of cases according to various reports in the literature (Schroeder et al. 1976). Lymphedema of the low extremities is a rare complication of lymphadenectomy. Fortunately incontinence can be efficiently treated with the artificial urinary sphincter, as has been shown by Barrett and Furlow (1983). Sexual impotence after radical prostatectomy remains a problem, but according to Walsh and Donker 1982, it can be reduced by applying the nerve-sparing technique.

Radiotherapy

Radiotherapy is applicable to the same group of patients as radical prostatectomy with the theoretical possibility that a number of patients with locally more extensive disease and/or early lymphatic involvement may be cured by radiotherapy. This possibility has, however, not been confirmed in patients with N+ disease, as indicated by the experience of Smith et al. (1984) and Paulson et al. (1984). The latter found, in a series of 73 patients, no difference in time to progression between a pelvic radiotherapy group of 40 patients and a delayed hormonal therapy group of 33 patients.

For some time there has been the suspicion that prostatic carcinoma may not be radiosensitive. Definite proof that prostatic carcinoma can be completely eliminated by radiotherapy has been presented by Bagshaw et al. (1965), who reported on six patients who had died from other causes after external beam radiotherapy for clinically manifest prostatic carcinoma. In these six patients no evidence of histologically identifyable prostatic carcinoma could be found. The tumors had apparently been completely eradicated by radiotherapy.

The technique of radiotherapy, which is applicable in various schemes and approaches, will not be reviewed in this chapter. Usually, doses of 6–7 Gy are applied to the prostate with 4–4.5 Gy to the regional lymph nodes. Besides external beam radiotherapy, interstitial radiotherapy using radioactive gold, iodine, or iridium has been applied by various researchers. Recently, the ^{125}I implantation, which can be carried out through the retropubic route as an open operation or by means of ultrasound manipulation using a perineal approach, has become more and more popular.

Results of Radiotherapy

The same restrictions apply to the interpretation of results of radiotherapy of prostatic carcinoma as were described in the sections on the natural history and on radical prostatectomy. There is clear evidence that in the presence of lymph node metastases, the prognosis is poor and cannot be improved by radiotherapy (Paulson et al. 1984; Bagshaw 1980). Results by local tumor extension (T category, stage) are remarkably uniform, as shown by the 5-, 10- and 15-year survival figures presented in Table 4. Considering the strong impact of competing causes of death on good survival figures, these data may not reflect any differences in effectiveness of the three forms of treatment. The remarkable uniformity of these data, which could be confirmed by the results of many other studies, may also mean that the natural history of the different stages of this disease is the most prominent determining factor. The results and complications of several large series of patients treated by means of external beam radiotherapy with curative intent have been reported by Gibbons et al. (1979). These authors showed that satisfactory dis-

Table 4. Overall survival by T category, external beam radiotherapy (Bagshaw (1984), interstitial 125 iodine implantation (Whitmore 1984), and total perineal prostatectomy (Schroeder and Belt 1975)

Survival (years)	(*n*)	5 (%)	10 (%)	15 (%)
Bagshaw (1984)				
T1	225	75	58	46
T2	119	75	50	36
T3	242	61	42	30
T4	32	23	±16	0
Whitmore (1984)				
T1	103	93	–	–
T2	52	76	–	–
T3	70	69	–	–
T4	15	13	–	–
Schroeder and Belt (1975)				
B	132	76	61	39
C	213	64	36	20

ease control could be achieved in 209 patients with a stage D adenocarcinoma of the prostate. Of these patients, 92% required no further management of urethral obstruction. Complications were mild, in 8% of cases strictures were observed. The well-documented large series of Stanford University was last reported upon by Bagshaw in 1984. Long-term results show significant influence on prognosis of the presence of lymph node metastases, the stage, and grade. For stage C disease 5-, 10-, and 15-year survival rates of 60%, 36%, and 22%, respectively, were reported. The Canadian experience was summarized by McGowen and Hanson in 1985. The Rotterdam experience has recently been reported on by Van der Werf-Messing et al. (1984). Overall survival after 5 and 10 years amounted to roughly 50% and 35%, respectively. Corrected survival amounted to 65% after 5 and 10 years in 269 patients.

Treatment failures are usually identified as distant metastases by means of bone scans or biochemical parameters. The definition of a local recurrence after radiotherapy remains a difficult problem. It has been known for a long time that after radiotherapy a prostatic biopsy may remain positive for periods up to 2 years or more. The older data on this subject have been reviewed by Schroeder and Belt (1975). In 1977 Cox and Stoffel studied the possible relation of positive biopsies after radiotherapy with the development of metastatic disease. They could not detect a correlation and recommended that biopsy was of no benefit to the patient. More recently, a number of authors have shown a clear correlation between a positive biopsy result after radiotherapy at 6, 12, and 18 months and the later development of metastases (Kurth et al. 1977; Scardino et al. 1986; Van der Werf-Messing et al. 1984). In the series of Van der Werf-Messing et al., the incidence of metastatic disease was 30%–40% higher in those patients that had positive biopsies at 6 months or later. It is not possible at this time to decide whether these observations are based on a selection phenomenon or represent actual treatment failure. However, it does mean that a large group of patients with an unfavorable prognosis after radiotherapy can be identified.

The Uro-oncology Research Group (Paulson et al. 1982) reported on a randomized study of radical surgery versus radiotherapy for adenocarcinoma of the prostate. A total of 97 patients with clinical stage A or B tumors were randomly assigned to radiotherapy or radical prostatectomy. After 3 years there was a significant difference in the rate of progression in favor of the radical prostatectomy group. The study has been criticized mainly because of the very high progression rate of 35% in the radiotherapy group. This is higher than what could be expected on the basis of the natural history for this group of patients. This may indicate some problem in patient selection rather than a difference in effect of therapy.

Results of ^{125}I Implantation

Implantation of ^{125}I as an open surgical procedure has been introduced by Whitmore (1980) and his group at Memorial Sloan Kettering Cancer Center in New York. He reported on 5-year follow-up of the first 100 patients in 1980. The technique had been applied to lymph node-positive and lymph node-negative patients since 1970. Stage B and stage C patients were included. Mortality and morbidity was low. The prognosis was poor in 36 patients who were identified as having regional lymph node metastases. They had a 71% incidence of distant metastases at 5 years. Patients without lymph node metastases fared very much better. Overall 5-year survival rates for stage B1 were 100%, for stage B2 88%, for stage B3 66%, for stage C1 33%, and for stage C2 53%. Side effects in this series were reported by Herr (1979a) and were mild. Sexual potency was retained in 40 out of 41 patients who had been sexually active preoperatively. Grossman et al. (1982b) have reported on longer-term follow-up of the same series of patients. Other authors reporting on results obtained with the same technique are Lytton et al. (1979), who treated 77 patients with stage B and C disease, and Schellhammer et al. (1985), who reported on 367 patients with localized prostatic carcinoma. In a comparative study of external beam radiotherapy and

^{125}I implantation (El-Mahdi et al. 1985), external beam radiotherapy seems to be more effective than iodine implantation in poorly differentiated prostatic carcinoma.

Complications of radiotherapy amount to roughly 20% in the early stages and 5% on a long-term basis. These include gastrointestinal problems with prostatitis being most prominent, radiation cystitis, urethral stricture, impotence and, rarely, rectal stenosis.

Radiotherapy as Adjuvant and Palliative Management

It has been shown by Gibbons et al. (1986) that radiotherapy is beneficial in patients who have undergone incomplete resection of their prostatic carcinoma at the time of radical prostatectomy. Ray et al. (1984) present data that may indicate that early radiotherapy in cases of incomplete resection produces better results than radiotherapy applied to clinically manifest local recurrence. The complications reported in both papers are acceptable. In the author's own experience, however, very serious complications may occur.

Radiotherapy is useful in management of painful bone metastases and threatening spinal cord compression.

In concluding this section on regionally limited prostatic carcinoma, it should again be emphasized that all treatment decisions made in this disease are relative to the background of the natural history of this tumor and the age of patients. If, however, therapy aims at cure, the effectiveness of the treatment modality chosen in controlling the tumor locally is of crucial importance. The recent biopsy data after radiotherapy and their correlation with the development of metastatic disease indicate that radiotherapy does not effectively control the local lesion in a high percentage of cases. Local recurrence rates after radical prostatectomy compare favorably to these data.

Management of Advanced Disease

Endocrine Management

Endocrine management of prostatic carcinoma was introduced into clinical medicine by Huggins, Hodges, Scott, and Stevens in a series of papers in 1941 (Huggins and Hodges 1941; Huggins et al. 1941a; Huggins et al. 1941b). Their pioneering work was later honored with the Nobel Prize. In their studies, they described the effect of castration and estrogenic hormones on the primary tumor, metastases, and acid phosphatase plasma levels in patients with advanced prostatic carcinoma. They also showed that the application of testosterone propionate leads to an increase in acid phosphatase values. In the subsequent period, a large number of retrospective studies appeared, including those by Nesbitt and Baum (1950), Nesbitt and Plumb (1946), and the study by Emmett et al. (1960). These early studies were uncontrolled and the patient populations were poorly characterized by modern standards. In the study by Nesbitt and Baum (1950), higher 5-year survival rates were reported for patients treated with orchiectomy and stilbestrol in combination. These data were not confirmed by Emmett et al. (1960) and other authors. However, the combination of orchiectomy and estrogens in the management of this disease became common practice for many years. This was based on the belief that estrogens might exert a direct effect on prostatic cancer tissue. Emmett et al. (1960) reported 5- and 10-year survival rates in 355 cases with metastases of 13.5% and 3.2%, respectively. In the stilbestrol group, a 5-year survival rate of 35.4% was found. No difference was revealed between orchiectomy alone and orchiectomy plus stilbestrol. These data are exclusively of historical interest and show, more than anything else, the tremendous pitfalls of retrospective studies and the strong influence of prognostic factors that were not identified clearly at that time.

Endocrinological Background

The predominant endocrine factor influencing prostatic carcinoma is testosterone. The most active androgen on the prostate, however, is 5-α-dihydrotestosterone (DHT). Normal plasma testosterone at our own institution averages 20 nmol per liter, which is comparable with 5.8 ng/ml. The ranges within these normal values are 10–50 nmol per liter and 2.8–14.0 ng/ml. Castration lowers plasma testosterone by 90%–95%. The remaining circulating testosterone is of adrenal origin. At the moment, it has not been completely established whether or not adrenal androgens alone are capable of supporting the growth of hormone-dependent prostatic carcinoma cells. There is some experimental evidence supporting this possibility (Labrie et al. 1988); however, most available clinical evidence is not in favor of this interesting working hypothesis. DHT concentrations in prostatic tissue rarely stay above levels of non-androgen-dependent control tissue (2.5 ng/g) after castration. However, in a substantial number of patients reported by Geller et al. (1984), DHT levels in prostatic carcinoma tissue after castration were shown to remain well above the castration level of plasma DHT and testosterone. It is not known at present whether this finding has any clinical significance.

Although there is some experimental evidence that estrogens may have a direct effect on the human prostate and prostate carcinoma cell, no strong clinical evidence supports this possibility. The role of other hormones and tissue growth factors (somatostatin, epidermal growth factor, etc.) in supporting or counteracting the growth of human prostatic carcinoma cells has not been clearly defined at this moment.

Various principles are available at this moment to either suppress androgen production or to counteract the effect of androgens at the prostatic carcinoma target cell. In essence, apart from surgical castration, testosterone production in the Leydig cells can be eliminated by interfering with the pituitary testicular axis (LH) by means of estrogenic or gestagenic hormones, respectively, LHRH agonists or antagonists. Antiandrogens, substances that interfere with the action of androgens at the target cell level, have the advantage of potentially also eliminating the effect of adrenal androgens. Antiandrogens can be of the pure antiandrogenic type (flutamide) or may have antigonadotrophic effects like cyproterone acetate. The combination of a treatment principle that achieves castrate levels of circulating androgens with an antiandrogen permits a complete suppression of androgenic effects at the target cell level to be achieved.

The effect of endocrine management is limited by the presence of hormone-independent tumor cell populations within most human prostatic carcinomas. Cure of prostatic carcinoma by means of endocrine management has rarely occurred. Time to progression and rate of progression depend on factors like the size, the rate of growth, and the doubling time of the hormone-independent cell populations. The events that finally lead to the predominance of hormone-independent tumor masses probably include the origination of new hormone-independent populations due to genetic instability and the phenomena of clonal-selective growth. These factors have been reviewed by Isaacs and Coffey (1981).

It does not appear likely that the prognosis of disseminated prostatic carcinoma will improve with further sophistication of endocrine management. Only an effective cytostatic management together with endocrine management will improve the future prospects of our patients. In the meantime, it will be important to answer questions relevant to endocrine management, questions such as: is there an advantage in early or delayed endocrine treatment; what is the best endocrine treatment regimen?

Results of Endocrine Management

An important result of prospective randomized trials of prostatic carcinoma, locally advanced and metastatic, has been the experience that even in apparently homogeneous groups of patients prognostic factors play an important role. Some of these factors are tumor related, others may be tumor independent. In the studies of VACURG (Byar and Corle 1984), the size of the primary tumor, the amount of elevation of acid phosphatase, the presence or absence of ureteral dilatation, the presence or absence of visible metastases, and the grade of malignancy of the primary tumor were found to have significant impact on prognosis. The impact of these factors, singly or together, is usually stronger than the effects of treatment observed in the trials. This was also confirmed in recent EORTC GU Group studies reported by Smith et al. (1986) and Pavone et al. (1986). These observations indicated the necessity to correct progression and survival rates for prognostic factors even in prospective randomized trials with clearly defined criteria of entry. The lesson for all clinicians to be learned from such observations should be that historical comparison of results of nonprospective, noncontrolled studies should never be applied in this disease. Interpretation of such data is impossible and should not be attempted.

With the advent of well-organized, cooperative oncological groups in Europe and other parts of the world, a new spirit of carrying out carefully organized and supervised clinical trials has arisen, and the quality standards for clinical trial work set by these organizations represent large steps forward to a better understanding of the disease process and the influence of treatment modalities. For the reasons just mentioned, no attempt will be made in this context to review information on the treatment of prostatic cancer that is not related to prospective trials.

The studies of VACURG were a milestone in the development of a better understanding of endocrine management of prostatic carcinoma. In three large studies this group has compared various endocrine regimens including placebo and 5.0, 1.0, and 0.2 mg diethylstilbestrol (DES). Patients with locally extensive disease (stage 3) and metastatic disease (stage 4) were recruited. Some of the important results can be summarized as follows: progression rates were higher in all placebo groups. There was no difference in gross survival between the treatment groups, including placebo. The higher rate of cancer death in the placebo groups was more than compensated for by a higher incidence of cardiovascular death in the DES-treated groups of patients. In those patients of the placebo group who were later changed to endocrine treatment regimens, there was no difference in survival when compared to those patients who had initially been treated by endocrine means. This has led to the conclusion that endocrine management may be delayed in prostatic cancer until symptomatic metastases occur, without shortening overall survival. The palliative effect of endocrine treatment was superior to that of placebo.

The data of the VACURG studies have been reported and summarized in several publications, including those by VACURG (1967), Blackard et al. (1973), and Byar (1973, 1981). After the VACURG studies, significant contributions have been made by the prospective trials of the NPCP and the EORTC GU Group. This work has recently been reviewed by Murphy et al. (1984) for the NPCP and by Robinson and Hetherington (1986) for the EORTC. Of the various endocrine regimens studied, a clear disadvantage was shown only for medroxyprogesterone acetate (MPA) in a relatively low dosage. It is interesting that the large EORTC study 30 805, which included a complete androgen suppression arm (castration plus 150 mg cyproterone acetate), did not show any advantage in the patients treated in this way as compared to castration alone or 1 mg of DES per day.

In the older urological literature, response rates to endocrine management were often indicated as being in the range of 70%–80%. Once strict response criteria are used, response rates drop down to disappointing levels ranging between 25% and 40%. Some representative data are shown in Table 5. If "stabilization" is also included as a response, as in the trials of the NPCP, then response figures will go up to around 80%.

Recently, with the availability of potent LHRH agonists, a new principle of treatment has become available in the management of prostatic carcinoma and other steroid-dependent tumors. The major advantage of this new form of treatment seems to be the virtual absence of side effects. Representative for the large volume of literature which has become available are the papers by Roger et al. (1985) and Labrie et al. (1986). Several randomized studies have been completed in which the new treatment is compared to orchiectomy (Parmar et al. 1985) and to DES (Leuprolide Study Group 1984). No advantages, as far as tumor control was concerned, could be demonstrated by any of these trials.

Table 5. Response rates EORTC protocol 30 761 and 30 762 (DES 1 mg + i. d.) and NPCP protocol 500 (DES or castration). (Data from Smith et al. 1984; Murphy et al. 1984)

	Drug	(*n*)	CR (%)	PR (%)	SD (%)	Total
EORTC 30 761	DES	32	5	18	–	23
EORTC 30 762	DES	44	4	28	–	32
NPCP 500	DES or orchiectomy	83	12	29	40	81
						CR + PR = 41

The concept of Labrie et al. (1983) of applying regimens of "total androgen suppression" as an initial form of treatment has stimulated much clinical research effort. The decisive trials are still ongoing at the moment. Preliminary information on some of the early results by Brisset et al. (1988) and by Navratil (1988) seem to show that total androgen suppression as compared to standard forms of treatment is unfortunately not associated with a lower progression rate. There may be a slight advantage in the number of early responses seen with total androgen suppression. The future will have to show whether these advantages are great enough to justify this expensive form of management of metastatic prostatic carcinoma.

Second Line Management

Second line management of prostatic cancer is usually installed after progression occurs with first line treatment. Second line management can consist of endocrine measures such as secondary adrenal suppression, aromatase inhibition, or high-dose estrogen management. None of these regimens has been shown to be very successful. Extensive discussion in this context is not warranted.

Another possible alternative consists of the drug estramustine phosphate, a chemical compound that combines the 17 phosphorylated estradiol molecule with nitrogen mustard. Reported response rates from phase II and phase III studies average 25%–30% in hormone-unresponsive cases as reported by Nilsson (1980). The effect of estramustine phosphate in the primary management of prostatic carcinoma is probably identical to that of standard endocrine management as shown by the result of a prospective randomized study by Andersson et al. (1980).

Cytostatic drugs have been investigated in a number of phase II and phase III studies carried out by the NPCP and the EORTC GU Group. These include methotrexate, *cis*-platinum, 5-fluorouracil, cyclophosphamide, methyl-CCNU, dacarbazine, hydroxyuria, procarbazine, mitomycin C, vindesine, and adriamycin. Response rates strongly depend on the response criteria employed and tend to be slightly higher in the American studies than in the European studies. The most effective agents identified are mitomycin C, methotrexate, *cis*-platinum, 5-fluorouracil, and cytoxan. The NPCP trials have been reviewed by Murphy et al. (1984), the EORTC GU Group chemotherapy studies have been reviewed by Jones et al. (1984). The mitomycin C study of the EORTC has also been recently published by Jones et al. (1986). This trial reports an objective response rate of 29% in patients with measurable lesions.

Future Developments

Obviously, the future of our patients with prostatic carcinoma will depend on finding a cure for hormone-independent prostatic carcinoma. In the meantime, important questions, such as initial combination of endocrine management and cytostatic drugs and early versus delayed endocrine treatment, are important issues to be solved.

References

Ackermann R, Frohmüller HGW (1983) Complications and morbidity following radical prostatectomy. World J Urol 1: 62–67

Ackermann R, Müller HA (1981) Der Wert der perinealen Stanzbiopsie zur Beurteilung des histologischen Differenzierungsgrades des Prostata-Carcinoms. In: Frohmüller H (ed) Verhandlungsbericht der Deutschen Gesellschaft für Urologie, vol 32. Springer, Berlin Heidelberg New York, pp 79–81

Akazaki K, Stemmermann GN (1973) Comparative study of latent carcinoma of the prostate among Japanese in Japan and Hawaii. JNCI 50 (5): 1137–1144

American Cancer Society (1975) Cancer facts and figures. ACS, Philadelphia

Andersson L, Berlin T, Boman L, Collste L, Edsmyr F, Esposti PL, Gustafsson H, Hedlund PO, Hultgren L, Leander G, Nordle O, Norlen H, Tillegard P (1980) Estramustine versus conventional estrogenic hormones in the initial treatment of highly or moderately differentiated prostatic carcinoma – a randomized study. Scand J Urol Nephrol 55 [Suppl]: 143–145

Bagshaw MA (1980) External radiation therapy of carcinoma of the prostate. Cancer 45 (8): 1912–1921

Bagshaw MA (1984) Radiotherapy of prostatic cancer: Stanford University experience. In: Kurth KH, Debruyne FMJ, Schroeder FH, Splinter TAW, Wagener TDJ (eds) Progress and controversies in oncological urology. Liss, New York, pp 493–512

Bagshaw MA, Kaplan HS, Sagerman RH (1965) Linear accelerator super voltage radiotherapy VII. Carcinoma of the prostate. Radiology 85: 121

Barrett DM, Furlow WL (1983) Radical prostatectomy incontinence and the AS 791 artificial urinary sphincter. J Urol 129: 528–530

Belt E, Schroeder FH (1972) Total perineal prostatectomy for carcinoma of the prostate. J Urol 107: 91–96

Belt E, Egbert CE, Surber AC Jr (1939) New anatomic approach in perineal prostatectomy. J Urol 48: 287

Benson MC, Walsh PC (1986) The application of flow cytometry to the assessment of tumor cell heterogeneity and the grading of human prostatic cancer: preliminary results. J Urol 135: 1194–1198

Bhat DJ, Karwa GL, Bard RH, Freed SZ (1981) Serum acid phosphatases after rectal examination of prostate gland. Urology 18: 464–466

Björk P, Forsgren B, Gustafsson J-A, Pousette A, Högberg B (1982) Partial characterization and "quantitation" of a human prostatic estramustine-binding protein. Cancer Res 42: 1935–1942

Blackard CE, Byar DP, Jordan WP (1973) Orchiectomy for advanced prostatic carcinoma. Urology 1 (6): 553–560

Bosch RJLH, Schroeder FH (1986) Current problems in staging and grading prostatic carcinoma with special reference to T3 carcinoma of the prostate. World J Urol 4: 141–146

Bosch RJLH, Kurth KH, Schroeder FH (1987) Surgical treatment of locally advanced (T3) prostatic carcinoma – early results. J Urol 138: 816–822

Brawn PN (1982) Adenosis of the prostate. A dysplastic lesion that can be confused with prostate adenocarcinoma. Cancer 49: 826–833

Brendler CB, Cleeve LK, Everett Anderson E, Paulson DF (1980) Staging pelvic lymphadenectomy for carcinoma of the prostate: risk versus benefit. J Urol 124: 849–850

Brendler CB, Follansbee AL, Isaacs JT (1985) Discrimination between normal, hyperplastic and malignant prostatic tissues by enzymatic profiles. J Urol 133: 495–501

Breslow N, Chan CW, Dhom G, Drury RAB, Franks LM, Gellei B, Lee YS, Lundsberg S, Sparke B, Sternby NH, Tulinius H (1977) Latent carcinoma of prostate at autopsy in seven areas. Int J Cancer 20: 680–688

Brisset J-M, Boccon-Gibod L, Botto H, Camey M, Crious G, Duclos J-M, Duval F, Gontiès D, Jorest R, Lamy L, Le Duc A, Mouton A, Petit M, Prawerman A, Richard F, Savatovsky I, Vallencien G (1988) Anandron (RU 23908) associated to surgical castration in previously untreated stage D prostate cancer: a multicenter comparative study of two doses of the drug and of a placebo. In: Khoury S, Murphy GP (eds) Cancer of the prostate. Liss, New York (in press)

Byar DP (1973) The Veterans Administration Cooperative Urological Research Groups studies of cancer of the prostate. Cancer 32: 1126–1130

Byar DP, Corle DK (1984) Analysis of prognostic factors for prostate cancer in the VACURG studies. In: Denis L, Murphy GP, Prout GR, Schroeder FH (eds) Controlled clinical trials in urologic oncology. Raven, New York, pp 147–169

Byar PB, Mostofi FK, Veterans Administration Cooperative Urological Research Group (1972) Carcinoma of the prostate: prognostic evaluation of certain pathologic features in 208 radical prostatectomies. Cancer 30: 5–13

Byar DP, Corle DK, Veterans Administration Cooperative Urological Research Group (1981) VACURG randomized trial of radical prostatectomy for stage I and II prostate cancer. Urology 12 [Suppl 4]: 7–11

Cantrell BB, DeKlerk DP, Eggleston JC, Boitnott JK, Walsh PC (1981) Pathological factors that influence prognosis in stage. A prostatic cancer: the influence of extent versus grade. J Urol 125: 516–520

Catalona WJ, Stein AJ, Fair WR (1982) Grading errors in prostatic needle biopsies: relation to the accuracy of tumor grade in predicting pelvic lymph node metastases. J Urol 127: 919–952

Centraal bureau voor de statistiek (1979) Kanker – morbiditeit en mortaliteit 1975/1976, pp 42–43

Chisholm GD, Stone AR, Beynon LL, Merrick MV (1982) The bone scan as a tumour marker in prostatic carcinoma. Eur Urol 8: 257–260

Chodak GW, Schoenberg HW (1984) Early detection of prostate cancer by routine screening. JAMA 252 (23): 3261–3264

Chodak GW, Wald V, Parmer E, Watanabe H, Ohe H, Saitoh M (1986) Comparison of digital examination and transrectal ultrasonography for the diagnosis of prostatic cancer. J Urol 135: 951–954

Chu TM, Murphy GP (1986) What's new in tumor markers for prostate cancer? Urology 27: 487–491

Cohen P, Dix D (1985) On the role of aging in cancer incidence: an interpretation of the prostate cancer anomaly with implications for screening routine screening. Prostate 6: 437–443

Cox JD, Stoffel TJ (1977) The significance of needle biopsy after irradiation for stage C adenocarcinoma of the prostate. Cancer 40: 156–160

Dähnert WF, Hamper UM, Eggleston JC, Walsh PC, Sanders RC (1986) Prostatic evaluation by transrectal sonography with histopathologic correlation: the echopenic appearance of early carcinoma. Radiology 158: 97–102

Diamond DA, Berry SJ, Umbricht C, Jewett HJ, Coffey DS (1982) Computerized image analysis of nuclear shape as a prognostic factor for prostatic cancer. Prostate 3: 321–332

Donohue RE, Earl Fauver H, Whitesel JA, Augspurger RR, Pfister (1981) Prostatic carcinoma. Influence of tumor grade on results of pelvic lymphadenectomy. Urology 17, 5: 435–440

Elder JS, Catalona WJ (1984) Management of newly diagnosed metastatic carcinoma of the prostate. Urol Clin North Am 11: 283

Elder JS, Jewett HJ, Walsh PC (1982) Radical perineal prostatectomy for clinical stage B2 carcinoma of the prostate. J Urol 127: 704–706

El-Mahdi AM, Kuban DA, Schellhammer PF (1985) The treatment of choice for localized poorly differentiated adenocarcinoma of the prostate. Am J Clin Oncol 8: 477–480

Emmett JL, Greene LF, Papantoniou A (1960) Endocrine therapy in carcinoma of the prostate gland: 10-year survival studies. J Urol 83 (1): 471–484

Esposti PL (1971) Cytologic malignancy grading of prostatic carcinoma by transrectal aspiration biopsy. Scand J Urol Nephrol 5: 199–209

Faul P (1983) Diagnostische und prognostische Bedeutung des zytologischen Differenzierungsgrades beim Prostatakarzinom. Urologe 22: 127–133

Flanders WD (1984) Review: prostate cancer epidemiology. Prostate 5: 621–629

Flocks RH (1973) The treatment of stage C prostatic cancer with special reference to combined surgical and radiation therapy. J Urol 109: 461–463

Foti AG, Fenimore Cooper J, Herschman H, Malvaez RR (1977) Detection of prostatic cancer by solid-phase radioimmunoassay of serum prostatic acid phosphatase. N Engl J Med 297 (25): 1357–1361

Franzen S, Giertz G, Zajicek J (1960) Cytological diagnosis of prostatic tumours by transrectal aspiration biopsy: a preliminary report. Br J Urol 32: 193–196

Freiha FS, Pistenma DA, Bagshaw MA (1979) Pelvic lymphadenectomy for staging prostatic carcinoma: is it always necessary? J Urol 122: 176–177

Gaeta JF (1981) Glandular profiles and cellular patterns in prostatic cancer grading. Urology 17 [Suppl 3]: 33–37

Garnett JE, Oyasu R, Grayhack JT (1984) The accuracy of diagnostic biopsy specimens in predicting tumor grades by Gleason's classification of radical prostatectomy specimens. J Urol 131: 690–693

Geller J, Albert JD, Nachtsheim DA, Loza D (1984) Comparison of prostatic cancer tissue dihydrotestosterone levels at the time of relapse following orchiectomy or estrogen therapy. J Urol 132: 693–696

Gibbons RP, Tate Mason J, Correa RJ Jr, Cummings KB, Taylor WJ, Hafermann MD, Richardson RG (1979) Carcinoma of the prostate: local control with external beam radiation therapy. J Urol 121: 310–312

Gibbons RP, Correa RJ Jr, Brannen GE, Tate Mason J (1984) Total prostatectomy for localized prostatic cancer. J Urol 131: 73–76

Gibbons RP, Cole BS, Richardson RG, Correa RJ Jr, Brannen GE, Tate Mason J, Taylor WJ, Hafermann MD (1986) Adjuvant radiotherapy following radical prostatectomy: results and complications. J Urol 135: 65–68

Gittes RF, Chu TM (1976) Detection and diagnosis of prostate cancer. Semin Oncol 3: 123–130

Gleason DF, Mellinger GT, Veterans Administration Cooperative Urological Research Group (1974) Prediction of prognosis for prostatic adenocarcinoma by combined histological grading and clinical staging. J Urol 111: 58–64

Gleason DF, Veterans Administration Cooperative Urological Research Group (1977) Histological grading and clinical staging of prostatic carcinoma. In: Tannenbaum M (ed) Urologic pathology: the prostate. Lea and Febiger, Philadelphia, pp 171–198

Goldenberg DM, DeLand FH, Bennett SJ, Primus FJ, Nelson MO, Flanigan RC, McRoberts JW, Bruce AW, Mahan DE (1983) Radioimmunodetection of prostatic cancer. JAMA 250 (5): 630–635

Göthlin JH, Höiem L (1981) Percutaneous fine-needle biopsy of radiographically normal lymph nodes in the staging of prostatic carcinoma. Radiology 141 (2): 351–354

Grayhack JT, Assimos DG (1983) Prognostic significance of tumor grade and stage in the patient with carcinoma of the prostate. Prostate 4: 13–31

Greene LF, Farrow GM, Ravits JM, Tomera FM (1979) Prostatic carcinoma of ductal origin. J Urol 121: 303–305

Grossman HB (1986) Hormonal therapy of prostatic carcinoma: is there a rationale for delayed treatment? Urology 27: 199–204

Grossman HB, Batata M, Hilaris B, Whitmore WF (1982) ^{125}I implantation for carcinoma of prostate. Urology 20: 591–598

Guinan P, Bush I, Ray V, Vieth R, Rao R, Bhatti R (1980) The accuracy of the rectal examination in the diagnosis of prostate carcinoma. N Engl J Med 303 (9): 499–502

Gutman EB, Sproul EE, Gutman AB (1936) Significance of increased phosphatase activity of bone at the site of osteoblastic metastases secondary to carcinoma of the prostate gland. Am J Cancer 28: 485–495

Haenszel W (1961) Cancer mortality among the foreign-born in the United States. JNCI 26: 37–132

Haenszel W, Kurihara M (1968) Studies of Japanese migrants. I. Mortality from cancer and other diseases among Japanese in the United States. J Natl Cancer Inst 40: 43–68

Harmer MH (ed) (1982) TNM classification of malignant tumours, 3rd edn. UICC, Geneva

Hellman L, Fishman J (1970) Oestradiol production rates in man before and after orchiectomy for cancer. J Endocrinol 46: 113–114

Hermanek P, Sobin LH (1987) TNM classification of malignant tumours. Springer, Berlin Heidelberg New York

Herr HW (1979a) Complications of pelvic lymphadenectomy and retropubic prostatic ^{125}I implantation. Urology 14: 226–229

Herr HW (1979b) Preservation of sexual potency in prostatic cancer patients after pelvic lymphadenectomy and retropubic ^{125}I implantation. J Urol 121: 621–623

Herr HW (1983) The patient, disease status and treatment options for prostate cancer: stages B1 and B2. Prostate 4: 447–459

Hoekstra WJ, Schroeder FH (1981) The role of lymphangiography in the staging of prostatic cancer. Prostate 2: 433–440

Huben RP, Schellhammer PF (1982) The role of routine follow-up bone scans after definitive therapy of localized prostatic cancer. J Urol 128: 510–512

Huggins C, Hodges CV (1941) Studies on prostatic cancer. I. The effect of castration, of estrogen and of androgen injection on serum phosphatases in metastatic carcinoma of the prostate. Cancer Res 1: 293–297

Huggins C, Stevens RE Jr, Hodges CV (1941a) Studies on prostatic cancer. II. The effect of castration on advanced carcinoma of the prostate gland. Arch Surg 43: 209–223

Huggins C, Scott WW, Hodges CV (1941b) Studies on prostatic cancer. III. The effects of fever, of desoxycorticosterone and of estrogen on clinical patients with metastatic carcinoma of the prostate. J Urol 46: 997–1006

Isaacs JT, Coffey DS (1981) Adaptation versus selection as the mechanism responsible for the relapse of prostatic cancer to androgen ablation therapy as studied in the Dunning R-3327-H adenocarcinoma. Cancer Res 41: 5070–5075

Jacobs SC (1983) Spread of prostatic cancer to bone. Urology 11: 337–344

Jewett HJ (1956) Significance of the palpable prostatic nodule. JAMA 160: 838–839

Jewett HJ (1975) The present status of radical prostectomy for stages A and B prostatic cancer. Urol Clin North Am 2: 105

Jöbsis AC, de Vries GP, Anholt RRH, Sanders GTB (1978) Demonstration of the prostatic origin of metastases. Cancer 41: 1788–1793

Jones WG, Members of the EORTC Genitourinary Cancer Cooperative Group (1984) EORTC phase II chemotherapy studies in prostate cancer. In: Denis L, Murphy GP, Prout GR, Schroeder FH (eds) Controlled clinical trials in urologic oncology. Raven, New York, pp 181–185

Jones WG, Fossa SD, Bono AV, Croles JJ, Stoter G, de Pauw M, Sylvester R, Members of the EORTC Genito-urinary Tract Cancer Co-operative Group (1986) Mitomycin-C in the treatment of metastatic prostate cancer: report on an EORTC phase II study. World J Urol 4: 182–185

Kane RD, Mickey DD, Paulson DF (1976) Serial carcinoembryonic antigen assays in patients with metastatic carcinoma of prostate being treated with chemotherapy. Urology 8: 559–562

Kastendieck H (1980) Prostatic carcinoma, aspects of pathology, and therapy. J Cancer Res Clin Oncol 96: 131–156

Kastendieck H, Altenähr E, Hüsselmann H, Bressel M (1976) Carcinoma and dysplastic lesions of the prostate. Z Krebsforsch 88: 33–54

Kirk D, Hinton CE, Shaldon C (1979) Transitional cell carcinoma of the prostate. Br J Urol 51: 575–578

Kramer SA, Cline WA, Farnham R, Carson CC, Cox EB, Hinshaw W, Paulson DF (1981) Prognosis of patients with stage D1 prostatic adenocarcinoma. J Urol 125: 817

Kroes R, Beems RB, Bosland MC, Bunnik GSJ, Sinkeldam EJ (1986) Nutritional factors in lung, colon and prostate carcinogenesis in animal models. Fed Proc Inst CIVO Toxicology and Nutrition TNO 45: 136–141

Kuriyama M, Wang MC, Lee CL, Killian CS, Papsidero LD, Inaji H, Loor RM, Lin MF, Nishiura T, Slack NH, Chu TM (1982) Multiple marker evaluation in human prostate cancer with the use of tissue-specific antigens. JNCI 68: 99–105

Kurth KH, Altwein JE, Skoluda D, Hohenfellner R (1977) Follow up of irradiated prostatic carcinoma by aspiration biopsy. J Urol 117: 615–617

Labrie F, Dupont A, Belanger A, Lacoursiere Y, Raynaud JP, Husson JM, Gareau G, Faekas ATA, Sandow J, Monfette G, Girard JG, Emond J, Houle JG (1983) New approach in the treatment of prostate cancer: complete instead of partial withdrawal of androgens. Prostate 4: 579–594

Labrie F, Dupont A, Belanger A, St-Arnaud R, Giguere M, Lacoursiere Y, Emond J, Monfette G (1986) Treatment of prostate cancer with gonadotropin-releasing hormone agonists. Endocr Rev 7: 67–74

Labrie F, Luthy I, Veilleux R, Simard J, Belanger A, Dupont A (1988) In: Murphy G (ed) Proceedings of the International Symposium on prostate cancer. Liss, New York (in press)

Lepor H, Gregerman M, Crosby R, Mostofi FK, Walsh PC (1985) Precise localization of the autonomic nerves from the pelvic plexus to the corpora cavernosa: a detailed anatomical study of the adult male pelvis. J Urol 133: 207–212

Leuprolide Study Group (1984) Leuprolide versus diethylstilbestrol for metastatic prostate cancer. N Engl J Med 311: 1281–1286

Lieskovsky G, Skinner DG, Weisenburger T (1980) Pelvic lymphadenectomy in the management of carcinoma of the prostate. J Urol 1980: 635–638

Luciani L, Piscioli F (1983) Accuracy of transcutaneous aspiration biopsy in the definitive assessment of nodal involvement in prostatic carcinoma. Br J Urol 55: 321–325

Lytton B, Collins JT, Weiss RM, Schiff M Jr, McGuire EJ, Livolsi V (1979) Results of biopsy after early stage prostatic cancer treatment by implantation of ^{125}I seeds. J Urol 121: 306–309

Mattila S (1969) Further studies on the prostatic tissue antigens. Invest Urol 7: 1–9

McGowan DG, Hanson J (1985) The National Canadian study of the prostate treated by external beam radiation (1970–1978). J Assoc Can Radiol 36: 216–222

McNeal JE (1969) Origin and development of carcinoma of the prostate. Cancer 23: 24–34

McNeal JE (1981) Origin and evolution of prostatic carcinoma. In: Ablin RJ (ed) Prostatic cancer. Dekker, New York, pp 43–50

McNeal JE, Bostwick DG, Kindrachuk RA, Redwine EA, Freiha FS, Stamey TA (1986) Patterns of progression in prostate cancer. Lancet 8472: 60–63

Mettlin C, Natarajan N, Murphy GP (1982) Recent patterns of care of prostate cancer patients in the United States: results from the surveys of the American College of Surgeons Commission on Cancer. Int Adv Surg Oncol 5: 277–321

Middleton RG, Smith JA Jr, Melzer RB, Hamilton PE (1986) Patient survival and local recurrence rate following radical prostatectomy for prostatic carcinoma. J Urol 136: 422–424

Milford Ward A, Cooper EH, Houghton AL (1977) Acute

phase reactant proteins in prostatic cancer. Br J Urol 49: 411–418
Moss AJ, Bissada NK, Boyd CM, Hunter WC (1979) Significance of protein-bound neuraminic acid levels in patients with prostatic and bladder carcinoma. Urology 13: 182–184
Mostofi FK (1975) Grading of prostatic carcinoma. Cancer Treat Rep 59: 111–117
Murphy GP, Slack NH (1980) Response criteria for the prostate of the USA National Prostatic Cancer Project. Prostate 1: 375–382
Murphy GP, Slack NH, and participants in the National Prostatic Cancer Project (1984) Current status of the National Prostatic Cancer Project treatment protocols. In: Denis L, Murphy GP, Prout GR, Schroeder FH (eds) Controlled clinical trials in urologic oncology. Raven, New York, pp 119–134
Navratil H (1987) Double-blind study of anandron versus placebo in stage D prostate cancer patients receiving buserelin. In: Khoury S, Murphy GP (eds) Cancer of the prostate. Liss, New York (in press)
Nesbit RM, Baum WC (1950) Endocrine control of prostatic carcinoma: clinical and statistical survey of 1818 cases. JAMA 143: 1317–1320
Nesbit RM, Plumb RT (1946) Prostatic carcinoma: a follow up on 795 patients treated prior to the endocrine era and a comparison of survival rates between these and patients treated by endocrine therapy. Surgery 20: 263–272
Nilsson T (1980) Estracyt – clinical experiences. Scand J Urol Nephrol 55 [Suppl]: 135–138
Oosterom R, Leijnse B, Bogdanowicz J, Schroeder FH (1986) Evaluation of an enzyme-immunoassay for prostatic acid phosphatase utilizing monoclonal antibodies. World J Urol 4: 153–158
Papsidero LD, Wojcieszyn JW, Horoszewicz JS, Leong SS, Murphy GP, Chu TM (1980) Isolation of prostatic acid phosphatase-binding immunoglobulin G from human sera and its potential for use as a tumor-localizing reagent. Cancer Res 40: 3032–3035
Parmar H, Phillips RH, Lightman SL, Edwards L, Allen L, Schally AV (1985) Randomised controlled study of orchidectomy vs. long-acting D-Trp-6-LHRH microcapsules in advanced prostatic carcinoma. Lancet 8466: 1201–1205
Paulson DF, Lin GH, Hinshaw W, Stephanis S, Uro-oncology Research Group (1982) Radical surgery versus radiotherapy for adenocarcinoma of the prostate. J Urol 128: 502–504
Paulson DF, Byron Hodge G, Hinshaw W, Uro-oncology Research Group (1984) Radiation therapy versus delayed androgen deprivation for stage C carcinoma of the prostate. J Urol 131: 901–902
Pavone Macaluso M, De Voogt HJ, Viggiano G, Barasolo E, Lardennois B, De Pauw M, Sylvester R (1986) Comparison of diethylstilbestrol, cyproterone acetate and medroxyprogesterone in the treatment of advanced prostatic cancer: final analysis of a randomized phase III trial of the European Organization for Research and Treatment of Cancer Urological Group. J Urol 136: 624–631
Pearson JC, Dombrovskis, Dreyer J, Williams RD (1983) Radioimmunoassays of serum prostatic acid phosphatase after prostatic massage. Urology 21: 37–41
Peeling WB, Griffiths GJ (1984) Imaging of the prostate by ultrasound, review article. J Urol 132: 217–224
Pollen JJ, Schmidt JD (1979) Diagnostic fine needle aspiration of soft tissue metastases from cancer of the prostate. J Urol 121: 59–61
Ray GR, Bagshaw MA, Freiha F (1984) External beam radiation salvage for residual or recurrent local tumor following radical prostatectomy. J Urol 132: 926–930
Rifkin MD, Friedland GW, Shortliffe L (1986) Prostatic evaluation by transrectal endosonography: detection of carcinoma. Radiology 158: 85–90
Robinson MRG, Hetherington J (1986) The EORTC studies: is there an optimal endocrine management for M1 prostatic cancer? World J Urol 4: 1–5
Roger M, Duchier J, Lahiou N, Nahoul K, Schally AV (1985) Treatment of prostatic carcinoma with D-Trp-6-LH-RH: plasma hormone levels after daily subcutaneous injections and periodic administration of delayed-release preparations. Prostate 7: 271–282
Segalowsky AI, Milam H, Reveley LR, Silva FG (1982) Prediction of lymphatic metastases by Gleason histologic grading in prostatic cancer. J Urol 128: 951–952
Scardino PT, Frankel JM, Wheeler TM, Meacham RB, Hoffman GS, Seale C, Wilbanks JH, Easley J, Carlton CE Jr (1986) The prognostic significance of post-irradiation biopsy results in patients with prostatic cancer. J Urol 135: 510–515
Schellhammer PF, El-Mahdi AE, Ladaga LE, Schultheiss T (1985) ^{125}Iodine implantation for carcinoma of the prostate: 5-year survival free of disease and incidence of local failure. J Urol 134: 1140–1145
Schmidt JD, Slack NH, Ming Chu T, Murphy GP (1982) Placenta-like isoenzyme of alkaline phosphatase in prostatic cancer. J Urol 127: 457–459
Schroeder FH (1980) Prostatic carcinoma: comments on radical surgical treatment. Scand J Urol Nephrol 55 [Suppl]: 181–185
Schroeder FH (1982) Prostatic cancer: prognostic factors of importance in patients management. In: Proceedings of the Sociétée Internationale d'Urologie, San Francisco, 1982
Schroeder FH, Belt E (1975) Carcinoma of the prostate: a study of 213 patients with stage C tumors treated by total perineal prostatectomy. J Urol 114: 257–260
Schroeder FH, Jellinghaus W, Frohmüller H (1976) Behandlung des lokal begrenzten Prostata-Carcinoms: Bestrahlung oder totale Prostatektomie? Urologe [A] 15: 67–72
Schroeder FH, Blom JHM, Hop WCJ, Mostofi FK (1984 a) Incidental carcinoma of the prostate treated by total prostatectomy. The prognostic impact of microscopic tumor extension and grade. World J Urol 1: 15–23
Schroeder FH, European Organization for Research and Treatment of Cancer Urological Group (1984 b) Treatment response criteria for prostatic cancer. Prostate 5: 181–191
Schroeder FH, Hop WCJ, Blom JHM, Mostofi FK (1985) Grading of prostatic cancer. III. Multivariate analysis of prognostic parameters. Prostate 7: 13–20
Siddall JK, Cooper EH, Newling DWW, Robinson MRG, Whelan P (1986) An evaluation of the immunochemical measurement of prostatic acid phosphatase and prostatic specific antigen in carcinoma of the prostate. Eur Urol 12: 123–130
Silverman LM, Chapman JF, Jones ME, Dermer GB, Pullano T, Tökes ZA (1981) Creatinine kinase BB and other markers of prostatic carcinoma. Prostate 2: 109–119
Smith JA, Seaman JP, Gleidman JB, Middleton G (1983) Pelvic lymph node metastasis from prostatic cancer: influence of tumor grade and stage in 452 consecutive patients. J Urol 130: 290–292
Smith JA Jr, Haynes TH, Middleton RG (1984) Impact of external irradiation on local symptoms and survival free of disease in patients with pelvic lymph node metastases from adenocarcinoma of the prostate. J Urol 131: 705–707

Smith PH, Pavone Macaluso M, Viggiano G, De Voogt HJ, Lardennois B, Robinson MRG, Richards B (1984) EORTC protocols in prostatic cancer. In: Denis L, Murphy GP, Prout GR, Schroeder FH (eds) Controlled clinical trials in urologic oncology. Raven, New York, pp 107–117

Smith PH, Suciu S, Robinson MRG, Richards B, Bastable JRG, Glashan RW, Bouffioux C, Lardennois B, Williams RE, De Pauw M, Sylvester R (1986) A comparison of the effect of diethylstilbestrol with low dose estramustine phosphatase in the treatment of advanced prostatic cancer: final analysis of a phase III trial of the European Organization for Research and Treatment of Cancer. J Urol 136: 619–623

Snowdon DA, Phillips RL, Choi W (1984) Diet, obesity and risk of fatal prostate cancer. Am J Epidemiol 120: 244–250

Ten Kate FJW, Gallee MPW, Schmitz PIM, Joebsis AC, van der Heul RO, Prins MEF, Blom JHM (1986) Problems in grading of prostatic carcinoma: interobserver reproducibility of five different grading systems. World J Urol 4 (3): 147–152

Tomlinson RL, Currie DP, Boyce WH (1977) Radical prostatectomy: palliation for stage C carcinoma of the prostate. J Urol 117: 85–87

Van Aubel OGJM, Hoekstra WJ, Schroeder (1985) Early orchiectomy for patients with stage D1 prostatic carcinoma. J Urol 134: 292–294

Van der Werf-Messing BPH, Menon RS, Van Putten WLJ (1984) Prostatic cancer treated by external irradiation at the Rotterdam Radiotherapy Institute. Strahlentherapie 160: 293–300

Veterans Administration Co-operative Urological Research Group (1967) Treatment and survival of patients with cancer of the prostate. Surg Gynecol Obstet 124: 1011–1017

Veterans Administration Cooperative Urological Research Group (1968) Factors in the prognosis of carcinoma of the prostate: a cooperative study. J Urol 100: 50–65

Vihko P, Kontturi M, Lukkarinen O, Vihko R (1985) Immunoreactive prostatic acid phosphatase in prostatic cancer: diagnosis and follow up of patients. J Urol 123: 979–982

Wajsman Z, Chu TM, Bross D, Saroff J, Murphy GP, Johnson DE, Scott WW, Gibbons RP, Prout GR, Schmidt JD (1978) Clinical significance of serum alkaline phosphatase isoenzyme levels in advanced prostatic carcinoma. J Urol 119: 244–246

Walsh PC (1981) Randomized study of prostatic cancer. Letter to the editor. Urology 18: 219

Walsh PC (1986) Radical retropubic prostatectomy. In: Walsh PC, Gittes RE, Perlmutter AD, Stamey TA (eds) Campbell's urology, vol 3. Saunders, Philadelphia, pp 2754–2775

Walsh PC, Donker PJ (1982) Impotence following radical prostatectomy: insight into etiology and prevention. J Urol 128: 492–497

Webb KS, Lin GH (1980) Urinary fibronectin. Invest Urol 17: 401–404

Whitmore WF (1973) The natural history of prostatic cancer. Cancer 32: 1104–1112

Whitmore WF (1980) Interstitial radiation therapy for carcinoma of the prostate. Prostate 1: 157–168

Whitmore WF (1984) Interstitial I-125 implantation in the management of localized prostatic cancer. In: Kurth KH, Debruyne FMJ, Schroeder FH, Splinter TAW, Wagener TDJ (eds) Progress and controversies in oncological urology. Liss, New York, pp 513–527

WHO (1979) Handbook for reporting results in cancer treatment, WHO offset publication no 48. World Health Organization, Geneva

Wilson JWL, Morales A, Bruce AW (1983) The prognostic significance of histological grading and pathological staging in carcinoma of the prostate. J Urol 130: 481–483

Wynder EL, Mabuchi K, Whitmore WF (1971) Epidemiology of cancer of the prostate. Cancer 28: 344–360

Yagoda A, Watson RC, Natale RB, Barzell W, Sogani P, Grabstald H, Whitmore WF (1979) A critical analysis of response criteria in patients with prostatic cancer treated with *cis*-diamminedichloride platinum II. Cancer 44 (5): 1553–1562

Young HH (1945) The cure of cancer by radical perineal prostatectomy. J Urol 53: 188

Zaridze DG, Boyle P, Smans M (1984) International trends in prostatic cancer. Int J Cancer 33: 223–230

Zincke H, Farrow GM, Myers RP, Benson RC Jr, Furlow WL, Utz DC (1982) Relationship between grade and stage of adenocarcinoma of the prostate and regional pelvic lymph node metastases. J Urol 128: 498–501

Zincke H, Utz DC, Taylor W (1986) Bilateral pelvic lymphadenectomy and radical prostatectomy for clinical stage C prostatic cancer: role of adjuvant treatment for residual cancer and in disease progression. J Urol 135: 1199–1205

Carcinoma of the Penis

J. P. Blandy

Definition

Cancer of the penis is usually a primary squamous cell carcinoma arising from the foreskin or glans penis, but secondary tumours and other primary growths are occasionally encountered.

Classification

1. Primary
   - Carcinoma in situ (Queyrat's erythroplasia, Bowen's disease)
   - Squamous cell cancer

- Basal cell carcinoma
- Melanoma
- Sarcoma – fibrosarcoma, endothelioma, leiomyosarcoma, rhabdomyosarcoma, Kaposi's sarcoma

2. Secondary
   - Nodular, from carcinoma of bladder or prostate
   - Intraurethral/intradermal from carcinoma of bladder

Epidemiology, Risk Factors

Race, Geography and Circumcision

It is impossible today to disentangle the three factors: race, geography and circumcision. There is a very considerable difference in the reported incidence of carcinoma of the penis in different parts of the world: Ceylon and the East Indies having the most, and white citizens of the United States the least.

Some of these differences may be genetic, but there are anomalies, for example, mainland Chinese are said to have widely disparate incidences of penile cancer varying from 17.5% of all cancers in the male in Peking, 15.2% in Java, 5.7% in Canton, 3.6% in Malaysia, but only 1.9% in Singabore (Hu and Yang 1959; Muir 1962; Marsden 1958). To some extent, genetic or racial differences in susceptibility must be obscured by the differing practices in circumcision, for example, in Africa, Dodge (1965) observed considerable differences in incidence of penile cancer between adjacent tribes who did and did not circumcise their children.

For centuries it has been recognised that cancer of the penis is virtually never seen in Jews ritually circumcised in infancy: indeed Boczko and Freed (1979) believe that only nine such cases have ever been reported. There are of course no control studies of large numbers of uncircumcised Jews to permit one to conclude that circumcision is a true prophylactic rather than a coincidence. However, in India Paymaster and Gangadharan (1967) reported 910 cases amongst those whose religions did not enforce circumcision versus 12 cases among Muslims and none amongst Jews. Interestingly, they suggested that the 12 Muslim cases might reflect the slight delay in performing circumcision in these children – a practice which varies from 3 to 12 years in different societies – whereas the Jewish rite is performed on the 8th day after birth (Reddy and Indira 1963). It is not clear why circumcision does protect men from cancer of the penis in later life. Two explanations are usually advanced: (a) that in removing the foreskin one removes the major part of the skin in which cancer usually arises; Marcial et al. (1962) suggested that carcinoma arose from the foreskin in at least one-third of their cases; (b) it permits the patient to keep the glans penis clean, and, in particular, free from the accumulation of smegma, although the role of smegma as a carcinogen has been doubted by Reddy and Baruah (1963).

In a careful study of the topic, the Fetus and Newborn Committee of the Canadian Pediatric Society (1982) pointed out that there were wide differences in the incidence of penile cancer among African tribes who practised circumcision, and that in Sweden, where circumcision is seldom performed, penile cancer was very rare.

There is no doubt that in every large series, authors comment on the association of penile cancer with phimosis and retained smegma, sometimes so severe as to lead to the formation of calcified concretions under the irretractible prepuce.

There is, however, another factor, in the writer's opinion, which is more likely to have an aetiological significance, namely the frequent association of recurrent inflammation and healing under the phimosis. Recurrent balanitis is often seen in little boys between the ages of 2 and 5 with foreskins that do not retract easily, and on performing circumcision it is common to find the glans penis denuded of epithelium. In elderly men these changes can be even more marked, and the repeated loss and regeneration of epithelium would seem, by analogy with Marjolin's ulcer, a more probable carcinogenic influence.

Repeated inflammation of the penis with a more specific aetiology has also been incriminated. Previous syphilis and chancroid are often cited in large series, with an incidence that varies from 10% to 66.5% (Paymaster and Gangadharan 1967; Staubitz et al. 1955; Howard and Holtham 1950; Furlong and Uhle 1953; Lenowitz and Graham 1946). However, Lenowitz and Graham (1946) warn against the too ready acceptance of previous venereal disease as an aetiological agent, pointing out that the incidence was actually higher in men from the same population but not having penile cancer.

In England it has often been stated that cancer of the penis is a disease of old men who do not retract their foreskins or wash their penises, but in recent years the writer has been obliged to treat a number of highly intelligent and well-educated men, scrupulously clean in their person, who have developed penile cancer, and one must speculate whether there is not some other precancerous aetiological agent at work.

The most obvious culprit is some infective virus, e.g. human papilloma- or herpesvirus. Graham et al. (1979) have point out that the incidence of cervical cancer was unexpectedly high in the wives of 227 men in New York with cancer of the penis, and Cartwright and Sinson (1980) have reported an amazing coincidence of three men with cancer of the penis living in the same street, the wives of two of whom also having cervical cancer.

Balanitis Xerotica Obliterans

Often held to be a benign condition, we were disturbed to find in a recent review of our own cases (El Demiry et al. 1984) that 22% had a previous history of balanitis xerotica. In the writer's series of some 50 men requiring meatoplasty or urethroplasty for balanitis xerotica, no fewer than three have developed squamous cell carcinoma of the urethra over a period of some 20 years. No careful prospective long-term follow-up of this condition has yet been reported, but it may be time to revise our notion of its innocence.

Histopathology

Primary Neoplasms

In Situ Cancer

In situ cancer was first described by Paget (1874) as "a persistent rawness of the glans penis, like a long-standing balanitis ... followed after more than a year's duration by cancer of the substance of the glans". It was not until 1911 that Queyrat referred to four similar cases with raw flat red areas on the glans; two were later found to have invasive cancer.

Bowen's disease – dry brownish encrusted lesions – occurs on the penis as it does elsewhere in the skin: this is also an intradermal carcinoma, and though Brown (1966) considered it to be identical with Queyrat's erythroplasia, Mostofi and Price (1973) advance arguments for considering them to be distinct entities.

Squamous Cell Cancer of the Penis

Macroscopically this may present in three forms – a proliferative lesion, a nodular infiltrating lesion, or an ulcer that may arise in the sulcus of the glans and invade deeply into the corpora and actually lead to disappearance of the entire penis. As with other squamous cell cancers of the skin, they show a spectrum of degrees of differentiation which may be classified into three or four grades according to the numbers of mitoses present, or, more usefully, according to whether they show a "solid" or a "cord" pattern of growth, for this correlates very closely with the clinical behaviour of the growth (Frew et al. 1967; Salaverria et al. 1979; El-Demiry et al. 1984).

Buschke-Loewenstein Tumour

Special care must be taken with this tumour, so often believed in the past to be benign. In the writer's experience, as in that of Schmauz et al. (1977), these massive lesions, which resemble giant condylomata acuminata clinically and may have a benign microscopic appearance in a superficial biopsy, are by no means benign: they invade deeply, they recur after timid surgery, and they spread to the inguinal nodes. They are of great interest because it is tempting to see in them a tumour of virus origin that undergoes malignant transformation (Oriel and Almeida 1970; Kovi et al. 1970; Lowe and McKee 1983).

Basal Cell Cancer

Basal cell cancer occurs on the penis, but excessively rarely. Staubitz et al. (1955) reported one among 204 cases of cancer and Fegen et al. (1970) reviewed ten cases in the literature. As with basal cell carcinoma elsewhere, they do not spread in lymphatics, and it is only necessary to remove them locally to effect cure.

Melanoma

Melanoma of the penis is very rare. In the United States Armed Forces Institute of Pathology (USAFIP), Dixon and Moore (1952) could only find 25 cases among 2500 examples of penile cancer (1%), and in Bombay, Paymaster and Gangadharan (1967) found only two among 1055 penile cancers (0.2%). Compared with other sites for a melanoma to occur, the penis is very uncommon – Cascinelli (1969) found only one in the penis in a series of 720 melanomas. Melanomas are usually pigmented. They have a very bad prognosis, with early invasion of the inguinal lymph nodes, but as with other examples of this unpredictable tumour, an occasional prolonged survival is reported (Reid 1957; Wheelock and Clark 1943).

Sarcoma

Probably first described by Jonathan Hutchinson in 1855, Abeshouse et al. (1962) have published a comprehensive review of these uncommon tumours: 72 cases were 36 fibrosarcomas, 21 endotheliomas, eight myosarcomas and seven Kaposi's sarcomas. A myxosarcoma was reported by Frazer (1965). In most of the reported cases it appears that the correct treatment is a wide initial local excision.

One unusual presentation of these tumours is priapism, caused by an endothelial or haemangioendothelial sarcoma: Hodgins and Hancock (1970) reviewed nine such cases. Lymphoma and reticulosis may occasionally be confined to the penis (Gough 1970).

Secondary Tumours

Secondary tumours occur in two clinical forms. The most common, which is often seen in advanced cases of cancer of the prostate and bladder, presents as a woody infiltration of the corpora, not unlike the fibrosis of Peyronie's disease. The diagnosis is confirmed by a Trucut needle biopsy. The writer has one such patient with infiltration of the penis by transitional cell cancer of the bladder with a 2-year complete response to combination chemotherapy, and another with cancer from the prostate which responded (for 1 year) to orchidectomy.

In the less common clinical form there is an intradermal infiltration of the glans penis with bladder tumour that has spread along the urethral lymphatics to produce a shiny pink change in the glans, around the external meatus, comparable to Paget's disease of the nipple. The writer has seen this in one 50-year-old male with extensive recurrent tumour of the bladder that also encircled the rectum and caused intestinal obstruction: both lesions responded (temporarily) to single-agent vinblastine.

Natural History

The typical carcinoma of the penis is seen in an elderly, unintelligent poor man, whose prepuce does not retract and issues a foul-smelling discharge. A mass is easily felt involving the glans and prepuce, which is often ulcerated and always infected. The inguinal lymph nodes are inflamed and swollen.

If the disease is confined to the prepuce, circumcision is enough to effect a cure, but very few patients come up at such an early stage. If limited to the glans, it may be destroyed by local irradiation or partial amputation. The prognosis depends on whether the tumour has invaded the inguinal lymph nodes. At first, the clinical swelling of the nodes is usually caused by secondary infection, so it is wise to wait, after circumcision and removal of the primary tumour, to control infection with a few weeks of chemotherapy. If induration and enlargement of the lymph nodes persist, then they should be biopsied. If positive, a proportion of patients can be cured by radical node dissection, but the majority return with distant metastases.

Staging

Baker and Watson (1975) have reviewed the half-dozen proposed staging systems and have offered a way of reconciling them with each other. The TNM system is shown in Table 1. In practice the TNM system is not very relevant to the clinical situation and the writer prefers a system adapted from Jackson (1966) (Table 2). This classification lends itself to the selection of patients for radiotherapy with the iridium mould as only patients with stage I and II disease can be fitted with a mould.

Johnson (1982) uses an equally simple system that lends itself to a policy of amputation:

Stage I Malignant disease confined to the penis

Stage II Clinical suspicion of tumour extension

Table 1. Staging of cancer of the penis

T – Primary Tumour	
TX	Primary tumour cannot be assessed
T0	No evidence of primary tumour
Tis	Carcinoma in situ
Ta	Non-invasive verrucous carcinoma
T1	Tumour invades subepithelial connective tissue
T2	Tumour invades corpus spongiosum or cavernosum
T3	Tumor invades urethra or prostate
T4	Tumour invades other adjacent structures
N – Regional Lymph Nodes	
NX	Regional lymph nodes cannot be assessed
N0	No regional lymph node metastasis
N1	Metastasis in a single superficial inguinal lymph node
N2	Metastasis in multiple or bilateral superficial inguinal lymph nodes
N3	Metastasis in deep inguinal or pelvic lymph node(s), unilateral or bilateral
M – Distant Metastasis	
MX	Presence of distant metastasis cannot be assessed
M0	No distant metastasis
M1	Distant metastasis

Table 2. Staging of cancer of the penis. (From Jackson 1966)

Stage I	Confined to foreskin or glans penis
Stage II	Extending to the shaft of the penis
Stage III	Inguinal nodes positive, but operable
Stage IV	Fixed inoperable inguinal nodes, or primary tumour invading the perineum or scrotum, or distant metastases

beyond the penis but not beyond the regional ilioinguinal lymphatic drainage

Stage III Disseminated disease as seen in generalised abdominal (visceral) or pulmonary metastases

Staging Investigations

One of the main limitations of the TNM system is the uncertainty of the state of the inguinal nodes, which are almost always inflamed when the patient is first seen. Biopsy of such an infected mass is clearly pointless, and lymphangiography is difficult to interpret in the presence of acute inflammation and apt to be followed by oedema and cellulitis. Nor is the diameter of the initial lesion very relevant since quite large fungating tumours may be confined to the prepuce of the glans and have a good prognosis. The crucial issues for therapy are (a) whether the tumour has or has not invaded the vascular spaces of the corpora spongiosum or cavernosa; (b) whether the tumour can be ablated by radiation or partial amputation; and (c) whether inguinal lymph nodes are removable or not.

Prognosis

The most important guides to prognosis are tumour grade and tumour stage.

Tumour Grade

In the writer's series (El Demiry et al. 1984) the most important factor was undoubtedly tumour grade. When tumours were categorised according to G1, 2 and 3 grades, the overall 5-year survival rate for G1 tumours was 91%, for G3 only 51%. In the favourable "solid" pattern of tumour growth there was a 96% 5-year survival rate, compared with the unfavourable "cord" pattern of growth which had a 73% 5-year survival rate.

Tumour Stage

In stage I, where the tumour was limited to the glans penis or foreskin, the 5-year survival rate was 80%. In stage II, where the corpora had been invaded, it was 56%. In stage III, where there was invasion of the perineum or scrotum and the inguinal nodes, if present, were operable, the survival was 59%. There were no survivors in more advanced cases.

In our series, when the local lesion was very large, it was almost always severely infected, and the inguinal lymph nodes were almost always enlarged, but after a period of observation and treatment with antibiotics, only 42% of these nodes proved to be positive.

In contrast, when the original lesion was small and confined to the prepuce or the glans, the finding of enlarged lymph nodes was of much more significance. When the inguinal nodes were found to be swollen in these patients at the time of presentation, no fewer than 80% were later proved to harbour cancer. Enlargement of inguinal nodes in an "early" case is obviously a very important prognostic feature.

In a tumour as uncommon as cancer of the penis, which presents as a rule in elderly men, many other factors contribute to prognosis, and intercurrent respiratory or vascular disease often rules out the use of adjuvant chemotherapy or wide surgical excision.

Screening of Asymptomatic Disease

If the prepuce cannot be retracted to allow a boy to wash his glans penis and keep it clean, he should undergo circumcision. If this simple rule were adhered to, the incidence of neglected cancer of the penis would be considerably reduced.

In parts of the world where soap and water is in short supply, one can make a case out for routine circumcision, but it is doubtful if it can be justified in affluent countries of the West. In view of our own findings of preceding balanitis xerotica obliterans in 22% of our cases (El-Demiry et al. 1984), it would seem wise to follow up all these patients indefinitely.

Diagnosis of Symptomatic Disease

The only safe rule is to insist upon a biopsy of every suspicious lesion of the penis. This is particularly necessary in the elderly man who presents with a weeping inflamed fissure in the sulcus of the glans penis, while any exfoliative lesion except for the obvious condyloma acuminatum should always be biopsied.

In most of our patients it has been necessary to perform a circumcision in order to see the lesion and obtain a biopsy. Very occasionally the growth has been entirely confined to the foreskin, and this initial circumcision has been sufficient to effect a cure.

For the same reason, the foreskin of any middle-aged or elderly man taken at circumcision should always be carefully examined histologically. All too often the opportunity for making an early diagnosis is missed because the specimen has been discarded, and the condition is not diagnosed or treated until the patient returns months later with inoperable inguinal metastases.

Staging Investigations

When the inguinal nodes are enlarged, a 2–3-week course of appropriate antibiotics is given to treat the secondary infection in the inguinal lymph nodes. If they remain persistently enlarged, it is our practice to perform a needle aspiration of the nodes for cytological examination. If this is positive, a CT examination of the pelvic lymph nodes is supplemented by a bilateral pedal lymphangiogram, paying particular attention to the iliac and para-aortic nodes.

Treatment

Carcinoma In Situ

Having established the diagnosis by means of a biopsy, carcinoma in situ may be safely treated by one of a number of techniques. One simple method is that of Mantell and Morgan (1969) who made a sheath for the penis from silicone elastomer impregnated with yttrium oxide and converted in a nuclear reactor to yttrium 90, a beta particle emitter. The sheath was applied for 10 min on two occasions 1 week apart, giving a surface dose of 1500 rad on each occasion.

An alternative is to apply topical 5-fluorouracil (Goette 1976). This is available as a 5% cream and is applied by the patient to the affected area twice daily for 2 weeks and, thereafter, daily for 1 month. It produces an intense local desquamation which is often very uncomfortable (Johnson 1982).

Carcinoma Limited to the Foreskin

It is enough to perform a careful circumcision with a good clear margin. If the carcinoma is entirely confined to the prepuce no further treatment is needed, but the patients must be carefully followed up.

Carcinoma Confined to the Glans Penis (Stage I)

Since excellent results may be obtained by a variety of techniques, the one that gives the best functional and cosmetic result is to be preferred. Of the methods that are available, that in use at the London Hospital (Hope-Stone 1975) has certain advantages: it is painless, easy to apply, gives good results and is safe for the patient and the nursing staff.

A mould is prepared which consists of an inner Perspex cylinder that is worn over the penis. Over this fits an outer cylinder, which is armed with iridium 192 wire and is kept beside the patient in a leaden box. In the privacy of his room the patient is taught to place the outer cylinder over the inner one and make a note of the time it is in place. The timing of the applications, and the length of the iridium 192 wire is calculated to give 6000 rad to the tumour, but only 5000 rads to the urethra. The applicator is removed by the patient when he wishes to urinate and in practice is worn for about 12 h a day for 1 week.

The technique does demand the cooperation of the patient. Some elderly and confused patients have been unable to understand what they are expected to do or to handle the applicator correctly.

Delclos (1982) describes an alternative way of delivering irradiation by transfixing the glans penis with a series of radium, iridium or tantalum needles. Using this method Haile and Delclos (1980) claimed to have preserved the penis in 16 out of 20 cases (80%), but no details were given of the long-term results or recurrence rates. Delclos admits to having had local necrosis, urethral stenosis and fistulae among the complications of this technique.

In contrast, the complications of Hope-Stone's iridium mould method are negligible: no patient developed necrosis or fistulae. Four patients out of 27 (14.8%) developed a minor stenosis of the meatus which was easily remedied by a meatoplasty. One must, however, be aware that local recurrence may develop in about 20% of these cases and be prepared to biopsy any suspicious lesion and perform a partial amputation if needed. When, for one reason

Table 3. Comparison of results using different treatment procedures in stage I disease. (From El-Demiry et al. 1984)

Method	(*n*)	Local recurrence (%)	Deaths from metastases (%)	Five-year survival rate (%)
Iridium mould	23	21.7	8.6	89
Cobald 60	10	70	20	76
Partial amputation	7	29	14.2	71
	40	35	13	80

Table 4. Comparison of results using different treatment procedures in stage II disease

Method	(*n*)	Recurrence rate (%)	Deaths from metastases (%)	Five-year survival rate (%)
Iridium	4	75	25	75
Cobald 60	5	80	0	75
Amputation	9	33	33	56
	18	56	22	56

or another, the use of the iridium mould was not considered appropriate, partial amputation was performed, or teletherapy given with cobalt 60, Grafstald and Kelley (1980) and Duncan and Jackson (1972) having reported cures in 90% with this form of irradiation.

The results in Stage I with this policy are shown in Table 3. This experience emphasises the considerable risk of local recurrence after any form of treatment and the need for careful follow up. Our local failure rate is much higher than that claimed by Johnson (1982) for amputation (two recurrences in > 250 patients).

One advantage of the iridium mould method is that if there is a local failure, a later partial amputation can easily be performed: healing does not seem to be impaired by the previous irradiation, even if the line of incision passes through irradiated tissue.

Carcinoma Invading the Corpora (Stage II)

Here the results of radiotherapy are far less good, and the chance of local recurrence makes partial amputation necessary in most cases. However, the survival figures suggest that preliminary radiation may improve the long-term cure rate: the results for amputation alone seem, in these small numbers, to have been worse (Table 4).

Partial Amputation

The technique of partial amputation is important because one of the distressing complications that used to be seen very commonly was a stenosis at the new meatus. This can be easily avoided by a simple manoeuvre in which the urethra is spatulated and an n-shaped flap of penile skin is inserted as in a meatoplasty to prevent subsequent stenosis (Blandy 1986). To avoid the risk of local recurrence, at least a 2-cm clear margin should be taken, especially in the urethra, where subepithelial spread is so apt to occur (Baker et al. 1976).

Stage III

Here we have not felt that local irradiation is appropriate and have favoured early radical amputation. In the usual elderly patient, when the growth is invading the scrotum, we have preferred a very wide excision of all the scrotal contents as well as the entire penis, with both corpora cavernosa and the entire urethra except for about 5 cm of the bulb (Blandy 1986). With this very radical excision we have had eight out of nine 5-year survivors.

Inguinal Nodes

Once cancer has invaded the inguinal lymph nodes, the outlook is bad but not entirely hopeless. It depends very much on how far up the successive barriers in the lymphatic catchment system the tumour has progressed. Cabanas (1977) pointed out that if only one "sentinel" node (at the foramen ovale where the saphenous joins the femoral vein) were involved, the 5-year survival rate could be as good as 70%, falling to 50% if more than one inguinal node were involved, and as little as 20% if the iliac nodes were affected. Unfortunately, a negative sentinel node does not exclude involvement of nodes higher up (Perinetti et al. 1980).

The price for survival after successful block dissection is a high one: delayed healing of the inguinal incision is common, and when it does heal, there is permanent and distressing lymphoedema of the lower limb. There is no case for routine prophylatic inguinal node dissection (Baker et al. 1976; Johnson 1982).

Because the inguinal incision is so slow to heal after block dissection and the wound so apt to be infected, there is a real danger that the femoral artery, lying naked in the floor of a patch of infected granulation tissue, may rupture. To avoid this it is wise to protect the vessel by swinging the sartorius muscle over it (Blandy 1986).

In an attempt to improve the poor results of surgery alone for inguinal node involvement, we have used adjuvant chemo- and radiotherapy, monitoring the iliac and inguinal lymph nodes by CT and lymphangiography. The use of preoperative chemotherapy and radiation does not make the block dissection of the groin much more difficult or the postoperative course significantly worse, and in our own small series has allowed a 67% 5-year survival rate for men with positive inguinal nodes, which may be compared with the rates reported in the literature of 15% Narayana et al. (1982), and 20%–50% by Schellhammer and Grabstald (1979).

In many centres the block dissection of the inguinal nodes is carried up into the pelvis, with removal en bloc of the iliac nodes through a long vertical incision or a second oblique abdominal one. The chance of cure, if these iliac nodes are involved, is very slender – Hardner and Woodruff (1967) believed it was nil. The already formidable morbidity of inguinal node dissection is made worse, and, in the writer's view, surgical dissection of these pelvic nodes should only be considered if chemotherapy and radiation have been tried and have failed.

Adjuvant Treatments

When Ichikawa et al. (1969) announced their results with bleomycin for carcinoma of the penis, urologists were quick to adopt this promising new therapy but were quickly disappointed. Sklaroff and Yagoda (1979, 1980) have had promising results with single-agent platinum and methotrexate, and more recently we have had two complete responses (up to 18 months) with widespread pelvic and inguinal node disease using combination chemotherapy with *cis*-platinum, vinblastine and methotrexate.

Treatment of Disseminated Disease

The terminal stage of the patient for whom treatment of cancer of the penis has failed is unbearably distressing for all concerned. All too often there is a local recurrence after heroic surgery in the groin, with an unhealed, infected and discharging wound, adding to the distress of swollen limbs which are subject to repeated attacks of cellulitis. Cancer *en cuirasse* is common. Localised to the lower part of the body, spreading so slowly, and without the mercy of spread to the liver or brain, death comes with cruel slowness. The terminal care of these unfortunate men calls for the utmost skill of the physician to relieve pain and maintain hope.

Follow-up

Although the superficial primary tumours have an excellent prognosis, local recurrence is common and must be watched for. Hence, regular follow-up is an important part of treatment of every penile cancer. Any suspicious lesion, any suture line that does not heal kindly, must be biopsied, and the surgeon must not be slow to perform a re-amputation. The inguinal nodes must be regularly checked and, if there is any suspicious node, carefully aspirated for cytological examination.

Treatment of Recurrence

Local recurrence in the penis after radiotherapy can usually be managed by partial amputation 2 cm proximal to the recurrence. If the scrotum or perineum is involved, the wide and radical excision used in Stage III can be employed. In younger patients the scrotal contents may be spared so long as it does not compromise a wide excision (Johnson 1982).

Results

In Stage I disease it should be possible to obtain > 90% 5-year survival either with partial amputation or using iridium or some other form of radiation therapy, but local recurrence can be expected in about 20% of cases which will call for late local amputation. In Stage II disease, where the vascular spaces of the corpora cavernosa have been invaded, complete control of the disease by radiation is less likely, but with a combination of preoperative radiotherapy and amputation one should be able to obtain prolonged survival in about 80%, though this will be reduced in G3 tumours with a "cord" pattern.

In very bulky disease (Stage III) early and radical excision is the only effective therapy and may give

> 80% 5-year survival if the inguinal nodes are uninvolved and the tumour has a favourable histological grade. When the inguinal nodes are involved, therapy today calls for the deployment of every means at our disposal, including radiotherapy, combination chemotherapy and surgical excision.

Rehabilitation

It does not need a study of Freud to remind a doctor that the fear of losing his penis is one of the most ancient of all the nightmares of man and of immense psychological importance. To break the news to the patient is not easy for the surgeon, but it is the writer's conviction that this must not be delegated to anyone else: firm, kindly and gentle explanation will make the mutilation easier for the patient to bear.

If part of the penis can be preserved, these patients can nearly always resume intercourse, achieving penetration, orgasm and ejaculation in a way that would surprise many who have not had the privilege of discussing this matter with them.

Hardly less distressing is the oedema of the lower limb or limbs after block dissection of the lymph nodes. From the 1st day after the operation the limbs are bound in crepe bandages or supportive stockings. Diuretics may help get rid of some of the oedema, and the patient is encouraged to keep the legs elevated as much as possible during the day and to sleep with the foot of the bed raised at night.

The swollen limbs often itch, readily become secondarily infected, and cellulitis and eczema add to the discomfort. Mild infections must be treated promptly with antibiotics, and any minor breach of the skin must be carefully dressed and well supported.

Future Development

Since small cancers of the penis can usually be completely cured by very minor measures, the most important advance in the future would follow an improvement in the education of the next generation of patients to report minor ailments of the penis, and of their doctors to insist on a biopsy of anything that is in the least suspicious.

Universal circumcision is often advocated, but the logistics of making it available to every male child are formidable. In a former generation Gairdner (1949) estimated that in Britain about 20% of boys were being circumcised at the price of an annual mortality rate of 16. Even if the technique of circumcising the 500 000 neonates in Britain were to be made as safe as it is in the hands of experienced mohelim (Snowman 1962), it would still not be entirely without risk, for, as Shulman et al. (1964) pointed out, even in Jerusalem, about one in 800 children had to be admitted to hospital after circumcision, usually from excessive bleeding, but also because of necrosis of the glans, septicaemia, laceration of the scrotum, fistulae, and even accidental removal of the entire penile skin. Since all the evidence suggests that soap and water are just as effective a remedy, it is perhaps in the field of simple hygiene and education that more effective advances might be made.

Once the cancer has appeared, it does seem that before long a judicious combination of minimal radiation, minimal chemotherapy, and limited surgery may permit the maximal preservation of structure and function in the penis, and heroic resection may no longer be required.

References

Abeshouse BS, Abeshouse GA, Goldstein AE (1962) Sarcoma of the penis: a review of the literature and a report of a new case; and a brief consideration of melanoma of the penis. Urol Int 13: 273–293

Baker BH, Watson FR (1975) Staging carcinoma of the penis. J Surg Oncol 7: 243

Baker BH, Spratt JS, Perez-Mesa C, Watson FR, Leduc RJ (1976) Carcinoma of the penis. J Urol 116: 458–461

Blandy JP (1986) Operative urology, 2nd edn. Blackwell Scientific, Oxford, pp 198–199

Boczko S, Freed S (1979) Penile carcinoma in circumcised males. NY State J Med 79: 1903–1904

Brown PB (1966) Erythroplasia of Queyrat. Br J Plast Surg 19: 378–382

Cabanas RM (1977) An approach for the treatment of penile carcinoma. Cancer 39: 456–466

Cartwright RA, Sinson JD (1980) Carcinoma of the penis and cervix. Lancet 1: 97

Cascinelli N (1969) Melanoma maligno del pene. Tumori 55: 313–314

Delclos L (1982) Interstitial irradiation of the penis. In: Johnson DE, Boileau M (eds) Genitourinary tumors: fundamental principles and surgical techniques. Grune and Stratton, New York, pp 219–225

Dixon FJ, Moore RA (1952) Tumors of the male sex organs. Atlas of tumor pathology VIII. USAFIP, Washington

Dodge OG (1965) Carcinoma of the penis in East Africans. Br J Urol 37: 223–226

Duncan W, Jackson SR (1972) The treatment of early cancer of the penis with megavoltage X-rays. Clin Radiol 23: 246–248

El-Demiry MIM, Oliver RTD, Hope-Stone HF, Blandy JP (1984) Reappraisal of the role of radiotherapy and surgery

in the management of carcinoma of the penis. Br J Urol 56: 724–728
Fegen JP, Beebe D, Persky L (1970) Basal cell carcinoma of the penis. J Urol 104: 864–866
Fetus and Newborn Committee, Canadian Pediatric Society (1982) Benefits and risk of circumcision: another view. Can Med Assoc J 126: 1399
Frazer GA (1965) Myxosarcoma of the penis: a case report. Br J Urol 37: 465–467
Frew IDO, Jefferies JD, Swinney J (1967) Carcinoma of the penis. Br J Urol 39: 398–404
Furlong JH, Uhle CH (1953) Cancer of the penis: a report of 88 cases. J Urol 69: 550
Gairdner D (1949) The fate of the foreskin. Br Med J 2: 1433–1437
Goette DK (1976) Review of erythroplasia of Queyrat and its treatment. Urology 8: 311–315
Gough J (1970) Primary reticulum cell sarcoma of the penis. Br J Urol 42: 332–339
Grabstald H, Kelley CD (1980) Radiation therapy of penile cancer. Urology 15: 575–576
Graham S, Schotz W (1979) Epidemiology of cancer of the cervix in Buffalo, New York. J Natl Cancer Inst 63 (1): 23–27
Haile K, Delclos L (1980) The place of radiation therapy in the treatment of carcinoma of the distal end of the penis. Cancer 45: 1980–1984
Hardner GJ, Woodruff MW (1967) Operative management of carcinoma of the penis. J Urol 98: 487–492
Hodgins TE, Hancock RA (1970) Hemangio-endothelial sarcoma of the penis: report of a case and review of the literature. J Urol 104: 867–870
Hope-Stone HF (1975) Carcinoma of the penis. Proc R Soc Med 68: 777–779
Howard HH, Holtham WH (1950) Epidermoid carcinoma of the penis: a statistical study of 106 cases. Urol Cutan Rev 54: 45–49
Hu C-H, Yang C (1959) A decade of progress in morphologic pathology. Chin Med J [Engl] 79: 409–422
Hutchinson J (1855) Fibrocellular tumor excised from prepuce of a boy. Trans Path Soc Lond 6: 228–229
Ichikawa T, Nakano I, Hirokawa I (1969) Bleomycin treatment of the tumors of penis and scrotum. J Urol 102: 699–707
Jackson SM (1966) The treatment of carcinoma of the penis. Br J Surg 53: 33–35
Johnson DE (1982) Carcinoma of the penis: overview. In: Johnson DE, Boileau MA (eds) Genitourinary tumors, fundamental principles and surgical techniques. Grune and Stratton, New York
Kovi J, Tillman RL, Lee SK (1970) Malignant transformation of condyloma acuminatum. Am J Clin Pathol 61: 702–710
Lenowitz H, Graham AP (1946) Carcinoma of the penis. J Urol 56: 458–484
Lowe D, McKee PH (1983) Verrucous carcinoma of the penis (Buschke-Loewenstein tumour): a clinical pathological study. Br J Urol 55: 427–429
Mantell BS, Morgan WY (1969) Queyrat's erythoplasia of the penis treated by beta particle irradiation. Br J Radiol 42: 855–857
Marcial VA, Figueroa-Colon J, Marcial Rojas RA, Colon JE (1962) Carcinoma of the penis. Radiology 79: 209–220
Marsden ATH (1958) Geographical pathology of cancer in Malaya. Br J Cancer 12: 161–176
Mostofi FW, Price EB (1973) Tumors of the male genital system. USAFIP, Washington DC
Muir CS (1962) Male and female genital tract cancer in Singapore. Cancer 15: 354–363
Nayarana AS, Olney LE, Leoning SA, Weimar GW, Culp DA (1982) Carcinoma of the penis: analysis of 219 cases. Cancer 49: 2185–2191
Oriel JD, Almeida JD (1970) Demonstration of virus particles in human genital warts. Br J Vener Dis 46: 37–42
Paget J (1874) On disease of the mammary areola preceding cancer of the mammary gland. St Barts Hosp Rep 10: 87–89
Paymaster JC, Gangadharan P (1967) Carcinoma of the penis in India. J Urol 97: 110–113
Perinetti E, Crane DB, Catalona WJ (1980) Unreliability of sentinel lymph node biopsy for staging penile carcinoma. J Urol 124: 734–735
Queyrat L (1911) Erythroplasie du gland. Bull Soc Fr Dermatol Syphiligr 22: 378–382
Reddy DJ, Baruah IKSM (1963) Carcinogenic action of human smegma. Arch Pathol 75: 414–420
Reddy DJ, Indira C (1963) Some aspects of the pathology carcinoma penis. J Indian Med Assoc 41: 277–280
Reid JD (1957) Melanocarcinoma of the penis: report of a case. Cancer 10: 359–362
Salaverria JC, Hope-Stone HF, Paris AMI, Molland EA, Blandy JP (1979) Conservative treatment of carcinoma of the penis. Br J Urol 51: 32–37
Schellhammer PF, Grabstald H (1979) Tumors of the penis and urethra. In: Harrison JH, Gittes RF, Perlmutter AD, Stamey TA, Walsh PC (Eds) Campbell's urology, vol 2. pp 1171–1199. Saunders, Philadelphia
Schmauz R, Findlay M, Lalwak A, Katsumbira N, Buxton E (1977) Variations in the appearance of giant condyloma in an Ugandan series of cases of carcinoma of the penis. Cancer 40: 1686–1689
Shulman J, Ben-Hur N, Neuman Z (1964) Surgical complications of circumcision. Am J Dis Child 107: 149–154
Sklaroff RB, Yagoda A (1979) *Cis*-diaminodichloride platinum II (DDP) in the treatment of penile carcinoma. Cancer 44: 1563–1565
Sklaroff RB, Yagoda A (1980) Methotrexate in treatment of penile carcinoma. Cancer 45: 214–216
Snowman J (1962) The surgery of ritual circumcision, 3rd edn. Weinberg, London
Staubitz WJ, Lent MH, Oberkircher OJ (1955) Carcinoma of the penis. Cancer 8: 371–378
Wheelock MC, Clark PJ (1943) Sarcoma of the penis. J Urol 49: 478–481

Cancer of the Testis

G. Pizzocaro

Definition

Cancer of the testis is a relatively rare disease, but it was the commonest cause of cancer death in young adults until a few decades ago. Nowadays cancer of the testis is a potentially curable disease. This dramatic improvement started in the 1950s with a better knowledge of pathology and natural history, which led to an accurate use of surgery and radiotherapy. This improvement exploded in the 1970s with more sophisticated staging techniques and the introduction of *cis*-platinum combination chemotherapy.

Epidemiology and Risk Factors

The annual incidence of cancer of the testis ranges from two to three cases per 100 000 males in the United States to over six cases in Denmark. The incidence of the disease seems to be increasing. Caucasians are six to eight times more frequently affected than Negroes and Asians. Cancer of the testis is a disease of young adults. The major incidence for nonseminomatous tumours is in the third decade, for pure seminoma it is in the fourth and fifth decades. Bilaterality, familiarity and HLA studies suggest that a genetic origin of cancer of the testis may exist, but it has not yet been proved. Infertility is very common among patients with cancer of the testis, but it may recover after cure. The only well-recognized risk factor is cryptorchidism (Mostofi 1973).

Pathology

Cancer of the testis is a multifaceted disease. Approximately 95% of the tumours are germinal in origin (Mostofi 1980). The remainder are derived from the gonadal stroma, the mesenchyma or from paratesticular structures.

Germ Cell Tumours (Mostofi 1980)

Pure seminoma accounts for 40%–50% of all testicular tumours. It appears as a solid intratesticular nodule with a protruding, pale grey cut surface. Typical seminoma is composed of monomorphic regular round cells with large nuclei and evident nucleoli. Lymphocytic infiltration is frequent. Anaplastic seminoma is characterised by at least three mitoses in each of ten consecutive high-power fields. Anaplastic cells, increased vascularity and some haemorrhagic areas may also be present. Trophoblastic seminoma is characterised by the presence of scattered giant syncytial cells with positive staining for human chorionic gonadotropin (HCG) immunoperoxidase. Spermatocytic seminoma is a very rare disease of the elderly and is made up of cells resembling spermatogonia.

Embryonal carcinoma is the most indifferentiated germinal tumour of the testis, made up of poligonal anaplastic cells which sometimes tend to form glandular or papillary structures. Areas of haemorrhagic necrosis are often found and they cause the characteristic variegated appearance of the cut surface of the tumour. Embryonal carcinoma is often mixed with areas of teratoma, and this combination is usually called "teratocarcinoma". When embryonal carcinoma and seminoma are present in the same testis, they are two separate entities.

Teratoma is considered to be the result of the somatic differentiation of totipotent embryonal carcinoma. The tumour is defined as "immature" or "mature" according to the degree of somatic differentiation into epithelial or mesenchymal structures. Small and large cystic areas are typical of teratoma and give the characteristic gross appearance of multiloculated tumour. Mature teratoma can undergo cancerisation of some of its differentiated components.

Yolk sac tumour is a typical infantile germinal testis tumour. It is rare as a pure tumour in adults, but it is often mixed with embryonal carcinoma and teratoma. It produces alpha-fetoprotein (AFP), and its cells typically stain with AFP immunoperoxidase.

Choriocarcinoma is extremely rare as a pure tumour in the testis, but areas of choriocarcinoma can be found in several nonseminomatous germinal tumours of the testis. The simultaneous presence of the syncytial and of the trophoblastic components is necessary to make the diagnosis of choriocarcinoma. Scattered giant cells cannot be considered as areas of choriocarcinoma.

Other Tumours

Gonadal stroma tumours (Sertoli-Leydig cell tumours) are very rare. They usually produce steroid sex hormones and can give rise to pseudopuberty in infants and feminisation in adults. They appear as intratesticular well-defined yellow-red nodules. Approximately 10% of the tumours metastatise, but it is usually impossible to differentiate benign from malignant gonadal stroma tumours on a histological basis only. They can be mixed with seminoma, then they are called "gonadoblastoma", a typical tumour associated with the Klinefelter's syndrome.

Adenoma and adenocarcinoma of the rete testis as well as intratesticular sarcomas are extremely rare.

Non-Hodgkin's lymphomas are not uncommon.

Paratesticular tumours are usually embryonal rhabdomyosarcoma of infants and young adults, or malignant mesothelioma of the tunica vaginalis. They are aggressive soft-tissue sarcomas.

Natural History

Germ Cell Tumours

Germinal tumours grow as a testicular mass and they can infiltrate the tunica albuginea, the rete testis, the epididymis and the spermatic cord. The infiltration of the scrotum is extremely rare. Microvascular invasion and lymphatic permeation are common.

Retroperitoneal nodes are characteristically involved by cancer of the testis. The landing zone for the left testicle is close to the origin of the left spermatic vessels, in the angle between the left renal vein and the aorta. The landing zone for the right testicle is in the interaortocaval nodes, from the renal vein down to the aortic bifurcation. Tumours in cryptorchid testis can metastatise to the pelvic nodes. The bilateral inguinal nodes can be primarily involved following inguinal surgery. Pulmonary metastases are present in approximately 50% of patients with nonseminomatous histology and retroperitoneal metastases. They will develop in approximately 10% of patients with negative nodes. The metastatic potential of embryonal carcinoma is much higher than that of teratoma. Pure choriocarcinomas and infantile yolk sac tumours characteristically metastatise through the blood stream. On the other hand, pure seminoma tends to be confined in the lymph nodes for a long time before developing haematogenous spread. Mediastinal and supraclavicular nodes are involved in approximately 5%–10% of all germ cell tumours, usually following retroperitoneal metastases. The liver and the brain can be involved in disseminated disease. The bone and the skin are rarely affected. Death is usually due to obstructive uropathy or to widespread metastases.

Other Tumours

Other malignant tumours have a similar natural history. Malignant epithelial tumours usually metastatise primarily to the retroperitoneal nodes. Paratesticular sarcomas have a high potential for distant dissemination. Malignant lymphoma of the testis behaves as an extranodal lymphoma.

Tumour Markers

A great variety of markers has been studied in testicular tumours, but AFP, HCG and lactate dehydrogenase (LHD) are the most commonly used markers for germ cell tumours (Barzell and Whitmore 1979).

Alpha-Fetoprotein

AFP is a glycoprotein which is normally secreted by the yolk sac, the fetal liver and the intestine. It is usually elevated in the newborn and infants, but the normal serum value is less than 15–40 ng/ml in adults. AFP can be produced by nonseminomatous tumours only. The half-life kinetic of the marker is 5 days.

Human Chorionic Gonadotropin

HCG is normally produced by the giant syncytial cells of the placenta. It is a glycoprotein composed of two chains. The alfa chain is common to other pituitary gonadotropins, the beta subunit is specific. The marker is not only produced by choriocarcinoma but also by scattered giant syncytial cells present in both seminomatous and nonseminomatous tumours. Normal serum levels do not exceed 5 mIU/ml. The half-life kinetic of HCG is 24–48 h.

Lactate Dehydrogenase

LDH is a proteolytic enzyme which arises in the serum following cytolytic phenomena. It is not characteristic of the tumour, but it is an expression of the tumour mass. Normal serum levels do not exceed 240 mIU/ml at 25 °C (320 mIU/ml at 30 °C).

Staging

Clinical Staging Systems

The *TNM system* (Table 1) is very useful in staging the primary tumour, but it is not as good for nodes and distant metastases.

The *traditional staging system* is as follows:

Stage I No evidence of metastases
Stage II Metastases to retroperitoneal nodes only
Stage III Mediastinal, supraclavicular or distant metastases

Peckham et al. (1979) suggested a highly detailed clinical staging which is reported in Table 2.

Table 1. TNM classification of cancer of the testis (1978)

T	Primary tumor
	In the absence of orchidectomy the symbol TX must be used.
T0	No evidence of primary tumour
T1	Tumour limited to the body of the testis
T2	Tumour extending beyond the tunica albuginea
T3	Tumour involving the rete testis or epididymis
T4	Tumour invading the spermatic cord and/or scrotal wall: T4 a Invasion of spermatic cord; T4 b Invasion of scrotal wall
N	Regional and juxtaregional lymph nodes
N0	No evidence of involvement of lymph nodes
N1	Involvement of a single homolateral regional lymph node, which, if inguinal, is mobile
N2	Involvement of contralateral or bilateral or multiple regional lymph nodes, which, if inguinal, are mobile
N3	A palpable abdominal mass is present, or there are fixed inguinal lymph nodes
N4	Involvement of juxtaregional lymph nodes
M	Distant metastases
M0	No evidence of distant metastases
M1	Distant metastases present

Table 2. Clinical staging system. (After Peckham et al. 1979)

Stage I	No evidence of metastases
Stage II	Metastases confined to retroperitoneal nodes
	II-A Maximal diamter < 2 cm
	II-B Maximal diameter 2–5 cm
	II-C Maximal diameter > 5 cm
Stage III	Metastases to supradiaphragmatic nodes without extralymphatic metastases
	Suffixes A, B, C for retroperitoneal nodes as in stage II
Stage IV	Extralymphatic metastases
	Suffixes A, B, C for retroperitoneal nodes as for stage II
	Lung status L1 < 3 Metastases present, < 2 cm
	L2 Multiple metastases < 2 cm
	L3 Multiple metastases > 2 cm
	Liver status H + : liver involvement

From a practical point of view, cancer of the testis can be divided into:

- *Locoregional disease:* stage I and nonbulky stage II
- *Disseminated disease:* bulky stage II and stage III

The division of stage II into small volume and large volume disease is not univocal. The proposed landmarks are 5–10 cm in diameter for pure seminoma and 2–5 cm for nonseminomatous tumours (Pizzocaro 1987). Disseminated disease is nowadays divided into minimal, moderate (bulky) and advanced (very bulky) disease (Table 3).

Table 3. Classification of disseminated disease

	INT, Milano (Pizzocaro et al. 1985b)	Indiana University (Birch et al. 1986)
Minimal	HCG and or AFP only.	Idem
	Cervical, mediastinal or retroperitoneal metastases <5 cm	Cervical or nonpalpable unresectable retroperitoneal metastases
	No more than 5 metastases per lung field, none > 2 cm	Idem
Moderate (bulky)	Lymph node metastases between 5 and 10 cm	Palpable abdominal mass only
	More than five metastases per lung field or at least one metastasis between 2 and 5 cm	Five to ten metastases per lung field, none > 3 cm, or a mediastinal mass < 50% of the intrathoracic diameter
Advanced (very bulky)	Lymph node metastases > 10 cm	Mediastinal mass > 50% of the intrathoracic diameter
	Invasion of > 50% of lung fields or at least one pulmonary metastasis > 5 cm	More than ten metastases per lung field or multiple pulmonary metastases > 3 cm
	Hepatic, osseous, CNS metastases	Idem

Examinations for Clinical Staging

The *primary tumour* is only staged pathologically (Table 1).

The *retroperitoneal nodes* can be staged by palpation, bipedal lymphangiography (LAG), echography, computed tomography (CT) and magnetic resonance (MR). Intravenous pyelography (IVP) and vascular examinations have been practically abandoned. Echography is the least precise technique for the staging of retroperitoneal nodes, while LAG and CT are complementary (Tesoro-Tess et al. 1985). LAG can individualise small intranodal defects, but can miss large nodes completely filled by the tumour. CT shows enlarged nodes very well, but it can miss small intranodal deposits. The role of MR has yet to be defined, but it seems to be similar or even superior to CT. We advise CT or MR as first choice, followed by LAG in patients with negative reports. LAG is also useful for the follow-up of the retroperitoneal nodes during treatment.

Distant metastases are usually checked by clinical examination (neck) and chest X-ray. Scalene node biopsy, full-lung tomograms or CT or the chest are not mandatory. Other examinations (CT or MR of the skull, bone survey, etc.) are usually carried out only on clinical indication.

Table 4. Pathological staging of resected retroperitoneal nodes

Subgroup	Vugrin et al. 1981a	Pizzocaro et al. 1984
Stage I	Negative nodes	Idem
Stage II-A	No more than five nodes involved, none > 2 cm, no capsular invasion	Idem
Stage II-B	More than five nodes; at least one node > 2 cm; capsular invasion	More than five nodes; at least one node > 2 cm; microscopic capsular invasion
Stage II-C	(B2 = extracapsular invasion)	Mass > 5 cm, macroscopic extranodal invasion; invasion of retroperitoneal veins

The half-life kinetics of AFP and HCG are important in staging locoregional nonseminomatous tumours. Serum determinations must be done just before surgery and regularly after the operation. Persisting elevated values or half-life kinetics longer than 5 days for AFP or 2 days for HCG are signals of persisting disease, even in patients with negative radiological work-up.

Pathological Staging

Retroperitoneal nodes are staged pathologically following lymphadenectomy as depicted in Table 4.

Prognosis

Histology, extent of the disease, disease localisations and tumour marker levels are the most important prognostic factors for cancer of the testis.

Locoregional Pure Seminoma

In locoregional pure seminoma the most important prognostic feature is the stage of the disease. The higher metastatic potential of anaplastic seminoma is reflected in a higher stage at disease presentation, while an elevated HCG titre does not change the results of radiotherapy for either stage I or stage II disease (Swartz et al. 1984).

Stage I Nonseminomatous Tumours

In clinical stage I nonseminomatous tumours, metastases occur more frequently in patients with embryonal carcinoma, vascular invasion and high T categories (Peckham 1985; Pizzocaro et al. 1986c).

Resected Stage II Nonseminoma

In resected stage II nonseminoma the occurrence of distant dissemination is proportional to the involvement of the retroperitoneal nodes (Vugrin et al. 1981a; Pizzocaro et al. 1984).

Disseminated Disease

In disseminated disease the most important prognostic features are the extent of the disease (tumour mass and disease localisations) and postorchiectomy tumour marker values (Bosl et al. 1983; Birch et al. 1986). Very large tumour masses in multiple organ sites and highly elevated serum titres of AFP, HCG and LDH are the poorest prognostic features.

Screening of Asymptomatic Disease

Self-examination of the testicle is the best screening for asymptomatic disease and should be carried out by all young adults. Serum AFP and HCG cannot be used for screening programmes, because only 30% of pure seminomas produce HCG and 10%–20% of nonseminomatous tumours do not produce any marker. Furthermore, the disease is too rare to justify a screening programme with expensive techniques such as immersion echography. Routine testicular biopsy in infertile males can reveal in situ cancer in approximately 5% of cases, and 50% of these patients will develop a testicular tumor within 5 years.

Diagnosis of Symptomatic Disease

Intrascrotal Mass

Testicular cancer is a nontransilluminable testicular mass which is characteristically heavy and insensitive. However, over 20% of testicular tumours are painful. Furthermore, it is not always possible to recognise a normal epididymis. Therefore, misdiagnosis with epididymitis is not rare. Serum AFP and HCG levels are to be determined, but they are diagnostic only when they are positive. Echography is an excellent diagnostic procedure to study an intrascrotal mass, but whenever an intrascrotal mass cannot be diagnosed with certainty as benign by clinical means, it deserves surgical exploration.

Surgical Exploration

Surgical exploration for an intrascrotal mass must be performed through an inguinal incision. The spermatic cord is isolated at the external inguinal ring and the testis is exteriorised within its envelopes. The exposed testis is isolated with sponges from the surgical field and the tunica vaginalis is opened. Usually, a testicular tumour appears as a firm intratesticular mass deforming the testis and accompanied by pathological vascularisation of the overlying tunica albuginea. These signs are diagnostic. However, if only a very small or a very regular nodule is found, an open biopsy and a frozen section may be necessary.

In such cases it is mandatory to clamp the spermatic cord and to protect the surgical field before the testis is opened. Once cancer has been diagnosed, the testis is enveloped with sponges, the inguinal canal is opened and the cord is divided at the level of the internal inguinal ring. In the case of a scrotal incision these manoeuvres cannot be performed correctly, and the chance of local and distant dissemination is increased (Pizzocaro et al. 1986c).

Metastases as First Sign

Metastases may be the first sign of testicular cancer in a small proportion of cases. Gynaecomastia, back pain, abdominal mass, enlarged supraclavicular nodes and intrathoracic metastases can occasionally be found. If any of these signs appears in a young adult, the testes must be carefully examined and serum AFP and HCG levels determined. Furthermore, one must consider the possibility of a primary extragonadal germ cell tumour.

Staging

The search for metastatic disease (staging) in a patient with cancer of the testis is completed after orchiectomy. Before surgical exploration, only a complete physical examination and a chest X-ray are performed and a blood sample for AFP and HCG is taken. Expensive procedures to check the retroperitoneal nodes (LAG, CT, MR) are performed only after orchiectomy, when the diagnosis is sure.

Surgical and Combined Treatment of Locoregional Disease

Stage I, II-A and II-B (Table 2) pure seminomas and stage I and II-A nonseminomatous tumours can be considered as locoregional disease and can be successfully treated with locoregional treatment in a high proportion of cases. Stage II-C pure seminoma and II-B nonseminoma are in a borderline situation, but in our opinion they are better treated with chemotherapy as the first choice, because the likelihood of cure with locoregional treatment alone is not very high.

Management of the Primary Tumour

The treatment of choice for the primary tumour is high inguinal orchiectomy as described above. The testis must also be removed in the occasional patient in whom the diagnosis of disseminated testicular cancer has been made by a biopsy of secondary deposit because the testis is a sanctuary for systemic chemotherapy.

Management of Retroperitoneal Nodes

The treatment of choice for the retroperitoneal nodes in locoregional disease is different for pure seminoma and for nonseminomatous tumours.

Stage I pure seminoma is usually treated with 25–30 Gy high-energy irradiation to the retroperitoneal nodes. Bilateral para-aortic and homolateral iliac nodes are treated over a 3-week programme. We do not advise surveillance following orchiectomy alone in stage I pure seminoma because the good tolerance of radiotherapy does not justify a long and difficult follow-up.

Stage II-A and II-B pure seminoma are usually treated with 30–40 Gy high-energy irradiation to the retroperitoneal nodes over 4 weeks. Prophylactic irradiation of the mediastinum and of the neck has been abandoned because of the low incidence of recurrence in such regions and their high curability with delayed therapy (Thomas et al. 1982).

Stage I nonseminoma can be treated with either retroperitoneal lymphadenectomy or surveillance. High-energy irradiation has been practically abandoned. The untoward side effect of radical lymphadenectomy is loss of antegrade ejaculation which occurs in approximately 70% of patients. The advantage of the operation is that a pathological staging is obtained and unsuspected microscopic retroperitoneal deposits are removed. The advantages of surveillance following orchiectomy alone are that major surgery is avoided, and 70% of patients will need no further treatment, but the follow-up of retroperitoneal nodes is very difficult, and CT and LAG must be repeated for at least 3 years (Pizzocaro et al. 1986c). We now advise unilateral retroperitoneal lymphadenectomy (Pizzocaro et al. 1985c). It is not followed by retroperitoneal recurrence, antegrade ejaculation is lost by a few patients only, pathological staging is obtained and only the chest X-rays and markers must be repeated during the follow-up.

Stage II-A and II-B nonseminoma can be treated with either primary retroperitoneal lymphadenectomy or primary *cis*-platinum based chemotherapy. If surgery is performed first, a pathological staging is obtained, and patients with positive retroperitoneal nodes can be treated with either adjuvant chemotherapy or surveillance for distant dissemination (Williams et al. 1986). If chemotherapy is administered first, surgery is performed only in partial responders and it is avoided in complete responders (Peckham and Hendry 1985). In our experience with primary lymphadenectomy (Pizzocaro 1987) we found that 40% of clinical stage II-A patients actually had negative nodes, and 67% of clinical stage II-B cases needed successive chemotherapy. Therefore, we advise primary chemotherapy for patients with stage II-B disease, and primary lymph node dissection for clinical stage II-A.

Management of Non-Germ Cell Tumours. In gonadal stroma tumours, retroperitoneal lymphadenectomy is indicated only if there is a sound radiological suspicion of nodal involvement. On the rare occasion of a carcinoma of the rete testis, retroperitoneal lymphadenectomy must be performed. In the case of a paratesticular sarcoma, excision of the primary tumour must be radical, and lymphadenectomy is mandatory when there is a radiographic suspicion of nodal involvement (Exelby 1980). Testicular lymphomas must be treated as extranodal lymphomas.

Table 5. PVB schedule (vinblastine = 0.3 mg/kg, q. 3 weeks)

Drugs	Dosages	Days of administration						
		1,	2,	3,	4,	5	9	16
Vinblastine	0.15 mg/kg i.v.	X	X					
Cis-platinum	20 mg/m^2 i.v.	X	X	X	X	X		
Bleomycin	30 units i.v.		X				X	X

Vigorous hydration prior to and after *cis*-platinum is necessary to avoid nephrotoxicity.

Adjuvant Treatments

Systemic adjuvant chemotherapy has been routinely used in resected stage II nonseminomatous germ cell tumours and in paratesticular sarcomas.

Pathological Stage II Nonseminoma

Long-term (2-year) adjuvant treatments without *cis*-platinum have not been successful in reducing the relapse rate following orchiectomy and radical retroperitoneal lymphadenectomy (Vugrin et al. 1981a; Pizzocaro et al. 1984). Only *cis*-platinum-based chemotherapy was able to avoid recurrences in resected stage II nonseminomatous tumours (Vugrin et al. 1981b). In a randomised study comparing two courses of the adjuvant *cis*-platinum, vinblastine and bleomycin combination (PVB, Table 5) versus observation followed by four courses of PVB in the event of relapse (Williams et al. 1986), no significant difference could be found and survival approached 100% in both arms. Pizzocaro et al. (1984) were able to select a subgroup of pathological stage II patients with a very high risk of relapse (pathological stage II-C, Table 4) and advise immediate postoperative *cis*-platinum-based chemotherapy in these patients only. *Cis*-platinum adjuvant chemotherapy is advisable in pathological stage II-A and II-B patients only if they cannot attend a close follow-up.

Paratesticular Sarcomas

As the risk for haematogenous spread of these tumors is very high, adjuvant chemotherapy is indicated both in stage I following orchiectomy alone and in stage II following orchiectomy and lymphadenectomy (Exelby 1980).

Treatment of Disseminated Disease

Disseminated cancer of the testis is the only disseminated solid tumour of the adult which can be cured by chemotherapy in a high proportion of patients. Surgery is important in removing residual masses after induction chemotherapy. Debulking surgery performed before induction chemotherapy has been practically abandoned.

Cis-platinum Combination Chemotherapy

The introduction of *cis*-platinum in the vinblastine and bleomycin combination (Table 5) resulted in a 70% complete remission rate, and another 10%–15% of patients were rendered tumour free with postchemotherapy surgery (Einhorn and Donohue 1977). Maintenance chemotherapy was not necessary after four courses of therapy (Einhorn et al. 1981), and the reduction of the dosage of vinblastine from 0.4 to 0.3 mg/kg did not change the results and reduced toxicity (Einhorn and Williams 1980). Also, the introduction of high-dose *cis*-platinum in the vinblastine, actinomycin D and bleomycin (VAB) combination resulted in an overall 60% complete remission rate (Reynolds et al. 1981). Results improved from VAB-3 to VAB-6 (Vugrin et al. 1983) because the proportion of patients rendered tumour free with postchemotherapy surgery increased from 10%–15% to 30%–35%.

The Role of Surgery in Disseminated Disease

Surgery is useful in removing residual masses following induction chemotherapy. In most patients a retroperitoneal lymphadenectomy is needed, and in a few cases it is necessary to remove intrathoracic metastases (Pizzocaro 1985). Supraclavicular masses can be easily removed at the same time as the retroperitoneal lymphadenectomy. The simultaneous removal of intrathoracic metastases and of retroperitoneal nodes is possible with a sternotomy plus a xiphopubic incision, but in the case of metastases in the posteroinferior mediastinum, a posterolateral thoracotomy is needed, and the two operations are usually performed at different times.

Results of postchemotherapy surgery depend on complete excision of the residual pathological tissue, histological findings and on preoperative serum tumour marker levels (Pizzocaro 1985). Usually, patients with negative markers are operated, and fibrosis-necrosis is found in approximately 40% of cases, mature teratoma in another 40% and residual cancer in the remaining 20%. The cure rate in the first two groups is 80%–90%. It is only 40%–50% when residual cancer is present in the resected tissue. The prognosis is usually poor when patients with elevated markers or unresectable cancer are operated on.

Follow-up

Follow-up of Disease-free Patients

The follow-up of disease-free patients must be compulsory, because relapses can be cured in a significant proportion of cases. Following radical treatment of locoregional disease, relapses usually occur in the chest or in the neck. Following successful treatment of disseminated disease, relapses are rare but can occur anywhere. The great majority of relapses occur within 1 year from starting therapy, and the remainder usually occur within 3 years. For pure seminoma the time to relapse can be longer, but relapses after more than 5 years are exceptional. During these periods of time, visits must be at short intervals: every 1–2 months during the first years and every 2–3 months thereafter. AFP, HCG and a chest X-ray must be repeated at each visit. A CT scan of the abdomen must be repeated every two to three visits. Echography can be substituted for CT in these patients. It is not necessary to repeat CT scans of the abdomen at frequent intervals after a properly executed lymphadenectomy because retroperitoneal recurrences are rare following such an operation. LAG is very useful to follow the retroperitoneal nodes after both radiotherapy and chemotherapy. In surveillance following orchiectomy alone, LAG must be repeated after reabsorption of the contrast material.

Follow-up of Incomplete Responders to Chemotherapy

A small proportion of patients have unresectable residual masses with negative markers at the end of induction chemotherapy. These masses can be completely necrotic or can contain residual cancer. These patients must be followed very closely and very carefully until documented complete regression or progression of the disease. On the other hand, residual teratoma is usually resectable.

False Positive Rise of AFP and HCG during Follow-up

As the measurement of marker levels is repeated frequently during the follow-up, false positive values of either AFP or HCG can occur. The examination must be repeated immediately. If a technical error can be ruled out and the value has not increased substantially, a biological cause of false positivity can be documented. HCG increases falsely in patients with low testosterone, and AFP increases if the liver function is impaired. Only progressively increasing levels of serum markers are sure signals of relapse.

Treatment of Recurrence

The treatment of recurrence following locoregional therapy can be planned as treatment of primarily advanced disease, while patients who relapse or do not enter complete remission following systemic therapy for disseminated disease are candidates for salvage therapy.

Relapses Following Radiotherapy

The main problem with patients with relapses following radiotherapy is the reduction of the bone marrow reserve following irradiation. It is very difficult to treat these patients with full doses of PVB or VAB-6. Peckham et al. (1983) substituted vinblastine with etoposide (VP-16) in the PVB regimen for these patients (BEP, Table 6). The 5 days treatment with 120 mg/m^2 VP-16 was poorly tolerated, but the 3-day regimen was feasible, and it was particularly well tolerated by patients who had received only subdiaphragmatic irradiation. The standard dosage of VP-16 is nowadays 100 mg/m^2 for 5 consecutive days in the not pretreated and for 3 days in the pretreated patient.

Recurrence of Disseminated Disease

Cis-platinum and VP-16 combination chemotherapy is a successful treatment, particularly in patients who have not been pretreated with the two drugs, but it is also successful in approximately 30% of patients pretreated with *cis*-platinum (Williams et al. 1980). The addition of ifosfamide to *cis*-platinum and VP-16 increases toxicity but does increase the response rate in patients pretreated with *cis*-platinum (Loeh-

Table 6. BEP schedule (q. 3–4 weeks)

Drugs	Dosages	Days of administration						
		1,	2,	3,	4,	5	9	16
VP-16	100 mg/m^2 i.v.	X	X	X	X	X		
Cis-platinum	20 mg/m^2 i.v.	X	X	X	X	X		
Bleomycin	30 units i.v.		X				X	X

VP-16 is withheld on days 2 and 4 in patients pretreated with radiotherapy.

rer et al. 1986). Responders to salvage therapy were usually responders to previous *cis*-platinum combination chemotherapy. The few patients who progressed during the first treatment with *cis*-platinum, were usually unresponsive to salvage therapy too. New agents and high-dose regimens are being tried, but no convincing results have yet been achieved.

The Role of Surgery in Recurrent Disseminated Disease

The proportion of patients requiring postchemotherapy resection of intrathoracic or other distant metastases is very high in this set of cases. Furthermore, the majority of cases still have residual cancer in the resected tissue. However, if the surgical excision of the residual masses is complete, approximately 40%–50% of patients rendered tumour free with surgery will be permanently cured (Pizzocaro 1985).

Freedom from Disease and Survival

The overall prognosis of patients with testicular cancer is excellent today.

Pure Seminoma

The prognosis of pure seminoma was good even before sophisticated staging techniques and *cis*-platinum based chemotherapy were available. Thomas et al. (1982) reported an overall 5-year survival rate of 87% in 444 patients treated with high-energy irradiation between 1958 and 1976. In particular, the 5-year survival of stage III patients was 36%.

Low-stage pure seminoma are much better staged today, and the results of subdiaphragmatic radiotherapy are consequently improved. Thomas (1985) reported 98% 3-year disease-free survival in 166 consecutive patients treated for either stage I or nonpalpable stage II disease between 1977 and 1981.

Bulky stage II seminoma can be successfully treated with radiotherapy alone in 60% (Thomas 1985) to 85% (Smalley et al. 1985) of cases. Results of primary *cis*-platinum chemotherapy are also excellent (Pizzocaro et al. 1986a), and it is very difficult to state which treatment should be given first.

Disseminated seminoma is currently treated with *cis*-platinum combination chemotherapy. Complete remission is achieved in 80% of cases, and 70% are definitely cured (Pizzocaro et al. 1986a; Stanton et al. 1985). The best results are usually achieved in patients who have not been pretreated with radiotherapy, or in those who received subdiaphragmatic irradiation only. Extensively irradiated patients cannot be adequately treated with chemotherapy because haematological toxicity is too severe, and results are usually poor.

Nonseminomatous Tumours

Prognosis is excellent in low stages and in disseminated disease with good prognostic features. Results are not so good only in advanced disease with poor prognosis.

Stage I Nonseminoma. The long-term results of lymphadenectomy in pathological stage I disease show a 10%–15% relapse rate and an approximately 98% long-term survival rate (Pizzocaro 1985). More recent results on the surveillance studies show a 25%–30% relapse rate and the same 98% survival rate (Peckham 1985; Pizzocaro et al. 1986c).

Nonbulky stage II Nonseminoma. Peckham and Hendry (1985) reported two deaths in 54 patients treated with primary chemotherapy followed by surgery in partial responders. Pizzocaro (1985) reported only one death in 75 patients treated with primary surgery followed by chemotherapy in pathological stage II-C disease and patients who had a relapse. The Testicular Cancer Interstudy Group (Williams et al. 1986) randomised 197 patients to either adjuvant chemotherapy or to observation. Relapses were 46% in patients assigned to observation and 6% in patients assigned to adjuvant chemotherapy, but following treatment of relapses, the survival rates were 98% and 99%, respectively. In conclusion, whatever treatment policy in stage I and nonbulky stage II nonseminoma, the long-term survival rate will be approximately 98%.

In advanced nonseminoma results depend on the extent of the disease and on serum tumour marker levels. The results of the VAB, PVB and BEP combinations are comparable (Einhorn et al. 1981; Peckham et al. 1983; Vugrin et al. 1983). The last two combinations have recently been compared in a randomised study (Williams et al. 1985), and BEP was superior to PVB only in advanced disease with poor prognosis. Approximately 90%–100% of patients with minimal or intermediate disease enter complete remission following chemotherapy and eventually surgery (Birch et al. 1986; Pizzocaro et al. 1985 b). Less toxic regimens are being studied in these patients with good prognosis. Bosl et al. (1986) have successfully compared etoposide and *cis*-platinum alone to the more toxic VAB-6 combination. Pizzocaro et al. (1986 b) have successfully reduced vinblastine in the PBV combination. The cure rate of poor-prognosis far-advanced disease is less than 50% with either PVB or VAB-6 (Bosl et al. 1983; Birch et al. 1986; Pizzocaro et al. 1985 b). In our experience (Pizzocaro et al. 1985 a), BEP and surgery succeeded in achieving a 92.5% complete remission rate and a 82.5% continuous disease-free survival in 40 consecutive patients with far-advanced disease. These results are competitive with those of high-dose aggressive regimens (Ozols et al. 1983; Daugaard and Rorth 1985). Einhorn is comparing normal-dose versus high-dose *cis*-platinum in the BEP combination, and preliminary results show no advantage for the high-dose regimen.

Paratesticular Rhabdomyosarcoma

Prognosis of infantile paratesticular rhabdomyosarcoma has improved dramatically in recent years. None of 12 children treated at the Memorial Hospital prior to 1960 survived, versus six out of 13 treated between 1960 and 1969 (Exelby 1980). Since 1970, 14 more children with the same tumour have been treated. Ten out of 12 patients with locoregional disease were cured. The two patients with advanced disease died. In our Institute, 14 patients with paratesticular rhabdomyosarcoma were treated with planned surgery, radiation and chemotherapy from 1970 to 1984. Eleven out of 13 patients with locoregional disease are alive and disease free. One patient with disseminated disease died. More active chemotherapy is needed to treat disseminated disease. But results of the combined treatment modality are excellent for locoregional disease.

Rehabilitation

Nearly all patients who are rendered disease free after cancer of the testis are able to recover and readjust to life within 2–6 months after ending therapy. The time to recovery is longer after chemotherapy than after surgery, but retroperitoneal lymphadenectomy may subsequently evolve into psychological problems linked to the loss of antegrade ejaculation (Tamburini et al. 1986).

Future Development

The future development in the management of cancer of the testis will be in several directions.

Early diagnosis can be achieved by self-examination and close follow-up of cryptorchid and infertile patients.

Low morbidity treatment is the goal to be achieved in patients with a good prognosis. Less toxic chemotherapy regimens have proved to give results which are comparable with standard therapy in selected patients with good prognostic features (Bosl et al. 1986; Pizzocaro et al. 1986 b). Similarly, modifications of retroperitoneal lymphadenectomy can spare antegrade ejaculation in stage I patients (Pizzocaro et al. 1985 c; Richie and Garnick 1985).

More aggressive treatments are under investigation to improve prognosis in patients with a poor prognosis. It is very difficult to find a truly unresponsive germ cell testicular tumour, but it is very important to individualise patients who will be incomplete responders or who will relapse. These patients probably need more intensive treatments.

Knowledge of the correct management of cancer of the testis must be widespread, but patients should be treated and followed up in specialised centres. The disease is relatively rare, and it is practically impossible to get enough experience treating occasional patients.

References

Barzell WE, Whitmore WF (1979) Clinical significance of biologic markers. Semin Oncol 6: 48–52
Birch R, Williams S, Cane A et al. (1986) Prognostic factors

for favorable outcome in disseminated germ cell tumors. J Clin Oncol 4: 400–407
Bosl GA, Geller NL, Cirrincione C et al. (1983) Multivariate analysis of prognostic variables in patients with metastatic testicular cancer. Cancer Res 43: 3404–3407
Bosl GJ, Bajorin D, Leitner S et al. (1986) A randomized trial of etoposide plus cisplatin versus VAB-6 in good risk patients with germ cell tumor. Am Soc Clin Oncol 5: 104 (Abstract 405)
Daugaard G, Rorth M (1985) High dose cisplatin and VP.16 in patients with poor risk prognosis germ cell cancer. Am Soc Clin Oncol 4: 99 (Abstract C-385)
Einhorn LH, Donohue JP (1977) *Cis*-diammine dichloroplatinum, vinblastine and bleomycin combination chemotherapy in disseminated testicular cancer. Ann Intern Med 87: 293–298
Einhorn LH, Williams SD (1980) Chemotherapy of disseminated testicular cancer: a random prospective study. Cancer 46: 1339–1344
Einhorn LH, Williams SD, Troner M et al. (1981) The role of maintenance therapy in disseminated testicular cancer. N Engl J Med 13: 727–731
Exelby PR (1980) Testicular cancer in children. Cancer 45: 1803–1809
Loehrer PJ, Einhorn LH, Williams SD (1986) VP.16 plus ifosfamide plus cisplatin as salvage therapy in refractory germ cell cancer. J Clin Oncol 4: 528–536
Mostofi PFK (1973) Testicular tumours: epidemiologic, etiologic and pathologic features. Cancer 32: 1186–1201
Mostofi FK (1980) Pathology of germ cell tumors of the testis. A progress report. Cancer 48: 1735–1754
Ozols RF, Deisseroth AB, Javadpour N et al. (1983) Treatment of poor prognosis nonseminomatous testicular cancer with a high dose platinum combination chemotherapy regimen. Cancer 51: 1805–1807
Peckham MJ (1985) Surveillance following orchiectomy for clinical stage I testicular germ-cell malignancy. Acta Urol Belg 53: 155–164
Peckham MJ, Hendry WF (1985) Clinical stage II nonseminomatous germ-cell testicular tumors. Results of management by primary chemotherapy. Br J Urol 57: 763–768
Peckham MJ, McElwain TJ, Barret A, Hendry WF (1979) Combined management of teratoma of the testis. Lancet 2: 267–269
Peckham MJ, Barret A, Liew KH et al. (1983) The treatment of metastatic germ-cell testicular tumors by bleomycin, etoposide and cisplatin (BEP). Br J Cancer 47: 613–619
Pizzocaro G (1985) Primary, secondary and salvage surgery in the management of germinal testis cancer. In: Jones WG, Milford Ward A, Anderson CK (eds) Germ cell tumours. Pergamon, Oxford, pp 395–402
Pizzocaro G, Piva L, Salvioni R et al. (1984) Adjuvant chemotherapy in resected stage II nonseminomatous germ cell tumours of testis. Eur Urol 10: 151–158
Pizzocaro G, Piva L, Salvioni R et al. (1985a) Cisplatin, etoposide, bleomycin first-line therapy and early resection of residual tumor in far-advanced germinal testis cancer. Cancer 56: 2411–2415
Pizzocaro G, Salvioni R, Pasi M et al. (1985b) Early resection of residual tumor during cisplatin, vinblastine, bleomycin combination chemotherapy in stage III and bulky stage II nonseminomatous testicular cancer. Cancer 56: 249–255
Pizzocaro G, Salvioni R, Zanoni F (1985c) Unilateral lymphadenectomy in intraoperative stage I nonseminomatous germinal testis cancer. J Urol 134: 485–489
Pizzocaro G, Salvioni R, Piva L et al. (1986a) Cisplatin combination chemotherapy in advanced seminoma. Cancer 58: 1625–1629
Pizzocaro G, Salvioni R, Zanoni F et al. (1986b) Successful treatment of good-risk disseminated testicular cancer with cisplatin, bleomycin and reduced-dose vinblastine. Cancer 57: 2114–2128
Pizzocaro G, Zanoni F, Milani A et al. (1986c) Orchiectomy alone in clinical stage I nonseminomatous testis cancer: a critical appraisal. J Clin Oncol 4: 35–40
Pizzocaro G (1987) Retroperitoneal lymph node dissection in clinical stage II A and II B nonseminomatous germ-cell tumours of the testis. Int J Androl 10: 269–275
Reynolds TF, Vugrin D, Cvitkovic E et al. (1981) VAB-3 combination chemotherapy of metastatic testicular cancer. Cancer 48: 888–898
Richie JP, Garnick MB (1985) Limited retroperitoneal lymphadenectomy for patients with clinical stage I testicular tumours. J Urol 133–247 A (Abstract 534)
Smalley SR, Evans RG, Richardson RC et al. (1985) Radiotherapy as initial treatment for bulky stage II testicular seminoma. J Clin Oncol 3: 1333–1338
Stanton GF, Bosl GJ, Whitmore WF et al. (1985) VAB-6 as initial treatment of patients with advanced seminoma. J Clin Oncol 3: 336–339
Swartz DA, Johnson DE, Hussey DH (1984) Should an elevated human chorionic gonadotropin titer alter therapy for seminoma? J Urol 131: 63–65
Tamburini M, Filiberti A, Barbieri A et al. (1986) Psychosocial measurement of testicular cancer therapy. Preliminary data of a prospective study. International Workshop Quality of Life. 13 December 1985, Milano
Tesoro Tess JD, Pizzocaro G, Zanoni F, Musumeci R (1985) Lymphangiography and computed tomography in testicular carcinoma: how accurate is early stage disease? J Urol 133: 967–970
Thomas GM (1985) Controversies in the management of testicular seminoma. Cancer 55: 2296–2302
Thomas GM, Rides WD, Dembo AJ et al. (1982) Seminoma of the testis: results of treatment and patterns of failure after radiation therapy. Int J Radiat Oncol Biol Phys 8: 165–174
Vugrin D, Whitmore WF, Cvitkovic E et al. (1981a) Adjuvant chemotherapy combination of vinblastine, actinomycin D, bleomycin and clorambucil following retroperitoneal lymph node dissection in stage II testis tumour. Cancer 47: 840–844
Vugrin D, Whitmore WF, Cvitkovic E et al. (1981b) Adjuvant chemotherapy with VAB-3 of stage II-B testicular cancer. Cancer 48: 233–237
Vugrin D, Whitmore WF, Golbey RB (1983) VAB-6 combination chemotherapy without maintenance in the treatment of disseminated cancer of the testis. Cancer 51: 211–215
Williams SD, Einhorn LH, Greco FA et al. (1980) VP.16.213 salvage therapy for refractory germinal neoplasms. Cancer 46: 2154–2158
Williams SD, Einhorn LH, Greco FA et al. (1985) Disseminated germ cell tumors: a comparison of cisplatin plus bleomycin plus either vinblastine (PVB) or VP.16 (BEP). Am Soc Clin Oncol 4: 100 (Abstract C-390)
Williams SD, Muggia F, Einhorn LH et al. (1986) Resected stage II testicular cancer: immediate adjuvant chemotherapy versus observation. Am Soc Clin Oncol 5: 98 (Abstract 380)

Cancer of the Ovary

F. di Re and R. Fontanelli

Epidemiology and Statistics

Over the past 40 years ovarian cancer has shown a slight but gradual increase in incidence and at present it makes up 5% of all female malignancies and 20% of female genital tumours (Waterhouse et al. 1982). The highest incidence rate is seen in northern Europe (11–15 per 100 000) and the lowest in Japan (2.8 per 100 000). As in breast cancer, epidemiological studies suggest an environmental influence which is not just racial, in fact the mortality rate in second-generation Japanese immigrants in the United States has increased to reach the level of the local population (Bennington et al. 1968).

Ovarian cancer is rare before menarche and increases proportionally with age, with a peak incidence in the age group between 40 and 70. In contrast, germ cell ovarian tumours occur mostly in children and in young women.

Little is known about the aetiology and pathogenesis of ovarian cancer. A higher incidence of ovarian carcinoma is seen in nulliparous women and more generally in women with few and relatively late pregnancies or infertility (Franceschi et al. 1982; McGowan et al. 1979). Although not clearly established (Rosenberg et al. 1982; Dicker et al. 1983), the administration of oral contraceptives seems to exert a prophylactic effect against this tumour.

The role of hormonal contraceptives and the role of pregnancies could be explained by Fathalla's theory about "incessant ovulation" in the genesis of ovarian carcinoma (Fathalla 1971; Henderson et al. 1982). This concept suggests that the risk of developing cancer is correlated to the number of ovulations in the reproductive life of a woman, due to epithelial microtrauma or inclusion cyst formation, and the subsequent differentiation and proliferation of entrapped epithelium.

In analogy with asbestos in the pathogenesis of pleural mesothelioma and bronchogenic carcinoma (Selikoff 1977), the identification of talc particles in ovarian cancer tissue has lead to the hypothesis of carcinogenesis by foreign body stimulation (Henderson et al. 1979).

The association between irradiation and cancer of the ovary has not been proved, although women who have previously been irradiated have a higher than expected frequency of late ovarian carcinoma (relative risk 1.6; $P < 0.05$) (Kleinerman et al. 1982). These observations point out the importance of environmental risk factors, and further data are necessary to clarify the role of these factors.

Studies of viral association have so far been inconclusive; the protective effect of mumps has not been confirmed, nor has the supposedly higher risk in subjects with rubella virus exanthem (Weiss et al. 1981; McGowan et al. 1979).

There have been reports in the literature of familial association, and cases of ovarian carcinoma in multiple relatives of various generations are known (Piver et al. 1982; Lynch et al. 1985). This familiar carcinoma is bilateral in 75% of cases, with a higher frequency of serous and undifferentiated histotype (Scully 1970), and it has been correlated to genetic as well as hormonal and dietary factors (King et al. 1980; Lynch et al. 1978). In addition, various genetic diseases (Peutz-Jeghers syndrome, gonadal dysgenesis), endocrine disorders and alimentary habits seem to predispose women to ovarian cancer, but no proven association has been established (De Palo 1980).

Pathology

The classification of malignant ovarian tumours adopted by the World Health Organization and the Federation of Gynecology and Obstetrics (FIGO) is presented in Table 1. Epithelial tumours are generally classified according to whether they are benign, malignant (invasive) or "of low malignant potential" (borderline). Ovarian carcinoma accounts for 80%–90% of ovarian malignancies and originates from the ovarian mesothelium; and since coelomic epithelium has a multipotential differentiation capacity, it may have endometrioid, serous or mucinous characteristics (Serov et al. 1973). The frequency of invasive carcinoma by histotype is shown in Table 2.

The cell type has prognostic significance and survival is correlated to histotype and grading of differentiation. Survival in mucinous and endometrioid adenocarcinoma is better than in serous adenocarcinoma (Barber et al. 1974; Bush 1979). Our data are in agreement with these results, although no statistically significant difference has been seen among different cell types.

Grading generally ranges from G1 to G3–4 in relation to the least differentiated area, if present in

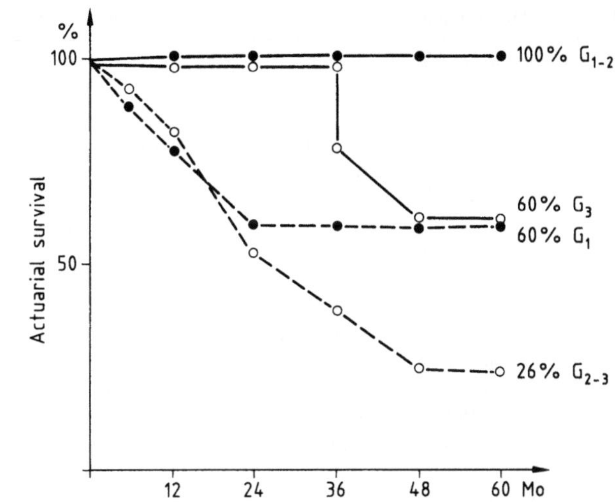

Fig. 1. Survival in relation to stage and grade – 136 patients. *Solid line*, stage I; *broken line*, stage III

more than 10% of all sections examined. There are several cellular and histological criteria applicable in grading (number of mitoses, nucleo/cytoplasm, lymphoid infiltration, etc.) (Russel 1979; Broders 1976), which mean that the evaluation of this parameter is rather subjective. The value of the grading as a prognostic factor (Ozols et al. 1980) has been confirmed in a clinical series of the Istituto Nazionale Tumori, Milan (Fig. 1).

The incidence of borderline epithelial tumours in 2412 patients was shown to be 15% (De Palo 1980). This group is characterised by the absence of stroma invasion, and the tumour has a less aggressive clinical course. The best treatment for borderline tumours is controversial. Surgical resection gives excellent results in early stages; however, in advanced stages treatment should be similar to that used in invasive tumours because of the fact that about 15% of these patients will die of the disease within 5 years of diagnosis.

Some other features of ovarian carcinoma regarding the DNA content of cells (polyploidy, aneuploidy, hyperdiploidy) are detected by flow cytometry and seem to be a prognostic factor independent of histotype and grading (Friedlander 1984). Lastly, the dosage of hormonal receptors has shown promising results, but up to now no actual prognostic or therapeutic significance has been demonstrated.

Diagnosis

Symptoms indicating ovarian cancer are rare in the earlier stages of the disease and routine pelvic examination remains the most reliable way to detect

Table 1. Histological classification of ovarian tumours (WHO 1973)

I. Common "epithelial" tumours
A. Serous tumours
1. Benign
a. Cystadenoma and papillary cystadenoma
b. Surface papilloma
c. Adenofibroma and cystadenofibroma
2. Of borderline malignancy (carcinomas of low malignant potential)
a. Cystadenoma and papillary cystadenoma
b. Surface papilloma
c. Adenofibroma and cystadenofibroma
3. Malignant
a. Adenocarcinoma, papillary adenocarcinoma and papillary cystadenocarcinoma
b. Surface papillary carcinoma
c. Malignant adenofibroma and cystadenofibroma
B. Mucinous tumours
1. Benign
a. Cystadenoma
b. Adenofibroma and cystadenofibroma
2. Of borderline malignancy (carcinomas of low malignant potential)
a. Cystadenoma
b. Adenofibroma and cystadenofibroma
3. Malignant
a. Adenocarcinoma and cystadenocarcinoma
b. Malignant adenofibroma and cystadenofibroma
C. Endometrioid tumours
1. Benign
a Adenoma and cystadenoma
b. Adenofibroma and cystadenofibroma
2. Of borderline malignancy (carcinomas of low malignant potential)
a. Adenoma and cystadenoma
b. Adenofibroma and cystadenofibroma
3. Malignant
a. Carcinoma
(i) Adenocarcinoma
(ii) Adenoacanthoma
(iii) Malignant adenofibroma and cystadenofibroma
b. Endometrioid stromal sarcomas
c. Mesodermal (müllerian) mixed tumours, homologous and heterologous
D. Clear cell (mesonephroid) tumours
1. Benign: adenofibroma
2. Of borderline malignancy (carcinomas of low malignant potential)
3. Malignant: carcinoma and adenocarcinoma
E. Brenner tumours
1. Benign
2. Of borderline malignancy (proliferating)
3. Malignant
F. Mixed epithelial tumours
1. Benign
2. Of borderline malignancy
3. Malignant
G. Undifferentiated carcinoma
H. Unclassified epithelial tumours
II. Sex cord stromal tumours
A. Granulosa-stromal cell tumours
1. Granulosa cell tumour
2. Tumours in the thecoma-fibroma group
a. Thecoma
b. Fibroma
c. Unclassified
B. Androblastomas: Sertoli-Leydig cell tumours
1. Well differentiated
a. Tubular androblastoma; Sertoli cell tumour (tubular adenoma of Pick)
b. Tubular androblastoma with lipid storage; Sertoli cell tumour with lipid storage (folliculoma lipidique of Lecene)
c. Sertoli-Leydig cell tumour (tubular adenoma with Leydig cells)
d. Leydig cell tumour; hilar cell tumour
2. Of intermediate differentiation
3. Poorly differentiated (sarcomatoid)
4. With heterologous elements
C. Gynandroblastoma
D. Unclassified
III. Lipid (lipoid) cell tumours
IV. Germ cell tumours
A. Dysgerminoma
B. Endodermal sinus tumour
C. Embryonal carcinoma
D. Polyembryoma
E. Choriocarcinoma
F. Teratomas
1. Immature
2. Mature
a. Solid
b. Cystic
(i) Dermoid cyst (mature cystic teratoma)
(ii) Dermoid cyst with malignant transformation
3. Monodermal and highly specialized
a. Struma ovarii
b. Carcinoid
c. Struma ovarii and carcinoid
d. Others
G. Mixed forms
V. Gonadoblastoma
A. Pure
B. Mixed with dysgerminoma or other form of germ cell tumour
VI. Soft tissue tumours not specific to ovary
VII. Unclassified tumours
VIII. Secondary (metastatic) tumours

this form of neoplasia. The presence of a palpable or fixed ovary in postmenopausal women should raise the suspicion of ovarian neoplasm and induce the planning of further investigations. Cell samples obtained by needle culdocentesis have diagnostic accuracy in about 66%–96% of cases examined, but this method can only be used in patients with a palpable mass, in advanced stages and in the follow-up of treated patients, but not as a screening test or in preclinical diagnosis (Bolandgray et al. 1972).

Table 2. Frequency of invasive carcinoma by histotype

	(%)
Serous adenocarcinoma	52–48
Undifferentiated carcinoma	18–16
Endometrioid adenocarcinoma	17–14
Mucinous adenocarcinoma	13–11
Clear cell adenocarcinoma	0–5

[Collected series (Kent and McDay 1960; Greenspan 1975)].

Table 3. Ovarian tumour markers

Trophoblastic	
Human placental alkaline phosphatase (PAP)	
Human chorionic gonadotrophin (HCG)	
Human placental lactogen (HPL)	
Pregnancy-specific beta-1 globulin (SP1)	
Embryonic	
Carcinoembryonic antigen (CEA)	
Embryonic prealbumin (EPA)	
Beta-oncofetal antigen (βOFA)	
Alpha-fetoprotein (αFP)	
Miscellaneous	
Pregnancy-associated macroglobulin (PAM, PZP)	
Tumour polypeptide antigen (Björklund)	
Enzymes	
Urokinase	
Glycosyl transferases	
Glycosidases	
Ovarian antigens	
OCAA	
OCAA-1	
OVC-1	
OVC-2	
OCA	
Immune complexes (various)	
Ca 125 – Ca 199	
Ovarian antigen reacting with	MoV1, MoV2, MoV18 ID3 DU-PAN 2 F 36/22

Ultrasound may be helpful in discriminating ovarian masses: the presence of solid elements or papillary projections or the involvement of adjacent organs suggests ovarian malignancy (Samuels 1975). Ultrasound may also be useful in direct percutaneous fine needle aspiration of a pelvic mass or enlarged lymph nodes (Berkowitz et al. 1974). The diagnostic accuracy of CT scanning is similar to that of ultrasound, but gives a better view of the diffusion of disease in the liver, lymph nodes and lungs (Solomon et al. 1983).

A new diagnostic method is nuclear magnetic resonance, the results of which are evaluable mostly in the bone marrow and the brain. The preliminary data obtained in gynaecological malignancies allow a good discrimination and evaluation of the borders of pelvic and abdominal masses (Bies et al. 1984).

Laparoscopy is used to identify pelvic tumours (uterine or ovarian) and in the preoperative staging of disease; it also allows the inspection of the pelvis, peritoneal surfaces and diaphragm. Unfortunately, it cannot distinguish benign disease from an encapsulated malignant neoplasm. Biopsy of an encapsulated ovarian cyst may cause intraperitoneal spilling of malignant cells and must be absolutely avoided.

Barium enema cannot reveal serosal involvement but may nevertheless be advisable in order to detect deep infiltration of the intestine wall.

Pyelography is helpful in excluding the presence of disease in adjacent pelvic structures.

Lymphangiography has been proposed for the detection of lymph node involvement. Although lymph node metastases have been found from 10% in stage I to 30% in stage III with 80%–90% accuracy (Musumeci et al. 1977), the sensitivity of the method is too low for safe therapeutic planning.

Many efforts have been directed towards the identification of tumour markers which can detect early ovarian cancer. Up to now a number of markers have been proposed (Table 3) with varying but usually inadequate results. For pure choriocarcinoma and yolk sac tumours, beta human chorionic gonadotrophin (β-HCG) and alpha-fetoprotein (αFP) have been found to be reliable for diagnosis, response monitoring and follow-up (Kurman and Norris 1976; Goldstein and Piro 1972). They can also be used in malignant mixed cell teratoma, although in this tumour the presence of cells not producing markers invalidates the interpretation of the results. αFP and β-HCG are not significant markers for epithelial ovarian cancer.

Carcinoembryonic antigen (CEA) has been found in the serum of 60%–80% of patients with ovarian carcinoma in stage III–IV, with a higher frequency in the mucinous type (Di Saia et al. 1977). Although the sensitivity and specificity are too low for it to be used for diagnostic purposes, serum CEA measurement may be useful in monitoring the disease when elevated levels have been detected before treatment.

Placental alkaline phosphatase is another substance found in the serum of 40%–50% of patients with ovarian carcinoma (Fishman et al. 1975).

Ovarian cystoadenocarcinoma-associated antigen (OCAA) and ovarian carcinoma antigen (OCA) are present in approximately 70% of patients with ovarian carcinoma and correlate with the clinical course of disease in 60%–70% of cases (Bhattacharya and Barlow 1979; Piver et al. 1975).

In recent years the monoclonal antibody technique (Kohler and Milstein 1975) has been applied in the development of antibodies against human epithelial ovarian cancer. The monoclonal antibody OC 125 was developed, recognising multiple determinants expressed on a high molecular weight glycoprotein. The antigen is not found in normal ovarian tissue but it is expressed in approximately 80% of nonmucinous ovarian carcinoma. A good correlation is seen between the clinical course of disease and antigen levels, but a minimal amount of tumour is usually not revealed by this marker (Kabawat et al. 1983).

Another promising monoclonal antibody is MoV (Tagliabue et al. 1985; Colnaghi et al. 1985), which recognises a glycoprotein antigen associated with ovarian epithelial tumours. Among the primary malignancies tested, MoV2 immunostained 100% of mucinous, 81% of serous and 73% of endometrioid carcinomas. The capacity of the monoclonal antibody MoV2 to detect the antigen was also seen in the serum of patients with ovarian carcinoma.

More recently the new monoclonal antibodies MoV18 and MoV19 seem to be of particular interest because of their restricted tumour specificity. The soluble antigen is present in the serum of 30% of patients with ovarian carcinoma, whereas only one out of 100 sera from healthy donors was found to be borderline positive. In urine samples the levels of the marker were found to undergo a considerable increase (Tagliabue et al. 1987).

A new, promising diagnostic procedure is immunoscintigraphy using monoclonal antibodies, but this technique is still under investigation (Epenetos et al. 1982).

Diffusion and Surgical Staging

Spread is mostly peritoneal by continuity or cell implants on the visceral and parietal peritoneum. This spread is favoured by the circulation of physiological peritoneal free fluid which is moved from the pelvis to the diaphragm by the changing abdominal pressure during respiration. Lymphatic spread is a less common but still quite important pathway of diffusion. The main lymphatic drainage of the ovary follows the ovarian vessels, reaching the para-aortic nodes. Another group of efferent lymph vessels crosses the cardinal ligament to reach the upper external iliac nodes. A third, less important draining route follows the round ligament to the external and inguinal nodes (Plentl and Friedman 1971). Haematological diffusion is less frequent; distant metastases (liver, lung, pleura) are present in about 10% of patients at diagnosis.

Table 4. Surgical staging procedures

Vertical xiphopubic incision
Aspiration of ascites or peritoneal free fluid or peritoneal washings
Examination of visceral and parietal peritoneum
Total abdominal hysterectomy – bilateral salpingo-oophorectomy[a]
Omentectomy
Retroperitoneal lymph node dissection
Excision of ovarian vessels at their origin
Appendectomy
Biopsy of Douglas' cul-de-sac, paracolic gutters, diaphragm, mesentery

[a] In selected cases of stage IA, the uterus and contralateral ovary may be spared. In these cases ovarian biopsy and endometrioid curettage should be performed.

The identification of the sites of initial involvement and the staging of ovarian carcinoma are done by accurate primary surgery which is the keystone of further management of the patients. All the procedures that should be performed are shown in Table 4.

A longitudinal midline incision extending from the xiphoid to the pubis is necessary to allow adequate exploration of the entire abdominal cavity including the domes of the diaphragm. Any peritoneal free fluid must be collected, even in early clinical stages. In the absence of peritoneal fluid, the peritoneal surfaces should be washed with Hanks solution or 200 cc saline, to be collected from the pelvis and paracolic gutters. Tumour cells are present in 2%–36% of cases of apparent stage I–II disease (Creasman and Rutledge 1971; De Palo et al. 1981).

The opposite ovary is generally removed because of the possibility of microscopic tumour involvement reported in 6%–43% of cases (De Palo et al. 1981; Fuks 1980). As the disease progresses the incidence of bilateral involvement increases as well, in relation to histological types.

Out of 291 cases of surgical staging performed at the Istituto Nazionale Tumori, Milan, bilateral ovarian involvement was demonstrated in 45.8% of stage II, 71.4% of stage III and 68.2% of stage IV disease, but only 2.4% of all cases proved to be real stage IB.

Since the endometrium and Fallopian tubes are potential sites of occult metastases or synchronous/metachronous adenocarcinoma, hysterectomy and salpingectomy should be performed routinely, even when the serosa is not involved (Buchsbaum and Lifshitz 1984).

The infracolic omentum below the transverse colon must be removed routinely due to the presence of microscopic metastases reported in 8.9% of patients in whom it seemed to be macroscopically free (Buchsbaum and Lifshitz 1984). When the omentum is macroscopically involved, removal of the gastrocolic ligament is also recommended. The appendix is routinely removed.

All peritoneal surfaces (mesentery, serosa of small and large intestine) are carefully explored and biopsies of any suspicious areas are taken, as well as biopsies from the paracolic gutter, Douglas's cul-de-sac, pelvic walls, bladder serosa and diaphragm. In a study by the Gynecologic Oncology Group of the National Cancer Institute (GOG) (Buchsbaum and Lifshitz 1984), 4.2% of patients with ovarian carcinoma had malignancy demonstrated in random biopsies of clinically negative diaphragm.

To complete accurate surgical staging, a retroperitoneal lymph node dissection may be performed. Although retroperitoneal involvement has been reported for many years (Abrams 1950; Bergman 1966), the incidence and clinical significance of lymph node metastases in ovarian carcinoma have been underestimated. More recently (Chen and Lee 1984; Di Re et al. 1982), lymph node metastases have also been reported in early stages of disease. At the Istituto Nazionale Tumori in Milan retroperitoneal lymph node dissection has been performed routinely during surgical staging from 1974 onwards. Until December 1986, 129 radically operable patients underwent complete lymphadenectomy, while lymph node biopsies were performed on a further 72 patients.

The retroperitoneal space is exposed up to the renal vessels by incision of the posterior peritoneum from the hepatocolic ligament to Treitz's ligament, and by turning back the caecum and the ascending colon, following which the descending colon is moved aside. Lymphadenectomy starts with the isolation of the renal pedicle; the ovarian vessels are bisected at their origin. Then dissection of the caval and aortic lymph nodes is performed, preserving the inferior mesenteric artery. Finally, the bilateral common and external iliac nodes are removed.

The incidence of lymph node metastases in relation to stage of disease (classified according to FIGO and TNM criteria) and to histotype is shown in Table 5. From these data it is evident that serous adenocarcinoma also has a clear tendency to spread by the lymphatic route in earlier stages. The incidence of lymph node metastases in relation to grade of differentiation (studied in 175 patients) shows significant difference only for stage I (9.7% – G1–G2; 27.3% – G3) (Table 6). The sites of lymph node metastases were: only para-aortic in 18.2% of cases, only pelvic in 31.4% and both pelvic and para-aortic in 50.4% of cases, which is not in agreement with the anatomical study of Plentl and Friedman (1971) on the subject of preferential drainage to para-aortic groups.

Table 6. GRADE of tumour differentiation and incidence of lymph node metastases ($n = 175$)

Stage	Cases	G1		G2		G3	
	(n)	(n)	(%)	(n)	(%)	(n)	(%)
I	94	3/33	9.0	4/39	10.2	6/22	27.3
II	19	2/4	50.0	3/10	30.0	2/5	40.0
III	52	3/4	75.0	15/25	60.0	12/23	52.2
IV	10	–	–	2/2	100.0	4/8	50.0
	175	8/4	19.5	24/76	31.6	24/58	41.4

Table 5. Incidence of retroperitoneal lymph node metastases by stage and histotype ($n = 201$)

Stage		Serous	Mucinous	Endometrioid	Clear cell	Undifferentiated	Mixed	Adenocarcinoma	Unspecified
I	(n)	10/34	0/22	1/20	1/6	–	0/5	2/11	14/98
	(%)	29.4	0.0	5.0	16.6	–	0.0	18.2	14.3
II	(n)	3/12	1/4	0/4	0/1	–	0/1	–	4/22
	(%)	25.0	25.0	0.0	0.0	–	0.0	–	18.2
III	(n)	24/35	5/10	5/12	–	2/3	–	4/8	40/68
	(%)	68.6	50.0	41.6	–	66.6	–	50.0	58.8
IV	(n)	2/3	1/3	2/3	–	–	1/2	0/2	6/13
	(%)	66.6	33.3	66.6	–	–	50.0	0.0	46.1
	(n)	39/84	7/39	8/39	1/7	2/3	1/8	6/21	64/201
	(%)	46.4	17.9	20.5	14.3	66.6	12.5	28.6	31.8

Treatment

Surgery

Surgery plays a major role in the management of patients with ovarian cancer, both in establishing the extent of disease (as previously described in the section on staging) and in performing radical or partial tumour removal. Radical surgery may be performed in stage I A, I B, II A and in a few cases of II B or III for omentum or for retroperitoneal lymph nodes only. Except in selected cases of stage I A, in which survival is about 90% (Istituto Nazionale Tumori, Milan, series), surgery alone does not provide adequate treatment and adjuvant therapy is necessary.

Unilateral oophorectomy may be performed in young women in tumour stage I A G1–2, with an intact capsule, without capsule invasion and no intraoperative spilling, provided that there is no evidence of disease in any other site. In these cases a biopsy should be taken from the opposite ovary for frozen section examination to exclude presence of tumour. For the same reason, endometrial curettage should be performed whenever conservation of the uterus is considered.

Out of 27 cases of conservative surgery, six subsequent pregnancies have been observed (22%), and all patients are alive (Istituto Nazionale Tumori, Milan series) and free of tumour (median follow-up 58 months).

Cytoreductive Surgery

Clinical observations of palliation and prolongation of survival by removal of tumour masses were already reported a decade ago; these favourable results were probably due to reduction of the tumour damage subsequent to the improvement of the metabolic and nutritional status of the patient. At present the aim of surgical cytoreduction is the resection of tumour masses to enable the eradication of residual tumour by complementary treatment (radiotherapy or chemotherapy). On the other hand, debulking surgery carries the implication of a synergistic effect between reduction in the number of tumour cells and secondary therapy; in experimental terms, such combined treatment is supported by the concept that tumour excision increases the growth fraction of the tumour cells, which become more susceptible to cytotoxic agents (Skipper 1978; Goldie and Coldman 1979).

Using a multivariate analysis, Griffiths (1975) found that the diameter of the largest residual primary tumour was a significant determinant of survival. The survival time decreased in patients with residual tumours larger than 1.0 ± 0.5 cm, regardless of other prognostic or therapeutic variables. In addition, patients in whom the tumour mass was surgically reduced to less than 1.5 cm did just as well as those with small metastases of less than 1.5 cm before surgery.

Table 7. Survival in relation to residual tumour diameter following surgery in patients with stage III and IV disease

Author	Diameter of residual tumour (cm)	Cases (*n*)	Median survival (months)	Actuarial survival (%)
Griffiths 1975	<1.5	47	22	20 (80 months)
	>1.5	26	11	0 (38 months)
Smith and Day 1979	<2	161	-	37.3 (5 years)
	>2	453	-	4.5 (5 years)
Wharton and Hersen 1981	≤2	45	27.6	-
	>2	59	15.3	-
Hacker et al. 1983	<0.5	7	40 }	29.1
	<1.5	24	18 }	
	>1.5	16	6	0
Van Lindert et al. 1984	<0.5	27	-	68 (3 years)
	>0.5	26	-	13 (3 years)

Several other studies have demonstrated a correlation between survival and volume of disease after primary surgery, and, although not clearly established, the concept of "minimal residual disease" is now generally accepted (Table 7) (Hacker et al. 1983; Wharton and Herson 1981; Van Lindert et al. 1984; Smith and Day 1979). From these reports it appears that the size of residual nodules is more important than primary stage and extension of disease.

Disease volume following surgery is also correlated with findings at second-look surgery subsequent to chemotherapy, as reported by Smith and Schwartz (1980), who noted a negative second look in 30% of patients with residual tumour of less than 2 cm and in 16% of cases with gross residual disease. The same data have been reported by other authors (Griffiths 1986) and are confirmed by the experience of the Istituto Nazionale Tumori, Milan, of 140 cases in which second-look surgery was performed.

Many problems regarding cytoreductive surgery remain, in particular:

- The fact that some tumours of similar grade and stage are operable and others are not may be related to an unknown biological factor conditioning the response to treatment as well as survival.

- Even if we acknowledge the fact that cytoreductive surgery may have a therapeutic value when performed before any other treatment, the role of debulking surgery after two or three cycles of chemotherapy or at the end of an induction course of chemotherapy is not clear.

An increase in survival is reported by debulking surgery following primary radiotherapy or chemotherapy (Smith and Schwartz 1980; Berek et al. 1983); even in these cases, improved survival is related to a diameter of residual disease of less than 2 cm. These findings are contradictory to those of other authors (Joyeux et al. 1986; Vogl et al. 1984) who have reported that further debulking at second look did not improve survival expectancy. Nevertheless, due to the lack of data from randomised studies and the poor results of second-line chemotherapy, the choice of repeated surgery is reserved to selected patients.

Cytoreductive surgery requires good surgical knowledge because all the abdominal structures are often involved by peritoneal carcinomatosis.

The retroperitoneal approach has been recommended (Hudson 1973) for the mobilisation of fixed ovarian masses and the excision of the Douglas's cul-de-sac and pelvic implants, exposing the iliac vessels and the ureter, which are rarely invaded by the tumour.

Tumour masses involving the sigmoid or rectum require bowel resection; tumours infiltrating bladder serosa may be dissected, although cystectomy is absolutely to be avoided. When massively involved, the omentum is usually removed without ligating the gastroepiploic vessels if possible and subsequent dissection along the transverse colon or from the greater curvature of the stomach. If the splenic pedicle is involved splenectomy may be performed. In general not more that two segments of the small intestine or colon should be excised. Radical lymphadenectomy is performed only if optimal debulking is achieved in the peritoneal cavity, otherwise only retroperitoneal biopsies are taken. Metastases in the liver parenchyma or hilus, positive lymph nodes above the origin of the renal vessels and multiple masses infiltrating the mesentery or the diaphragm are usually not resectable. Optimal cytoreduction is obtained in 30%–80% of patients and seems independent of histotype and grade (Griffiths 1986; Chen and Bochner 1985; Di Re et al. 1986; Delgado et al. 1983).

The postoperative complication rates vary from 13.3% to 43% (Griffiths 1986; Chen and Bochner 1985; Di Re et al. 1986). In any case, it is necessary to keep in mind that all these patients require postoperative chemotherapy and that surgical procedures and complications may delay postoperative treatment to such an extent that tumour regrowth may occur.

Second-Look Operations

The concept of a "second-look laparotomy", formulated by Wangensteen et al. (1951) and originally performed in patients with colon cancer, is now an important step in the management of ovarian cancer. The term is generally used to define a surgical procedure which is performed subsequent to radio- or chemotherapy in patients without clinical evidence of disease in order to confirm complete remission and plan further treatment. Surgical exploration should be carried out in the same way as primary surgery.

The abdomen is opened by a xiphopubic incision and peritoneal washing for cytology is performed; biopsies are obtained from the pelvic peritoneum, paracolic gutters, diaphragm, residual omental tissue and mesentery. All adhesions should be excised and sent for pathological examination. If not performed during primary surgery, hystero-oophorectomy and retroperitoneal lymph node dissection should be done.

Laparoscopy has been proposed as a second-look procedure (Berek et al. 1981); actually, if this demonstrates persistent tumour, it is not necessary to perform laparotomy for the planning of further treatment. Negative laparoscopy does not provide sufficient evidence for complete remission of the disease; in fact, in about 50% of cases complete pelvic examination is impossible due to multiple adhesions. Moreover, there are reports in the literature of 17%–70% of persistent tumour at laparotomy in patients without clinical evidence of disease: different degrees of reliability are in relation to stage of disease, timing of the procedure and type of primary chemotherapy (Phillips et al. 1979; Smith and Schwartz 1980; Roberts et al. 1982; Barnhill et al. 1984; Lusley et al. 1984).

At the Istituto Nazionale Tumori, Milan, from 1974 to 1986 out of 81 patients (stages IC–IV) in complete clinical remission and with no evidence of disease at preoperative diagnostic procedures (including laparoscopy and peritoneal washing), 26 were found to have persistent tumour at laparotomy (i.e. 32%).

The sites of microscopic and macroscopic disease are illustrated in Table 8: as reported by other authors, the peritoneum was the most common site, but in 58.8% of cases the retroperitoneal lymph nodes were also positive. Findings at second look

Table 8. Localisations revealed at second look – 26/81 cases in complete clinical remission

Site	(*n*)	(%)		Unique	(%)	
Peritoneum	13	50.0		3	11.5	
Omentum	7	26.9		–	–	
Lymph nodes[a]	7	58.8		4	22.2	
Ovary[b]	7	43.7	62.5	3	18.7	31.2
Opposite ovary[b]	3	18.7		2	12.5	
Ovarian pedicle[a]	4	–		2	–	
Sigmoid	4	15.4		1	3.8	
Liver	2	7.7		1	3.8	
Cytology	7	26.9		2	7.7	

[a] Eighteen patients not submitted to lymphadenectomy at primary surgery.
[b] Sixteen patients not submitted to oophorectomy at primary surgery.

Table 9. Randomised trials comparing combination chemotherapy in advanced ovarian cancer

	Chemotherapy	CR + PR (%)	CR (%)	Median survival (months)
Young et al. (1978)	HEXA-CAF	75	33	29
	L-PAm	54	16	17
Vogl (1982)	CHAP	61	38	20
	L-PAm	40	21	19
Cormo-Pereira (1983)	PAH	38	19	11
	C	66	29	12
Williams (1985)	PAC	68	26	13
	Cb	26	15	11

CR, complete remission; PR, partial remission; C, cyclophosphamide; Cb, chlorambucil; A, doxorubicin; H, hexamethylmelamine; L-PAM, melphalan; P, cisplatin; HEXA-CAF, H + C + 5-fluorouracil + methotrexate.

are a good prognostic factor, in fact patients in complete remission have a good chance of prolonged survival (88% 3-year survival in Istituto Nazionale Tumori series).

Unfortunately, in a very high proportion of cases with initial stage III–IV the tumour will recur in 2–5 years after a negative second-look procedure (Ozols et al. 1981; Phillips et al. 1979). These data show that a negative second look is not synonymous with "cure" and suggest a possible need for additional treatment.

If second look has a place in the management of ovarian carcinoma, the role of third-look surgery has not been established.

Chemotherapy

Chemotherapy has been used increasingly in the treatment of ovarian cancer because:

1. This neoplasm is highly sensitive to cytotoxic drugs.
2. Two-thirds of all patients present with surgically noncurable advanced disease.
3. It provides an opportunity of adjuvant treatment also in radically operated patients in whom recurrence is seen to occur in about 40% of cases.

Alkylating agents have been the most frequently used chemotherapeutic drugs with an objective response rate of 35%–65%, as quoted in published reports of more that 1000 patients, with a median survival of 17–20 months in responders against 6–13 months in nonresponders (Young et al. 1985). In addition to alkylating agents, doxorubicin, *cis*-platinum and hexamethylmelamine have been used extensively, as single agents or in combination, with response rates of 25%–40%. Over the past decade a number of retrospective or prospective and randomised studies have been published, reporting the results of single or combined treatment. A few of these randomised studies are listed in Table 9. These trials provide good evidence for the increased effectiveness of combinations compared to single agents, as shown by the response rates (Trope 1981; Decker et al. 1982; Williams et al. 1985).

Although other studies do not support these results (MRC Working Party on Ovarian Cancer 1981; Cormo-Pereira et al. 1981), and there is no ideal trial available so far, the consensus is that the best chance for achieving complete remission in advanced carcinoma is produced by cis-platinum-containing combination regimens administered at full dose. The benefit of combinations with respect to overall survival remains somewhat controversial. At present, single agent chemotherapy is only given to old patients or patients with metabolic disease or poor performance status and sometimes as adjuvant treatment in early stages of disease.

Some questions still remain as to the application of chemotherapy in advanced stages:

- How long should it be given?
- Should administration be intraperitoneal or systemic?
- What are the possibilities of second-line chemotherapy?

The current trend in the treatment of ovarian cancer is towards shorter courses of chemotherapy: the reason for this policy is that no difference in response has been demonstrated during 6–12 months of treatment. In accordance with the Goldie-Coldman hypothesis of tumour cell mutation (Goldie and Coldman 1979), it is likely that over several months of therapy tumour cells will become resistant to drugs; accurate trials in other tumours show that a short treatment course is as effective as long-term therapy. Recently experimental and clinical studies have provided insight into the pharmacokinetic pattern of intraperitoneal drug administration (Myers and Collins 1983). As expected, following intraperitoneal administration local drug concentration is seen to be higher than systemic drug concentration, and this fact should be translated into an improved therapeutic index.

Some data emphasise the need for drug administration in fluid volumes high enough to guarantee complete distribution into the peritoneal contents (belly bath) and the use of drugs with a clear dose-response relationship and no peritoneal toxicity.

Because of possible adhesions and peritoneal sac in patients submitted to repeated laparotomies, the distribution of fluid in the abdominal cavity may be inhibited. This can be assessed by CT scan or peritoneography of the entire abdominal cavity after intraperitoneal instillation of 2000 cc of saline with contrast medium (Myers 1984). The use of a semipermanent Tenckhoff catheter allows a more simple delivery of dialysate and chemotherapy. General toxicity is almost the same as in systemic chemotherapy. Catheter-related side effects may involve wound infection, peritonitis and abdominal distress. Several drugs have been administered intraperitoneally with varying results and *cis*-platinum seems at present the most attractive (Brenner 1980).

While this kind of therapy is not indicated in bulky disease, it may have a role as a substitute for intraperitoneal radioisotopes in early ovarian cancer, or as a component of first-line therapy in the subgroup of patients with minimal residual disease after primary surgery, or as second-line chemotherapy for remission consolidation in patients with no or minimal residual disease after systemic treatment.

In all forms of ovarian cancer, second-line chemotherapy has been very disappointing so far, and when an effective drug combination is used and fails, there is virtually no chance of obtaining significant response with secondary chemotherapy. For this reason it is mandatory to continue the efforts in identifying alternatives to current therapy.

New cytotoxic agents, such as platinum compounds, ifosfamide and mitomycin, have been found to have some activity in recurrent or persistent ovarian carcinoma.

At present, hormonal therapy does not offer any valid approach in the treatment of this neoplasm.

New studies are directed towards the development of the human tumour stem cell assay to test the in vitro sensitivity of the drugs, towards the evaluation of the role of biological response modifiers and towards increasing tolerable drug doses or enhancing drug effectiveness.

Radiotherapy

For many decades, external radiation has been widely employed in the management of ovarian carcinoma, but the evaluation of the results is virtually impossible because of the differences between the reported series, in radiation fields and in doses; as a result, the efficacy of the treatment cannot be demonstrated. Moreover, the need to irradiate large abdominal fields and at the same time reduce the dose due to the limited tolerance of the kidney, liver, bone marrow and small intestine to radiation (with frequent occurrence of adhesive peritonitis) has led to the substitution of postoperative radiotherapy by chemotherapy both in early and advanced disease.

Pelvic irradiation seems to be inappropriate as adjuvant therapy even in stage I A because relapses are seen to occur at the same rate as in control cases; recurrences are seen all over the peritoneal cavity, as demonstrated by Dembo et al. (1979) in a prospective randomised study. The same conclusions are reported by the GOG study in which patients with stage I ovarian carcinoma were randomised to no further therapy, melphalan, or pelvic radiation, and no difference in relapse was seen in the three patient arms (Hreshchyshyn et al. 1980).

Although neither the Princess Margaret Hospital (PMH; Dembo et al. 1979) nor the GOG study (Hreshchyshyn et al. 1980) demonstrates any survival benefits from postoperative radiotherapy in stage I, it must be emphasised that not all patients in these studies were subjected to complete surgical staging so that an indeterminate number of relapses probably occurred in patients with more advanced disease that had remained unrecognised. Also, in more advanced stages the results of postoperative radiation treatment are not clear.

Nevertheless, some conclusions can be drawn from the studies of PMH (Dembo 1985) and M.D. Anderson Hospital and Tumor Institute (Delclos and Dembo 1980) comparing pelvic vs. abdomino-pelvic irradiation vs. single agent chemotherapy: the efficacy of radiation therapy is directly related to residual tumour and grade, the fields of irradiation should always include the whole peritoneal cavity, the moving strip and open field techniques seem to be equally effective.

From these experiences it appears that radiotherapy may be curative in selected patients and may have its own role as primary postoperative treatment in patients with minimal or no residual disease or as part of sequential multimodality therapy in patients with no macroscopic residual tumour following surgery and chemotherapy.

The intraperitoneal instillation of radioactive colloidal ^{198}Au and ^{32}P has been employed in the treatment of ovarian cancer with the aim of sterilising microscopic peritoneal implants. The advantages of radionuclide therapy consist in a high dose applied to the peritoneal surface (6000–7000 rad), with a limited depth dose, given in one short, single treatment session. For this reason, it is indicated primarily as adjuvant treatment in stages IAii and IC and in cases with no macroscopic residual disease following surgery (and chemotherapy).

Intraperitoneal administration of radioisotopes presents the same problems as intraperitoneal chemotherapy, and it should be ascertained that there is a proper distribution of fluids. In a recent series of stage I patients treated with intraperitoneal radioisotopes, excellent survival rates were reported, i.e. between 85% and 95%, and improved survival was shown in comparison with patients treated with pelvic irradiation (Young 1983). Due to the lack of randomised trials, the results of this kind of treatment cannot yet be considered to be clearly established and frequent complications (small bowel obstruction and stenosis) make radionuclide therapy not very attractive for the moment (Peznec et al. 1978; Kolstad et al. 1977).

Sex Cord Stromal Ovarian Tumours

Sex cord stromal tumours account for approximately 6% of all ovarian tumours and for the majority of functioning tumours with clinical endocrine manifestations. Management of patients with neoplasms at an early stage is usually limited to conservative surgery, whereas treatment of patients with advanced disease remains controversial, largely due to the limited number of patients seen in one institution over a short period of time.

The histological classification is presented in Table 1; the most frequent types are granulosa cell tumours, thecoma-fibroma group and Sertoli-Leydig cell tumours.

Granulosa cell tumours represent about 2% of all ovarian tumours. They occur primarily in postmenopausal women, and the most frequent symptom is bleeding, due to uninhibited estrogen secretion by the tumour cells, resulting in endometrial hyperplasia; moreover, approximately 5% of patients also develop adenocarcinoma of the endometrium (Bjorkholm and Silfersward 1981). When occurring prior to puberty (5% of cases), granulosa cell tumour is frequently associated with sexual pseudoprecocity.

Granulosa cell tumours usually present as stage I disease; factors such as tumour size, degree of differentiation and histological patterns are of uncertain prognostic importance (Bjorkholm and Silfversward 1981; Stenwig et al. 1979). The current management of these tumours involves bilateral salpingo-oophorectomy and hysterectomy; proper surgical staging is needed in order to decide upon the most appropriate postoperative treatment approach. In young patients unilateral oophorectomy may be performed in stage I A when no further therapy is needed. In advanced cases aggressive treatment is required and debulking surgery recommended. Postoperative chemotherapy comprises vincristine, actinomycin D and cyclophosphamide combined (VAC) and cisplatinum, vinblastine and bleomycin combined (PVB). The effect of alkylating agents has not been particularly noteworthy, although some tumour regressions have been reported. Long-term follow-up of these patients is imperative, as tumours may recur late. Hormonal therapy may be useful in the management of recurrences although experience with this kind of treatment is limited (Schwartz et al. 1983). A variant of granulosa cell tumour occurs in young females and is associated with distinct microscopic features (high degree of nuclear atypia and mitotic activity) (Scully 1977). Thus juvenile granulosa cell tumor is associated with rapid growth and spread throughout the abdomen (Takenchi et al. 1983). Radiotherapy and chemotherapy have been unsuccessful in the treatment of this kind of tumour.

Tumours of the thecoma-fibroma group originate from the gonadal stroma, comprising a spectrum of cases ranging from the typical fibroma to the typical thecoma. They represent 5% of all ovarian tumours and occur most often in perimenopausal and postmenopausal women. Thecomas may be associated with endometrial hyperplasia and adenocarcinoma of the endometrium due to their estrogen production. Tumours larger than 10 cm in diameter may be associated with Meigs' syndrome with ascites and hydrothorax.

These tumours have an excellent prognosis although rare malignant examples occur. Their management requires unilateral oophorectomy, although in older women total abdominal hysterectomy and bilateral salpingo-oophorectomy are recommended (Bjorkholm and Silfersward 1980).

Sertoli-Leydig cell tumours (androblastoma) account for less than 0.2% of ovarian neoplasms. Their peak occurrence is at 25–28 years. Approximately 50%–70% of patients present with virilisation, hirsutism, oligo-amenorrhoea and defeminisation as Sertoli-Leydig cell tumours secrete a variety of androgens. Elevated αFB levels have been reported in rare cases. The most important factor in the prognosis and management of Sertoli-Leydig cell tumours is stage of disease. Tumour size has no clear prognostic significance (Roth et al. 1981). Stage I Ai may be treated by means of unilateral oophorectomy if preservation of fertility is desired. Patients with stage I B–IV disease should undergo total abdominal hysterectomy and bilateral oophorectomy as well tumour debulking.

Experience with chemotherapy for recurrent metastatic tumours is limited although CDDP, VP16 and bleomycin combined (PEB), VAC and other combined regimens have given good results.

Germ Cell Tumours

Germ cell tumours are rare malignancies occurring mostly in young women. They may have a mixed histological pattern, and in this case the most malignant component of the tumour should be decisive for the choice of treatment. Dysgerminoma, which accounts for approximately 45% of primary malignant germ cell tumours, has a high cure rate (10-year survival of more that 90% in stage I A). It is bilateral in 10%–20% of cases, and metastases occur mainly by the lymphatic route; in fact, lymph node involvement is present in about 15% of cases in apparent stage I (Di Re et al. 1987). It can be considered as the classic radiosensitive ovarian neoplasm; nevertheless, radiotherapy has an important role even when preservation of the reproductive function is desired.

Conservative surgery is possible in stage I A provided that complete staging is performed and a negative wedge biopsy has been obtained from the contralateral ovary. In these cases ipsilateral radical pelvic and para-aortic lymphadenectomy should be performed; when lymph node involvement can be excluded, no further treatment is necessary. However, if positive nodes are found, a dose of 2500–3000 rad should be delivered to the ipsilateral pelvic and para-aortic sites, shielding the contralateral ovary. Patients with advanced disease should be submitted to aggressive debulking surgery followed by total abdominal irradiation. Recently, advanced and recurrent dysgerminoma have been treated successfully with chemotherapy regimens (vincristine-bleomycin, doxorubicin-cyclophosphamide, PVB, VAC), but more data are necessary before the role of systemic treatment can be defined.

Endodermal sinus tumour, immature teratoma, embryonal carcinoma and choriocarcinoma are mostly unilateral and if so, surgical treatment of stage I A may be conservative, sparing the contralateral ovary.

However, these tumours have an extremely poor prognosis and surgery alone offers long-term survival only in a small percentage of patients. The management of these tumours should, therefore, always include postoperative combination chemotherapy, even in early stages; this treatment policy has significantly improved the survival rates.

The reports of Smith and Rutledge (1975) and Slayton et al. (1978) demonstrated the efficacy of prolonged treatment (21 months) with the VAC regimen. Creasman et al. (1978) reported an effective protocol employing methotrexate, actinomycin D and cyclophosphamide (MAC) with or without radiotherapy. Improved results in the management of germ cell tumours of the testis led to the introduction of the PVB regimen, first employed by Wiltshaw (1982) who successfully treated seven out of eight patients with endodermal sinus tumours.

Serum αFP and β-HCG are present in those tumours which reproduce extraembryonic structures or contain syncytiotrophoblast cells. In these patients, chemotherapy is generally administered until biological markers are negative (often one additional course is given after the first negative titre). Second-look surgery is recommended only if the tumour is biomarker negative.

References

Abrams HR, Spiro R, Goldstein N (1950) Metastases in carcinoma. Cancer 3: 74–85

Barber HRK, Sommer SC, Snyder R et al. (1974) Histologic and nuclear grading and stromal reactions as indices for prognosis in ovarian cancer. Am J Obstet Gynecol 2: 795–807

Barnhill DR, Haskins WJ, Heller PB et al. (1984) The second-look surgical reassessment for epithelial ovarian carcinoma. Gynecol Oncol 19: 148–194

Bennington JL, Ferguson BR, Haber SL (1968) Incidence and relative frequency of benign and malignant ovarian neoplasms. Obstet Gynecol 32: 627–632

Berek JS, Griffiths CT, Leventhal JM (1981) Laparoscopy for second-look evaluation in ovarian cancer. Obstet Gynecol 58: 192–198

Berek JS, Hacker NF, Lagasse LD et al. (1983) Survival of patients following secondary cytoreductive surgery in ovarian cancer. Obstet Gynecol 61: 189–193

Bergman F (1966) A clinicopathological study of 86 autopsied cases with special reference to mode of spread. Acta Obstet Gynecol Scand 45: 211–231

Berkowitz RS, Leavitt T Jr, Knopp RC (1974) Ultrasound-directed percutaneous aspiration biopsy of periaortic lymph nodes in cervical carcinoma recurrence. Am J Obstet Gynecol 131: 100–105

Bhattacharya M, Barlow JJ (1979) Ovarian cystoadenocarcinoma-associated antigen (OCAA). In: Herberman RB (ed) Compendium of assays for immunodiagnosis of human cancer. Elsevier North Holland Biomedical, Amsterdam, pp 327–431

Bies JR, Ellis JH, Kopecky KK et al. (1984) Assessment of primary gynecologic malignancies: comparison of 0,15 – T resistive MRI with CT. AJR 143: 1249–1257

Björkholm E, Silfverswärd C (1980) Theco-cell tumors – clinical features and prognosis. Acta Radiol Oncol Radiat Phys Biol 19: 241–244

Björkholm E, Silfverswärd C (1981) Prognostic factors in granulose-cell tumor. Gynecol Oncol 11: 261–274

Bolandgray A, Mahallati KA, Ardekany MS (1972) Early detection of ovarian malignancy by culdocentesis. J Reprod Med 9: 32–34

Brenner DE (1980) Intraperitoneal chemotherapy: a review. J Clin Oncol 4: 1135–1147

Broders AC (1976) Carcinoma grading and practical application. Arch Pathol 2: 367–381

Buchsbaum HL, Lifshitz S (1984) Staging and surgical evaluation of ovarian cancer. Semin Oncol 11: 227–237

Bush RS (1979) Malignancies of the ovary, uterus and cervix. Arnold, New York

Chen SS, Bochner R (1985) Assessment of morbidity and mortality in primary cytoreductive surgery for advanced ovarian carcinoma. Gynecol Oncol 20: 190–195

Chen SS, Lee L (1984) Prognostic significance of morphology of tumor and retroperitoneal lymph nodes in epithelial carcinoma of the ovary. I. Correlation with lymph node metastases. Gynecol Oncol 18: 87–93

Colnaghi MI, Canevari S, Della Torre G (1985) Tumor detection by immunochemical and radioimmunometric methods. In: Pinchera A, Dorio G, Dammaco F, Bargellesi A (eds) Monoclonal antibodies: biological and clinical application. Kurtis, Milano

Cormo-Pereira J, Costa FO, Henriques E et al. (1981) Advanced ovarian carcinoma. A prospective and randomized clinical trial of cyclophosphamide versus combination cytotoxic chemotherapy (Hexa-CAF). Cancer 48: 1946–1951

Creasman WT, Rutledge F (1971) The prognostic value of peritoneal cytology in gynecologic malignant disease. Am J Obstet Gynecol 100: 773–781

Creasman WT, Fetter BF, Hammond CP et al. (1978) Germ cell malignancies of the ovary. Obstet Gynecol 53: 226

Decker DG, Fleming TR, Makasian GD et al. (1982) Cyclophosphamide plus cisplatinum in combination: treatment program for stage III or IV ovarian carcinoma. Obstet Gynecol 60: 481–487

Delclos L, Dembo AJ (1980) Ovaries. In: Fletcher GH (ed) Textbook of radiotherapy. Lea and Febiger, Philadelphia, pp 834–851

Delgado G, Oram DH, Petrilli ES (1983) Stage III Epithelial ovarian cancer: the role of maximal surgical reduction. Gynecol Oncol 18: 293–298

Dembo AJ (1985) Abdominopelvic radiotherapy in ovarian cancer – a 10 year experience. Cancer 59: 2285–2290

Dembo AJ, Bush RS, Beale FA et al. (1979) The Princess Margaret study of ovarian cancer stage I, II and asymptomatic III presentations. Cancer Treat Rep 63: 248–254

De Palo G (1980) Il carcinoma ovarico: quasi uno sconosciuto I. Argom Oncol 1: 59–84

De Palo G, Musumeci R, Spinelli P et al. (1981) Radiologic peritoneoscopy and cytologic assessment of ovarian carcinoma diffusion. Proceedings of the American Society of Clinical Oncology vol 22. Washington DC (Abstr C-218)

Dicker RC, Webster LA, Loyde DM et al. (1983) Oral contraceptive use and the risk of ovarian cancer. JAMA 249: 1596–1599

Di Re F, Fontanelli R, Benedetti-Panici P et al. (1982) Lymphatic metastases in ovarian carcinoma: analysis of 109 cases. Proceedings of the first congress of the European Society of Surgical Oncology, Athens, November 26–27, 1982, p 210

Di Re F, Fontanelli R, Raspagliesi F et al. (1986) Chirurgia di second-look nei tumori dell'ovaio. In: Veronesi U, Candiani GB, Di Re R, Santoro A (eds) XXVII Corso Superiore di Oncologia: neoplasie ginecologiche. Progressi Terapeutici. Ambrosiano, Milano

Di Re F, Raspagliesi F, Fontanelli R (1987) Chirurgia conservativa nel disgerminoma ovarico. Simposio di aggiornamento internationale Italo-Austriaco. 22–28 February 1987, Merano

Di Saia PJ, Morrow CP, Hoverback BJ et al. (1977) Carcinoembryonic antigen in cancer of the female reproductive system: serial plasma values correlated with disease status. Cancer 39: 2365–2370

Epenetos AA, Matthew S, Granowsha M et al. (1982) Targeting of iodine 123-labelled tumour-associated monoclonal antibodies to ovarian, breast and gastrointestinal tumours. Lancet 2: 999–1004

Fathalla MF (1971) Incessant ovulation: a factor in ovarian neoplasia. Lancet 2: 163–165

Fishman WH, Inglis NR, Vaitukaitis JL et al. (1975) Regan isoenzyme and human chorionic gonadotrophin in ovarian cancer. Natl Cancer Inst Monogr 42: 63–73

Franceschi S, La Vecchia C, Helmrich SP et al. (1982) Risk factors for epithelial ovarian cancer in Italy. Am J Epidemiol 115: 714–719

Friedlander ML, Medley DW, Taylor IW (1984) Influence of cellular DNA content on survival in advanced ovarian cancer. Cancer Res 44: 397–400

Fuks Z (1980) Patterns of spread of ovarian carcinoma: relation to therapeutic strategies. In: Newman CE, Ford CHJ, Jordan JA (eds) Proceedings of the international symposium on ovarian cancer. Pergamon Birmingham

Goldie JH, Coldman JA (1979) A mathematic model for relating the drug sensitivity of tumors to their spontaneous mutation rate. Cancer Treat Rep 63: 1727–1733

Goldstein DP, Piro AJ (1972) Combination chemotherapy in the treatment of germ cell tumors containing choriocarcinoma in males and females. J Surg Gynecol Obstet 134: 61–66

Greenspan EM (1975) Ovarian cancer. In: Greenspan EM (ed) Clinical cancer chemotherapy. Raven P, New York, pp 207–220

Griffiths CT (1975) Surgical resection of tumor bulk in the primary treatment of ovarian carcinoma. NCI Monogr 42: 101–104
Griffiths CT (1986) Surgical cytoreduction for stage III–IV carcinoma of the ovary. In: Three postgraduate gynecology courses: advanced gynecologic oncology. Department of Continuing Education, Harvard Medical School and Vincent Memorial Hospital, Boston, September 5–14, 1986
Hacker NF, Berek JS, Lagasse LD et al. (1983) Primary cytoreductive surgery for epithelial ovarian cancer. Obstet Gynecol 61: 413–420
Henderson BE, Ross RK, Pike MC et al. (1982) Endogenous hormones as a major factor in human cancer. Cancer Res 42: 3232–3239
Henderson WJ, Hamilton TC, Griffiths K (1979) Talc in normal and malignant ovarian tissue. Lancet 1: 499
Hreshchyshyn MM, Park RC, Blessing JA et al. (1980) The role of adjuvant therapy in stage I ovarian cancer. Am J Obstet Gynecol 138: 139–145
Hudson CN (1973) Surgical treatment of ovarian cancer. Gynecol Oncol 1: 370–378
Joyeux H, Szawlowski AW, Saint-Aubert et al. (1986) Aggressive regional surgery for advanced ovarian carcinoma. Cancer 37: 142–147
Kabawat SE, Bast RC Jr, Welch WR et al. (1983) Immunopathologic characterization of a monoclonal antibody that recognizes common surface antigens of human ovarian tumors of serous, endometrial and clear cell type. Am J Clin Pathol 79: 98–104
Kent SW, McDay DG (1960) Primary carcinoma of the ovary. An analysis of 349 cases. Am J Obstet Gynecol 80: 430–438
King M, Go RCP, Elston RC et al. (1980) An allele increasing susceptibility to human breast cancer may be linked in the glutamate-pyruvate transaminase locus. Science 208: 406–408
Kleinerman RA, Curtis RE, Boice JD et al. (1982) Second cancers following radiotherapy for cervical cancer. J Natl Cancer Inst 69: 1027–1033
Kohler G, Milstein C (1975) Continuous cultures of fused cells secreting antibody of predefined specificity. Nature 250: 495–497
Kolstad P, Davy M, Hoeg K (1977) Individualized treatment of ovarian cancer. Am J Obstet Gynecol 128: 617–625
Kurman RJ, Norris HJ (1976) Endometrial sinus tumor of the ovary: a clinical and pathological analysis of 71 cases. Cancer 38: 2404–2419
Lusley DM, Chan KK, Fielding JWL et al. (1984) Second-look laparotomy in management of epithelial ovarian carcinoma: an evaluation of fifty cases. Obstet Gynecol 64: 421–426
Lynch HT, Harris RE, Guirgis HA et al. (1978) Familial association of breast/ovarian carcinoma. Cancer 41: 1543–1549
Lynch HT, Schnelke GS, Wells IC (1985) Hereditary ovarian carcinoma – Biomarkers studies. Cancer 55: 410–415
McGowan L, Parent L, Lednar W et al. (1979) The woman at risk for developing ovarian cancer. Gynecol Oncol 7: 325–344
MRC Working Party on Ovarian Cancer (1981) Medical Research Council study on chemotherapy in advanced ovarian cancer. Br J Obstet Gynecol 88: 1174–1185
Munnell EW (1968) The changing prognosis and treatment in cancer of the ovary. Am J Obstet Gynecol 100: 790–805
Musumeci R, Banfi A, Bolis et al. (1977) Lymphangiography in patients with ovarian epithelial cancer: an evaluation of 289 consecutive cases. Cancer 40: 1444–144
Myers C (1984) The use of intraperitoneal chemotherapy in the treatment of ovarian cancer. Semin Oncol 11: 275–284
Myers CE, Collins JM (1983) Pharmacology of intraperitoneal chemotherapy. Cancer Invest 1: 395–407
Neijt JP, Van der Burg MEL, Vriesendorp R et al. (1984) Randomized trial comparing two combination chemotherapy regimens (HEXO-CAF vs. CHAP-S) in advanced ovarian carcinoma. Lancet 2: 594–600
Ozols RF, Garvin AJ, Costa J et al. (1980) Advanced ovarian cancer: correlation of histologic grade with response to therapy and survival. Cancer 45: 572–581
Ozols RF, Fisher RI, Anderson T et al. (1981) Peritoneoscopy in the management of ovarian cancer. Am J Obstet Gynecol 140: 611
Pezner RD, Stevens KR Jr, Tong D et al. (1978) Limited carcinoma of the ovary treated with curative intent by intraperitoneal installation of radiocolloids. Cancer 42: 2563–2671
Phillips BR, Bushbaum HJ, Lifshitz S (1979) Re-exploration after treatment for ovarian cancer. Gynecol Oncol 8: 339–345
Piver MS, Barlow JJ, Bhattacharya M (1975) Treatment and immunodiagnosis of advanced ovarian adenocarcinoma: a preliminary report. Cancer Treat Rep 3: 265–267
Piver MS, Barlow JJ, Sawyer DM (1982) Familial ovarian cancer: increasing in frequency? Obstet Gynecol 60: 397–400
Plentl AA, Friedman EA (1971) Lymphatic system of the female genitalia. Saunders, Philadelphia
Roberts WS, Hodel K, Rich WH, Di Saia PJ (1982) Second-look laparotomy in the management of gynecologic malignancy. Gynecol Oncol 13: 345–355
Rosenberg L, Shapiro S, Slone D et al. (1982) Epithelial ovarian cancer and combination ovarian contraceptives. JAMA 247: 3210–3212
Roth LM, Anderson MC, Govers ADT et al. (1981) Sertoli-Leydig cell tumors: a clinicopathologic study of 34 cases. Cancer 48: 187–197
Russel PP (1979) The pathological assessment of ovarian neoplasm. III. Malignant epithelial tumors. Pathology 11: 493–532
Samuels BI (1975) Usefulness of ultrasounds in patients with ovarian cancer. Semin Oncol 2: 229–233
Schwartz PE, MacLusky N, Sokomoto H et al. (1983) Steroid receptor proteins in non-epithelial malignancies of the ovary. Gynecol Oncol 15: 305–315
Scully E (1970) Recent progress in ovarian cancer. J Hum Pathol 1: 73–98
Scully RE (1977) Ovarian tumours. Am J Pathol 87: 686–720
Selikoff IJ (1977) Cancer risk of asbestos exposure. In: Hiatt HH, Watson JD, Winstein JA (eds) Origin of human cancer. Cold Spring Harbor Laboratory, New York, pp 1765–1784
Serov SF, Scully RE, Sobin LA (1973) International histological classification of tumors. World Health Organization, Geneva, pp 17–18
Skipper HE (1978) Adjuvant chemotherapy. Cancer 41: 930–940
Slayton RE, Hreshchyshyn MM, Silverberg SC et al. (1978) Treatment of malignant ovarian germ cell tumors: response to vincristine, dactinomycin and cyclophosphamide (preliminary report). Cancer 42: 390
Smith JP, Day TG (1979) Review of ovarian cancer at the University of Texas Center – MD Anderson Hospital and Tumor Institute. Am J Obstet Gynecol 135: 984–993
Smith JP, Rutledge F (1975) Advances in chemotherapy for gynecologic cancer. Cancer 36: 669
Smith JP, Schwartz PE (1980) Second-look laparotomy and prognosis related to extent of residual disease. In: Van Oosterom AT, Muggia FM, Cleton FJ (eds) Therapeutic

progress in ovarian cancer, testicular cancer and the sarcoma. Nijhoff, The Hague

Solomon A, Brenner HJ, Rubinstein Z et al. (1983) Computerized tomography in ovarian cancer. Gynecol Oncol 18: 48–55

Stenwig JT, Hazekamp JT, Beecham JB (1979) Granulose cell tumors of the ovary. A clinico-pathological study of 111 cases with long-term follow up. Gynecol Oncol 7: 136–152

Tagliabue E, Menard S, Della Torre G et al. (1985) Generation of monoclonal antibodies reacting with human epithelial ovarian cancer. Cancer Res 45: 379–385

Tagliabue E, Mantovani L, Morelli D et al. (1987) Production of monoclonal antibodies against tumor-associated circulating antigens. Second Conference on Immunity to Cancer, Williamsburg, Virginia, November 9–11

Takenchi H, Hamada H, Sodemoto Y et al. (1983) Juvenile granulosa cell tumor with rapid distant metastases. Acta Pathol Jpn 33: 537–545

Trope C (1981) A prospective randomized trial comparison of melphalan vs adriamycin-melphalan in advanced ovarian carcinoma. Proceedings of the American Society of Clinical Oncology, vol 22: Washington DC, pp 469

Van Lindert ACM, Alsbach GPJ, Barentz J et al. (1984) The abdominal radical tumor reduction procedure. In: Heintz APM, Griffiths CT, Trimbos JB (eds) Surgery in gynecological oncology. Nijhoff, The Hague, pp 275–287

Vogl SE, Pagano M, Kaplan B (1982) Diamminedichloroplatinum(D)based combination chemotherapy (CT) is superior to melphalan (m) for advanced ovarian cancer (OvCa) when age is ⩾50 and tumor diameter > 2 cm. Proceedings of the American Society of Clinical Oncology. Washington DC (Abstr c-462)

Vogl SE, Seltzer V, Calanog A et al. (1984) "Second-effort" surgical resection for bulky ovarian cancer. Cancer 34: 2220–2225

Wangensteen OH, Lewis FJ, Tongen LA (1951) The "second look" in cancer surgery: a patient with colic cancer and involved lymph nodes negative on the sixth look. Lancet 2: 303–307

Waterhouse J, Muir L, Shaumugaratnam K, Powell J (eds) (1982) Cancer incidence in five continents. International Agency for Research on Cancer Scientific Publication No. 42, Lyon

Weiss NS, Lyon JL, Liff JM et al. (1981) Incidence of ovarian cancer in relation to the use of oral contraceptives. Int J Cancer 28: 669–671

Wharton JT, Herson J (1981) Surgery for common epithelial tumors of the ovary. Cancer 48: 582–589

Williams CJ, Mead GM, Macbeth FR et al. (1985) Cisplatin combination chemotherapy versus chlorambucil in advanced ovarian carcinoma: mature results of a randomized trial. J Clin Oncol 3: 1455–1466

Wiltshaw E, Stuart-Harris R, Barker GH et al. (1982) Chemotherapy of endodermal sinus tumour (yolk sac tumour) of the ovary: preliminary communication. J R Soc Med 79: 888

Young RC, Chabner BA, Hubbard SP et al. (1978) Advanced ovarian adenocarcinoma: a prospective clinical trial of melphalan (L. PAM) versus combination chemotherapy. N Engl J Med 299: 1261–1266

Young RC, Walton L, Decker D et al. (1983) Early stage ovarian cancer: preliminary results of randomized trials after comprehensive initial staging. Proceedings of the American Society of Clinical Oncology, vol 148. Washington DC (Abstr c-578)

Young RC, Fuks Z, Knapp RC et al. (1985) Cancer of the ovary. In: De Vita VT, Hellman S, Rosenberg SA (eds) Cancer – principles and practice of oncology. Lippincott, Philadelphia, p 1086

Cancer of the Uterus

J. P. Wolff

Introduction – Definition

Carcinoma of the cervix is the gynecological cancer for which the most progress has been achieved in recent years, and the most progress can be expected in the near future. It is not unrealistic to hope for complete eradication of this disease in the forseeable future.

The *cervix* is the lower part of the uterus and is situated in the vagina. Cervical cancers include both exocervical and endocervical lesions. The exocervix is covered with stratified squamous epithelium resting on a basal membrane; the epithelium is continuous with the vaginal epithelium which is of the same type. The endocervix is lined with a glandular epithelium consisting of a single layer of cells, containing numerous glands, evaginations of the epithelium itself; below, it is marked off from the exocervical epithelium by a "squamocolumnar junction." The *corpus* is lined with a glandular epithelium of a single layer of cells (endometrium). It is in continuity with endocervical epithelium. The term "*carcinoma in situ*" (CIS) designates a lesion which is considered to be precancerous.

The progress achieved in reducing the morbidity and the mortality from cervical cancer is believed to be related to the availability of a simple and reliable technique of early screening, namely cytological diagnosis. For cancer of the corpus, reducing the mortality is related to early diagnosis and more satisfactory treatment. Nevertheless, while the treatment itself is currently more simple, better adapted, and produces fewer complications, the survival rates for each stage have not improved much.

Epidemiology – Risk Factors

An obvious starting point is to examine how the incidence of uterine cancer varies among different countries, with different methods of recording, according to whether morbidity (frequency, incidence) or mortality is studied, according to whether or not invasive cervical cancer is distinguished from carcinoma in situ and from endometrial carcinoma.

Variations with Time

The incidence of invasive *cervical* cancer has been decreasing in the developed countries (e.g., from 42.4 to 17.8 per 100000 in the USA between 1957 and 1973; Cutler and Young 1975). Carcinoma in situ and endometrial carcinoma, on the other hand, have been very much on the increase (Fig. 1) (Kim et al. 1978). The distribution of the different stages is also shifting, with a relative increase of stage I cases and a concomitant decline in the numbers of stage II and stage III patients (Fig. 2).

The incidence of cancer of the *corpus* remained stable until 1970 and then began to rise, especially in the developed countries. The ratio of cancer of the corpus to cervical cancer has increased from 1:10 to 1:2 in the United States. The progression involved mainly the oldest age groups (Barber and Sommers 1981).

Age-Related Incidence

The incidence of *cervical* carcinoma increases steadily from age 20 (it is exceptional before this age) until 50–60 years, after which, depending on the author,

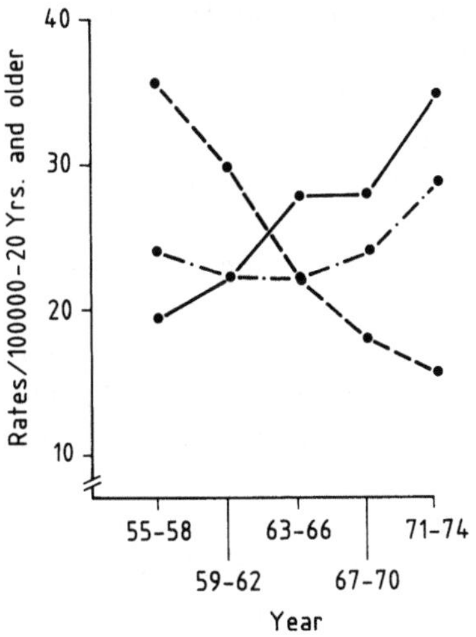

Fig. 1. Average annual age-adjusted incidence rate trends for carcinoma *in situ* and invasive squamous carcinoma of cervix and endometrial carcinoma by five time periods (1955–1974) *Solid line,* carcinoma in situ; *broken/dotted line,* endometrial carcinoma; *broken line,* invasive cervical carcinoma

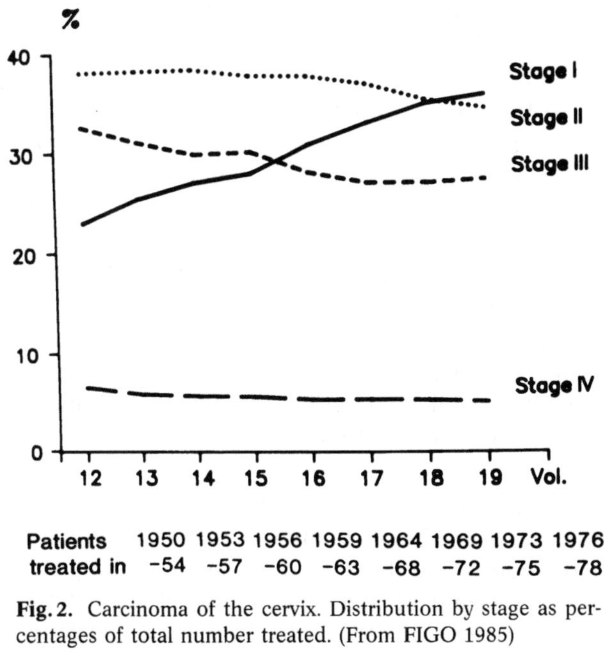

Fig. 2. Carcinoma of the cervix. Distribution by stage as percentages of total number treated. (From FIGO 1985)

it either decreases slightly (Christopherson et al. 1976), increases slightly (Silverberg 1975) or levels off. This pattern has serious implications, namely that screening by vaginal smears must not be discontinued after menopause. The maximal incidence for invasive carcinoma occurs between the ages of 45 and 55. For CIS the maximal rate occurs between the ages of 25 and 35 years and declines rapidly after age 40. In other words, the age-related incidence does not show the same pattern for the two conditions.

In cancer of the *corpus,* 80%–90% of the cases occur after menopause, with maximal incidence during the sixth decade, 10–15 years after menopause, and decreases after the seventh decade (Mahboui et al. 1982).

Socioeconomic Level

There is a definite link between the incidence of *cervical* carcinoma in a community and the socioeconomic level (Gardner and Lyon 1977 and many other publications). The incidence of *corpus* carcinoma is not connected with the socioeconomic level.

Sexual Factors

Certain sexual factors have long been suspected of being implicated in the etiology of *cervical* carcinoma. The incidence of cervical cancer is influenced by (Rotkin 1973): age of first sexual intercourse; large number of sexual partners (promiscuity); marital status; husband's profession, with frequent and/or long absences from home (Beral 1974).

The frequency of sexual activity or intercourse, however, does not seem to make any difference. Moreover, other risk factors (the number of pregnancies, age at marriage, and age at first pregnancy) seem to be related to those listed above. Tobacco, as a risk factor, seems to have its own specific carcinogenic effect on the cervical epithelium.

Oral contraceptives, too, has been suspected of playing a part in the emergence or development of cervical cancer. Current opinion holds that there is no definite connection between the two phenomena; oral contraception tends to go hand in hand with a certain permissiveness, which in turn heightens the risks. But, on the other hand, women who use oral contraceptives represent a better monitored and hence a somewhat better protected subpopulation.

Cancer of the *corpus* occurs in patients with few or no children, early puberty, and late menopause. Ovarian dystrophy is often associated with this cancer, as are anovulatory disorders. Finally, the patients are often obese with an increase in fatty tissue. All these features tend to incriminate hyperestrogenemia not counterbalanced by progestogens; this can be either endogenous (hormonal disturbance, obesity) or exogenous (prolonged estrogen treatment). But the hyperestrogenic factor seems to be neither necessary nor sufficient. Oral contraceptives seem to have a protective influence, especially for nulliparous women and if taken for more than 12 consecutive months.

Viral Factors

Epidemiological evidence converges towards the hypothesis that cervical cancer can be considered as a possible venereally transmitted disease, which would presumably imply the existence of some transmissible agent. And indeed, numerous studies have demonstrated an association between cervical cancer and viral factors, initially the herpes simplex virus 2 (HSV2), then the papilloma virus; certain types of which (types 16, 18) seem to be associated with certain types of lesions. More recently, the part played by oncogenes (genes carried by certain retroviruses) has come to light, but the mechanisms of action are poorly understood. It would appear that cooperation takes place between viral genes and cell oncogenes which become activated as a result of mutation, amplification or gene rearrangement (Riou et al. 1984; zur Hausen 1982).

Moreover, these viruses often seem to be associated with other microorganisms (e.g., chlamydiae) making it impossible to know for certain if they are present merely as markers, or if they intervene or play a real part in the initiation of malignancy. Viral factors do not seem to play any role in the etiology of endometrial adenocarcinoma.

Histopathology

Cervix

Epidermoid Cancer (Squamous Cell Carcinoma). It is composed of cells resembling squamous cells. The cells are grouped together in sheets or strands arranged without any discernible pattern and separated by a more or less fibrous stroma. Three principal types of malignancy can be distinguished on the basis of the appearance and the arrangement of the cells: keratinizing epidermoid cancers, large cell nonkeratinizing epidermoid cancers, small cell nonkeratinizing epidermoid cancers. Two particular forms should be set apart: spindle cell carcinoma (resembling sarcoma) and verrucous carcinoma. In practice, it is important to note the exact degree of maturation (keratinization) of the cells and, particularly, the grade of differentiation (nil, moderate, or marked).

Glandular Cancer or Adenocarcinoma. This neoplasm develops at the expense of the endocervical mucosa. Representing some 5%–10% of the cervical cancers, its incidence seems to be increasing and the mean age of onset decreasing. Two different types can be distinguished:

- The adenocarcinomas, comprising cells resembling the columnar cells of the endocervix. They can be poorly, moderately, or well differentiated. Two particular varieties are recognized: malignant adenoma, a highly differentiated form, and mucous adenocarcinoma.
- The adenocarcinomas, whose cells are different from the endocervical type. They can be either endometrioid or clear cell adenocarcinomas.

Mixed Cancers. These are the mucoepidermoid and adenoepidermoid cancers in which the two components are associated.

Others. Cylindroma is extremely rare.

Carcinoma In Situ (Intraepithelial, Preinvasive, Stage 0). The lesion consists of abnormal squamous epithelium, with intact basal membrane, and is separated from normal epithelium by a distinct straight-line border. Cell division goes on at all levels, with the cells spreading out in all directions in a disordered fashion. The nuclei are hyperchromatic and anisochromatic, crudely structured, irregularly shaped, and almost always larger than normal. The nucleocytoplasmic ratio is increased, abnormal multipolar mitoses are seen, and the number of chromosomes is variable. The lesion shows the characteristics of a malignant lesion, except that it is not invasive and does not metastasize.

Microinvasive Carcinoma. This implies a breakthrough of the basal membrane by the CIS at one or more points, and the invasion of the underlying stroma to a depth of 5 mm (definition of the International Federation of Gynecology and Obstetrics (FIGO).

Corpus

Highly Differentiated Adenocarcinomas. These resemble in different ways the appearance of endometrial tissue; the structure becomes disordered and all the more atypical as the tumor is less differentiated and more disorganized. Mucosecreting and papillary forms can be distinguished (de Brux 1982).

Undifferentiated Adenocarcinomas. These comprise sheets or strands separated by thin connective tissue, sometimes with slight differentiation.

Rearranged Carcinomas. Characteristic of rearranged carcinomas is the epithelial rearrangement with epidermoid metaplasia (adenoacanthoma).

Clear Cell Carcinomas. These form 5% of all cancers and are more or less papillary. *Grading* is very important, on the basis of the operative specimen if possible: it is taken into consideration in the staging.

Sarcomas. Cancers in this category can represent any one of the sarcomas in general or uterine sarcoma in particular (leiomyosarcoma, chorionic sarcoma, cytogenic sarcoma).

Natural History

Cervix

Dysplasia and CIS (CIN 1, 2, 3 in American Terminology)

Current oncogene and virus research has brought us closer to the starting point of cancer, but not all the way to knowing exactly *when* the cancer begins. Most authors agree with the sequence: mild dysplasia →moderate dysplasia →severe dysplasia →carcinoma in situ →invasive epithelioma. But no-one can tell precisely when the lesions become irreversible. It is generally accepted that mild dysplasia (CIN 1) is certainly reversible, and that severe dysplasia and CIS (CIN 3) are not. But the future evolution of a moderate dysplasia (CIN 2) cannot be foretold. Similarly, no-one can attest that all CIS become invasive lesions, nor that all invasive cancers first go through an in situ stage, although the probability is very strong.

A further problem is knowing *where* the malignancy begins. It is currently admitted that the cytogenetic and cytological transformations occur at the squamocolumnar junction, at the expense of its basal cells.

Microinvasive Carcinoma

After CIS has breached the basal membrane at one or more points, the malignant plugs join up together to form a single focus (Burghardt 1984). Thus two types of lesions can be described, namely microinvasion by incipient and by confluent invasion (Kolstad 1969). Several issues concerning microinvasive carcinoma remain unresolved:

1. What is the proportion of microinvasive carcinomas compared to CIS? According to different authors 5%–7% of CIS are actually microinvasive carcinomas.
2. What are the chances of lymph node involvement with lesions not exceeding 5 mm? Morgan and Nelson (1982) reported a rate of 1.1% (13/1210). Lymph node involvement seems to be related to the extent of stromal invasion and to the presence of vascular emboli.
3. How common are vascular emboli? For Morgan and Nelson (1982) the overall mean was 12.7%, ranging from 3.5% to 57%.

Cervical Extension

The lesions gradually spread over the cervix, according to different patterns: exophytic, with budding and hemorrhage; endophytic, by infiltration, eventually producing a barrel-shaped cervix; ulcerating, crateriform, often associated with cervical infiltration. Not enough is known about endocervical progression, which seems to be more common in the infiltrating or ulcerating forms.

Endometrial Extension

Purportedly rare (Pujol and Prade 1979), it may actually be more common than hitherto believed, as suggested by recent studies (Perez et al. 1975).

Vaginal Extension

It occurs frequently, in the form of invasive or preinvasive lesions.

Extrauterine Extension

The lesions spread to pelvic tissue, involving the parametria laterally or the sacrogenital ligament anteroposteriorly. Progression to the bladder is gradual, but the mucous membrane remains intact for a long time. Invasion of the rectum seems to be related to lymphatic embolization. The urinary tract is the first to be affected by repercussion of the cancer, with compression of the ureters; this results in alterations in kidney function and structure which it is important to recognize because of the implications on management and prognosis. The frequency of ureteral complications can be estimated as 2%–3% in stage I, 5%–10% in stage II, but as much as

20%–25% in stage III, and even 50%–55% in stage IV.

Nodes

Frequency of Lymph Node Involvement. A great number of studies have made it possible to determine the following rates of lymph node involvement: stage I – 15%–20%; stage II – 30%–35%; stage III – 45%–55%; stage IV – 50%. Lymph node involvement is related to tumor volume and appears to be more common in the infiltrative forms and in adenocarcinomas.

Invasion of Para-aortic Nodes. The frequency is difficult to establish with certainty (it is exceptional in the case of negative pelvic nodes): stage I – 0%–7%; stage II – 8%–22%; stage III – 30%–40%; stage IV – 40%–50%.

Invasion of Supraclavicular Nodes. If prescalenic biopsies are systematically taken, supraclavicular invasion is found more commonly than expected, namely in half of the cases with lumboaortic involvement (Ketcham et al. 1973).

Distant Metastases

Distant metastases are relatively rare in the early stages of this disease which is essentially locoregional. Bone metastases are the most common, closely followed by lung metastases.

Time course

The course of cervical carcinoma seems to be progressive: there are, however, phases of more rapid development as well as chronic spread. The time it takes for dysplasia to become CIS and for CIS to become invasive has been the object of numerous computations, all of which have been distorted by our inability to know the precise progression status at the time of diagnosis. Each of the phases is roughly estimated to last some 5–10 years (Boyes et al. 1970).

Corpus

Hyperplasia

Be it simple (or adenomatous cystic), adenomatous (rare, localized), or atypical (cellular or architectural atypia), hyperplasia is considered to be a precursor of endometrial cancer. Whether there is any connection between the three types is unclear. It is very likely that atypical hyperplasia develops into invasive cancer, but this is not invariable and can be reversed by progestogens (Kistner 1982).

Uterine Cavity

A lesion in the uterine cavity originates at some point in the cavity (most often the fundus) and spreads (a) toward the isthmus, the endocervix, and then the exocervix; (b) interiorly, within the myometrium, toward the serosa.

Extrauterine Extension

Extrauterine extension can take a number of directions: to the vagina and/or the parametria, by contiguity; within the pelvic and abdominal cavity, following perforation of the serosa, late in the course; to the bladder and/or rectum, also occurring late.

Lymph Node Extension

Lymph node extension is seen in 5%–15% of stage I cases (Rochet 1977). Para-aortic invasion without pelvic involvement occurs in 10% of cases. Lymph node involvement seems to be related to grade, intramyometrial infiltration, and extension of the lesion to the lower part of the uterine cavity.

Distant Metastases

Distant metastases, rare with limited lesions, occur in the lungs and, more rarely, the bones. It is worth noting that ovarian metastases are not exceptional.

Staging

The clinical staging of uterine carcinoma was meticulously regulated by FIGO and by the International Union Against Cancer (UICC); but their rules are not immutable and indeed they have evolved since the initial classification in 1928 by the League of Nations.

FIGO Classification

Cervix (Table 1)

Notes to the Staging

Stage 0 comprises those cases with full thickness involvement of the epithelium with atypical cells, but with no signs of invasion into the stroma.

Table 1. Definition of the clinical stages in carcinoma of the cervix (correlation between the FIGO, UICC and AJCC nomenclatures). (From FIGO 1985)

Stage 0	Carcinoma in situ, intraepithelial carcinoma Cases of Stage 0 should not be included in any therapeutic statistics for invasive carcinoma
Stage I	The carcinoma is strictly confined to the cervix (extension to the corpus should be disregarded)
Stage I a	Microinvasive carcinoma (early stromal invasion)
Stage I b	All other cases of Stage I. Occult cancer should be marked "occ"
Stage II	The carcinoma extends beyond the cervix, but has not extended on to the pelvic wall. The carcinoma involves the vagina, but not as far as the lower third
Stage II a	No obvious parametrial involvement
Stage II b	Obvious parametrial involvement
Stage III	The carcinoma has extended on to the pelvic wall. On rectal examination there is no cancer-free space between the tumour and the pelvic wall The tumour involves the lower third of the vagina. All cases with a hydronephrosis or nonfunctioning kidney should be included, unless they are known to be due to other causes.
Stage III a	No extension on to the pelvic wall, but involvement of the lower third of the vagina
Stage III b	Extension to the pelvic wall or hydronephrosis or nonfunctioning kidney
Stage IV	The carcinoma has extended beyond the true pelvis or has clinically involved the mucosa of the bladder or rectum
Stage IVa	Spread of the growth to adjacent organs
Stage IVb	Spread to distant organs

Stage I a (microinvasive carcinoma) represents those cases of epithelial abnormalities in which histological evidence of early stromal invasion is unambiguous. The diagnosis is based on microscopic examination of tissue removed by biopsy, conization, portio amputation, or removal of the uterus. Cases of early stromal invasion should thus be allotted to stage I a. Modification of stage I a is under discussion.

In the interest of accuracy, it is recommended that cases staged I a on the basis of punch biopsy material be sufficiently sampled to rule out a more advanced histology. In most instances conization and examination of the lesion in its entirety is to be preferred. The remaining stage I cases should be allotted to stage I b. As a rule, these cases can be diagnosed by routine clinical examination. Occult cancer is a histologically invasive cancer that cannot be diagnosed by routine clinical examination. As a rule, it is diagnosed either on the basis of a cone or the amputated portio, or on the removed uterus. Such cancers should be included in stage I b and should be marked "stage I b, occ."

As a rule, it is impossible to estimate clinically whether a cancer of the cervix has extended to the corpus or not. Extension to the corpus should therefore be disregarded.

A patient with a growth fixed to the pelvic wall by a short and indurated but not nodular parametrium should be allotted to stage II b. It is impossible, at clinical examination, to decide whether a smooth and indurated parametrium is truly cancerous or only inflammatory. Therefore the case should be placed in stage III only if the parametrium is nodular out on the pelvic wall or if the growth itself extends out on the pelvic wall.

The presence of hydronephrosis or nonfunctioning kidney due to stenosis of the ureter by cancer permits a case to be allotted to stage III even if, according to the other findings, the case should be allotted to stage I or stage II.

The presence of bullous edema, as such, should not permit a case to be allotted to stage IV. Ridges and furrows into the bladder wall should be interpreted as signs of submucous involvement of the bladder if they remain fixed to the growth at palposcopy (i.e., examination from the vagina or the rectum during cystoscopy). A finding of malignant cells in cytological washings from the urinary bladder requires further examination and biopsy from the wall of the bladder.

Corpus (Table 2)

Histopathology – Degree of Differentiation

Cases of carcinoma of the corpus should be grouped with regard to the degree of differentiation of the adenocarcinoma as follows:

G 1 Highly differentiated adenomatous carcinoma
G 2 Moderately differentiated adenomatous carcinoma with partly solid areas
G 3 Predominantly solid or entirely undifferentiated carcinoma
GX Grade not assessed

TNM Classification (UICC)

The TNM classification roughly matches the FIGO system. The tumor is designated T and classified much the same as in the FIGO system. N refers to the lymph nodes; since their involvement cannot be

Table 2. Definition of the clinical stages in carcinoma of the corpus (correlation of the FIGO, UICC and AJCC nomenclatures)

Stage 0	Atypical endometrial hyperplasia, carcinoma in situ. Histological findings are suspicious of malignancy (cases of Stage 0 should not be included in any therapeutic statistics)
Stage I	The carcinoma is confined to the corpus
Stage Ia	The length of the uterine cavity is 8 cm or less
Stage Ib	The length of the uterine cavity is more than 8 cm
Stage II	The carcinoma has involved the corpus and the cervix, but has not extended outside the uterus
Stage III	The carcinoma has extended outside the uterus, but not outside the true pelvis
Stage IV	The carcinoma has extended outside the true pelvis or has obviously involved the mucosa of the bladder or rectum. A bullous oedema as such does not permit a case to be alloted to Stage IV
Stage IVa	Spread of the growth to adjacent organs such as urinary bladder, rectum, sigmoid or small bowel
Stage IVb	Spread to distant organs

determined with certainty in uterine carcinoma, they are labeled Nx. Metastases are termed M, with M0 signifying no distant metastases, and M1 the presence of secondary metastases.

Screening of Asymptomatic Disease

Cervix

Primary prevention aims at preventing risk factors from appearing or joining forces (see "Epidemiology"). This type of prevention is difficult if not impossible to apply in the case of cervical carcinoma since much depends on life style, moral attitudes, and social context, which the physician cannot hope to influence. But in the future, routine detection, and thus the treatment of viral infection, may prevent the initiation of premalignant lesions.

Secondary prevention aims at preventing the establishment of malignant lesions by screening and treating premalignant lesions (dysplasia and CIS). The different aspects of screening need to be scrutinized: feasibility, reliability (sensitivity and specificity), ease of application, efficiency (effects on morbidity and mortality), cost-effectiveness for the community.

Definition of "screening": "application of a relatively simple, inexpensive test to a large number of persons in order to classify them as likely or unlikely to have the cancer that is the object of the screen" (Cole and Morrison 1980).

Feasibility

Two facts make screening for cervical carcinoma possible:
- The existence of lesions exhibiting the cytological and architectural characteristics of malignant lesions
- The ability of the lesions to desquamate cells which can be found in the vagina and on the cervix

Reliability

The validity of a screening test is defined as the rate of subsequent confirmation by acceptable diagnostic methods (Walton et al. 1976). Sensitivity and specificity are measures of the reliability of a test.

Sensitivity is the ability of a test to give positive results for truly positive cases; the fewer false negative results it gives, the better is the sensitivity. The number of false positives in cervical carcinoma screening is low (but not nil); the sensitivity of the test can be considered satisfactory.

Specificity is the ability of a test to give negative results for truly negative cases; the specificity is best when the number of false positive is lowest. The specificity of screening tests can be considered satisfactory.

Ease of Application

The ease of application hinges on certain characteristics of the test itself: *simplicity* and *acceptability* by the patients concerned. Furthermore, certain conditions must be strictly fulfilled if the interpretation of the tests is to be meaningful [technics of preparation, qualification of cytotechnicians (Riotton 1979)].

Effectiveness (Effects on Morbidity and Mortality)

Numerous reports have been unable to reach complete agreement about the effectiveness of screening because of events such as the following:
- The decreased incidence of cervical carcinoma preceded large-scale screening.
- Improved living conditions in the developed countries have diminished certain risk factors.

- Inversely, changes in life style have increased certain risk factors.
- Evasion of the screening programs by high-risk females.

Incidence (Morbidity). In the Scandinavian countries, except Norway, the incidence of cervical carcinoma has decreased considerably since 1965; yet it has been demonstrated that a section of the high-risk population escaped screening (Asvall and Eker 1974). For Canada the figures are even more striking: in most provinces the decrease in morbidity has been directly proportional to participation in screening. It therefore seems reasonable to conclude that screening is effective in reducing cervical carcinoma morbidity.

Mortality. The evidence as regards mortality is much more difficult to interpret in spite of the numerous studies published. In Canada the overall mortality has declined, although unevenly among the provinces, with sharper declines in the provinces with more intensive screening; in some instances, mortality has diminished by as much as 50%. However, according to some authors (e.g. Walton et al. 1976) whose findings did not show such a marked decline, there is a danger of screening overlooking high-risk women (subpopulations of low socioeconomic level) and missing high-risk cervical cancers (rapid evolution and/or short preclinical period).

Cost-Effectiveness

The issue of cost-effectiveness is even more controversial than the efficacy of screening. Profitability must, of course, be calculated independently of ethical considerations. The cost aspect comprises administrative expenses (secretarial, postal, etc.) and technical expenditure (sampling, staining, mounting, interpretation).

The benefit aspect includes: the lower cost of treating CIS, or even microinvasive carcinomas, than invasive lesions; considerably less time lost off work; benefits to younger women, an economically important group; the better cure rate for preinvasive forms, namely 99%, compared to an average of 50% for the invasive forms. While the financial costs of screening can be roughly estimated, the benefits cannot, especially since it is impossible to put a price on human life. In the near future, however, both the administrative and technical burdens will be considerably lightened and made less expensive by the intensive use of computers. The current policy trend is, therefore, to direct screening efforts selectively at high-risk groups.

Timing

The frequency of smears depends on the degree of risk:

1. For low- or moderate risk women, an annual smear for 2 years, followed by a smear every 2–3 years if the results of the first tests are negative.
2. For high-risk women (first intercourse before age 17, numerous partners, early first pregnancy), active seeking out of these women who do not come forward on their own (Walton et al. 1976).

The cervical smear should *begin* at the time of first sexual intercourse. Contrary to widespread opinion, it should not stop at menopause or at age 60, since the risks persist, and the prognosis becomes poorer (West 1977).

Corpus

Primary prevention of endometrial carcinoma consists mainly in endeavoring to limit the administration of exogenous estrogens and in simultaneously prescribing progestogens.

Secondary prevention – there is no sufficiently reliable, effective, and simple technique which could permit generalized screening for premalignant lesions of the endometrium.

Diagnosis of Symptomatic Disease

Uterine carcinoma is diagnosed in three steps: clinical examination, radiological and cytohistological analysis, and investigation to delineate the spread of the disease.

Cervix

Clinical Diagnosis

It is generally metrorrhagia that raises the possibility of cervical carcinoma. The bleeding can be more or less abundant, recurring, intermenstrual, spontaneous, or especially brought on by intercourse or washing. Metrorrhagia can have other causes (e.g., cervical polyp), and can vary considerably in intensity, sometimes even presenting as micrometrorrhagia. Alternatively, the vaginal discharge can be in the form of leukorrhea which is frequent, recurrent, and irritating. Other symptoms may be observed, but they are indicative of more extensive lesions: pelvic pain, venous problems, rectal complaints. As for signs of impairment of general condition, they show up later. Finally, cervical cancer can also be latent and asymptomatic.

Clinical Examination

Speculum examination is the first step; it shows either a budding irregular lesion (cauliflower like) protruding in the vagina, bleeding spontaneously or on contact; or irregular ulceration centered on the cervix and prone to bleeding; or overall increased cervical volume with normal morphology and subnormal mucosa. Two actions should follow discovery of the lesion: vaginal smear for cytological study and punch biopsy within the middle of the lesion, avoiding necrotic tissue. The biopsy should be taken at the end of the clinical examination.

Vaginal examination confirms the type of the lesion. Above all, its extension to the vaginal fornix and to the vagina is determined. The size, position, and mobility of the uterus are also appreciated.

Rectal examination and bidigital rectovaginal examinations are essential for judging the condition of the parametria, the sacrogenital ligament, possibly the nodes adhering to the pelvic wall, the state of the rectal mucosa, and the rectovaginal septum.

The clinical examination should be done under the best possible conditions: the patient should be relaxed, with bladder and rectum empty. In fact, it requires general anesthesia, which permits the best appreciation of the condition of the parametria. The clinician must avoid being misled by inflammatory disease, abnormal pelvic configuration, or unusual cervical or uterine volume. The examination under anesthesia also enables the different specialists involved in the treatment to agree on the staging and evaluate the therapeutic possibilities.

Cyto- and Histological Diagnosis

There is no such thing as cytological diagnosis: indeed, it is impossible to establish a diagnosis on the basis of vaginal smears. They can furnish grounds for suspicion, but never a sufficient foundation for formal diagnosis. Histology, on the other hand, is both necessary and sufficient for diagnosing cervical cancer: it is impossible to establish diagnosis and undertake a course of treatment without formal pathological proof.

Evaluation of Extension

Local, regional, and general extension is assessed.

Urinary Evaluation

The appearance of the whole vesical mucosa is examined by *cystoscopy.* The trigone and the ureteral meatus can appear raised, deviated, or edematous. Edema of the mucosa is noted if present, as are retroparietal or protruding granulation, irregular budding, ulceration, or bleeding. If there is the slightest doubt, the presence of malignancy should be verified by biopsy.

The ureter is examined over its different segments for deviation, compression, or invasion by *intravenous pyelography,* without compression, with delayed pictures, and by cystography. Examination of the renal cavities can show delayed or absent secretion and unilateral or bilateral dilatation, in which case the thickness of the renal parenchyma must be subject to particular scrutiny.

Rectal Evaluation

The rectal mucosa can be examined for congestion, edema, rigidity, budding, ulceration, infiltration, or stenosed lumen by *proctoscopy.*

The extension of the lesion can be delineated by barium enema, which is particularly useful when external radiation is considered.

Lymph Node Evaluation

The frequency, extent, precocity, and significance of lymph node involvement are such that the advent of lymphangiography had raised great hopes. However, important limitations affect its interpretation (Musumeci 1984). Anatomical variations, the impossibility of detecting small lesions, sources of error related to infection or to the presence of adipose lacunae, render the interpretation restrictive for cervical cancer. While the number of false positives is fairly low and of no serious consequence, the number of false negatives is relatively high (14.5% according to Musumeci 1984). In practice, a positive lymphangiogram can modify the treatment scheme, but a negative lymphangiogram must not.

Uterine Evaluation

Hysterography is of limited help in evaluating cervical cancer. It is useful for judging the upward extension of endocervical cancer and for confirming the endocervical rather than endometrial origin of adenocarcinoma (which could change the treatment).

Regional Evaluation

Pelvigraphy, phlebography, and arteriography are not very useful for regional assessment. In contrast, ultrasonography, computer-assisted tomography – and possibly nuclear magnetic resonance in the near future – can help delineate the extent of some lesions and palliate the shortcomings of other examinations.

General Condition

The general condition is assessed by radiography (chest, skeleton) in a search for metastases and by biological tests (hemogram; ionogram; liver function; markers, especially carcinoembryonic antigen) to check the repercussions of the disease on the overall condition.

Exploratory Laparotomy

The difficulties of the clinical examination and the divergent interpretations about lesion extension and the limited reliability of complementary examinations had led a number of authors to recommend initial surgery on a routine basis in order to establish more precise staging and to judge better the actual extension of the lesions and of lymph node involvement. But the risk of digestive complications in patients irradiated subsequently is sufficient reason for opposing this practice, at least as a routine measure (Rutledge et al. 1976).

Diagnosis of Infraclinical Disease

When faced with abnormal cells on vaginal smears or metrorrhagia with no apparent cause, the clinician should suspect subclinical disease. Cytology does not supply a diagnosis. Clinical examination affords no corroborating evidence and colposcopy should be resorted to. *Colposcopy* – using a magnification of 10–40, acetic acid followed by Lugol's solution, natural or green light – cannot furnish a diagnosis either. The abnormalities that can be discovered by colposcopy are in no way specific (Kolstad and Stafl 1977) (except for the so-called exophytic nodular type). The abnormalities can represent benign lesions or CIS of varying degrees. What can be accomplished with the colposcope, however, is viewing of the junction, in the vicinity of which the lesion where the abnormal cells originate may be located. Thus colposcopy can serve to pinpoint the location where the biopsy, which is the only dependable basis for diagnosis, should be taken.

Cytology Alerts, Colposcopy Pinpoints, Histology Proofs

If the cervix looks normal at colposcopy or if the junction cannot be seen, the examination is not conclusive, and the endocervix needs to be explored.

- Endocervicoscopy or microendocervicoscopy can be helpful, but the technique is delicate and difficult to use routinely.
- That is why *diagnostic conization or amputation* is often done instead. By study of the specimen, the lesion can be diagnosed, either as dysplasia, CIS, microinvasive cancer, or occult invasive cancer.

Corpus

Clinical Diagnosis

Metrorrhagia (generally postmenopausal) is the only symptom. The bleeding is sparse, recurrent, brownish-colored, spontaneous, and painless. Other symptoms are much rarer.

Clinical Examination

See Cervix.

Cytological Diagnosis

If the cervix appears normal, endometrial smears should be taken. The results of the examination, except when positive, are subject to caution.

Radiological Diagnosis

Hysterography has met with some acceptance and extensive objection, but it does yield a considerable amount of information about abnormalities requiring biopsy and about the tumor itself.

Histological Diagnosis

The tissue is obtained either by biopsy guided by hysterogram, or curettage under general anesthesia. Histology is the only completely reliable basis for a sound diagnosis.

Hormonal Diagnosis

Dosage of estrogen receptors and progesterone receptors is available in this hormone-dependent tumor. The level of receptors is all the more increased as differentiation is higher.

Evaluation of Extension

In addition to the procedures outlined for the cervix, hysterography can help delimit tumor size, localization, and intrauterine extension, as well as the size of the uterus.

Treatment

Surgery and radiotherapy are the two main forms of treatment for uterine cancer, with chemotherapy occupying a secondary position at this time. While there is general agreement against the advisability of surgery when extensive disease is present, this is not the case for the more limited lesions (Dargent et al. 1979).

Cervix

Types of Treatment

Surgery

Colpohysterectomy. The usual surgical procedure for cervical cancer is radical colpohysterectomy with lymphadenectomy. It includes removal of a wide vaginal cuff, the pelvic cellular tissue, the parametria, and the external iliac nodes; the node dissection commences immediately above the anulus femoralis, with exeresis of the first hypogastric nodes. Opinions vary concerning the level to which the iliac nodes should be taken out, ranging from dissection limited by the nodes immediately above the iliac bifurcation, to excision of all the common iliac nodes. Some surgeons do not remove the common iliac nodes when the external iliac nodes are negative (Pilleron et al. 1972). Another matter of controversy is the associated removal of the para-aortic nodes, but this increases intestinal complications, particularly if radiation is given later.

Other Surgery. Simple hysterectomy with bilateral adnexectomy is rarely performed, except when the general condition is poor. However, simple hysterectomy with repositioning of the ovaries away from subsequent vaginal irradiation, with a view to preserving ovarian function, is sometimes carried out in younger patients. Vaginal hysterectomy, too, is rarely done, since it yields no information about the condition of the pelvis and the pelvic nodes.

Pelvic Exenteration (Pelvectomy). Pelvic exenteration consists of a radical colpohysterectomy associated with either bladder resection in anterior exenteration, or exeresis of the rectum for posterior exenteration. It is of necessity accompanied by urinary diversion and/or colostomy. Exenteration can be total, partial or atypical. Different types of contraindications can limit its possibilities: general (poor general condition), malignant (distant metastases), locoregional (inoperable lesions), psychosocial factors.

Surgery Confined to the Cervix (CIS). Exeresis or destruction are the surgical procedures of choice. *Exeresis* comprises conization and amputation, both of which are restricted to the limited forms. Conization can be done by: sharp-knife dissection, electric scalpel, diathermo-resection, CO_2 laser. Amputation is more extensive than conization and thus gives better assurance of total removal of the involved tissue.

Destruction is achieved by: electrocoagulation, cryotherapy, CO_2 laser. Following laser treatment, healing is remarkably swift, the return to normal is habitual, without bleeding or pain. Cryotherapy is also effective, but the destruction is not so deep with electrocoagulation, healing takes longer, and it is necessary to ensure that no inflammation or infection is present which could become reactivated.

Aims of Surgery
- Complete evaluation of lesions.
- Excision of the primary lesion and the adjacent tissues.
- Dissection of satellite lymph nodes.
- Furthermore, surgery does not preclude subsequent radiotherapy.

Disadvantages of Surgery
- Treatment-associated *mortality* is reported to be between 0% and 3% (Dargent 1979) and can currently be considered negligible.
- *Complications:* see p. 799.

Radiotherapy

Brachytherapy. In this therapy, continuous radiation is delivered by a source close to the tumor. The principal radioisotopes in current use are cesium 137, iridium 192 and, less commonly, cobalt 60. The doses delivered are expressed in grays (Gy). Many techniques of application have been described and the devices used are numerous. They can associate, simultaneously or in succession, vaginal and endometrial application by the use of uterine inserts, ovoids, and customized moulds. In some cases brachytherapy can be delivered by implantation.

External Irradiation. External irradiation requires sources of high-energy radiation (telecobalt, betatron, linear accelerator). The optimal voltage is 20 MV which enables high doses to be delivered to target organs. The *fields irradiated* include the uterus, vagina, parametria, external and common iliac nodes. It is limited above by the upper edge of L5, below by the lower part of the vagina, and laterally by the cotyloid cavities. The fields measure from 15 cm × 15 cm to 17 cm × 17 cm, depending on the technique. Usually the box technique is used, with anterior, posterior, and two lateral fields.

Total *doses* of 40–50 Gy are delivered (8–10 Gy per week). Dosage, timing, and fractioning vary with different techniques. In any event, the overall radiation scheme must be based on the anatomical parameters of the lesion (Fletcher 1979).

Association of External Radiation with Brachytherapy. This approach is becoming widespread, generally in the form of preliminary external irradiation by the box technique, followed by an intracavitary uterovaginal booster to the primary tumor.

Aims of Radiotherapy
- Sterilize the primary lesion, its vaginal and/or parametrial extensions and the iliac nodes.
- Treat all patients, regardless of general condition, since there are no contraindications.
- Avoid mutilating surgery and postoperative complications.
- Permit subsequent surgery, following moderate doses.

Disadvantages of radiotherapy. Pertherapeutic mortality is nil. Complications: see p. 799.

Combined Irradiation and Surgery

Combined therapy originated with the idea of pooling the advantages of both techniques and reducing the disadvantages to a minimum. In practice, this association consists of:

- First, radiotherapy either by preliminary brachytherapy of the uterus and the vagina, or external irradiation of the pelvis with moderate doses (20–30 Gy over 2 weeks), followed by complete brachytherapy.
- Secondly, 6 weeks later, radical colpohysterectomy with lymphadenectomy. By this time the post-radiation hyperemia has practically disappeared and post-radiation sclerosis has not yet set in. Immediate surgery is nevertheless preferred by some surgeons.

Aims of Radio-Surgical Treatment
- Sterilization of the cervix and pericervical lesions.
- Surgical excision of possibly unsterilized lesions and nodes, and precise evaluation of the extent of the malignancy.
- Avoidance of external irradiation for a considerable number of patients with negative nodes.
- Minimization of therapeutic complications.

Chemotherapy

Although its role in treating cervical cancer is secondary, chemotherapy does have its uses. Certain drugs have demonstrated their effectiveness against metastases, particularly in the lungs (Chauvergne et al. 1980).

Drugs. Numerous agents have been tested, the most helpful being chlorambucil, mitomycin C, vincristine, and especially *cis*-platinum.

Drug Combinations. These have been found particularly effective. Some of the most widely used and most effective combinations are: endoxan, adriamycin, *cis*-platinum (CAP); vindesin, bleomycin, mitomycin C, cis-platinum (BEMP); methotrexate, vincristine, chlorambucil, cis-platinum (Mevicol).

Aims of Chemotherapy
- To sterilize metastases when no other treatment can be employed.
- To sterilize subclinical lesions, either as the main treatment or as an adjunct to radiation (see below) and/or surgery (Blake et al. 1984).

Combining Chemotherapy with Radiotherapy and/or Surgery

The combination of chemotherapy with radiotherapy and/or surgery is currently impossible to evaluate conclusively. The association of chemotherapy with irradiation or surgery seems to be an attractive proposition, holding out the promise of reducing distant lesions. However, while its feasibility has been demonstrated, so far its efficacy has not (Wolff et al. 1985).

Therapeutic Indications. Different types of situations can be described:
- Operable lesions.
- Inoperable disease.
- Special cases.
- Incipient forms (CIS and microinvasive).

In *operable lesions* (stage I and limited stage II), the superiority of either of the techniques described has never been demonstrated statistically. The apparently better results reported for some surgical series were in fact based on selected patients (operable). This bias does not occur in the series treated by irradiation.

Surgery alone is employed in many institutions. In institutions where limited cervical cancers are habitually irradiated, surgery is nevertheless used for younger patients, certain histological (adenocarcinoma) or anatomical types (barrel-shaped cervix with poor radiosensitivity). In some countries, for cases with associated inflammatory or benign lesions (di Saia 1981), surgery by the vaginal route is relatively common, with or without extraperitoneal lymphadenectomy.

Radiotherapy alone is used mostly in the Anglo-Saxon countries and in a number of European centers. Tolerance is good and the results comparable to surgery alone.

Radiosurgical treatment is still relatively uncommon, but it is becoming more widespread, particularly in the Scandinavian countries (Einhorn et al. 1980), Europe, and the United States. Postoperative pelvic irradiation is given only in case of histologically proven iliac node invasion. When the para-aortic nodes are involved, pelvic and para-aortic irradiation can be considered, possibly backed up by chemotherapy. In some institutions surgery is done first (simple hysterectomy with repositioning of the ovaries) with younger patients (under 40) who have tumors smaller than 1 cm at their largest diameter.

Special cases
- When the general and/or medical condition contraindicates surgery, radiotherapy alone is given.
- With patients whose general and/or medical condition precludes both surgery and external radiation (very old patients), brachytherapy alone is used.

In the case of *inoperable disease* (extended stage II, stages III and IV), there is broad consensus against the advisability of surgery for the more advanced stages, but rather for their treatment by irradiation, possibly completed by chemotherapy. *Radiotherapy* consists of initial external pelvic irradiation followed by intracavitary brachytherapy.

Patients with urinary repercussions (stage III "urinary") are particularly vulnerable:
- The picture is dominated by the state of the kidneys (hypercreatininemia, anuria, etc.): initial ureterostomy or percutaneous nephrostomy is followed by standard treatment.
- Unilateral or bilateral uretero-hydronephrosis (or one silent kidney) with normal renal function: the usual treatment is administered, with particular attention paid to the urinary condition: urinary deviation is performed in case of alert.

Stage IV management is more difficult to schematize.
- In cases of definite involvement of the *bladder and/or rectum* (stage IVa), surgery is required: anterior, posterior, or total exenteration; at least urinary and/or intestinal deviation, which is imperative in cases of fistula. Involvement of the vulva may call for associated vulvectomy. After surgical time, it is possible to irradiate.
- When *distant metastases* are present (stage IVb) the first line of attack is systemic chemotherapy. If the results are good, it can be followed by locoregional treatment.

Special cases include *cancer of the cervical stump.* Here the therapeutic problems differ little from those encountered in cervical cancer with "in place" uterus, except that:
- Surgery can be more difficult because of the previous operation.
- Brachytherapy may be limited to intravaginal since it may be impossible to insert a device in what remains of the cervix.

In *cervical cancer during pregnancy* the basic problem is to reduce the cervical cancer to what it would be in the absence of pregnancy. It should be noted that staging is difficult, particularly as the pregnancy progresses (Lutz et al. 1979).

During the *first trimester* maternal considerations predominate.

- Operable cases: treatment in two steps: surgery and irradiation, with the order to be determined.
- Inoperable cases: irradiation alone after extraction of the embryo by curettage.

During the *second trimester* the decision rests with the mother as much as, if not more than, the physician. If the fetus is sacrificed, the procedure becomes the same as for the first trimester. Otherwise viability is awaited and the third semester scheme applies.

During the *third trimester* the viability of the fetus is the main consideration.

- Operable cases: treatment in two phases: cesarian section with colpohysterectomy and lymphadenectomy, followed by intravaginal irradiation, external pelvic irradiation and brachytherapy if the lymph nodes are involved.
- Inoperable cases: cesarian section followed by external pelvic irradiation and brachytherapy.

For *cervical sarcoma* see treatment procedure for the uterine corpus.

In cases of *preinvasive (CIS) and microinvasive carcinoma* two therapeutic approaches are debated: excision or destruction.

Excision is carried out by: conservative surgery or radical surgery (hysterectomy). Whatever the procedure, examination of the operative specimen is of paramount importance:

- If the entire lesion is removed, no complementary treatment is needed.
- When the resection is not "in sano" to the endocervix, the treatment should be supplemented by hysterectomy.
- When the resection is not "in sano" to the vagina, opinion ranges from recommending simple surveillance to intravaginal irradiation or laser. Reoperating is fraught with technical difficulties.

The main advantages of excision are two-fold:

- It can be employed in all cases (junction visible or not).
- It permits histological study of the operative specimen.

Its drawbacks include relative cumbersomeness, the need to hospitalize patients, and the patient's fear of surgery.

Destruction imperatively requires that the junction be seen in its entirety on colposcopy.

The results are the same (see below) for the two approaches, namely excision or destruction. In any event, prolonged surveillance is imperative by clinical examination, colposcopy, and cytology. The consequences on the possibility of pregnancy and the obstetrical prognosis are also the same (except with hysterectomy). Complications, too, are equally uncommon with both forms of treatment.

Corpus

Types of Treatment

Surgery is the same as for cervical cancer, but often tends to be more limited, comprising radical hysterectomy with pelvic lymph node sampling.

Radiotherapy is also the same as for cervical cancer, consisting of vaginal or uterovaginal brachytherapy and external pelvic irradiation.

Chemotherapy has not really proven its efficacy. Hormonotherapy with progestogens, with or without tamoxifen, has been widely recommended, but its usefulness is not apparent.

Therapeutic Indications

Operable Lesions and Operable Patients (Stages I and II)

Surgery alone is widely employed without any complementary treatment.

Brachytherapy in association with surgery, which considerably diminishes the rate of local recurrence, is becoming more widely used, either immediately before surgery or postoperatively. For the same indications, some therapists give pre- or postoperative external pelvic irradiation (Chassagne et al. 1977).

Complementary external irradiation is given in case of positive lymph nodes or infiltration of more than half of the myometrium, or grade 3 lesions.

Inoperable Lesions and/or Patients

The most effective treatment is the association of external irradiation (box technique) with a course of booster brachytherapy.

When the general condition and/or age require less aggressive treatment, a full course of brachytherapy alone or external irradiation alone is administered.

When distant metastases are present, the practicable treatment is supplemented by intensive hormonotherapy which improves the general condition and can temporarily stabilize the lesions, especially if they are localized in the lungs.

Special Cases: Sarcomas

Surgery is the basic treatment in cases of sarcomas, either colpohysterectomy or simple hysterectomy, depending on the circumstances. It is worth noting that it is not rare for sarcoma to be diagnosed on the basis of the surgical specimen. Opinions vary as to which of the following complementary treatments are advisable: no treatment, radiotherapy, chemotherapy, or combined radio-chemotherapy. The poor prognosis prompts the use of aggressive combination therapy, selected on the basis of the extension of the lesions, the histological type, and the degree of malignancy (number of mitoses per field).

Recurrence and Metastasis

Cervix

Recurrence

Recurrence of uterine carcinoma can be:
- Local (cervix, vagina);
- Regional (pelvis, pelvic nodes);
- Distant (metastases).

Timewise, recurrence can be:
- Early (less than 1 year; it actually represents continuing evolution and accounts for some 60% of recurrences (Kurohara et al. 1971);
- Intermediate (1–5 years);
- Late (over 5 years).

Management depends on localization, time of occurrence, and previous treatment. Furthermore, several of the different types of recurrences can appear simultaneously.

Local Recurrence

Prognosis is best for local recurrence confined to the centre of the pelvis; it should be treated aggressively to maximize the chances of success (Munnel 1961).

Clinical Symptoms. The clinical symptom which should arouse suspicion of local recurrence is metrorrhagia, sometimes moderate, and also pain, or urinary or rectal complaints suggestive of extension or fistula. Diagnosis will be based on clinical, cytological, and histological evidence, but histological proof is necessary before treatment can be undertaken. These local recurrences are noted in 6%–12% of cases, more often after treatment of extended lesions, and more often after surgery than radiotherapy.

Early Local Recurrence. When vaginal recurrence appears following brachytherapy and surgery in a zone which received large doses of radiation the treatment is surgery, which is often hampered by the discovery of a larger lesion than expected and by long and complicated healing. After irradiation alone, the treatment of recurrent lesions is also surgery if possible, but it is likely to be extensive and mutilating.

Intermediate or Late Local Recurrence. If previous irradiation was not too intensive, either combination radiotherapy and surgery or surgery alone can be envisaged.

Surgery Alone as Initial Treatment. Whatever the time of onset, if the initial therapy was surgery alone, local recurrence should be treated by irradiation.

Regional Recurrence (Often Locoregional)

Regional recurrence can be at the origin of a wide variety of clinical profiles:
- *Metrorrhagia* occurs when both local and pelvic lesions are present.
- A wide variety of *pelvic symptoms* can occur, such as unilateral or bilateral pelvic pain which spreads to the lumbar, gluteal, sciatic, or crural regions.
- *Urinary pathology* (dysuria, hematuria, incontinence, retention, and, very rarely, anuria) should be responded to with intravenous pyelogram (to check for uretero-pyelo-dilatation) and cystoscopy.
- *Rectal and intestinal pathology* (tenesmus, proctorrhagia) should be investigated by proctoscopy and/or colonoscopy and barium enema.
- When *circulatory problems* are observed (edema essentially from compression), urography should be done.

A clinical picture which associates pelvic pain, leg edema, and alteration of the ipsilateral pyelogram suggests a diagnosis of pelvic recurrence, generally in the lymph nodes, which should be verified by ultrasonography or, better still, by computerized tomography. In some instances, a simple pelvic X-ray will show changes compared to the previous lymphangiogram.

The *treatment* of pelvic recurrence is surgery, namely exploratory laparotomy with excision as required, opening possible obstructions, urinary or intestinal deviation if required. Prudent reirradiation can also be given if previous doses were not too high. Chemotherapy, however, is rarely effective on previously irradiated lesions (Chauvergne 1980).

Recurrence in the *para-aortic nodes* is a special case, often accompanied by other distant metastases. It is manifested by pain (nerve compression) and diagnosed by simple X-ray (alteration of lymphangiogram), by computerized tomodensitometry, or by evidence indicating spread to the vertebral corpus by contiguity. The lesions can be treated by radiotherapy if the region has not yet been irradiated. This can be supplemented by chemotherapy. For previously irradiated patients, chemotherapy alone is administered, but its chances of success are slim.

Metastases

Whether metastases occur at the outset, which is rare, or during the post-therapeutic course, the clinical management is not fundamentally different. The metastases themselves do not exhibit features by which they can be distinguished from those of other cancers.

Pulmonary metastasis is manifested by progressive dyspnea or discovered by routine follow-up X-ray. It may be confirmed by bronchial fibroscopy and by biopsy. If a single focused metastasis is present, surgery can be successful or, less commonly, irradiation. This treatment should be followed by a 6-month course of chemotherapy, or, for corpus carcinoma, by hormonotherapy.

Bone metastasis is signalled by pain and confirmed by X-ray and/or scintiscanning. Certain cases can be operated on, but the treatment is radiotherapy if the metastases are not too numerous, or extended. Backup chemotherapy can be helpful.

Brain metastases produce a wide variety of clinical pictures, and diagnosis is based on tomodensitometry. Surgery with radiotherapy is the preferred treatment, or irradiation alone can be used. Chemotherapy is generally not effective.

For *hepatic metastases*, chemotherapy can be attempted, although its usefullness is uncertain.

Corpus

Problems are the same as in cervical carcinoma. Local recurrences are more frequent (mostly in nonirradiated patients) than pulmonary metastases. Hormonotherapy may give some stabilization.

Complications of Treatment

A great number of patients have been cured of uterine carcinoma, permitting in-depth study and statistical analysis of the complications resulting from the treatment itself. The harsh prognosis does justify aggressive therapy, and the complications resulting from the treatment are neither more frequent nor more severe than for other cancers. They do, however, sometimes entail problems which can be tantamount to veritable infirmity, are occasionally life treatening, and can pose particulary troublesome diagnostic enigmas.

It is customary to distinguish between complications arising from surgery and from irradiation. The distinction is purely arbitrary: the same complications can have different causes, just as different complications can have the same causes. Nevertheless, surgical treatment does generate mainly urinary complications, radiotherapy mainly digestive complications, and chemotherapy mainly hematological complications. Surgical complications generally tend to appear soon after treatment, whereas radiological complications occur later; chemotherapy produces immediate complications or, much less often, delayed reactions. Some of the complications are produced by a combination of causes (Chassagne 1980).

In recent years, a decline has been universally reported in the rate of complications, particularly the serious ones (Einhorn et al. 1985; Perez et al. 1986). Yet differential diagnosis between complications and recurrences is one of the thorniest problems that arise during follow-up.

Urinary Complications

Bladder

Functional Disturbances. Dysuria, pollakiuria, even hematuria, and cystalgia can appear singly or in various combinations. The symptoms can be accompanied by urinary incontinence (sometimes simply stress incontinence). With early onset the cause is usually surgical, and the symptoms generally regress spontaneously. With intermediate or late onset, radiotherapy or a combination of causes are to blame. The frequency of urinary disturbances is difficult to determine and is estimated at about 25% of the patients treated.

Cystoscopic examination can indicate the course to follow. If no lesion is found, the problems are most likely related to postsurgical alterations of the vascular and nerve supply of the bladder and are difficult to treat. If a shrunken bladder is seen, it can be treated with intravesical instillations, variously repeated. At worst, repeated and/or severe hematuria (hemorrhagic bladder) may warrant definitive urinary deviation. Finally, a fistula may be discovered.

Vesical Fistula. This is a much rarer complaint (rates of 0%–5% have been reported) and is manifested by urinary incontinence. Definitive diagnosis is based on clinical symptoms, cystoscopy and/or intravenous pyelography. Early fistulas have surgical origins; later appearance incriminates irradiation or combined radio-surgical treatment. Fistulas are corrected surgically, but operating on irradiated tissues can be delicate.

Ureteral Fistulas

Ureteral fistulas are rare (0%–10%). They are indicated either by urinary incontinence or vaginal leakage of urine with micturition partially conserved. The diagnosis is suggested by clinical features, confirmed by the methylene blue test, and corroborated by intravenous pyelogram and/or retrograde ureteropyelogram. Cystoscopy verifies the absence of vesical pathology.

Ureteral fistulas generally appear early and are the result of surgery; their formation is enhanced by previous irradiation, but they rarely occur after radiotherapy alone. The incidence varies directly with the scope of the surgery: the more radical the surgery, the higher the rate.

The treatment is surgical correction. Simple suturing may suffice if the fistula is far from the bladder. But the more usual solution is reimplantation, with or without an artificial implant, for fistulas adjacent to the bladder, which is the most common site. At worst, intestinal or cutaneous deviation, or even nephrectomy, may be necessary.

Ureteral Stenosis and Ureterohydronephrosis

Of intermediate or late onset, the pathology of ureteral stenosis and ureterohydronephrosis is due to irradiation, or rather to combined irradiation and surgery. It is, in fact, most often related to recurrence, and the rare cases of early onset are due to radical surgery.

The symptomatology is minimal or even nonexistent, comprising lumbopelvic pain and heaviness, often connected with attendant urinary infection or lymphocele (see below). These conditions are usually discovered by routine urological examination.

Treatment will depend on how the ureterorenal pathology affects urinary function. If it is not affected, no more than monitoring is required. If creatinine and urea excretion are altered and if the renal parenchyma appears too reduced, exploratory surgery with urinary deviation is indicated. When renal function is very much diminished or even destroyed, or worse, if pain is experienced, nephrectomy is unavoidable.

Digestive Complications

Except for certain rectovaginal fistulas which occur fairly soon after surgery, digestive complications can all be ascribed to irradiation. During the course of radiotherapy, a picture of functional pathology is observed which includes nausea, anorexia, meteorism, and diarrhetic phenomena. These disorders are of mild to moderate severity and can be palliated by symptomatic treatment. Post-therapeutic intestinal complications are due to obliterating endarteritis and resist treatment. They can appear moderately (12–18 months) or very late, after developing over a long period.

Rectum

Rectal complications are becoming rarer with improving dosimetry in brachytherapy. Three types can be described:

- Ulcerative proctitis characterized by tenesmus and glaireous discharge. Rectoscopic examination reveals a pale and ulcerated mucosa, particularly the anterior wall.
- Hemorrhagic proctitis: rectoscopy shows the presence of multiple superficial telangiectases on a fragile mucosa which bleeds readily on contact.
- Microrectitis, with constipation, painful defecation, and narrow stools. Rectoscopy shows more or less extended stenosis which is sometimes annular.

Colon

Subobstructive phenomena are seen, including alternation of diarrhoea and constipation, meteorism, melena and/or proctorrhagia, and abdominal pain. Proctoscopy yields little information: normal or subnormal mucosa, with stenosis which is occasionally impassable at about 15 cm. On colonic X-ray, the stenosis exhibits irregular outlines, variable extension with undefined borders, and smooth colonic mucosa, all of which is confirmed by colonoscopy.

Small Intestine

Intestinal complications give rise to the most serious and occult of the digestive troubles: diarrhoea and subocclusive episodes, with asthenia, anorexia, and weight loss. The repetition of such episodes can alter the general condition. Occasionally, intestinal occlusion occurs and requires aggressive treatment.

Course

These disorders develop in irregular, capricious fashion, over a period of years, often after a symptom-free interval of 12–18 months. At times the episodes decrease in frequency and intensity; at others, they become more frequent and more severe, with hemorrhage, fistula, occlusion by single colonic stenosis or multiple stenoses of the small intestine.

Treatment

Minimum measures are dietary supervision and prevention of constipation; local rectal treatment can be given (corticoids, vitamin A), with antispasmodic medication in the case of subocclusive episodes. The most drastic treatment is surgery: iliac anus for severe proctorrhagia or sigmoid stenosis; resection of various portions of the small intestine, with transileal or transjejunal anastomosis.

Lymphocysts

The complication of lymphocysts is common after radical surgery. It is asymptomatic in most cases and is discovered by follow-up pyelography (compression of ureters, bladder). It tends to regress spontaneously, but kidney state and function should nevertheless be monitored. In some instances, clinical manifestations (lumbar and/or pelvic pain) reflect serious superinfection or renal pathology. The effusion should then be drained, and a favorable outcome can be expected.

Bone

Complications which affect the bones are all due to external irradiation and occur relatively late. They include:

- *Fractures* of the femoral neck or the fundus of the acetabulum.
- *Coxarthrosis*, sometimes in association with progressive necrosis of the femoral caput.
- *Osteolytic or osteodystrophic* lesions of the rest of the pelvis or of lumbar vertebrae; asymptomatic or expressed by more or less specific pain.

Fractures and some coxarthroses are treated by orthopedic surgery, generally with satisfactory results. The other lesions call for symptomatic treatment; they should not be mistaken for metastases and, above all, must not be reirradiated.

Vascular Complications

Vein and lymphatic compression is relatively common, resulting in chronic edema of one or both legs. Treatment is difficult.

Sexual Complications

Dyspareunia is common after uterine cancer treatment, whatever the therapy (Wolff and Cachelou 1985). This complaint is not always related to the treatment nor to ensuing anatomo-physiological changes, but is most often connected with the patient's anxiety and guilt feelings, mainly concerning her previous sexual tractus. The ailment may be attributable to indifference, rejection, lack of desire, anorgasmy, or genuine pain, superficial or deep, on penetration. Treatment is difficult and is above all preventive.

Corpus

Problems are identical to those seen with cervical cancer, but complications are less frequent – except the side effects on general status and/or preexistent disease in elderly patients.

Follow-up

Follow-up after treatment for uterine carcinoma is a crucial phase in the management, and also one of the most difficult. It has a number of objectives:

- At the earliest possible time, spot any recurrence or metastasis.
- Detect complications of treatment and distinguish them from recurrences.

- Be on the alert for possible other cancers.
- Ensure best possible rehabilitation.

Means of Surveillance

- Clinical: general and gynecological examination (including palpation of supraclavicular region).
- Vaginal smears, one of the best methods of local surveillance.
- Cystoscopic examination and urinary X-rays at the least suspicion.
- Proctoscopy, colonoscopy, barium enema in case of digestive complaints.
- Chest X-ray yearly, hemogram, ionogram, liver function, and the whole range of special tests as required.
- There are no specific *markers* for uterine carcinoma. One of the most frequently positive markers is the carcinoembryonic antigen (CEA) which is present in about 50% of the cases. It diminishes to normal levels after treatment, increasing again in case of recurrence or metastasis (in 80% of initially positive cases; C/Kjorstad and Orjaseter 1978), before the emergence of any clinical symptoms.

Management for Different Clinical Profiles

Metrorrhagia

On clinical examination, postirradiation cervical and vaginal mucosa appears pale, hypovascular (or hyperemic), fragile, bleeding on contact. Locate an abnormal zone by inspection or colposcopy.

Vaginal smears and, often, colposcopy are indispensable. If an abnormal zone is seen, a biopsy should be taken. It is important to note that in *postirradiation dysplasia* the cells are difficult to differentiate from the malignant cells of recurrent disease. *Pelvic symptoms* are more often associated with recurrence than with treatment complications. *Pain* may be due to osteoarticular lesions, but is most often indicative of regional recurrence, particularly if it is associated with other pelvic pathology. Management is by X-ray examination. *Urinary pathology* can be related to complications or recurrence. Management is by cystoscopy, intravenous pyelogram, kidney function (Photopulos et al. 1977).

The symptoms of *intestinal and rectal pathology* are more often indicative of complications than recurrence. Management is by proctocolonoscopy and X-ray of the colon.

Circulatory pathology includes leg edema, related to pelvic vessel compression, due to recurrent disease or to sclerosis resulting from treatment. Management is by intravenous pyelography and CT scan.

It is worth emphasizing that a number of different complaints often occur in association, which, to a certain extent, makes the diagnosis easier.

Any *abnormal clinical symptom* may indicate metastasis or recurrent disease, just as it can indicate a *second cançer*. The organs most often affected following cervical cancer are the genitalia, the colon, and the breast (Boice et al. 1985).

Sexual problems are rarely reported by the patients and should be sought out during interview. About 2 years after treatment, the patients are more willing to admit to problems, when they no longer feel their life to be threatened.

Timing of Surveillance

The majority of deaths from uterine carcinoma occur within 2 years after treatment. After 7 years, the survival curve for cervical cancer patients becomes parallel to that of the general population (Pejovic et al. 1981). Hence the surveillance should be intensive at the beginning, with examination every 3 months during the first year, then every 6 months for another 4 years. After 5 years, an annual examination suffices, and after 10 years, an examination every 2 years. But it is important to continue the follow-up for a long time (Fig. 3).

Rehabilitation

Rehabilitation after uterine carcinoma treatment must address all the aspects, including personal, family, sexual, social, and professional. It presupposes that the disease is cured, or at least stabilized. It must start before treatment. Satisfactory readjustment hinges on two conditions:
- Pluridisciplinary cooperation (clinicians, psychologists, nurses, social workers).
- Aggressivity of treatment reduced to the unavoidable minimum: less is best.

It must also be borne in mind that this cancer strikes organs which are particularly sensitive psychologically, and so the disease will have a major emotional impact on subsequent mental health.

Personal. Explain, explode myths, allay anxiety, assuage guilt feelings: all this should be tackled before

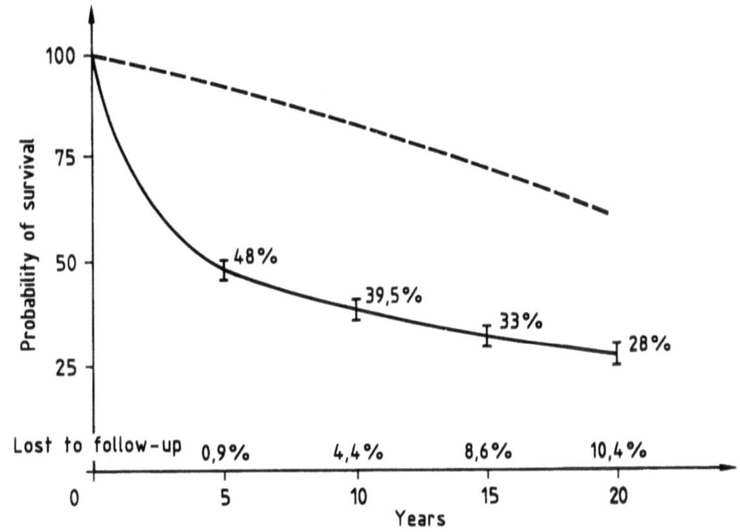

Fig. 3. Reference population survival curve *(broken line)* and patient population actuarial survival curve *(solid line)* (2 SD): all stages

treatment. Giving the patient "the whole truth" is a delusion. Only frankness "adjusted" to what the patient can understand and endure is advisable, diverging the farther from the strict facts the more serious the condition.

Family Circle. The immediate family should, as far as possible, understand the situation. It should therefore be explained to family members, who should also be warned against overreacting or underreacting towards the patient.

Sex Life. Sexual adjustment is an important component of general well-being. It is essential to explode myths, ease guilt, and advise the patient to resume intercourse as soon as possible after treatment. This will also help to strengthen the patient's optimistic view of the future. Explain the consequences on hormone function and make plain that subsequent pregnancy is impossible. The prevention of troubles is one way of avoiding them.

Social Context. The impairment attendant on treatment is inconspicuous. The less it is known outside the family circle and the less it is discussed, the easier it will be for the patient to regain her place in the community. Since cancer still has such an appalling reputation, it is preferable to avoid community reactions which can only be negative.

Employment. The problem is extremely complex. A patient in a satisfactory condition after treatment should return to normal employment. The solution depends on countries, on type of employment, and on the age of the patient.

Results of Treatment – Survival

Cervix

Reports on survival require very careful reading. While several claim that 5-year survival rates have increased considerably, no such rise is brought out in the FIGO Annual Report (Figo 1985). Two preliminary observations can be made:

- The distribution by stage has shifted towards more cases in the earlier stages.
- Survival by stage has increased very little in spite of improvements in treatment.

Survival Rates

The rates of survival from the FIGO Annual Report are listed in Tables 3 and 4. Overall 5-year survival is 55%. Survival varies with a number of factors (see "Prognosis"). Survival rates also vary considerably from one institution to another (5-year survival: stage I 60%–90%, stage II 35%–65%, stage III

Table 3. Carcinoma of the cervix uteri – 5-year result. Patients treated in 1976–1978 (From FIGO 1985)

	Patients	
	(*n*)	(%)
Alive at 5 years	17843	55.0
Died of carcinoma of the cervix	11650	35.9
Lost to follow-up	1762	5.5
Died from intercurrent disease	1173	3.6
	32428	100.0

Table 4. Carcinoma of the corpus uteri – 5-year result. Patients treated in 1976–1978. (From FIGO 1985)

	Patients (n)	(%)
Alive at 5 years	9192	67.7
Died of carcinoma of the corpus	3048	22.4
Lost to follow-up	514	3.8
Died from intercurrent disease	827	6.1
	13581	100.0

Table 5. Carcinoma of the cervix uteri. Distribution by stage and 5-year survival in the different stages. Patients treated in 1976–1978

Stage	Patients treated		Five year survival	
	(n)	(%)	(n)	(%)
I	10791	33.3	8430	78.1
II	11599	35.8	6610	57.0
III	8623	26.6	2671	31.0
VI	1377	4.3	107	7.8
No stage	9	0.0	4	–
	32428	100.0	17843	55.0

Exact data taken from the FIGO Annual Report (FIGO 1985).

15%–55%, stage IV 0%–20%. The differences are partly due to different appreciation of clinical stage, and also to different treatment modalities, on which it is impossible to elaborate from present evidence.

Causes of Mortality. The causes of death have changed: whereas until the 1970s, two-thirds of the deaths could be blamed on locoregional recurrence and one-third on metastasis, the proportions are becoming reversed, and most deaths now result from metastasis. This confirms the progress that has been made in controlling local disease and highlights the need for associated systemic chemotherapy.

Corpus

Survival Rates

The rates are shown in Table 5 from the FIGO Annual Report. The following points are worthy of note:
- The overall survival rate is 67.7%.
- The rate varies with a number of factors (see "Prognosis").
- Survival rates have not increased much between the 1962–1968 series and the 1976–1978 series, and the gains which have been observed may be related to the greater number of stage I cases.

Correspondingly, numerous studies report 5-year survival rates of 80%–85% for operable stage I cases (which comprise the majority), but the rates decline rapidly for older and/or inoperable patients.

Prognosis

Cervix

Prognosis is particularly difficult to determine in cervical carcinoma. Moreover, the evidence we do have is applicable only to series of patients and cannot be extrapolated to individual cases. Three sorts of prognostic indicators can be of use: anatomical and histological factors related to the tumor itself, dynamic factors of host-tumor interaction, and factors concerning the host. Factors relating to the treatment are operative only at the end of the therapy.

Static Factors

Anatomy

Extension and tumor volume are the basis for any concept of prognosis. Table 5 illustrates the importance of stage for prognosis. The following complementary anatomical variables can be taken into account.

Tumor Size in Stages I and II. The 3-year survival rate falls from 92% to 70% in stage I, and from 76% to 64% in stage II when the tumor diameter becomes larger than 2 cm (Wolff et al. 1965). Tumor size is also known to be related to lymph node involvement (Dargent et al. 1985).

Endometrial Extension in Stage I.

The Extent of Parametrial Involvement in Stages II and III. The 5-year survival rate of 32% when only one parametrium is involved falls to 15% when both are involved.

The Extent of Vaginal Involvement, particularly in Stage III. The 5-year survival rate is 50%, 32% or 8% according to whether the vagina shows no involvement, involvement confined to the upper two-thirds, or involvement of the whole organ.

Combination of Vaginal/Parametrial Extension. 3-year survival rates of stage III patients are 44% in the case of no vaginal involvement (one or both par-

Table 6. Carcinoma of the corpus uteri, 1976–1978. Distribution by stage and 5-year survival in the different stages. (From FIGO 1985)

Stage	Patients treated		Five year survival	
	(*n*)	(%)	(*n*)	(%)
I	10285	75.7	7729	75.1
II	1885	13.9	1089	57.8
III	844	6.2	253	30.0
IV	452	3.3	48	10.6
No stage	115	0.9	73	63.5
	13581	100.0	9192	67.7

ametria) and 10% in the case of total vaginal involvement + both parametria.

Involvement of Pelvic Lymph Nodes. Pelvic node involvement is a major prognostic indicator, especially when the lesions are small. In stage I b the 5-year survival rates are, respectively, 51.8% and 84.6% for cases with or without histologically documented pelvic lymph node involvement (based on 2279 cases, FIGO 1985). The *number* of nodes involved should be taken into consideration. When a single node is involved, the *size* of the metastasis is relevant: metastases smaller than 5 mm (clandestine or micrometastases) have little effect on survival. Rupture of the *capsule* is significant: 5-year survival rate of 59% or 22% respectively. The *site* of the positive nodes is also relevant to survival: the rate is 53% or 21% depending on whether the site is below or above the bifurcation of the common iliac artery (van Vorhis 1970).

Invasion of the *para-aortic nodes* considerably worsens the prognosis, with survival rates of 0%–20% (depending on the author) for cases of proven para-aortic involvement. For *scalene node* involvement the prognosis is even worse.

The repercussions of cervico-parametrial lesions and/or node involvement on the *urinary tract* (without actual invasion) considerably worsen prognosis, particularly in stage III: the 5-year survival is 18% or 48% depending on whether or not there are changes in the intravenous pyelography (Fenton and Decroix 1979).

Histology

The histological type of the lesion plays an important role in its spread. The prospects in cervical adenocarcinoma are less favorable than in epidermoid carcinoma: the FIGO Annual Report (1985) gave the 5-year survival rate for epidermoid carcinoma as 76.2% (6484 cases) and for adenocarcinoma as 68.8% (823 cases). The histological grade does not have as much significance here as in endometrial carcinoma.

Dynamic Factors (Delay)

It would seem reasonable to expect that the length of the *interval* between first symptoms and diagnosis could give some indication as to the type of evolution of a carcinoma. However, not only is the length of this interval difficult to determine with any degree of precision, but studies with long series of patients have been unable to find any statistically significant correlation between the interval and survival. The survival rates were not better for the shorter intervals, nor poorer when the delays were longer. Yet a certain relation between the two variables becomes apparent when the series of patients are studied by stage. A combination of the two factors (stage and delay) does supply some evidence about the type of development, but the findings are meaningful only in a statistical sense and cannot be translated into individual terms.

Host-Related Factors

Age. Current opinion is virtually unanimous in affirming that survival rates decrease with age. This conclusion is not obvious from studies comparing patients by stage; but the distribution of patients by stage and age does show that the proportion of stage III and IV patients compared to the number of stage I and II patients increases correspondingly to age: hence the poorer survival rates.

Factors Related to Treatment

Radioresistance can be estimated only at the end of treatment or after treatment: it is an "a posteriori" factor. Nevertheless, it can be affirmed that while radiosensitive cancer cannot always be cured, radioresistant cancer is never cured (even by surgery).

Corpus

Stage is an important prognostic factor. As in all cancers, survival rates decrease with more extended lesions (Table 6). Moreover, the *size of the uterus* is an important prognostic indicator (Gusberg and Yonnopoulos 1964), hence the subdivision of stage I into I a and I b: 5-year survival in I a is 85% and in I b it is 67% (Berman et al. 1980).

Tumor size also has prognostic significance, but not as much as the localization: survival is poorer when lesions extend to the isthmus or are implanted low in the cavity.

Intramyometrial penetration is universally accepted as an important prognostic factor and is related to grade and to lymph node involvement. The 5-year survival rate for stage I, with intramyometrial penetration less than two-thirds, is 91%; with intramyometrial penetration of more than two-thirds it is 85%; and with total infiltration it is 56% (Rochet 1977).

Lymph node involvement has the same significance as in cervical cancer: thus in stage I the 5-year survival rate of 94% for cases with no lymph node involvement falls to 28% for cases where the lymph nodes are involved (Berman et al. 1980).

Histological differentiation is an important element of the prognosis (Gusberg and Yonnopoulos 1964); it is recognized in the FIGO classification and should be evaluated from the surgical specimen. The 5-year survival rate for stage I, grade 1 is 77%, grade 2: 73%, and grade 3: 58% (FIGO 1985).

Age is undeniably a prognostic factor, and mortality increases with age. It may be related to general condition, associated pathology and/or intramyometrial penetration, and histological grading.

Future Prospects

Future developments in uterine carcinoma can be expected from three main directions: etiology and detection, diagnosis, treatment.

Cervix

Etiology and Detection

Etiology and detection are related. Indeed, progress in very early detection can be expected to follow from oncogene research (with monoclonal antibodies). We can also hope to learn to "label" different types of lesions and thus treat only truly precancerous lesions and ignore the risk-free ones. Cytological detection, too, should see improvement:

- With the use of monoclonal antibodies, rendering the method more reliable and more selective.
- With the wide use of computers, making screening possible on a vast scale.

Diagnosis

A powerful new diagnostic tool will be specific markers for cervical carcinoma that can be expected to emerge from progress in immunology reasearch. In the nearer future, medical imaging (nuclear magnetic resonance and metastasis detection by labeled monoclonal antibodies) should provide more precise delineation of the extent of disease and thus lead to improved therapeutic indications.

Treatment

Treatment Techniques

Brachytherapy will change towards either more intense and shorter courses, or more fractionated application (trials in progress). More individualized interstitial brachytherapy, perhaps peroperative, can be envisaged. A similar evolution can be expected for external irradiation (trials in progress).

For both types of radiotherapy, radiosensitizers (misonidazole and similar agents) should improve the radiosensitivity of lesions by increasing the oxygenation (trials in progress). Associated hyperthermia may increase the efficiency of irradiation still further (trials in progress).

Chemotherapy will play a more important role with better drugs and drug combinations (numerous trials in progress), with efficacy possibly enhanced by the transport and fixation of the drugs at the lesions.

Treatment Modalities

Combined radio-surgical treatment will become more widespread with theoretic progress in radiotherapy (see above), including peroperative external irradiation (trials in progress) and brachytherapy. Combining chemotherapy with irradiation and/or surgery will be more common, or even the norm (trials in progress). Thus the number of metastases can be expected to diminish and their treatment to become more effective.

Corpus

Primary prevention can be improved only by better adapting estrogen treatments and associating them with progestogens. *Secondary prevention* (screening) is currently difficult to improve and cannot be implemented on a large scale. Endometrial hyperplasia must never go untreated, and hysterectomy can even be performed in cases of atypical hyperplasia. *Early diagnosis* can be promoted by improved endouterine cytology and the development of hysteroscopy.

Improvement of current techniques in *treatment* does not seem to be in the offing. The therapeutic program itself needs to be tailored as much as possible to individual patients, in particular by a better understanding of the prognostic factors and their interplay. A better knowledge of hormone receptors should promote better adapted hormone treatments. More effective drugs or drug combinations can be anticipated, be it for chemotherapy alone or in association with other treatments (numerous trials in progress).

References

Asvall JE, Eker R (1974) Cervical cancer screening. Cancer control in Norway. Universitetsforlaget, Oslo, pp 24–27

Barber HK, Sommers LC (1981) Carcinoma of the endometrium. Masson, New York

Beral V (1974) Cancer of the cervix: a sexually transmitted disease? Lancet 1: 1037–1040

Berman M, Ballon SC, Lagarre LD, Watring WG (1980) Prognosis and treatment of endometrial cancer. Am J Obstet Gynecol 9: 1–5

Blake PR, Lambert HE, MacGregor WG, O'Sullivan JC, Dowdell JW, Anderson T (1984) Surgery following chemotherapy and radiotherapy for advanced carcinoma of the cervix. Gynecol Oncol 19: 198–203

Boice JD, Day NE, Anderson A et al. (1985) Second cancers following radiation treatment for cervical cancer. An international collaboration among cancer registries. J Natl Cancer Inst 74: 955–975

Boyes DA, Worth AJ, Fidler HK (1970) The results of treatment of 4389 cases of preclinical cervical squamous carcinoma. J Obstet Gynecol Br Commonwealth 77: 769

Burghardt E (1984) Micro-invasive carcinoma in gynecological pathology. Clin Obstet Gynecol 11: 239–257

Chassagne D (1980) Cancer du col utérin. Glossaire ou lexique des complications. Bull Cancer (Paris) 67: 120–125

Chassagne D, Gerbaulet A, Wolff JP, Michel G, Prade M (1977) Techniques et indications de la curiethérapie et de la radiothérapie transcutanée dans les cancers de l'endomètre. In: L'endomètre. Masson, Paris, pp 403–414

Chauvergne J, Durant M, Cappelaere P, Gary Bobo J, Guerrin J, Hoerni B (1980) La chimiothérapie des cancers du col utérin. Bilan de 267 traitements palliatif et orientation actuelle. Bull Cancer (Paris) 67: 78–89

Christopherson WW, Lundiu FE, Mendez WW, Parker JE (1976) Cervical cancer control. A study of morbidity and mortality trends over a twenty-one year period. Cancer 38: 1357–1366

Cole P, Morrison AS (1980) Basic issues in population for cancer. J Natl Cancer Inst 64: 1263–1272

Cutler SJ, Young JL Jr (1975) Third national cancer survey: incidence data. DHEW Public. (NIH) 75–787, US Gov Print Off (National Cancer Institute Monograph 41)

Dargent D, Gerbaulet A, Le Floch O (1979) Cancer du col utérin. Encycl Med Chir (Paris) 597–600

Dargent D, Frobert JC, Bear G (1985) Factor (tumor volume) and T factor (FIGO classification) in the assessment of cervix cancer prognosis is the risk of lymph node spread. Gynecol Oncol 22: 15–22

De Brux J (1982) Histopathologie gynécologique. Masson, Paris

Di Saia PJ (1981) Surgical aspects of cervical carcinoma. Cancer 48: 548–559

Einhorn N, Bygdeman M, Sjöberg B (1980) Combined radiation and surgical treatment for carcinoma of the uterine cervix. Cancer 45: 720–723

Einhorn N, Patek E, Sjöberg B (1985) Outcome of different treatment modalities in cervix carcinoma stage Ib and IIa. Observations in a well defined Swedish population. Cancer 55: 949–955

Fenton J, Decroix Y (1979) Radiothérapie exclusive des épithéliomas du col utérin de stade II distal et III. Résultats et complications thérapeutiques de 393 cas traités à l'Institut Curie. Bull Cancer (Paris) 66: 542–548

FIGO Annual report on the results of treatment in gynecological cancer. FIGO Radium Hemmet, Stockholm, no. 19

Fletcher GH (1979) Predominant parameters in the planning of radiation therapy of carcinoma of the cervix. Bull Cancer (Paris) 66: 561–572

Gardner JW, Lyon JL (1977) Low incidence of cervical cancer in Utah. Gynecol Oncol 5: 68–80

Gusberg S, Yannopoulos D (1964) Therapeutic decision in corpus cancer. Am J Obstet Gynecol 88: 157–162

Hermanek P, Sobin LH (eds) (1987) TNM classification of malignant tumors. Springer, Berlin Heidelberg New York

Ketcham D, Chretien P, Hoye R, Harrah J, Deckers P, Sugarbaker E, Taylor P, Rabson A (1973) Occult metastases to the scalene lymph nodes patients with clinically operable carcinoma of the cervix. Cancer 31: 80–183

Kim K, Rigal RD, Pahick JR (1978) The changing trends of uterine cancer and cytology. A study of morbidity and mortality trends over a twenty year period. Cancer 42: 2439–2449

Kistner RW (1982) Treatment of carcinoma in situ of the endometrium. Clin Obstet Gynecol 5: 1166

Kjörstad KE, Orjaseter H (1978) Carcinoembryonic antigen levels in patients with squamous cell carcinoma of the cervix. Obstet Gynecol 51: 536–540

Kolstad P (1969) Carcinoma of the cervix stage Ia. Am J Obstet Gynecol 104: 1015–1022

Kolstad P, Stafl A (1977) Atlas of colposcopy. Universitetsforlaget, Oslo

Kurohara SS, Vongtama VY, Webster JH, George FW (1971) Post irradiational recurrent epidermoid carcinoma of the uterine cervix. Am J Roentgenol 111: 249–259

Lutz MH, Underwood PB, Rozier JC, Putney FW (1979) Genital malignancy in pregnancy. Am J Obstet Gynecol 129: 536–542

Mahboui E, Eyler N, Wynder EL (1982) Epidemiology of cancer of the endometrium. Clin Obstet Gynecol 25: 5–17

Morgan LS, Nelson JH (1982) Surgical treatment of early cervical cancer. Semin Oncol 9: 312–330

Munnel E (1961) Can recurrent cervical carcinoma be successfully managed? Am J Gynecol Obstet 81: 521–525

Musumeci R, de Palo G (1984) Radiological assessment of gynecological malignancies. In: Whitehouse JM, Williams C (ed) Cancer of the female reproductive system, Wiley, Chichester

Pejovic MH, Wolff JP, Kramar A, Goldfarb E (1981) Cure rate estimation and long term prognosis of uterine cervix carcinoma. Cancer 47: 203–206

Perez C, Zivnuska F, Askin F, Kumar B, Camel H, Powers W (1975) Prognostic significance of endometrial extension from primary carcinoma of uterine cervix. Cancer 35: 1493–1504

Perez CA, Camel HM, Kuske RP, Kao MS, Galakatos A, Hederman MA, Powers WE (1986) Radiation therapy alone in the treatment of carcinoma of the uterine cervix: a 20 year experience. Gynecol Oncol 23: 127–140

Photopulos GY, Shinley RE, Ansbocher R (1977) Evaluation of conventional diagnostic tests for detection of recurrent carcinoma of the cervix. Am J Obstet Gynecol 129: 533–535

Pilleron JP, Durand JC, Lenoble JC (1972) Carcinoma of the uterine cervix stages I and II treated by radiation therapy and extensive surgery (1000 cases). Cancer 29: 593–596

Pujol H, Prade M (1979) Extension aux trompes des cancers du col utérin. Bull Cancer (Paris) 66: 503–514

Riotton G (1979) Evaluation du dépistage du col utérin. Bull Cancer (Paris) 66: 404–406

Riou G, Barrois M, Tordjman I, Dutronquay V, Orth G (1984) Présence de génomes de papilloma virus et amplification des oncogénes C-myc et C-HA-RAS dans les cancers envahisants du col de l'utérus. CR Acad Sci Paris (III) 299 (14): 575–580

Rochet Y (1977) Indications thérapeutiques dans les cancers de l'endomètre. In: L'endomètre. Masson, Paris, pp 467–476

Rotkin ID (1973) A comparison review of key epidemiological studies in cervical cancer related to current searches for transmissible agents. Cancer Res 33: 1353–1367

Rutledge F, Wharton JJ, Fletcher GH (1976) Clinical studies with adjunctive surgery and irradiation therapy in the treatment of carcinoma of the cervix. Cancer 38: 596–602

Silverberg E (1975) Gynecologic cancer: statistical and epidemiological information. American Cancer Society Professional and Educational Publications

Van Vorhis LW (1970) Carcinoma of the cervix. I. Therapeutic and patient factors affecting survival. Am J Obstet Gynecol 108: 105–114

Walton RJ, Blanchet M, Boyes DA, Carmichael J, Marshall KG, Miller AB, Thompson DW (1976) Dépistage du cancer du col utérin. Union Med Can 105: 997–1052

West R (1977) Cervical cancer: age at registration and age at death. Br J Cancer 35: 236–241

Wolff JP, Cachelou P (1985) Sexualité chez les hystérectomisées pour cancer gynécologique. Contrac Fertil Sexual [Suppl] 13: 211–215

Wolff JP, Rouquette C, Danon J (1965) The value of clinical examination for the prognosis of cancer of the uterine cervix. Am J Obstet Gynecol 93: 472–478

Wolff JP, George M, Haie C, Pejovic MH, Horiot JC, Fenton F, Lefloch O, Heron JP (1985) Phase II study of combination of radiotherapy and chemotherapy in the primary treatment of advanced uterine cervix carcinoma. Arch Gynecol [Suppl] 237: 281

Zur Hausen H (1982) Humour genital cancer: synergism between two virus infections or synergism between a virus infection and initiating events. Lancet 2: 1370–1372

Primary Adult Vaginal Cancer

G. Michel and A. Gerbaulet

Definition

In a patient presenting with vaginal malignancy two features are essential to confirm its origin:

1. The cervix must be healthy, for any concomitant malignant involvement of the cervix and of the vagina suggests the diagnosis of cervical cancer with vaginal extension.
2. Where the vagina is still intact following uterine hysterectomy or cervicotomy, whether surgery occurred more or less than five years previously, knowledge of the histology of the operative specimen is mandatory. The latter must differ from the vaginal tumour, otherwise the diagnosis is that of a recurrence.

We will only deal here with primary vaginal tumours. Secondary vaginal tumours require special consideration. This chapter is devoted to adult vaginal cancer.

Epidemiology and Risk Factors

Incidence

Vaginal cancer, if strictly defined as above, is rare. In the literature its incidence is between 1% and 3% of gynaecological malignancies (only 2,5% of 3000 cases of gynaecological malignancy seen at the Institut Gustave-Roussy).

Age

The incidence of vaginal cancer increases with age. It tends to affect the older woman. The mean age from different series varies between 60 and 65 years. In 80%–85% of cases the patients are postmenopausal.

Risk Factors

Different risk factors have been described but there is no consensus upon their relative importance. A previous hysterectomy is noted in 15%–50% of patients with vaginal cancer. Several explanations for the role of surgery in the genesis of this tumour have been suggested. First, could a total hysterectomy and partial colpectomy change the local anatomy, shorten the vagina and increase repeated minor local trauma from sexual intercourse? Secondly, could bilateral annexectomy in a woman who was still menstruating suppress ovarian function with consequent effects on the vagina, one of its target organs? Thirdly, could the hysterectomy have been carried out when the uterus was the site of undiagnosed occult malignancy associated with a latent subclinical vaginal lesion which came to light subsequently? Dargent (1980) suggests that vaginal malignancy may be induced by therapeutic ionising radiation.

The second most commonly cited risk factor is the pessary. This is used to support a prolapsed uterus and is often worn for many years without regard to adequate local hygiene. According to various publications, about 10% of patients with vaginal cancer have pessaries in place. A previous gynaecological or obstetric history, often cited in cervical cancer, is thought to play only a very minor role in vaginal cancer. There is no racial predisposition, although the incidence is higher among some black African women who are, in general, young.

Histopathology

Among the primary tumours of the vagina, two histological types must be distinguished, carcinoma in situ and invasive carcinoma.

Carcinoma In Situ

Very rare as a primary lesion, carcinoma in situ is much more often an extension of an adjacent invasive cancer of the cervix or of the vulva. Patients can be identified as being at risk: thus a previous history of cervical cancer necessitates close follow-up examination of the vagina. The site of in situ change is most often at the vaginal vault. Systematic use of Schiller's test remains the diagnostic method of choice. A smear may lead to diagnosis, but only biopsy, which is sometimes difficult, proves the diagnosis. The histological features of vaginal carcinoma in situ are the same as those of the cervix.

Invasive Carcinoma

Site

The common site of origin is the upper third of the vagina, in particular the posterior vaginal wall. However, extensive lesions, as well as multicentric ones, are frequent.

Macroscopic Appearance

Macroscopic features are similar to those of cervical cancer, namely an ulcerating, exophytic and infiltrative lesion. A very accurate diagram must be made of the lesion before any therapeutic procedure. The imprint of the tumour on an alginate paste provides precise information on its surface topography.

Microscopic Appearance

In more than 90% of cases one is dealing with a squamous cell carcinoma which is usually well differentiated. Murad et al. (1975) distinguish three types: spreading in situ, papillary and submucous. Adenocarcinoma of the vagina, in the absence of any previous oestrogen therapy, is reported in 5%–10% of publications. To confirm its primary vaginal origin one must exclude malignant vaginal extension from an adjacent organ (uterus, rectum) or indeed a distant metastasis (kidney and, in particular, ovary). Malignant melanoma of the vagina only represents 1%–3% of vaginal malignancy. It presents as a pigmented lesion with an overlying mucosa which is often normal in appearance. Primary vaginal sarcomas in adults are equally rare, in contrast to their frequency in childhood.

Natural History

Spread of vaginal cancer, as in cervical cancer, is initially locoregional. Anterior lesions invade the periurethral region, then the trigone of the bladder. Posterior lesions may involve the rectum, and paravaginal extension may occur laterally. In addition to this direct extension of the primary, a search must be made for evidence of blood-borne and, especially, lymphatic spread. The lymphatic drainage of the vagina is explained by its dual embryological origin from the muellerian duct (upper two-thirds) and urogenital sinus (lower third). The first stage of lymphatic drainage from the upper third is that of the external iliac nodes; from the middle third: the external iliac and hypogastric nodes, and from the lower third: the inguinal nodes. The posterior vaginal wall has, in addition, a preferential lymphatic drainage to the superior haemorrhoidal and presacral nodes.

Staging: FIGO Stages

0 Carcinoma in situ
I Confined to vaginal mucosa
IIa Subvaginal infiltration, not into the parametrium
IIb Parametrial invasion, not extending to the pelvic wall
III Tumour extending to the pelvic wall, no distant metastases
IV Tumour extending to the bladder or rectum (IVa), or distant metastases (IVb)

Prognosis and Prognostic Factors

The main prognostic factors in primary adult vaginal carcinoma are tumour size, nodal involvement and histology.

Tumour Size

Although lymph node involvement correlates with the size of the primary, tumour size alone is an important prognostic factor. Table 1 shows the 5-year survival rate by FIGO stage.

Nodal Involvement

Inguinal nodes, as in cancer of the vulva, are hard to assess clinically. Lymphography or CT scanning are useful for pelvic and pancreatic node evaluation. Review of the literature shows a strong correlation of survival with lymph node invasion: for all stages combined, 5-year survival is 50%–60% without and 15%–20% with nodal involvement.

Pathological Characteristics

Exophytic and well-differentiated squamous carcinomas are more radioresponsive and radiocurable. Poorly differentiated or anaplastic tumours present more often with nodal invasion. Sarcomas and melanomas have a poor prognosis. In sarcomas, differentiation is a predictive feature for survival and, according to some authors, for chemosensitivity. For melanomas the prognosis correlates with the characteristics described in cutaneous melanoma according to Hasumi (1970) and McGovern (1970).

Screening of Asymptomatic Disease

Two approaches need to be considered in the screening of asymptomatic disease, namely prevention and screening. Prevention consists of detecting precancerous lesions at a stage when they can be treated before they become malignant. Screening remains a problem of health education, both of the general public and, indeed, of the medical profession. It is also, however, an economic problem. Any mass screening requires qualified personnel, health care facilities, and established channels of communication. In both prevention and screening, insofar as action cannot be taken on the whole of the population, it is necessary to be selective. This selection is based upon known risk factors (previous hysterectomy, annexectomy, pessary, old age).

Diagnosis of Symptomatic Disease

Symptoms

The symptoms of vaginal cancer are comparable to those of cervical cancer: spontaneous or contact bleeding, vaginal discharge, pain, urinary and rectal symptoms. Frank inguinal adenopathy, although rare, must be noted.

Physical Signs

A gynaecological examination enables the tumour to be seen and its local extent appreciated. This examination must be carried out with the utmost care. One must insist upon the whole of the vaginal cavity being examined, rotating the sides of the speculum since they may obscure part of the tumour. The vaginal impression plays an important role since the paste injected into the vagina flattens the mucosa and gives an accurate picture of the vaginal cavity and of the surface topography of the tumour.

Vaginal and rectal examinations, if necessary under a general anaesthetic, enable the vaginal, paravaginal, parametrial and vulval extension of the tumour to be assessed. This examination must be accompanied by an accurate diagram describing the lesions. Such a diagram, while always useful, is essential when external beam and curietherapy are combined. It will serve as a basis for planning the target volume to be irradiated by curietherapy. The inguinal regions are routinely palpated. Particularly detailed examination is required when the lower vagina is involved.

Histology

The formal diagnosis will only be made on the histological evidence of a biopsy. Cytology is indicative, but only biopsy is confirmatory. For lesions of significant size, biopsy presents no difficulty, but in other cases it is facilitated by colposcopy.

Investigations

Apart from any special tests required by virtue of any concomitant diseases, the investigations for vaginal cancer are principally radiological and endoscopic.

Radiology

Radiological investigation should include chest X-ray; intravenous urogram (without compression) to look for urinary tract obstruction and bladder compression due to invasion and uretero-hydronephrosis. Lymphography is useful if positive. Nodal involvement is detectable if metastases are greater than 5 mm in diameter. They are seen as lacunae (seen on the late films). They are not crossed by lymphatic channels (seen in the first phase of the examination). Ultrasound, CT scanning and magnetic resonance imaging complete the radiological work-up, providing additional information on tumour extension and on the character of the lymph nodes.

Endoscopy

Cystoscopy and rectoscopy are required.

Surgical and Combined Treatment of Locoregional Disease

The choice of therapy is governed by the site and local extent of the tumour, the age of the patient and her general medical condition. The main methods of treatment are surgery and radiotherapy, predominantly the latter. Either may be the sole treatment, although the use of surgery alone is rare. Alternatively, they may be combined. We will deal in turn with the methods of treatment that can be recommended for the different stages of vaginal cancer.

Carcinoma In Situ

By definition, these are lesions confined histologically to the superficial layers of the epithelium. Their distribution is not always well defined, and their spread over the vaginal mucosa may be extensive. It is always particularly difficult in a young woman with a localised lesion to suggest a total colpectomy, or vaginal brachytherapy, where the dose of radiation to the ovaries could arrest reproductive endocrine function. Curietherapy must be limited to menopausal women with particularly extensive in situ lesions. Thanks to the modern techniques of brachytherapy in current use, to which we will return later when we consider treatment of invasive vaginal cancer, treatment can be individualised.

For extensive carcinoma in situ, a total colpectomy is a major and mutilating procedure. It can, in some cases, be completed by a graft from the bowel or skin. The current trend is towards conservative brachytherapy, limited surgery or laser therapy. We would stress, however, the difficulties and, sometimes, the hazardous nature of laser therapy in the management of vaginal cancer.

Invasive Cancer

Surgery

Surgery can be limited, with conservation of the ovaries, for lesions confined to the upper third of the vagina in young women. The operative procedure is comparable to that for localised cancer of the cervix (lesions less than 1 cm in diameter) in women under the age of 40. This involves a total extended colpohysterectomy with bilateral external iliac lymphadenectomy. The upper half of the vagina is removed but the ovaries are conserved by transposing them superiorly and laterally to the position of the anterosuperior iliac spines. Such lesions are rare and the few advocates of a surgical approach favour a very extensive operation (Dargent 1980), namely a total colpectomy with a hysterectomy, annexectomy and bilateral ilio-obturator lymphadenectomy. Lesions lower in the vagina could require a vulvo-colpo-hysterectomy with annexectomy and bilateral inguino-cruro-iliac lymphadenectomy. Finally, a total anterior, posterior or modified pelvic exenteration can be proposed, depending on the involvement of bladder or rectum.

Having mentioned the different types of operation, one is well aware of the morbidity and particularly the mortality that they may carry, and that the indications for surgery in vaginal cancer are rare as many authors favour radiotherapy (Perez and Camel 1982; Pirtoli and Santoni 1980; Fletcher 1980; Rousseau et al. 1977; Gerbaulet 1981, 1986).

Radiotherapy

External Radiotherapy

External beam irradiation is carried out using high-energy equipment. Although cobalt 60 is the main treatment source in many centres, a linear accelerator, where available, is preferable because of its higher photon energy which allows shorter treatment times, greater homogeneity of dose distribution, depth dose and, consequently, less frequent complications.

Three target areas for irradiation can be defined, depending on the site of the tumour and of nodal involvement. The basic target area, which is always irradiated in vaginal cancer, is the pelvis. This includes the whole of the vagina, the uterus, adnexa and pelvic nodes. For tumours involving the lower third or lower half of the vagina, this vaginal area is supplemented by fields covering both inguino-crural lymph node chains. This inguinal irradiation is most frequently carried out in separate fields using electrons. The energy level is chosen according to the depth of the tissues to be irradiated. The third area comprises the lumbo-aortic nodes, either irradiated prophylactically if the pelvic nodes are involved, or of necessity if the lumbo-aortic nodes are involved.

The doses delivered are between 45 Gy to the pelvis and 45–55 Gy to the lumbo-aortic and inguino-crural nodes. To these basic doses can be added boosts of localised irradiation of between 5 and 10 Gy. The daily dose varies from 6 to 9 Gy per week and is delivered in four to five daily fractions. The overall duration of external beam therapy is thus between 5 and 7 weeks.

Brachytherapy

The considerable progress made in this area has enabled the indications for brachytherapy in the management of malignant disease to be expanded, particularly in the treatment of vaginal cancer. Radium has virtually disappeared from modern centres, but its use since the beginning of the century enabled considerable experience to be built up. This served as a basis for the brachytherapy practised today. In vaginal cancer two major types of brachytherapy are used: intracavitary and interstitial.

Intracavitary. Numerous standardised applicators of varying adaptability are widely used. However, as

Dargent (1980) writes: "The ideal method is that practised at Institut Gustave-Roussy, based on the use of a vaginal mould". Our method consists of inserting into the vagina a soft, fast-setting paste which hardens in a few minutes. This is then removed from the vagina and enables an impression to be taken which corresponds to the particular anatomy of the patient and accurately delineates the topography of the tumour. From this impression a tailor-made vaginal applicator is fashioned containing the tubes which will later be loaded with the radioactive sources.

Interstitial. Most often combined with intracavitary therapy, interstitial implantation involves incorporating the tumour in a sandwich and irradiating it selectively (Prempree et al. 1977). The nonradioactive preparations used include: guide gutters for periurethral and paravaginal lesions, plastic tubes for lesions involving the posterior and lateral vaginal walls, the latter adapted to different types of applicators for high and circumferential tumours.

The radioactive sources are caesium 137 and iridium 192 for intracavitary therapy and iridium for interstitial therapy. The caesium sources are in the form of a set of blades and iridium as flexible wire. The small diameter, flexibility and the variety of length and activity of these blades or wires and the ease with which other areas can be protected against radiation allow therapy to be individualised for each patient.

The last step in treatment is obviously the calculation of the (prescribed) dose. With computerised dosimetry it is now possible to calculate the dose to precise points (tumour, bladder, rectum, etc.) lymphatic planes, pelvic side walls and to the chosen target volume. Each patient should be given the chance of benefitting from a computerised calculation of the dose, the last but vital step in individualised therapy. This will enable better local tumour control and a much lower rate of complications.

By convention, the dose delivered by curietherapy is 60 Gy. This is reduced when combined with external beam irradiation. In practice, 60 Gy is the minimal dose given to the isodose which encompasses the tumour volume, as long as the dose to the critical organs is compatible with an acceptable risk of complications.

The indications for treatment in a young woman with a tumour confined to the upper third of the vagina can be summarised as follows: colpohysterectomy, lymphadenectomy and transposition of the ovaries, followed by external pelvic irradiation and vaginal curietherapy if the nodes are involved, or by curietherapy alone in the absence of nodal involvement. Other forms of vaginal tumour may benefit from combined external beam irradiation and curietherapy with the proviso that the necessary high-energy equipment, moulded applicators and computerised dosimetry are available.

Adjuvant Treatment

Chemotherapy, as in cervical cancer, has not proved to be of value in vaginal cancer. On the other hand, it may be indicated in patients presenting with nodal involvement. Indeed, if one analyses the causes of death in such patients, 30% are because of secondary metastases. It is logical to suggest adjuvant chemotherapy in patients whose chances of local pelvic control are high, but who are at risk of metastatic disease. Chemotherapy is most often given with a combination of drugs, for example cyclophosphamide (600 mg/m^2) adriamycin (45 mg/m^2). CIS-platinum (50–100 mg/m^2) in monthly cycles can be used equally well, but the various combinations usually also include CIS-platinum.

Treatment of Disseminated Disease

Chemotherapy

The development of metastatic disease is an indication for chemotherapy, of necessity rather than as an adjuvant. If used alone, it is often only used palliatively. For most patients it involves combination chemotherapy, including CIS-platinum.

Radiotherapy

Unfortunately, radiotherapy often has only a palliative role in the treatment of metastatic disease, particularly of bone, brain and lung. For bony metastases, however, it can result in a reduction in the level of analgesics required for pain control.

Surgery

Surgery is indicated for the removal of certain accessible isolated metastases. Overall, surgery, radiotherapy and chemotherapy can be combined in the more favourable cases. Otherwise, chemotherapy can be used alone.

Follow-up

Follow-up visits are made every 3 months for the first 2 years, then every 6 months. Each visit should involve a thorough gynaecological examination and a vaginal smear. Six months after the end of treatment, reassessment should be carried out, including chest X-ray, intravenous urogram, and follow-up lymphogram, with additional tests according to symptoms. The need to maintain the patency of the vagina, particularly in elderly patients, must be stressed, to allow satisfactory follow-up examinations.

Treatment of Recurrence

Surgery plays an essential role in the treatment of recurrence; salvage surgery is, however always a difficult procedure. In patients previously irradiated and in whom the local vaginal recurrence is well localised, conservative resection by an inferior approach or by laser therapy may be considered. These recurrences may be treated by salvage curietherapy as a last resort. A low-dose rate is used to obtain local control without significantly increasing complications.

Unfortunately, recurrences are most often massive, involving the pelvis and the vagina. Insofar as the patient's general medical condition permits it, exploratory laparotomy may be considered. If the recurrence is not associated with distant metastases, anterior, posterior, total or modified pelvic exenteration may be considered. These are major and difficult procedures, more so because they are carried out on irradiated tissues and carry a substantial postoperative morbidity.

For patients previously treated by surgery alone, where the recurrence is well localised, curietherapy or surgical resection by an inferior approach may be indicated. Most often the treatment of choice will be external pelvic or lumbo-aortic irradiation combined with a boost by brachytherapy.

There remains chemotherapy, which at the moment only has a limited effect in the treatment of recurrent disease. It is, however, often the sole feasible means of treatment. Its efficacy will be hampered by the impaired vascular supply within tissue which has been previously irradiated.

Freedom from Disease and Survival

Primary adult vaginal cancer is rare; there are no large published series of patients. We therefore need to pool data from small series in order to compare treatments in terms of disease-free survival and also in terms of therapeutic morbidity.

The Stockholm Report (volume 18, 1973–1975), with 55 reports covering 541 patients, shows an overall survival at 5 years for all stages and treatments of 37,5%. The FIGO 1976 annual report, with 1075 patients, gives a disease-free survival at 5 years of 33.5%. At the Institut Gustave-Roussy we have compared three series (164 patients) of three periods: 1949–1967, 1961–1971 and 1970–1976. The 5-year disease-free survivals were 21%, 30% and 40%, respectively. Finally, an analysis of 24 individual studies published between 1962 and 1983 and comprising 2146 patients, gives an overall 5-year survival of 40.6% (range: 17.1%–51.6%). (Gerbaulet 1981, 1986).

When results are separated according to the type of treatment, however, a different picture emerges. Surgical results from four reports seem much better, with 5-year disease-free survivals of 84% for stage I, 58% for stage II, 38% for stage III and 25% for stage IV (Table 1). Radiotherapy (Table 2) gives 5-year survivals of 58%, 41%, 31% and 9%, respectively. However, a glance at the number of patients for each stage demonstrates the importance of patient selection and the small number suitable for surgery. In addition, most surgically treated patients, especially those with locally advanced disease, have been secondarily irradiated.

Treatment morbidity is an essential consideration. To be useful, surgery must involve complete excision of the primary tumour and the lymph nodes. The minimal surgical procedure is hysterectomy and partial vaginectomy, but more often total vaginectomy or anterior, posterior or total pelvic exenteration

Table 1. Five-year survival by stage after surgical treatment

Reference	Stage				
	I	II	III	IV	Overall
Herbst et al. (1970)	8/10	0/1	4/11	—	12/22 (55%)
Al Kurdi and Monaghen (1981)	5/6	—	—	2/7	7/13 (54%)
Ball et al. (1982)	16/19	5/8	1/2	0/1	22/30 (73%)
	29/35	5/9	5/13	2/8	41/65 (63%)

Table 2. Five-year survival by stage after radiotherapy

	I		II		III		IV		Overall	
	(*n*)	(%)	(*n*)	(%)	(*n*)	(%)	(*n*)	(%)	(*n*)	(%)
Brown et al. (1971)	17/27	63	26/47	55	10/27	37	0/6	0	53/107	50
Rousseau et al. (1977)	9/15	60	10/24	42	8/24	33	1/3	33	28/66	42
Pride et al. (1979)	9/66	14	22/97	23	4/25	16	0/8	0	35/196	18
Kucera (1980)	40/53	75	38/79	48	41/113	36	8/46	17	127/291	44
Pirtoli and Santoni (1980)	8/18	44	0/1	0	2/4	50	0/1	0	10/24	42
Mohlen (1980)	14/19	74	12/29	41	3/25	12	0/9	0	29/82	35
Prempree (1982)	7/9	78	21/37	57	10/26	38	0/8	0	38/80	48
Perez et al. (1982)	34/39	87	26/70	37	4/12	33	1/8	12	65/129	50
Nori (1983)	10/14	71	4/6	67	1/3	33	0/13	0	15/36	42
Benedet et al. (1983)	20/28	71	12/24	50	2/13	15	0/10		34/75	45
	168/288	58	171/414	41	85/272	31	10/112	9		

must be performed. With such extensive surgery and postoperative irradiation, the rate of severe complications ranges from 40% to 50%. In our own most recent series (37 patients, 1970–1976; Gerbaulet 1981, 1986), our severe complication rate for radiotherapy alone was 22%. Minimal complications occurred in 52% and none in 26% of the patients. All patients treated by combined surgery and irradiation died.

Conclusions

Primary adult vaginal carcinoma is rare but serious. The mean age of patients is over 60, and the patients often have poor general medical status. The therapeutic option is usually limited to external irradiation and brachytherapy. To improve treatment results, we feel that a combination of improved radiological techniques of tumour imaging, refinements in external irradiation and especially in brachytherapeutic techniques is essential. With an improvement in tumour localisation, these techniques offer the hope of better local control and survival with a reduction in the complication rate.

References

Al Kurdi M, Monaghan JM (1981) Carcinoma of the vagina. Br J Obstet Gynaecol 88: 1145

Ball HG, Berman ML (1982) Management of primary vaginal carcinoma. Gynaecology 14: 154–163

Benedet JL, Murphy KJ, Fairey RN, Boyes DA (1983) Primary invasive carcinoma of the vagina. Obstet Gynecol 62: 715–719

Brown GR, Fletcher GH, Rutledge FN (1971) Irradiation of in situ and invasive squamous cell carcinomas of the vagina. Cancer 28: 1278–1283

Dargent D (1980) Tumeurs du vagin. Encyclopédie Medico-Chirurgicale, Paris, 530 A 10, 4

FIGO (1976) Annual report on the results of treatment in carcinoma of the uterus, vagina and ovary (ed. Kottmeier HL). Radiumhemmet, Stockholm, vol 16

Fletcher GH (1980) Text book of radiotherapy, 3rd edn. Lee and Febiger, Philadelphia

Gerbaulet A (1981) Le cancer primitif du vagin de l'adulte. Cours de perfectionnement post-universitaire de la Société française de radiologie, 5 November 1981, Paris pp 1–11

Gerbaulet A (1986) Cancer primitif du vagin de l'adulte. Stratégie thérapeutique en cancérologie. Doin, Paris

Hasumi L (1978) Vaginal carcinoma. Cancer 42: 2677–2686

Herbst AL, Green TH, Ulfelder H (1970) Primary carcinoma of the vagina. Am J Obstet Gynecol 106: 210–217

Kucera H, Langer M, Smekal G, Weghaupt K (1983) Zur Klinik und Radiotherapie des primären vaginal Karzinoms. Geburtsh U Frauenheil 43: 443–447

McGovern VJ (1970) The classification of melanoma and its relationship with prognosis. Pathology 2: 85–98

Murad TM, Durant JR, Maddox WA (1975) The pathologic behavior of primary vaginal carcinoma and its relationship to cervical cancer. Cancer 14: 353–358

Möhlen KH et al. (1980) Primary carcinoma of the vagina. An analysis of 82 cases of squamous cell carcinoma. J Cancer Res Clin Oncol 97: 199–204

Nori D, Hilaris BS, Stanimir G et al. (1983) Radiation therapy of primary vaginal carcinoma. Int J Radiat Oncol Biol Phys 9 (10): 1471–1475

Perez CA, Camel H (1982) Long term follow-up in radiation therapy of carcinoma of the vagina. Cancer 49: 1308–1315

Pirtoli L, Santoni N (1980) Radiation therapy of primary vaginal carcinoma. Acta Radiol Oncol Radiat Phys Biol 19: 353–359

Prempree T, Viravathuna T, Slawson R, Wizenberg M, Cascia C (1977) Radiation management of malignant tumor of the vagina. Cancer 40: 109–118

Prempree T (1982) Role of radiation therapy in the management of primary carcinoma of the vagina. Acta Radiol [Oncol] 21 (3): 195–201

Pride GL, Buchler DA (1977) Carcinome of the vagina 10 or more years following pelvic irradiation therapy. Am J Obstet Gynecol 97: 635–649

Pride GL, Schultz AE, Cuprevich TW, Buchler DA (1979) Primary invasive squamous carcinoma of the vagina. Obstet Gynecol 53: 218–225

Rousseau J, Fenton J, Mathieu G, Taleb M (1977) Les cancers vaginaux primitifs de l'adulte. A propos de 72 cas traités à la Fondation Curie de 1956 à 1968. Bull Cancer 64, 3: 429–442

Cancer of the Vulva

G. Michel and A. Gerbaulet

Definition

Malignant tumours of the vulva constitute a heterogeneous group comprising several different histopathological types whose natural history and treatment differ appreciably. In the vast majority of cases, one is dealing with squamous carcinomas. Adenocarcinomas, sarcomas and secondary deposits are rare. These tumours are relatively uncommon (about 4% of gynaecological tumours).

Classification

The most recent classification is the one established by the International Society of Gynaecological Pathologists (Table 1).

Table 1. Classification of malignant tumours of the vulva

1. *Intraepithelial neoplasia*
   A. Squamous intraepithelial neoplasia
      1. (VIN I) Mild dysplasia
      2. (VIN II) Moderate dysplasia
      3. (VIN III) Severe dysplasia or carcinoma in situ
   B. Non-squamous intraepithelial neoplasia
      a. Paget's disease
      b. Tumours of melanocytes, non-invasive

2. *Invasive tumors*
   A. Epithelial tumours of skin and mucosa
      1. Squamous cell carcinoma
         a. Epidermioid carcinoma
         b. Verrucous carcinoma
      2. Basal cell carcinoma
      3. Malignant melanoma
      4. Adenocarcinoma
   B. Malignant tumours of urethra
   C. Bartholin gland carcinoma
      a. Squamous cell carcinoma
      b. Adenocarcinoma
      c. Adenoid cystic carcinoma
      d. Adenosquamous carcinoma
      e. Transitional cell carcinoma
      f. Other carcinomas
   D. Carcinoma and sarcoma of ectopic breast tissue
   E. Soft-tissue sarcomas
      a. Embryonal rhabdomyosarcoma
      b. Leiomyosarcoma
      c. Malignant fibrous histiocytoma
      d. Epithelial sarcoma
      e. Others
   F. Other malignant tumours
      a. Endodermal sinus tumour (yolk sac tumour)
      b. Neuroectodermal tumours
      c. Lymphomas
      d. Others
   G. Secondary and metastatic tumours
   H. Unclassified tumours

Epidemiology and Risk Factors

Cancer of the vulva is very rare in young premenopausal women. The average age of patients is between 60 and 65 years. It is therefore a tumour of menopausal women, a finding confirmed in over 90% of cases.

Among the symptoms with which women present, the most frequently noted and most characteristic of cancer of the vulva is pruritus which may have been present for months or even years. Pruritus is, however, a nonspecific symptom and can occur in simple dystrophic states. Much rarer and indicating a more advanced lesion are symptoms of pelvic or perineal pain or even bleeding.

It is possible that the patient may not have any symptoms but presents because she has noticed a vulvar lesion. This can be an erosion, ulcer or exophytic tumour. It develops most frequently at the level of one of the labia majora, sometimes with extension towards the fourchette and the clitoris. It can arise primarily from the clitoris. One must emphasise that the delay between the lesion being noticed and the time of first presentation may be long since it tends to occur in prudish women of low intelligence.

A certain number of risk factors have been established in 30%–40% of cases: patients have often undergone a premature artificial menopause (40%–50%). Lack of ovarian function, resulting in a deprivation of oestrogen is one of the aetiological factors most commonly cited. Furthermore, in nonmenopausal women, it is common to find clinical signs of hypo-oestrogenism in relation to the external genitalia. The recognition and measurement of hormonal receptors in the vulva has confirmed these clinical observations.

The frequently observed fact that venereal disease has preceded cancer of the vulva prompts one to speculate on the aetiological role of venereal agents, but to date no formal proof has been brought to bear to support this hypothesis. At present, viral factors are being considered in the aetiology of lesions in the vulva.

Cancer of the vulva develops under very special conditions, namely in patients who are elderly and suffering from organic diseases including hypertension, cardiovascular or renal disease, arteritis, obesity, or diabetes mellitus. Numerous authors (e.g. Podratz et al. 1983) have found a higher frequency of diabetes mellitus in women with invasive carcinoma of the vulva than in the normal population.

Cancer of the vulva often develops in pre-existing dystrophic lesions, considered by some to be precancerous, such as atrophic vulvitis, leucoplakia, lichen sclerosus or other dermatoses. The key to diagnosis is, however, histological examination. This necessitates a biopsy of every vulvar lesion, whether or not it is clinically suspicious.

Cancer of the vulva can also be associated with other primary tumours diagnosed either previously or subsequently. Podratz et al. (1983) has noted such an association in 27% of cases. These tumours essentially involve other genital organs, in particular the cervix, and the breast.

Histopathology

Intraepithelial Epithelioma (Bowen's Disease)

Intraepithelial epithelioma is most often a solitary lesion, of variable size, with polycyclic margins, slightly raised, and it is coloured reddish brown. It can affect the cutaneous as well as the mucosal side of the vulva. Histological examination shows that the lesion remains confined to the epithelium without breaching the basement membrane or invading the underlying chorion. Lymphatic invasion does not occur. Colposcopic examination of the cervix must be carried out routinely since it is quite frequent to find associated intraepithelial lesions on both the cervix and the vulva. Where there is invasion of the chorion, not exceeding 5 mm in depth, this is defined as "microinvasive epithelioma", and it is possible to find lymphatic invasion.

Invasive Squamous Cell Carcinoma

Invasive squamous cell carcinoma is the type which usually affects the vulva, representing 90% of malignant tumours of the vulva. From the histological point of view, the tumour can be divided into three subtypes according to the presence or absence of keratinisation and the size of the tumour cells:
- Keratinising
- Nonkeratinising large cells
- Nonkeratinising small cells

This division has been adopted by the World Health Organisation because it appears to be more closely related to prognosis than the standard classification according to degree of differentiation: well, moderately and poorly differentiated.

Nodal metastases are very frequent, the more so the poorer the differentiation.

Verrucous carcinoma or giant condyloma acuminatum (tumours of Buschke-Loewenstein) is a rare type. It presents as a slowly developing exophytic tumor mass and results, after years of growth, in destruction of the anogenital region. A viral aetiology for this lesion is often suspected: its growth remains essentially localised, nodal metastases being exceptional.

Glandular Epithelioma (Adenocarcinoma)

This is rare and develops most often from Bartholin's gland. The histological diagnosis is easy since it is well differentiated. It can be misdiagnosed when the histology is atypical. Its prognosis is very guarded.

Extramammary Paget's disease can be included in this category. It presents in the form of an eczematous or erythematous lesion, greyish-white in colour, well-defined and sometimes ulcerated. Histology shows the presence of large rounded cells with clear and vacuolated cytoplasm with large nuclei in a hyperacanthotic epithelium. PAS staining, even after digestion, is positive. These elements, still called "Paget's cells", are either isolated or en masse. They originate in an intracanalicular epithelioma of the sweat glands and represent, as in the breast, the epithelial extension of the underlying carcinoma. In fact, this epithelial extension is only found in 30% surgical specimens. Its prognosis is similar to intraepithelial epithelioma. It only gives rise to nodal metastases in cases where there is an underlying adenocarcinoma.

Basal Cell Carcinoma

Based cell carcinoma develops slowly on the cutaneous border of the labia majora, never metastasises and has the same histological structure and behaviour as its cutaneous counterpart at other sites.

Sarcoma

Sarcomas are rare and occur in children as well as adults. For the most part, they are fibroblastic sarcomas, liposarcomas or sarcomas with giant polymorphic cells. Their prognosis is poor because they give rise to distant metastases which are essentially to the lungs.

Malignant Melanoma

Malignant melanoma is a highly malignant tumour developing from an abnormal proliferation of pigment-producing cells: the melanocytes. It is a rare tumour appearing after the fifth decade in the form of a brown or black lesion, usually ulcerated and bleeding easily. These tumours rapidly give rise to metastases, both locoregional and distant (peritoneum, lung, liver, heart, brain, breast, kidney, etc.).

Metastatic Tumours

Metastatic tumours are rare. Usually they form an extension to the vulva from a neighbouring tumour of uterine origin. A few cases of vulvar metastasis of hydatidiform mole, chorion carcinoma, malignant melanoma or of renal cell carcinoma have been described (Krupp 1981).

Natural History

The spread of cancer of the vulva occurs at three levels: locoregional, lymphatic and distant sites.

Locoregional Spread

It is the labia majora that are most commonly affected. Lesions of the labia minora and of the clitoris are rarer. Then come bilateral lesions of the labia majora and minora. Lesions involving the whole of the vulva are now extremely uncommon.

Spread is either superficial or deep towards the vaginal mucosa, the urethral meatus, the anterior extension of the ischiorectal fossa and the genitocrural groove, with extension to the mons veneris and to the skin of the root of the thigh. The posterior fourchette and anal canal are invaded later. This locoregional extension is one of the most serious features of the spread of cancer of the vulva.

Lymphatic Spread

Cancer of the vulva is very lymphophilic. Lymphatic spread occurs towards the superficial and deep inguinal nodes and then to the external iliac and para-aortic nodes. For lesions arising in the clitoris, the external iliac nodes can be involved first. Inguinal node involvement occurs, on average, in 50% of cases. Two features characterise this spread:

- Clinical appearance is deceptive. Indeed, nonpalpable inguinal nodes can be histologically invaded. On the other hand, palpable, mobile clinically suspicious nodes can be inflammatory. However, fixed or ulcerated nodes are, in general, positive.
- The frequency of bilateral inguinal node involvement is 60% for bilateral vulvar tumours, and 20%–30% for unilateral lesions.

Distant Spread

Distant spread with visceral or bony metastasis is rare because the locoregional growth and the advanced age of these patients does not often allow tumours to reach this stage.

Staging

The clinical classification most widely used is the TNM classification adopted by FIGO (Table 2). In practice, accurate clinical assessment of local tumour extension is made more difficult by obesity, which is frequent in these patients, and by the almost constant inflammatory nature of vulvar tumours. The presence of nonpalpable metastatic nodes or en-

Table 2. TNM classification

T Primary tumour		
Tis	(Stage 0)	Carcinoma in situ
T0	(Stage 0)	No evidence of primary tumour
T1	(Stage 1)	Tumour confined to the vulva – 2 cm or less in diameter
T2	(Stage 2)	Tumour confined to the vulva, more than 2 cm in diameter
T3	(Stage 3)	Tumour of any size with adjacent spread to the urethra and/or vagina and/or perineum and/or to the anus
T4	(Stage 4)	Tumour of any size infiltrating the bladder mucosa and/or the rectal mucosa or both, including the upper part of the urethral mucosa and/or fixed to the bone
N Regional lymph nodes		
N0	N0 nodes palpable	
N1	Nodes palpable in either groin not enlarged, mobile (not clinically suspicious of neoplasm)	
N2	Nodes palpable in either one or both groins enlarged, firm and mobile (clinically suspicious of neoplasm)	
N3	Fixed or ulcerated nodes	
M Distant metastases		
M0	No clinical metastases	
M1	Palpable deep pelvic lymph nodes	
M1b	Other distant metastases	

Table 3. Staging of cancer of the vulva. (From Krupp and Bohm 1978)

Stage 0	"In situ" cancer
	A Single site
	C Central (clitoral only)
	L Lateral (labial, including fourchette)
	CL Combined
	B Multiple sites: C, L, CL
Stage I	Invasive lesions (3 cm or less in greatest diameter)
	A Single site C, L or CL
	B Multiple sites C, L, CL
Stage II	Invasive lesions (greater than 3 cm)
	A Single site
	B Multiple sites
Stage III	Invasive lesion with extension to superficial or deep inguinal lymph nodes (histologically proven)
	A Unilateral lymph node involvement
	B Bilateral lymph node involvement
Stage IV	Vulvar lesions with involvement of contiguous organs and/or metastases beyond regional lymph nodes
	A Contiguous organ involvement
	B Bony or distant metastases
	A–B Both of the above

larged noninvolved inflammatory nodes is an example of the difficulties encountered in trying to achieve accurate preoperative clinical staging. The size of the tumour can be enlarged by the presence of oedema, and therefore the appraisal of the involvement of the vulva and vagina can be very difficult.

The percentage error in clinical assessment increases progressively with the stage of the disease, from 10% for stages I and II to 30% for stages III and IV. The results of postoperative staging show a constant upgrading of clinically staged I or II patients, and it is not uncommon to downstage stages III and IV when the histopathology is available. This is the reason why a surgical and histological staging procedure seems to be more accurate. The staging method used by Krupp and Bohm (1978) can be recommended (Table 3).

Prognosis – Prognostic Factors

The main prognostic factors are lymphatic invasion, size of the tumour and histological features of the tumour.

Lymphatic Invasion

Inguinal Nodes

It is nearly impossible to assess lymphatic invasion clinically. On average 20% of nonpalpable inguinal nodes are histologically positive, and equally, 20% of palpable and clinically suspect nodes are negative. That is why only nodal dissection can provide histological proof of lymphatic invasion.

In 40%–50% of cases, there is inguinal node involvement, and in this population the risk of recurrence and of death is multiplied three-fold. The 5-year survival rate decreases from 80% for patients with negative nodes to 30% for patients with positive nodes.

Pelvic Nodes

Authors who have carried out a routine pelvic lymphadenectomy (Krupp 1981; Hacker et al. 1988; Franklin and Rutledge 1971; Monaghan and Hammond 1984) have shown that:

- Pelvic nodal invasion is rare (< 3%).
- In the absence of inguinal nodal invasion, the risk of invasion of the pelvic nodes is very slight.
- As a result, involvement of the pelvic nodes is only seen when the inguinal nodes are involved and, more commonly, when there is a higher number of positive inguinal nodes (> 3).
- The only site prone to accompanying isolated pelvic nodal invasion is the clitoris.
- Finally, invasion of the pelvic nodes in patients with positive inguinal nodes does not worsen the prognosis.

Size of the Tumour

The size of the tumour is a prognostic factor which is directly correlated with nodal invasion. The frequency of inguinal node involvement increases with the size of the tumour and thus with the stage. For tumours between 2 and 4 cm, one finds about 35% positive nodes. For tumours over 4 cm, 50% or more have nodal invasion.

Characteristics of the Tumour

The characteristics of the tumour constitute another prognostic factor which correlates with nodal involvement. Indeed, its frequency is much higher the deeper the invasion of the stroma and the poorer the differentiation. The percentage of positive nodes is much higher in anaplastic tumours than in well-differentiated tumours. It is in this respect that grade has a prognostic significance.

Screening of Asymptomatic Disease

Routine examination of the vulva must be an integral part of every gynaecological examination. It is in this way that asymptomatic vulvar lesions, such as intraepithelial carcinomas can be detected. More than 10% of invasive tumours have no warning symptoms. The diagnosis could be suggested by cytology, but only routine biopsy of every vulvar lesion can prove the diagnosis. Biopsy can be guided by the fluorescent induction test with tetracycline, which often shows lesions extending beyond the visible clinical limits, and by colposcopy, which can provide substantial diagnostic help.

Diagnosis of Symptomatic Disease

The vast majority of vulvar tumours are accompanied by symptoms dominated by pruritus. Examination of the vulva will enable one to discover a lesion which is already clinically very suggestive, whether it be an ulcer, an exophytic, or an exophytic and ulcerating lesion. The diagnosis depends upon routine biopsy of such lesions.

The inguinal regions will be systematically palpated. As for the pelvic nodes, information can be derived from lymphography and from CT scanning, but these examinations are generally little used in the pretreatment work-up of cancer of the vulva.

Surgical and Combined Treatment

Surgery is always the treatment of choice in malignant tumours of the vulva.

Squamous Cell Carcinoma

Invasive Form

Three reasons justify the choice of surgery:
- The locoregional spread is the main mode of growth of cancer of the vulva.
- There is often multifocal spread. In 20% of cases, secondary microscopic foci are found, occurring at any site on the vulva. As a result the vulva can be considered as an organ which must be excised in its entirety. This condemns any partial vulvectomy. Total vulvectomy is thus the minimal treatment for the primary tumour.
- The frequency of inguinal nodal invasion (about 50% of cases) has as its corollary the necessity of carrying out an inguinal node dissection which, ideally, must be bilateral given the anatomical cross-over of the nodal chains (the frequency of bilateral nodal involvement is 60% for bilateral tumours of the vulva and 20%–30% for unilateral lesions) and the impossibility of confirming their involvement or noninvolvement by simple clinical examination.

Lymphatic dissection will include:
- The superficial supra-aponevrotic inguinal nodes
- The sub-aponevrotic deep inguinal nodes

In addition, some authors (Krupp and Bohm 1978) have recommended carrying out a routine pelvic lymphadenectomy. However, it is not acceptable in the absence of inguinal nodal involvement or, in particular, of Cloquet's node, where involvement of the pelvic nodes is very improbable. Under these conditions, the only site that can justify routine bilateral pelvic lymphadenectomy is the clitoris. This is because this can drain directly to the external iliac nodes via the pedicle of the round ligament (the superior pedicle of Basset). This pelvic lymphadenectomy will be carried out by an extraperitoneal approach.

As a result, in the majority of cases the ideal treatment will consist of a simultaneous total vulvectomy with bilateral inguinal node dissection: inguinal node dissection will be performed through separate incisions beginning 2 cm inside the anteriosuperior iliac spine, crossing the inguinal ligament and stopping 2 cm outside the middle of the lateral vulvar incision.

Unfortunately, the indications for such surgery are limited since it involves a long and destructive operation which can only reasonably be proposed for relatively young women and those free of the general medical diseases usually encountered. However, cancer of the vulva develops most often in elderly women, who are, moreover, often suffering from various organic diseases: obesity diabetes, renal or cardiovascular disease.

For the purposes of treatment one can distinguish three groups of patients (Michel and Lacour 1981; Gerbaulet and Michel 1986).

- Patients who are still young and in good general medical condition who justify a total vulvectomy and routine bilateral inguinal node dissection, knowing that the vulvectomy can be enlarged, according to the extent of the vulvar lesion: (a) either to the inferior part of the urethra or to the skin of the genitocrural groove laterally which may necessitate a skin flap or graft; (b) or to the anus and to the anal sphincter if the tumour lies posteriorly (posterior exenteration with permanent colostomy).
- Elderly patients and those in poor medical condition should only undergo a simple total vulvectomy. Lymph nodes confirmed by needle cytology or limited biopsy will be treated by radiotherapy if they are positive.
- Finally, the patients in between these extremes who cannot undergo radical surgery without very considerable risks, but whose general condition allows a total vulvectomy and elective unilateral or bilateral nodal sampling.

In the latter category, several therapeutic options are possible depending upon the clinical state of the lymph nodes:
- There are no palpable nodes: avoidance of any nodal dissection.
- There are palpable nodes: a simple node sampling with frozen section examination initially to avoid nodal clearance if the lymph nodes are purely inflammatory. If the nodes are involved, a unilateral inguinal node dissection is carried out by a separate incision or a bilateral inguinal node dissection by two separate incisions where the nodes are positive bilaterally.

Finally, in certain cases of large, infected and painful tumours, whatever the age and general condition of the patient, a "toilet" vulvectomy under epidural anaesthesia can be suggested.
This surgery results in:
- An operative mortality rate which varies between 2% and 10% according to different authors (Podratz et al. 1983; Michel and Lacour 1981; Michel et al. 1978) and which reflects the particularly unfavourable conditions in which these tumours develop.
- A significant morbidity dominated by local complications which become more serious as the extent of the operation increases.
- Almost invariably necrosis of skin flaps, most often with superinfection which prolongs hospitalisation because wound healing is very slow.
- Frequent but transient lymphorrhoea despite routine aspiration drainage.
- Transient resolving oedema of the lower limbs.
- Massive haemorrhage due to necrosis of the femoral artery, very rare.

These complications can result in the following sequelae:
- Chronic oedema of the lower limbs which can result in substantial functional incapacity.
- Painful retractile scarring.
- Vaginal prolapse and urinary stress incontinence are rare.

The indications for radiotherapy are limited:
1. At the level of the vulva in the following circumstances:
- Preoperatively, usually by electrons, with the aim of reducing a very bulky tumour and allowing its excision.
- Peroperatively in the form of interstitial curietherapy allowing the indications for pelvectomy to be curtailed.
- Postoperatively, when histological examination shows that the excision is insufficient, using either external beam irradiation or interstitial curietherapy according to the degree of residual tumour.

2. At the level of the nodes by external beam irradiation:
- Where the nodes are fixed.
- In all cases without palpable nodes where lymph node dissection has been contraindicated or where positive nodes have only been biopsied.
- Postoperatively if there are several nodes invaded or a single node invaded but with capsular rupture.

The indications for supplementary radiotherapy must always be considered with circumspection since the risk of complications is increased in cases where radiotherapy and surgery are combined, and these complications may become very incapacitating by virtue of the sclerosis added by radiotherapy.

Finally, there is a limited group of patients whose general medical state is so precarious and in whom the local or locoregional extent is so substantial that only radiotherapy alone can be attempted.

As for chemotherapy, bleomycin has been tried but without showing any great benefit.

Verrucous Epithelioma. Its treatment is purely surgical: total vulvectomy, extended, if necessary, to the skin, neighbouring organs and inguinal nodes. In these circumstances, radiotherapy would be ineffective or even harmful.

Preinvasive Form

Surgery can be conservative: simple excision of the lesion or partial superficial vulvectomy with histological verification of the resection margins by frozen section and without lymph node dissection.

Other types of treatment have been suggested (George et al. 1985):

1. Applications of 5-fluorouracil (5FU) or dinitrochlorobenzene (DNCB) with variable results.
2. Destruction by vaporisation using CO_2 laser, which can be carried out on an outpatient basis and on several occasions if the lesions are multifocal. This form of treatment would appear to be indicated in particular in young women on two conditions:
   - That the absence of microinvasion has been previously confirmed by one or more biopsies
   - That the patients have been informed of the risk of recurrence and the need for strict follow-up.

Other Histopathological Types Requiring Surgery

Glandular Carcinoma (Adenocarcinoma)

If it is a tumour of Bartholin's gland, the treatment is surgical with combined total vulvectomy and routine bilateral inguinal node dissection.

If it is Paget's disease, we have recourse to a routine total vulvectomy. The need for a supplementary inguinal node dissection will be dictated by histological examination of the operative specimen. Node dissection is indicated if there is an underlying adenocarcinoma.

Basal Cell Carcinoma

The treatment of basal cell carcinoma is surgical, but one is satisfied with a superficial partial vulvectomy, ensuring that the vulval resection, taking a wide margin around the lesions, is checked histologically by frozen section of the skin margins. Under these conditions recurrences can always be avoided.

Sarcoma

Treatment of sarcomas is again surgical and combined with chemotherapy.

Malignant Melanoma

Surgery of malignant melanomas will involve a standard total vulvectomy. Lymphatic dissection is only indicated in the presence of palpable inguinal nodes. Radiotherapy is ineffective, and chemotherapy has now been abandoned for the same reasons.

Metastatic Tumours

In cases of metastatic tumours palliative resection of the metastasis may be indicated.

Adjuvant Treatment

Innovations that may improve results include chemotherapy to reduce extensive lesions, eradicate occult nodal metastases or control advanced disease. The single agent that has been most extensively investigated for chemotherapy of squamous cell carcinoma of the vulva is bleomycin. Some objective responses have been reported (Blum et al. 1973). Bleomycin in combination with radiotherapy tends to give more complete responses and a longer duration of response than bleomycin alone.

Reports on combination chemotherapy are few: the European Gynecological Cancer Group Study (1987) have assessed combination chemotherapy with bleomycin, methotrexate and lomustine for locally advanced inoperable disease in order to study response rate and operability after chemotherapy and also the sideeffects of the chemotherapeutic regimen. Early analysis of the 20 fully evaluable patients showed a complete response in two and partial response in ten (a response rate of 60%). Of particular interest was the fact that in seven of these patients, disease became amenable to radical surgery of major therapeutic benefit and producing the only possibility of cure. However, the level of toxicity of this schedule was high. It was therefore proposed to study the efficacy and toxicity of a modified schedule.

Treatment of Disseminated Disease

Cancer of the vulva mainly spreads locoregionally. Distant metastases are rare. In these cases chemotherapy can be tried, but in general one is limited to treatment aimed at pain relief.

Follow-up

Regular and unlimited follow-up is essential following treatment of any malignant lesion of the vulva. Even with carcinoma in situ, which has an excellent prognosis, there is always the risk of local recurrence which remains surgically curable. Any suspicious vulvar lesion appearing after treatment of an invasive lesion must be biopsied. Any palpable inguinal node must be needled for cytological examination.

Recurrences generally occur during the first 2 years following treatment. Their frequency is related to nodal invasion and to the number of nodes involved. According to Hacker et al. (1983), the rates of vulvar and inguinal recurrences are, respectively 6% and between 3% and 33% when there are more than three nodes involved. Franklin and Rutledge (1971) found a 20% inguinal recurrence rate in node-positive cases. Månaghan and Hammond (1984) gave rates of vulval and inguinal recurrence at 60% and 20%, respectively, in node-positive patients. At the Institut Gustave-Roussy, the risk of local recurrence is increased by a factor of 2.5 in patients who are node positive. In addition, all authors agree that the risk of recurrence is greatly increased (on average three-fold) when lymphatic dissection has not been carried out.

Treatment of Recurrence

Treatment of recurrence is palliative. If it occurs in the vulva, it is sometimes possible to contemplate an exenteration or to combine a limited resection with peroperative interstitial implantation. If it occurs in the inguinal region, a second operation is rarely possible, and often the only possibility is palliative external irradiation, combined with chemotherapy.

Survival

The 5-year survival rate is a function of the size of tumour and the nodal status. Overall 5-year survival for stages I and II is good, varying between 75% and 80% according to different authors (Monaghan and Hammond 1984; Podratz et al. 1983; Hacker et al. 1983; Franklin and Rutledge 1971; Michel and Lacour 1981; Michel et al. 1978). The survival rate for stage III is, on average, 60% and for stage IV 0%–20%.

The overall 5-year survival rate for patients without nodal invasion is, on average, between 85% and 90%. By contrast, patients who are node positive have a 5-year survival rate of about 40%–45%. In this latter category, the number of nodes involved is the critical factor. Generally, where there are more than two nodes involved, the 5-year survival rate is about 20%.

Finally, the results are clearly related to the type of treatment. Patients who have benefitted from a vulvectomy and bilateral inguinal node clearance have a 5-year survival which is twice that of patients treated by radiotherapy alone. This latter group, however, includes the most advanced tumours in the most elderly women.

Rehabilitation

Vulvectomy is a mutilating procedure but is nonetheless generally well tolerated by patients, as long as one explains that the operation has an immediate analgesic effect and that sexual intercourse remains possible. Naturally, the operation is much more difficult for younger patients to accept than older ones.

In cases where an exenteration is indicated, the surgeon ought previously to have discussed at length and in detail with the patient the nature of the mutilation to which she will be subjected and to obtain her firm acceptance and cooperation. These patients will be managed by a department which has specialist experience in looking after the proper function of stomas.

The possible late complications are oedema of the lower limbs related to nodal clearance which can be particularly incapacitating. It may involve the thigh alone, more rarely the leg, sometimes extending to the whole operative site, reaching the abdomen and the perivulvar region. Sometimes it can result in substantial functional impairment. Crural hernias are uncommon. Prolapse and urinary stress incontinence are rare but can require surgical correction if they cause a significant handicap. Finally, one can see painful retractile scarring, particularly when radiotherapy and surgery are combined. It may require surgical repair.

Future Developments

The only hope of no longer seeing advanced tumours of the vulva rests with better education of patients and doctors. As a result, preinvasive forms, which we know can be cured without mutilation or sequelae, could be diagnosed. The development of contraceptive methods ought to permit the eradication of invasive tumours due to the regular follow-up required for these women, on the condition that doctors include routine examination of the vulva in every gynaecological examination.

References

Blum RH et al. (1973) A clinical review of bleomycin. A new antineoplastic agent. Cancer 31: 903–914

Franklin EW, Rutledge FD (1971) Prognostic factors in epidermoid carcinoma of the vulva. Obstet Gynecol 37 (6): 892–901

George M, Avril MF, Duvillard P, Michel G, Wolff JP (1985) Epithelioma intraepithelial de la vulve. Etude de 19 cas traités à l'Institut Gustave-Roussy de 1970 à 1984. Gynécologie 36 (3): 243–245

Gerbaulet A, Michel G (1986) Le cancer de la vulve. Stratégie thérapeutique en cancérologie. Doin, Paris, pp 273–278

Hacker NF, Berek JS, Lagasse LD, Leuchter RS, Moore JG, Hacker NF (1983) Management of regional lymph nodes and their prognostic influence in vulvar cancer. Obstet Gynecol 61 (4): 408–412

Krupp PJ (1981) Invasive tumours of vulva: clinical features and management. In: Coppleson M (ed) Gynecologic oncology, vol 1. Churchill Livingstone, Edinburgh, pp 329–338

Krupp PJ, Bohm JW (1978) Lymph gland metastases in invasive squamous cell cancer of the vulva. Am J Obstet Gynecol 130 (8): 943–952

Michel G, Lacour J (1981) Les vulvectomies pour cancer invasif de la vulve. Encyclopedie Medico-Chirurgicale Paris, 4.7.07, 41890

Michel G, Lacour J, Frydmann R, Chassagne D, Wolff JP, Prade M (1978) Epithélioma épidermoïde de la vulve. Gynécologie 29: 671–676

Monaghan JM, Hammond IG (1984) Pelvic node dissection in the treatment of vulval carcinoma; is it necessary? Br J Obstet Gynecol 91: 270–274

Podratz KC, Richard PD, Symmonds E, Taylor WF, Williams PD, Williams TJ (1983) Carcinoma of the vulva: analysis of treatment and survival. Obstet Gynecol 61 (1): 63–74

Cancer of the Breast

U. Veronesi, A. Costa, and P. Veronesi

Epidemiology and Prevention

Every year some 800000 women throughout the world develop a carcinoma in their breast. Out of these, some 180000 occur in Europe, where breast cancer is the most common type of cancer among women, representing 20% of all female malignancies. Also in North America, in Australia and in many Latin American countries, breast cancer is the most frequent cancer in women. Breast cancer is exceptional before the age of 20 and is rare below 30, but then the incidence rises very steadily up to the age of 50, after which the rate of increase slows down considerably, although the incidence continues to rise (Fig. 1). This difference in the shape of the age-specific curves has suggested that there may be two types of breast cancer, one hormonally induced in the early decades and one nutritionally induced in the late decades (De Waard 1980). The difference in the age-specific incidence curve in Japanese women, which shows no increase in incidence rates after the age of 50, has been explained by a "cohort" effect, with women of younger ages having a greater expected breast cancer risk than the women from earlier birth cohorts (Stevens et al. 1982). Mortality rates for breast cancer in western Europe are in the order of 15–25 per 100000 women, i. e. 30%–50% of the incidence rates, which are around 50–60 per 100000 women.

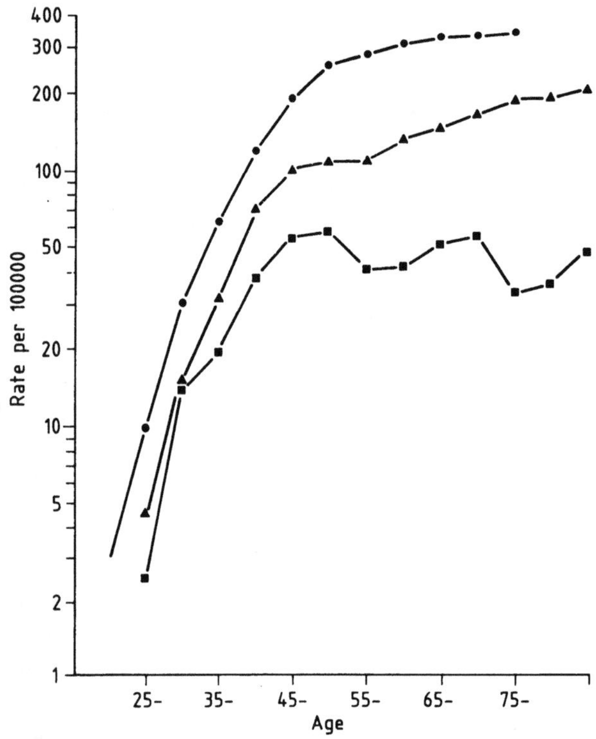

Fig. 1. Examples of age-specific incidence curves for breast cancer. *Circles,* Los Angeles whites; *triangles,* Finland; *squares,* Miyagi, Japan

Time Trends

The incidence of breast carcinoma is increasing in most countries in the world, at an average of 1%–2% annually (Table 1). It is interesting to note that this trend is, in general, more pronounced in low-risk populations than in high-risk populations with a tendency, therefore, to a levelling off in a distant future. For instance, it appears likely that the big difference in incidence between women living in western countries and those living in Japan will decrease

Table 1. Breast cancer incidence per 100000 in some European countries and mean annual rate of increase

Registry and country	Year	Rate	Year	Rate	Annual increase (%)
Denmark	1955	43.8	1974/1975	58.5	1.8
FRG – Hamburg	1961	37.8	1975	55.7	3.4
FRG – Saarland	1970	50.6	1975	57.2	2.6
Finland	1960	26,3	1973/1974	40.1	3.9
GDR	1965	28.6	1975	37.4	3.1
Hungary – Szabolcs	1964	17.3	1975	20.6	1.7
Israel	1963	44.9	1974	59.9	3.0
Norway	1960	39.0	1975	49.6	1.8
Poland – Warsaw	1965/1966	28.4	1975	36.5	3.0
Spain – Saragossa	1970	30.6	1975	36.5	3.9
Sweden	1960	29.1	1973	55.2	6.9
Switzerland – Geneva	1971	70.6	1975	76.1	2.0
UK – Birmingham	1961	46.8	1974/1975	56.4	1.5
UK – Sheffield	1964/1965	46.4	1968/1969	49.6	1.7
Yugoslavia – Slovenia	1958	21.3	1974/1975	34.2	3.7

Table 2. Breast cancer mortality per 100 000 in some European countries and mean annual rate of increase

Country	Rate 1950–1951	Rate 1978–1979	Mean annual increase (%)
Austria	14.28	18.71	1.7
Belgium	19.04	25.49	2.5
Denmark	24.36	24.74	0.1
England and Wales	23.19	27.74	1.1
Finland	10.73	14.87	2.1
France	12.73	18.10	2.3
FRG	14.72	20.52	2.2
Israel	16.89	23.20	2.1
Italy	12.27	18.48	2.9
Netherlands	23.28	25.79	0.6
Norway	17.32	19.05	0.6
Portugal	10.54	14.54	3.2
Scotland	22.01	27.61	1.4
Sweden	15.83	18.07	0.8
Switzerland	21.24	23.78	0.7

with time. In Europe the highest increase in incidence rates has occurred in Sweden (6.9% annually between 1960 and 1973), in Spain, Saragossa (3.9% annually between 1970 and 1975), in Finland (3.9% annually between 1960 and 1974), while the lowest rates were observed in Norway and Denmark (1.8% annually between 1965 and 1975). The mortality rates are also increasing in Europe (Table 2), but at a lower pace, with the lowest values in Denmark, the Netherlands, Norway, Sweden and Switzerland (0.1%–0.8% increase annually) and the highest values in Belgium, France, Germany, Italy, Portugal (2.2%–3.2% increase annually) between 1950 to 1979.

Geographical Variations

As with most cancer types, breast cancer shows a wide variation in incidence and mortality in different countries. The highest incidence rates have been observed among white Americans in Hawaii, among women living in British Columbia (Canada) and among white inhabitants of California. In these areas, the annual incidence rate is around 80–90 per 100 000 women. On the opposite side, the lowest incidence has been observed in some areas of Japan with an incidence rate around 12–15 per 100 000 women. Western Europe shows rates which range from 40–60 cases per 100 000 women annually, whilst Indian, African and Chinese women show figures which are intermediate between European and Japanese women. Latin American women show incidence rates either close to the European ones in some areas (Sao Paulo, Brazil), or close to the Indian ones in other areas (Puerto Rico). Among European countries the highest incidence has been observed in Switzerland (Geneva) and the lowest in Spain (Saragossa), in Yugoslavia (Slovenia) and in Poland (Cracow). Apart from these examples, in general, the incidence rates in Europe decrease from the north to the south and from west to east. Inside each country, breast cancer incidence correlates well with the per capita income of the population in the various districts. A recent analysis on cancer mortality in Finland (Pukkala et al. 1986) shows that the high-risk areas for breast cancer are those in which there is a high proportion of women in the higher social classes. In Italy the mortality rates for breast cancer in the northern regions are twice those of the southern areas (Cislaghi et al. 1986).

Studies conducted among Japanese migrants to California (Dunn 1977) have clearly shown a tendency of these populations to reach the incidence rates of the women living in the host countries, thus confirming within a couple of generations the great importance of the environment, meaning with this term all external factors, including life style.

Family Factors

A number of studies conducted in many countries in the last few decades have shown a uniform two- to three-fold increase of risk of breast cancer among first-degree relatives of patients with cancer of the breast (Wassink 1935; Martynova 1937; Penrose et al. 1948; Smithers 1948; Bucalossi et al. 1954; Macklin 1959; Tulinius et al. 1982). In particular, the Milan study (Bucalossi et al. 1954) showed an increased risk in relatives of patients with bilateral breast carcinoma. More detailed studies by Anderson published in the early 1970s (Anderson 1972, 1976) showed that relatives of breast cancer patients in whom the onset of the disease was in premenopause had a three-fold higher risk of breast carcinoma, whilst relatives of patients with bilateral carcinoma had a five-fold higher risk. If the two variables were associated (premenopausal onset and bilaterality) and it was a first-degree relationship, the risk increased to nine-fold.

A more recent study conducted in Sweden by Adami et al. (1981) drastically reduced the importance of the familial factor, showing a relative risk of 1.7 times higher in mothers and sisters of breast cancer patients compared to the risk of mothers and sisters of controls. When the carcinoma was bilateral and the onset of the disease occurred in premenopause, the risk increased to 2.4 and 2.2, respectively. It is impossible to establish how much of this increased familial risk is due to a common life style, including diet, among the members of the same family and how much is due to a genetically inherited factor which might increase the susceptibility to breast carcinoma.

Benign Breast Disease

Apart from particular types of benign breast proliferations like diffuse papillomatosis and atypical hyperplasia, it is generally accepted that the most common types of benign breast diseases (fibroadenomas, cystic disease) do not bear an important increase in the risk of breast carcinoma. The fact that many studies (Table 3) have shown a two-fold increased risk of breast carcinoma among patients with cystic disease (Veronesi and Pizzocaro 1968; Donnelly et al. 1975; Kodlin et al. 1977; Page et al. 1978; Hutchinson et al. 1980) may be partly explained by other factors which are associated with cystic disease, like pauci-parity, which in turn increase the risk of breast cancer.

Endocrine Factors

The facts that nulliparous women are at increased risk of breast cancer (Mustacchi 1961), that, on the contrary, a full-term pregnancy before the age of 20 protects women from the disease (MacMahon et al. 1970) and that women who have had their ovaries removed or inactivated before the age of 40 years have a reduced risk of breast cancer (Lilienfeld 1956) clearly show that a relationship must exist between reproductive hormonal factors and breast carcinoma. However, which specific hormones may be involved in this process and by which mechanisms has not been clarified.

The estrogenic hypothesis is one of the oldest and is mainly based on experimental evidence in laboratory animals and on the progression of the disease in women during estrogenic stimulation. The reproductive history of women with breast cancer is not completely in favour of the estrogen hypothesis, since repeated full-term pregnancies at an early age, with the consequent long-lasting increase of estrogen levels, are associated with a decreased risk of breast cancer and since prolonged lactations, which suppress the estrogenic exposure, do not reduce the risk. Moreover, administration of estrogens in old women with breast cancer often results in a long-lasting regression of the breast carcinoma and of its metastases.

The hypothesis that the amount of estriol (E_3) relative to estrone (E_1) and estradiol (E_2) produced in the early years after menarche is inversely correlated to subsequent breast cancer risk (Cole and MacMahon 1969; Lemon 1969) has been challenged on several grounds by many authors (Marmosten et al. 1965; Zumoff et al. 1975).

A variation of the estrogen hypothesis is the "two windows" one which postulates that there are two periods (early pubertal years and perimenopausal years) during which the breast tissue is exposed to estrogens without adequate exposure to progesterone (Korenman 1980).

Table 3. Comparison between prospective studies of patients who had biopsies and later had cancer and the number of cancers predicted by the 1970 and 1976 surveys of the NCI

Study	Patients (*n*)	Average follow-up (years)	Incidence reported in paper			Recalculated incidence			
						1970 NCI survey		1976 NCI survey	
			Cancers observed	Cancers predicted	Increased risk	Cancers predicted	Increased risk	Cancers predicted	Increased risk
Kodlin et al. (1977)	2900	7	67	23.8	2.69	20.4	3.13	23.0	2.78
Veronesi and Pizzocaro (1968)	875	8.75	16	10.1	1.58	10.5	1.52	11.9	1.34
Donnelly et al. (1975)	370	17.5	14	8.5	1.64	7	2	8	1.75
Page et al. (1978)	925	20	31	22.6	1.37	25.3	1.22	29.1	1.06
Hutchinson et al. (1980)	1441	12.9	66	31.5	2.10	26.6	2.48	30.8	2.15
	6511		191	96.5	1.98	89.8	2.13	102.8	1.86

A protective action of progesterone has been suggested, and it has also been proposed that the full differentiation of the breast tissue due to pregnancy allows the breasts of parous women to respond to progesterone, whilst the mammary gland of nulliparous women are unable to incorporate it. However, the epidemiological evidence in support of the protective hypothesis of progesterone is very weak.

It has also been shown that women with breast cancer often have anovulatory cycles, due to the fact that estrogen secretion is accompanied by an inadequate progesterone formation (Grattarola 1978).

Increased levels of androgens have also been proposed as a possible carcinogenic factor for breast cancer. This hypothesis is mainly supported by the fact that incidence of breast cancer is considerably higher in postmenopausal women, when estrogenic levels are low and androgenic levels are high, that administration of androgens for cystic disease has been shown to increase the risk of breast cancer (Veronesi and Pizzocaro 1968) and that increased levels of androgenic metabolites and low levels of progesterone have been found in premenopausal women with breast cancer compared to controls (Secreto et al. 1984). Moreover, Japanese women, who are at a lower risk of breast cancer than British women, have lower plasma androgen levels.

Recent studies have shown that elevated levels of sex hormone-binding globulin (SHBG), a protein present in human serum capable of binding to both androgens and estrogens, reduce the availability of estrogens to the mammary epithelium (Siiteri et al. 1981). The SHBG would therefore play a fundamental role in any possible type of endocrine carcinogenesis, either in the estrogen or in the androgen hypothesis.

Although old studies suggested that the use of dopamine antagonist could increase the breast cancer risk (Jick et al. 1974), due to an increased production of prolactin, more recent investigations have failed to confirm these data, and the present opinion is that increased levels of prolactin do not cause an increased incidence of breast cancer (Boyns et al 1973; Wagner and Mantel 1978).

An important issue is the possible association between chronic use of oral contraceptives and increased risk of breast cancer as suggested by some studies (Paffenbarger et al. 1977; Kelsey et al. 1978). More recent investigations (Ravnihar et al. 1979; Kelsey et al. 1981; Harris et al. 1982; Rosenberg et al. 1984) conducted on large populations exposed for a considerable length of time have shown that the use of oral contraceptives is not associated with an increased risk but more likely to a decreased incidence of breast cancer.

Finally, the risk of breast cancer associated with postmenopausal estrogen replacement therapy has been repeatedly investigated, but the results are controversial: a number of studies reveal an increased risk of breast cancer whereas several others have failed to find any correlation between the two events (Hoover et al. 1976; Sartwell et al. 1977; Jick et al. 1980; Sobin and Sherif 1980; Brinton et al. 1981; Hulka et al. 1982).

Diet

The first suggestion of an association between high-fat diet and breast cancer comes from experimental studies in laboratory animals, which have repeatedly shown that the incidence of spontaneous mammary tumours in mice is increased by the administration of a high-fat diet. This has also been proved for dimethylbenzanthracene (DMBA)-induced mammary tumours in rats (Carroll and Hopkins 1979).

A second type of evidence lies in the epidemiological data in human populations, showing that countries with high incidence and mortality rates of breast cancer also have a diet with high fat intake (Buell 1974). In Japan breast cancer is increasing progressively, paralleling the average increase of daily fat intake, whilst the offspring of Japanese migrants to the United States increase their incidence rates of breast cancer with the progressive adaptation to the high-fat diet of the Americans (Dunn 1977). The same phenomenon has been observed in Iceland, while among some religious groups, like the Seventh Day Adventists, who have a low fat intake, the incidence rates of breast cancer are particularly low (Philips et al. 1980). Studies on these religious groups have also shown an interesting fact, that the cohorts who entered the religious group in adult life did not show a reduction of breast cancer rates, suggesting that the dietary factors operate before adult life.

The effect of high-fat diet on breast cancer has been explained by various mechanisms, such as the increased introduction into the body, through the fat, of chemical carcinogens from the environment; an increase in the amount of adipose tissue which in turn increases the level of circulating estrogens; or the indirect anticipation of the age of menarche; or the alteration of the composition of the intestinal microflora with an increased production of potentially carcinogenic substances.

Table 4. Relationship of age at exposure to atomic bomb radiation (>10 rad) and breast cancer risk in Japanese women. (Data from Tokunaga et al. 1984)

Age	Relative risk
0- 9	2.4
10-19	2.0
20-29	1.6
30-39	1.2
40-49	1.1
>50	1.2

Radiation

Evidence of increased risk of breast cancer in women exposed to various doses of radiation has been shown in Japanese atomic bomb survivors (Tokunaga et al. 1984) (Table 4), in patients receiving radiotherapy for postpartum mastitis (Land et al. 1980) and in patients who have had multiple fluoroscopies during treatment of pulmonary tuberculosis (A. B. Miller, G. R. Howe, G. J. Sherman et al. unpublished). Although, in these studies, a linear dose-response relationship was found, it has been observed that sensitivity to radiation is mainly concentrated in the first two or three decades of life. In the atomic bomb survivors study, it appears that the relative risk is 2.4 in women who were exposed to the radiation when in the first decade of life, 2.0 in women exposed during the second decade and 1.6 in women exposed during the third decade. Women who were more than 30 when irradiated did not show any increase in breast cancer risk. Identical results were obtained in the recent Canadian Fluoroscopy Study (Miller et al. 1986). This fact is especially important as regards the issue of the hypothetical breast carcinogenic risk in repeated mammograms.

Finally, it must be recorded that in a large review of patients irradiated for treatment of cancer of the cervix, no increased risk of breast cancer was noted (IARC Working Group 1986).

Other Factors

The papers by Wolfe (1976 a, b) on mammographic patterns suggested that an intensively dense, dysplastic breast parenchyma is associated with an increased risk of breast cancer, but his data were not unanimously confirmed, and recent results (Tabar et al. 1985) are in conflict with the original Wolfe data.

Comparing the alcohol intake of women with breast cancer with that of other women, an excess of drinkers among breast cancer patients was shown, but this finding may reflect the effects of other dietary factors associated with alcohol intake. Case-control studies evaluating the possible effect of hair dyes in increasing the breast cancer risk have produced conflicting results, and no firm conclusions can be drawn at present (Hennekens et al. 1979; Nasca et al. 1980).

Possible Preventive Measures

The causes of breast cancer are unknown. In laboratory animals, breast cancer can be induced by viruses, radiation, chemical carcinogens and hormones. In humans, breast cancer may be induced by radiation, but the number of cases due to such exposure are certainly well below 1% of the total number of cases. Neither is it possible to verify in humans any hypothesis based on viral or chemical factors, whilst for hormones many conflicting opinions have been recorded. Nevertheless, breast cancer is mainly an enviromental disease as has been proved by the great variability in incidence in different geographical areas and by the studies on migrant populations. However, what the main environmental factor responsible is, is not known.

For this reason, any plan for a reduction of breast cancer in the population by preventive measures cannot be but extremely weak in its premises. A simple and empirical type of approach would be to analyse the life style of the populations with low breast cancer incidence (for instance the Japanese women) and recommend the high-risk populations (like the western European and the American) to conform their life style to the former. Along this line, the United States project for reducing breast cancer incidence by 25% by the year 2000 is mainly based on dietary modifications. The reduction of fat consumption to 100 g per day per capita and the reduction of obesity are the main objectives of the plan (Greenwald and Sondik 1986).

A second type of promising prevention action refers to the intervention trials aimed at the evaluation of a possible effect of prolonged administration of antiestrogens (tamoxifen) or differentiating agents (retinoids) on breast cancer incidence.

In conclusion, the feasibility of breast cancer prevention depends first on the knowledge of the exact proportion of breast carcinomas attributable to various factors, and, secondly, on the extent to which women can be persuaded to modify their exposure to these factors. Both aspects require extensive research on the biology of breast cancer, on its causative factors and on the socioeconomic conditions linked to them as well as on the psychological reactions and behavioural characteristics of women faced with the risk of breast cancer.

Pathology of the Breast

Morphological Precursors of Cancer

For a long time fibrocystic disease was considered a condition which increased the risk of developing a cancer of the breast. Many clinical prospective or cohort studies indicated an average increasing risk of 2.0 (Stevens et al. 1982). A 1982 review by Love et al. (1982), reevaluating 654 cases from five major studies, concluded that the overall increased risk of 1.86 could be due more to the selection of the patients than to the real malignant potentiality of the disease.

More recently, a number of studies have demonstrated that the most important pathological risk for the subsequent development of carcinoma from a benign lesion is the degree of epithelial proliferation and its atypical nature (Fig. 2) (Black et al. 1972; Page et al. 1978; Dupont and Page 1985; Page et al. 1985). Dupont and Page, in their recent review on 3303 benign lesions, could state that the risk of developing cancer in non-proliferative cases was less than the expected incidence rates, whilst in proliferative cases it was twice the expected rates. The relative risk was, however, not very high (1.6) in proliferative disease without atypia, but if the hyperplasia was atypical, the risk was higher (4.4) and much higher if the finding was associated with a family history of breast cancer (8.9 relative risk).

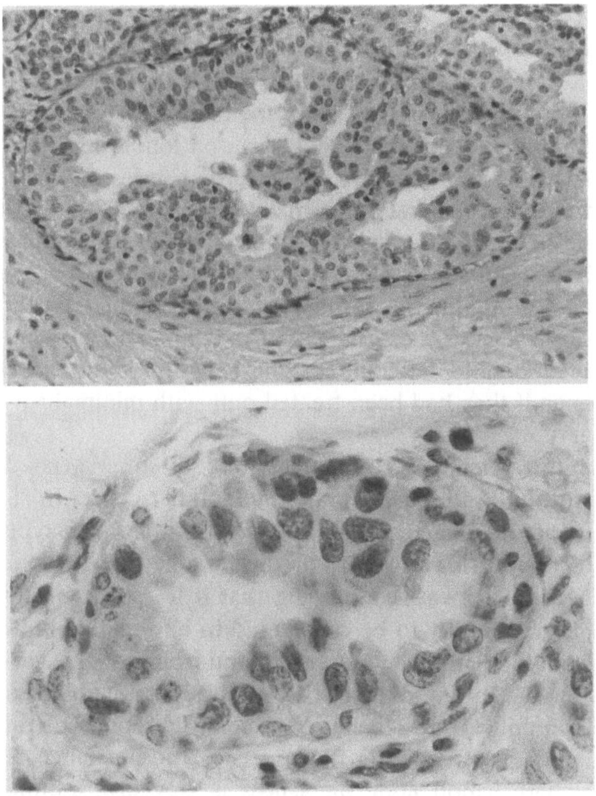

Fig. 2. Atypical epithelial hyperplasia

Among benign lesions at high risk of developing cancer, multiple intraductal papillomas must be considered. A recent study, in which surgically excised specimens were subjected to three-dimensional reconstruction showed that the association with carcinoma was present in 37.5% of the cases. On the other hand, solitary central papillomas showed no higher risk of undergoing malignant transformation than normal breast tissue (Ohuchi et al 1984).

Non-invasive Breast Carcinoma

Lobular Carcinoma In Situ

The term "acinar carcinoma" was introduced by Muir in 1941 to define lesions in which carcinoma involved the mammary lobules. Foote and Stewart (1941) defined as "lobular carcinoma in situ" (Fig. 3) mammary carcinoma originating in the lobules without invasion of the basement membrane. They also described the lobular-terminal duct complex, considered as an anatomic unit, the multicentricity, the "pagetoid" extension and the central mucoid globules in the cells. They also stressed the "occult" clinical character of the lesion. The same type of lesion was then defined with various terms such as "epitheliosis", "small cell neoplasia", and "lobular neoplasia".

Lobular carcinoma in situ occurs at an earlier age than duct carcinoma and affects mainly premenopausal women. Lobular carcinoma in situ is multicentric in 50%–70% of the cases and is often bilateral. The evaluation of bilaterality is, however, mainly based on contralateral biopsy, which is of limited value. A number of studies have tried to evaluate the incidence of invasive breast carcinoma in patients with lobular carcinoma in situ not treated by mastectomy. McDivitt et al. (1967) showed a 15% risk of developing a homolateral invasive carcinoma at 10 years and 35% at 20 years, with figures somewhat lower for the contralateral breast. Wheeler et al. (1974) showed a risk of 9.7% at 10 years, without dif-

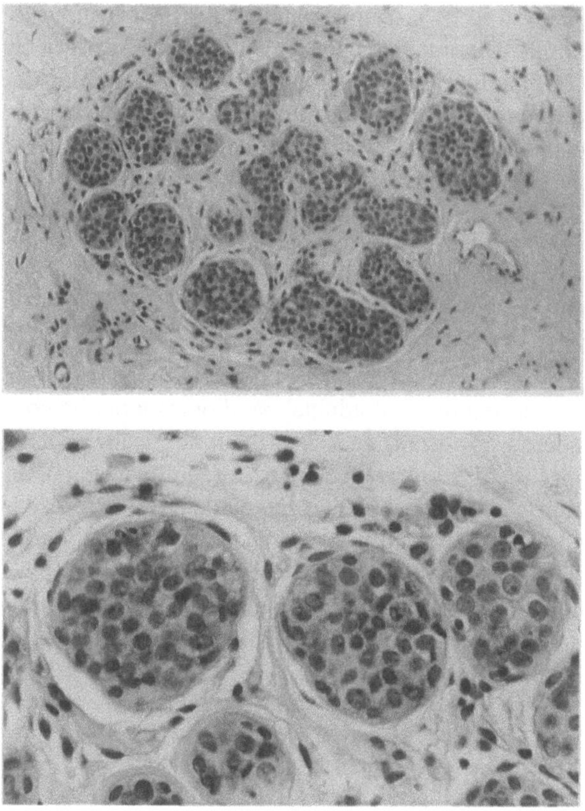

Fig. 3. Lobular carcinoma in situ

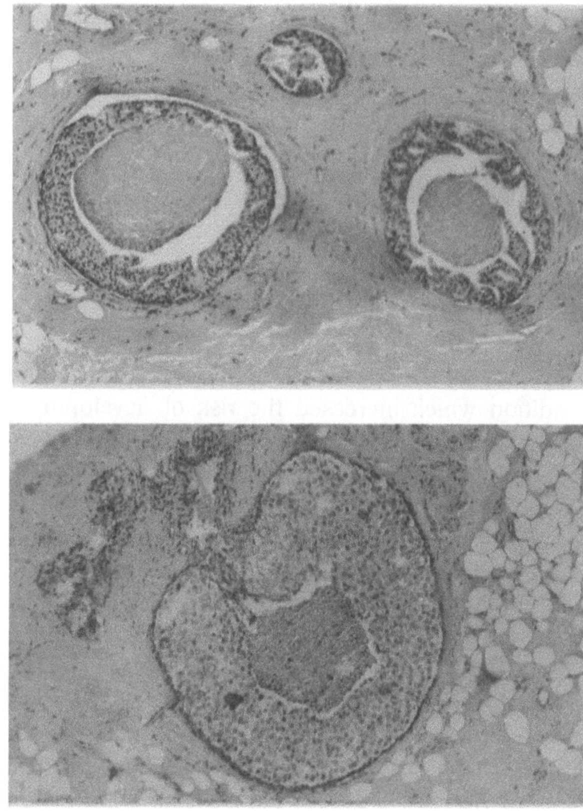

Fig. 4. Intraductal carcinoma

ferences of a homolateral vs. a contralateral invasive carcinoma.

An extensive review of 99 cases with lobular carcinoma in situ followed up for an average of 24 years was published by Rosen et al. (1978). All cases had a limited resection of the breast without other treatments, and the frequency of invasive carcinomas was compared to the expected rates in the general population as per the data of the Connecticut Tumor Register. In 28 of the 99 cases subsequent cancers occurred, whilst the expected rate was 3.1, with a risk nine times higher than in the general population. There was no difference in the incidence of subsequent cancers between the homolateral and the contralateral breast.

In 1978 Haagensen et al. (1978) reported the results of a long-term follow-up of 209 patients with lobular carcinoma in situ (defined by the authors as "lobular neoplasia") not treated by mastectomy. The total number of invasive carcinomas observed was 35, whereas the expected number of breast cancers in the general population was 4.85 for this time period, thus yielding a risk seven times that of a normal woman. The incidence of contralateral cancers appeared to be of the same order as the homolateral.

Non-infiltrating Intraductal Carcinoma

There is less information on the natural history of intraductal carcinoma (Fig. 4) than on lobular carcinoma in situ as there are no important series in which the lesion has been minimally treated and followed up. The great majority of intraductal carcinomas have been submitted to some sort of radical surgery and, although the results appear excellent (10-year survival rates close to 100%) it is not known what the possible outcome of these cases would have been if they had been treated only with minimal surgery.

Intraductal carcinoma is more often associated with infiltrating carcinoma than lobular cancer in situ, and its dimension may be 2 cm or more. This type of tumour may grow to a considerable size without becoming invasive, showing that it is a biologically different entity to be considered to be separate both from lobular carcinoma in situ and from invasive carcinoma. In one-third of cases, intraductal carcinoma is multifocal, foci being present in the contralateral breast in one-quarter of the cases. The incidence of axillary lymph node metastasis is very low, around 2%–3% (Murad and Scapelli 1967; Ashikari et al.

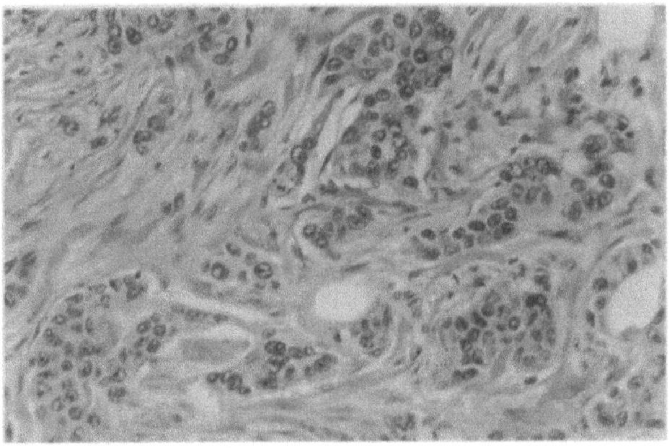

Fig. 5. Infiltrating ductal carcinoma

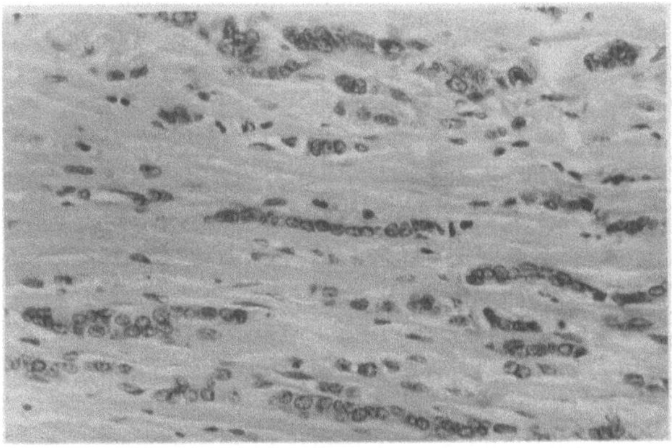

Fig. 6. Infiltrating lobular carcinoma

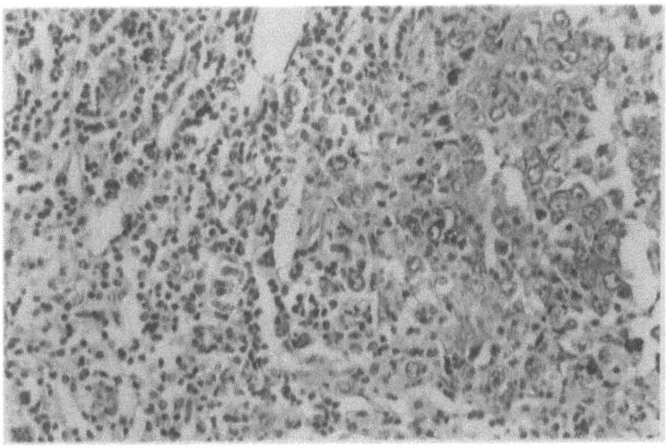

Fig. 7. Medullary carcinoma

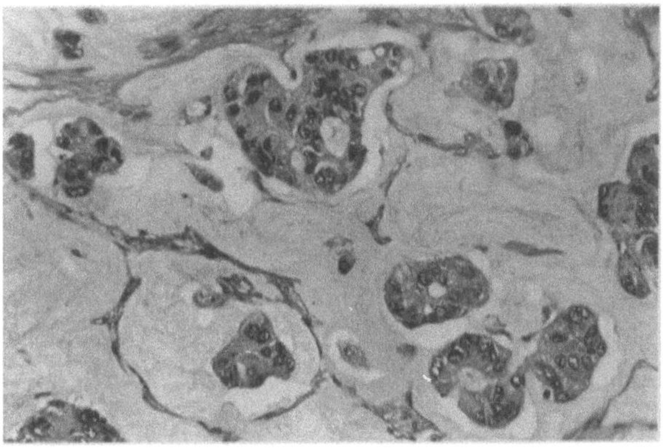

Fig. 8. Mucinous carcinoma

1971; Gallagher and Martin 1971; A. Veronesi et al. 1981; Fisher et al. 1986).

Invasive Breast Carcinoma

Invasive ductal carcinoma (Fig. 5) accounts for 70%–80% of all cases and includes the tumours that were formerly defined as "scirrhous carcinoma", "carcinoma simplex", "comedocarcinoma", "infiltrating carcinoma not otherwise specified (NOS)". Ductal invasive carcinoma was found to be multicentric in 10%–30% of cases. Ductal invasive carcinoma may contain a component of intraductal carcinoma that may be so extensive as to be predominant.

Invasive lobular carcinoma (Fig. 6) represents 10%–20% of all breast cancers and it is considered multicentric in 20%–50% of cases.

The other types of carcinomas are less common. Medullary carcinoma (Fig. 7) has sharp tumour borders and lymphoid infiltration, mucoid carcinoma is characterised by the presence of large amounts of extracellular mucus (Fig. 8), papillary carcinoma

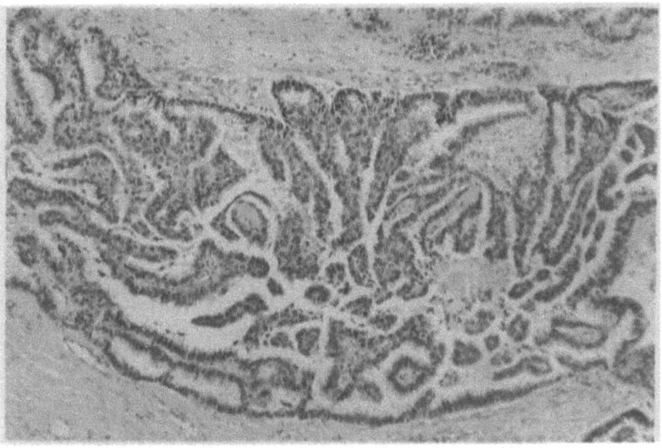

Fig. 9. Papillary carcinoma

(Fig. 9) by a well-differentiated papillary structure. There are also entities which represent only pathological curiosities, such as adenoid cystic carcinoma, apocrine carcinoma and carcinoma with squamous metaplasia.

Inflammatory carcinoma is not specifically recognisable on histological examination. It has the mor-

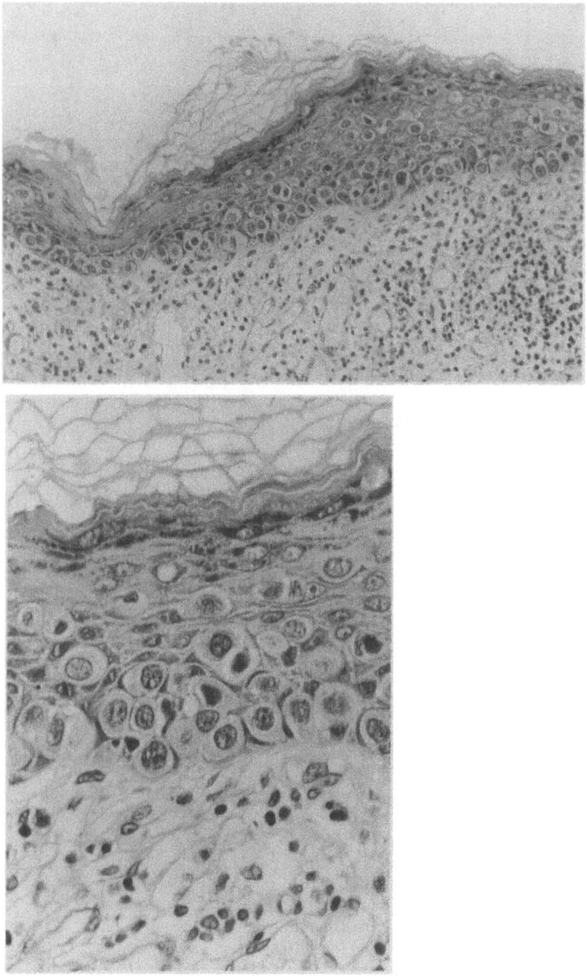

Fig. 10. Mammary Paget's disease

phology of an invasive ductal carcinoma with extensive invasion of lymphatic vessels of the dermis.

The so-called Paget's disease of the nipple (Fig. 10), better defined as "epidermotropic intraductal carcinoma" (Veronesi et al. 1955), is a variant of intraductal carcinoma with cells invading the ducts without infiltrating the base membrane, reaching the major ducts of the nipple and extending into the epidermis of the areola, always with a non-infiltrating character. Only later on in the development does an invasive carcinoma often appear in the mammary gland.

A controversial point in breast cancer pathology is represented by the grading. Grading may be histological, cellular or nuclear, or a mixture of all three. There are many grading schemes, based on various parameters such as differentiation, size of cells, size of nuclei, chromasia, mitotic index, nuclear atypia, nuclear crowding and others. All have in common a good correlation between grade and survival rates, but the disturbing fact about grading is low interobserver reproducibility (Bloom and Richardson 1957; Scarff and Torloni 1968; Rilke 1984).

Local and Regional Spread of Breast Cancer

Intraductal Extension

Paget's disease is the most spectacular example of the spread of breast cancer through the ductal tree. However, today, the presence of diffuse microcalcifications at mammography frequently reveals many instances in which intraductal invasion is considerable, either around a well-defined mass, or without any palpable lump. The frequency of the peritumoral intraductal spread is difficult to assess as minor signs of this extension are very common, but "important" extension may be given a different meaning by different pathologists (E. R. Fisher et al. 1975). It has also been noted, that when the intraductal component in a tumour is abundant, the prognosis is more favourable and nodal metastases less common (Silverberg and Chitale 1973).

Patients with a carcinoma with an extensive prominent intraductal component frequently also have intraductal peritumoral spread, as well as multicentric breast carcinomas (E. R. Fisher et al. 1975). The peritumoral extension of intraductal spread is important for the modern surgeon as it seems to be correlated to the risk of recurrence after lumpectomy or limited breast resection (Schnitt et al. 1984).

Peritumoral Vascular Invasion

An important histological characteristic of primary breast cancer is its ability to invade surrounding lymphatic and blood vessels. Peritumoral intralymphatic invasion is present in 20%–40% of cases, according to various series (E. R. Fisher et al. 1975; Nime et al. 1977; Rosen et al. 1981) and represents an unfavourable prognostic factor. Blood vessel invasion is not uncommon, although it has been found in totally different percentages of cases, from 4% to 45%, by various pathologists. As with intralymphatic invasion, tumour emboli in the blood vessels seem to be associated with a poor prognosis (Friedell et al. 1965).

Multicentricity

In many cases breast cancers are multicentric. However, there is considerable discrepancy in the percentage of cases displaying multicentricity and on the clinical significance of multicentricity. In an extensive case review (Popkin and De Feo 1976), multicentric primary carcinomas were found in 13.4% of the cases, but the majority (70%) were non-invasive. In the contralateral breasts, too, the incidence of occult primaries is of the order of 15% (Van Scott 1979; Sanderson and MacKie 1979). This high incidence reported by the pathologists is, however, in contrast with the common clinical observation of the infrequent finding of a double carcinoma in the same breast and of a simultaneous bilateral carcinoma. It has been reported that the incidence of occult carcinomas in the breast of patients over 70 who had died from causes other than mammary carcinoma is 19 times greater than the incidence of clinical breast cancer (Sage and Casson 1976). Therefore, it may well be that many occult foci of carcinoma will never progress to overt disease, as in the case of the thyroid and the prostate.

However, the notion of the presence of foci of carcinoma in the breast, independently of the primary tumour, is of great importance in the development of a policy of conservative treatment of breast cancer. A fundamental paper was recently published by Holland et al. (1985) who studied a series of 399 mastectomy specimens with invasive cancer, with characteristics comparable to those eligible for breast conserving therapy. The specimens were macroscopically sectioned at 5 mm, and a radiograph was made of each macrosection. Any radiologically suspicious area was carefully examined histologically, with an average of 20 blocks per breast specimen. In 37% of the specimens there were no tumour foci around the primary tumour, in 20% tumour was found within 2 cm and in 43% tumour foci were found beyond 2 cm (27% non-invasive, 16% invasive). Invasive carcinoma was found at 3 cm in 9% of the cases and in 7% at 4 cm. It is possible, therefore, to predict the risk of local recurrence according to the size of the normal tissue removed around the primary mass.

Axillary Node Metastases

Axillary nodes are invaded by metastases from breast carcinoma with a frequency which varies according to the size of the primary and its histological and biological characteristics. The location of the primary in the breast has limited significance, with only a somewhat higher incidence in tumours of the outer upper quadrants. The percentage of axillary involvement is related to the completeness of the surgical dissection and to the degree of pathological analysis (Wilkinson et al. 1982). The axillary lymph nodes are conventionally subdivided by most pathologists into three levels: the first including the nodes external to the lateral margin of the minor pectoralis muscle; the second, the nodes posterior to the minor pectoralis muscle; and the third level including the nodes medial to that muscle. In a recent study of 539 cases with positive nodes (Veronesi et al. 1987b), 11082 lymph nodes were removed, with an average of 20.5 nodes per patient. The average number of lymph nodes at the first level was 13.8, at the second level 4.5 and at the third level 2.2. The number of nodes was 20.7 in cases treated with Halsted mastectomy, 20.9 with modified radical mastectomy, 20.3 with quadrantectomy and axillary dissection. In 96.2% of the cases, the distribution by level showed a regular orderly progression of the metastatic spread from the first to the third levels: in 58% the first level only was involved, in 22% the first and the second levels were involved and in 16% all three levels were sites of metastases. Only in fewer than 4% of the cases was an irregular distribution observed, with metastases skipping the first level (1.2%) or the first and the second levels (0.4%).

It appears, therefore, that the predicting value of the information which may be obtained from the first level is excellent. When the nodes of the first level are clear the chances of metastatic nodes being present at the second and third levels are negligible. When the first level is positive, the chances of metastases being present at the second and the third levels are high, in the order of 40%. The risk of cancer at higher levels when the first is positive changes according to the number of nodes involved at the first level and according to the size of primary tumour (Table 5).

Internal Mammary Node Metastases

In the 1960s, dissection of the internal mammary nodes became popular, with results that seemed to improve survival compared to the classic Halsted mastectomy (Giacomelli and Veronesi 1952; Urban and Baker 1952). However, a multicentric international randomised clinical trial, started in 1962,

Table 5. Risk of metastases at level II and/or level III when level I is invaded, according to the size of primary tumour at pathological evaluation. (From Veronesi et al. 1987b)

Tumour size	Risk (%)
T1	28.4
T2	51.3
T3	67.9
All cases	41.1

Table 6. Probability of metastases at level II and/or III when level I is invaded, according to the number of metastatic nodes at level I. (From Veronesi et al. 1987 b)

Metastatic nodes at level I (*n*)	Probability of metastases at level II and/or III (%)
1	8.0
2	25.3
3	30.2
4 or more	65.8

Table 7. Disease-free and overall 10 year survival related to type of surgery. (From Veronesi and Valagussa 1981)

	Halsted mastectomy		Extended mastectomy	
	(*n*)	(%)	(*n*)	(%)
Disease-free survival				
Total	374	49.7	342	47.3
Node-positive	200	27.0	181	25.4
Node-negative	174	75.8	161	72.1
Overall survival				
Total	374	60.7	342	57.0
Node-positive	200	43.2	181	38.1
Node-negative	174	80.4	161	79.5

showed that prognosis was not improved by the radical dissection of the internal mammary chain (Lacour et al. 1983; Veronesi and Valagussa 1981). The data on the survival rates among the patients randomised at the Milan Cancer Institute are reported in Table 7.

The results of the trial opened a number of questions on the approach to primary cancer of the breast regarding both the need for surgical or radiological treatment of internal mammary nodes and the usefulness of the information on their involvement for prognostic evaluation (Veronesi et al. 1983).

In a series of 1119 cases treated with mastectomy plus internal mammary dissection, the probability of metastatic involvement of internal mammary nodes according to the characteristics of the primary tumour was evaluated. Table 8 shows the frequency of metastases to internal mammary nodes according to the quadrant where the primary tumour is located. All quadrants have a similar frequency of internal mammary metastases, although a slightly higher incidence is present in the central quadrant (22.1%) compared with the internal (19.0%) and the external ones (18.0%). The common belief that internal mammary node metastases are frequent for tumours of the internal quadrants and rare for tumours of the external ones is, therefore, disproven.

Table 8. Frequency of metastases to internal mammary chain according to quadrant of origin of breast cancer. (From Veronesi et al. 1985 a)

Quadrants	Patients (*n*)	Metastases	
		(*n*)	(%)
Inner	620	118	19.0
Central	122	27	22.1
Outer	377	68	18.0
	1119	213	19.0

Chi-square = 0.67; distribution of freedom = 2; $P = 0.71$.

Table 9. Risk of internal mammary chain metastases according to the age of patient, pathological diameter of primary and positivity of axillary nodes. (From Veronesi et al. 1985 a)

Age	Size (cm)	Risk (%)
Positive axillary nodes		
Less than 40	>2	44.3
	<2	36.0
41–50	>2	34.9
	<2	27.5
More than 50	>2	28.6
	<2	22.1
Negative axillary nodes		
Less than 40	>2	17.0
	<2	12.7
41–50	>2	12.2
	<2	8.9
More than 50	>2	9.4
	<2	6.8

The dimension of the primary tumor accounts for a significant difference in incidence of internal mammary node metastases. The subdivision of the total number into two groups according to the pathological size (up to and more than 2 cm) shows a considerable difference of involvement of internal mammary nodes. The age of the patient is another important factor: the younger the patient, the more likely the risk of internal mammary metastases. The presence or absence of axillary metastases is a fundamental factor affecting the involvement of internal mammary nodes: out of the 563 cases without axillary metastases, 51 (9,1%) showed internal mammary involvement, while out of 556 with axillary node metastases, 162 (29.1%) had internal mammary node metastases.

If the three major characteristics affecting the incidence of internal mammary node metastases (i.e. the size, the presence of axillary metastases and the age) are evaluated simultaneously, the risk of a breast cancer patient having occult metastases in the internal mammary nodes can be calculated (Table 9).

Natural History of Breast Cancer

A proper knowledge of its natural history is a mandatory background for approaching every neoplastic disease. For breast cancer, moreover, all the new data from experimental research can potentially influence all aspects of the disease leading the oncologists to modify their priorities or to change their approaches. It is exactly our improved understanding of its natural history that has brought us to fight breast cancer today by looking for a very early diagnosis, to reduce our surgical aggressiveness and to take into consideration new hypotheses such as chemoprevention. The surgeon has almost always the privilege, and the responsibility, of making the first diagnosis of breast cancer: all that will happen to that specific patient will depend, in good part, on how the lump in her breast was interpreted by her surgeon and on how deep his awareness of the extreme complexity of this disease is.

Experimental Mammary Carcinogenesis

Mammary Carcinogenesis in Mice

The use of strains of mice carrying the so-called "milk factor", which was later identified as a "murine mammary tumour virus" (MMTV) gave rise to a large number of research projects (Fekety 1938; Huseby and Bittner 1946) which produced information of great importance on the interaction between the genetic characteristics, the endocrine factors and the presence or absence of the Bittner virus (Bittner 1936). From the histogenetic point of view, the mammary tissue of mice bearing the virus revealed the presence of hyperplastic alveolar nodules which were shown to be preneoplastic (DeOme et al. 1959), endocrine dependent and age dependent: these preneoplastic nodules were not expressed in the absence of the MMTV. However, in mice not carrying the virus, similar nodules may be induced by chemical carcinogenesis, provided that this is associated with an intense hormonal stimulation (Faulkin 1966).

Mammary Carcinogenesis in Rats

The first results on the induction of mammary carcinomas in rats by DMBA were published by Huggins et al. in 1961. The advantages of DMBA-induced mammary carcinomas in rats are the short time needed to produce them, the specificity of DMBA, the high incidence and the histological and endocrine similarity with the mammary carcinomas in humans (Shellabarger 1972). However, their biological properties are different from the human ones as they are much less aggressive and have little metastatising activity. More recently, the use of nitrosomethylurea (NMU) as a chemical carcinogen has resulted in the induction of a mammary adenocarcinoma which is more similar to human breast cancer as it tends to metastatise to liver, lung and spleen (Gullino et al. 1975).

Attempts to induce mammary carcinomas in rats with ionising radiation have shown that the potency of radiation as a carcinogenic agent, although it can elevate the incidence of mammary adenocarcinomas moderately, is very low, especially if compared with the potency of the chemical carcinogens (Shellabarger et al. 1980).

Histopathogenesis of Breast Cancer in Humans

Although there are a number of benign proliferative lesions that are associated with carcinoma of the breast, their preneoplastic character is uncertain. Some of these lesions are more common in cancer-bearing breasts than in glandular samples taken from random autopsies. However, the hyperplastic lesions are more common in the age period between 35 and 50 years and are less extensively found after the menopause, whilst breast cancer increases in incidence after the menopause. Moreover, epidemiological studies have shown that the risk of developing a breast cancer in women with fibrocystic disease is not much higher than in normal women, with the exception of subjects with atypical hyperplasia (Dupont and Page 1985). Furthermore, there is evidence that in many cases breast cancer arises de novo without any premalignant phase.

It has been extensively demonstrated that the neoplastic transformation occurs mainly in the terminal ductal/lobular unit of the breast. According to some authors (Squartini and Sounelli 1981), the first appearance of the cancer process is in situ, but how long the proliferation would remain intraepithelial before becoming infiltrating has never been elucidated. In addition to the in situ condition as a first proliferative disorder, Wellings (1980) has classified other non-neoplastic proliferative preneoplastic lesions, according to their site of origin, into type A atypical lobules, in which the proliferative changes are in the terminal ducts; and the type B atypical lobules, in which the anomalous proliferation is within the lobules themselves (Wellings et al. 1975). The type A lobules would represent the very early stages of the in situ ductal carcinoma, whilst the type B lobules would precede the lobular carcinoma in situ (Wellings 1980).

Cellular Heterogenicity of Mammary Carcinoma

The extensive heterogenicity of malignant cells in human breast cancer has been documented in a great variety of phenotypic expressions and it is most likely due to the existence of different clonal cell subpopulations in some tumours. Histology itself has been shown not to be uniform within breast carcinomas, this finding being confirmed by intrastructural studies (Tseng 1980). Biochemical markers of differentiation, like casein, are irregularly distributed, as are many tumour-associated antigens and hormone receptors (Johnson et al. 1983a; Horan Hand et al. 1983; Natali et al. 1983; Oxenhandler et al. 1984). The introduction of flow cytometry has allowed a better study of the chromosomal variability of tumours, and differences in ploidy within single breast carcinomas have been reported. One of the most obvious signs of heterogeneity of breast carcinomas in humans is the common clinical observation of a mixed response to endocrine, chemotherapeutic or radiological treatments. In disseminated breast carcinoma, for instance, bilateral oophorectomy induces mixed responses in a percentage of cases varying between 10% and 20%; some metastases may disappear completely, whilst others may remain stable or continue their progression. Sometimes the primary tumour regresses, whilst distant metastases may progress, and it is also not infrequent to observe a regression of a portion of the tumour and a progression of the others in large bulky primary carcinomas.

The cell heterogeneity of breast carcinoma may be explained either by its polyclonal origin or by a progressive emergence of variant cell populations as the cancer develops. The monoclonal origin of cancer (i.e. that it arises from a single transformed cell) is a commonly accepted dogma (Fialkow 1979). However, if the origin of breast cancer may be multifocal, and if in a single restricted area of the normal breast, under the action of a carcinogenic agent particularly concentrated in that area, many normal cells undergo the neoplastic transformation simultaneously, the resulting carcinoma may be composed of different clonal cell subpopulations. According to the second hypothesis, the cancer cells are genetically unstable (Nowell et al. 1976). This instability is the cause of the tumour "progression", with appearance of new phenotypic characteristics due to the generation of new cell subpopulations. However, which type of modification at genomic level is responsible for the appearance of the new cellular variants is not known. On the other hand, the differentiation process is often kept to the same degree by many breast carcinomas, and a certain variability in the expression of differentiation may be considered a normal physiopathological characteristic.

Finally, it is difficult to state whether some modifications of the biological behaviour of breast carcinoma (for instance, a sudden rapid tumour growth) may be due to the appearance of a new variant of cell populations or to the sudden failure of the immune defence mechanisms in the host.

Local Development of Breast Carcinoma

The most common type of local spread of breast carcinoma is represented by the infiltration of the surrounding parenchymatous breast tissue giving rise to a palpable mass which is particularly hard if compared to the surrounding normal tissues. If the tissues are homogeneously dense, the shape of the tumour is spheric, with irregular margins which are generally stellate due to the retraction of the interstitial breast tissue. If the malignant process has started in an irregular tissue with different degrees of density, as may happen in fibrocystic breasts, the shape is often very irregular, with extensions along the planes where the tissues are softer. This is the reason why after the menopause, in a substantially fatty breast, the clinical and mammographic shape of breast cancer is always that of a round, moderately stellate, mass, whilst in young, dense, often fibrotic breasts its appearance is much more variable.

A less common type of local spread is represented by the intraductal extension. This extension may be an occasional pathological finding at the edges of any infiltrating breast carcinoma, whilst, on occasions, it represents the exclusive or the major component of the proliferative process. In these cases, the mass is often impalpable although its extension (which is generally indicated by microcalcifications at mammography) may be very large, occupying a significant portion of the breast tissue.

In a limited percentage of cases, the spread may occur by direct invasion (or permeation) of lymphatic vessels, which creates the clinical picture of skin oedema and, if particularly aggressive and rapidly growing, the clinical picture of the inflammatory carcinoma.

The majority of breast carcinomas originate in the upper parts of the breast, some 50% of the total being located in the upper outer quadrant. Relatively infrequent (5%–10%) are the cases originating in the lower inner quadrants, whilst some 15% arise in the central portion of the breast.

The time from the orginal cell transformation to the clinical appearance has been at the centre of many investigations. In their original article in 1956, Collins et al. assumed an exponential model for tumour growth and observing a median volume doubling time of 78 days, concluded that the time required for a simple malignant cell to grow to a 1 cm mass would be around 6–7 years. Other studies have shown, in cases of breast carcinomas, average doubling times of 120 days (Gerschon-Cohen et al. 1963), of 212 days (Fournier et al. 1980) and of 105 days (Kusama et al. 1972).

It must be considered, however, that the conclusions which may derive from these studies, are valid only if one assumes a constant growth rate and an exponential model. On the other hand, if the growth rate is variable at different stages of tumour development and if the human tumour growth is better described by a gompertzian model rather than by an exponential one, the results may be totally different. As a matter of fact, the tumour doubling time is the result of a complex relationship between the length of the cell cycle (generally of 1–3 days), the percentage of cycling cells (growth fraction) and the "cell loss fraction". The last fraction is a fundamental one and it is represented by the newly formed cells which will never be able to divide again, either because of differentiation or natural death.

Distant Spread of Breast Carcinoma

The most common site of distant metastases from breast cancer are the lungs, the bones, the liver (Warren and Whitman 1937; Veronesi et al. 1957; Haagensen 1986). Metastases may, rarely, be present at the time of first diagnosis of breast cancer, whilst in the majority of cases they will appear years after the treatment of the primary. The risk of metastases occurs mainly in the 3rd and the 4th years after treatment. During the 1st year, as well as after the 5th, after primary treatment, the patients are relatively free of risk of metastases. However, differences exist according to the loco-regional conditions at the time of primary treatment. Cases with an aggressive type of disease and extensive regional metastases will show an early appearance of distant metastases. However, if these cases are free of metastases after 8 or more years, the likelihood of further dissemination is scarce. On the other hand, in patients with less aggressive types of carcinoma, without any involvement of the axillary nodes at the time of primary treatment, the appearance of distant metastases will be somewhat delayed, though even after many years the likelihood of developing metastases remains present to a certain degree.

Whether the distribution of distant metastases is regulated purely by biological factors or possibly influenced by haematodynamic factors remains to be clarified. The fact that liver and bone metastases may be present in the absence of macroscopic lung metastases suggests that the malignant cells may easily overcome the lung "filter". However, an analysis on postmortem material by Veronesi et al. (1957) showed that when lung metastases were present, liver metastases were present in 64% of the cases, whilst if the lungs were macroscopically free of metastases, the rate of liver metastases was lower (41%). Another problem which is not clear is the type of metastases in the bone system as they occur with the greatest frequency in the spine and pelvis, whilst the long bones are relatively untouched. This singular distribution has suggested that the invasion of the bones might occur mainly by way of a retrograde venous invasion through the paravertebral vein system (Batson 1940). Although this hypothesis is not convincing, no other explanation for the peculiar metastatic distribution in bones has been put forward.

As regards the timing of distant spread, no clear data are available. The fact that at the time of first diagnosis of breast cancer the great majority of patients are free from overt distant metastases leads one to assume that the metastatic growth in distant organs starts at variable times after the initial development of the primary carcinoma.

Prognostic Factors

Age

In general, age does not appear to be an important prognostic factor. Although in many studies younger women show a better prognosis than older ones (Langlands 1979; Hibbert et al. 1983), very young women under 30 years seem to have a worse prognosis than women in other age groups (Noyes et al. 1982). According to another series, women in the age group 50–54 years have a better prognosis than women of other ages.

Histology

Some histological types of breast carcinoma show a better prognosis than the common infiltrating carcinomas (ductal and lobular): medullary carcinomas (Richardson 1956), mucoid carcinomas (Veronesi and Gennari 1960) and papillary carcinomas (Veronesi et al. 1964) definitely have a better prognosis than other types. Histological grading shows a significant correlation with prognosis (Bloom and Field 1971). Nuclear grading, lymphoid reactions and sinus histiocytosis have also been reported to be correlated with prognosis (Black and Spur 1950; Cutler et al. 1969). However, a recent study in which different pathologists reviewed the same specimen showed a very low rate of agreement on the evaluation of the nuclear grade and of the sinus histiocytosis (Gilchrist et al. 1985), and the difficulty in obtaining reproducible scores represents a clear limitation to the practical applications of this prognostic factor. The importance of the doubling time as an indicator of prognosis has been reported in many papers (Gershon-Cohen et al. 1963; Kusama et al. 1972; Fournier et al. 1980; Galante et al. 1986).

Growth Rate

One of the most extensive studies on the importance of the rate of growth (evaluated by a comparison of subsequent mammographic findings) was published by Lundgren (1983). Out of 280 evaluable cases, 139 were diagnosed by repeated screening, but on a prior mammogram an obvious cancer had been overlooked, and their average doubling time was 12.4 months, whilst 114 cases were diagnosed between screenings with an average doubling time of 2.2 months. There was a clear relationship between doubling time and survival: patients with a doubling time of less than 3 months had a 56% 5-year survival rate, whilst patients with a doubling time of more than 3 months were all alive at 5 years.

An interesting study was published in 1986 by Galante et al. on a series of 196 breast cancer patients, who received two preoperative mammographic examinations at an interval of 20 or more days. The cases were divided into slow-growing (doubling time more than 90 days: 81 patients), intermediate-growing (30–90 days: 84 patients), fast-growing (less than 30 days: 31 patients), and their survival was evaluated according to the number of axillary nodes involved. The data showed that the prognostic value of doubling time was present only in the cases with extensive nodes and showed no differences in survival in the three subgroups with different growth rates. Taking the extensive axillary involvement as a sign of the metastasising power, the data of Galante et al. would suggest that the growth rate and the ability to metastasise are, at least partly, two independent variables. When both are present (high growth rate, extensive axillary metastases) the prognosis is bad, but when only one is present, the prognosis is much better. This conclusion, which, however, needs confirmation, would imply that the biological factors which sustain the local growth are quite different from the factors which are responsible for the metastatic implant.

Cell Kinetics

The aspect which has been most extensively investigated to study the potential proliferative activity of cell population is the fraction of S-phase cells. The two approaches mainly pursued are the autoradiographic evaluation of 3 H-thymidine-labelled cells (labelling index, LI) and flow cytometric determination of DNA content.

Studies on the cell kinetics of breast cancer have been carried out independently by different groups (Meyer et al. 1983; Tubiana et al. 1984; Silvestrini et al. 1985). The results have consistently shown that LI is not related to axillary nodal invasion and slightly related to pathological tumour size, but it represents an important prognostic factor. This finding is evident mainly in patients with node-negative resectable tumours given only locoregional treatment (Table 10) and in locally advanced diseases (Silvestrini et al. 1987), whereas it is less evident in patients in whom systemic therapy may have modified the natural history of the tumour.

Recently, flow cytometry has been used to define DNA, and the relationship between aneuploidy and clinical outcome has been investigated. Patients with diploid carcinomas have been found to have a better prognosis than patients with carcinoma composed largely of aneuploid cells (Hedley et al. 1984; Coulson et al. 1984).

Size of the Primary

The clinical size of the primary carcinoma is a parameter of great importance in the prognostic assess-

Table 10. Clinical outcome as a function of cell kinetics in patients with resectable node-negative tumours. (Data from Silvestrini et al. unpublished)

Labelling index	Cases (n)	Outcome at 5 years			
		Regression-free survival		Overall survival	
Low	214	82	$P<0.0001$	96	$P<0.0001$
High	200	61		86	

ment. In a recent study by Russo et al. (1987) on a multivariate analysis of different characteristics of 646 breast carcinomas, the size of the primary tumour appeared as one of the most important independent prognostic variables. Another study by Koscielny et al. (1984), based on data from 2648 cases followed up for 10–25 years, showed a direct relationship between tumour size and prognosis. In a study of the 30-year survival rates Adair et al. (1974) found a great difference in survival both in patients with negative and with positive nodes, according to the size of the primary carcinoma.

Regional Node Metastases

The prognostic significance of axillary involvement is well established. The 10-year survival rate according to the number of nodes involved has recently been reviewed, in a series of patients treated surgically only, by Cascinelli et al. (1987), who found that whilst patients with more than three axillary nodes involved have a poor prognosis, patients with a single metastatic node show a 10-year survival rate of 70%. Similar data were reported by Salvadori et al. (1983). Also the level of axillary invasion plays an important role, the prognosis being much worse when the third level is involved (Schottenfeld 1976).

As the metastatic involvement is a function of the size of the primary carcinoma, it is sometimes difficult to dissociate the two variables as regards their relative prognostic value. From many studies it appears, however, that the two factors have a certain independent prognostic value. For instance, the data of Valagussa et al. (1978) showed that the 5-year relapse rate was 37% in patients with positive nodes and small primary tumours (< 2 cm) and 79% in patients with positive nodes and large primary tumours (> 5 cm).

The great prognostic significance of internal mammary node involvement has been stressed in several recent papers (Veronesi et al. 1983, 1985; Lacour et al. 1987 a). The overall 10-year survival rate was evaluated in 1119 patients, treated by dissection of internal mammary nodes, by Veronesi et al. (1985 a), showing that the prognosis, when either the axillary nodes or the internal mammary nodes are involved separately, is similar. On the other hand, the prognosis is excellent when both nodal stations are free of metastases and it is ominous when both are involved (Fig. 11).

Receptor Status

Receptor assays have been largely utilised to identify the responsiveness of breast carcinomas to endocrine treatment. However, besides their predictive role, receptor assays have also been employed as prognostic factors. Estrogen receptor- (ER) positive tumours, in fact, show a low proliferative potential, and are associated with marked morphological evidence of differentiation and have a less aggressive biological behaviour. Data from many studies has shown an improved prognosis in patients with ER-positive tumours (Walt et al. 1976; Knight et al. 1977; Osborne et al. 1981), although in some others this finding has not been found clearly (Howat et al. 1983; Hilf et al. 1980; Bloom and Degenshein 1980; Pichon et al. 1980).

Also the presence of progesterone receptors (PR) has been found to be associated with an improved prognosis (Saez et al. 1983; Mason et al. 1983; Clark et al. 1983) although, again, some studies have not found the same correlation (Stewart et al. 1983; Allegra et al. 1979). The largest series of patients evaluated for the predictive value of hormone receptors has recently been reported by Di Fronzo et al.

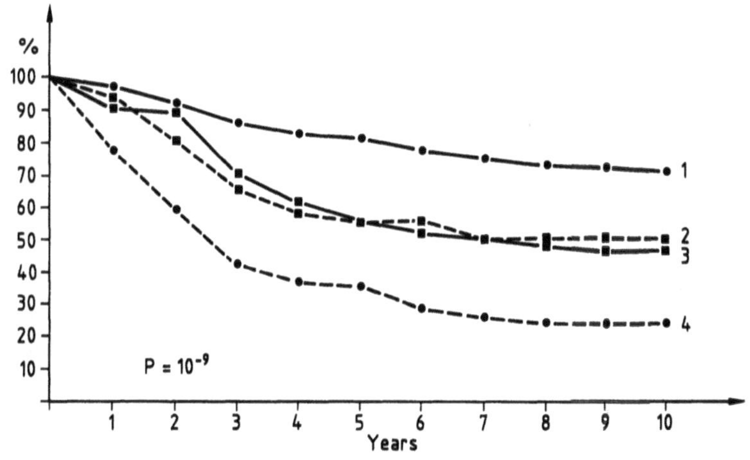

Fig. 11. Disease-free survival of 1119 breast cancer patients according to axillary and internal mammary nodes status. *1*, N– N– (512 patients); *2*, N+ axillary, N– mammary (394 patients); *3*, N– axillary, N+ mammary (51 patients); *4*, N+ N+ (162 patients)

(1986). This group of investigators, from the Milan Cancer Institute and Baylor College of Medicine in Houston, pooled the data from the two centres totalling the extraordinary number of 10 613 patients who had the ER data available. Of these patients 7035 were also examined for PR values. Apart from a number of interesting observations on this case series, amongst which the most important was the progressive trend towards higher levels in the baseline values for both estrogen and progesterone receptors, in time, in both centres, the long-term disease-free survival of patients showed a significant difference between patients who were ER- and PR-positive and patients who were ER- and PR-negative, whilst patients who were ER-positive and PR-negative showed intermediate values. However, when node-negative patients were evaluated separately according to ER status or PR status, although the disease-free survival of both ER-negative and PR-positive patients was somewhat better than that of ER- and PR-negative patients, the difference was not statistically significant.

Biomolecular Factors

The availability of information on molecular biological data in a retrospective series of patients has allowed prognostic studies on a number of parameters. The most significant investigation was reported in 1987 by Slamon et al. who evaluated the long-term survival of breast cancer patients according to the *new* oncogene amplification.

Staging

The grouping of patients according to the extent of the disease is an essential need in clinical research to compare results and to identify the most appropriate choices of treatment. The most widely used staging system is the one adopted by both the UICC and the AJC, based on the TNM system (Hermanek and Sobin 1987). This classification, agreed by both organisations in 1987, is reported in Tables 11–13.

Table 11. TNM clinical classification

T – Primary tumour	
TX	Primary tumour cannot be assessed
TO	No evidence of primary tumour
Tis	Carcinoma in situ: intraductal carcinoma, or lobular carcinoma in situ, or Paget's disease of the nipple with no tumour
Note:	Paget's disease associated with a tumour is classified according to the size of the tumour.
T1	Tumour 2 cm or less in greatest dimension
	T1 a 0.5 cm or less in greatest dimension
	T1 b More than 0.5 cm but not more than 1 cm in greatest dimension
	T1 c More than 1 cm but not more than 2 cm in greatest dimension
T2	Tumour more than 2 cm but not more than 5 cm in greatest dimension
T3	Tumour more than 5 cm in greatest dimension
T4	Tumour of any size with direct extension to chest wall or skin
Note:	Chest wall includes ribs, intercostal muscles and serratus anterior muscle but not pectoral muscle.
	T4 a Extension to chest wall
	T4 b Oedema (including peau d'orange), or ulceration of the skin of the breast, or satellite skin nodules confined to the same breast
	T4 c Both 4 a and 4 b above
	T4 d Inflammatory carcinoma
Notes:	Inflammatory carcinoma of the breast is characterized by diffuse, brawny induration of the skin with an erysipeloid edge, usually with no underlying palpable mass. If the skin biopsy is negative and there is no localized, measurable primary cancer, the T category is pTX when pathologically staging a clinical inflammatory carcinoma (T4 d). When classifying pT the tumour size is a measurement of the *invasive* component. If there is a large in situ component (e.g. 4 cm) and a small invasive component (e.g. 0.5 cm) the tumour is coded pT1 a. Dimpling of the skin, nipple retraction or other skin changes, except those in T4, may occur in T1, T2 or T3 without affecting the classification.

Detection and Diagnosis

The last 30 years have witnessed an extensive change in our concepts and methodologies for the diagnosis of breast cancer. What was once an elementary method of diagnosis based on a simple physical examination (inspection and palpation) has been transformed into a highly sophisticated complex of technologies which allow the recognition of lesions of minimal size, often not palpable. The advances in breast cancer diagnosis methods have opened up a new area of investigation with the objective of searching for and screening occult early carcinomas among the normal general population. This line of development, which followed the already established one in the detection of cervical cancer with the Pap test, was initiated in the United States more than 20 years ago and has been followed by a number of new studies, in Europe and the United States.

Table 12. TNM clinical classification

N – Regional lymph nodes
NX Regional lymph nodes cannot be assessed (e.g. previously removed)
N0 No regional lymph node metastasis
N1 Metastasis to movable ipsilateral axillary node(s)
N2 Metastasis to ipsilateral axillary node(s) fixed to one another or to other structures
N3 Metastasis to ipsilateral internal mammary lymph node(s)

M – Distant metastasis
MX Presence of distant metastasis cannot be assessed
M0 No distant metastasis
M1 Distant metastasis (includes metastasis to supraclavicular lymph nodes)

The category M1 may be further specified according to the following notation:

Pulmonary	PUL	Bone marrow	MAR
Osseous	OSS	Pleura	PLE
Hepatic	HEP	Peritoneum	PER
Brain	BRA	Skin	SKI
Lymph nodes	LYM	Other	OTH

Table 13. pTNM pathological classification

pT – Primary tumour
The pathological classification requires the examination of the primary carcinoma with no gross tumour at the margins of resection. A case can be classified pT if there is only microscopic tumour in a margin.

The pT categories correspond to the T categories.

pN – Regional lymph nodes
The pathological classification requires the resection and examination of at least the low axillary lymph nodes (level I). Such a resection will ordinarily include six or more lymph nodes.

pNX Regional lymph nodes cannot be assessed (not removed for study or previously removed)
pN0 No regional lymph node metastasis
pN1 Metastasis to movable ipsilateral axillary node(s)
- pN1a Only micrometastasis (none larger than 0.2 cm)
- pN1b Metastasis to lymph node(s), any larger than 0.2 cm
  - pN1bi Metastasis in one to three-lymph nodes, any more than 0.2 cm and all less than 2.0 cm in greatest dimension
  - pN1bii Metastasis to four or more lymph nodes, any more than 0.2 cm and all less than 2.0 cm in greatest dimension
  - pN1biii Extension of tumour beyond the capsule of a lymph node metastasis less than 2.0 cm in greatest dimension
  - pN1biv Metastasis to a lymph node 2.0 cm or more in greatest dimension

pN2 Metastasis to ipsilateral axillary lymph nodes that are fixed to one another or to other structures
pN3 Metastasis to ipsilateral internal mammary lymph node(s)

pM – Distant metastasis
The pM categories correspond to the M categories.

Breast Cancer Screening

The three major areas for the control of breast cancer are prevention, detection and treatment. As preventive measures are difficult to identify and, in any case, would take decades before being able to make a major impact, and as the results of the present means of treatment, in the absence of major advances, seem to have reached a ceiling, screening represents the most rational and potential way of reducing breast cancer mortality. As the early experiences with the screening programmes go back to the 1960s, the information now available on the efficacy of breast cancer screening is sufficient to make an early assessment on risk-benefits and cost-benefits.

Screening Methods

Different modalities may be used to screen for breast cancer, including clinical examination of the breast by a doctor, by a nurse and by the patient herself, by imaging techniques (like mammography, xeromammography, ultrasonography), by perception of heat production in the breast (such as with distant or contact thermography) and by detection of a cancer marker in the serum.

The screening test must fulfil five major requirements: it must be sensitive, specific, simple, safe and economic. Sensitivity is the power of the test to identify the disease and it is measured by the proportion of true positive tests out of the total number of the people with the disease. The lower the percentage of false negative tests (i.e. cases with the disease which the test was unable to identify), the higher the overall sensitivity. Specificity is the power of the test to detect *only* the disease and therefore to classify as negative all persons without the disease. The lower the percentage of false positive tests (i.e. cases without the disease but indentified as positive or suspicious by the test), the higher the overall specificity.

Clinical examination, the oldest method of screening, is not a very sensitive test. According to various studies, the sensitivity is around 50%, meaning that the interval cases, appearing within 1 year from a negative screen, equal the cases detected at screening. Also, specificity is low, as palpation detects a large number of cysts and other benign conditions which may require a biopsy to be confirmed as non-malignant.

Although, by tradition, clinical examination was considered to be only that performed by a doctor, recent studies, especially in the United Kingdom, have shown that well-trained nurses may well perform the examination with similar results. The examination of the breast by the woman herself (breast self-examination, BSE) is certainly the most simple, repeatable and economic measure of cancer screening, based on the assumption that today the great majority of the patients present themselves to the doctor because they have found a lump in their breast by occasional palpation. If one could convince women to change the "occasional" palpation into a periodic "systemic" examination, one would logically expect an increased number of early cases detected by the women themselves. However, there is a psychological barrier against BSE in many women, and the percentage of those who perform BSE regularly varies from 15% to 30% of the population, a rate too low to be effective in a screening programme. As a matter of fact, BSE may create a condition of anxiety in many women and, if the breasts are nodular in character, may produce more uncertainties than certainties. In any case, BSE has never been appropriately evaluated and it may have more potential applicability than other screening tests for breast cancer because it does not need the auxiliary high technology (Miller et al. 1985).

Mammography today fulfils the criteria for screening better than all other tests. The sensitivity varies from 80% to 95%, according to various reports, and its specificity is also high. In the Swedish experience only 0.2% of subjects with non-malignant conditions needed to be biopsied.

In the late 1970s, widespread publicity was given to the carcinogenic risk of mammography (Bailar 1976) which led to diffuse public concern which, in turn, resulted in a fall in the acceptability of this technique by women, especially as a detection procedure in the absence of clinical signs. This fear appears unjustified as with the low-dose film-screen combination now available a mammography exposes the breast to a dose of 0.2–0.5 rad per examination. If one considers that the carcinogenic risk of radiation exists only for women exposed before the age of 30 (see "Epidemiology and Prevention"), the radiation risk of mammography in adult women is very minimal and infinitely inferior to the benefit of the early discovery of an occult carcinoma.

Ultrasonography for visualising breast tissue has been developed recently, and its performance is improving year by year. So far it has been used only in symptomatic patients to distinguish benign (especially cystic) lesions from malignant ones. The limitations of this method lie in an inability to detect cancers of less than 5 mm in size and an inability to identify microcalcifications, which, when detected by mammography, are an important indicator of early malignant intraductal lesions.

Thermography measures the heat emitted from the breast. Although many carcinomas produce more heat compared to the surrounding normal tissue, many others are undetectable by thermography, and therefore sensitivity remains low. At the same time, specificity is also low, and a surgeon would not perform a biopsy only on the basis of a positive thermograph in the absence of any clinical or mammographic sign.

The possibility of utilising as a screening procedure a circulating breast cancer marker by taking a small blood sample from the female population appears to be a very appealing objective, but, for the moment, no tests with sufficient specificity and sensitivity are available to warrant an extensive trial.

Feasibility

The feasibility of a screening programme, apart from the availability of an appropriate test, is linked to two main variables; the first being a good social and logistic organisation to call up the participation of the chosen segment of the population, to perform the test, to ask for rescreening, to follow up the women, etc.; the second being a good level of acceptability by the female population, which in turn is linked to the fear of facing a possible unpleasant truth, the fear of mutilation, the anxiety produced by the waiting time until the test and until the final results. The first variable shows that a screening programme may be performed only in well-developed, well-organised and rich countries. In the case of breast screening, contrary to what happens in cervical cancer, there is coincidence between the high level of development of a country and the high incidence of breast cancer. The second variable shows that great attention must be paid to publicising the screening programme and to convincing the women to participate in it, dissolving by appropriate communication the fears linked with the programme. Certainly the introduction of conservative treatments for carcinomas of small size has been a great tool in persuading women to participate in screening programmes. In the first New York trial the compliance was already, on the whole, rather good, 65% of the 31000 women allocated to the study group attended one or more of the four annual screening examinations scheduled (Shapiro 1977).

Evaluation of Efficacy

In principle, the mere fact that screening will yield an increased number of early cases compared to the normal community health care would suggest that it is effective and to be recommended. However, as always in good medical practice, the results of a programme of breast cancer screening must be evaluated with great care and objectivity, especially considering the many pitfalls that one can encounter in the assessment process. There are, in fact, four major areas of bias in evaluating mass detection, and diagnostic procedures in general: lead time, length time, selection, overdiagnosis (Miller 1986).

Lead time is the time at diagnosis that has been advanced by the screening test. The survival will automatically be prolonged by this interval by the simple fact that the diagnostic procedure is applied earlier in the natural history of the disease, but this longer survival time must obviously not be considered an improvement. Lead time for breast cancer screening has been evaluated to be of the order of 1–4 years, shorter for younger than for older women.

Length time bias is due to the fact that the growth rate of the tumour may create a selection, as rapidly growing tumours are less likely to be detected by screening tests applied at periodic intervals (1 or 2 years) than slowly growing ones. Therefore the cases detected inside a screening plan will have a better prognosis than the ones detected by conventional methods.

The selection bias reflects the unavoidable self-selection in attending the screening programme, as the more informed women and those who are more careful about their health are more liable to participate.

Finally, the overdiagnosis bias is due to the fact that the screening might detect a number of lesions of borderline malignancy (like in situ carcinomas) that otherwise would never have been diagnosed.

The difficulties in assessing the efficacy of breast screening are therefore considerable, both in the four areas of bias mentioned and in the need for a very long follow-up, and it appears essential that a control group forms an integral part of the design and that the end point for the evaluation is the mortality rate on a population basis.

The Health Insurance Plan Study (Shapiro et al. 1982)

In this study, which started in 1963 supported by the Health Insurance Plan of Greater New York (HIP), 62 000 women were randomly allocated to a study group and to a control group. The age of the women was 40–64. The women of the group under examination were asked to submit to an annual screening by clinical examination and by mammography on four successive occasions at yearly intervals. A difference in mortality between the study group and the control group became evident 5 years from the date of entry, and after 14 years the number of deaths in the study group was 218 compared with 262 in the control group. This difference (24%) at 14 years appears remarkable, although at year 5 it was much higher (38%), considering that the screening continued only for the first 4 years, compliance was not very high (50%–60%) and the quality of mammography was poor compared to that currently available. It was estimated that if the screening had continued for 10 years, the study group would have had 32% less breast cancer mortality. The difference in mortality was concentrated in women diagnosed after the age of 50, with no benefit to women below this age.

The Breast Cancer Detection Demonstration Projects

Ten years after the beginning of the HIP trial, the American Cancer Society, in association with the National Cancer Institute (NCI) launched a large project for breast cancer detection, the Breast Cancer Detection Demonstration Projects (BCDDP), recruiting some 10 000 women between the ages of 35 and 75 in each of 28 centres throughout the United States (Baker 1982). The women were screened by physical examination, by mammography and by thermography, but no control group was contemplated. The analysis of the malignant tumours detected during the 5 years of the BCDDP showed that the ability of mammography to identify breast carcinomas was considerably higher than the physical examination and that, contrary to the results of the HIP study, its efficacy was also maintained in women under 50.

However, a panel of pathologists who reviewed the collected material was able to show a high rate of false positive cases, suggesting, in addition, that some minimal cancers could never have progressed and could have remained occult and innocuous for the total life span (Beahrs et al. 1979).

The Swedish Trials

Four large trials on mammography alone have been in progress in Sweden for some years. Three of them use single-view mammography and one uses double-view mammography. In each trial there is a control group selected by randomisation based on a cluster sampling basis (two trials) and by randomisation of individuals (two trials). Results were recently reported from the first two studies in the areas of Koffarberg and Ostergotland, which were initiated in 1977

(Tabar et al. 1985). Compliance was very good (90%) among women between 40 and 74, but was very low (< than 50%) among older women. The estimate of relative risk in the two areas combined was 0.69, but there was no reduction in breast cancer mortality in women younger than 50. In women over 50, the reduction in breast cancer mortality in the screened group compared to the controls was around 40%, confirming the ability of mammography alone to reduce drastically the mortality rates for breast carcinoma.

Other studies have been started in recent years in the Netherlands (de Waard et al. 1984), the United Kingdom (UK Trial of Early Detection 1981) and Canada (Baines 1984), but the final results will only be available in a few years' time.

Economic Factors

For many public health authorities the decision to implement or not implement a breast cancer screening project depends in part on the cost-benefit evaluation. The calculations obviously vary considerably when computed in different countries. In a recent calculation by Miller (1983) it was shown, for instance, that a 5-year screening programme for 100000 women, aged 50–59, with a double-view mammography plus a biennial physical examination, would cost some 5 million US dollars, (with 2558 person-years of life saved, with a cost of some 2000 US dollars per year of life saved).

Breast Cancer Diagnosis

A preoperative diagnosis of breast cancer may be obtained by a number of means, three of which are at present considered of fundamental importance to give a complete picture of the breast disease before treatment. The three methods are: (a) physical examination; (b) mammography; (c) fine needle biopsy; and they represent a basic "triplet" with which accuracy of diagnosis becomes very high.

Physical Examination

The examination starts with the patient lying supine, with her arms raised above her head. A first inspection gives an immediate evaluation of the conditions of the skin and of the nipples. For a right-handed doctor, it is better to examine both breasts standing at the left of the bed and using the left hand for palpation as, in general, the left hand is more sensitive than the right one. The palpation must be very delicate and superficial with two separate evaluations, first with the palm of the hand and then with the finger tips. The palpation must be performed without hurting the patient, as many patients have very sensitive breasts, and a rough or heavy palpation may be painful. The entire breast must be accurately palpated and all types of lumps, nodules, recesses and irregularities must immediately be mentally evaluated for their risk of being malignant. It must be said that with the arms raised above the head, the judgement tends to be somewhat pessimistic, and sometimes a suspicious judgement may become more optimistic when the patient is asked to lower her arms. In this position, palpation is less easy, but it is important as a complement to the one performed in the previous position. Then the patient is requested to contract the pectoralis muscles by pressing her hips firmly with her hands. This makes an additional useful examination possible.

The patient must then be examined in a sitting position. When the patient raises the arms upwards, alterations in the lower part of the breast and in the intramammary fold may easily become apparent, and the contraction of the pectoralis muscles may demonstrate an otherwise inapparent skin retraction. Inspection is completed by looking at asymmetries, modifications of the shape or changes in colour or thickness of the skin.

The obvious suspicious signs are skin ulceration, retraction, oedema and erythema. As regards retraction, one must, however, recall that in postmenopausal women and in women who have recently lost weight, there may be false retractions due to localised areas of fat and breast tissue atrophy, especially in the lower parts of the breast. The oedema of the breast skin is a very grave sign of dermal lymphatic involvement, but sometimes may be due to massive axillary lymph node involvement. If the patient has had an axillary dissection, the breast may easily have areas of skin oedema, especially if she has had radiotherapy on the breast, a condition which is becoming more and more common after the introduction of conservative treatments. Erythema of the skin is also an ominous sign and, although it may due to an inflammatory process, inflammatory carcinoma must always be suspected.

As regards the nipple, apart from the relatively frequent introflection, often bilateral and congenital, but not uncommon in women after the menopause as a result of a progressive hypotrophy of the breast, one must look carefully at any sign of superficial erosion or ulceration. This may be a sign of an early stage of Paget's disease, otherwise defined as "epidermothropic intraductal carcinoma", which may commence with a strictly limited area of itching erithema around one lactiferous porus of the nipple and without any other sign.

The discharge of fluid from the nipple is not infrequent and is generally a benign sign. Milky, aqueous, green or brown discharges have no pathological relevance. On the other hand, yellow and red (serous and bloody) discharges must be given careful attention as they may be the sign of a papilloma of the ducts or, very rarely, of an intraductal carcinoma.

The axillary fossae are then carefully examined holding the patient's arms to allow the chest-wall muscles to relax. The minor pectoralis muscle is sometimes contracted and may give a false impression of nodal involvement. The physician must evaluate the number, the site, the size and the consistency of the palpable nodes and mentally form a judgement on the ones involved. This mental process must consider the age of the patient, her professional history (women who have had their arms exposed to rough manual work are likely to have large lymph nodes) and the history of previous inflammatory processes in the breasts or in the arms. The supraclavicular fossae and both sides of the neck must also be examined in the upright position in a search for any suspicious lymph node.

Mammography

Soft-tissue radiography of the breast is the method of choice for identification of a breast carcinoma today. Its superiority over the physical examination in detecting small carcinomas has been unequivocally shown by the BCDDP in the United States. Not infrequently, a mammography may detect a non-palpable small carcinoma, whilst carcinomas detected by palpation and not visible by mammography are less frequent, with the exception of cases of cancer in young, dense, dysplastic breasts.

In most cases a carcinoma may be distinguished from a benign lesion, the two main direct signs being the presence (a) of an opacity; and (b) of microcalcifications. The typical malignant opacity is nonhomogeneous and has irregular margins. However, in some instances the margins may be smooth (like in colloid carcinoma and in medullary carcinoma) and may simulate benign lesions. The microcalcifications that indicate the presence of a carcinoma are very fine, punctated and elongated, frequently with irregular margins. The calcifications may be the only sign of malignancy, as in many intraductal carcinomas, or they may be associated with an opacity. In this case, they may be found inside, adjacent to, or at a distance from the opacity. When a large number of fine calcifications are present in a *limited* area of the breast, the diagnosis of cancer is almost certain. Secondary signs of malignancy may be the hypervascularity, the structural alterations of the breast tissue and thickening of the skin. Skin retraction may also be seen.

Some benign lesions, such as plasma cell mastitis, fat necrosis and sclerosing adenosis, may simulate a small breast carcinoma and are the main causes for false positive diagnosis.

Finally, it must be recorded that the radiographic size of the carcinoma is usually smaller than the clinical size due to the presence of a hard oedema around the tumour, radiographically invisible but palpable. The difference is sometimes considerable, and in our experience some 30% of cases clinically defined as T2 were classified as T1 by mammography.

Fine Needle Biopsy

The refinement of the techniques of aspiration with a fine needle has made it possible, in many istances of breast carcinoma, to avoid an open biopsy, either preoperative or extempore. Large studies with fine needle biopsy have shown that the risk of false positive diagnosis is extremely low and almost non-existant in the hands of experienced cytologists.

On the other hand, false negative cases are not infrequent and they become more and more common as the tumours to be detected become smaller. Therefore, a negative cytological diagnosis should not be considered if a clinical or mammographic suspicion exists. Cytology cannot demonstrate that the tumour is invasive, and therefore a cytological diagnosis of malignant cells could not fully justify a radical surgical procedure. However, if the clinical and mammographic evidence of cancer offers no doubts, the adjunctive evidence of malignant cells justifies definitive surgery without an open biopsy, with the advantage of operating in an intact breast. This is particularly useful in the case of conservative surgery.

Open Biopsy

Histology is the final and recognised proof of malignancy, and the biopsy remains, therefore, an important step before definitive radical treatment, although cytology may replace it in many cases. Open biopsy is performed by the removal of all the primary tumour (excisional) or of a part of it (incisional). The choice between the first and the second procedures depends on the dimension of the mass. If the tumour is large, an excisional biopsy is impractical because it would remove such a large portion of the mammary gland as to create difficulties for the surgeon who performs the final operation and might also increase the risk of seeding cancer cells. On the other hand, a lump of limited size is better removed by total excision, as an incisional biopsy would provide the pathologist with too small an amount of tissue. Masses of intermediate size may be biopsied by both techniques, although many surgeons would prefer the excisional biopsy.

As regards the timing of biopsy, the extempore biopsy with frozen section is performed less and less, both because a fine needle biopsy has already provided the proof of malignancy and because the two-stage approach is gaining ground among many surgeons. According to this approach, an adequate preliminary biopsy, which may even be performed in the doctor's surgery under local anaesthesia, provides considerable information on the biological and histological characteristics of the primary tumour making it possible to establish a better plan of the final treatment.

Preoperative Localization of Clinically Occult Lesions

The introduction on a large scale of mammography has led to the frequent appearance of suspicious lesions which are not palpable. Very often the suspicious sign is only the presence of a number of microcalcifications. A very rough way to obtain a diagnosis is a large excision of the breast tissue, such as a quadrantectomy including the suspicious area, but this procedure appears unacceptable today. On the other hand, it is generally possible to localise the position of the lesion with great accuracy by inserting a needle under double-view mammographic control. The needle may leave in place either a coloured substance to be recognised by the surgeon or a spring-hook wire which provides a stable, anchored guide for the surgeon. In this way, it is possible to remove only a limited portion of tissue around the lesion, which, in any case, must be submitted to a specimen radiography to document the complete removal of the suspicious area. The specimen radiography must obviously be performed whilst the patient is under anaesthesia so that in case of error, a re-excision may be made immediately.

Other Diagnostic Techniques

Ultrasonography utilises high-frequency sound waves produced by piezoelectric crystals and stimulated by electronic pulses. Although ultrasonsography has the ability to differentiate between cystic and solid masses, its sensitivity to detect small size carcinomas is poor.

Thermography enjoyed a certain success at the end of the 1970s when the fear of a possible induction of cancer by ionising radiation from mammography strongly urged research towards alternative methodologies. Although some breast cancers increase the local temperature which may be revealed by thermography, both the specificity and sensitivity of thermography are low and certainly very low in the case of the minimal cancerous lesions. We believe that this diagnostic procedure will soon disappear from clinical practice.

CT scanning and magnetic resonance imaging are also under evaluation, but from the preliminary data it appears that they cannot compete, in accuracy, simplicity and cost, with mammography.

Treatment

The two major dogmas which were at the basis of the Halstedian theory were (a) that since the lymphatic network of the breast was richly anastomosed, a cancer cell that escaped from a primary cancer would rapidly reach any point in the mammary gland; and (b) that cancer cells very often invaded the major lymphatic trunks by way of a "permeation" process, i.e. "filling" the lymph vessels. According to these principles, in order to obtain locoregional control of the cancer process, it is necessary to remove all the mammary tissue with all the intermediate lymphatic vessels together with the axillary lymph nodes. In recent decades the Halsted procedure has been subjected to a number of criticisms. The first was that the classic Halsted technique was inadequate and not sufficiently extensive because of the failure to remove internal mammary nodes. In fact, around the 1960s, a number of procedures were developed for a more "radical" approach: extended surgical techniques with removal of the internal mammary nodes, superradical operations with dissection of internal mammary, supraclavicular and mediastinal nodes and aggressive postsurgical regional radiotherapy. Controlled trials conducted mainly in the 1960s showed, however, that neither very extensive surgical operations, nor intensive postoperative radiotherapy were able to improve the prognosis of breast cancer.

An opposing criticism considered the radical mastectomy an unnecessarily mutilating operation since equally good results could be obtained with more conservative techniques, either surgical or radiotherapeutic, or a combination of the two. The sporadic attempts by a few pioneers of the 1950s and 1960s encountered, however, a hostile reaction on the part of many surgeons, but were later encouraged by newer information on the natural history of breast cancer. The new concepts postulate that the fate of breast cancer patients is linked more to the presence or absence of occult metastases than to the extent of locoregional surgery. Therefore, efforts should be particularly directed to the avoidance (early detection of breast cancer) and the control of distant metastases, which in fact are the main cause of failure, whereas locoregional control can be obtained with more limited procedures.

Objectives of Locoregional Treatment

The first objective of the surgical treatment of breast cancer is complete locoregional control of the disease. It would be unfair to expose the fraction of patients who do not have disseminated disease to the risk of locoregional recurrence. Every patient must, in principle, be considered as potentially curable with locoregional treatment and must benefit from a treatment that assures maximal local control of the disease. If prognostic data show that the risk of recurrence of the disease is high, the treatment may be supplemented, but not substituted, with other measures aimed at controlling occult distant metastases.

The second objective is to obtain as much information as possible from the surgical act on the spread of the disease, both for a prognostic evaluation and the planning of adjunctive treatments. The third objective is to limit the mutilation as much as possible, so as to reach results that will be acceptable from the cosmetic and the functional point of view. Sometimes, it is difficult to fulfil the three objectives simultaneously and they have been enumerated according to logical priority.

The Breast Cancer Patient

The implementation of many breast cancer detection programmes, the increased information on breast cancer problems among the general population, the publicity on self-examination and the large-scale introduction of mammography have all contributed to an increased consciousness of the importance of early diagnosis among the female public in most western countries. As a result, there has been a considerable increase of women presenting themselves with a small breast cancer.

At the National Cancer Institute in Milan, the proportion of cases with primary carcinomas of less than 2 cm in diameter has increased considerably over the last 10 years, reaching nearly 50% in the last few years. Certainly, the awareness that small cancer may be treated without the loss of the breast has stimulated many women to follow a policy of accurate and regular control of their breast and of participation in community cancer detection programmes.

Moreover, the opinion of the patient herself has become an important component in the choice of treatment. There has been a burst of interest among the public about the problem of breast cancer and, in particular, the breast conservation issue. The controversy concerning the avoidance of mastectomy has generated articles in the medical and lay press with passionate public debates on the most acceptable and appropriate breast cancer treatment. What women ask the surgeon today is for complete information on the type of treatment, possible alternatives and related risks.

Treatment of Primary Breast Cancer

Surgery of Primary Breast Cancer

Halsted Mastectomy. Although the treatment of choice in breast cancer surgery for nearly a century (and still widely practised), Halsted mastectomy has gradually been substituted by a variety of different operations. It was the type of operation most extensively applied to breast cancer patients in the last century. The first was performed by Halsted in 1882, and the preliminary results were published in 1894. In the same year, Meyer (1894) reported his results with a very similar operation. This mastectomy involved an en bloc removal of the breast, both pectoralis muscles and the content of all axillary fossa. Important modifications such as the vertical type of incision, the extensive skin excision, the very thin skin flaps and the removal of the thoraco-dorsal nerve and vessels, were introduced by Haagensen (1986).

Total Mastectomy and Axillary Dissection. In the late 1930s, Patey and Dyson (1948) in Great Britain introduced a less mutilating operation, preserving the major pectoralis muscle and its neurovascular bundle. Although, for a few decades, this variation was not considered by most surgeons as appropriate to fulfil the dogmas which were at the root of the so-called radical breast surgery, in the last 15 years it has gained widespread acceptability and is today the type of operation practised most. Many variations have been introduced by Scanlon and Caprini (1975), Maier et al. (1977), Roses et al. (1977) and Anderson et al. (1979).

Extended Mastectomy. The extended types of mastectomy have as their major objective the inclusion in the surgical act of the regional node areas which are neglected by the Halsted mastectomy, in particular the internal mammary nodes. The first attempts were made by W. S. Handley in 1927 and were then followed by his son R. S. Handley (Handley and Thackray 1954), in London, and by many other European (Margottini and Bucalossi 1949; Giacomelli and Veronesi 1952; Redon and Lacour 1955; Veronesi 1963) and American surgeons (Urban and Baker 1952). Superradical operations, including the dissection of internal mammary nodes, supraclavicular nodes and, optionally, the mediastinal nodes, were devised and performed by Wangensteen (1949) in the United States and by Dahl-Iversen (1952) and Veronesi and Zingo (1967) in Europe.

Quadrantectomy. This term was coined by U. Veronesi at the beginning of the 1970s to describe an operation which involved the removal of a quadrant of the breast including the skin, the subcutaneous fat tissue, the mammary gland and the fascia of the major pectoralis muscle (Veronesi 1977; Veronesi et al. 1977). The aim of this operation is the radical elimination of the primary carcinoma, provided it is of limited extent, which may be obtained by the removal of a breast quadrant without the need of total mastectomy.

Large Mammary Resection. This definition describes a more limited operation, without removal of the skin or the pectoralis fascia, but with margins of normal tissue of at least 2 cm from the edge of the tumour. This operation represents an intermediate type of conservative surgery, a sort of compromise between the quadrantectomy (whose aim is a radical removal of the tumour) and the lumpectomy (which has only a debulking aim). Synonyms are "wide excision", "tylectomy", "segmental mastectomy" and "wedge resection".

Narrow Mammary Resection. This is an operation which provides for the removal of the tumour mass without the objective of local radicality. It is a reduced debulking operation to improve the effectiveness of radiotherapy which, in this case, is the main treatment procedure. Synonyms: "lumpectomy", "tumourectomy", "excisional biopsy" and "excision".

The Problem of Resection Margins. In protocol no. 06 of the National Surgical Adjuvant Breast Program (NSABP) study in North America, one of the requirements for the conservative procedure was that the margins of the breast resection should be free from cancer cells. In fact, some 10% of the cases treated with limited surgery were found to have positive margins and were immediately submitted to mastectomy. However, out of the remaining 90% of cases with free margins, one-third had a local recurrence showing that the fact that the margins were found free from cancer cells had very limited value in predicting the risk of recurrence (B. Fisher et al. 1985 c).

Radiotherapy of Primary Breast Cancer

The possibility of treating breast cancer with radiotherapy goes back to the 1920s, when in 1927 Hirsch reported 22 cases treated with lumpectomy plus radiotherapy between 1914 and 1924, with a survival rate of more than 90% at 3 years. In Great Britain, Keynes began to study the use of radiotherapy in breast cancer in 1924 and developed an original technique for implanting radium needles into the breast. In 1937 he reported on a series of 250 patients treated with this technique, showing results no different from those obtained by surgery regarding both the local control and survival (Keynes 1937).

Pfahler (1932) in the United States showed a 5-year survival rate of 80% in a small series of patients with early breast cancer treated with radiotherapy alone. In 1939 Peters (1967), a radiotherapist in Toronto, treated 184 patients with T1-T2 tumours with radiation (after a local excision) yielding results similar to those observed in matched patients treated by conventional surgery. Beginning around 1940, Mustakallio (1972), in Helsinki, treated negative-node patients with lumpectomy plus radiotherapy, with a dose of 21 Gy in six fractions to the breast and the axillary nodes. In his series of patients, 26% developed locoregional recurrence within 10 years, but, despite this high local recurrence rate, a 10-year survival rate of 71% was observed.

A great effort to use radiotherapy as primary treatment of breast cancer was developed in France, following the pioneering studies of Baclesse (1949). This radiotherapist in Paris developed a sophisticated technique for primary radiotherapy as the sole treatment of breast cancer, showing an 82% complete response in tumours of less than 6 cm in diameter. Baclesse was aware of the need for the large doses required for the total elimination of the cancer cells in the breast (60 Gy) and the need for fractionation. Baclesse's teaching in France stimulated a number of radiotherapy centres to treat primary breast cancer with radical irradiation.

Pierquin et al. (1980), also in Paris, introduced a combined modality, adding to the external irradiation with cobalt and the boosting by electrons to the axilla and internal mammary nodes, an interstitial implantation with iridium 192. Lumpectomy was performed in patients with small tumours. The results were excellent, and the 5-year survival rate was 93% in T1 cases, 85% in T2 cases and 70% in T3 cases, with a very low rate of local recurrences.

Calle et al. reported in 1978 a series of 700 cases treated at the Fondation Curie, Paris, with external radiotherapy using high-energy doses of 65 Gy in the tumour area after lumpectomy (small tumours) and of 80 Gy if lumpectomy was not performed (large tumours). The entire breast received 50 Gy, and the same dosage was given to the regional nodes. The overall survival rate for patients with tumours of less than 3 cm was 85% at 5 years and 75% at 10 years.

In 1977, Spitalier et al. (1977), in Marseille, published the 5-year results of 400 cases treated with radiotherapy between 1960 and 1970 with a survival rate of 87% in T1 cases, 75% in T2 cases and 42% in T3 cases. However, 29% of patients were subsequently submitted to salvage mastectomy for suspected local recurrence which, however, in one-third of the cases was not confirmed by histology.

In the United States, the largest experience has been accumulated by the Boston group (Joint Center for Radiation Therapy, JCRT) (Harris et al. 1978), who have recently published the results on the treatment of 525 stage I–II patients treated between 1968 and 1980 (Recht et al. 1986). At 5 years the local control was 90%, which increased to 94% for stage I patients treated with excisional biopsy followed by whole breast irradiation and a boost to the primary site. The survival rate was 93% in clinical stage I and 82% in clinical stage II.

A number of other centres in the United States and Canada have devoted much effort to the treatment of primary breast cancer with radiotherapy, all with similarly statisfactory results: Clark et al. (1982) in Toronto, 87% 5-year survival in T1 N0 patients; Montague et al. (1984), in Houston, 85% 5-year survival in stage I.

Primary Chemotherapy and Endocrine Therapy

Primary chemotherapy or induction chemotherapy was introduced in the early 1970s to treat locally advanced breast carcinomas, in combination with radiotherapy, surgery, or with both. Primary chemotherapy showed its ability to reduce the tumour mass to allow radical surgery in cases which looked inoperable at the original examination. The response rates after chemotherapy with adriamycin-containing drugs appeared very high: De Lena et al. (1978) reported a complete or partial response of 86% to four cycles of adriamycin and vincristine; Hortobagyi et al. (1983) reported an overall response rate of 83% with a combination of cyclophosphamide, adriamycin and 5-fluorouracil CAF; and Sorace et al. (1985) reported a 33% complete response rate with treatment with CAF plus methotrexate (M), leucovorin rescue plus Premarin and tamoxifen. However, the impact of primary chemotherapy on long-term local control and survival seems to be of limited importance. The 5-year survival rate of patients treated at JCRT in Boston with either radiation only or radiation with single agent chemotherapy (38%) was inferior to that obtained with radiation following CMF or adriamycin (51%), but the difference was not statistically significant. The median survival in the various studies varied from 30 to 65 months, not much superior to that obtained with radiotherapy alone or radiotherapy plus surgery (Harris et al. 1983).

The use of hormones as the sole primary treatment for locally advanced breast cancer was reported by A. Veronesi et al. (1981). Tamoxifen was administered as the only primary treatment in 46 postmenopausal women with locally advanced breast cancer with a response rate of only 30% and a median survival of 17.5 months.

More recently, a possible use of chemotherapy as a primary treatment (with the bizarre name of "neoadjuvant") has been suggested in early breast cancer, stages I and II. The objective would be to exploit the local action of chemotherapy in addition to its general action, which would increase the spectrum of possibilities of conservative treatments and possibly reduce the rate of local recurrences. Although interesting scattered reports have been published by many authors (Forrest et al. 1986; Jacquillat et al. 1987), no clear evidence of the advantages of this new approach is at present available.

Review of Clinical Trials on Less Mutilating and Conservative Treatments

Evaluating Less Mutilating Types of Mastectomy

The introduction of the so-called modified radical mastectomy, which consists of total mastectomy with dissection of axillary nodes but sparing of the pectoralis major muscle, was not the result of any controlled study. Only after the procedure had become popular, were the results of clinical trials made available. Paradoxically, the two available trials did not totally encourage the lesser procedure.

In the United States Maddox et al. (1983) reported the results of a prospectively randomised trial comparing standard (Halsted) radical mastectomy with a modified radical mastectomy. A total of 311 patients with primary operable carcinoma of the breast were entered into a surgical and adjunctive chemotherapeutic trial in the state of Alabama between 1975 and 1978. A total of 91 surgeons participated. After a median follow-up of 5 years, there was no significant difference in disease-free survival or in overall survival between the two groups. However, there was a trend in favour of Halsted mastectomy (84% 5-year survival) compared to the modified one (76%).

Another randomised trial, conducted by Turner et al. (1981) in the United Kingdom, compared 534 patients undergoing either modified radical or radical mastectomy. No difference in disease-free or overall survival was noted, but a trend of improved survival at 5 years was observed in the radical mastectomy group (85%), compared to the modified radical mastectomy (78%). Moreover, there was an increased incidence of local wound recurrence in those patients who had undergone modified radical mastectomy (*P* 0.03).

Trials Evaluating Conservative Procedures

The Guy's Hospital Trial. This was the first attempt to evaluate the role of conservative treatments through a randomised control study (Hayward 1977). A total of 370 stage I and II patients aged over 50 were randomised from 1961 to 1971 into two groups. Halsted mastectomy with postoperative radiotherapy (24 Gy with orthovoltage) to axillary, supraclavicular and internal mammary nodes was performed in 188 patients. Breast resection with radiotherapy to the breast residual tissue (35 Gy by linear accelerator) and to the regional nodes was performed in 182 patients. Until 1969, both groups received three doses of thiotepa up to a total dose of 0.7 mg/kg body weight over 4 days. In stage I patients (without palpable nodes), local excision was followed by a higher incidence of local and axillary recurrence, but the survival rates were not significantly different from those obtained in the Halsted mastectomy group. By contrast, in stage II patients with clinically palpable nodes, the 10-year survival rate was lower than in the mastectomy group.

A second series of 253 patients with stage I disease was studied between 1971 and 1975. The patients were randomly allocated to either wide excision or radical mastectomy. In both cases, radiotherapy was administered with a dosage similar to that used for the first series. In this second series of patients, there was a significantly higher local and distant recurrence rate after wide excision, with reduced survival. The excess of local recurrences after wide excision occurred mostly in the axilla and was probably due to an insufficient dose of radiation therapy. According to Hayward (1983), the increased distant recurrence rate and the diminished survival appear to be the direct result of the axillary recurrences, suggesting that effective local control of disease is essential in the management of patients with early breast cancer.

The Milan Trial. A randomised trial, known as the "QUART" study, (QUART is an abbreviation of "quadrantectomy, axillary dissection, radiotherapy") was designed in 1969 and implemented at the Milan Cancer Institute 3 years later (Veronesi and Costa 1982; Veronesi et al. 1981). The principle of the quadrantectomy was that a complete radical removal of all cancer cells in the breast in small cancers does not require total mastectomy but may be obtained with a less mutilating surgical technique. This would involve excision of a good amount of normal tissue around the tumour, including the overlying skin and the underlying muscular fascia. In the quadrantectomy technique, the shape of the incision was elliptical with the major axis radial from the nipple. A margin of at least 3 cm was kept from the biopsy incision. If the axillary dissection could be performed in continuity, a peripheral extension of the incision was made to give adequate exposure of the axilla (Fig. 12). The en bloc operation was generally possible when the primary tumour was situated in the upper quadrants. In the other situations the axillary dissection was carried out with a separate incision. Radiotherapy on the operated breast was given in all cases, with either positive or negative axillary nodes. It started 3–6 weeks after the operation according to the condition of the operated breast. The breast tissue was irradiated with a linear accelerator or with a cobalt 60 unit. The two opposed tangential fields

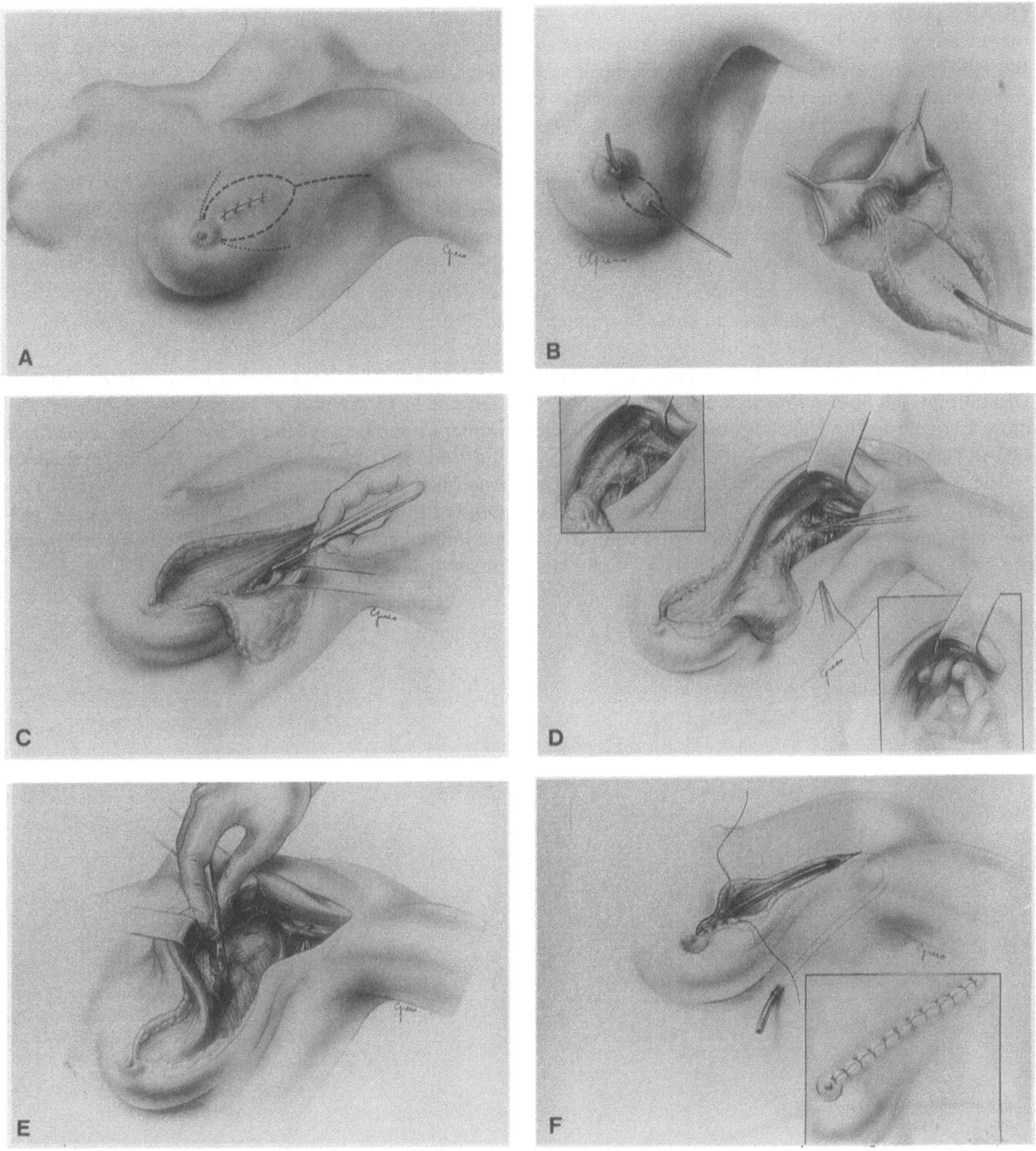

Fig. 12 A–F. Surgical procedure of a quadrantectomy

had an extension wide enough to cover the breast and the adjacent tissue. Moreover, since January 1976, all patients with positive nodes have been treated with 12 cycles of chemotherapy with the CMF regimen according to the following schedule: cyclophosphamide, 100 mg/m^2 of the body surface area per day for 14 days per month; methotrexate, 40 mg/m^2; and 5-fluorouracil, 600 mg/m^2, on days 1 and 8 i.v.

From June 1973 to May 1980, 701 evaluable patients were accrued in the trial: 349 were treated by Halsted mastectomy and 352 with the conservative procedure (QUART). Comparison of the two groups according to age, menopausal status, tumour site, dimensions of the primary cancer and previous biopsy showed no statistically significant differences.

After 15 years from the beginning of the trial, seven patients in the Halsted group and eight in the

QUART group showed local recurrence of the primary cancer as the first sign of failure. Moreover, in the conservative group seven more cases developed a second primary cancer in the ipsilateral breast that had been treated with quadrantectomy and radiotherapy.

The number of contralateral breast carcinomas was 36; 18 occurred in patients treated with Halsted mastectomy and 18 in those treated with QUART.

In the conservative group, it appears that the incidence of a second primary carcinoma in the ipsilateral breast is lower than that in the contralateral breast, suggesting that the radiotherapy given to the ipsilateral breast may have had a protective effect. Distant metastases, as a first sign of recurrence, were more frequent in the Halsted group (72) than in the QUART patients (57).

The long-term results of the trial showed similar 10-year relapse-free and overall survival rates in the two groups of patients: relapse-free survival: 77.1% in the conservative treatment and 75.7% in the Halsted mastectomy group; overall survival: 81.1% in the first group and 77.0% in the second group (Figs. 13, 14).

In conclusion, the QUART technique is compatible with acceptable cosmetic results in most cases and appears to be the first conservative treatment scientifically proven in a controlled study to be an alternative to mastectomy. However, these results are limited to carcinomas of less than 2 cm, which account for 30%–40% of all breast cancers in most hospital series in western countries. The quadrantectomy procedure, although suitable for carcinoma of very limited extent (less than 2 cm), is less suitable for tumours of a larger size. In fact, the need to remove a large portion of normal tissue around the primary tumour may lead to poor cosmetic results if the tumour is larger than 2 cm. This is particularly true for patients with small breasts. Therefore, for tumours of more than 2 cm in diameter, the quadrantectomy technique may be indicated only when the breast is large.

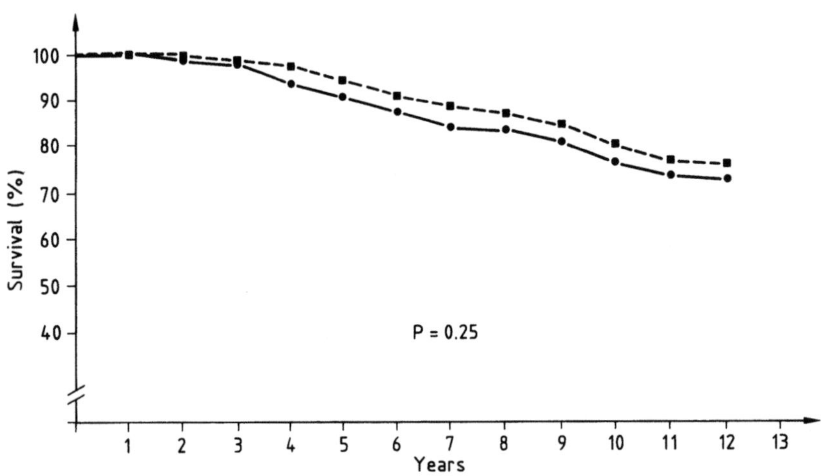

Fig. 13. Overall survival curves according to type of treatment (Milan trial I). *Solid line*, Halsted mastectomy; *broken line*, QUART

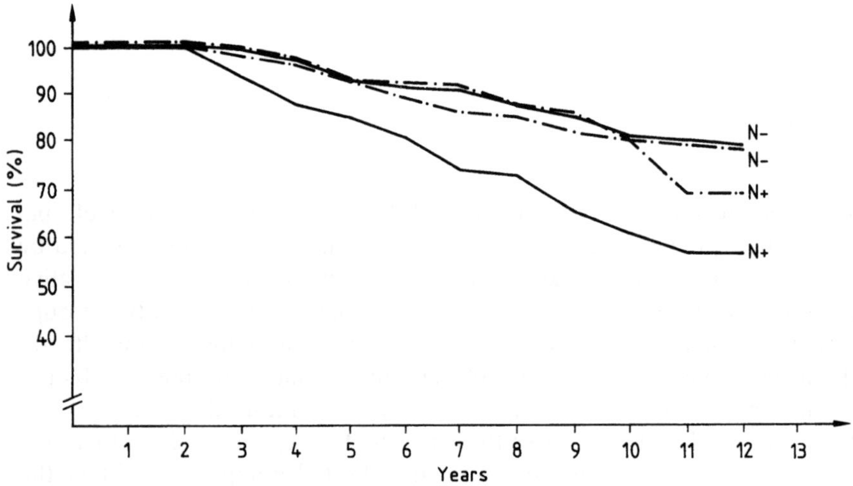

Fig. 14. Overall survival curves of patients treated with Halsted mastectomy *(solid line)*, axillary dissection and radiotherapy (QUART; *broken line*), according to absence ($N-$) or presence ($N+$) of axillary node metastases (Milan trial I)

The Gustave Roussy Institute Trial. The results of a trial carried out at the Gustave Roussy Institute in Paris from 1972 to 1979 were published by Sarrazin in 1983. Patients with breast cancer of less than 2 cm (at macroscopic evaluation), with negative or positive mobile axillary nodes (N0 N1), were randomised to mastectomy or local excision plus irradiation. In both groups, low axillary dissection and histological extempore examination of the nodes were performed. If node metastases were present, complete axillary dissection was performed.

The surgical technique for the primary tumour consisted of a breast resection. Radiotherapy to the breast was delivered with cobalt 60 teletherapy (45 Gy) plus a boost to the tumour bed of 15 Gy with the same apparatus or with an electron beam giving a total dose of 60 Gy in 6 weeks. Altogether 179 patients were randomised into the two main arms; 88 to the conservative and 91 to the mastectomy group.

The 5-year results showed no difference either in terms of locoregional recurrences or distant metastases. The overall and disease-free curves showed a slight advantage for conservatively treated patients compared to the mastectomised patients. The actuarial 5-year disease-free survival rates were 94% for the breast resection group and 91% for the mastectomy group, whereas the overall survival rates were 84% and 72% for the conservative and mastectomy groups, respectively.

A total of 72 node-positive patients were further randomised for regional radiotherapy: 41 received nodal irradiation and 31 did not. Postoperative regional radiotherapy failed to show any advantage; patients who did not receive regional radiotherapy had an overall five year survival of 96 per cent whereas in patients who were irradiated to regional nodes the survival was 83%.

The NSABP Trial. In 1976, the NSABP in North America started a randomised trial that compared total mastectomy with two conservative treatments (Fisher et al. 1985a). The three arms to which the patients were allocated were: (a) total mastectomy with axillary dissection; (b) wide mammary resection with axillary disssection; and (c) wide mammary resection, axillary dissection and radiotherapy (45 Gy) to the ipsilateral breast.

Patients with primary breast cancer up to 4 cm in diameter were considered eligible for the study. The extension of the breast removal was not defined in the protocol, but may be considered as a "wide mammary resection". However, if the specimen submitted to the pathologist showed breast cancer cells at the margins of the resected mammary tissue, a total mastectomy was performed. The skin overlying the primary cancer was not, in general, excised.

It is important to note that in this trial the removal of the primary cancer was performed with a minor surgical act which was little more than a lumpectomy, with the minimal extension necessary for tumour-free margins. The preliminary results published in 1985 (Fisher et al. 1985a) showed no difference in survival among the three groups. However, the differences in local recurrences were striking. Patients who had been treated with partial resection without radiotherapy experienced a 28% rate of breast recurrences, whilst 10% of the patients who had had the resection plus radiotherapy had local recurrences. True local recurrences and new primary carcinomas were computed together. Patients submitted to modified radical mastectomy had some 5% local recurrences.

The NCI Trial. A randomised trial which compared total mastectomy and axillary dissection with lumpectomy plus radiotherapy and axillary dissection was begun in 1979 at the NCI (Bethesda) (Lichter 1983). Patients were assigned either to a total mastectomy plus axillary dissection or to lumpectomy followed by external radiotherapy up to a dose of 45–50 Gy to the breast, internal mammary and supraclavicular nodes with a 4- or 6-MeV linear accelerator and implantation radiotherapy (20–30 Gy using iridium or caesium to the tumour bed in an interstitial implant). Patients with positive nodes, from both groups in the study, were treated with two-drug combination chemotherapy, using doxorubicin and cyclophosphamide, for a total cumulative dose of 330 mg/m^2 of doxorubicin. A total of 250 are expected to enter the study.

The EORTC Trial. Between 1980 and 1985 the Breast Group of EORTC conducted a study on conservative treatment of breast cancer. Patients with stages I and II breast cancer, with a tumour mass of less than 5 cm, were randomised to undergo a radical mastectomy (Halsted or Patey) or local excision of the tumour plus axillary dissection and radiotherapy to the breast. Beginning within 6 weeks of surgery, radiotherapy of 50 Gy in 5 weeks was administered to the whole breast. Moreover, radiotherapy of 50 Gy to the internal mammary nodes was given to all patients in both groups, if the tumour was located medially or centrally. Within 2–6 weeks after completion of external radiotherapy, ^{192}Ir implantation was done, the target volume including the whole excisional bed with a 1-cm margin. Adjuvant chemotherapy with CMF was administered to patients with positive axillary nodes. Altogether 903 patients were entered into the study, of whom 148 were in stage I and 755 were in stage II. The 6-year disease-free survival, evaluated by the log rank test, was similar in both groups ($P = 0.927$). At stage I, local recurrences, including supraclavicular adenopathies and ipsilateral tumours, were absent in the radical group and occurred at a rate of 5% in the conservative one; at stage II the rates were 5% in both groups (van Dongen 1987).

The Second Milan Trial. At the Milan Cancer Institute, between 1985 and 1987, a second randomised trial was conducted with the aim of comparing the classic QUART technique with a more reduced surgical intervention followed by aggressive radiotherapy treatment consisting of 45 Gy by external high-energy source plus an implant of ^{192}Ir wires which would deliver an additional 14–17 Gy to the tumour bed. The operation consisted in a simple "tumourectomy", which removed the tumour mass with a very limited amount of peripheral normal tissue. Altogether 713 cases, all with a carcinoma of less than 2.5 cm at macroscopic examination, were entered into the trial, 355 of whom were treated with QUART and the other 358 were treated with TART (tumourectomy, axillary dissection, radiotherapy). Two per cent of the QUART cases and 14% of the TART cases were found to have positive resection margins, but no modification of treatment was introduced in these cases.

In November 1987, two new trials were initiated at the Milan Cancer Institute, the aim of the first being to compare the classic QUART with quadrantectomy and axillary dissection alone, followed by radiotherapy only in case of a local recurrence. The possible advantages of the breast conservation with surgery alone are: (a) that treatment is easier and cheaper; (b) that a local recurrence is easier to discover as there is not the fibrosis due to radiotherapy; (c) that possible late effects of radiotherapy (such as pulmonary fibrosis and cardiac damage as well as any hypothetical oncogenic risk) are avoided.

The fourth Milan trial, which also started at the end of 1987, has the objective of evaluating the efficacy of intensive radiotherapy after tumourectomy without the radioactive iridium implant. The TART technique previously described is, therefore, compared with a similar technique, the only difference being that the boost is administered through external irradiation with photons or electrons with a dosage of 10 Gy.

At least three trials are in progress in the United Kingdom, comparing different conservative techniques. In the Scottish trial the patients treated with breast resection plus low axillary dissection are randomised between breast radiotherapy and no further treatment. A trial in progress in Manchester randomises stage I patients treated with breast resection (without axillary dissection) between radiotherapy to all breast tissue and radiotherapy by direct field limited to the area of the breast where the primary carcinoma was located. Finally, in the West Midlands trials the patients are randomised to breast resection and no axillary dissection, and radiotherapy and breast resection, no axillary dissection and no radiotherapy.

Treatment of Regional Nodes

Axillary Nodes

As already mentioned, the axillary lymph nodes are the ones more exposed to the risk of metastases from a breast carcinoma. The spread starts from the first level and then progresses to the second and to the third. Therefore, if a single axillary lymph node is involved, it is *always* at the first level, and if the first level is not involved by metastases, the risk that cancer cells are present at the higher levels is negligible. On the other hand, if the first level is involved, the chances that the other two levels are also involved are in the order of 40%, with great variations according to the number of nodes involved at the first level and to the size of the primary tumour (Veronesi et al. 1986). As a general order of probabilities, one may say that in T1 cases, one-third of the patients have occult or overt axillary metastases, that in T2 cases nearly half of the patients have axillary involvement and that in T3 cases this goes up to nearly two-thirds of the patients. The clinical diagnosis is good in the case of clinically positive nodes with some 20% of false positivity, and less good in case of clinically negative nodes, with some 30% of false negativity.

The treatment of axillary nodes has been the object of many prolonged controversies. In the case of clinically positive nodes, most surgeons agree that the nodes must be removed, but the type of surgical dissection suggested is often different. In the case of clinically negative nodes, the major question is the real need for the dissection, as in early breast cancer the chances that the nodes are negative are high.

That clinically positive nodes should be treated is then a unanimous principle. However, although surgical dissection appears the most widely accepted form of treatment, for a long period of time axillary radiotherapy has been considered the treatment of choice, especially in the United Kingdom and in northern Europe. This procedure was supported especially by McWhirter (1955) in Edinburgh, who was able to show that total mastectomy plus axillary radiotherapy may produce results similar to the Halsted mastectomy.

Moreover, in a large randomised trial in the United Kingdom by the Cancer Research Campaign (1980), 2268 patients in stages I and II were randomised between mastectomy plus radiotherapy (including the axilla) and mastectomy followed by a watch policy. At 5 years there was no evidence that radiotherapy increased survival, although the rate of local recurrences was lower in the irradiated patients. The value of axillary radiotherapy was proved by a clinical randomised trial conducted by the NSABP in the United States between 1971 and 1974 (Fisher et al. 1985c). In this study 1665 patients with stage II disease (with suspicious palpable nodes) were randomised between Halsted mastectomy and total mastectomy with or without radiotherapy. The study showed that at 10 years there was no significant difference between the two treatments in terms of locoregional and distant failures and survival.

It must be said, however, that although axillary radiotherapy appears to be equally as effective as surgery in the control of the disease, it has been gradually abandoned, principally because of its inability to provide useful information on the state of the axillary nodes. In fact, the prognostic value of the axillary node involvement is considerable, and the advantage of the surgical axillary dissection is to have access to this information, which in turn may be important in making a decision on possible adjunctive treatments.

The "staging" aim of the axillary dissection has often been considered the main reason for justifying the dissection in clinically negative-node patients. In fact, when the axillary nodes are negative at clinical examination, immediate dissection does not show any superiority, in terms of survival, compared to dissection, performed only on the appearance of clinical metastases (Fisher et al. 1985b). Therefore, the only justification of the dissection is to provide information on the status of the axillary nodes. This staging aim of dissection has led many surgeons to reduce the extent of the dissection to the removal of the first level only, as the absence or presence of metastases at the first level is highly predictive of higher axillary involvement (Veronesi et al. 1986).

The need for axillary dissection in clinically node-negative patients has recently been questioned on the following grounds: (a) that in early breast cancer the chances that the axillary nodes are healthy is in the order of 75%–80%, in these cases dissection is useless and most likely dangerous; (b) a dissection performed at the time of the appearance of clinical metastases does not change the survival rates and avoids an unneccessary operation and its unpleasant consequences like arm oedema; (c) in postmenopausal patients, in whom the indication of adjunctive treatment is mainly limited to tamoxifen, this may be applied in all patients without the need to know the state of the axillary nodes; (d) in premenopausal patients the application of adjunctive chemotherapy or endocrine therapies may be deferred to the time of the clinical evidence of axillary metastases, as the timing of its application does not seem very important (Glucksberg et al. 1982; Taylor et al. 1985); (e) alternatively, prognostic indications to be decided for adjunctive treatments may be derived from the primary tumour (growth rate, ploidy, ER status, peritumoral lymphatic invasion, etc.) without the need for axillary dissection.

Certainly, on the lines of a progressive reduction of surgery in the treatment of early breast cancer, these considerations must be carefully evaluated as it is likely that in the near future the present policy of axillary dissection will be largely revised.

If the need of axillary dissection in clinically node-negative patients is under discussion, even more uncertain is its extent and the technique to be adopted.

The "sampling" technique advocated by many surgeons (Davies et al. 1980; Pigott et al. 1984) with which only the first level (or a portion of it) is removed has some disadvantages. The main problem is that if the sampling shows an involvement of the first axillary level, the second and/or the third are likely to be involved, and therefore the problem of the treatment of these occult metastases must be faced. It is important to underline that the recurrences in the axilla are very difficult to detect early, are painful and often create a paralysis of the arm, due to the invasion of the brachial plexus. The treatment of the occult residual disease should, therefore, aim at the total destruction of the cancer cells in this site. This can be obtained either by another operation, such as total axillary dissection, or with radiotherapy. However, both procedures have certain disadvantages. Surgical dissection is not easy when a portion of the axilla has already been resected, as the fibrosis may expose the axilla vein to possible lesions. Radiotherapy, on the other hand, may create late lymphoedema of the arm and, in radioresistant cases, may have no efficacy.

These complications may be easily avoided if the axillary dissection is a total one, including all three levels of lymph nodes. The advantages of this operation are (a) that the prognostic information is excellent, as the distribution by level will give the maximum for evaluation; (b) that no additional treatment is needed; and (c) that the risk of a local recurrence in the axillary fossa is practically nil. As the difference between the dissection of the nodes of the first level and the total axillary dissection is only a matter of an extra few minutes, there are no reasons for foregoing total axillary dissection.

As regards the technique for axillary dissection, it must be stressed that the number of nodes which can be removed by the Halsted mastectomy, Patey mastectomy and quadrantectomy with en bloc or in-discontinuity axillary dissection are the same. Moreover, the conservation of the minor pectoralis muscle appears to be compatible with a complete dissection of the axillary nodes.

Adjunctive radiotherapy on the axilla after axillary dissection was practised for many years, but has been gradually abandoned, both because of its inefficacy and because of the considerable increase of arm lymphoedema.

Treatment of Internal Mammary Nodes

Internal mammary nodes as a possible site of metastases from breast cancer were neglected by surgeons until Handley and Thackray (1954) in London inaugurated a surgical technique which included, after the classic radical mastectomy, the removal of the internal mammary nodes from the second to the fifth intercostal spaces, a technique which was immediately followed by a number of European surgeons. The first reports showed a rate of metastatic spread to the internal mammary nodes of around 20%–30%, confirming the importance of this nodal basin in the natural history of breast cancer. Urban and Baker (1952) in New York developed a more extensive procedure removing en bloc a good portion of the chest wall, including part of the sternum and anterior portion of four ribs. With this operation Urban and Baker claimed long-term results superior to the Halsted mastectomy and advocated an extensive use of the extended procedure. A randomised international clinical trial was then designed and implemented by five different institutions and the results were published in 1976 and in 1983 with clear evidence of the overall inefficacy of the extended procedure to the traditional mastectomy (Lacour et al. 1976; Lacour et al. 1983).

The Milan series, which was part of the study, was analysed separately with a survival rate at 10 years of 60.7% for the Halsted mastectomy and 57% for the extended mastectomy (Veronesi and Valagussa 1981). An analysis according to the size and the site of the primary tumour and to the axillary involvement did not identify any subset of patients who would benefit from the extended procedure. The radical removal of the internal mammary nodes appeared, therefore, very clearly a procedure incapable of improving the prognosis of breast cancer. However, we recently reanalysed a large series of our 1000 patients treated with extended mastectomy, showing that the information on the status of the internal mammary nodes is very important from the prognostic point of view and that, in a refined staging process, this information should not be ignored. We suggested, therefore, that every effort should be made to obtain this information, possibly by non-invasive methods (such as computerised tomography or magnetic resonance), or by a delicate biopsy at the second intercostal space (Veronesi et al. 1983). It was also shown in this review that the traditional belief that internal mammary node metastases are more frequent in the case of tumours in the inner quadrants than in the outer quadrants of the breast is not true (Veronesi et al. 1985 a). If the radical surgical removal of the internal mammary nodes appeared to be a procedure incapable of improving control over breast cancer, the total consequence is that their irradiation would be equally ineffective. Therefore, the traditional "postoperative or adjuvant" radiotherapy on the internal mammary and supraclavicular nodes, which, for many decades, was a treatment widely applied in many parts of the world, has gradually lost its popularity. At the Milan Cancer Institute postoperative radiotherapy (which was previously given on the axillary, internal mammary and supraclavicular regions) was abandoned some 20 years ago, when surgery of the internal mammary nodes showed its inefficacy: the positive effects were that the rate of arm lymphoedema dropped dramatically and the cases with late paresis of the arm disappeared completely.

In the same period of time, a number of clinical trials comparing Halsted mastectomy with Halsted mastectomy plus postoperative radiotherapy were conducted in many countries. The first was effected at the Christie Hospital of Manchester, beginning in 1949 (Paterson and Russell 1959). By 1955, 1461 cases had been analysed, half of them receiving surgery alone and the other half receiving, after the Halsted mastectomy, postoperative radiotherapy, in part limited to the chest wall and axilla, and another part including the supraclavicular and internal mammary area. Radiotherapy was given with an orthovoltage technique. The patients treated with surgery alone were submitted to radiotherapy only in the case of local recurrence. Long-term results reported over 30 years did not show any advantage of radiotherapy on regional nodes compared to the watch policy (Palmer and Ribeiro 1985).

Other trials were then designed and conducted in the United States (B. Fisher et al. 1970), in Oslo (Høst et al. 1986) and in Stockholm (Wallgren et al. 1986) without any clear advantages in the cases treated with postoperative radiotherapy as regards the overall survival compared to surgery alone. Cuzick et al. (1987) assembled the results of different randomised trials (Manchester, Oslo, Stockholm, Heidelberg) and concluded that postoperative radiotherapy was not effective; on the contrary, at 15 years there was a statistically significant lower survival rate associated with the use of radiotherapy ($P = 0.005$).

Postmastectomy Reconstruction

It is only in recent years that the importance of reconstruction after ablative cancer surgery has been recognised by breast surgeons. Indeed, it was common opinion that reconstruction could either promote the risk of recurrence or make the detection of possible local recurrences difficult. Furthermore, the cosmetic results, often unsatisfactory, contributed to the growing scepticism among surgeons.

The new trends in breast cancer treatment with the replacement of the standard Halsted mastectomy by the modified radical mastectomy, have given great impulse to the development of the practice of breast reconstruction: in fact, by preserving the pectoral muscles, the modified mastectomy offers a basis for thorax symmetry after a breast reconstruction with appropriate techniques. The conservative treatment with quadrantectomy or lumpectomy have introduced the principle that a breast harbouring a cancer may be preserved, thus influencing the general trend towards more attention to the problems of women after breast mutilation. Moreover, today, the survival of breast cancer patients is longer than in the past, thus putting more emphasis on the importance of the psychological condition of the patients and their quality of life, and, in turn, bestowing a substantial role on reconstructive surgery.

Indications

Selection of patients and timing of reconstruction are at present not strictly defined but often based on the surgeons' experience and preferences. All patients operated on for breast cancer are possible candidates. Actually, breast reconstruction is possible following any kind of cancer surgery (Bohmert and Strombeck 1986).

The patient must be informed of the choices of reconstruction available to her and of the possible results; she has to understand that the reconstructed breast can never become completely normal. The patient herself, however, must decide on whether further surgery is worthwhile to restore her personal image. As well as the wish of the patient, the general health and the anaesthetic risk are obviously decisive factors concerning a further surgical opportunity.

As regards the timing of reconstruction, there are many trends. Primary reconstruction after mastectomy for cancer is still an uncommon procedure and is performed especially on those patients who refuse to have a mastectomy unless a reconstruction is done simultaneously. This procedure is technically possible, but the number of patients operated on is too small to allow any conclusions to be drawn. In order to plan this procedure, the tumour should not be too large and the breast should be of normal size. But two arguments go against this technique: doubts concerning the rotating of the skin flaps and the absence of accurate staging. To avoid these difficulties there is the possibility of a delayed primary reconstruction until 5 days after mastectomy.

Better results, however, are obtained when breast reconstruction is done at least 6 months after mastectomy, when the skin cover has become soft and elastic. If the patient has to have chemotherapy or radiation, reconstruction must wait at least until the adjuvant therapy is completed.

In the case of the presence of distant metastases, reconstruction is not usually performed. But it should be done if the patient, in spite of the poor prognosis, urgently wishes it in order to improve her quality of life, even if only for a relatively short period of time.

Methods of Breast Reconstruction

Many techniques of breast reconstruction after cancer surgery are available (Bostwick 1987). A choice between the different techniques depends on the prerequisites at hand following ablative surgery. The mastectomy deformity may range from mild asymmetry after lumpectomy, to an irradiated ulcer containing locally recurrent tumour following an extended radical mastectomy. Also, the appearance of the opposite breast influences the choice of a reconstructive method. For simple deformities, such as those resulting from a modified radical mastectomy, a breast reconstruction with a silicone breast implant

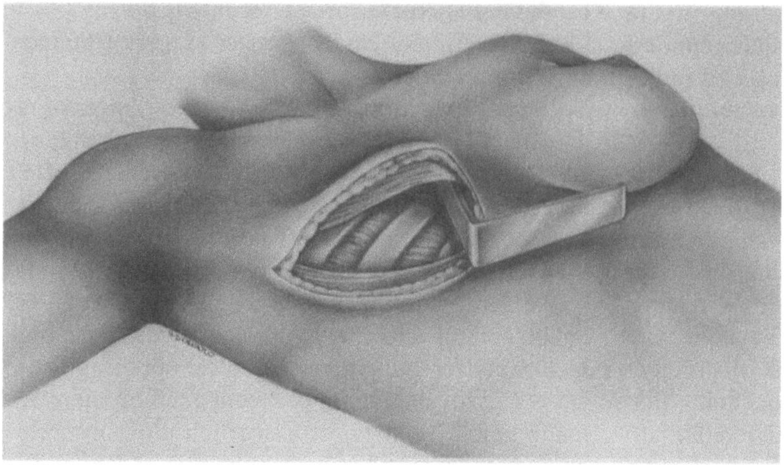

Fig. 15. The prosthesis is placed beneath the musculofascial layer of the chest wall

may be satisfactory. In other cases, with larger defects and ulceration, distant flaps either pedicled into the area or transferred by microvascular techniques are necessary.

Submuscular Implantation

In patients who have had a modified radical mastectomy, with preservation of the pectoralis muscles, the submuscular implantation of a prosthesis is the method of choice. This technique is suitable to achieve symmetry with the opposite breast that is not large and does not have significant ptosis (Dowden and Dinner 1984). The size of the silicone breast implant is chosen for its symmetry with the opposite breast. It is placed under the total mastectomy site beneath the musculofascial layer of the chest wall (Fig. 15).

To avoid additional scars, the incision usually follows the mastectomy scar. The tight tissues are gradually stretched by the silicone breast implant, so the final result is achieved several months after operation. If there is a deficiency of the local skin cover, it is possible to use an upper abdominal advancement flap (Lewis 1979). When the mastectomy has been done with a horizontal incision, the old scar is excised and the abdominal skin mobilised, usually, up to the level of the umbilicus. The mobilised skin cover is advanced cranially and fixed at the periosteum of the ribs at the level of the inframammary fold (Ryan 1982).

In patients with vertical or oblique scars, it is necessary to make an incision in the inframammary crease in order to attach the upper abdominal flap in its new position. If the patient has had radiation therapy, the skin circulation might be impaired, and this procedure is, therefore, usually unpractical.

The most common complication in the use of a silicone breast implant is the development of a fibrous capsule around it. A certain fibrosis in order to provide a support for the prosthesis is favourable; but the capsular contraction may distort the reconstructed breast, leading to an eventual asymmetry. This asymmetry may require an additional operation to review, or change, the silicone breast implant.

Use of a Tissue Expander

When, after total mastectomy, the local tissues are either deficient or too tight for a silicone breast implant, it is possible to use the recent skin expanders (Fig. 16) (Argenta 1984; Radovan 1984). These are silicone shell prostheses placed beneath the musculofascial layer and inflated daily during the postoperative period by injecting saline solution through a subcutaneous valve. When the local tissues have been expanded satisfactorily, the skin expander is exchanged for a permanent silicone breast implant making use of the scar of its implantation. This further operation is avoidable by using a new type of expander, called "Becker's expander". After the ideal dimension has been achieved, this prosthesis is left in place and the filling device is removed.

The technique of using tissue expanders in breast reconstruction allows the use of available tissue and obviates the need for more complex reconstruction that involves distant flaps and additional scars. This technique is suitable for patients with ptosis and also permits the reconstruction of large breasts.

In addition to the complications of the reconstruction experienced with a silicone breast implant, the specific complications of this technique include valve failure and secondary infection following the introduction of bacteria at the time of expansion.

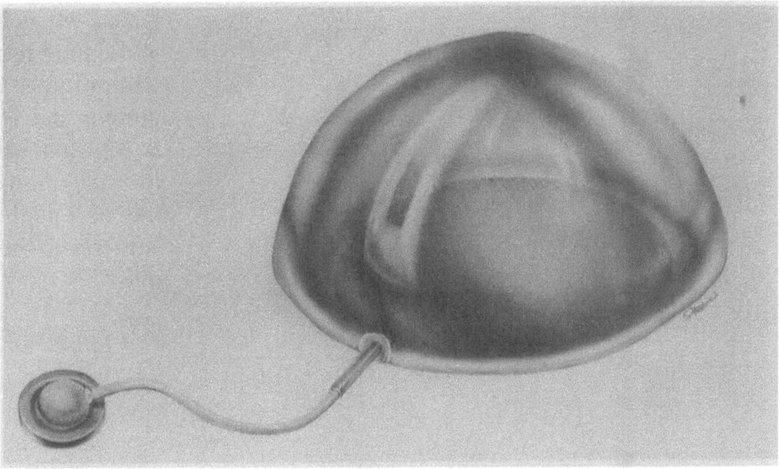

Fig. 16. A classic skin expander

Use of Skin Flap

The thoracoepigastric flap can, in certain reconstructive cases, be the method of choice. In selected cases it can correct the skin deficit, especially when oblique or vertical postmastectomy scars create a horizontal skin deficit (Bohmert 1980). The infraclavicular contour defect in the medial-cranial area and the contour defect in the axilla with loss of the anterior axillary fold cannot be corrected by this flap. In the axillary area, it might be possible to insert a distally de-epithelialised skin flap that, in combination with a special prosthesis, can eliminate the contour defect.

The surgical techniques consist in marking the flap from the middle of the rectus muscle to the mid-axillary line of the homolateral hemithorax (Fig. 17) and then mobilising it, starting at its apex. The flap is dissected off the muscles. The postmastectomy scar is excised and the edges are widely undermined, so the flap can be transposed into position (Fig. 18) and the donor area can in all cases be closed primarily following mobilisation (Fig. 19). This flap will supply the extra skin that is needed to rebuild the breast contour with silicone implants. The advantage in comparison with other flap techniques is that this procedure is technically simple and safe.

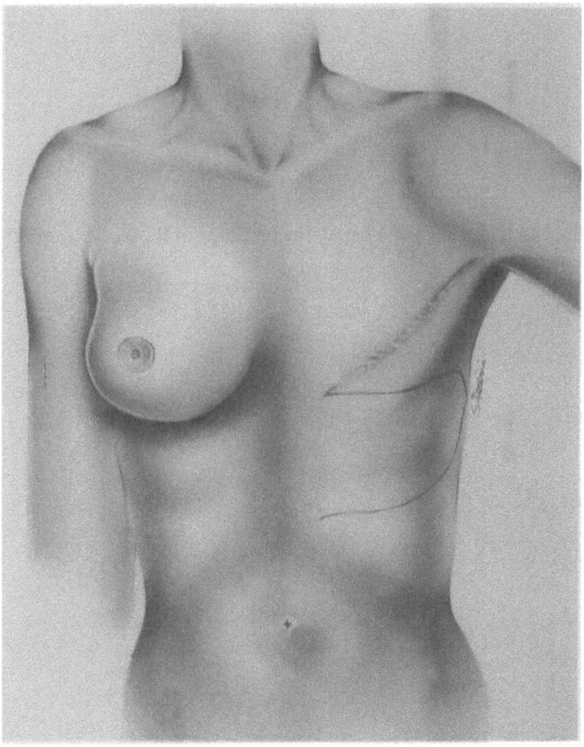

Fig. 17. The design of the thoracoepigastric flap

Use of Musculocutaneous Flaps

Many techniques using musculocutaneous flaps to rebuild the breast contour after mastectomy are available. The most common utilise the latissimus dorsi musculocutaneous flap, the lower transverse rectus abdominis musculocutaneous flap and the gluteus maximus musculocutaneous free flap.

The latissimus dorsi musculocutaneous flap and the lower transverse rectus abdominis musculocutaneous flap are usually selected for patients who have undergone a Halsted radical mastectomy in whom additional tissue is needed to fill the infraclavicular region, as well as to recreate the anterior axillary fold. The latissimus dorsi myocutaneous flap method is usually indicated when the tissue requirements are not too great, whilst the transverse rectus abdominis myocutaneous flap technique, which provides the largest amount of autogenous tissue, is se-

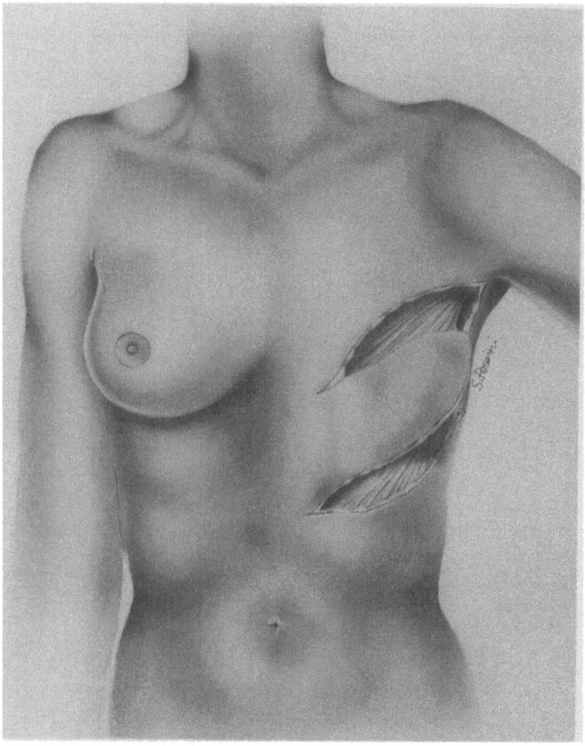

Fig. 18. The flap is elevated toward the midline and rotated upward

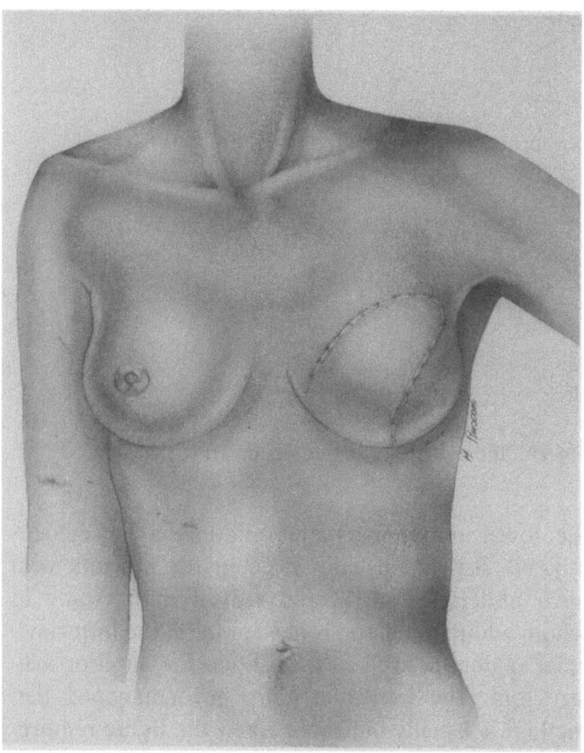

Fig. 19. The donor area is closed primarily and a silicone implant is inserted

lected when the patient has an abundance of lower abdominal tissue and desires a breast reconstruction without the use of a silicone breast implant. The gluteus maximus musculocutaneous flap technique is selected when the abdominal site is not suitable for the transverse rectus abdominis myocutaneous flap method. This method naturally requires the surgeon to be experienced in microvascular techniques.

The Latissimus Dorsi Musculocutaneous Flap Method. The main indication for this method is in patients who have undergone Halsted radical mastectomy, especially when the prominent ribs form an obvious deformity. This flap provides tissue to substitute not only the missing pectoral major muscle, but also breast skin, giving a natural shape to the reconstructed breast and an adequate cover for an implant should this be required (Biggs and Cronin 1981).

As regards the operative technique, the first step is to be sure that the nerve and blood supply of the muscle have not been damaged by the mastectomy. Before starting surgery, the borders of the muscle are outlined and the skin island is designed in order to fit into the postmastectomy scar area (Fig. 20). When the musculocutaneous flap is raised, it is brought to the postmastectomy scar area through a subcutaneous tunnel and sutured by layers. Before the closure is completed, a silicone breast implant is placed beneath the flap to give the reconstructed breast the proper size. The skin on the donor area is closed directly, without any skin graft.

This flap is one of the most reliable and safest flaps to use in reconstructive surgery. Its use is associated with a very low incidence of necrosis of the flap, infections and haematoma. Other possible complications include capsular contraction around the silicone prosthesis and insufficient reconstruction in cases in which more tissue is needed than is supplied by the flap.

The Lower Transverse Rectus Abdominis Musculocutaneous Flap Method. This technique has its main indication in patients with a major tissue deficit in the mastectomy area and a fair amount of surplus skin and fat in the lower abdomen (Hartrampf 1982). An ellipse of lower abdominal skin and fat is pedicled as a musculocutaneous flap on the upper rectus abdominis muscle (Fig. 21). With adequate rotation, the flap is brought through a subcutaneous tunnel to the postmastectomy scar area that has been excised. The abdominal wound in the donor area is closed as in an abdominoplasty. In selected patients, this reconstructive procedure may be accomplished by using

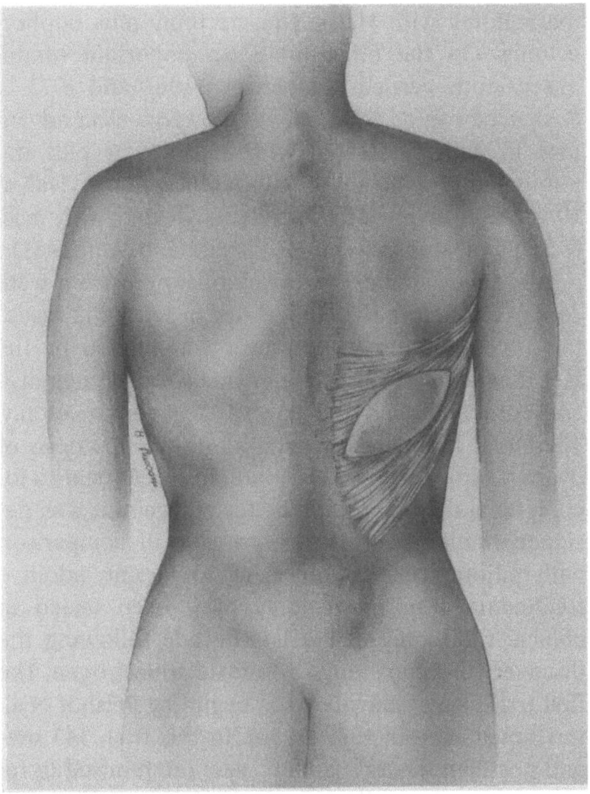

Fig. 20. The skin island is designed to fit into the postmastectomy scar area

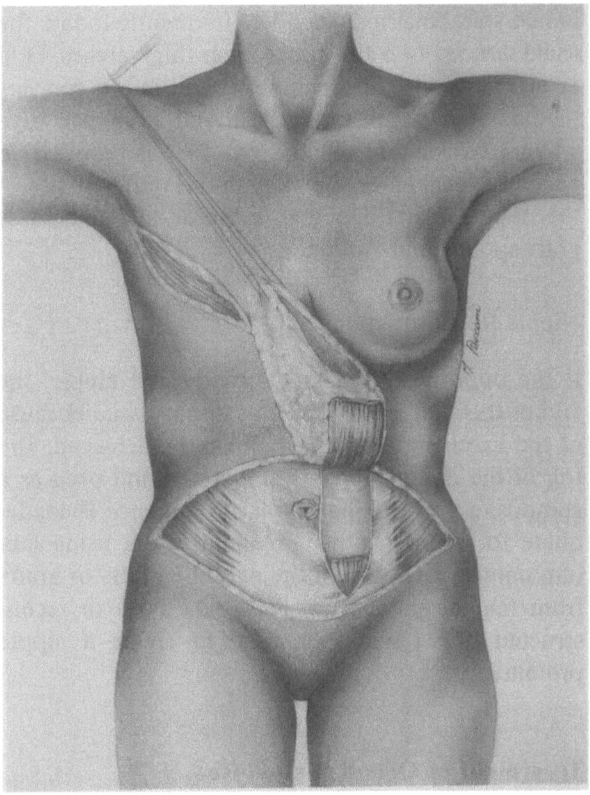

Fig. 21. Dissection of the pedicle based on the upper rectus muscle

the excess lower abdominal tissue and without the use of a silicone breast implant.

The potential complications of this method are more numerous than those associated with less complex methods of breast reconstruction. The patient must have excellent microcirculation, because fat necrosis may develop if a relative decrease in blood flow to the fat of the flap occurs. This may result in a thickening in the fat of the reconstructed breast, which may mimic a tumour. In addition, the abdominal wall may also be weakened by the transfer of the rectus abdominis muscles.

Free Flap Method of Breast Reconstruction. In this procedure the gluteus maximus musculocutaneous flap is transferred from the buttocks to the breast area and the gluteal vessels are anastomosed with a microvascular technique to the internal mammary vessels dissected deep to the fourth and fifth medial costal cartilages (Shaw 1983). The advantages of this method are that abundant tissue is available and that the donor scar is practically out of sight. Potential complications are failure of the flap and haematomas or infection of the donor site.

Nipple-Areolar Complex Reconstruction

The nipple-areolar complex reconstruction is the last phase of breast reconstruction and it is done after symmetry of the reconstructed breasts is achieved. This usually takes 3–6 months after the reconstruction. The goal is to reconstruct a nipple-areolar complex that is symmetrically positioned and similar in appearance to the opposite nipple-areolar complex. This operation is done for the sake of appearance only as there is no sensation other than the minimal sensation that is present on postmastectomy skin flaps. The technique for reconstruction of the areola and nipple is selected on the basis of the type of breast reconstruction and the configuration of the opposite nipple-areolar complex.

Areolar Reconstruction

The donor skin area is selected to match the colour of the contralateral areola. Therefore, the best method is that of using the areola of the opposite breast. If the contralateral areola is sufficiently large, a part of it can be used for reconstruction. Available methods are the concentric circle method and the conjoined spiral method, used less frequently today. The usual donor site is the upper inner thigh crease. Other areola donor sites include labium minus for very pigmentated areolas and the retroauricular area when an areola of a lighter pink tone is required. In all these techniques the skin in the outlined site of the new areola is denuded in the dermis and a free graft applied and sutured.

Nipple Reconstruction

If the opposite breast has a good-sized nipple, the end of this nipple is selected as donor tissue because of the excellent symmetry that can be achieved. The top of the donor nipple is amputated and used as a composite graft. If the nipple prominence is inadequate for sharing, other possibilities are using labium minus grafts, composite ear lobe grafts or grafts from the toe pulp. Also, local skin flaps of reconstructed breast might be used to create a nipple prominence.

Treatment of Occult Metastases

Endocrine Treatment

The first attempts at treating occult distant metastases with systemic therapy go back to the years immediately after the Second World War, when a number of trials were designed to verify whether the early removal of the ovaries would improve the overall control of the disease.

The first trial of this type was initiated in 1948 at the Christie Hospital in Manchester (Cole 1970, 1975), where 598 premenopausal and perimenopausal women were randomised either to Halsted mastectomy or to Halsted mastectomy plus ovarian irradiation. At 15 years, 45% of the patients treated with radiological castration and 40% of the patients treated with mastectomy alone were alive, the statistical significance being borderline.

In a large study conducted in Toronto, 308 premenopausal patients above 45 years of age were randomised either to ovarian irradiation, to ovarian irradiation plus prednisone, or to mastectomy alone (Meakin et al. 1979, 1983). At 15 years, 72% of the patients treated with ovarian inactivation, plus prednisone were alive, compared to only 44% of the control group ($P = 0.02$). Women below 45 did not show any advantage by the ovarian suppression.

As regards surgical oophorectomy, an NSABP study (Ravdin et al. 1970) did not show any significant difference in a 1961 trial comparing the Halsted mastectomy with Halsted mastectomy plus oophorectomy. On the other hand, an important randomised study carried out between 1964 and 1973 in Saskatchewan on 359 patients showed a clear advantage in patients treated with mastectomy plus oophorectomy, with an 11% difference in survival at 10 years in favour of the patients treated with mastectomy plus oophorectomy (Bryant and Weir 1981).

All these studies on ovarian suppression were conducted before the clinical use of hormone receptors, and therefore their power was limited by the fact that some 50% of the patients were ER negative and probably not responsive to oophorectomy. Therefore, it appears essential that the hypothesis of ovarian suppression as an adjunctive treatment to locoregional therapy should be tested again in well-designed randomised studies, possibly in comparison with adjunctive chemotherapy. Endocrine additive treatments after mastectomy have been tested in clinical trials only in the last decade following the discovery of tamoxifen, a non-toxic antiestrogen. The first trial using tamoxifen was begun by Palshof et al. in Copenhagen in 1975 (1980). In this trial, 343 pre- and postmenopausal patients were randomised to receive either tamoxifen or no further treatment. At 8 years the disease-free survival in postmenopausal patients was much higher in women receiving tamoxifen (70%) compared to that of women without further treatment (44%). Most of the following trials produced similar results, but the overall survival, although mainly in favour of the tamoxifen treatment, did not show any statistical significance (Henderson 1987a). One important exception is represented by the Nolvadex Adjuvant Treaty Organization (NATO) investigation, conducted on 1129 women, pre- and postmenopausal, node-positive and node-negative (Baum 1985). The study, which started in 1977, has produced long-term results which show a clear statistically significant advantage, in terms of disease-free and of overall survival of the 2-year treatment with tamoxifen. The favourable effect of tamoxifen was documented not only in patients with positive estrogen receptors, but also in those with negative estrogen receptors. The results of the NATO trial were recently confirmed by a large trial conducted by the Scottish group (Scottish Cancer Trial Office 1987).

Chemotherapy

At the end of the 1950s, the diffuse notion that the surgical treatment of cancer could produce a release of cancer cells in the blood stream led to the first attempts to counteract this fact by chemotherapeutic treatment given at the time of the mastectomy.

A number of trials were then implemented using chemotherapy perioperatively, i.e. in the days immediately following the mastectomy (B. Fisher et al. 1968; B. Fisher et al. 1975b; Nissen-Meyer et al. 1978). The regimens were of very short duration (1 or 2 weeks), and in some trials the drug was administered while the patient was in the operating theatre and then continued during the postoperative days. The two perioperative trials which accrued the largest number of patients were the NSABP and the Scandinavian trials. The former showed at 10 years a limited advantage with the thiotepa treatment in the subset of patients who were premenopausal and with four or more positive nodes. The updated results of the Scandinavian trial were recently published by Nissen-Meyer et al. (1984). After a 15-year follow-up, a significant increase in disease-free and overall survival was reported in patients receiving the cyclophosphamide perioperative treatment compared to the controls.

The new information acquired on the mechanism of action of chemotherapy, which destroys cancer cells by first-order kinetics, has led to new schedules in its use as an adjunction to locoregional treatment.

The recognition that maximal tumour cell reduction requires many courses of chemotherapy induced many centres to design clinical trials employing regimens lasting from 6 to 24 months. The first pioneer study was initiated in 1962 in Japan by Koyama et al. (1980), who randomised 551 patients into a 9-month postoperative treatment with mytomicin C and cyclophosphamide and local therapy alone. The results showed a significant advantage of adjuvant chemotherapy in patients with one to three lymph nodes involved, whilst the effectiveness of chemotherapy was much less in patients without nodal metastases and with four or more nodes involved.

In 1972 the NSABP (B. Fisher et al. 1975a; Glass et al. 1981) and in 1973 the Milan Cancer Institute (Bonadonna et al. 1976, 1977) initiated two randomised trials which have largely influenced studies in subsequent years. The two trials had many common characteristics, such as selection of patients (only node-positive patients) and stratification, but differed substantially in the choice of the drugs and in the duration. The NSABP used monochemotherapy (L-PAM) given orally for 2 years, whilst the Milan trial used a polychemotherapeutic regimen (CMF) for 1 year. The first chemotherapy regimen was chosen for its minimal toxicity and the second for its higher activity compared to L-PAM. The results obtained by these two studies, which have at present the longest follow-up, are remarkably similar. In brief, the two studies showed that adjunctive chemotherapy significantly improves the prognosis of premenopausal breast cancer patients and has little or no advantage after menopause, and that in premenopausal women the greatest effect is concentrated in patients with fewer than four axillary nodes involved. As expected, the CMF regimen proved to be somewhat superior to the L-PAM regimen. It must be added that, although the overall survival (and therefore the prognosis) was improved only in the above-mentioned subsets, the interval before the appearance of recurrence was prolonged in all subgroups of patients, without statistical significance in postmenopause.

Many other trials have been conducted in the subsequent years, substantially confirming the NSABP and Milan trials (Kaufmann et al. 1980; Rubens et al. 1983; Howell et al. 1984). However, the largest of these trials, the Danish one, conducted on 1029 pre- and perimenopausal patients, although confirming the increase in the rate of disease-free patients, especially in ER-negative tumours, failed to find a statistically significant overall survival rate (Brincker et al. 1985).

The fact that the efficacy of adjunctive chemotherapy is limited to premenopausal patients has inevitably led to the hypothesis that the effect of chemotherapy is mediated through the ovarian inactivation and may, therefore, act as a chemical oophorectomy. As a matter of fact, the majority of premenopausal patients who receive adjunctive chemotherapy undergo transient or permanent amenorrhoea. However, although many trials (Danish, ECOG, Guy's, Manchester, West Midlands) showed a better survival in patients who underwent amenorrhoea, supporting the chemical oophorectomy hypothesis, the NSABP and Milan trials were unable to show any advantage in patients who had amenorrhoea compared to the patients who did not have amenorrhoea. Moreover, patients who underwent amenorrhoea after chemotherapy responded nearly as well to oophorectomy as the patients who did not (Veronesi et al. 1987a). Finally, if chemotherapy acted only through an ovarian suppression, patients with negative ER status would not be favourably affected by the adjunctive chemotherapy, but this does not seem to be the case. In conclusion, present data suggest that the effect of chemotherapy may be partly due to the inactivation of the ovaries, but that it is unlikely that this is the only mechanism of action. New clinical trials should be designed to give an answer to this open question.

As regards the length of the adjunctive treatment, the Milan study clearly showed that a 6-month schedule was equally effective, if not superior, to the 12-month one (Bonadonna et al. 1986). Another aspect is the timing of the initiation of chemotherapy. In an accurate review of 460 patients treated with adjunctive combination chemotherapy, Buzdar et al. (1982) were unable to find differences in patients in whom the treatment was initiated earlier than 10 weeks from mastectomy and in patients in whom it was initiated at a later date, 10–17 weeks and more than 18 weeks from mastectomy. Similar results were reported by the Southwest Oncology Group and by ECOG in USA (Glucksberg 1982).

Finally, the toxicity of adjunctive chemotherapy must be considered. Contrary to the case in which chemotherapy is administered for a disseminated disease, in the adjunctive condition the patients are asymptomatic and, moreover, are potentially cured by the primary locoregional treatment. The proportion of these patients may be as high as 70%, for example in the case of patients with only one axillary lymph node involved.

The toxicity varies according to the type(s) of drug(s) used. Most of them cause myelosuppression, thrombocytopenia, nausea and vomiting, and some cause alopecia, mucositis and stomatitis. Specific toxic effects are unique for some drugs: cardiotoxicity (doxorubicin), neurotoxicity (vincristine) and cystitis (cyclophosphamide). The toxic effects may produce serious psychological reactions, which in occasional cases may lead to the discontinuation of the treatment. The most serious aspect of toxicity is the long-term one, in particular the increased incidence of leukaemia, as most of the chemotherapeutic agents are carcinogens. In the NSABP study with L-PAM an 11-fold increase in the risk of developing leukaemia and a 24-fold increase in the risk of developing acute myelogeneous leukaemia were reported (Fisher et al. 1985c). Although many other studies have not shown, with different drugs, the same level of increased risk, a leukaemogenic activity of cyclophosphamide has recently been reported by Haas et al. (1987) with a correlation between the dose and the level of risk: patients receiving cyclophosphamide for ovarian or breast cancer showed a relative risk of from 1.5 to 10 times, according to the dose administered.

Biological Substances

Although the repeated attempts to introduce bacille Calmette-Guerin (BCG) as a component in a combination adjunctive treatment has failed to show any advantage, a trial, conducted at the Villejuif Cancer Institute by Lacour et al. (1980) on stage II breast cancer patients using a combination of ribonucleotides (polyadenilic acid and polyuridilic acid, Poly A/Poly U) showed better survival rates in the patients treated with adjunctive Poly A/Poly U than in the patients treated with mastectomy alone.

More recently, between March 1982 and December 1985, the Federation of French Cancer Centres conducted a randomised trial comparing two different regimens in node-positive patients treated with mastectomy and axillary dissection: (a) postoperative radiotherapy and Poly A/Poly U for 6 weeks; and (b) CMF for 6 months. With a median follow-up of 3 years, there were no differences either in disease-free survival or overall survival between the two groups (Lacour et al. 1987b).

Treatment of Overt Metastases

Endocrine Treatment

Oophorectomy was introduced into clinical practice nearly a century ago, by Beatson in 1896. Since then it has been widely practised either as the first treatment in recurrent or disseminated disease in premenopausal women, or as an immediate adjunctive treatment after mastectomy. The overall response rate following oophorectomy is between 30% and 35% and is more pronounced in the 10 years before the menopause, whilst it is much less in women under 35 (Veronesi and Pizzocaro 1968; Veronesi U. et al. 1975). This may be a reflection of the low rate of ER content in tumours of younger women. The major problems regarding oophorectomy are: (a) what its efficacy in relation to endocrine receptors is; (b) what the indications of choice in disseminated disease are; (c) what the indications of oophorectomy in patients previously treated with chemotherapy are. A recent paper dealing with these questions, based on an analysis of 601 patients treated at the Milan Cancer Institute (Veronesi et al. 1987a), showed that the ER values, as predicting factors of the efficacy of oophorectomy, are important when determined on recurrences or metastases at the time of oophorectomy, whilst the ER determination done at the time of mastectomy is less important. Oophorectomy should be the treatment of choice in all premenopausal women with disseminated disease and positive ER values and may also be indicated in patients who have had previous chemotherapy, even if menstrual periods were suppressed. The study was unable to answer the question on the use of oophorectomy as an adjunctive treatment after local regional therapy. The overall response rate was 31.2% with 10.5% complete regression of all lesions. It was higher in women around 50 (38.4%), in cases with lung metastases only (41.6%) and with a free interval of more than 5 years (44.8%). The response rate increased to 47.8% in patients with positive ER values evaluated on a recurrent lesion.

Adrenalectomy and hypophysectomy were largely practised in the 1960s, especially in postmenopausal women, with regression rates of 30%–40% (Hayward et al. 1970; Robin and Dalton 1977). The regressions were in general more lasting than those obtained with the administration of hormones. However, operative mortality was not negligible (around 4%–5%), and the patients needed a carefully monitored substitution therapy. The advent of less toxic forms of endocrine therapy (tamoxifen, aminoglutethimide) (Ingle et al. 1981; Santen et al. 1982) have gradually reduced the use of this type of surgical endocrine treatment. Estrogens and androgens were also used extensively during recent decades, especially in postmenopausal women, with satisfactory results (20%–30% remissions). However, the side effects were considerable, with unpleasant masculinising symptoms in androgenic therapy and nausea, fluid retention and vaginal bleeding in estrogenic therapy. The discovery of tamoxifen at the beginning of the 1970s has considerably improved the possibilities of endocrine treatment of breast cancer patients. Tamoxifen is an antiestrogen that suppresses DNA polymerase activity, inhibits tritiated thymidine incorporation, reduces total DNA content and total cell numbers in tissue culture of MCF-7 cells and, in animals, decreases the levels of estrogens, prolactine and gonadotrophines. In rats, tamoxifen reduces or prevents the appearance of tumours, either induced by chemical carcinogens or spontaneous, if applied before the first evidence of a tumour (Jordan et al. 1980; Maltoni, unpublished data).

Tamoxifen has been tested in many clinical trials against conventional forms of additive endocrine therapy showing, in general, an equal or greater activity without serious side effects (Ingle et al. 1981). The use of tamoxifen has been largely employed in postmenopausal patients with disseminated disease, but recently a certain activity has also been observed in premenopausal patients. Recently, in two randomised trials, tamoxifen was shown to produce response rates not much different from those produced by oophorectomy (Hoogstraten et al. 1982; Planting et al. 1985). Medroxyprogesterone acetate has been used quite extensively, mainly in Europe, with satisfactory results (Johnson et al. 1983b; Cavalli et al. 1984). The overall response rate is more than 30% and, when employed in high dosages, it has been shown to be superior to tamoxifen (Pannuti et al. 1980). However, high dosages of medroxyprogesterone acetate are associated with an increased incidence of side effects (weight gain, fluid retention, cushingoid facies, hypertension, amenorrhoea and, if given intramuscularly, abscesses).

Aminoglutethimide, an anticonvulsant that was found to suppress corticosteroid synthesis, was introduced as an anticancer drug because it was thought to produce medical adrenalectomy. Aminoglutethimide is an effective type of endocrine treatment in postmenopausal women with an overall response rate of 31%, and its activity is comparable to that of tamoxifen. However, aminogluthetimide seems more likely to induce response in bone metastases (Lipton et al. 1982; Smith et al. 1982). Aminogluthetimide, which should be administered together with hydrocortisone, is, however, more toxic than tamoxifen. Toxicity is mainly neurological, with lethargy, dizziness and ataxia as the main symptoms. Cutaneous rash and vomiting are also not rare.

Chemotherapy

Patients who present with overt metastatic disease or who develop recurrent or metastatic disease after primary treatment have a very poor prognosis and are all virtually destined to die from their tumour. In disseminated breast cancer, therefore, as it is an incurable disease with our present methods of treatment, the major objective of patient management must be the palliation of symptoms and the maintenance of a good quality of life. The prolongation of survival is, of course, another important objective, but should not be obtained at the expense of a good quality of life. This concept is important, as chemotherapy may have very toxic side effects, and the quality of life during its administration may be very poor. Therefore, the prolongation of survival time must be "net", that is superior to the time during which chemotherapy is administered to the patient.

The number of cytotoxic drugs tested on patients with disseminated breast cancer is very high, but the number of active drugs are between 20 and 30. Looking at their overall efficacy, the objective response rate to first-line chemotherapy may be placed at between 50% to 60%, but complete response is around 10%. Unfortunately, the average duration of response is less than 1 year and the average survival of the patients who responded is around 2 years. The more frequently used drugs, all discovered between 1950 and 1970 are doxorubicin, cyclophosphamide, 5-fluorouracil, methotrexate, vincristine, L-PAM, mitomycin C. Doxorubicin (adriamycin) is the single most active agent, but it may be cardiotoxic at high dosages, above 400 mg/m^2, whilst cyclophosphamide is probably the most frequently used drug due to its simplicity of administration, both orally and intravenously. However, most of the above-mentioned drugs are associated in a large variety of combinations, the most common of which are CMFUP, CMF, CMFP, AV, CA, CAF (Table 14).

A number of new drugs have been tested recently, but they have shown only a limited improvement as compared to the classic ones. 4-Epidoxorubicin has an activity similar to doxorubicin but is less cardiotoxic (Brambilla et al. 1986). Mitoxantrone has been shown to be less active than doxorubicin, but its side effects are very mild (Henderson et al. 1985), prednimustine is even less active (with a response rate of 23%), but is practically a non-toxic agent (Lober et al. 1983), elliptinium is an active drug without bone marrow toxicity, although it may induce haemolysis in some patients (Rouëssé et al. 1985).

Choice of Treatment

In the absence of endocrine receptor data, patients with slowly growing disseminated disease and who have skin, nodal and bone involvement after a long disease-free interval should preferably be treated with endocrine therapy. On the other hand, patients with highly aggressive cancer and with visceral involvement will often be treated first with chemother-

Table 14. Combination chemotherapy regimens commonly used to treat metastatic breast cancer. (From Henderson 1987b)

Regimen	Dose	Route	Frequency	Cycle Length
"Cooper": [a] CMFVP				
Cyclophosphamide	2.5 mg/kg	p.o.	Daily	
Methotrexate	25-50 mg	i.v.	Weekly	
5-Fluorouracil	12 mg/kg	i.v.	Daily × 4	
	500 mg	i.v.	Weekly	8 Weeks induction
Vincristine	35 mg/kg	i.v.	Weekly	
Prednisone	0.75 mg/kg	p.o.	Daily, then taper	
CALGB CMFVP				
Induction phase				
Cyclophosphamide	80 mg/m^2	p.o.	Daily	
Methotrexate	30–40 mg/m^2	i.v.	Weekly	
5-Fluorouracil	500 mg/m^2	i.v.	Weekly	5 Weeks induction
Vincristine	1 mg/m^2 (max = 1.5 mg)	i.v.	Weekly	
Prednisone	40 mg/m^2	p.o.	Daily × 21 then taper	
Maintenance				
Cyclophosphamide	100 mg/m^2	p.o.	Days 1–14	
Methotrexate	30–40 mg/m^2	i.v.	Weekly	
5-Fluorouracil	500 mg/m^2	i.v.	Weekly	4 Weeks
Vincristine	1 mg/m^2 (max = 1.5 mg)	i.v.	Days 1 + 8	
Prednisone	40 mg/m^2	p.o.	Days 1–14	
CMF (P)				
Cyclophosphamide	100 mg/m^2	p.o.	Days 1–14	
Methotrexate	40–60 mg/m^2	i.v.	Days 1 + 8	4 Weeks
5-Fluorouracil	600–700 mg/m^2	i.v.	Days 1 + 8	
Prednisone	40 mg/m^2	p.o.	Days 1–14	
IV CMF				
Cyclophosphamide	600 mg/m^2	i.v.	Day 1	
Methotrexate	40 mg/m^2	i.v.	Day 1	3 Weeks
5-Fluorouracil	600 mg/m^2	i.v.	Day 1	
AV				
Adriamycin	75 mg/m^2	i.v.	Day 1	3 Weeks
Vincristine	1.4 mg/m^2	i.v.	Days 1 + 8	
CA				
Cyclophosphamide	200 mg/m^2	p.o.	Days 3–6	3–4 Weeks
Adriamycin	40 mg/m^2	i.v.	Day 1	
CAF				
Cyclophosphamide	400–500 mg/m^2	i.v.	Day 1	
Adriamycin	40–50 mg/m^2	i.v.	Day 1	3 Weeks
5-Fluorouracil	400–500 mg/m^2	i.v.	Day 1 + 8	

[a] This is the original Cooper induction regimen. Doses were reduced by unspecified amounts after the induction period.

apy. Of course, knowledge of the endocrine receptor status will make the choice easier.

Acknowledgements. The author wishes to thank Dr. Lucia Racca for her valuable cooperation and assistance in the preparation of the manuscript and Miss Sheila McGrath for the manuscript revision.

References

Adair F, Berg J, Joubert L (1974) Long term follow-up of breast cancer patients: the thirty year report. Cancer 33: 1145–1150
Adami HO, Hanse J, Hung B et al. (1981) Characteristics of familial breast cancer in Sweden. Absence of relation of age and unilateral versus bilateral disease. Cancer 48: 1688–1695
Allegra JC, Lippman ME, Thompson EB et al. (1979) Relationship between progesterone, androgen, and glucocorticoid receptor and response rate to endocrine therapy in metastatic breast cancer. Cancer Res 39: 1973–1979
Anderson DE (1972) A genetic study of human breast cancer. J Natl Cancer Inst 48: 1029–1034
Anderson DE (1976) Genetic study of breast cancer – identification of high risk group. Cancer 34: 1090–1097
Andersson I, Andren L, Hildell J et al. (1979) Breast cancer screening with mammography. A population-based randomised trial with mammography as the only screening mode. Radiology 132: 273–276
Argenta LC (1984) Reconstruction of the breast by tissue expansion. Plast Reconstr Surg 11: 247
Ashikari R, Hajdu SI, Robbins GF (1971) Intraductal carcinoma of the breast (1960–1969) Cancer 28: 1182–1187
Baclesse F (1949) Roentgen therapy as the sole method of treatment for cancer of the breast. Am J Roentgenol Radium Ther Nucl Med 62: 311–319
Bailar JC III (1976) Mammography: a contrary view. Ann Intern Med 84: 77–84
Baines CJ (1984) Impediments to recruitment in the Canadian National Breast Screening Study: response and resolution. Controlled Clin Trials 5: 129–140
Baker LH (1982) Breast cancer detection demonstration program. Five-year summary report. CA 32: 194–201
Batson OV (1940) The function of the vertebral veins and their role in the spread of metastasis. Ann Surg 112: 138–149
Baum M (1985) Nolvadex Adjuvant Trial Organization: controlled trial of tamoxifen as single adjuvant agent in management of early breast cancer; analysis at six years. Lancet 1: 836–839
Beahrs O, Shapiro S, Smart C (1979) Report of the working group to review the National Cancer Institute American Cancer Society Breast Cancer Detection Demonstration Projects. J Natl Cancer Inst 62: 640–709
Beatson GW (1896) On the treatment of inoperable cases of carcinoma of the mamma: suggestions for a new method of treatment with illustrative cases. Lancet 2: 104
Biggs TM, Cronin ED (1981) Technical aspects of the latissimus dorsi flap in breast reconstruction. Ann Plast Surg 6: 381
Bittner JJ (1936) Some possible effects of nursing on the mammary gland tumour incidence in mice. Science 84: 162
Black MM, Spur FD (1950) Sinus histiocytosis of lymph nodes in cancer. Surg Gynecol Obstet 106: 163–175
Black MM, Barclay THC, Cutler SJ et al. (1972) Association of atypical characteristics of benign breast lesions with subsequent risk of breast cancer. Cancer 29: 338–343
Bloom HJG, Degenshein GA (1980) Estrogen receptors and disease-free interval: a dissenting opinion. Breast 6: 25–27
Bloom HJG, Field JR (1971) Impact of tumour grade and host resistance on survival of women with breast cancer. Cancer 28: 1580–1589
Bloom HJG, Richardson WW (1957) Histological grading and prognosis of breast cancer. A study of 1409 cases of which 359 have been followed for 20 years. Br J Cancer 9: 359–377
Bohmert H (1980) Experience in breast reconstruction with thoracoepigastric and advancement flaps. Acta Chir Belg 79: 105
Bohmert H, Strömbeck JO (1986) Postmastectomy reconstruction. In: Strömbeck JO, Rosato FE (eds) Surgery of the breast. Thieme, Stuttgart, pp 243–266
Bonadonna G, Brusamolino E, Valagussa P et al. (1976) Combination chemotherapy as an adjuvant treatment in operable breast cancer. N Engl J Med 294: 405–410
Bonadonna G, Rossi A, Valagussa P et al. (1977) The CMF program for operable breast cancer with positive axillary nodes: updated analysis on the disease-free interval, site of relapse and drug tolerance. Cancer 39: 2904–2915
Bonadonna G, Valagussa P, Rossi A et al. (1985) Ten-year experience with CMF-base adjuvant chemotherapy in resectable breast cancer. Breast Cancer Res Treat 5: 95–115
Bostwick J (1987) Breast reconstruction after mastectomy. In: Harris JR, Hellman S, Henderson IC, Kinne DW (eds) Breast diseases. Lippincott, Philadelphia, pp 668–683
Boyns AR, Cole EN, Griffiths K et al. (1973) Plasma prolactin in breast cancer. Eur J Cancer 9: 99–102
Brambilla C, Rossi A, Bonfante V et al. (1986) Phase II study of doxorubicin versus epirubicin in advanced breast cancer. Cancer Treat Rep 70: 261–266
Brincker H, Mouridsen HT, Rank F et al. (1985) Evidence of a castration-mediated effect of adjuvant chemotherapy (CT) in a randomized trial of cyclophosphamide monotherapy versus CMF in premenopausal stage II breast. Proc Am Soc Clin Oncol 4: 56
Brinton LA, Hoover RN, Szklo M et al. (1981) Menopausal estrogen and risk of breast cancer. Cancer 47: 2517–2522
Bryant AJ, Weir JA (1981) Prophylactic oophorectomy in operable instances of carcinoma of the breast. Surg Gynecol Obstet 153: 660–664
Bucalossi P, Veronesi U, Pandolfi A (1954) Il problema dell'ereditarietà neoplastica nell'uomo. Il cancro della mammella. Tumori 40: 365–402
Buell P (1974) Changing incidence of breast cancer in Japanese American women. J Natl Cancer Inst 51: 479–487
Buzdar AU, Smith TL, Powell KD et al. (1982) Effect of timing of initiation of adjuvant chemotherapy on disease-free survival in breast cancer. Breast Cancer Res Treat 2: 163–169
Calle R, Pilleron JP, Schlieger P, Vilcoq JR (1978) Conservative management of operable breast cancer. Cancer 42: 2045–2053
Cancer Research Campaign Working Party (1980) Cancer research campaign (King's Cambridge) trial for early breast cancer. Lancet 2: 55–60
Carroll KK, Hopkins GJ (1979) Dietary polyunsaturated fat versus saturated fat in relation to mammary carcinogenesis. Lipids 14: 155

Cascinelli N, Greco M, Bufalino R et al. (1987) Prognosis of breast cancer with axillary node metastases after surgical treatment only. Eur J Cancer Clin Oncol 23: 795–799

Cavalli F, Goldhirsch A, Jugi F et al. (1984) Randomized trial of low- versus high-dose medroxyprogesterone acetate in induction treatment of postmenopausal patients with advanced breast cancer. J Clin Oncol 2: 414–419

Cislaghi C, Decarli A, La Vecchia C (1986) Dati, indicatori e mappe di mortalità tumorale. Italia 1975/1977. Pitagora Editrice, Bologna

Clark GM, McGuire WL, Hubay CA et al. (1983) Progesterone receptors as a prognostic factor in stage II breast cancer. N Engl J Med 309: 1343–1347

Clark RM, Wilkinson RH, Mahoney LJ et al. (1982) Breast cancer: a 21-year experience with conservative surgery and radiation. Int J Radiat Oncol Biol Phys 8: 967–975

Cole MP (1970) Prophylactic compared with therapeutic X-ray artificial menopause. In: Joslin CAF, Gleave EN (eds) The clinical management of advanced breast cancer, 2nd Tenovus Workshop. Alpha Omega Alpha, Cardiff, Wales, pp 2–11

Cole MP (1975) A clinical trial of an artificial menopause in carcinoma of the breast. Inserm 55: 143–150

Cole P, MacMahon P (1969) Oestrogen fractions during early reproductive life in the aetiology of breast cancer. Lancet 1: 604–606

Collins V, Loeffler RK, Tivey H (1956) Observations on growth rates of human tumors. AJR 76: 988–1000

Coulson PB, Thornthwaite JT, Woolley TW et al. (1984) Prognostic indicators including DNA histogram type, receptor content, and staging related to human breast cancer patient survival. Cancer Res 44: 4187–4196

Cutler SJ, Black MM, Mork T et al. (1969) Further observations on prognostic factors in cancer of the female breast. Cancer 24: 653–667

Cuzick J, Stewart, Peto R et al. (1987) Overview of randomized trials of post-operative adjuvant radiotherapy in breast cancer. Cancer Treat Rep 71: 7–14

Dahl-Iversen E (1952) Recherches sur les metastases microscopiques des cancers du sein dans les ganglions lymphatiques parasternaux et sousclaviculaires. Mem Acad Clin 78: 651–663

Davies GC, Millis RR, Hayward JL (1980) Assessment of axillary lymph node status. Ann Surg 192: 148–151

De Lena M, Zucali R, Viganotti G et al. (1978) Combined chemotherapy-radiotherapy approach in locally advanced (T3b–T4) breast cancer. Cancer Chemother Pharmacol 1: 53–59

De Ome KB, Faulkin LJ, Bern HA et al. (1959) Development of mammary tumours from hyperplastic alveolar nodules transplanted into gland free mammary fat pads of female C3H mice. Cancer Res 19: 515–520

de Waard F (1980) Premenopausal and postmenopausal breast cancer. One disease or two? J Natl Cancer Inst 65: 559

de Waard F, Collette HJA, Rombach JJ et al. (1984) The DOM project for the early detection of breast cancer. Utrecht, the Netherlands. J Chronic Dis 37: 1

Di Fronzo G, Clemente C, Cappelletti V et al. (1986) Relationship between ER-ICA and conventional steroid receptor assays in human breast cancer. Breast Cancer Res Treat 8: 35–43

Donnelly PK, Baker KW, Carney JA et al. (1975) Benign breast lesions and subsequent breast carcinoma in Rochester, Minnesota. Mayo Clinc Proc 50: 650

Dowden RV, Dinner MI (1984) Breast reconstruction without skin flaps. Clin Plast Surg 11: 265

Dunn JE (1977) Breast cancer among American Japanese in the San Francisco Bay area. Natl Cancer Inst Monogr 47: 157–160

Dupont WD, Page DL (1985) Risk factors for breast cancer in women with proliferative breast disease. N Engl J Med 312: 146–151

Faulkin LJ (1966) Hyperplastic lesions of mouse mammary glands after treatment with 3-methylcholanthrene. J Natl Cancer Inst 36: 289–297

Fekety EA (1938) A comparative morphological study of the mammary gland in a high and low tumor strain of mice. Am J Pathol 14: 557–578

Fialkow PJ (1979) Clonal origin of human tumors. Annu Rev Med 30: 135–143

Fisher B, Ravdin RG, Ausman RK et al. (1968) Surgical adjuvant chemotherapy in cancer of the breast: results of a decade of cooperative investigation. Ann Surg 168: 337–356

Fisher B, Slack NH, Cavanaugh PJ et al. (1970) Postoperative radiotherapy in the treatment of breast cancer: results of the NSABP clinical trial. Ann Surg 172: 711-730

Fisher B, Carbone P, Economou S et al. (1975a) L-Phenylalanine mustard (L-PAM) in the management of primary breast cancer. N Engl J Med 292: 117–121

Fisher B, Slack NH, Katrych D et al. (1975b) Ten-year follow-up results of patients with carcinoma of the breast in a co-operative clinical trial evaluating surgical adjuvant chemotherapy. Surg Gynecol Obstet 140: 528–534

Fisher B, Bauer M, Margolese R et al. (1985a) Five-year results of a randomised clinical trial comparing total mastectomy and segmental mastectomy with or without radiation in the treatment of breast cancer. N Engl J Med 312: 665–673

Fisher B, Redmund C, Fisher ER et al. (1985b) Ten-year results of a randomized clinical trial comparing radical mastectomy and total mastectomy with or without radiation. N Engl J Med 312: 674–681

Fisher B, Rockette H, Fisher ER et al. (1985c) Leukemia in breast cancer patients following adjuvant chemotherapy or postoperative radiation: the NSABP experience. J Clin Oncol 3: 1640–1658

Fisher ER, Gregorio RM, Fisher B et al. (1975) The pathology of invasive breast cancer. A syllabus derived from findings of the National Surgical Adjuvant Breast Project (Protocol no 4). Cancer 36: 1–85

Fisher ER, Sass RR, Fisher B, Wickerham L, Paik SM and collaborating NSABP Investigators (1986) Pathologic findings from the National Surgical Adjuvant Breast Project (Protocol no 6). I. Intraductal carcinoma (DCIS). Cancer 57: 197–208

Foote FW, Stewart FW (1941) Lobular carcinoma in situ. A rare form of mammary cancer. Am J Pathol 17: 491–509

Forrest APM, Chetty U, Miller WR et al. (1986) A human tumour model. Lancet 2: 840-842

Fournier DV, Weber E, Hoeffken W et al. (1980) Growth rate of 147 mammary carcinomas. Cancer 45: 2198–2207

Friedell GH, Betts A, Sommers SC (1965) The prognostic value of blood vessel invasion and lymphocytic infiltrates in breast carcinoma. Cancer 18: 164–66

Galante E, Gallus G, Guzzon A et al. (1986) Growth rate of primary breast cancer and prognosis: observations on 3 to 7 year follow-up in 180 breast cancers. Br J Cancer 54: 833–836

Gallager HS, Martin JE (1971) An orientation to the concept of minimal breast cancer. Cancer 28: 1505–1507

Gershon-Cohen J, Berger SM, Klickstein HS (1963) Roentgen-

ography of breast cancer moderating concept of "biological predeterminism". Cancer 16: 961–964
Giacomelli V, Veronesi U (1952) Internal mammary nodes as a site for metastatic spread of breast cancer. Tumori 38: 376–393
Giacomelli V, Veronesi U (1952) I linfatici mammari interni come sede e via di diffusione metastatica nel cancro della mammella. Tumori 4: 375–393
Gilchrist KW, Kalish L, Gould VE et al. (1985) Interobserver reproducibility of histopathological features in stage II breast cancer. Breast Cancer Res Treat 5: 3–10
Glass A, Wieand S, Fisher B et al. (1981) Acute toxicity during adjuvant chemotherapy for breast cancer: the National Surgical Adjuvant Breast and Bowel Project (NSABP) experience from 1717 patients receiving single and multiple agents. Cancer Treat Rep 65: 363–376
Glucksberg H, Rivkin SE, Rasmussen S et al. (1982) Combination chemotherapy (CMFVP) versus L-phenylalanine mustard (L-PAM) for operable breast cancer with positive axillary nodes: a Southwest Oncology Group Study. Cancer 50: 423–434
Grattarola R (1978) Anovulation and increased androgenic activity as breast cancer risk in women with fibrocystic disease of the breast. Cancer Res 38: 3051–3054
Greenwald P, Sondik E (1986) Division of cancer prevention and control. Cancer Control. Objectives for the nation 1985–2000. National Cancer Institute Monogr, no 2, Bethesda, MD
Gullino PM, Pettigrew HM, Grantham HF (1975) *N*-Nitrosomethylurea as mammary gland carcinogen in rats. J Natl Cancer Inst 54: 401–414
Haagensen CD (1986) Diseases of the breast, 3rd edn. Saunders, Philadelphia, p 426, pp 864–871
Haagensen CD, Lane N, Lattes R et al. (1978) Lobular neoplasia (so-called lobular carcinoma in situ) of the breast. Cancer 42: 737–769
Haas JF, Killelmann B, Mehnert WH et al. (1987) Risk of leukaemia in ovarian tumour and breast cancer patients following treatment by cyclophosphamide. Br J Cancer 55: 213–218
Halsted WS (1894–1895) The results of operations for the cure of cancer of the breast performed at the Johns Hopkins Hospital from June, 1889 to January, 1894. Johns Hopkins Hosp Bull 4: 297
Handley WS (1927) Parasternal invasion of the thorax in breast cancer and its suppression by the use of radium tubes as an operative precaution. Surg Gynecol Obstet 45: 721
Handley RS, Thackray AC (1954) Invasion of the internal mammary lymph nodes. Br Med J 1: 61
Harris JR, Leven MB, Hellman S (1978) The role of radiation therapy in the primary treatment of carcinoma of the breast. Semin Oncol 5: 403–416
Harris NV, Weiss NS, Francis AM et al. (1982) Breast cancer in relation to patterns of oral contraceptive use. Am J Epidemiol 116: 643
Harris JR, Sawicka J, Gelman R et al. (1983) Management of locally advanced carcinoma of the breast by primary radiation therapy. Int J Radiat Oncol Biol Phys 9: 345–349
Harthampf CR, Scheflan M, Black PW (1982) Breast reconstruction following mastectomy with a transverse abdominal island flap. Anatomical and clinical observations. Plast Reconstr Surg 69: 216–224
Hayward JL (1977) The Guy's trial of treatment of early breast cancer. World J Surg 1: 314–316
Hayward JL (1983) Prospective studies, the Guy's Hospital trials on breast conservation. In: Harris JR, Hellman S, Silen WJB (eds) Conservative management of breast cancer. Lippincott, Philadelphia
Hayward JL, Atkins HJB, Falconer MA et al. (1970) Clinical trials comparing transfrontal hypophysectomy with adrenalectomy and with transethmoidal hypophysectomy. In: Joslin CAF, Gleave EN (eds) The clinical management of advanced breast cancer. Alpha Omega Alpha, Cardiff, Wales, pp 50–53
Hedley DW, Rugg CA, Ng ABP et al. (1984) Influence of cellular DNA content on disease free survival of stage II breast cancer patients. Cancer Res 44: 5395–5398
Henderson IC (1987a) Adjuvant systemic therapy of early breast cancer. In: Harris JR, Hellman S, Henderson IC, Kinne DW (eds) Breast diseases. Lippincott, Philadelphia, pp 324–353
Henderson IC (1987b) Chemotherapy for advanced disease. In: Harris JR, Hellman S, Henderson IC, Kinne DW (eds) Breast diseases. Lippincott, Philadelphia, p 444
Henderson IC, Wolff S, Allegra J et al. (1985) A randomised trial comparing mitoxantrone and doxorubicin in patients with metastatic breast cancer. In: Coltman CA Jr (ed) The current status of novantrone. Wiley, New York, pp 45–53
Hennekens CH, Speizer FE, Rosner B et al. (1979) Use of permanent hair dyes and cancer among registered nurses. Lancet 1: 1390–1393
Hermanek P, Sobin LH (eds) (1987) TNM classification of malignant tumours, 4th edn. Springer, Berlin Heidelberg New York
Hibberd AD, Harwood IJ, Wells JE (1983) Long term prognosis of women with breast cancer in New Zealand: study of survival to 30 years. Br Med J 286: 1777–1779
Hilf R, Feldstein ML, Gibson SL et al. (1980) The relative importance of estrogen receptor analysis as a prognostic factor for recurrence or response to chemotherapy in women with breast cancer. Cancer 45: 1993–2000
Hirsch J (1927) Radiumchirurgie des Brustkrebses. Dtsch Med Wochenschr 34: 1419–1421
Holland R, Veling SHJ, Mravunac M, Hendriks JHCL (1985) Histologic multifocality of Tis, T1–2 breast carcinomas. Implications for clinical trials of breast-conserving surgery. Cancer 56: 979–990
Hoogstraten B, Fletcher WS, Gad-el-Mawla N et al. (1982) Tamoxifen and oophorectomy in the treatment of recurrent breast cancer. Cancer Res 42: 4788–4791
Hoover R, Gray LA Sr, Cole P et al. (1976) Menopausal estrogens and breast cancers. N Engl J Med 295: 401–405
Horan Hand P, Nuti M, Colcher D et al. (1983) Definition of antigenic heterogeneity and modulation among human mammary carcinoma cell populations using monoclonal antibodies to tumor-associated antigens. Cancer Res 43: 728–735
Hortobagyi GN, Blumenschein GR, Spanos W et al. (1983) Multimodal treatment of locally advanced breast cancer. Cancer 51: 763–768
Høst H, Brennhovd IO, Loeb M (1986) Post-operative radiotherapy in breast cancer. Long-term results from the Oslo study. Int J Radiat Oncol Biol Phys 12: 727–732
Howat JMT, Barnes DM, Harris M et al. (1983) The association of cytosol oestrogen and progesterone receptors with histological features of breast cancer and early recurrence of disease. Br J Cancer 47: 629–640
Howell A, Bush H, George WD et al. (1984) A controlled trial of adjuvant chemotherapy with cyclophosphamide, methotrexate and fluorouracil for breast cancer. Lancet 2: 307–311

Huggins C, Grand LC, Brilantes FP (1961) Mammary cancer induced by a single feeding of polynuclear hydrocarbons and its suppression. Nature 189: 204–207

Hulka BS, Chambless LE, Deubner DC et al. (1982) Breast cancer and estrogen replacement therapy. Am J Obstet Gynecol 143: 638–644

Huseby RA, Bittner JJ (1946) A comparative morphological study of the mammary glands with reference to known factors influencing the development of mammary carcinoma in mice. Cancer Res 6: 240–255

Hutchinson WB, Thomas DB, Hamlin WB et al. (1980) Risk of breast cancer in women with benign breast disease. J Natl Cancer Inst 65: 13–20

IARC Working Group (1986) Cancer, causes and control. Available from World Health Organization, Geneva

Ingle JN, Ahmann DL, Green SJ et al. (1981) Randomised clinical trial of diethylstilbestrol versus tamoxifen in postmenopausal women with advanced breast cancer. N Engl J Med 304: 16–21

Jacquillat C, Baillet F, Auclerc G et al. (1987) Pre-operative (Neoad) chemotherapy (Chem) and radiotherapy in breast cancer (BC). EORTC Breast Cancer Cooperative Group, 4th Working Conference, June 30–July 3, 1987 London p 4.8

Jick H, Slone D, Shapiro S et al. (1974) Reserpine and breast cancer. Lancet 2: 669–671

Jick H, Walker AM, Watkins RN et al. (1980) Replacement estrogens and breast cancer. Am J Epidemiol 112: 586

Johnson ML, Levy J, Rosen JM (1983a) Isolation and characterization of casein-producing and nonproducing cell populations from 7,12-dimethylbenz(a)anthracene-induced rat mammary carcinomas. Cancer Res 43: 2199–2209

Johnson PA, Bonomi PD, Wolter JM et al. (1983b) Megestrol acetate versus tamoxifen in advanced breast cancer: a retrospective study. Proc Am Assoc Cancer Res 24: 172

Jordan VC, Allen KE, Dix CJ (1980) Pharmacology of tamoxifen in laboratory animals. Cancer Treat Rep 64: 745–759

Kaufmann M, Fournier DV, Sievers H et al. (1980) Adjuvant chemotherapy with chlorambucil and 5-fluorouracil in primary breast cancer (Cooperative Study Heidelberg). In: Mouridsen HT, Palshof T (eds) Breast cancer – experimental and clinical aspects. Pergamon, Elmsford, NY, pp 157–160

Kelsey JL, Holford TR, White C et al. (1978) Oral contraceptives and breast disease: an epidemiological study. Am J Epidemiol 107: 236

Kelsey JL, Fisher DB, Holford TR et al. (1981) Estrogenous estrogens and other factors in the epidemiology of breast cancer. J Natl Cancer Inst 67: 327–333

Keynes G (1937) Conservative treatment of cancer of the breast. Br Med J 2: 643–647

Knight WA III, Livingston RB, Gregory EJ (1977) Estrogen receptor as an independent prognostic factor for early recurrence in breast cancer. Cancer Res 37: 4669–4671

Kodlin D, Winger EE, Morgenstern NL et al. (1977) Chronic mastopathy and breast cancer. A follow-up study. Cancer 39: 2603–2607

Korenman SG (1980) Oestrogen window hypothesis of the aetiology of breast cancer. Lancet 1: 700–701

Koscielny S, Tubiana M, Lê MG et al. (1984) Breast cancer: relationship between the size of the primary tumour and the probability of metastatic dissemination. Br J Cancer 49: 709–715

Koyama H, Wada T, Takahashi Y et al. (1980) Surgical adjuvant chemotherapy with mitomycin C and cyclophosphamide in Japanese patients with breast cancer. Cancer 46: 2373–2379

Kusama S, Spratt JS, Donegan WL et al. (1972) The gross rates of growth of human mammary carcinoma. Cancer 30: 594–599

Lacour J, Bucalossi P, Caceres E et al. (1976) Radical mastectomy versus radical mastectomy plus internal mammary dissection. Cancer (Suppl) 37: 206–214

Lacour J, Spira A, Petit JY et al. (1980) Adjuvant treatment with polyadenylic-polyuridylic acid (Poly A, Poly U) in operable breast cancer. Lancet 2: 161–164

Lacour J, Lê M, Caceres E et al. (1983) Radical mastectomy versus radical mastectomy plus internal mammary dissection. Ten-year results of an international cooperative trial in breast cancer. Cancer 51: 1941–1943

Lacour J, Lê MG, Hill C et al. (1987a) Is it useful to remove internal mammary nodes in operable breast cancer? Eur J Surg Oncol 13: 309–314

Lacour J, Laplanche A, Delozier T et al. (1987b) Comparison of the adjuvant value of polyadenylic-polyuridylic acid (Poly A, Poly U) + radiotherapy (Rx) versus chemotherapy with CMF, in operable breast cancer. Preliminary results of a randomised trial of the French Federation of Cancer Centers (FFCC). 4th European Conference on Clinical Oncology and Cancer Nursing, November 1–4, 1987, Madrid, p 114 (Abstr 431)

Land CE, Boice JD Jr, Shore RE et al. (1980) Breast cancer risk from low-dose exposure to ionizing radiation: results of parallel analysis of three exposed populations of women. J Natl Cancer Inst 65: 353–376

Langlands AO, Popock SJ, Kerr GR et al. (1979) Long term survival of patients with breast cancer: a study of the curability of the disease. Br Med J 2: 1247–1251

Lemon HM (1969) Endocrine influences on human mammary cancer formation. A critique. Cancer 23: 781–790

Lewis JR (1979) Use of a sliding flap from the abdomen to provide cover in breast reconstructions. Plast Reconstr Surg 64: 491

Lichter A (1983) Mastectomy and axillary dissection versus excisional biopsy, axillary dissection and definitive radiotherapy for stage I–II breast carcinoma. In: Compilation of experimental cancer therapy protocol summaries, 7th edn. US Department of Health, Education and Welfare, Bethesda, p 33

Lilienfeld A (1956) The relationship of cancer of the female breast to artificial menopause and marital status. Cancer 9: 927–934

Lipton A, Harvey HA, Santen TJ et al. (1982) Randomised trial of aminoglutethimide versus tamoxifen in metastatic breast cancer. Cancer Res 42: 3434–3436

Lober J, Mouridsen HT, Christiansen IE et al. (1983) A phase III trial comparing prednimustine (LEO 1031) to chlorambucil plus prednisolone in advanced breast cancer. Cancer 52: 1570–1576

Love SM, Gellman RS, Silen W (1982) Fibrocystic "disease" of the breast – a nondisease? N Engl J Med 307: 1010–1014

Lundgren B (1983) The growth rate of breast cancer as a dynamic indicator of prognosis. Australas Radiol 27: 178–180

Macklin MT (1959) Comparison of the number of breast cancer deaths observed in relatives of breast cancer patients, and the number expected on the basis of mortality rates. J Natl Cancer Inst 22: 927–951

MacMahon B, Cole P, Lin TM et al. (1970) Age at first birth and cancer of the breast. A summary of an international study. Bull WHO 43: 209

Maddox WA, Carpenter JT, Laws HL et al. (1983) A randomised prospective trial of radical (Halsted) mastectomy

versus modified radical mastectomy in 311 breast cancer patients. Ann Surg 198: 207–212
Maier WP, Leber D, Rosemond GP et al. (1977) The technique of modified radical mastectomy. Surg Gynecol Ostet 145: 69–74
Margottini M (1952) Recent developments in the surgical treatment of breast carcinoma. Acta Unio Int Contra Cancrum 8: 176
Margottini M, Bucalossi P (1949) Le metastasi linfoghiandolari mammarie interne nel cancro della mammela. Oncologia 23: 70–83
Marmosten J, Crowley LG, Myers SM et al. (1965) Urinary excretion of estrone, estradiol and estriol by patients with breast cancer and benign breast disease. Am J Obstet Gynecol 92: 460–467
Martynova RP (1937) Studies in the genetics of human neoplasms. Cancer of the breast, based on 201 family histories. Am J Cancer 29: 530–540
Mason BH, Holdaway IM, Mullins PR et al. (1983) Progesterone and estrogen receptors as prognostic variables in breast cancer. Cancer Res 43: 2985–2990
McDivitt RW, Hutter RVP, Foote FW, Stewart FW (1967) In situ lobular carcinoma of the breast. A prospective follow-up study indicating cumulative patient risks. JAMA 201: 82–86
McWhirter R (1955) Simple mastectomy and radiotherapy in the treatment of breast cancer. Br J Radiol 28: 128–139
Meakin JW, Allt WEC, Beale FA et al. (1979) Ovarian irradiation and prednisone therapy following surgery and radiotherapy for carcinoma of the breast. Can Med Assoc J 120: 1221–1228
Meakin JW, Allt WEC, Beale FA et al. (1983) Ovarian irradiation and prednisone following surgery and radiotherapy for carcinoma of the breast. Breast Cancer Res Treat (Suppl) 3: 45–48
Meyer JS, Friedman E, McCrate MM et al. (1983) Prediction of early course of breast carcinoma by thymidine labeling. Cancer 51: 1879–1886
Meyer W (1894) An improved method of the radical operation for carcinoma of the breast. Med Rec 46: 746
Miller AB (1983) Screening for breast cancer. Breast Cancer Res Treat 3: 143–156
Miller AB (1986) Early detection of breast cancer. In: Harris JR Jr, Hellman S, Henderson IC, Kinne DW (eds) Breast diseases. Lippincott, Philadelphia, pp 122–134
Miller AB, Chamberlain J, Tsechkovski M (1985) Self-examination in the early detection of breast cancer. A review of the evidence, with recommendations for further research. J Chronic Dis 38: 527
Montague ED, Ames FC, Schell SR et al. (1984) Conservative surgery and irradiation as an alternative to mastectomy in the treatment of clinically favorable breast cancer. Cancer 54: 2668–2672
Muir R (1941) The evolution of carcinoma of the mamma. J Pathol Bacteriol 52: 153
Murad TH, Scarpelli DG (1967) The ultrastructure of medullary and scirrhous mammary duct carcinoma. Am J Pathol 50: 335–360
Mustacchi P (1961) Ramazzini and Rigoni-Stern on parity and breast cancer. Arch Intern Med 108: 195
Mustakallio S (1972) Conservative treatment of breast carcinoma. A review of 25 years of follow-up. Clin Radiol 23: 110–116
Nasca PC, Lawrence CE, Greenwald P et al. (1980) Relationship of hair dye use, benign breast disease, and breast cancer. J Natl Cancer Inst 64: 23–28
Natali PG, Giacomini P, Bigotti A et al. (1983) Heterogeneity in the expression of HLA and tumour-associated antigens by surgically removed and cultured breast carcinoma cells. Cancer Res 43: 660–668
Nime FA, Rosen PP, Thaler HT, Ashikari R, Urban JA (1977) Prognostic significance of tumour emboli in intramammary lymphatics in patients with mammary carcinoma. Am J Surg Pathol 1: 25–30
Nissen-Meyer R, Kjellgren K, Malmio K et al. (1978) Surgical adjuvant chemotherapy. Cancer 41: 2088–2098
Nissen-Meyer R, Host H, Kiellgren K et al. (1984) Scandinavian trials with one single postoperative course vs. 12 courses. Recent Results Cancer Res 96: 48–54
Nowell PC (1976) The clonal evolution of tumour cell populations. Science 194: 23–28
Noyes RD, Spanos WJ, Montague ED (1982) Breast cancer in women aged 30 and under. Cancer 49: 1302–1307
Ohuchi N, Abe R, Kasai M (1984) Possible cancerous change of intraductal papillomas of the breast. A 3-D reconstruction study of 25 cases. Cancer 54: 605–611
Osborne CK, Knight WA III, Yochmowitz MG et al. (1981) Estrogen receptor and prognosis in breast cancer. In: McGuire WL (ed) Breast cancer. Plenum, New York, pp 33-49 (Advances in research and treatment, vol 4)
Oxenhandler RW, McCune R, Subtelney A et al. (1984) Flow cytometric determination of estrogen receptors in intact cells. Cancer Res 44: 2516–2523
Paffenbarger RS, Fasal E, Simmons ME et al. (1977) Cancer risk as related to use of oral contraceptives during fertile years. Cancer 39 (Suppl): 1887–1891
Page DL, Vanderzwagg R, Rogers LW et al. (1978) Relationship between component parts of fibrocystic disease complex and breast cancer. J Natl Cancer Inst 61: 1055–1063
Page DL, Dupont WD, Rogers LW et al. (1985) Atypical hyperplastic lesions of the female breast: a long-term follow-up study. Cancer 55: 2698–2708
Palmer MK, Ribeiro GG (1985) Thirty-four year follow-up of patients with breast cancer in a clinical trial of postoperative radiotherapy. Br Med J 291: 1088–1091
Palshof T, Mouridsen HT, Daehnfeldt JL (1980) Adjuvant endocrine therapy of breast cancer – a controlled clinical trial of oestrogen and anti-oestrogen: preliminary results of the Copenhagen breast cancer trials. In: Henningsen B, Linder F, Steichele C (eds) Endocrine treatment of breast cancer, a new approach. Springer, Berlin Heidelberg New York, pp 185–189
Pannuti F, Martoni A, Fruet F et al. (1980) Hormone therapy in advanced breast cancer: high-dose medroxyprogesterone acetate (MPA) vs. tamoxifen (TMX). Preliminary results. In: Mouridsen HT, Palshof T (eds) Breast cancer – experimental and clinical aspects. Pergamon, Oxford, pp 93–98
Paterson R, Russel MH (1959) Clinical trials in malignant disease. III. Breast cancer: evaluation of postoperative radiotherapy. J Fac Radiol 10: 175
Patey DH, Dyson WH (1948) The prognosis of carcinoma of the breast in relation to the type of operation performed. Br J Cancer 2: 7
Penrose LS, MacKenzie HJ, Karn MNA (1948) Genetical study of human mammary cancer. Ann Eug 14: 234–266
Peters V (1967) Wedge resection and irradiation. An effective treatment in early breast cancer. JAMA 200: 134–135
Pfahler GE (1932) Results of radiation therapy in 1022 private cases of carcinoma of the breast from 1902 to 1928. Am J Roentgenol Radium Ther Nucl Med 27: 497–508
Philips RL, Garfinkel L, Kuzoma JW et al. (1980) Mortality

among California Seventh-Day Adventists for selected cancer sites. J Natl Cancer Inst 65: 1097–1107

Pichon MF, Pallud C, Brunet M et al. (1980) Relationship of presence of progesterone receptors to prognosis in early breast cancer. Cancer Res 40: 3357–3360

Pierquin B, Owen R, Maylin C et al. (1980) Radiation therapy of breast cancer. Int J Radiat Oncol Biol Phys 6: 17–24

Pigott J, Nichols R, Maddox WA et al. (1984) Metastases to the upper levels of the axillary nodes in carcinoma of the breast and its implications for nodal sampling procedures. Surg Gynecol Obstet 158: 255–259

Planting AST, Alexieva-Figusch J, Blonk-v d Wijst J et al. (1985) Tamoxifen therapy in premenopausal women with metastatic breast cancer. Cancer Treat Rep 69: 363–368

Popkin GL, De Feo CP Jr (1976) Basal cell epithelioma. In: Andrade R, Gumport SL, Popkin GL et al. (eds) Cancer of the skin. Biology – diagnosis – management. Saunders, Philadelphia, pp 821–844

Pukkala E, Gustavsson N, Teppo L (1986) Atlas of cancer incidence in Finland 1953- 1982. Cancer Society of Finland. Helsinki, no 37

Radovan C (1984) Tissue expansion in soft-tissue reconstruction. Plast Reconstr Surg 74: 482–492

Ravdin RG, Lewison EF, Slack NH et al. (1970) Results of a clinical trial concerning the worth of prophylactic oophorectomy for breast carcinoma. Surg Gynecol Obstet 131: 1055–1064

Ravnihar B, Siegel DG, Lindtner J (1979) An epidemiologic study of breast cancer and benign breast neoplasia in relation to the oral contraceptive and estrogen use. Eur J Cancer 15: 395–405

Recht A, Conolly JL, Schnitt SJ et al. (1986) Conservative surgery and primary radiation therapy for early breast cancer: results, controversies, and unresolved problems. Semin Oncol 13: 434

Redon H, Lacour J (1955) La place du curage parasternal dans le traitement du cancer du sein. Presse Méd 63: 1173–1176

Richardson WW (1956) Medullary carcinoma of the breast. A distinctive tumour type with a relatively good prognosis following radical mastectomy. Br J Cancer 10: 415

Rilke F (1984) Influence of pathologic factors on management. In: Bonadonna G (ed) Breast cancer diagnosis and management. Wiley, New York, pp 35–62

Robin PE, Dalton GA (1977) The role of major endocrine ablation. In: Stoll BA (ed) Breast cancer – early and late. Yearbook Medical Publishers, Chicago, pp 147–156

Rosen PP, Lieberman PH, Braun DW, Kosloff C, Adair F (1978) Lobular carcinoma in situ of the breast. A detailed analysis of 99 patients with average follow-up of 24 years. Am J Surg Pathol 2: 225–239

Rosen PP, Saigo PE, Braun DW Jr, Weathers E, De Palo A (1981) Predictors of recurrence in stage I (T1NOMO) breast carcinoma. Ann Surg 93: 15–25

Rosenberg L, Miller DR, Kaufman DW et al. (1984) Breast cancer and oral contraceptive use. Am J Epidemiol 119: 167

Roses DF, Harris MN, Gumport SL (1977) Total mastectomy with axillary dissection. Am J Surg 134: 674–677

Rouëssé JG, Le Chevalier T, Caille P et al. (1985) Phase II study of elliptinium in advanced breast cancer. Cancer Treat Rep 69: 707–708

Rubens RD, Knight RK, Fentiman IS et al. (1983) Controlled trial of adjuvant chemotherapy with melphalan for breast cancer. Lancet 1: 839–843

Russo J, Frederick J, Ownby HE et al. (1987) Predictors of recurrence and survival of patients with breast cancer. Am J Clin Pathol 88: 123–131

Ryan JJ (1982) A lower thoracic advancement flap in breast reconstruction after mastectomy. Plast Reconstr Surg 70: 153–160

Saez S, Cheix F, Asselain B (1983) Prognostic value of estrogen and progesterone receptors in primary breast cancer. Breast Cancer Res Treat 3: 345–354

Sage HH, Casson PR (1976) Squamous cell carcinoma of the scalp, face, and neck. In: Androde R, Gumpport SL, Popkin GL et al. (eds) Cancer of the skin. Saunders, Philadelphia, pp 899–915

Salvadori B, Greco M, Clemente C et al. (1983) Prognostic factors in operable breast cancer. Tumouri 69: 477–484

Sanderson KV, Mackie R (1979) Tumours of the skin. In: Rook A, Wilkinson DS, Ebling FJS (eds) Textbook of Dermatology, 3rd edn. Blackwell Scientific, London, pp 2171–2179

Santen RJ, Worgul TJ, Lipton A et al. (1982) Aminoglutethimide as treatment of postmenopausal women with advanced breast carcinoma. Ann Intern Med 96: 94–101

Sarrazin D, Lê MG, Fontaine MF et al. (1983) Conservative treatment versus mastectomy in T1 or small T2 breast cancer: a randomised trial In: Harris JR, Hellman S, Silen W (eds) Conservative management of breast cancer. Lippincott, Philadelphia, pp 101–114

Sartwell PE, Arthes FG, Tonascia JA (1977) Estrogenous hormones, reproductive history, and breast cancer. J Natl Cancer Inst 59: 1589–1592

Scanlon EF, Caprini JA (1975) Modified radical mastectomy. Cancer 35: 710-713

Scarff RW, Torloni H (1968) Histological typing of breast tumours. International histological classification of tumours, no 2. World Health Organization, Geneva

Schnitt SJ, Connolly JL, Harris JR et al. (1984) Pathologic predictors of early local recurrences in stage I and II breast cancer treated by primary radiation therapy. Cancer 53: 1049–1057

Schottenfeld D, Nash AG, Robbins GF et al. (1976) Ten-year results of the treatment of primary operable breast carcinoma. Cancer 38: 1001–1007

Scottish Cancer Trial Office (MRC) (1987) Adjuvant tamoxifen in the management of operable breast cancer: the Scottish Trial. Report from the Breast Cancer Trials Committee, Edinburgh. Lancet II: 171–175

Secreto G, Toniolo P, Berrino F et al. (1984) Increased androgen activity and breast cancer risk in premenopausal women. Cancer Res 44: 5902–5905

Shapiro S (1977) Evidence on screening for breast cancer from a randomised trial. Cancer 39: 2772–2782

Shapiro S, Venet W, Strax P et al. (1982) Ten to fourteen-year effects of screening on breast cancer mortality. J Natl Cancer Inst 69: 349–355

Shaw WW (1983) Breast reconstruction by superior gluteal microvascular free flaps without silicone implants. Plast Reconstr Surg 72: 490–499

Shellabarger CJ (1972) Mammary neoplastic response of Lewis and Sprague-Dawley female rats to 7,12-dimethylbenz(a)anthracene or X-ray. Cancer Res 32: 883–885

Shellabarger CJ, Chmelevsky D, Kellerer AM (1980) Induction of mammary neoplasms in the Sprague-Dawley rat by 430 keV neutrons and X-ray. J Natl Cancer Inst 64: 821–833

Siiteri PK, Hammond GL, Nisker JA (1981) Increased availability of serum estrogens in breast cancer: a new hypothesis. In: Pike et al. (eds) Banbury Report no 8: Hormones and cancer. Cold Spring Harbor Laboratory, Cold Spring Habour, NY, p 87

Silverberg SG, Chitale AR (1973) Assessment of significance

of proportions of intraductal and infiltrating tumour growth in ductal carcinoma of the breast. Cancer 32: 830–837
Silvestrini R, Daidone MG, Gasparini G (1985) Cell kinetics as a prognostic marker in node negative breast cancer. Cancer 56: 1982–1987
Silvestrini R, Daidone MG, Valagussa P, Salvadori B, Rovini D, Bonadonna G (1987) Cell kinetics as a prognostic marker in locally advanced breast cancer. Cancer Treat Rep 71: 375–379
Slamon DJ, Clark GM, Wong SG et al. (1987) Human breast cancer: correlation of relapse and survival with amplification of the HER-2/new oncogene. Science 235: 177–182
Smith IE, Harris AL, Morgan M et al. (1982) Tamoxifen versus aminoglutethimide versus combined tamoxifen and aminoglutethimide in the treatment of advanced breast carcinoma. Cancer Res 42: 3430–3433
Smithers DW (1948) Family histories of 459 patients with cancer of the breast. Br J Cancer 2: 163–167
Sobin LH, Sherif M (1980) Relation between male breast cancer and prostate cancer. Br J Cancer 42: 787–790
Sorace RA, Bagley CS, Lichter AS et al. (1985) Management of nonmetastatic locally advanced breast cancer using primary induction chemotherapy with hormonal synchronization followed by radiation therapy with or without debulking surgery. World J Surg 9: 775
Spitalier J, Brandone H, Ayme Y et al. (1977) Cesium therapy of breast cancer: a five-year report on 400 consecutive patients. Int J Radiot Oncol Biol Phys 2: 231–235
Squartini F, Sounelli R (1981) Structure, functional changes, and proliferative pathology of the human mammary lobule in cancerous breasts. J Natl Cancer Inst 67: 33–46
Stevens RG, Moolgavkar SH, Lee JH (1982) Temporal trends in breast cancer. Am J Epidemiol 115: 759
Stewart JF, Rubens RD, Millis RR et al. (1983) Steroid receptors and prognosis in operable (stage I and II) breast cancer. Eur J Cancer Clin Oncol 19: 1381–1387
Tabar L, Fagerberg CJG, Gad A et al. (1985) Reduction in mortality from breast cancer after mass screening with mammography: randomised trial from the breast cancer screening working group of the Swedish National Board of Health and Welfare. Lancet 1: 829–832
Taylor SG, Kalish LA, Olson JE et al. (1985) Adjuvant CMFP versus CMFP plus tamoxifen versus observation alone in postmenopausal, node-positive breast cancer patients: three-year results of an Eastern Cooperative Oncology Group study. J Clin Oncol 3: 144–154
Tokunaga M, Land CE, Yamamoto T et al. (1984) Breast cancer among atomic bomb survivors. In: Boice JD Jr, Fraumeni JF Jr (eds) Radiation carcinogenesis. Epidemiology and biological significance. Raven, New York, pp 45–46
Tseng MT (1980) Ultrastructure of the hormone-dependent *N*-nitrosomethylurea-induced mammary carcinoma of the rat. Cancer Res 40: 3112–3115
Tubiana M, Pejovic MH, Chavaudra N et al. (1984) The long term prognostic significance of the thymidine labeling index in breast cancer. Int J Cancer 33: 441–445
Tulinius H, Day NE, Bjarnason O et al. (1982) Familial breast cancer in Iceland. Int J Cancer 29: 365–371
Turner L, Swindell R, Bell WGT (1981) Radical versus modified radical mastectomy for breast cancer. Ann R Coll Surg Engl 63: 239
U.K. Trial of early detection of breast cancer group (1981) Trial of early detection of breast cancer: description of method. Br J Cancer 44: 618–627
Urban JA, Baker HW (1952) Radical mastectomy in continuity with en bloc resection of the internal mammary lymph-node chain. Cancer 5: 992–1008
Valagussa P, Bonadonna G, Veronesi U (1978) Patterns of relapse and survival following radical mastectomy. Cancer 41: 1170–1178
Van Dongen E (1987) Breast conserving therapy in operable breast cancer. EORTC Working Conference on Breast Cancer, 1–3 July 1987, London
Van Dongen JA; Bartelink H, Aaronson N et al. (1987) Randomised clinical trial to assess the value of breast conserving therapy in stage I and II breast cancer (trial 10801). EORTC Breast Cancer Cooperative Group, 4th Working Conference, June 30–July 3, 1987, London p 1.1
Van Scott EJ (1979) Basal cell carcinoma. In: Fitzpatrick TB, Eisen AZ, Wolff K et al. (eds) Dermatology in general medicine, 2nd edn. McGraw-Hill, New York, pp 377-383
Veronesi A, Frustaci S, Tirelli U et al. (1981) Tamoxifen therapy in postmenopausal advanced breast cancer: efficacy of the primary tumour site in 46 evaluable patients. Tumori 67: 235–238
Veronesi U (1963) Removal of internal mammary nodes in cancer of the breast. Report of 350 cases. Acta Unio Int Contra Cancrum 19: 1560–1565
Veronesi U (1977) New trends in the treatment of breast cancer at the Cancer Institute of Milan. AJR 128: 287–289
Veronesi U, Costa A (1982) The role of surgery in the management of primary breast cancer. Clin Oncol 1: 853–873
Veronesi U, Gennari L (1960) Il carcinoma gelatinoso della mammella. Tumori 46: 119–155
Veronesi U, Pizzocaro G (1968) Breast cancer in women subsequent to cystic disease of the breast. Surg Gynecol Obstet 126: 529–532
Veronesi U, Valagussa P (1981) Inefficacy of internal mammary nodes dissection in breast cancer surgery. Cancer 47: 170–175
Veronesi U, Valagussa P (1983) Internal mammary node involvement. Results of a prospective randomised study comparing two different surgical procedures. In: Harris JR, Hellman S, Silen W (eds) Conservative management of breast cancer. New surgical and radiotherapeutic techniques. Lippincott, Philadelphia, pp 201–209
Veronesi U, Zingo L (1967) Extended mastectomy for cancer of the breast. Cancer 20: 677–680
Veronesi U, Rabotti GC, Sirtori C (1955) Il carcinoma intraduttale epidermotropo della mammella (cosiadetto morbo di Paget). Tumori (Suppl) 41: 1–142
Veronesi U, Consolandi G, Briziarelli G (1957) The metastatic spread of breast cancer. Lav Anat Pat Perugia 17: 5–66
Veronesi U, Giarrusso AM, Guarino M (1964) Il carcinoma papillifero della mammella. Tumori 50: 421–429
Veronesi U, Pizzocaro G, Rossi A (1975) Oophorectomy for advanced carcinoma of the breast. Surg Gynecol Obstet 141: 569–570
Veronesi U, Banfi A, Saccozzi R et al. (1977) Conservative treatment of breast cancer. Cancer 39: 2822–2826
Veronesi U, Saccozzi R, Del Vecchio M et al. (1981) Comparing radical mastectomy with quadrantectomy, axillary dissection, and radiotherapy in patients with small cancers of the breast. N Engl J Med 305: 6–11
Veronesi U, Cascinelli N, Bufalino R et al. (1983) Risk of internal mammary lymph node metastases and its relevance on prognosis of breast cancer patients. Ann Surg 198: 681–684
Veronesi U, Cascinelli N, Greco M et al. (1985 a) Prognosis of breast cancer patients after mastectomy and dissection of internal mammary nodes. Ann Surg 202: 702–707
Veronesi U, Zucali R, Del Vecchio M (1985 b) Conservative

treatment of breast cancer with the QUART technique. World J Surg 9: 676–681
Veronesi U, Banfi A, Del Vecchio M et al. (1986) Comparison of Halsted mastectomy with quadrantectomy, axillary dissection, and radiotherapy in early breast cancer: long-term results. Eur J Cancer Clin Oncol 22: 1085–1089
Veronesi U, Cascinelli N, Greco M et al. (1987a) A reappraisal of oophorectomy in carcinoma of the breast. Ann Surg 205: 18–21
Veronesi U, Rilke F, Luini A et al. (1987b) Distribution of axillary node metastases by level of invasion: an analysis of 539 cases. Cancer 59: 682–687
Wagner S, Mantel N (1978) Breast cancer at a psychiatric hospital before and after the introduction of neuroleptic agents. Cancer Res 38: 2703–2708
Wallgren A, Arner O, Bergstrom J et al. (1986) Radiation therapy in operable breast cancer: results from the Stockholm trial on adjuvant radiotherapy. Int J Radiat Oncol Biol Phys 12: 533–537
Walt AJ, Singhakowinta A, Brooks SC et al. (1976) The surgical implications of estrophile protein estimations in carcinoma of the breast. Surgery 80: 506–512
Wangensteen OH (1949) Remarks on extension of the Halsted operation for cancer of the breast. Ann Surg 130: 315
Warren S, Witman EM (1937) Studies on tumour metastases: the distribution of metastases in cancer of the breast. Surg Gynecol Obstet 57: 81
Wassink WF (1935) Cancer et hérédité. Genetika 17: 103–144
Wellings SR (1980) Development of human breast cancer. Adv Cancer Res 31: 287–314
Wellings SR, Jensen HM, Marcun RG (1975) An atlas of subgross pathology of the human breast with special reference to possible precancerous lesions. J Natl Cancer Inst 55: 231–273
Wheeler JE, Enterline HT, Roseman JM, Tomasulo JP, McIvanic CH, Fitto WT, Kirschenbaum J (1974) Lobular carcinoma in situ of the breast. Long-term follow-up. Cancer 34: 554–563
Wilkinson EJ, Hause LL, Hoffman RG et al. (1982) Occult axillary lymph node metastases in invasive breast carcinoma: characteristics of the primary tumour and significance of the metastases. Pathol Annu 17: 67
Wolfe JN (1976a) Breast parenchymal patterns and their changes with age. Radiology 121: 545–552
Wolfe JN (1976b) Risk for breast cancer development determined by mammographic parenchymal pattern. Cancer 37: 2486–2492
Zumoff B, Fishman J, Bradlow HL et al. (1975). Hormone profiles in hormone-dependent cancers. Cancer Res. 35: 3365–3373

Thyroid and Parathyroid Carcinoma

P.-O. GRANBERG, M. BÄCKDAHL, B. CEDERMARK, B. HAMBERGER, G. LUNDELL, T. LÖWHAGEN, and G. WALLIN

Thyroid Carcinoma

Malignant neoplasms of the thyroid are rare and account for about 1% of all cancers. About 90% of the thyroid malignancies are differentiated carcinomas including papillary, follicular and medullary tumours. Differentiated thyroid carcinomas often appear in young individuals and have a peak incidence in the third or fourth decade. In contrast, the anaplastic thyroid carcinoma is largely a disease of the elderly.

According to Swedish autopsy studies (Bondeson and Ljungberg 1981; Nielsen and Zetterlund 1985) the prevalence of non-clinical thyroid cancer is around 8% with most tumours being of the papillary type. There are no differences in regard to sex and age distribution. In other studies prevalence figures as high as 35% have been recorded (Fukunaga and Yamati 1975, Harach 1985).

In Sweden the annual morbidity in thyroid cancer is around 4.6 per 100 000 inhabitants. The mortality rate shows a decreasing tendency and is now about 0.8 per 100 000 inhabitants per year. Anaplastic cancer, which constitutes around 10% of the thyroid malignancies, has a mortality of almost 100%. Thus, the annual mortality rate in differentiated thyroid cancer is only 0.4 per 100 000 inhabitants. The Swedish figures are in accordance with similar data from the United States. (Cutler and Young 1975; Thompson et al. 1978).

Colloid goitre often precedes thyroid carcinoma but should not be considered as a precancerous condition. However, a solitary nodule in the thyroid should always be regarded as potentially malignant as such a "solitoma" may harbour a carcinoma in up to 20% of cases (Psarras et al. 1972; Katz and Warren 1976). In patients younger than 25 years of age solitomas are malignant in about 50% of cases and in children below the age of 15 years the probability of malignancy may be as high as 75% (Harness et al. 1971). If a nodule is hyperfunctioning, it is almost never malignant. Irradiation to the neck, especially in childhood, increases the risk for later development of both malignant and benign lesions in the thyroid gland.

The epidemiology of thyroid cancer varies in different parts of the world (Fig. 1). Papillary thyroid cancer is more common in areas with a high iodine intake, such as the United States, Japan and Iceland, where up to 80% of thyroid carcinomas are of the papillary type (Woolner 1971; Cady et al. 1976; Maz-

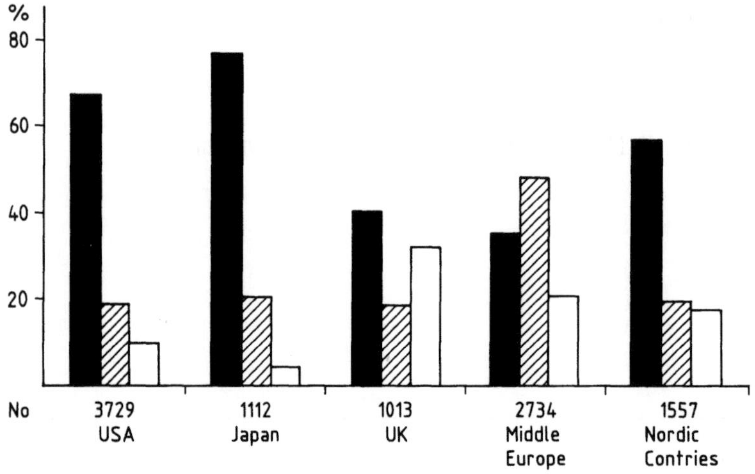

Fig. 1. Epidemiological differences in papillary *(solid bars)*, follicular *(hatched bars)* and medullary *(open bars)* carcinomas of the thyroid according to the WHO classification. (Data from Hedinger and Sobin 1979; Hirabayashi and Lindsay 1961; McKenzie 1971; Marruchi et al. 1971; Woolner 1971; Ranke et al. 1973; Neracher and Heding 1975; Beaugie et al. 1976; Cady et al. 1976; Heitz et al. 1976; Georgii 1977; Mazzaferri et al. 1977; Williams et al. 1977; Figg et al. 1978; Byar et al. 1979; Frauenhoffer et al. 1979; Staunton and Skeet 1979; Söreide et al. 1979; Ito et al. 1980; Taylor and Al-Wattar 1980; Franssila et al. 1981; Wanebo et al. 1981; Meybier et al. 1983; Ozaki et al. 1983; Christensen et al. 1984)

zaferri et al. 1977; Ito et al. 1980; Ozaki et al. 1983). In the United Kingdom and central Europe papillary carcinomas account for less than 40%. On the other hand, the frequency of follicular carcinoma is extremely high in these areas. In areas where iodine prophylaxis has been introduced, the incidence of papillary cancer has increased, while the incidence of follicular cancer has decreased. Throughout the world medullary carcinoma comprises about 5% of all thyroid carcinomas.

The incidence of anaplastic thyroid carcinoma is remarkably high in England and is more frequently encountered in endemic goitre areas. However, during the last two decades a decreasing frequency of this dreaded tumour has been recorded (Beaugie 1976; Staunton and Skeet 1979).

Differentiated Thyroid Carcinoma

Papillary thyroid carcinoma is the most common type of thyroid cancer in most parts of the world. With regard to diagnosis, treatment and prognosis, not only pure papillary, but also mixed papillary-follicular tumours should be considered papillary (Woolner 1971; Hedinger and Sobin 1974). The tumour is two to four times more frequent in females (Woolner 1971). For occult tumours (see below) there is no difference in sex ratio. Although papillary thyroid carcinoma may occur at any age, it accounts for at least 80% of the thyroid tumours in children and young adults. As mentioned earlier it is less frequent in endemic goitre areas and rises in frequency with increased iodine intake. Most irradiation-induced thyroid carcinomas are of the papillary type (Mazzaferri 1981).

Papillary thyroid carcinomas vary in size from microscopic tumours to large cancers invading the thyroid capsule and contiguous structures. Depending on how extensively the gland is examined, 20%–80% of the papillary carcinomas are reported to be multifocal (Black et al. 1960; Cady et al. 1976; Mazzaferri et al. 1977). This finding has been interpreted as an intrathyroidal spread but probably merely reflects a multicentric origin of the cancer.

Frequently, papillary tumours harbour follicular areas. This fact has resulted in many papillary carcinomas being diagnosed as follicular tumours. Earlier these mixed forms were considered as an intermediate group – papillary-follicular tumours. However, these tumours have the same biological behaviour as the pure papillary cancers and should, according to the WHO classification, be classified as such. If there are difficulties in classification, determination of intermediate filament proteins (cytoskeleton) by immuno-histochemical techniques can differentiate the tumours from each other. Papillary cancer reveals both cytokeratin and prekeratin, while follicular cancer lacks the prekeratin (Miettunen et al. 1984).

Papillary carcinomas metastasise mainly via the lymphatics and about half of the patients already have cervical lymph node involvement at the time of surgery. In fact, an enlarged lymph node in the neck is sometimes the first clinical sign of the disease.

Distant metastases, mainly to the lungs, skeleton and soft tissue, are seen in less than 1% of the patients at the time of diagnosis (Woolner et al. 1961; Mazzaferri et al. 1977).

Most *occult* thyroid cancers are of the papillary type. By definition, occult carcinomas are less than 1.5 cm in diameter (Woolner et al. 1961). By meticulous microscopic investigation of 100 thyroid glands removed at autopsies, Harach et al. (1985) found no less than 36% occult papillary carcinomas with a median diameter of 0.44 mm (0.15–14.0 mm).

Follicular thyroid carcinoma is more common in endemic goitre areas and comprises between 20%–45% of all malignant thyroid tumours (Beaugie et al. 1976; Löhrs et al. 1980). It may occur at any age but has a peak incidence in the third and fourth decades. Females are affected three times as frequently as males.

In general, follicular thyroid cancer presents as a solitary, encapsulated tumour with a pink, reddish-yellowish or grey cut surface. Histologically, the degree of vascular invasion varies, and the microscopic structure usually contains some small follicles as evidence of differentiation. Sometimes the tumour has a brown-coloured cut surface and a histological picture revealing big oxyphilic cells. This type of tumour, often referred to as "Hürthle cell carcinoma", is considered to be a more malignant form of the follicular carcinoma.

Regional lymph node metastases will be found in only 2%–3% of patients with follicular cancer. However, in some studies the frequency of nodal involvement has been reported to be between 15% and 28%. These high figures certainly reflect an admixture of papillary cancers. Therefore, a follicular carcinoma with regional lymph node metastases should be reevaluated on the suspicion of being a papillary carcinoma. Distant metastases from a follicular carcinoma most commonly affect the lungs and the skeleton, and distant spread is sometimes the first clinical sign of the disease.

Medullary thyroid carcinoma was first defined as a specific entity by Horn (1951). The tumour consists of endocrine cells, derived from the parafollicular cells or the C cells of the thyroid, and fewer than 5% of thyroid carcinomas belong to this group. The familial occurrence of medullary thyroid carcinoma in connection with other manifestations such as pheochromocytoma and hyperparathyroidism was first suggested by Sipple (1961) and was later termed "multiple endocrine neoplasia" (MEN) type II.

The different types of medullary thyroid carcinoma are:

1. The sporadic form which is the most common type and usually detected because of a palpable tumour in the neck.
2. MEN type II A with medullary thyroid carcinoma, pheochromocytoma and hyperparathyroidism.
3. MEN type II B with medullary thyroid carcinoma, pheochromocytoma, multiple mucosal neurimonas and a marfanoid habitus.

Not all MEN patients do develop all the components of the syndrome, but almost invariably medullary thyroid carcinoma is present in MEN patients (Cance and Wells 1985).

When presenting as a lump in the neck the diagnosis of medullary thyroid carcinoma is similar to other thyroid tumours (see below). However, medullary thyroid carcinoma contains and secretes a number of hormones and peptides which can be used as tumour markers during the diagnostic work-up (Lloyd et al. 1983; Clark 1985). Most widely used is calcitonin which is present in increased levels in the serum of patients with medullary thyroid carcinoma. For early detection of MEN II, stimulation of calcitonin release with pentagastrin and/or calcium should be used as such stimulation markedly increases the sensitivity. Screening of all possibly affected members of a kindred is recommended (Sizemore et al. 1980; Telenius-Berg et al. 1984; Cance and Wells 1985) as early detection and treatment will reduce mortality.

Diagnosis

The most important aspect of detecting a thyroid carcinoma is a meticulous clinical examination of the neck. The harder and firmer a thyroid nodule, the greater the probability of malignancy. However, also a soft and/or cystic lesion can occasionally harbour a carcinoma, whereas a rock-hard nodule may represent a degenerated and calcified colloid goitre. The diagnostic policy for thyroid nodules at the Karolinska Hospital in Sweden is presented in Fig. 2.

Aspiration Biopsy Cytology

Fine needle aspiration biopsy cytology (ABC) is the method of choice in selecting patients with suspect thyroid nodules for surgery (Löwhagen et al. 1979, 1981; Granberg et al. 1983). The availability of a cytological diagnosis within minutes makes this technique an excellent tool for preoperative investigation of all tumour and tumour-like conditions in the thy-

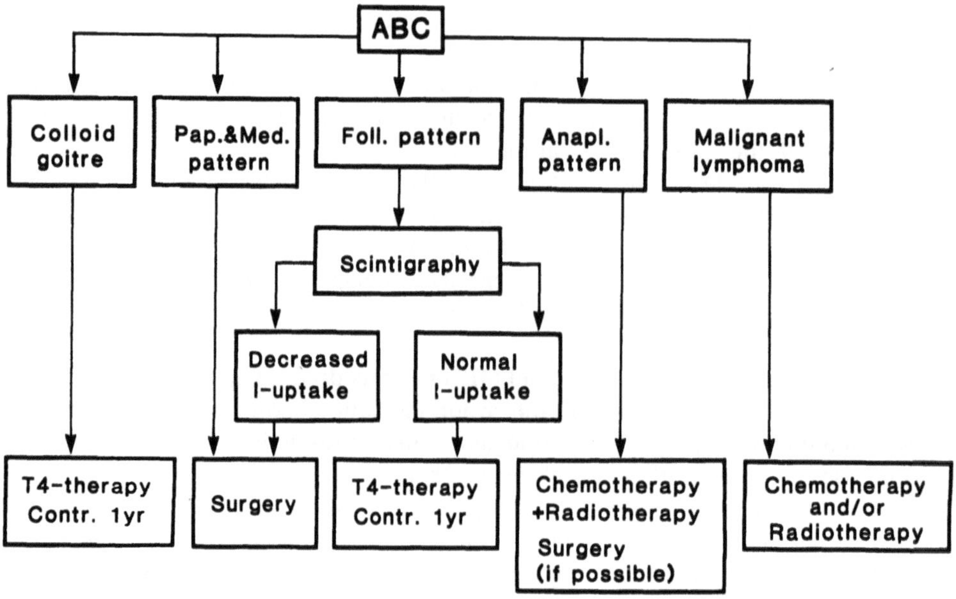

Fig. 2. Flow chart for evaluation of solitary thyroid nodules according to the principles at the Karolinska Hospital

roid. Technical details have been described elsewhere (Löwhagen et al. 1981). In general, thyroid neoplasms yield a cell-rich aspirate, and the cell patterns are usually characteristic for the various types of tumours:

Papillary carcinoma is recognised by the papillary form of the tumour fragments. In more than two-thirds of the tumours, the nuclei contain cytoplasmic inclusions – "pseudonucleoli". Psammoma bodies are rare but helpful in the diagnosis when present. Ropy strands of dense colloid are other characteristic features of these tumours (Fig. 3).

Follicular tumours reveal monotonously repeated microfollicular cell clusters. The cells generally have monomorphous nuclei and resemble normal follicular cells in their cytoplasmic characteristics (Fig. 4). Some tumours consist of large oncocytic cells with fine granulated cytoplasm. These tumours constitute a special group of follicular lesions which has been called "Hürthle cell tumours".

Medullary carcinoma displays a typical dispersed cell pattern, where the cells tend to be elongated and the cytoplasm may be speckled with small red granules. Amyloid is a common finding (Fig. 5).

Papillary and medullary carcinomas are readily diagnosed with ABC, and in these two forms the absolute sensitivity approaches 100%. The differences in cytological appearance between follicular adenomas and carcinomas are subtle. Thus, on the cellular level, there are no reliable criteria distinguishing the two conditions. Therefore, a tumour with a follicular cytological pattern should be referred to as a "follicular neoplasm" on the understanding that surgery should be performed for histopathological examination of the tumour. Special attention should then be paid to capsular and blood vessel invasion. This policy is also valid for Hürthle cell tumours, where cytological separation of benign and malignant tumours is particularly difficult. Even histopathology may err in this respect as a few patients with a supposedly benign follicular tumour will later develop metastases, consistent with follicular carcinoma (Lang et al. 1980).

Cystic lesions represent a difficult diagnostic problem and ABC must be interpreted with caution. When a cyst has been evacuated, the fluid should be centrifuged and the sediment smeared. After emptying the cyst, it is important to check for any residual mass which must then be reaspirated. Aspiration with the guidance of ultrasound may prove valuable in these instances. Ashcraft and van Herle (1981) reviewed 2290 cystic lesions in the thyroid of which 10% had been operated on for histopathological investigation. According to ABC, eight cases were diagnosed as malignant, but definitive histopathology revealed 21 cancers, i.e. 9% of the surgically treated tumours.

ABC usually provides more direct information about the underlying pathology than can be obtained by other available techniques. By beginning

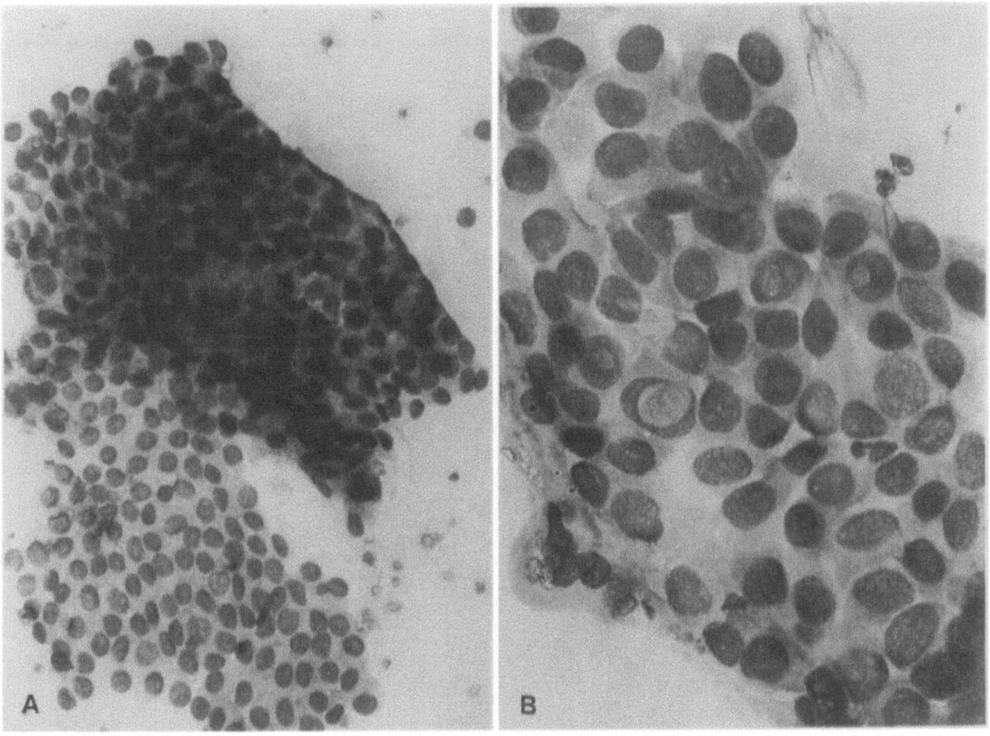

Fig. 3 A, B. Papillary carcinoma. **A** Partly folded monolayer sheet of medium-sized tumour cells with well-defined cellular borders. **B** Several nuclei with cytoplasmic inclusions. ABC, air-dried May-Grünewald-Giemsa (MGG)-stained smear

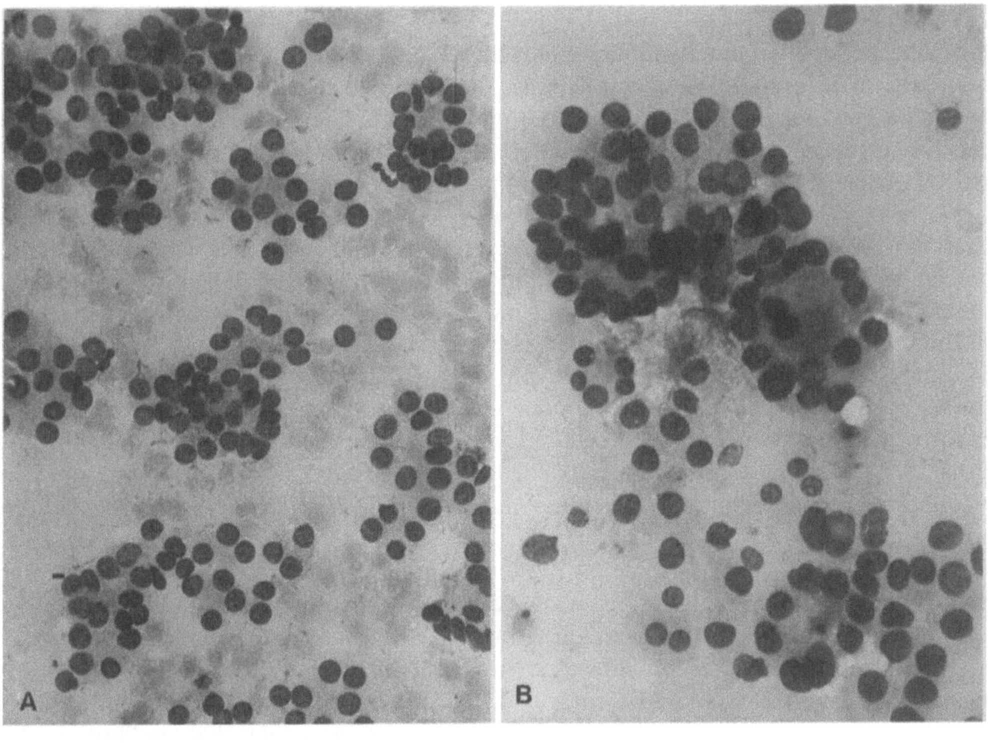

Fig. 4 A, B. Follicular neoplasm. Numerous equi-sized groups in annular formations indicating follicular growth. ABC, air-dried MGG-stained smear. Note that ABC does not enable differential diagnosis between adenoma and carcinoma

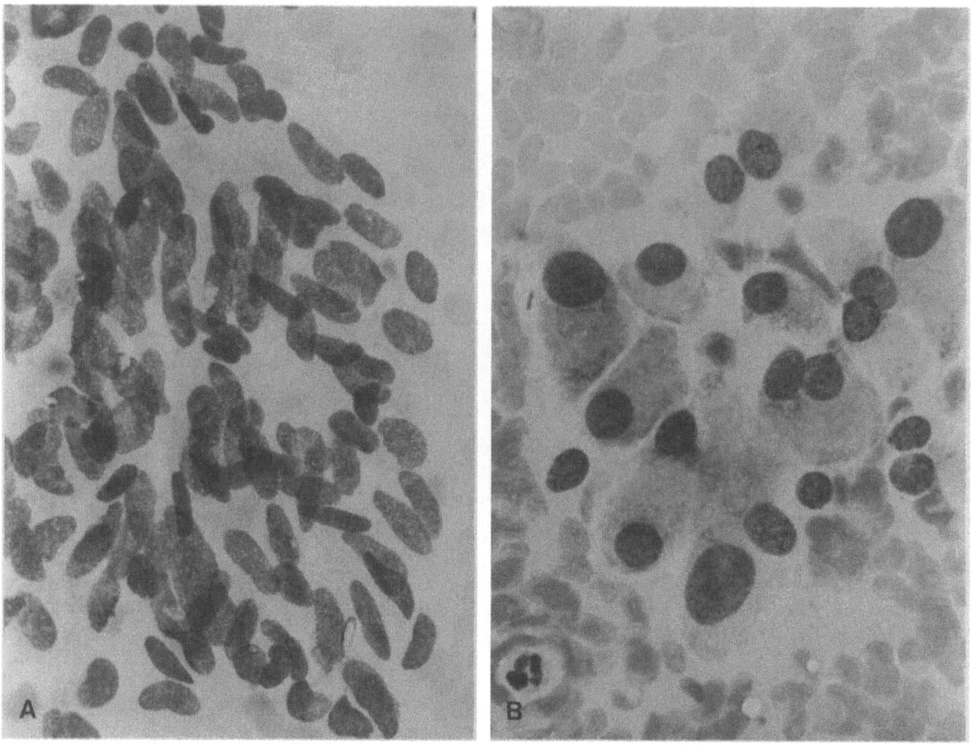

Fig. 5 A, B. Medullary carcinoma, two common morphological patterns. **A** Cluster of predominantly elongated cells. **B** Cells of plasmocytoid and triangular shape. ABC, air-dried MGG-stained smear

the clinical evaluation of a thyroid nodule with ABC, the cost can be reduced by up to 50% as ABC reduces the need for diagnostic surgery and other expensive investigations. Furthermore, the method gives valuable information as to what complementary investigations should be done, when surgery is necessary for a definite diagnosis, which surgical procedure is necessary or whether the disease should be treated with non-surgical modalities.

The false negative rate with ABC ranges between 5% and 10% (Löwhagen et al. 1981). This figure compares favourably with all other preoperative diagnostic methods (van Herle et al. 1982; Hamberger et al. 1982). Most false positive results encountered in published material concern the differential diagnosis between follicular adenoma and follicular carcinoma (Boey et al. 1984). In some institutions, large needle biopsies for histological evaluation are preferred (Wang et al. 1976). This technique is associated with a higher complication rate than ABC but does not improve the diagnostic accuracy.

Thyroid Scan

In most institutions scintigraphy precedes the fine needle aspiration biopsy in the evaluation of thyroid nodules. However, it is our opinion that ABC should be the first examination performed on thyroid nodules in patients who are not suspected of suffering from hyperthyroidism.

As ^{123}I is produced by a cyclotron and still remains relatively unavailable in many countries, ^{131}I and ^{99m}Tc (technetium) are the isotopes mostly used in thyroid imaging. Despite the fact that no increase in the occurrence of thyroid malignancies has been seen after diagnostic use of ^{131}I (Holm 1982), the radiation dose should always be kept at a minimum. Thus, routine thyroid scintigraphy should be made with ^{99m}Tc or ^{123}I, at least in young patients.

The scintigraphic examinations are performed with either a gammacamera or a rectilinear scanner. The importance of the scintigraphy lies in the fact that a thyroid nodule showing a normal or an increased uptake of iodine is almost invariably benign. However, in clinical practice it is important to realize that with ^{99m}Tc this is not always true. Therefore, thyroid nodules that are "hot" on ^{99m}Tc scans should be re-examined with radioiodine (Freitas et al. 1985). The probability of malignancy in a solitary "cold" thyroid nodule is less than 20%.

Treatment

Surgery

In general, surgery is the first step in the treatment of differentiated thyroid carcinoma. However, there are different opinions concerning the extent of the operation. In particular, there is disagreement as to whether a *papillary carcinoma* clinically confined to one lobe should be removed by a total thyroidectomy or a less radical procedure (Clark et al. 1966; Block 1977; Cady 1981). In contrast to lobectomy, total thyroidectomy is accompanied by significant postoperative morbidity in the form of recurrent nerve lesions and hypoparathyroidism occurring in 3%–27% of cases (Clark et al. 1959; McKenzie 1971; Attie et al. 1979).

When the tumour is confined to the thyroid, functioning recurrent laryngeal nerves should, whenever possible, be spared and not deliberately sacrificed. This is true even when the primary tumour or lymph node metastases are growing close to the nerve. In most instances the nerve can be dissected without influencing the radicality of the operation. However, when unilateral vocal cord paralysis is present, and tumour invasion in the surroundings of the homolateral recurrent nerve is found, the nerve should be excised with the tumour. When the individual branches of the superior thyroid vessels are ligated, care should be taken to avoid lesions to the external branch of the superior laryngeal nerve.

When performing a total thyroidectomy, truncal ligation of the inferior thyroid artery should be avoided to prevent hypoparathyroidism. If none of the parathyroid glands can be preserved in situ, at least one gland should be cut into pieces of around 2 mm^3 and transplanted into separate pockets in the sternocleidomastoid muscle. Transplantation into the brachio-radial muscle should be preferred when postoperative irradiation to the neck is contemplated.

Addition of a "radical neck" to a thyroidectomy does not influence life expectancy and should not be used as a routine procedure (Mazzaferri 1978). When regional lymph node metastases are present, a modified neck dissection with extirpation of only the metastatic nodes is sufficient. Excision of the sternocleidomastoid muscle and/or the internal jugular vein is seldom necessary.

A preoperative ABC diagnosis of a *follicular neoplasm* should lead to no less than hemithyroidectomy to get a proper histological diagnosis. *Frozen* sections are often not reliable and should in general not be used. If the final histopathological diagnosis is follicular carcinoma, the remaining thyroid tissue should be extirpated in a second operation.

Before surgery for *medullary thyroid carcinoma* is contemplated, the presence of MEN II and a concurrent pheochromocytoma must be excluded as surgery on a patient with an undetected pheochromocytoma may be life threatening. The most widely used surgical treatment of medullary thyroid carcinoma is total thyroidectomy with removal of all lymph nodes in the central compartment. When macroscopic appearance suggests involvement of other lymph nodes in the neck, more extensive neck dissection should be undertaken. Less than total thyroidectomy cannot be recommended as bilateral tumours are also found in sporadic cases in about 20% (Russell et al. 1983). Following surgery, basal and stimulated calcitonin levels can be measured to find out whether the patient is disease free. In patients with postoperatively elevated calcitonin levels, reoperation with meticulous dissection of the whole neck may normalise the calcitonin levels (Tisell et al. 1986).

Whether such a strategy prolongs survival has not been established. Thus, the extent of primary surgery of medullary thyroid carcinoma has not yet been solved.

Radioiodine Therapy

It has now been clearly established that patients with metastatic disease and without radioiodine uptake in their metastases have a less favourable prognosis than those in whom the metastases can be treated with radioiodine. The use of systemic radioiodine therapy (^{131}I) in order to destroy remaining thyroid tissue and possible foci of tumour tissue has therefore been advocated (Mazzaferri et al. 1977; Young et al. 1980; Beierwaltes et al. 1984). However, in some studies no differences have been found in survival time or rate of recurrence between surgery alone and surgery plus radioiodine therapy, at least in patients with localised disease (Cady et al. 1976; Snyder et al. 1983; Christensen et al. 1984; Carcangiu et al. 1985b). Currently, it seems reasonable to recommend the use of postoperative radioiodine therapy in patients with either incomplete surgery, metastatic disease and/or tumour growth outside the thyroid capsule. However, awaiting results from randomised clinical studies of radioiodine therapy, the true indications for radioiodine therapy still remain unclear. Although conflicting reports occur, most authors agree that there is no place for radioiodine therapy in medullary carcinoma (Saad et al. 1983).

For the radioiodine therapy to be effective, the patient should be clinically hypothyroid after thyroid ablation. Exogenous administration of thyrotropin even in large doses is by no means as effective as the continuous thyrotropin stimulation seen in the hypothyroid state. Furthermore, thyrotropin stimulates not only the uptake of radioiodine, but also the growth of the tumour and any metastases. For patients who have been made hypothyroid, the capacity to perform physical work responds only slowly to thyroxine substitution. This capacity does not increase significantly until 6 months after full substitution (Hylander et al. 1983).

Radioiodine has been in use for nearly 40 years in the treatment of hyperthyroidism and thyroid cancer. The risk for radiation-induced tumours seems to be low, but recently a small excess of cancer in the urinary bladder and leukaemia has been found in a group of patients with thyroid cancer treated with radioiodine (Edmonds and Smith 1986).

External Irradiation

External irradiation occasionally exerts a notable effect on palpable differentiated thyroid cancer. In those cases an interval of several months or even 1 year must elapse before the effect becomes clinically manifest. Combinations of external radiotherapy and radioiodine are well tolerated. The major side effect of external irradiation is the dry mouth that most patients will experience.

Radiotherapy with 50 Gy or more given to patients who have had non-radical surgery results in a low incidence of local recurrence (Tubiana et al. 1985). Prophylactic postoperative external radiotherapy may sometimes be of benefit. We favour the use of external postoperative radiotherapy in patients above the age of 40 years who have had tumour growth outside the thyroid capsule into surrounding tissues and in patients who have had repeated local recurrences and where reoperation might be difficult.

There are no results available from randomised clinical studies aimed at evaluating the role of external radiotherapy in thyroid carcinoma. Therefore, the role of external irradiation in the treatment of thyroid carcinoma cannot as yet be defined.

Chemotherapy

The effect of chemotherapy, either in the form of single drug therapy or in combination has mostly been disappointing in patients with differentiated thyroid carcinoma. This is contrary to the results obtained in patients with malignant lymphoma of the thyroid gland where several chemotherapy regimens alone or in combination with external radiotherapy are effective.

The drug that has been tried most often is adriamycin, and partial responses have been reported in 15%–20% of patients treated (Stratton Hill 1983). Some complete responders have recently been reported after treatment with a combination of adriamycin and cisplatinum (Shimaoka et al. 1985). However, the side effects with this regimen can be severe.

Hormone Treatment

There is abundant evidence that thyroid-stimulating hormone (TSH) can stimulate the growth of papillary and follicular thyroid carcinoma (Clark 1985). Thyroid hormone given in adequate doses suppresses TSH to low or undetectable levels that will not rise in response to thyrotropin-releasing hormone (TRH). Recurrence rates of both papillary and follicular thyroid cancer are lower in patients treated postoperatively with thyroid hormone (Mazzaferri 1981). Therefore, all patients treated for papillary or follicular thyroid carcinoma should be given thyroid hormones in sufficient doses to suppress the TSH secretion, i.e. usually doses higher than those needed for substitution. In medullary thyroid carcinoma, TSH does not affect tumour growth, and thyroid hormone treatment is needed postoperatively in substitutional doses only.

Follow-up

Patients treated for differentiated thyroid carcinoma should be followed regularly. During the 1st and 2nd postoperative years, the patient should be examined at relatively short intervals; thereafter yearly. The examination should include a search for locoregional recurrence and distant metastases. Routine surveys with chest X-ray, bone scan, etc. are not indicated. A suspected lesion can be diagnosed by ABC. Laboratory investigations to evaluate the thyroid and parathyroid function are indicated during the first postoperative year. In patients treated for medullary carcinoma, the serum levels of calcitonin should be monitored.

Postoperative scintigraphy is of value to find out whether a thyroidectomy has been complete or not and may also be useful in detecting residual disease. The value of routinely repeated follow-up examinations with radioiodine in all patients treated for differentiated thyroid carcinoma has not been established. If at follow-up recurrent disease is suspected, a whole body scan is indicated to find out whether radioiodine-accumulating tissue is present or not.

Thyroglobulin (TG) is a glucoprotein which functions as a prohormone in the synthesis of thyroxin (T_4) and triiodothyronine (T_3). From the follicles of the thyroid gland, small quantities of TG are released into the circulation and can be detected by sensitive assays in most healthy individuals. Depending on the assay used, the serum concentrations of TG ranges from undetectable levels to 60 μg per litre (Bayer and McDougall 1984). Moderately increased concentrations are normally found in pregnancy and in the newborn. High concentrations of TG are found in patients with nodular goitre, hyperthyroidism, thyroiditis, physical injury to the thyroid gland and in patients with differentiated thyroid carcinoma. TG autoantibodies interfere with the determination of TG and, if present, cause thyroglobulin assays to have no clinical value.

In some patients with differentiated thyroid carcinoma the release of TG may be increased by TSH. Therefore, it is preferable to measure TG after thyroid hormone medication has been withdrawn for some period of time.

TG can also be measured in histological material by immunocytochemical techniques. This method is of clinical value to confirm a thyroid origin of a suspected lesion.

Papillary and follicular thyroid carcinomas and metastases thereof almost always have elevated TG levels while medullary thyroid carcinomas in general have no detectable or low levels of TG. The more aggressive the tumour, the lower the TG levels. Undifferentiated thyroid carcinomas mostly show very low TG levels in serum. According to some studies, TG is never present in anaplastic thyroid cancer cells (Carcangiu et al. 1985a).

The clinical importance of TG lies in its value as a tumour marker. After successful thyroidectomy for a differentiated thyroid cancer, serum TG should return to normal or undetectable levels. During follow-up, increasing TG levels in serum is an important sign of recurrent disease. Not least in patients with tumours without uptake of ^{131}I, measurement of TG in serum have proved to be of clinical value (Ericsson et al. 1984; Falk et al. 1984). The frequency of false negative as well as false positive measurement has been reported to be 5%–15%. However, it has been suggested that patients with appearently false positive TG measurements may represent a group with an increased probability of developing tumour recurrence (Falk et al. 1984).

Prognosis

Papillary thyroid carcinomas have a better prognosis than other thyroid malignancies, and the disease has a prolonged course in most patients. The mortality rate from this tumour is uncertain, but seems to be less than 10% over several decades. The prognosis depends mainly on the extent of the tumour, the age and the sex, with men over 40 and women over 50 years of age being at the highest risk (Halnan 1966; Franssila 1975). The presence of node metastases does not seem to have any significant effect upon the survival time (Mazzaferri 1981) but tends to predict more tumour recurrence, especially in patients above the age of 40.

Although occult papillary carcinomas sometimes present with regional lymph node metastases, the prognosis is very favourable. This is true even if local recurrence occurs. In two studies comprising 137 and 153 patients with occult tumours and followed for an average of 25 and 10 years, respectively, none of the patients developed distant metastases or died of thyroid cancer (Hubert et al. 1980; Mazzaferri and Oertle 1983).

The prognosis in *follicular carcinoma* also depends upon age, sex and extent of tumour growth (Cady et al. 1979). The distinctive mode of spread is via the blood stream to distant sites. In rare instances, the first clinical manifestation of the disease is due to distant metastases. Osseous metastases in particular have a poor outcome (Nêmec et al. 1979).

The prognosis for *medullary thyroid carcinoma* is generally worse than for papillary and follicular thyroid carcinomas. The mean 5-year survival rate is about 50%. The tumour status at the time of diagnosis is strongly related to the survival time. The presence of lymph node metastases at the time of primary surgery is an unfavourable prognostic factor. Asymptomatic patients diagnosed only because of increased calcitonin release upon stimulation have a favourable prognosis.

Nuclear DNA Content and Prognosis in Thyroid Cancer

Numerous cytochemical studies in clinical tumour material indicate a close correlation between ploidy level and grade of tumour malignancy as reflected by the clinical course (Auer et al. 1985). Thus, low-grade malignant tumours generally have euploid DNA content, i.e. DNA amounts predominantly in diploid or diploid and tetraploid regions (Fig. 6A, B) while high-grade malignant tumours are characterised by aneuploid DNA content, i.e. frequently increased and variable DNA values deviating from normal (Fig. 6 C). The differences in DNA distribution patterns can be demonstrated by means of slide-cytophotometric, slide-microspectrophotometric and flow-cytophotometric measurements. The main advantage of the slide method is the possibility of performing DNA measurements in morphologically identified cells, resulting in a high degree of tumour cell specificity. A major disadvantage is that the selection procedure is relatively time consuming, which limits the number of cells analysed per case. The flow method, on the other hand, offers the possibility of analysing large cell populations within a relatively short time period, but does not permit differentiation between non-neoplastic and neoplastic cells.

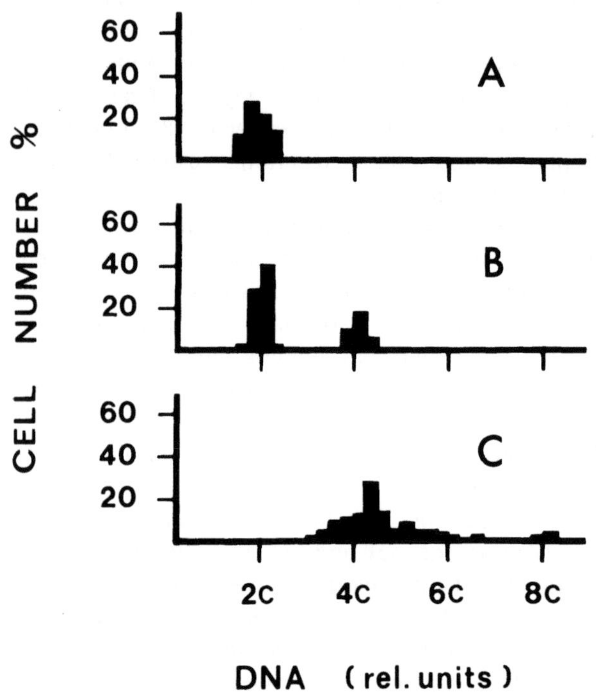

Fig. 6 A–C. DNA histograms from slide-cytophotometric measurements (cytology and sections) of (**A**) a diploid, (**B**) a polyploid and (**C**) an aneuploid thyroid carcinoma. The DNA values are expressed in relation to the median DNA values *(2c)* of the respective internal control cells

The DNA content of tumour cells has been compared retrospectively on differentiated thyroid cancers in patients with long survival and in patients who succumbed to their disease (Cohn et al. 1984; Bäckdahl et al. 1985, 1986 a). All the tumours from ten patients with *papillary thyroid cancer* who died from their disease within 12 years had increased nuclear DNA values (aneuploid), whereas 80 patients who were alive at least 10 years after the time of diagnosis had low (diploid) DNA levels (Fig. 7). As regards *follicular thyroid tumours* 17 out of 19 non-survivors (89%) with follicular carcinoma had tumours with aneuploid nuclear DNA profile, whereas 19 out of 20 survivors (95%) with follicular carcinoma and 25 out of 26 survivors (96%) with follicular adenoma had tumours with euploid DNA content. Of the 25 non-survivors with *medullary thyroid carcinoma* 21 (84%) had tumours with aneuploid tumour cell nuclear DNA pattern, whereas eight of the 11 survivors (73%) had diploid tumours.

A comparison of nuclear DNA content in neoplastic cells of primary thyroid tumours and corresponding recurrences showed similar DNA distribution patterns in both the primary and secondary lesions.

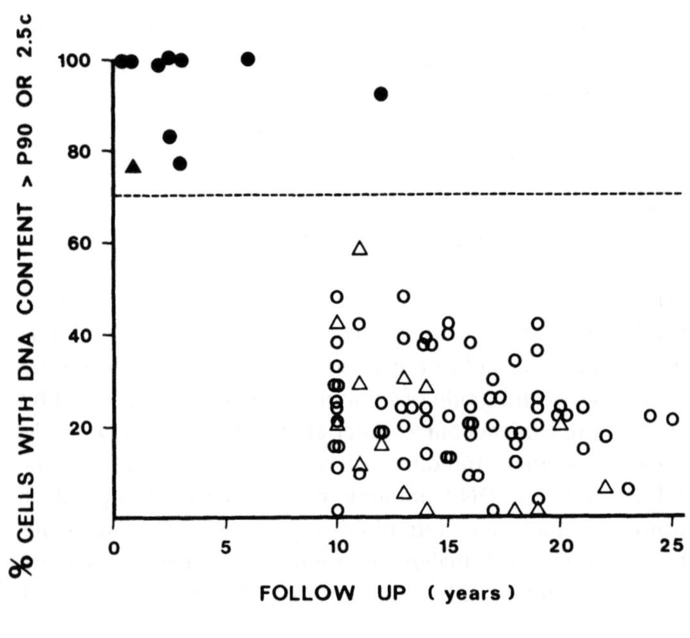

Fig. 7. Percentage cells with DNA content > P90 (histologic material; *solid circles* non-survivors; *open circles* survivors) or > 2.5 c (cytological material; *solid triangles* non-survivors; *open triangles*, survivors) in papillary thyroid carcinoma plotted against follow-up time ($n = 90$)

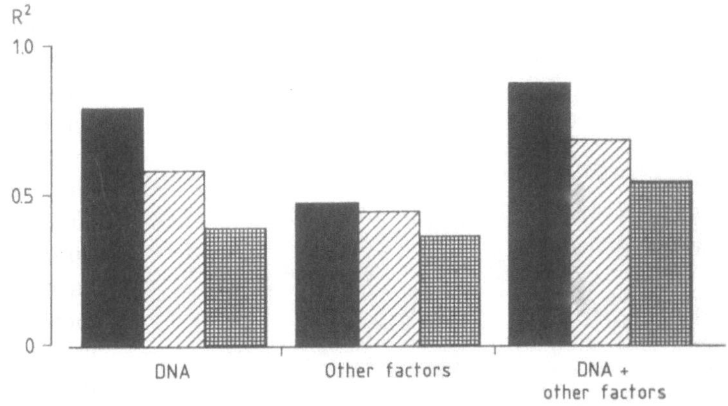

Fig. 8. The prognostic predictive power *(R)* of the tumour cell nuclear DNA content, other preoperative prognostic factors (age, sex, tumour size, preoperative TNM) and tumour cell nuclear DNA content plus other prognostic factors in papillary *(solid bars)*, follicular *(hatched bars)* and medullary *(squared bars)* thyroid carcinoma

The prognostic predictive power of the tumour cell nuclear DNA content was significantly greater in papillary and of similar magnitude in follicular and medullary thyroid carcinoma than that of all other preoperative prognostic factors combined (age, sex, tumour size, preoperative TNM). When the tumour cell nuclear DNA content was added to all other prognostic factors, a significant increase of the prognostic value was obtained (Fig. 8) (Bäckdahl et al. 1986 b).

As determination of the tumour cell nuclear DNA content in differentiated thyroid carcinoma can be performed preoperatively in fine needle aspirates, it should be a valuable prognostic indicator in these types of thyroid carcinoma.

Anaplastic Thyroid Carcinoma

Contrary to the relatively benign and non-aggressive course of the differentiated thyroid carcinomas, the undifferentiated, anaplastic variant is one of the most aggressive neoplasms encountered in humans. The mean age of patients suffering from this disease is between 60 and 66 years, and only very rarely are anaplastic thyroid carcinomas encountered in patients below the age of 50. The disease is more common in females, but the sex distribution difference is not as pronounced as in the differentiated thyroid neoplasms.

A significant number of anaplastic carcinomas are associated with a well-differentiated thyroid tumour. This fact has supported the view that an anaplastic transformation of a well-differentiated thyroid carcinoma may occur. The probability of such a transformation should be very low, less than 1% (Carcangiu et al. 1985 a). If a differentiated thyroid carcinoma were to precede an anaplastic tumour, the prevalence of anaplastic carcinoma should be correlated to the prevalence of differentiated thyroid carcinoma. However, the fact that the frequency of anaplastic forms decreases, and the frequency of differentiated carcinomas increases is contradictory to the theory of transformation.

Diagnosis

The most common manifestation of an anaplastic thyroid carcinoma is a rapidly growing mass in the neck. One-third of the patients have a history of a preexisting goitre. The combination of these clinical signs is rarely seen in patients with differentiated neoplasms.

The symptomatology is dominated by dysphonia, dysphagia and dyspnoea – the three Ds. Some patients also complain about cervical pain or irritating cough.

The histological features of anaplastic carcinoma include a mixture of different cell types. Giant and spindle cells are frequently encountered. Squamous cell and true small cell carcinomas, rarely found, have sometimes been considered to be anaplastic thyroid cancers as well (Carcangiu et al. 1985 a). Earlier, all small cell carcinomas were included in the group of anaplastic thyroid cancers. By employing monoclonal antibody techniques the nonepithelial origin of most of these tumours can be established and, in fact, almost all small cell tumors can be shown to represent malignant lymphomas (Tobler et al. 1984).

The differential diagnosis of anaplastic carcinoma includes not only other forms of malignant tumours of the thyroid, but also non-malignant disorders such as haemorrhage in a benign thyroid mass and acute thyroiditis. With ABC a haemorrhage can easily be excluded, while the other disorders may cause problems. Acute thyroiditis presents an aspirate filled with leucocytes. Rapidly growing anaplastic

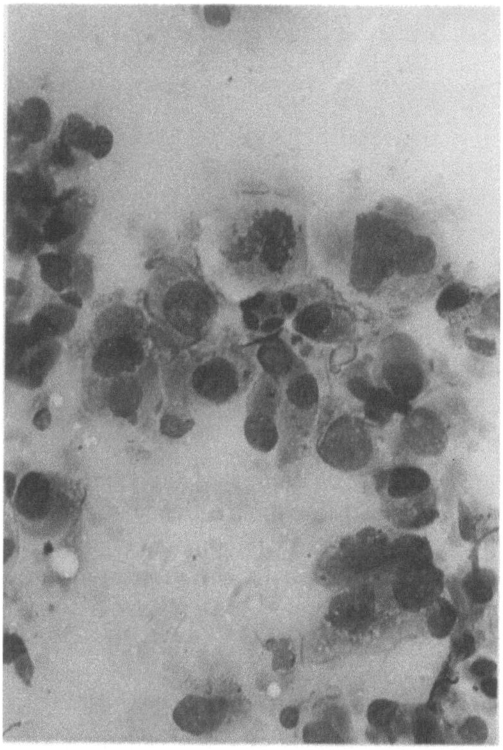

Fig. 9. Anaplastic giant cell carcinoma. Pleomorphic cells with bizarre nuclei and a mitotic figure. ABC, air-dried MGG-stained smear

carcinomas, especially those dominated by giant cells with central necrosis, can mimic acute thyroiditis. However, aspirates from the periphery of the tumour often show bizarre tumour cells with frequent mitotic figures typical of this kind of cancer (Fig. 9). Medullary carcinomas may be misinterpreted as anaplastic cancers of spindle cell type. However, anaplastic thyroid carcinoma does not produce calcitonin.

Treatment

When an anaplastic carcinoma is confined within the thyroid gland or has a limited local spread, there is a chance of cure. Total thyroidectomy is indicated only when the tumour involves both lobes of the thyroid gland. Otherwise, hemithyroidectomy should be sufficient as local recurrences do not occur in the opposite lobe. Extended surgery, such as laryngectomy and/or tracheal resection, is rarely indicated for these malignant tumours (Nel et al. 1985).

Before 1968, 79 patients with anaplastic thyroid carcinoma were treated at the Karolinska Hospital with thyroidectomy and (if possible) followed by external irradiation. The results were poor with a mean survival time of 2.5 months and with 38% of the patients requiring tracheostomy because of the progressive local growth (Jereb et al. 1975). Because of these disappointing results the treatment was changed (Werner et al. 1984). Up to now, 26 patients have been given pre- and postoperative hyperfractionated radiotherapy in combination with bleomycin, cyclophosphamide and 5-fluorouracil. The mean survival time increased and none of the patients required a tracheostomy. Three patients appeared to have been cured. Those who died did so from distant metastases and escaped strangulation. The combined chemo- and radiotherapy is, however, often strenous for the patients, with mucositis being the most frequent side effect. To improve the results and reduce the side effects, other modalities of combined therapy should be explored. Weekly low-dose adriamycin in combination with hyperfractionated radiotherapy has recently been given to five patients. One of these patients was still alive more than 2 years after diagnosis (Tallroth et al. 1987). However, in one patient a tracheostomy was required.

Prognosis

Anaplastic carcinoma of the thyroid gland is a lethal disease. Only sporadic reports of cure have been reported. Anaplastic tumours in patients surviving for an extended period of time should be reinvestigated as they may not represent true anaplastic carcinomas.

Parathyroid Carcinoma

Primary parathyroid carcinoma originates in the chief cells in the parathyroid gland and usually produces parathyroid hormone. Whether non-functioning parathyroid carcinoma exists has been a question of controversy. The rarity with which such tumours occur and the histological resemblance to other malignant tumours, such as follicular thyroid carcinoma and metastatic hypernephroma, make its existence difficult to prove. Metastatic disease to the parathyroid glands is a rare finding and should be of a negligible clinical significance. Nevertheless, frequencies as high as 12% have been reported from autopsy studies (Rivadeneyra et al. 1972; Cifuentes and Pickren 1979).

Epidemiology

The incidence of primary parathyroid carcinoma depends on the criteria employed in making the diagnosis. Thus, figures varying from less than 0.5% up to 4% of patients with parathyroid lesions have been stated (Woolner et al. 1952; Holmes et al. 1969; Schantz and Castleman 1972; Schane and Bilezikian 1982). As the increasing incidence of primary hyperparathyroidism recorded through the last decades has not been accompanied by any increase in reports on parathyroid cancer, the true incidence of the disease is likely to be less than 1% (Granberg et al. 1985).

The aetiology is unknown. There are scattered reports on carcinomas occurring within a parathyroid adenoma or in hyperplastic glands. It has also been described in connection with familial hyperparathyroidism, when concurrent chief cell hyperplasia or adenoma were found. (Woolner et al. 1952; Diunen et al. 1965; Golden et al. 1965; Mallete et al. 1974). Whether these findings indicate an increasing risk of malignant transformation in hyperfunctioning glands or in familial hyperparathyroidism, or whether they represent only random occurrence, cannot be stated (Granberg et al. 1985).

Parathyroid carcinoma is evenly distributed in men and women. This is in contrast to parathyroid adenoma which has a 3:1 preponderance in women. In addition, patients with parathyroid cancer tend to be younger than those with benign tumours. According to literature reviews, the mean age for patients with parathyroid cancer is between 44–50 years (Pollack et al. 1961; Holmes et al. 1969; Shane and Bilezikian 1982; Trigonis et al. 1984).

Histopathology

Parathyroid carcinoma usually presents as a large, multilobular parathyroid "tumour" with a firm consistency. It is often surrounded by a dense, fibrous capsule which gives the tumour a grey-tan to whitish colour. This is in contrast to parathyroid adenomas which are usually more brownish. The tumour often grows invasively and adheres to adjacent structures such as the thyroid, the muscles, the oesophagus and the recurrent laryngeal nerve. Regional lymph node metastases may be present but usually appear relatively late in the disease.

Microscopically, a parathyroid carcinoma is difficult to distinguish from a parathyroid adenoma. For the diagnosis of carcinoma the Armed Forces Institute of Pathology (AFIP) Fascicle emphasises the importance of a trabecular architecture, presence of mitotic figures in parenchymal cells, adherence to surrounding tissues, capsular and blood vessel invasion and extension of fibrous bands from the capsule into the tumour (Castleman and Roth 1978). Of these features, the presence of mitosis was considered the single most important criteria.

However, there are reports on parathyroid carcinomas lacking mitotic figures, and, according to Snover and Foucar (1981), mitotic activity may often be seen in adenomas and hyperplastic parathyroid glands. In a review of 14 cases, capsular invasion was seen in all instances while the mitotic activity varied (van Heerden et al. 1979). The trabecular pattern was found to be of limited value. Jacobi et al. (1986) have suggested that the mean nuclear diameter could be a useful discriminant between adenoma and carcinoma, and, according to the preliminary results of a retrospective multicentre study, the DNA nuclear pattern could prove to be of diagnostic importance (Granberg et al. 1987). Other features which may be seen are calcification and necrosis. Examination of the ultrastructural appearance of parathyroid carcinoma with electron microscopy has been undertaken in a few cases (Bichel et al. 1980; Holck and Tinggaard-Pedersen 1981). Although no firm differentiation between benign and malignant disease can be made by this method, it can still be of value in the rare cases of suspected non-functioning parathyroid carcinomas. By demonstration of secretory granules, glycogen particles and lipid material within the cytoplasm the parathyroid nature of a suspected lesion may be established.

Symptoms and Diagnosis

The symptomatology of parathyroid carcinoma depends on its hormonal activity. As the vast majority of the tumors are hyperfunctioning, the symptoms are mainly those of hypercalcaemia, and the clinical picture the same as in primary hyperparathyroidism. Since the serum calcium levels are usually markedly higher in patients with carcinoma than in those with benign parathyroid disease, the symptoms are often more severe. Shane and Bilezikian (1982) reviewed 41 patients reported in the literature and found all but one to have pronounced symptoms. The most frequent symptoms were polyuria and polydipsia occurring in over one-third of the patients, followed by general weakness, fatigue, anorexia, nausea, vomiting and weight loss. Renal involvement in the form of nephrolithiasis and renal function impairment is common. Also, skeletal disease is frequent, and, contrary to what is seen in benign hyperparathyroidism, renal and bone symptoms often occur concomitantly. Skeletal disease appears in the form of osteoporosis, subperiosteal bone resorption and osteitis fibrosa cystica with symptoms of pain and pathological fractures. Anaemia is more frequent in patients with carcinoma than in those with benign parathyroid disease, and sometimes acute, often recurrent, pancreatitis may occur. A palpable neck mass may be felt in 30%–50% of patients with parathyroid carcinoma (Holmes et al. 1969; Schantz and Castleman 1972; Shane and Bilezikian 1982). This is in contrast with the findings in benign parathyroid disease where a neck tumour can be felt in less than 10% of the patients (Flye et al. 1981). Paralysis of a recurrent laryngeal nerve in connection with hyperparathyroidism is another sign suggestive of cancer. In non-functioning parathyroid carcinoma, a palpable neck mass and/or unilateral recurrent laryngeal nerve paralysis could be the only symptoms of the disease.

Parathyroid carcinoma is almost never diagnosed preoperatively. In fact, the diagnosis is often not established even at the first operation but only at the time of tumour recurrence. The reason for this delay is the rarity of the disease, the symptomatic and clinical resemblance to benign parathyroid disease and the fact that there is no single diagnostic feature to prove the diagnosis. However, if a patient with a clinical diagnosis of primary hyperparathyroidism shows pronounced hyercalcaemia, usually with serum calcium levels above 3.5 mmol per litre, marked hypophosphataemia, very high levels of circulating parathyroid hormone and elevated alkaline phosphatases, the presence of parathyroid carcinoma should be suspected. Recurrent hypercalcaemia after previous operation for primary hyperparathyroidism is also suggestive of parathyroid cancer. This is particularly true if a single large "adenoma" was removed at the primary operation.

Treatment

The only curative treatment for parathyroid cancer is surgical removal of all the tumour. There has been some controversy regarding the extent of the surgical procedure, but most surgeons advocate radical excision of the lesion including ipsilateral hemithyroidectomy and the isthmus. Only when there is suspicion of regional lymph node metastases, should ipsilateral neck dissection be included in the procedure. Since most recurrent parathyroid carcinomas have primarily been misdiagnosed as adenomas and treated with local excision, such a limited operation is insufficient. During surgery, it is important to avoid rupture of the tumour capsule as spilling of tumour cells may give rise to recurrent disease.

Recurrent disease usually manifests itself through recurrent hypercalcaemia and develops in 30%–65% of the surgically treated patients. In most instances, recurrence will appear locally, but regional lymph node metastases occur in about 30% of the patients. Distant metastases, mainly to lungs, liver or skeleton, usually appear later in the disease. Patients with recurrent parathyroid carcinoma usually succumb to the effects of hypercalcaemia. Accordingly, treatment of recurrent disease must be primarily directed towards this condition. The best result is achieved by aggressive surgical excision of all recurrent, locoregional tumour and distant metastases, whereby the source of the parathyroid hormone can be removed or at least reduced. Although patients with recurrent parathyroid carcinoma will only rarely be cured, significant palliation can be achieved by this approach even if it has to be repeated.

When surgical treatment is impossible or without effect, the hypercalcaemia has to be controlled by other means, such as forced diuresis and administration of calcitonin, mithramycin, diphosphonates or inorganic phosphate (Mundy et al. 1983). Calcitonin should be the first choice as it has few toxic side effects. However, the calcium-reducing effect of calcitonin may sometimes be difficult to sustain for longer periods of time. Mithramycin is a cytotoxic antibiotic which inhibits RNA synthesis and inactivates osteoclasts despite the presence of parathyroid hormone. Apparently, mithramycin has no anti-tumour effect on parathyroid carcinoma but has proved to be very effective in the treatment of hypercalcaemia. The drug must be given intravenously and has several toxic side effects. Most commonly encountered are bone marrow depression, severe hypokalaemia and renal, hepatic, neurological and gastrointestinal toxicity. To minimise the toxicity, it is advisable to do a step-wise titration of a minimal effective dose. By this approach, the hypercalcaemia may be kept under control with mithramycin for long periods of time (Trigonis et al. 1984). Diphosphonates are hydrolysis-resistant analogues of pyrophosphate and inhibit bone resorption. Their value in the treatment of hypercalcaemia as a result of parathyroid carcinoma has so far not been defined but may prove to be significant (Shane et al. 1982). Intravenous administration of inorganic phosphate should be used with great care only in life-threatening situations when other treatment modalities have failed.

The experience with other chemotherapy regimens is limited. Nitrogen mustard, tried in two patients was without effect, while dacarbazine treatment, tried in one patient, induced a partial response (Cope et al. 1953; Pollack et al. 1961; Calandra et al. 1984). With a combination of fluorouracil, cyclophosphamide and dacarbazine, complete disappearance of pulmonary metastases and regression of hypercalcaemia for 5 months was achieved in one patient, and in another parietal disappearance of metastases was seen after administration of methotrexate, adriamycin, cyclophosphamide and 1-(-2-chloroethyl)-3-cyclohexyl-1-nitrosourea (CCNU) (Bukowski et al. 1984; Chahinian et al. 1981). Also, hormonal manipulation has been tried. Hypophysectomy was without effect in one patient while treatment of a male with a synthetic oestrogenic compound resulted in partial response and subjective improvement (Goepfert 1966).

Radiotherapy has been tried in a few patients with recurrent disease, but without significant effect (Holmes et al. 1969; Aldinger et al. 1982; Shane and Bilezikian 1982). It is currently being evaluated as a surgical adjuvant treatment (Lillemoe and Dudley 1985).

Prognosis

The 5- and 10-year survival rates of patients with parathyroid carcinoma are less than 50% and 35%, respectively. More gratifying results may be reached if surgeons keep the possibility of parathyroid carcinoma and its clinical appearance in mind. These rare tumours can then be detected and adequately resected at the primary operation.

References

Aldinger LA, Hickey RC, Ibanez ML (1982) Parathyroid carcinoma: a clinical study of seven cases of functioning and two cases of non-functioning parathyroid cancer. Cancer 49: 388–397

Ashcraft MW, van Herle AJ (1981) Management of thyroid nodules. II. Scanning techniques, thyroid suppressive therapy and fine-needle aspiration. Head Neck Surg 3: 297–322

Attie JN, Moskowitz GW, Margoeleff D, Levy LM (1979) Feasibility of total thyroidectomy in the treatment of thyroid carcinoma. Am J Surg 138: 555–560

Auer G, Bäckdahl M, Forsslund G, Askensten U (1985) Ploidy level in non-neoplastic thyroid cells. Ann Quant Cyt 7: 97–106

Bäckdahl M, Tallroth E, Auer G, Forsslund G, Granberg PO, Lundell G, Löwhagen T (1985) Prognostic value of nuclear DNA content in medullary thyroid carcinoma. World J Surg 9: 980–987

Bäckdahl M, Auer G, Forsslund G, Granberg P-O, Hamberger B, Lundell G, Löwhagen T, Zetterberg A (1986a) Prognostic value of nuclear DNA content in follicular thyroid tumours. Acta Chir Scand 152: 1–7

Bäckdahl M, Carstensen J, Auer G, Tallroth E (1986b) Statistical evaluation of the prognostic value of nuclear DNA content in papillary, follicular and medullary thyroid tumours. World J Surg 10: 974–980

Bayer MF, McDougall IR (1984) Differences in radioimmunoassay results for thyroglobulin that affect management of patients with thyroid cancer. Clin Chem 30 (1): 81–86

Beaugie JM, Brown CL, Doniach I, Richardson JE (1976) Primary malignant tumours of the thyroid: the relationship between histological classification and clinical behaviour. Br J Surg 63: 173–181

Beierwaltes WH, Rabbani R, Dmuchowski C, Lloyd RV, Malette S (1984) An analysis of "ablation of thyroid remnants" with I-131 in 511 patients from 1947–1984: experience at the University of Michigan. J Nucl Med 25: 1287–1293

Bichel P, Thomsen OF, Askjaer SAA, Nielsen HE (1980) Light and electronmicroscopic investigation of parathyroid carcinoma during dedifferentiation. Virshows Arch [A] 386: 363–370

Black BM, Kirk TA Jr, Woolner LB (1960) Multicentricity of papillary adenocarcinoma of thyroid: influence on treatment. J Clin Endocrinol 20: 130–135

Block MA (1977) Management of carcinoma of the thyroid. Ann Surg 185: 133–144

Boey J, Hsu C, Collins RJ, Wong J (1984) A prospective controlled study of fine-needle aspiration and Tru-cut needle biopsy of dominant thyroid nodules. World J Surg 8: 458–465

Bondesson L, Ljungberg O (1981) Occult thyroid carcinoma at autopsy in Malmö, Sweden. Cancer 47: 319–323

Bukowski RM, Sheeler L, Cunningham J, Esselstyn C (1984) Successful combination chemotherapy for metastatic parathyroid carcinoma. Arch Intern Med 144: 399–400

Byar DP, Green SB, Dor P, Williams ED, Colon J, v Gilse HA, Mayer M, Sylvester RJ, van Glabbeke M (1979) A prognostic index for thyroid carcinoma. A study of the EORTC thyroid cancer cooperative group. Eur J Cancer 15 (8): 1033–1041

Cady B (1981) Surgery of thyroid cancer. World J Surg 5: 3–14

Cady B, Sedgwick CE, Meissner WA, Bookwalter JR, Romagosa V, Werber J (1976) Changing clinical, pathologic, therapeutic and survival patterns in differentiated thyroid carcinoma. Ann Surg 184: 541–553

Cady B, Sedgwick C, Meisner W, Wool M, Salzman F, Werber J (1979) Risk factor analysis in differentiated thyroid cancer. Cancer 43: 810–820

Calandra DB, Chejfec G, Foy BK, Lawrence AM, Paloyan E (1984) Parathyroid carcinoma: biochemical and pathologic response to DTIC. Surgery 96: 1132–1137

Cance WG, Wells SA (1985) Multiple endocrine neoplasia type II A. Curr Probl Surg 22 No. 5

Carcangiu ML, Steeper T, Zampi G, Rosai J (1985a) Anaplastic thyroid carcinoma. A study of 70 cases. Ann J Clin Pathol 83: 135–138

Carcangiu ML, Zampi G, Pupi A, Castagnoli A, Rosai J (1985b) Papillary carcinoma of the thyroid: a clinicopathologic study of 241 cases treated at the University of Florence, Italy. Cancer 55: 805–828

Castleman B, Roth SI (1978) Tumours of the parathyroid glands. Atlas of tumour pathology. Armed Forces Institute of Pathology, Washington DC, pp 74–82

Chahinian AP, Holland J, Nieburgs HE (1981) Metastatic nonfunctioning parathyroid carcinoma: ultrastructural evidence of secretory granules and response to chemotherapy. Am J Med Sci 282: 80–84

Christensen SB, Ljungberg O, Tibblin S (1984) Thyroid carcinoma in Malmö, 1960–1977: epidemiologic, clinical and prognostic findings in a defined urban population. Cancer 53: 1625–1633

Cifuentes N, Pickren JW (1979) Metastases from carcinoma of mammary gland: an autopsy study, J Surg Oncol 11: 193–205
Clark O (1985) Medullary thyroid carcinoma. In: Clark O (ed) Endocrine surgery of the thyroid and parathyroid glands. Mosby, St. Louis, pp 91–103
Clark RL, White EC, Russel WO (1959) Total thyroidectomy for cancer of the thyroid: significance of intraglandular dissemination. Ann Surg 149: 858–866
Clark RL, Ibanez ML, White EL (1966) What constitutes an adequate operation for carcinoma of the thyroid? Arch Surg 92: 23–26
Cohn K, Bäckdahl M, Forsslund G et al. (1984) Prognostic value of nuclear DNA content in papillary thyroid carcinoma. World J Surg 8 (4): 474–480
Cope O, Nordi GL, Castleman B (1953) Carcinoma of the parathyroid gland. Four cases among 148 patients with hyperparathyroidism. Ann Surg 138: 661–671
Cutler SJ, Young JL (1975) Third national cancer survey incidence data. NCI Monogr 41: 775
Diunen JS, Greenwood RH, Jones JH, Wallser DA, Williams ED (1977) Parathyroid carcinoma in familial hyperparathyroidism. J Clin Pathol 30: 966–975
Edmonds CJ, Smith T (1986) The long-term hazards of the treatment of thyroid cancer with radioiodine. Br J Radiol 59: 45–51
Eriksson U-B, Tegler L, Lennquist S, Borup Christensen S, Stål E, Thorell JI (1984) Serum thyroglobulin in differentiated thyroid carcinoma. Acta Chir Scand 150: 367–375
Falk U, Schmidt-Gayk H, Hüfner M (1984) Radioimmunoassay for serum thyroglobulin designed for early detection of metastasis and recurrences in the follow-up of patients with differentiated thyroid carcinoma. J Clin Chem Clin Biochem 22: 661–670
Figg DM, Bratt HJ, van Vliet PD, Dean RE (1978) Thyroid cancer: diagnosis and management based on a review of 142 cases. Am J Surg 135: 671–674
Flye MW, Brennan MF (1981) Surgical resection of metastatic parathyroid carcinoma. Ann Surg 193: 425–435
Franssila KO (1975) Prognosis in thyroid carcinoma. Cancer 36: 1138–1146
Franssila KO, Saxén E, Teppo L, Bjarnason O, Tulinius H, Norrman T, Ringertz N (1981) Incidence of different morphological types of thyroid cancer in the Nordic countries. Acta Pathol Microbiol Scand [A] 89: 49–55
Frauenhoffer CM, Patchefsky AS, Cobanoglu A (1979) Thyroid carcinoma: a clinical and pathologic study of 125 cases. Cancer 43: 2414–2421
Freitas JE, Gross MD, Ripley S, Shapiro B (1985) Radionuclide diagnosis and therapy of thyroid cancer: current status report. Semin Nucl Med 15 (2): 106–131
Fukunaga FH, Yamati R (1975) Geographic pathology of occult thyroid carcinomas. Cancer 36: 1095–1099
Georgii A (1977) Die epithelialen Tumoren der Schilddrüse. Verh Dtsch Ges Pathol 61: 191–208
Golden A, Canary JJ, Kerwin DM (1965) Concurrence of hyperplasia and neoplasia of parathyroid glands. Am J Med 38: 562–578
Goepfert H, Smart CR, Rochlin DB (1966) Metastatic parathyroid carcinoma and hormonal chemotherapy. Case report and response to hexestrol. Ann Surg 164: 917–920
Granberg P-O, Cedermark B, Farnebo L-O, Hamberger B, Werner S (1985) Parathyroid tumors. In: Hickey RC (ed) Current problems in cancer, vol 9 (11). Year Book Medical Publishers, Chicago
Granberg P-O, Hamberger B, Lundell G, Löwhagen T, Willems J-S (1983) Preoperative evaluation of the solitary thyroid nodule. In: Kaplan E (ed) Surgery of the thyroid and parathyroid glands. Churchill Livingstone, Edinburgh, pp 3–17
Granberg P-O, Sandelin K, Bäckdahl M, Cedermark B, Grimelius L, Wallin G, Willems JS (1987) Determination of nuclear DNA content in parathyroid carcinoma (abstr). Presented at the 32nd Congress Soc Int Chir, Sydney 1987
Halnan KE (1966) Influence of age and sex on incidence and prognosis of thyroid cancer. Three hundred and fourty-four cases followed for ten years. Cancer 19: 1534–1536
Hamberger B, Gharib H, Melton LJ III (1982) Fine-needle aspiration biopsy of thyroid nodules: impact on thyroid practice and cost of care. Am J Med 73 (3): 381–384
Harness JK, Thompson NW, Nishijama RH (1971) Childhood thyroid carcinoma. Arch Surg 102: 278–284
Harach HR, Franssila KO, Wasenius VM (1985) Occult papillary carcinoma of the thyroid. Cancer 56: 531–538
Hedinger C, Sobin LH (1974) Histological typing of thyroid tumours. International histological classification of tumours, no 11. World Health Organization, Geneva
Heitz P, Moser H, Staub JJ (1976) Thyroid cancer: a study of 573 thyroid tumors and 161 autopsy cases observed over a thirty-year period. Cancer 37: 2329–2337
Hirabayashi RN, Lindsay S (1961) Carcinoma of the thyroid gland: a statistical study of 390 patients. J Clin Endocrinol Metab 21: 1596–1610
Holck S, Tinggaard-Pedersen N (1981) Carcinoma of the parathyroid gland. A light and electronmicroscopic study. Acta Pathol Microbiol Scand [A] 89: 297–302
Holm LE (1982) Carcinogenic and genetic risks of ionizing radiation with special reference to radioiodine. In: Becker C (ed) Thyroid diseases. pp 159:186
Holmes EC, Morton DL, Ketcham AS (1969) Parathyroid carcinoma. A collective review. Ann Surg 169: 631–640
Horn RC Jr (1951) Carcinoma of the thyroid: description of a distinctive morphological variant and report of seven cases. Cancer 4: 697–707
Hubert JP, Kiernan PD, Beahrs OH, McConahey WM, Woolner LB (1980) Occult papillary carcinoma of the thyroid. Arch Surg 115: 394–398
Hylander B, Ekelund L-G, Rosenquist U (1983) The cardiovascular response at rest and during exercise in hypothyroid subjects to thyroxine substitution. Clin Cardiol 6: 116–124
Ito J, Noguchi S, Murakami N, Noguchi A (1980) Factors affecting the prognosis of patients with carcinoma of the thyroid. Surg Gynecol Obstet 150 (4): 539–544
Jereb B, Stjernswärd J, Löwhagen T (1975) Anaplastic giant-cell carcinoma of the thyroid. A study of treatment and prognosis. Cancer 35: 1293–1295
Katz AD, Warren JZ (1976) The malignant "cold" nodule of the thyroid. Am J Surg 132: 459–462
Lance WG, Wells SA (1985) Multiple endocrine neoplasia type IIa. Curr Probl Surg 22 No. 5
Lang V, Georgii A, Staich G, Klenze E (1980) The differentiation of atypical adenomas and encapsulated follicular carcinomas in the thyroid gland. Virchows Arch [A] 385: 125–141
Lillemoe KD, Dudley NE (1985) Parathyroid carcinoma: pointers to successful management. Ann R Coll Surg Engl 67: 222–224
Lloyd RV, Sisson JC, Marangos PJ (1983) Calcitonin, carcinoembryonic antigen and neuron-specific enolase in medullary thyroid carcinoma: an immunohistochemical study. Cancer 51 (12): 2234–2239
Löhrs U, Permanetter W, Spelsberg F, Beitinger M (1980) Das

Schilddrüsencarcinom im bayerischen Strumaendemiegebiet. Klin Wochenschr 58: 415–424

Löwhagen T, Granberg P-O, Lundell G, Skinnari P, Sundblad R, Willems J-S (1979) Aspiration biopsy cytology (ABC) in nodules of the thyroid gland suspected to be malignant. Surg Clin North Am 59: 3–18

Löwhagen T, Willems J-S (1981) Aspiration biopsy cytology in diseases of the thyroid. In: Cos LG, Colman D (eds) Advances in clinical cytology. Butterworth, London, pp 201–231

Malette LE, Bilezikian JP, Ketcham AS, Aurbach GD (1974) Parathyroid carcinoma in familial hyperparathyroidism. Am J Med 57: 642–648

Maruchi N, Furihola R, Makivali M (1971) Population surveys on the prevalence of thyroid cancer in a non-endemic region, Negano, Japan. Int J Cancer 7: 575–583

Mazzaferri EL (1978) Thyroid cancer: an overview. Thyroid Today 1 (10): 1–6

Mazzaferri EL (1981) Papillary and follicular thyroid cancer: a selective approach to diagnosis and treatment. Annu Rev Med 32: 73–91

Mazzaferri EL, Oertel JE (1983) The pathology and prognosis of thyroid cancer. In: Kaplan E (ed) Surgery of the thyroid and parathyroid gland. Churchill Livingstone, Edinburgh

Mazzaferri EL, Young RL, Oertel JE, Kemmerer WT, Page CP (1977) Papillary thyroid carcinoma: the impact of therapy in 576 patients. Medicine (Baltimore) 56: 171–196

McKenzie AD (1971) The natural history of thyroid cancer. A report of 102 cases analyzed 10 to 15 years after diagnosis. Arch Surg 102: 274–277

Meybier H, Herfarth CH, Wahl RA, Abel U, Tschahanghane C (1983) Retrospektive klinische Studien als Basis für die Therapiewahl beim differenzierten Schilddrüsencarcinom. Chirurg 54: 203–210

Miettunen M, Franssila K, Leito VP, Paasivu R, Virtanen J (1984) Expression of intermediate filament proteins in thyroid gland and thyroid tumours. Lab Invest 50: 262–270

Mundy GR, Wilkinson R, Heath DA (1983) Comparative study of available medical therapy for hypercalcaemia of malignancy. Am J Med 74: 421–423

Nel CJC, van Heerden JA, Goellner JR, Gharib H, McConahey WM, Taylor WF, Grant CS (1985) Anaplastic carcinoma of the thyroid: a clinicopathologic study of 82 cases. Mayo Clin Proc 60: 51–58

Nêmec JV, Zamrazil V, Pohunkova D, Röhling S (1979) Radioiodine treatment of pulmonary metastases of differentiated thyroid cancer: results and prognostic factors. Nuclearmedizin 18: 86–90

Neracher H, Hedinger C (1975) Klassifizierung der Schilddrüsenmalignome nach der Nomenklatur der WHO 1974. Histologische Nachkontrolle von 327 bösartigen Schilddrüsentumoren. Schweiz Med Wochenschr 105 (32): 1000–1006

Nielsen B, Zetterlund B (1985) Malignant thyroid tumours at autopsy in a Swedish goitrous population. Cancer 55: 1041–1043

Ozaki O, Notsu T, Hirai K, Mori T (1983) Differentiated carcinoma of the thyroid gland. World J Surg 7 (2): 181–185

Pollack S, Golding RR, Cohen M (1961) Parathyroid carcinoma. Arch Intern Med 108: 139–143

Psarras A, Papadopoulos SN, Livadas D et al. (1972) The single thyroid nodule. Br J Surg 59: 545–548

Ranke E, Trieloft M, Wulsch E (1973) Intrathyreoidale Ausbreitung maligner Schilddrüsentumoren. Münch Med Wochenschr 115: 2016–2020

Rivadeneyra J, Lira-Puerto V, Aguilar-Parada E (1972) Metastases a glandulas endocrinas (revision de 1900 autopsias). Ginecol Obstet Mex 31: 139–150

Russell CF, van Heerden JA, Sizemore GW, Edis AJ, Taylor WF, ReMine WH, Carney JA (1983) The surgical management of medullary thyroid carcinoma. Ann Surg 197 (1): 42–48

Saad MF, Guido JJ, Samaan NA (1983) Radioactive iodine in the treatment of medullary carcinoma of the thyroid. J Clin Endocrinol Metab 57 (1): 124–128

Schantz A, Castleman B (1972) Parathyroid carcinoma. A study of 70 cases. Cancer 31: 600–605

Scisson JC (1983) Teaching editorial: applying the radioactive eraser: I-131 to ablate normal thyroid tissue in patients in whom thyroid cancer has been resected. J Nucl Med 24: 8, 743–745

Shane E, Bilezikian JP (1982) Parathyroid carcinoma: a review of 62 patients. Endocr Rev 3: 218–226

Shane E, Jacobs TP, Siris ES, Steinberg SF, Stoddart K, Canfield RE, Bilezikian JP (1982) Therapy of hypercalcemia due to parathyroid carcinoma with intravenous dichloromethylene diphosphonate. Am J Med 72: 939–944

Shimaoka K, Shoenfeld A, DeWys WD, Creech RH, DeConti R (1985) A randomized trial of doxorubicin versus doxorubicin plus cisplatin in patients with advanced thyroid carcinoma. Cancer 56: 2155–2169

Sipple JH (1961) The association of pheochromocytoma with carcinoma of the thyroid gland. Am J Med 31: 163–166

Sizemore GW, Heath III H, Carney JA (1980) Multiple endocrine neoplasia type 2. Clin Endocrinol Metab 9: 299–315

Sizemore GW, van Heerden JA, Carney JA (1983) Medullary carcinoma of the thyroid gland and the multiple endocrine neoplasia type 2 syndrome. In: Kaplan E (ed) Surgery of the thyroid and parathyroid gland, vol 6. Churchill Livingstone, Edinburgh, pp 75–102

Snover DC, Foucar K (1981) Mitotic activity in benign parathyroid disease. Am J Clin Pathol 75: 345–347

Snyder J, Gorman C, Scanlon P (1983) Thyroid remnant ablation: questionable pursuit of an ill-defined goal. J Nucl Med 24: 659–665

Söreide O, Varhaug JE, Heimann P (1979) Thyroid carcinoma: diagnosis and treatment in 106 patients. Acta Chir Scand 145: 137–141

Staunton MD, Greening WP (1976) Treatment of thyroid cancer in 293 patients. Br J Surg 63: 253–258

Straunton MD, Skeet RG (1979) Thyroid cancer: prognosis in 469 patients. Br J Surg 66: 643

Stratton-Hill J Jr (1983) Chemotherapy of thyroid cancer. In: Kaplan E (ed) Surgery of the thyroid and parathyroid glands, vol 6. Churchill Livingstone, Edinburgh, pp 120–126

Tallroth E, Wallin G, Lundell G, Löwhagen J, Einhorn J (1987) Multimodality treatment in anaplastic giant cell thyroid carcinoma. Cancer 60: 1428–1431

Taylor S, Al-Wattar K (1980) Surgical management. Cancer Res 73: 102–111

Telenius-Berg M, Berg B, Hamberger B, Tibblin S, Tisell L-E, Ysander L, Welander G (1984) Impact of screening on prognosis in multiple endocrine neoplasia type 2 syndromes: natural history and treatment results in 105 patients. Henry Ford Hosp Med J 32 (4): 225–231

Thompson NW, Harness JK, Nishiyama RH (1978) Thyroid carcinoma: current controversies. Curr Probl Surg 15: 1–67

Tisell L, Hansson G, Jansson S, Salander H (1986) Reoperation in the treatment of asymptomatic metastating medullary thyroid carcinoma. Surgery 99: 60–66

Tobler A, Maurer R, Hedinger CE (1984) Undifferentiated thyroid tumours of diffuse small cell type. Virchows Arch [A] 404: 117–126

Trigonis C, Cedermark B, Willems J, Hamberger B, Granberg P-O (1984) Parathyroid carcinoma – problems in diagnosis and treatment. Clin Oncol 10: 11–19

Tubiana M, Haddad E, Schlumberger M, Hill C, Rougier P, Sarrazin D (1985) External radiotherapy in thyroid cancers. Cancer 55: 2062–2071

van Heerden JA, Weiland LH, ReMine WH, Walls JT, Purnell DC (1979) Cancer of the parathyroid glands. Arch Surg 114: 475–480

van Herle AJ, Rich P, Ljung BME, Ashcraft MW, Salomon DH, Keeler EB (1981) The thyroid nodule. Ann Intern Med 96: 221–232

van Herle AJ, Rich P, Ljung BM et al. (1982) The thyroid nodule. Ann Intern Med 96: 221–232

Wanebo HJ, Andrews W, Kaiser DL (1981) Thyroid cancer: some basic considerations. Am J Surg 142: 474–479

Wang C, Vickery AL, Maloof F (1976) Needle biopsy of the thyroid. Surg Gynecol Obstet 143: 365–368

Werner B, Alveryd A, Ajörklund A, Franzén S, Granberg P-O, Landberg T, Lundell G, Löwhagen T, Sundblad R, Tennvall J (1984) Multinodal therapy in anaplastic giant cell thyroid carcinoma. World J Surg 8: 64–70

Williams ED, Doniach I, Bjarnason O, Michie W (1977) Thyroid cancer in an iodinerich area: a histopathological study. Cancer 39: 215–222

Woolner LB (1971) Thyroid carcinoma: pathologic classification with data on prognosis. Semin Nucl Med 1: 481–502

Woolner LB, Keating FR, Black BM (1952) Tumours and hyperplasia of the parathyroid glands. Cancer 5: 1069–1088

Woolner LB, Beahrs OH, Black WM, McConahey WM, Keating FR Jr (1961) Classification and prognosis of thyroid carcinoma. A study of 885 cases observed in a thirty year period. Am J Surg 102: 354–387

Young RL, Mazzaferri EL, Rahe AJ, Dorfman SG (1980) Pure follicular thyroid carcinoma: impact of therapy in 214 patients. J Nucl Med 21: 733–737

Gastrointestinal and Adrenal Tumours

F. Stadil and H. Kehlet

Gastrointestinal Tumours

The gastrointestinal tract is the largest endocrine organ in man. It was also the first to be investigated as endocrinology was founded in 1902 with the discovery by Bayliss and Starling of secretin and its mode of action. In spite of this the gastrointestinal tract has been treated with reluctance by clinical endocrinologists. The main reasons are the complex biology of gut hormones and the few gastrointestinal diseases which are of pure endocrinological origin. In the following chapter some basic aspects of the biology of gut hormones will be summarised prior to considering the clinical oncology.

Chemical Structure of Gut Hormones

Homology. Characteristic features of most peptide hormones are their grouping in families, in which members show considerable resemblance (homology) in structure and function. This resemblance is due to the development of the gene for a single stem hormone through gene duplication and ensuing diversion of daughter genes. The families established for gut hormones are indicated in Table 1. The homology is of clinical importance. The resemblance in structure means that related hormones may bind to the same receptor in the cell membranes. Hence, hypersecretion of one particular hormone may imitate secretion of another related hormone. Related hormones may also bind to the same antibodies which may invalidate interpretation of diagnostic immunoassays.

Heterogeneity. Other features of most hormones are the occurrence in tissue and circulation of molecular forms of different size and biological activity. The explanation of molecular heterogeneity is found in the process of biosynthesis. Protein and peptide hormones are first formed as a long polypeptide chain ("pre-pro-hormone"). The biologically active forms are released through a number of enzymatic modifications: post-translational processings. The modifica-

Table 1. The families of gut peptides

The secretin family	Secretin Glucagon Vasoactive intestinal polypeptide (VIP) Peptide histamine methionine (PHM) Gastric inhibitory polypeptide (GIP)
The gastrin family	Gastrin Cholecystokinin (CCK) Cerulein
The tachykinin family	Substance P Neurokinin A Neurokinin B
The pancreatic polypeptide family	Pancreatic polypeptide (PP) Peptide tyrosine tyrosine (PYY) Neuropeptide tyrosin (NPY)
The opioidpeptide family	Proopiomelanocortin peptides Proencephalin peptides Prodynorphin peptides

tions mainly consist in cleavage, but also in substitution and addition of various side groups. Each modification has a decisive influence on the function of the hormone. Heterogeneity is even more complicated as various cells will mature the same prohormones differently. As an example, the glucagon cells in the intestine will cleave proglucagon to a lesser extent than the glucagon cells in the pancreas. The resulting enteroglucagon molecules will be bigger than pancreatic glucagon and will have a totally different spectrum of action. A comparable cell-specific maturing of prohormones has been described for most gastrointestinal hormones. The clinical implications are considerable, particularly in the diagnosis of endocrine tumours which will often process peptides incompletely. Some of these immature peptides have no or only slight biological activity, which explains the considerable number of "non-functioning" or inactive endocrine tumours. In addition, the immunoreactivity of the immature peptides often differs from the active forms which creates diagnostic difficulties.

Hormone Measurements

Bioassays. So far bioassays have been of little clinical importance as the sensitivity and specificity are insufficient. In addition, bioassays are generally very complicated, expensive and time consuming.

Radioimmunoassays. Reliable radioimmunoassays may also be difficult to establish, but when the proper reactants are produced, the measurements are simple, sensitive, precise and cheap. Most radioimmunoassays are directed against the biologically active forms of the gut hormones, and this may create difficulties in detection of the inactive prohormones of some tumours. However, in contrast to bioassays it is possible to develop radioimmunoassays against inactive prohormones and fragments. A limited number of such assays is now available in special laboratories.

Classification of Gastrointestinal Endocrine Tumours

"APUD" is an acronym used by Pearse (1968) to describe a system of presumed endocrine cells with common cytochemical properties. The name refers to the amine-handling characteristics of the cells (amine precursor uptake and decarboxylation). The term "APUD-oma" was first used by Cszij et al. (1969) to describe neoplastic lesions arising in gastrointestinal endocrine cells (APUD cell system). The tumours share a number of morphological and cytochemical appearances which can assist the pathologist in identifying the lesions. At light-microscopic levels the cells are usually argyrophilic (Grimelius 1968), or they stain with lead haematoxylin (Service et al. 1976). Some argyrophilic cells are also argentaffinic and are called "enterochromaffin". Much confusion would be avoided if the term "carcinoid tumour" were restricted to enterochromaffinomas only. This is usually done in the German tradition, but the terminology varies from one country to another.

The APUD cells can be identified by histochemical methods. They will display fluorescence on treatment with formaldehyde ozone (Pitchet et al. 1976), and in some cases the content of specific peptides may be demonstrated immunohistochemically. Improper fixation or absence of storage granules may cause this method to fail. Many tumours contain neuron-specific enolase and all display neurosecretory granules at ultramicroscopy.

The secretory products of the cells can often be identified immunohistochemically. However, many tumours are of a mixed type and, in the case of non-functioning endocrine tumours, peptide content is usually prehormones which may fail to react with antibodies directed against the circulating peptides. Although most endocrine tumours of the gastrointestinal tract contain several cell types, the practical consequences are small. From a clinical point of view, the disease usually appears to be due to hypersecretion of a single substance. For this reason it is better to classify the tumours according to their clinical and biochemical features than according to their morphology (Larsson 1978). If a specific peptide is released into the circulation, the tumour is usually named after this peptide by adding "-oma" to it, e.g. "insulinoma". If more than one hormone is present, the tumour is named after the hormone responsible for the clinical symptoms. If no hormone release can be detected, the tumour is called "non-functioning" or "inactive endocrine tumour".

Non-functioning endocrine tumours of the pancreas and gastrointestinal tract have often been diagnosed in the past, but this label merely indicates the present state of ignorance and should become less frequent as diagnostic methods improve. Some authors may classify such tumours as "carcinoids". This term should preferably be restricted to enterochromaffinomas which are usually derived from the midgut and are argentaffinic because of their serotonin content.

Gastrointestinal endocrine tumours may be benign or malignant. They are often small but may grow to huge dimensions and can give rise to many clinical syndromes. The hypersecretion syndromes are relatively rare but are now diagnosed more frequently, which suggests that their true incidence is higher than thought in the past. Enterochromaffinomas (carcinoids) will not been included in this presentation.

Insulinomas

The insulinoma was first recognized in 1927; it is the best known of the endocrine pancreatic tumours. The estimated incidence is about 0.2 per 100 000.

Pathology

Insulinomas originate from the beta cells of the pancreatic islets. They are almost always solitary (90%) and rather small (2–50 mm in diameter). They can occur in all parts of the pancreas, including the uncinate process. In a survey of 951 patients with insulinomas, metastases were found in only 5% (Stefanini et al. 1974).

Clinical Features

The tumours are found equally in both sexes, and no age is exempt although insulinomas are extremely rare in young children and most are diagnosed in middle age. The symptoms are intermittent and are due to attacks of fasting hypoglycaemia. Symptoms usually occur in the morning after an overnight fast or after strenuous exercise. The patient may fail to notice the relationship betwen symptoms and fasting, although they are often aware of relief of symptoms by eating. The hypoglycaemia can develop quickly but is usually gradual, and the development of neuroglycopenia will give rise to bizarre symptoms with strange behaviour, confusion, epileptic fits, tremor, transient paralysis, or attacks of anger and violence. Patients are sometimes suspected of being drunk or psychotic. A diagnostic delay of several years is quite common (Christiansen et al. 1978). Repeated attacks of severe hypoglycaemia may lead to cerebral reduction.

Investigation

The diagnosis can be made if symptoms are provoked by hypoglycaemia and relieved by intravenous glucose. This is a basis for the classical fasting test (Whipple's triad). During the test the patients fast for up to 72 h under careful observation in hospital. In contrast to normal persons, patients with insulinomas will develop hypoglycaemic symptoms, usually during the first 24–28 h (Seyer-Hansen and Lundbaek 1979).

Constant hyperinsulinaemia is rare although a hyperinsulinaemia relative to the glucose level is quite frequent. When the blood glucose falls, insulin secretion normally decreases until it virtually stops when the glucose concentration falls below 1.7 mmol per litre. This does not occur in patients with insulinomas, where the morning concentration of plasma insulin prior to breakfast is often inappropriately high when related to the blood glucose concentration. The amended insulin/glucose ratio $\frac{\text{plasma insulin (mU per litre)}}{\text{(plasma glucose (mmol per litre)} - 1.7)}$ is usually > 50 in patients with insulinomas and < 10 in normal subjects (Turner et al. 1971).

Measurements of plasma proinsulin may also be diagnostic, as patients with insulinoma have relatively higher concentration of the prohormone (Creutzfeldt et al. 1978). Insulin and C-peptide are stored in islet cell granules and released into the circulation on an equimolar basis. The concentration of C-peptide in plasma indicates the endogenous insulin secretion and permits differentiation between insulinoma and factitious hypoglycaemia after exogenous insulin. If self-induced hypoglycaemia is suspected, analysis of the urine for sulphonyluria may also be required.

Localization of the Tumour

Ultrasonography and a CT scan may identify tumours bigger than 1 cm. In expert hands, arteriography may also result in the detection of many insulinomas (Madsen 1979; Rhys-Davies 1973), but ordinarily the best information is probably obtained by percutaneous transhepatic portal vein catheterisation with blood sampling for insulin determinations in samples drawn from the various branches of the portal system. It appears that selective catheterisation of the small pancreatic veins, although recommendable, is not strictly necessary for the identification of the part of the pancreas with abnormal insulin release (Burcharth et al. 1979; Ingemansson et al. 1975).

Differential Diagnosis

In children the differential diagnosis of hypoglycaemic states are complicated due to various inborn errors of metabolism. However, insulinomas are very rare in the very young.

In adults the differential diagnosis of fasting hypoglycaemia is usually easy. Some extrapancreatic tumours, including sarcomas and hepatocellular carcinomas, may, for other reasons, cause hypoglycaemia. Most such tumours are very large and easily detected. Alcohol-induced hypoglycaemia, liver failure, hypopituitarism and Addison's disease seldom give rise to diagnostic difficulties, but self-administration of insulin is difficult to detect, though it may be revealed by C-peptide estimations.

Treatment

Hypoglycaemia can be controlled by administration of glucose. For prolonged control, diazoxide can be tried. Diazoxide will inhibit the granular release of insulin and is effective if normal storage mechanisms are maintained. The starting dose is usually 150 mg, rising up to 900 mg daily in some patients. Side effects are frequent and include water retention, oedema, dyspepsia, diarrhoea, skin reaction and bone marrow depression. Cytostatic treatment with streptozocin alone or in combination with 5-fluorouracil may result in remission in around 60% of patients (Broder and Carter 1973) and is usually given intravenously in doses of 1–4 g every 6 weeks. Side effects include serious renal damage, which may be seen even after a first dose of only 1 g streptozocin.

The treatment of choice is surgical removal of the tumour which should be undertaken whenever possible. The tumour can be removed by enucleation or by pancreatic resection. If the tumour has not been located preoperatively, explorative operation with mobilisation of the entire pancreas may be tried. If the tumour cannot be found during surgery, blind resection is not advised, but further attempts at localisation 6–12 months later is recommended.

The operative mortality in insulinomas is low, and cure is usually achieved. In the case of multiple or malignant tumours, pancreatoduodenectomy may be required.

Without surgery insulinomas will prove fatal due to hypoglycaemia. The course is usually protracted, the patients having attacks for many years.

Glucagonomas

Symptoms from a glucagonoma were first reported by McGavran et al. in 1966. The full description of the clinical presentation came with the publication of nine cases by Mallinson et al. in 1974.

Pathology

Glucagonomas originate in the A cell of the pancreatic islets and is probably the rarest of the islet cell tumours. Most glucagonomas are malignant and metastatic when they present clinically (Mallinson et al. 1974). Immunohistochemically the cells react with most types of glucagon, but the tumours appear mainly to secrete pancreatic glucagon.

Clinical Features

The cardinal symptoms are wasting, mild diabetes and a chronic severe skin eruption called "necrotising migratory erythema". It consists of an epidermal bulbous lesion, which tends to heal in the centre and spread peripherally. The erythema moves from one area to another. It can be found anywhere but seems to prefer the lower abdomen, arms, legs and feet. The pathogenesis is unknown. Additional clinical symptoms include anaemia, mild diarrhoea, glossitis and cheilitis. The patients usually suffer from severe fatigue.

Investigation

The diagnosis can be made by the finding of an increase in plasma glucagon. The plasma insulin may also be increased. Slight hyperglycaemia and hypoaminoacidaemia are usually present. Glucagonomas can be localized as described for insulinomas.

Treatment

The skin lesion may respond to intravenous hyperalimentations. Long-acting somatostatin analogues may depress the tumour secretion, but probably have little therapeutical value. Unresectable tumours can be treated with streptozocin alone or in combination with 5-fluorouracil (Chandeker et al. 1979). Favourable responses to dacarbazine have also been reported (Valverde et al. 1976). Furthermore, preliminary reports of the use of interferon in the treatment of gastrointestinal endocrine tumours suggest that this drug could be tried in poor responders (Öberg et al. 1983).

Treatment of choice is surgical removal of the tumour with as much of the local and metastatic deposits as possible. Removal of tumour will normalise the blood sugar values and restore the skin condition rapidly. In non-resectable or metastatic tumours transcutaneous or intraoperative implantation of radioactive seeds can also be used for debulking (Holm et al. 1981).

Most tumours grow slowly, and patients with unresectable lesions can survive for several years.

VIP-omas

In 1958 Verner and Morrison described a clinical syndrome with severe diarrhoea, hypokalaemia and an islet cell tumour. The syndrome is caused by hyperproduction of vasoactive intestinal polypeptide (VIP). Some authors have speculated that other peptides may also cause similar syndromes.

Pathology

Most VIP-omas are found in the pancreas, but some neurogenic tumours can also produce VIP, i.e. phaeochromocytomas, neuroblastomas, ganglioneuroblastomas, neurofibromas, ganglioneurinomas. VIP-secreting neurinomas are most frequently found in the retroperitoneum and in the thorax. They are most often found in children. The pancreatic tumours are usually seen in the middle aged or the elderly. The VIP-omas are usually malignant and over half of the tumours have metastasised at the time of the diagnosis (Verner and Morrison 1974).

Clinical Features

The VIP-oma syndrome has also been called "pancreatic cholera" or "WDHA syndrome" (watery diarrhoea, hypokalaemia and achlorhydria). Both names are inappropriate as only half of the patients have achlorhydria, and the tumours are not always found in the pancreas. The incidence is about 0.1 per 100 000.

The main symptoms are watery diarrhoea, often intermittent and present for 1 or 2 years prior to the diagnosis. In active episodes, more than 10 litres of fluid stools may be passed per day, and the stools will resemble tea or urine. The potassium and bicarbonate content is high, and potassium loss may exceed 200 mmol per day. The resulting severe hypokalaemia is associated with metabolic acidosis due to loss of bicarbonate. Many patients have low secretion of gastric hydrochloric acid, and some have decreased glucose tolerance. Mild flushing is noted in many of the patients.

In patients with neurogenic tumours, the clinical findings are more varied and may be dominated by excess production of catecholamines or other substances.

Investigations

The diagnosis can be made by the finding of increased plasma VIP. When plasma concentrations are two to three times above normal, patients seem to develop the active phase of the disease with diarrhoea (Fahrenkrug 1980). The tumours may be localised as indicated for insulinomas. If the abdominal examinations are negative, X-rays of the chest or even bronchoscopy should be undertaken.

Differential Diagnosis

The main finding is diarrhoea which continues during fasting. Bacterial and parasitic causes can be excluded by culture and microscopy of stool. Crohn's disease and ulcerative colitis can be excluded by endoscopy and radiology. Biliary, gastro- and urocolonic fistulae, malabsorption of bile salts, villous intestinal adenomas, drug intake and laxative abuse must also be considered. A few endocrinopathies like Addison's disease, hyperthyroidism and hypoparathyroidism may also be associated with diarrhoea, as may other endocrine tumours such as gastrinomas, enterochromaffinomas (carcinoids) and medullary thyroid carcinomas.

Treatment

Fluid replacement can be difficult during severe attacks of diarrhoea, and the patients should be observed in a department for intensive care. Suppression of the diarrhoea has occasionally been observed after steroids, lithium, trifluoperazine and somatostatin, but most patients probably respond within a few days to 1–2 g streptozocin daily. Renal function should be followed carefully during such treatment. Prolonged remissions after streptozocin have been observed. The treatment is usually repeated at 6–12-week intervals with dosage from 1–4 g.

Cure by surgical excision is possible in only about one-third of the patients because of metastatic disease (Verner and Morrison 1974). Symptoms may also be controlled by debulking surgery, and as much tumour as possible should be removed. Alternatively, embolisation of the hepatic metastases of interstitial irradiation with percutaneous implantation of radioactive seeds guided by ultrasound can be tried (Holm et al. 1981).

Early diagnosis is essential for cure, but aggressive treatment of unresectable lesions will usually control the diarrhoea for long periods. The tumours grow slowly, and if hypersecretion is controlled, the patients may live many years with few symptoms.

Gastrinomas

The gastrinoma syndrome was described by Zollinger and Ellison in 1955. Gastrinomas are the most common type of islet cell tumour and occur with an incidence of 0.3 per 100 000. The condition is still underdiagnosed.

Pathology

Gastrinomas probably arise from the D_1 cells of the pancreatic islets (Larsson 1978) but might quite frequently be found in the duodenal mucosa and, rarely, in the antrum. The tumours are often small. Solitary gastrinomas are seen in fewer than one-third of the patients (Ellison and Wilson 1964). This may be an underestimation as metastases can be small and easily overlooked (Zollinger et al. 1976, 1984). Even small tumours of less than 2–3 mm can be associated with a full clinical syndrome.

Normally gastrin cells are not present in the adult pancreas, and circulating gastrin originates mainly from the antrum and duodenum.

Clinical Features

Gastrinomas occur at all ages and equally in both sexes. Approximately one-tenth of the patients are children (Ellison and Wilson 1964). The clinical picture varies. Mild forms of the disease are the most frequent (Deveney et al. 1978; Stage and Stadil 1979).

The main symptom is continuous or episodic dyspeptic abdominal pains, which is seen in approximately three-quarters of the patients. Two-thirds of the patients have diarrhoea, and in one-tenth of the patients this is the only complaint (Stage and Stadil 1979). A few patients may present with peptic oesophagitis. Except in advanced malignancy, all symptoms are due to the hypersecretion of gastric acid.

The diagnosis is frequently missed, and patients may be subjected to one or more ulcer operations. Most such patients will do quite well for one or several years after each operation, but eventually the ulcers will recur. In a minority, the disease presents differently with dramatic perforation, haemorrhage, oesophageal stricture, jejunal ulceration, or anastomotic breakdown, but in the majority the clinical presentation cannot be distinguished from ordinary ulcer disease.

Diagnosis

The main diagnostic features are hypergastrinaemia and hypersecretion of gastric acid.

Hypergastrinaemia in the fasting state is always present, but occasionally values at the upper normal limit may be found. The circulating gastrins are the same as in normal subjects, but in some patients a single component or prohormone may dominate. This stresses the importance of careful selection of diagnostic antisera.

Screening of all ulcer patients for circulating gastrins is simple and cheap and would lead to earlier diagnosis. When gastrin levels are elevated, gastric secretion of acid should be studied to rule out hypochlorhydria and achlorhydria as the underlying cause for the hypergastrinaemia. Gastrinoma patients will have hypersecretion of acid, but unfortunately no absolute criteria for the diagnosis can be based on the acid determination because of marked variations from patient to patient and from day to day (Stage and Stadil 1979; Aoyagi and Summerskill 1966). However, a spontaneous acid secretion of over 20 mmol H^+/h is highly suggestive of a gastrinoma.

When serum gastrin concentrations measured in the fasting state are borderline, various provocative tests, such as feeding, secretin, calcium and glucagon, may be used (Stage and Stadil 1979; Stage et al. 1978; Mignon et al. 1986; Poynard et al. 1986). The diagnostic value of these tests is, however, still open to argument. Alternatively, the patients are followed at regular intervals with measurements of serum gastrin after an overnight fast.

Ulcers are found in the duodenum, jejunum and stomach. Most patients will have a single duodenal ulcer in the bulb, but multiple or ectopic ulcers or erosions in the duodenum or the jejunum are very suggestive of the diagnosis and can quite often be seen at duodenoscopy.

Localisation

Tumours may be localised as indicated previously (see Insulinomas). By percutaneous transhepatic portography with venous blood sampling, the gastrin-producing parts of the pancreas can be located, and the presence of any normal part of the pancreas can be evaluated. Due to the frequent finding of multiple tumours, both kinds of information are essential for the planning of the surgical treatment. In gastrinomas, selective catheterisations of as many pancreatic veins as possible are essential.

Differential Diagnosis

Fasting hypergastrinaemia is seen in patients with pernicious anaemia and atrophic gastritis due to loss of the acid brake of antral gastrin release. These conditions are diagnosed by acid secretory studies. Hyperplasia of the G cells in the antrum is a very rare condition which may lead to hypergastrinaemia in the fasting state. These patients will have marked gastrin responses at feeding. Vagotomy operations will result in moderate hypergastrinaemia for unknown reasons, as will sustained and efficient suppression of gastric acid secretion by treatment with high doses of antacids, anticholinergics, histamine H_2 receptor antagonists and substituted benzimidazoles (Omeprazole).

The clinical differentiation from ordinary ulcer disease is impossible and can only be performed by gastrin measurements. In recurrence of ulcers or in the presence of ectopic ulcers in the jejunum or duodenum, gastrin studies should always be undertaken.

All patients should be examined for associated endocrinopathies. Familiar disease with multiple endocrine adenomatosis occurs in 20%–30% of the patients.

Treatment

Complete control of symptoms usually follows the complete suppression of acid secretion. This used to be achieved by total gastrectomy, but subsequently surgery was replaced by continuous treatment with histamine H_2 receptor antagonists (McCarty 1978). When histamine H_2 receptor antagonists are insufficient, substituted benzimidazoles (Omeprazole) can be employed. These drugs inhibit the potassium-dependent ATP-ase within the parietal cell (Bardram and Stadil 1986), and a single daily dose of 30–60 mg usually abolishes the acid secretion for 12–24 h, also in patients with Zollinger-Ellison syndrome. It may be an advantage to divide the dose into a morning and an evening dose. The long-term actions and unwanted effects of Omeprazole are still being assessed, but at present no direct side effects have been noted in humans. It is interesting that after sustained and efficient suppression of gastric acid, hyperplasia of gastric endocrine cells in the gastric body and fundus can be noted. In female rats treated continuously with Omeprazole for 2 years, formation of enterochromaffin-like (ECL) cell tumours was observed. This is a consequence of the resulting severe hypergastrinaemia and is not directly related to the drug. The phenomenon may be of little importance in humans but suggests that all patients with severe and constant hypergastrinaemia (gastrinoma patients, patients with pernicious anaemia, patients treated continuously with efficient inhibitors of gastric acid secretion) should have a gastric endoscopy with biopsy at annual intervals.

The treatment of choice is surgical excision of the gastrinomas before metastatic spread has occurred. If percutaneous transhepatic blood samplings locate the tumour area and demonstrate that the remaining pancreas is normal, pancreatic resection is indicated (Mignon et al. 1986; Stadil 1980). Tumours located in the pancreatic tail should probably always be resected when found as the risk of surgery is small. Blind pancreatic resection should be avoided.

With early diagnosis about one-quarter of the patients can be cured by surgery, the rest can obtain complete relief from symptoms by medical treatment and will usually live without symptoms for periods of several years. In some patients tumour progression is very slow, and they may live on symptomatic treatment for 10 or 15 years without signs of major progression. When tumour growth is progressing and symptomatic, cytostatic treatment with streptozocin alone or in combination with 5-fluorouracil may induce remissions in a substantial number of patients.

Somatostatinomas

Somatostatin was originally isolated from the hypothalamus and later from other parts of the central nervous system. It is found in the D cells of the pancreatic islets and in the mucosa of the upper gastrointestinal tract. Somatostatin inhibits the secretion of most gut hormones and the exocrine pancreatic and gastric secretion. More than 100 patients with somatostatinomas in the pancreas have been reported since the initial report in 1977 (Ganda et al. 1977; Larsson et al. 1977).

Pathology and Clinical Features

Most of the patients reported had metastatic disease at the time of diagnosis. The main clinical symptoms were mild diarrhoea, wasting, fatigue, anaemia, diabetes and malabsorption. At examination most patients had low secretion of gastric acid and gallstone disease.

The diagnosis can be made by the finding of elevated plasma concentration of somatostatin. The patients diagnosed so far had metastases at the time of diagnosis. Some had evidence of multiple endocrine neoplasia with increased concentration of calcitonin or adrenocorticotropic hormone (ACTH) in serum. Because of the uncharacteristic clinical picture, the recognition of early stages of the disease will probably depend on screening by somatostatin measurements of all patients with diabetes.

Treatment

Cure by surgical removal of the tumour may be possible when the diagnosis can be made early. Debulking surgery has relieved symptoms in a few patients. Alternatively, streptozocin treatment might be tried.

Adrenal Tumours

Adrenal carcinomas are rare tumours that may rise from any of the layers of the adrenal gland. The most important anatomically based subgrouping is adrenal cortical carcinomas and adrenal medullary carcinomas (phaeochromocytomas). The tumours may also be subgrouped according to their ability to secrete various steroids or catecholamines (functioning tumours) or inactive, non-functioning tumours.

Adrenocortical Carcinomas

Adrenocortical carcinoma is a rare tumour, with a yearly incidence of less than 0.2 per 100 000 (Richie and Gittes 1980). More than half of the tumours secrete one or more cortical steroids to produce a clinical syndrome [Cushing's syndrome, hyperaldosteronism (Conn's syndrome), virilising or feminising syndromes] classified as functioning, versus non-functioning tumours without clinically important secretion of steroids.

Functioning Tumours

The majority of functioning carcinomas occur before the age of 40 years with a female : male ratio of 4 : 1. The clinical features of the syndromes due to functioning adrenocortical carcinomas are similar to those due to benign tumours or hyperplasia, except that they usually progress rapidly with a history of less than 6 months.

Diagnosis

Diagnosis of the endocrine disorder is made in accordance with standard endocrine investigations, the only difference between patients with cancer and patients with benign disease being that adrenocortical carcinomas usually secrete large amounts of steroid precursor metabolites.

Cushing's syndrome is diagnosed on increased urinary cortisol excretion, and the tumour pathogenesis is suggested by non-suppressible urinary cortisol following high doses (2 mg/6 h) of dexamethasone and low/undetectable ACTH in plasma. Hyperaldosteronism due to a tumour is diagnosed on increased urinary aldosterone excretion, non-suppressible by fluorohydrocortisone 0.5 mg/day and low plasma renin. Virilising and feminising syndromes are diagnosed from clinical characteristics and elevated excretion of 17-ketosteroids, non-suppressible following high doses of dexamethasone.

Preoperative Localization Studies

Preoperative localisation studies should primarily include a CT scan, which may also demonstrate local invasion and distant metastases. ^{131}I cholesterol scanning is less suitable in adrenal malignancy because of an insufficient steroid metabolism per gram of the tissue as compared with normal adrenal tissue, and also because many tumours may be hormonally non-functional. Thus, the iodocholesterol scan usually shows non-visualisation of the tumour or adrenal gland on the affected side. Arteriography is only indicated to define the vascular anatomy to help in planning surgical excision. Venous catheterisation with sampling from the left adrenal vein and the right renal vein for aldosterone analysis is of help in localisation of small aldosterone-producing tumours.

Table 2. Staging of adrenocortical cancers

Stage	Size (cm)	Nodes[a]	Local invasion[a]	Metastases[a]
I	<5	–	–	–
II	>5	–	–	–
III	Any size	+	+	–
IV	Any size	+	+	+

[a] –, absent; +, present.

Staging

The staging should be performed in order to make a suitable comparison between different series and since it may aid in therapeutic and prognostic assessment. The most widely accepted system is shown in Table 2 (Sullivan et al. 1978).

Pathology

Adrenal cortical cancers are usually larger than 6 cm and with a weight exceeding 100 g (Scott et al. 1985; Neville and O'Hare 1982a). On gross appearance there are usually areas of necrosis, haemorrhage, cystic changes and calcification. The microscopic appearance may be difficult to distinguish from benign disease, but characteristically the tumour cells exhibit pleomorphism and marked nuclear vesicularity (Neville and O'Hare 1982a). Differential diagnosis between benign and malignant disease should be performed by an experienced pathologist with specific interest in the adrenal gland, but even so a postoperative follow-up may show that the initial benign tumour was in fact malignant. Aldosterone-producing carcinomas may show a more characteristic microscopic appearance with zona glomerulosa-type cells arranged in large trabeculae separated by prominent vascular sinusoids (Neville and O'Hare 1982b).

Metastases usually evolve in draining lymph nodes, bones, contralateral adrenal gland, lungs and liver.

Treatment

Fewer than 50% of adrenal carcinomas are resectable for cure at the time of diagnosis (Scott et al. 1985; Henley et al. 1983). The prognosis after surgical excision is poor since most patients with stage III and IV disease do not survive beyond 12–18 months and patients with stage I and II disease have a 5-year survival rate of 20%–40% (Scott et al. 1985; Henley et al. 1983; Didolkar et al. 1981). The success of adjuvant therapy with radiotherapy or chemotherapy has largely been disappointing (Henley et al. 1983; Percarpio and Knowlton 1976; Hajjar et al. 1975). Although the adrenolytic drug mitotane has been reported to give significant tumour regression (Hutter and Kayhoe 1966; Schteingart et al. 1982), the results are usually not impressive since survival is rarely extensively prolonged. For palliative relief of Cushing's syndrome, enzymatic blockers (aminoglutethimide, metyrapone) may be employed, as well as the antifungal agent ketoconanzole which may inhibit cortisol synthesis (Shepherd et al. 1985; Coontreras et al. 1985). Recently, a glucocorticoid antagonist (RU 486) has been reported of value in Cushing's syndrome (Nieman et al. 1985), but no information is available in malignant cortisol-secreting tumours.

Non-functioning Tumours

Due to the increased use of ultrasound and CT scanning, non-functioning adrenal nodules are being diagnosed with increased incidence. Such nodules have been reported to occur in 1%–15% of the patients in autopsy series (Neville and O'Hare 1982a). However, the risk of cancer in such an "incidentaloma" is very limited (less than 1%) (Abbecassis et al. 1985; Paes and Hunter-Craig 1985; Lewinsky et al. 1974). The indication for surgery in the incidentally diagnosed adrenal nodule has not been finally settled, but surgical excision is advocated in nodules larger than 3–6 cm due to the increased risk of malignancy with increasing volume (Geelhoed and Droy 1982; Seddon et al. 1985). In the published series, including patients with non-functioning tumours diagnosed before the widespread use of CT scans, the prognosis was poor, as fewer than 50% could be resected for cure (Paes and Hunter-Craig 1985). Adjuvant therapy for non-functioning tumours may be tried along the same lines as with functioning tumours, but the results have not been encouraging (Paes and Hunter-Craig 1985; Lewinsky et al. 1974).

Malignant Phaeochromocytoma

Malignant phaeochromocytoma is a very rare tumour with an incidence probably less than 0.1 per 100 000 (Lewi et al. 1985).

Diagnosis

The clinical presentation of a primary, recurrent or metastatic phaeochromocytoma is undistinguishable from its benign counterpart (Scott et al. 1982; ReMine et al. 1974). The biochemical diagnosis of the syndrome is similar to patients with benign phaeochromocytomas, i.e. elevated urinary excretion of metanephrine, vanillylmandelic acid (VMA) and free catecholamines. Plasma noradrenaline and adrenaline are elevated (see endocrine textbooks).

Localisation Techniques. The most valuable techniques are CT scanning and ^{131}I-metaiodobenzyl guanidine (^{131}I-MIBG) scanning (Scott et al. 1982; Thomphson et al. 1984; Chatal and Charbonnel 1985). Both techniques may be of equal value in localisation of an intradrenal tumour, while the ^{131}I-MIBG scan may be preferable in diagnosing metastatic disease (Thomphson et al. 1984; Chatal and Charbonnel 1985).

Staging

No commonly accepted system is available, but the staging system advised for adrenocortical cancers (see above) can be used.

Pathology

The microscopical distinction between a malignant and a benign phaeochromocytoma is often impossible as mitotic figures and vascular and capsular invasion may be seen in both benign and malignant neoplasms. In fact, malignancy can only be positively diagnosed when metastases have been demonstrated or local invasion is confirmed during surgery. It is important to notice that the time between initial operation for a suggested benign tumour and recurrence because of an initially unnoticed malignant condition may, in some cases, be up to 5 years (ReMine et al. 1974).

Treatment

The primary treatment is radical en bloc resection of the tumour and lymph nodes with subsequent resection of recurrences including palliative debulking of functioning metastases (Scott et al. 1982). The experience with chemotherapy is limited, but uncontrolled data suggest that cyclophosphamide and/or streptozocin may be of some value (Bukowsky and Widt 1984). Radiotherapy, otherwise ineffective, may be of some palliative value in painful osseous metastases. Recently, administration of therapeutic doses of ^{131}I-MIBG has been used in ten patients, with apparant success in five patients with objective responses including diminution of size of metastases and reduced catecholamine excretion (Thomphson et al. 1984).

Palliative symptomatic relief may be obtained by α- and β-blockade together with the synthesis inhibitor α-methyl paratyrosine.

Prognosis

Since most series are very small and because of the pronounced variability in growth, as well as the lack of a commonly accepted staging system, the available data cannot provide a uniform conclusion. However, on average the 5-year survival rate may be in the order of 30%–40% (Lewi et al. 1985; Scott et al. 1982; van Heerden et al. 1982). Information on risk and prognosis in malignant phaeochromocytoma in multiple endocrine neoplasia, types IIa and IIb is limited, but the risk may be significant since two out of four patients developed malignancy (van Heerden et al. 1984). Obviously, because of the limited experience, comparison of prognosis of malignant phaeochromocytomas with or without association with the MEN syndromes cannot be made.

References

Abbecassis N, McLoughlin MJ, Langer B, Kudlow JE (1985) Serendipitous adrenal masses: prevalence, significance, and management. Am J Surg 149: 783–788

Aoyagi I, Summerskill WHJ (1966) Gastric secretion with ulcerogenic islet cell tumour. Arch Intern Med 117: 667–672

Bardram L, Stadil F (1986) Omeprazole in the Zollinger-Ellison syndrome. Scand J Gastroenterol 21: 374–378

Bayliss WM, Starling EH (1902) The mechanism of pancreatic secretion. J Physiol (Lond) 28: 325–353

Broder LE, Carter SK (1973) Pancreatic islet cell carcinoma. Results of therapy with streptozocine in 52 patients. Ann Intern Med 79: 108–118

Bukowsky RM, Widt DG (1984) Chemotherapy trials in malignant pheochromocytoma: report of 2 patients and review of the literature. J Surg Oncol 27: 89–92

Burcharth F, Stage JG, Stadil F, Jensen LI, Fischerman K (1979) Localization of gastrinomas by transhepatic portal catheterization and gastrin assay. Gastroenterology 77: 444–450

Chandeker JD, Oyer D, Miller HJ, Vick NA (1979) Neurologic involvement in glucagonoma syndrome. Response to combination chemotherapy with 5-fluorouracil and streptozocine. Cancer 44: 2014–2016

Chatal JF, Charbonnel B (1985) Comparison of iodobenzylguanedine imaging with computed tomography in locating pheochromocytoma. J Clin Endocrinol Metab 61: 769–772

Christiansen LA, Nielsen OV, Stadil F, Stage JG (1978) Delay in the diagnosis of insulinomas. Scand J Gastroent [Suppl 53] 14: 15–18

Contreras P, Altieri E, Liberman C, Gac A, Rojas A, Ibarra A, Rawanal M, Seron-Ferre M (1985) Adrenal rest tumour of the liver causing surgical cure. J Clin Endocrinol Metab 60: 21–23

Creutzfeldt W, Arnold R, Frerihs H (1978) Insulinomas and

gastrinomas. In: Bloom SR (ed) Gut hormones. Livingstone, New York, pp 589–599
Cszij I, Csapo FA, Laszlo F, Kowacs K (1969) Medullary cancer of the thyroid gland associated with hypercorticism. Cancer 24: 167–173
Deveney CW, Deveney KS, Way LV (1978) The Zollinger-Ellison syndrome – 23 years later. Ann Surg 188: 384–393
Didolkar MS, Bescher RA, Elias EG, Moore RH (1981) Natural history of adrenal cortical carcinoma. Cancer 47 2153–2161
Ellison EH, Wilson SD (1964) The Zollinger-Ellison syndrome: reappraisal and evaluation of 260 registered cases. Ann Surg 160: 512–520
Fahrenkrug J (1980) Vasoactive intestinal polypeptide. Clin Gastroenterol 9: 633–643
Ganda OP, Weiss GC, Stewart-Soeld J, Legg MA, Crick WL, Patel YC, Ebeid AM, Gabbay KH, Reichlin S (1977) Somatostatinoma: a somatostatin containing tumour of the endocrine pancreas. N Engl J Med 286: 963–967
Geelhoed GW, Droy EM (1982) Management of the adrenal "incidentaloma". Surgery 92: 866–874
Grimelius L (1968) The argyrophil reaction in islet cells of adult human pancreas studied with a new silver nitrate procedure. Acta Soc Med Ups 73: 271–294
Hajjar RA, Hickey RC, Samaan NA (1975) Adrenal cortical carcinoma. Cancer 35: 549–554
Henley DJ, van Heerden JA, Grant CS, Carney JA, Carpenter PC (1983) Adrenal cortical carcinoma – a continuing challenge. Surgery 94: 926–931
Holm HH, Strøyer I, Hansen H, Stadil F (1981) Ultrasonically guided percutaneous interstitial implantation of iodine^{125} seeds in cancer therapy. Br J Radiol 54: 665–670
Hutter AM, Kayhoe DE (1966) Results of treatment with O,p'DDD in 138 patients. Am J Med 41: 581–592
Ingemansson S, Lunderquist A, Lunderquist J, Lovdahl R, Tibblin S (1975) Portal and pancreatic vein catheterization with radioimmunologic determination of insulin. Surg Gynecol Obstet 141: 705
Larsson L-I (1978) Classification of pancreatic endocrine tumours. Scand J Gastroenterol [Suppl 53] 14: 15–18
Larsson L-I, Hirsch MA, Holst JJ, Ingemansson S, Kühl C, Lindkær-Jensen S, Lundqvist G, Rehfeld JF, Schwartz TW (1977) Pancreatic somatostatinoma. Clinical features and physiological implication. Lancet 1: 666–668
Lewi HJE, Reid R, Mucci D, Davidson JK, Kylle KF, Macpherson SG, Semple P, Kaye S (1985) Malignant pheochromacytoma. Br J Urol 57: 394–398
Lewinsky BS, Grigor KM, Symington T, Neville AM (1974) The clinical and pathologic features of "non-hormonal" adrenocortical tumors. Report of 20 new cases and review of the literature. Cancer 33: 778–790
Madsen B (1979) Angiographic localization of B-cell tumours. Scand J Gastroenterol [Suppl 53] 14: 101–109
Mallinson CN, Bloom SR, Waren AP, Salmon PR, Cox B (1974) A glucagonoma syndrome. Lancet 2: 1–15
McCarty DM (1978) Report on the United States' experience with cimetidine in Zollinger-Ellison syndrome and other hypersecretory states. Gastroenterology 74: 453–458
Mc Gavran MH, Unger RH, Recant L, Polck HC, Kilo C, Levin ME (1966) A glucagon secreting alpha-cell carcinoma of the pancreas. N Engl J Med 274: 1408–1413
Mignon M, Ruszniewski P, Haffar S, Rigaud D, Rene E, Bonfils S (1986) Current approach to the management of tumoral process in patients with gastrinoma. World J Surg 10: 703–710
Neville AM, O'Hare MJ (1982a) The distinction between benign and malignant adrenocortical tumors causing Cushing's and/or the adrenogenital syndromes: structure and functional criteria. In: Neville AM, O'Hare MJ (eds) The human adrenalcortex. Springer Berlin Heidelberg New York, pp 186–201
Neville AM, O'Hare MJ (1982b) Hyperaldosteronism and related syndromes of mineralocorticoid excess. In: Neville AM, O'Hare MJ (eds) The human adrenal cortex. Springer, Berlin Heidelberg, New York, pp 202–241
Nieman LK, Chrousos GP, Kellner C, Spitz IM, Nisula BC, Cutler GB, Merriam GR, Bardin CW, Loriaux DL (1985) Successful treatment of Cushing's syndrome with a glucocorticoid antagonist RU 486. J Clin Endocrinol Metab 61: 536–538
Öberg K, Funa K, Alm G (1983) Effects of leucocyte interferon on clinical symptoms and hormone levels in patients with mid-gut carcinoid tumors and carcinoid syndrome. N Engl J Med 309: 129–132
Paes TRF, Hunter-Craig ID (1985) Carcinoma of the adrenal cortex. J R Soc Med 78: 408–409
Pearse AGE (1968) Common cytochemical properties of cells producing polypeptide hormones (the APUD series) and their relevance to thyroid and ultimobranchial C-cells and calcitonin. Proc R Soc Med [Biol] 170: 71–80
Percarpio B, Knowlton AC (1976) Radiation therapy of adrenal cortical carcinoma. Acta Radiol [Ther] (Stockh) 15: 288
Pitchet R, Rall I, Phelps P, Rutter J (1976) The neural crest and the origin of the insulin-producing and other gastrointestinal hormone-producing cells. Science 191: 191–192
Poynard T, Mignon M, Accary JP, Bonfils S (1986) Sensitivity, specificity, and predictive values of the secretin infusion test in the diagnosis of gastrinoma. Gastroenterol Clin Biol 10: 492–496
ReMine WH, Chong GC, van Heerden JA (1974) Current management of pheochromocytoma. Ann Surg 179: 740–747
Rhys-Davies E (1973) The radiological and scintigraphic investigation of spontaneous hypoglycaemia. Clin Radiol 24: 177–185
Richie JP, Gittes RF (1980) Carcinoma of the adrenal cortex. Cancer 45: 1957–1964
Schteingart DE, Motazedi A, Noonan RA, Thompson NW (1982) Treatment of adrenal carcinomas. Arch Surg 117: 1142–1146
Scott HW, Reynolds V, Green N, Page D, Oates JA, Robertson D (1982) Clinical experience with malignant pheochromocytomas. Surg Gynecol Obstet 154: 801–818
Scott HW, Abumrad NN, Orth DN (1985) Tumors of the adrenal cortex and Cushing's syndrome. Ann Surg 201: 586–594
Seddon JM, Baranetsky N, van Boxel PJ (1985) Adrenal "incidentaloma". Need for surgery. Urology 25:1–7
Service FJ, Dale JD, Elveback LR, Jiang NS (1976) Insulinoma: clinical and diagnostic features of 60 consecutive cases. Mayo Clin Proc 51: 417–429
Seyer-Hansen K, Lundbaek K (1979) The clinical diagnosis of insulinomas. Scand J Gastroenterol [Suppl 53] 14:39–42
Shepherd PA, Hoffert B, Evans WK, Emery G, Trachtenberg J (1985) Ketoconazole, use in the treatment of ectopic adrenocorticotopic hormone production and Cushing's syndrome in small cell lung cancer. Arch Intern Med 45: 863–864
Stadil F (1980) Gastrinomas. In: Glass GBJ (ed) Gastrointestinal hormones. Raven, New York
Stage JG, Stadil F (1979) The clinical diagnosis of the Zollinger-Ellison syndrome. Scand J Gastroenterol [Suppl 53] 14: 79–91
Stage JG, Stadil F, Rehfeld RF, Fahrenkrug J, Schaffalitzky

DE, Muckadell OB (1978) Secretin and the Zollinger-Ellison syndrome. Scand J Gastroenterol 13: 501–511
Stefanini P, Carboni C, Patrassi N, Basoil A (1974) Beta-islet cell tumours of the pancreas. Surgery 75: 597–609
Sullivan M, Boileace M, Hodges CV (1978) Adrenal cortical carcinoma. J Urol 120: 660–665
Thompson NW, Allo MD, Shapiro B, Sisson JC, Beierwalters W (1984) Extra-adrenal and metastatic pheochromocytoma: the role of ^{131}I-metaiodobenzylguanidine (^{131}I-MIBG) in localization and management. World J Surg 8: 605–611
Turner RC, Oakley NW, Nabarro JDN (1971) Control of the insulin secretion with special reference to the diagnosis of insulinomas. Br Med J 2: 132–135
Valverde J, Lemon HM, Kinsinger A, Unger RH (1976) Distribution of plasma glucagon immunoreactivity in a patient with suspected glucagonoma. J Clin Endocrinol Metab 42: 804–808
Van Heerden JA, Ships SG, Hamberger B, Sheeby PF, Paston JG, ReMine WH (1982) Pheochromocytoma: current status and changing trends. Surgery 91: 367–373
Van Heerden JA, Sizemore GW, Carney JA, Grant CS, ReMine WH, Ships SG (1984) Surgical management of the adrenal gland in the multiple endocrine neoplasia type II syndrome. World J Surg 8: 612–621
Verner JV, Morrison AB (1958) Islet cell tumour and a syndrome of refractory watery diarrhoea and hypokalaemia. Am J Med 25: 374–380
Verner JV, Morrison AB (1974) Endocrine pancreatic islet disease with diarrhoea. Arch Intern Med 133: 492–499
Zollinger RM, Ellison EH (1955) Primary peptic ulcerations of the jejunum associated with islet cell tumours of the pancreas. Ann Surg 142: 709–723
Zollinger RM, Martin EW Jr, Carey LC, Sparkes J, Menton JP (1976) Observations of the postoperative tumour growth behaviour of certain islet cell tumours. Ann Surg 184: 525–530
Zollinger RM, Ellison EH, O'Dorisio TM, Sparks J (1984) Thirty years' experience with gastrinoma. World J Surg 8: 427–435

Melanoma of the Skin

N. Cascinelli and C. Clemente

Definition

Melanoma is the malignant tumor of melanocytes. Even if it may appear wherever melanocytes are present, in the vast majority of cases it is located on the skin.

Epidemiology and Risk Factors

Geographical distribution of melanoma reveals some very peculiar features: the continent where the disease is most frequent is Oceania. In this area the incidence of the disease is about seven times that reported from the rest of the world: both in Australia and in New Zealand the incidence of melanoma in whites is over 32 per 100000 both in males and females (Waterhouse et al. 1982). The second highest frequency is reported from the United States where the rates per 100000 in the white population vary from 8.8 to 19.6 among males and from 7.0 to 17.4 among females (Waterhouse et al. 1982). In Europe the disease appears to be less frequent, the average incidence in males varies from 1.2 to 17.2 and in females from 1.2 to 10.4 (Waterhouse et al. 1982).

The observation that in both Australia and the United States the incidence of melanoma increases with the decreasing latitude gave strength to the hypothesis that sunshine may play an important role in the etiology of melanoma (Lancaster and Nelson 1957). This hypothesis was strongly supported in the 1960s, but in more recent papers this concept has been questioned because: (a) the north-south (or vice versa) trend is not always evident; in Europe, for example, the disease is more frequent in northern countries (Waterhouse et al. 1982); (b) people staying outdoors for occupational reasons, like fishermen, are those less affected by the disease (Holman et al. 1980); (c) melanoma is more frequent in covered areas of the body (Cascinelli 1983); (d) studies on immigrants in tropical countries indicate dissimilar results (Anaise et al. 1978; Holman et al. 1980; Wards et al. 1980); (e) melanoma occurs more frequently in people living in towns than in the country (Cascinelli 1983).

For all these reasons, sunlight should not be regarded as the major etiological factor of melanoma, even if some evidence of its role may be supported by recent studies indicating that sunburns during childhood are more frequently reported by melanoma patients (Holman et al. 1980). These findings need confirmation.

It is certainly an attractive hypothesis that protection can be procured by prolonged and continuous exposure to the sun, confirmed by the inferior incidence, worldwide, of melanoma in the rural population, in those persons who work outdoors, and in particular, in fisherman and sports instructors. However, in recent years much has changed with regard to the evaluation of the etiological role of ultraviolet (UV) irradiation and sunlight: the most recent data acquired concerning the natural history of melanoma (Veronesi et al. 1978), the identification of dysplastic lesions (Greene et al. 1985), a reassessment of the importance of ethnic groups (Cascinelli 1983), warnings regarding the potential risk of drugs, contraceptives (Beral et al. 1977), recognition of melanoma as a disease which is more frequent in the upper classes (Elwood et al. 1985), and the possible genetic implications (Greene et al. 1985; Pellegris et al. 1980; Privitera et al. 1985) have all certainly contributed to mitigating the drastic affirmation of the supporters of the high risk of UV irradiation, even if none of these has been proven. Thus it is that we no longer read such statements as, "One of the major causal factors – ultraviolet light – is known and theoretically it should be possible to reduce exposure to this causative agent, there is however, a series of complex medical, psychological and practical problems connected with the utilization of this knowledge in the control of the disease. It is surprising that so little attention has been paid to these problems in the past and this is a challenge for future preventive medicine" (Magnus 1977). Or "The influence of latitude on the incidence and mortality from malignant melanoma is the original and strongest evidence of the importance of exposure to sunlight by white people as a cause of malignant melanoma" (Lee 1972).

To consider exposure to sunlight as the most important risk factor most probably represents an excessive simplification of the problem (Lee 1982; Wards et al. 1980; Teppo et al. 1980). Experiments on animals do not support the hypothesis that UV irradiation causes melanoma; none of the experiments carried out caused this neoplasia, in only one experiment was UV irradiation involved in some way in its origin.

Epstein et al. (1967) induced a melanoma in a rat exposed to UV irradiation, originating from a benign nevus obtained by way of a powerful cancerogenous chemical, dimethylbenzanthracene (DMBA). This was, however, a unique melanoma and since it was not induced in an "inbred animal," it could not be transplanted. More recently, another experimental melanoma has been induced in a rat (Kripke 1979), but the modalities by which it was obtained (if extrapolated to man) lead one to believe that the present increase in melanoma is not to be imputed to UV irradiation but to one, or more, cancerogenous agents in the atmosphere. It can, therefore, be concluded, as Lee (1982) states, that "only further knowledge of the biology of melanoma can protect society from this uncertainty and from the real or imaginary dangers that it conceals."

A more biological approach can be attempted by considering the problem of the geographical distribution of the disease from a different point of view: only the white ethnic groups will be taken into consideration since, as is well known, melanoma is an extremely rare disease in the Black and the Asiatic, wherever they may reside. We must, therefore, commence from Europe because the Caucasian populations which today inhabit the Americans, Australia, and South Africa originate from there. Two ethnic groups can be identified in Europe: Latins and Caucasians. We should have a more detailed possibility of objective evaluation to present a further subdivision of this latter group since the populations have become so mixed during the course of the centuries as to make any distinction practically impossible. Even though there has obviously been considerable intermixing between Latins and Caucasians, it is possible to identify two sufficiently diverse ethnic groups on the basis of the genetic characteristics (HLA system).

A contrived distinction into three ethnic groups (Scandinavians, Central Europeans, and Latins) cannot be supported because the Scandinavians and the Central Europeans present the same frequency of the different antigens of the HLA system. On the other hand, comparison between Latins and Caucasians permits us to discover some differences, especially among the antigens of locus B. More fragmentary data, but of some interest, is also available regarding the HLA–DR system which reveals a frequency of different genetic expression in different populations: namely, for example, the DR5 gene is more frequently present in Spaniards and Italians (11.7% and 19.4%, respectively), less frequently in the British and the Germans (8.7% and 6.9%, respectively) and even less in the Scandinavians (4.9%). By using this information, we can acquire a better identification of the Caucasian ethnic groups of Europe. If we consider the migratory movements, we can affirm, quite generally, that the southern European populations emigrated prevalently to Central and South America, where the incidence of melanoma is low and does not differ greatly from that of Spain. It can be argued that this inferior incidence may be a contrivance bound to the poor efficiency of the registers, but if within the limits of the same register, the frequency of the disease is associated with the various ethnic groups, it can be observed that the disease is rarer in Spaniards everywhere and corresponds to that observed in Spain.

Furthermore, it is interesting to observe that in Quebec (Canada), where French immigration was the most consistent, incidence is among the lowest in Canada, and the figures are intermediary with respect to the two figures reported from France.

All this information must be considered very carefully, and results obtained by epidemiological studies should be considered by the epidemiologists together with the different aspects of this particular disease because, by relying too much on statistical analysis without taking into consideration the biology of melanoma, paradoxically insignificant correlations may be found and accepted.

Histopathology

The most important advances obtained in recent years in the study of malignant melanoma concern the possibility of defining a prognosis by means of histological parameters ("microstaging"). In particular, for a first stage malignant melanoma, the measurement on a histological slide of the thickness has been demonstrated to be the most important morphological characteristic. This fact has determined an ever-increasing interest in thin pigmented lesions of small sizes, thus refining both clinical and histopathological diagnostic capability, but also demonstrating just how difficult and exacting the differential diagnosis between such benign and malignant pigmented lesions can be.

Classification of Malignant Melanoma

The classification of malignant melanoma recommended by an international group of pathologists and epidemiologists in 1982 (McGovern et al. 1986) (Table 1) is still based on Clark's classification of 1967 and represents an extension and clarification of the classification adopted in 1972 by the International Group of Pathologists of Sydney (McGovern et al. 1973).

The different histotypes are classified histologically on the basis of the "presence or absence of a population of abnormal melanocyte-derived cells in the skin adjacent to the invading melanoma" (McGovern et al. 1986).

In the superficial spreading malignant melanoma the component adjacent to the invading portion is characterized by the presence of melanoma cells arranged in nests or isolated on the epidermal basal layer and also in the dermis. This proliferation may display morphological pseudopagetoid characteristics or can be of the dysplastic nevus type (McGovern and Murad 1985).

The lentigo type of malignant melanoma is characterized by the presence at the edges of the invading part of a lentiginous proliferation of atypical melanocytes, in particular in the basal layer and along the hair follicles, without pagetoid invasion of the epi-

Table 1. Classification of malignant melanoma (1982)

1. Malignant melanoma with an adjacent component of superficial spreading type
2. Malignant melanoma with an adjacent component of lentiginous malignant type
3. Malignant melanoma with a component of acral lentiginous type
4. Malignant melanoma with an adjacent component of mucosal lentiginous type
5. Malignant melanoma with no adjacent component
6. Malignant melanoma of unclassifiable histogenetic type

dermis. Occasionally the melanocytes are arranged in "clusters," while there is always epidermal atrophy and marked solar elastosis with homogenization of the dermis.

In the acral lentiginous type of malignant melanoma, besides the acanthosis of the epidermis, there is also an extension of the "rete ridges" and both basal and intraepidermal proliferation of atypical melanocytes, often with prominent branching of heavily pigmented dendritic processes, with the formation of nests that vary in size and shape and tend toward confluence.

The malignant melanoma of the mucosal lentiginous type has morphological characteristics similar to the acral lentiginous type, but it is considered separately because of the more serious prognosis.

In nodular malignant melanoma there is no component adjacent to the invading melanoma. The difference between nodular malignant melanoma and superficial spreading melanoma based on the extension of the adjacent component to more or less than three rete ridges has recently been criticized. In fact, it has been proposed that all those cases in which there is a definite and typical "adjacent component," identifiable both clinically and histologically, should be considered as superficial spreading malignant melanoma.

Macroscopic Description

The macroscopic description must be accurate and must, above all, aim to supply the indispensable information for the subsequent histopathological evaluation. It is important to indicate the size of the specimen to be removed, of the pigmented lesion, and of any raised areas present, the distance of the lesion from the nearest margin, the appearance of the edges (clear or faint), the shape of the lesion (flat, domed, polypoidal), the color of the surface and of the section to be cut, the possible presence and dimensions of ulceration, and the maximal thickness of the lesion on the surface to be cut. It may be useful to mark the edges of the resection with Indian ink, and when possible, it is advisable to take photographs (slides or prints) of the specimen of skin to be removed.

Frozen Section

Due to technical limitations and the fairly high number of false negative cases, rather than false positive, the frozen section method must be limited to the cases which are strictly necessary and it should be carried out by expert pathologists only. The area to be examined must be chosen without compromising the possibility of finding the point of maximal infiltration of the lesion in the definitive histological section. In any case, this examination should be avoided in the cases of small (diameter less than 5 mm) or very thin lesions, or those with extensive regression. An accurate check of the edges of the resection by frozen section may be required in the case of desmoplastic malignant melanoma since it may be difficult to identify clinically the transition between healthy and neoplastic tissue by inspection and palpation only. In our experience, the percentage of deferred cases is less than 10% and diagnostic accuracy reaches 100% (Clemente et al. 1981).

Cytology

This is a simple diagnostic tool with high sensitivity and predictive value (about 100%) in the case of malignant melanoma which is ulcerated, or in the process of ulceration, provided the surface necrotic and scab material is removed first. The examination is effected by placing a slide on the lesion which may be slightly scarified. The material collected must immediately be fixed in ethanol at 95% for staining by the Papanicolaou method, and one or more specimens should be dried in the air and then stained by the May-Grünwald-Giemsa method. Subcutaneous, lymphonodal, or parenchymal metastases may be diagnosed by means of fine needle aspiration, preparing cytological smears and embedding any small specimens in paraffin (Gupta et al. 1985).

Fixation, Sampling, Staining, and Immunohistochemistry

It is advisable to fix the skin specimens for 12 h on a cork bar in buffered 10% formaline before sampling the specimen. The lesion must be examined with parallel cuts according to the minor axis of the skin in such a way as to display and excise the point of deepest infiltration (dermal and hypodermal) of the melanoma. Special histochemical stains are not indispensable for the diagnosis of malignant melanoma, although the demonstration of the melanic pigment with the methods of Masson-Fontana, Schmorl, or Lillie in conjunction with the method of Perls (Prussian blue) for the differentiation of melanic and hemosiderinic pigment may be useful. More recently notable advantages, principally in the interpretation of metastatic lesions or of primary amelanotic malignant melanoma, have been obtained by using immunohistochemical methods with the protein S-100 (Cochran and Duan-Ren Wan 1985; Gatter et al. 1985), while the use of antimelanoma monoclonal antibodies on frozen sections or on fixed materials is still being studied (Clemente 1985; van Duinen et al. 1984).

Histopathological Parameters with Prognostic Significance

Level

Level was the first morphological parameter to be applied in prognostic evaluation. Five levels are distinguished according to the depth to which the skin has been invaded (Table 2). The major criticisms of the determination of the levels relate to the differences in the thickness of skin from person to person and to the anatomical site, but they mostly relate to the variations which may be encountered in the evaluation by different observers (Prade et al. 1980). Despite this, levels should be indicated with the thickness of the malignant melanoma since many surgeons still use this parameter as a guide to treatment and also because of the biological implications deriving, above all, from the involvement of the reticular dermis (Kelly et al. 1985).

Table 2. Levels of invasion of cutaneous malignant melanoma[a]

Level I	The malignant melanoma is confined to the epidermis (malignant melanoma intraepithelial or in situ)
Level II	The malignant melanoma infiltrates the papillary dermis without plugging it totally
Level III	The malignant melanoma plugs the papillary dermis totally and constricts the reticular dermis without infiltrating it[b]
Level IV	The malignant melanoma infiltrates the reticular dermis
Level V	The malignant melanoma infiltrates the adipose subcutaneous tissue

[a] The levels cannot be determined in the malignant melanoma of mucous membranes and in malignant melanoma with marked regression and evident fibrosis.

[b] The polypoidal malignant melanomas, even if they do not totally infiltrate the papillary dermis, are considered by definition to belong to level III.

Thickness

Measured histologically by means of an ocular micrometer, thickness is the most important morphological parameter for the prognostic assessment of malignant melanoma. The measurement is effected vertically from the upper level of the granular layer of the epidermis, or from the ulcerated surface, to the point of deepest invasion of the malignant melanoma. The measurement must not include deep nodules (satellite nodules) separated from the malignant melanoma (Day et al. 1981) or the extension of the malignant melanoma along the hair follicles. In the case of an associated nevus, it is often difficult to decide where the malignant melanoma finishes and where the nevus begins, and, therefore, it may be useful to give two measurements: one for the melanoma and one for the melanoma and nevus. In the case of regression, notable difficulties can also arise in identifying isolated malignant cells present in the dermis (McGovern et al. 1986).

Regression

Regression must always be noted and, where possible, assessed in quantitative terms as slight, moderate, or marked. Regression can be recognized as continuing or as completed and can involve the entire malignant melanoma or only a part of it (McGovern et al. 1986). Sometimes it may be difficult to decide whether a lesion with marked regression is a malignant melanoma; in these cases it may be indispensable to prepare numerous histological sections in the search for a residual focus of the malignant melanoma. The possibility of total regression would explain 2%–8% of the metastases of malignant melanoma in which a primary malignant melanoma is not demonstrable. It is still a matter of controversy whether regression has a negative effect on prognosis (Gromet et al. 1978) or has little prognostic importance (Cooper et al. 1985).

Ulceration

A number of studies have shown that ulceration in malignant melanoma is an independent prognostic parameter of unfavorable significance (McGovern et al. 1982). The presence of an ulcer must be indicated in both the macroscopic description and the histological diagnosis. Ulceration has been noted in association with mitotic activity; in fact, thin ulcerated lesions usually have a very high mitotic activity (McGovern et al. 1986).

Type of Growth (Profile)

Malignant melanoma can be flat, domed, or polypoid. Polypoid malignant melanomas have a more serious prognosis; nevertheless, this characteristic seems to be correlated with the thickness of the malignant melanoma (Reed et al. 1986). In the absence of the measurement of the thickness of the malignant melanoma, the profile could be useful as general prognostic information.

Inflammatory Reaction

The significance of the presence of lymphocytes within or on the periphery of the malignant melanoma is unknown, nevertheless, its indication is thought to be useful in attempting to evaluate infiltration in quantitative terms (slight, moderate, marked) and in qualitative terms (presence of lymphocytes, plasma cells, etc.).

Mitotic Activity

The prognostic significance of the evaluation of mitotic activity is controversial. In an attempt to reach agreement at least on the type of evaluation, it has been recommended to count the mitoses in an area not inferior to 1 mm in the portion of the histological section in which the mitoses are more numerous. In general, the nodular malignant melanoma which are thicker and ulcerated have a larger number of mitoses (McGovern and Murad 1985).

Pathology Report

The pathologist can supply a large amount of information together with the diagnosis of malignant melanoma; some is regarded as essential (histotype, thickness, level, ulceration, regression, radicality of the excision, vascular invasion), while other items have a prevalently descriptice character and may be of potential research interest (type of growth, cell type, melanogenesis, mitotic index, lymphocyte infiltration, dermal solar degeneration, associated nevus).

Differential Diagnosis

Table 3 shows the main histological characteristics of benign pigmented lesions to be taken into consideration in differential diagnosis of malignant melanoma, in particular "thin" melanoma (thickness less than or equal to 0.75 mm). The procedure for reaching a diagnosis entails a sequence of observations that begins with the examination of the architectural characteristics, using a panoramic magnification with particular attention to the so-called shoulder of the lesion, and goes right up to the study of the cytological characteristics of the neoplasia and subsequently of the so-called associated dermal characteristics. Obviously, the correct evaluation of such characteristics can only be carried out if a complete examination of the lesion is possible, and so incisional biopsies must be avoided.

The diagnosis of lentigo is based upon the presence of a proliferation of benign melanocytes without the formation of nests corresponding to the basal layer of the epidermis, with digitiform elongation of the rete ridges (lentiginous hyperplasia). In differential diagnosis we must take into account the dysplastic nevus and the noninvasive malignant melanoma which display atypical cytological features not encountered in a lentigo. Lentigo can create some diagnostic difficulties when it appears in particular sites, such as, for example, a gland.

In most cases, there are also no diagnostic difficulties with malignant melanoma and the diagnosis of junctional nevi or compound nevi. The fundamental points for the diagnosis of nevus are: symmetry, sharp lateral demarcation, the discontinuous presence of junctional nests, and, in compound nevi, melanocytic maturation in depth.

In the differential diagnosis between nevus and malignant melanoma McGovern and Murad (1985) point out, in particular, the presence in the former of cells with prevalently clear or colorless cytoplasm, which is rarely encountered in the malignant melanoma, and of fine granular melanic pigment, present in the nevus cells in the papillary dermis and absent in those of the reticular dermis, as well as the absence of lymphocyte infiltration.

The epithelioid and spindle cell nevus and the spindle cell nevus are the two benign pigmented lesions which can most frequently be confused with malignant melanoma (Sagebiel et al. 1984). The most important criteria for histological diagnosis are: the presence of symmetry in the nevi, clear lateral demarcation, dermal maturation with desmoplasia, nests of uniform cells with a fascicular appearance, and eosinophilic intraepidermal globules. It is also important to take into account the clinical appearance of the epithelioid and spindle cell nevi and, above all, the diagnosis of benign lesion must be formulated in an adult only after having excluded that of a malignant melanoma with great care. Finally, it is useful to recall that there are malignant melanomas that can resemble a nevus with epithelioid cells, and from which they may be differentiated, above

Table 3. Differential histopathological diagnoses

Characteristics	Lentigo	J/C nevus	E/S nevus	S nevus	H nevus	Pseudom	Dysplastic nevus	Thin MM
Dimensions less than 10 mm	Yes	Variable	Yes	Yes	Variable	Yes	No	No
Symmetry	Yes	Yes	Yes	Yes	No	No	No	No
Lateral demarcation	Yes	Yes	Yes	Yes	Yes	Yes	No	No
Lentiginous hyperplasia	Yes	No	No	No	No	No	Yes	Yes
Fusion of rete ridges	No	No	Yes	Yes	No	No	Yes	Yes
Intraepidermal invasion	No	Rare	Yes	Yes	Rare	Yes	No	Yes
Nests prevalent over single intra-epidermal cells	No	Yes	Yes	Yes	Yes	Variable	Yes	No
Maturation in the dermis	–	Yes	Yes	Yes	Yes	No	Yes	No
Cellular polymorphism	No	Rare	Yes	No	No	Yes	occasional	Yes
Mitosis	No	Rare	Variable	Rare	No	No	Rare	Variable
Melanic pigment	Abundant	Variable	Slight	Abundant	Variable	Variable	Variable	Variable
Eosinophilic globules	No	Rare (0.9%)	Yes (60%)	Yes	No	No	Rare	Rare (2%)
Inflammatory reaction	Rare	No	Yes Intratumoral	With perivascular foci	Intense	Perivascular foci	Perivascular foci	In bands
Epidermal hyperplasia	Rare	Variable	Yes	Yes	No	No	Rare	Variable
Desmoplasia	No	No	Frequent	Rare	Yes	Yes	Fibroplasia	Variable
Dermal macrophages	Yes	No	Variable	Yes	Yes	Yes	Variable	Variable
Regression	No	No	No	No	Yes	No	Rare (10%)	Yes (50%)

J/C nevus, junctional and compound nevus; E/S nevus, epithelioid and spindle cell nevus; S nevus, spindle cell nevus; H nevus, halo nevus; Pseudom, pseudomelanoma; Thin MM, thin malignant melanoma.

all, by a careful examination of the shoulder of the lesion.

The halo nevus and the pseudomelanoma can only rarely be wrongly interpreted as malignant melanoma if the clinical characteristics and case history of the patient are known.

There are many problems, on the other hand, in the differential diagnosis between dysplastic nevi, compound nevi, and junctional nevi and malignant melanoma, especially thin malignant melanoma. Table 4 summarizes the principal histopathological characteristics of the dysplastic nevus according to Friedman et al. (1985). The architectural characteristics are of primary importance for the diagnosis of dysplastic nevus, whereas the cytological criteria, though important, are much less reproducible.

Atypical cytological features in the dysplastic nevus are not indispensable for Ackerman and Mihara (1985) either, who affirm that the dysplastic nevus is a very common pigmented lesion and must be considered a variant of the compound or junctional nevus. In our opinion, to diagnose a dysplastic nevus, the atypical cytological features associated with the architectural characteristics described above are indispensable.

The biological significance of the dysplastic nevus is still under discussion and is obscure (Clark et al. 1984; Rigel et al. 1985; Cook and Robertson 1985;

Table 4. Histopathological characteristics of the dysplastic nevus

Architectural anomalies:
Intraepidermal melanocytic hyperplasia, limited to the deepest part of the epidermis
Fusion of the epithelial spurs
Badly defined lateral margins
Cytological anomalies:
Nuclear polymorphism
Nuclear hyperchromasia
Rare mitoses
Concentric eosinophilic fibroplasia
Lamellar fibroplasia
Vascular neogenesis
Inflammatory infiltrate with foci, perivascular
Nevic cells mature in the dermis

Greene et al. 1985; Elder 1985); however it seems to be useful to identify such a lesion histologically not only with the aim of selecting case histories to study, but also to identify a lesion which could be wrongly diagnosed as malignant.

Natural History

Melanoma may originate on normal skin or in association with a melanocytic nevus. A great deal of discussion and literature has been dedicated to the so-called precursors of melanoma, but no agreement has been reached so far. The main reason for the different points of view is the impossibility of carrying out adequate studies because of the extraordinary number of nevi: it was calculated that a white adult has a mean of 25 nevi, and it is practically impossible to investigate all these lesions over several years. As a matter of fact, practically all papers on this subject consider the association of nevi and melanoma in series of melanoma patients, and from this perspective it is impossible to assess any potential risk of a nevus. If one takes into consideration the high number of nevi per individual and the fact that the average incidence of skin melanoma is around 6 per 100 000, it can be seen that the risk of a nevus giving rise to a melanoma is very low. There is considerable consensus that the nevi should not be regarded as a potential precursor, and the discussion is limited to congenital nevi and so-called dysplastic nevi. I (N.C.) am personally strongly convinced that there is no relation between nevi and melanoma: certainly a melanoma may arise on a nevus but the relative risk is minimal.

Melanoma arises as such and, in 80% approximately of cases, grows slowly locally. Most of the patients state that a pigmented mole has been present for several years, increased slowly in diameter, and changed color without any symptoms. After this period a nodule appears within the pigmented mole that grows quickly, it is usually not pigmented and frequently bleeds. The remaining 20% of patients state that a nodule suddenly appeared on the skin and grew rapidly. Melanoma spreads both via the lymphatic and the blood stream.

To evaluate dissemination of the disease, one must evaluate the patients submitted to excision of primary tumor only, because if patients submitted to elective regional lymph node dissection are taken into consideration, the group of patients with concomitant dissemination to regional nodes and distant organs is underestimated. In a relatively recent study carried out on the WHO Melanoma Programme Register (Cascinelli et al. 1983a), it was evaluated that 50% of patients who have a recurrence of the disease show regional lymph node metastases as first evidence, and the remaining 50% show distant metastases with or without regional lymph node metastases. Hematogeneous metastases are more frequently observed in subcutaneous fat, lung, and liver. Relatively infrequent is the dissemination to the skeleton; the central nervous system is also a site of distant metastases in approximately 10% of patients as first evidence of relapse, but this localization is present in over 40% of patients with disseminated disease.

Local recurrences are rather infrequent: 2%–5% of patients experience such a recurrence. Their frequency is significantly associated with maximal tumor thicknes: 1% were observed in melanoma of less than 1 mm, up to 5% observed in tumors thicker than 4 mm. On the contrary, resection margins do not seem to be related to local recurrences (Cascinelli et al. 1980).

So-called in-transit metastases are considered a typical spread of cutaneous melanoma: this term defines a dissemination of cutaneous or subcutaneous nodules between the site of origin of the primary melanoma and a regional lymph node basin. It was generally accepted that the melanoma cells that flaked off from the primary tumor could penetrate into a lymphatic vessel, proceed a certain distance, and reemerge after a few centimeters once they had reached the subcutaneous tissue; if they found suitable conditions for growth they would give rise to a new separate colony. On the basis of the experience accumulated at the National Cancer Institute of Milan, we (Cascinelli et al. 1986a) have observed that this is not the usual pathogenetic mechanism. The in-transit metastasis has to be regarded as a hematogenous spread located by chance near the primary tumor.

Staging

The definition of the extent of metastatic spread of cutaneous melanoma is based upon very simple tests in asymptomatic patients. Over a careful clinical examination aimed at the detection of superficial spread (regional and nonregional nodes, and cutaneous and subcutaneous metastases), we habitually check lungs by means of two-dimensional chest X-ray examination and liver by means of echotomography as these are the most frequent sites of asymptomatic metastates. Other, more sophisticated, examinations (computed tomography, isotope scanning, etc.) are done according to clinical requirements only. Lymphography is no longer performed at our institute because: (a) the clinical judgement of the status of groin and cervical nodes is quite good; in our experience, the concordance between clinical and histological examination is over 90% (Cascinelli et al. 1984); (b) retroperitoneal lymph nodes are not usually involved if no superficial metastases are detectable (Cascinelli et al. 1984); (c) at the level of the axilla, the lymph nodes along the dorsal vessels are seldom reached by the contrast; (d) as nodal secondary deposit is originally located at the center of the lymph node, contrary to what is normally observed in metastatic epithelial tumors, the differential diagnosis between malignant and benign diseases of the lymph node (such as lipoma, sclerosis, etc.) may be difficult. Diagnostic confirmation of a suspicious lymph node can be obtained much better by cytology, by means of a fine needle biopsy.

Once the extent of melanoma has been assessed, it can be classified. The following are the most widely used classifications: the three-stage classification shown in Table 5, the so-called M. D. Anderson classification shown in Table 6, which is used mostly by perfusionists. The TNM classification is shown in Table 7: this classification is the most complete because it describes systematically the characteristics of the primary tumor (T), node status (N), and distant metastases (M). Moreover, this classification takes into consideration the histological characteristics that are of paramount importance in the assessment of the prognosis of these patients.

It has to be stressed, however, that since the computer has entered into normal practice, the need for detailed clinical classification is felt less and less because it seems more important to have agreement on factors which are relevant in the assessment of the prognosis which should be collected in a homogeneous way. On the basis of these items it will be easy to categorize patients according to different criteria.

Table 5. Clinical stage classification

Stage I	Melanoma without regional and/or distant metastases
Stage II	Melanoma with regional not distant metastases
Stage III	Melanoma with distant metastases, with or without regional metastases

Table 6. Clinical classification – M. D. Anderson Hospital

Stage I	No metastases a. Primary lesion previously removed b. Present primary lesion
Stage II	Metastases confined within a 3-cm area from the primary lesion (primary tumor with satellitosis)
Stage III	Regional metastases a. Cutaneous and subcutaneous in-transit metastases over 3 cm from the primary lesion b. Metastases at regional lymph nodes ab. Both previous
Stage IV	Distant metastases

Prognostic Factors

Prognosis of cutaneous melanoma is a matter that has been widely discussed and profoundly evaluated. The first attempt to assess the prognosis of these patients was performed in the 1940s (Ackerman and del Regato 1954): at that time the prognosis of the patients was estimated taking into consideration the major steps of the disease, such as regional nodes and distant metastases. The first attempt to obtain a more detailed evaluation on the basis of the characteristics of the primary tumor was done by Bodenham in 1968. This author divided stage I melanoma into two main categories: (a) good melanoma, that was flat with evident clinical regression, slowly growing; (b) bad melanoma, that was elevated, fast growing. A few years later, along this conceptual line, Clark et al. (1969) were the first to describe microstaging of the primary tumor that was divided into five levels; McGovern (1970) considered the growth pattern and regression; at the same time Breslow (1970) published the prognostic relevance of maxi-

Table 7. TNM classification proposed by UICC

T – Primary Tumour	
The extent of tumour is classified after excision, see pT.	
N – Regional Lymph Nodes	
NX	Regional lymph nodes cannot be assessed
N0	No regional lymph node metastasis
N1	Metastasis 3 cm or less in greatest dimension in any regional lymph node(s)
N2	Metastasis more than 3 cm in greatest dimension in any regional lymph node(s) and/or in-transit metastasis
	N2a Metastasis more than 3 cm in greatest dimension in any regional node(s)
	N2b In-transit metastasis
	N2c Both
Note:	In-transit metastasis involves skin or subcutaneous tissue more than 2 cm from the primary tumour not beyond the regional lymph nodes.
M – Distant Metastasis	
MX	Presence of distant metastasis cannot be assessed
M0	No distant metastasis
M1	Distant metastasis
	M1a Metastasis in skin or subcutaneous tissue or lymph node(s) beyond the regional lymph nodes
	M1b Visceral metastasis
pTNM Pathological Classification	
pT – Primary Tumour	
pTX	Primary tumour cannot be assessed
pT0	No evidence of primary tumour
pTis	Melanoma in situ (Clark's level I) (atypical melanocytic hyperplasia, severe melanocytic dysplasia, not an invasive malignant lesion)
pT1	Tumour 0.75 mm or less in thickness and invades the papillary dermis (Clark's level II)
pT2	Tumour more than 0.75 mm but not more than 1.5 mm in thickness and/or invades to the papillary-reticular dermal interface (Clark's level III)
pT3	Tumour more than 1.5 mm but not more than 4.0 mm in thickness and/or invades the reticular dermis (Clark's level IV)
	pT3a Tumour more than 1.5 mm but not more than 3.0 mm in thickness
	pT3b Tumour more than 3.0 mm but not more than 4.0 mm in thickness
pT4	Tumour more than 4.0 mm in thickness and/or invades subcutaneous tissue (Clark's level V) and/or satellite(s) within 2 cm of the primary tumour
	pT4a Tumour more than 4.0 mm in thickness and/or invades subcutaneous tissue
	pT4b Satellite(s) within 2 cm of the primary tumour
Note:	In case of discrepancy between tumour thickness and level, the pT category is based on the less favourable finding.
pN – Regional Lymph Nodes	
The pN categories correspond to the N categories.	
pM – Distant Metastasis	
The pM categories correspond to the M categories.	

mal tumor thickness measured microscopically by means of a micrometer. A number of other factors were later considered (van der Esch et al. 1981), but none of these was found to be as reproducible as those previously mentioned (Cascinelli et al. 1980). It is now clear that the prognosis of the patients with melanoma must be based upon the clinical stage, and, within each stage, specific factors have to be considered.

Stage I

Histological characteristics of primary melanoma are the only elements which can assess the prognosis of stage I melanoma patients: several studies have been published in the last 10 years, and there is overall agreement that among these factors the most important and reproducible is maximal thickness of primary melanoma (Cascinelli et al. 1985; Balch and Milton 1984). Local recurrences, regional nodes, and distant metastases increase, and the survival rates decrease with increasing maximal thickness. The other criteria, such as levels of invasion, growth pattern, spontaneous regression, which are actually significantly related to survival of stage I melanoma patients and were once considered as single factors, are no longer relevant when adjusted by maximal tumor thickness.

Ulceration of histologically evaluated primary melanoma is the second most important factor that has an independent impact on survival (Balch et al. 1984), thin melanomas have a poorer prognosis when ulcerated.

The sex of the patient is also significantly associated with survival: it is unanimously accepted that females have a significantly better prognosis than males (Cascinelli et al. 1980). The role of sex is not easy to explain, but it does not seem that the more favorable site of origin or the thinner melanoma in females fully explains the better prognosis of females themselves (Cascinelli et al. 1980).

It is important to state that no other criteria are relevant to the prognosis of stage I melanoma patients. Site of origin in particular does not have any impact on survival, in spite of the fact that it is generally asserted that melanoma of the lower legs has a more favorable behavior. A few years ago it was claimed (Day et al. 1982) that melanomas originating in a particular region of the body termed "BANS" (back, posterior part of the arm, of the neck, and of the scalp) were associated with a particularly bad prognosis, but this finding was not confirmed by subsequent studies carried out on larger patient series (Cascinelli et al. 1986b).

Stage II

The prognosis of melanoma patients with histologically proven regional node metastases is ruled out by prognostic criteria related to the metastatic growth. In fact, it is unanimously accepted that the number of nodes involved and the invasion of metastatic growth beyond the lymph node capsula are the key prognostic factors (Cascinelli et al. 1984). The 43.4% chance of cure of patients with a single node affected by a neoplastic growth that does not substitute it completely, falls to 26.0% when two or more nodes are involved and the metastatic nodule extends beyond the lymph node capsules.

There are indications that the biological aggressiveness of melanoma with regional node metastases may be evaluated on the basis of a labeling index: Costa et al. (1985) recently showed that prognosis of patients with a low labeling index was better than the one observed in patients with a high labeling index. These data are very preliminary and need confirmation, but are important because biological evaluation is considered instead of the usual morphological criteria.

The characteristics of the primary tumor do not seem to be important in the assessment of prognosis of this group of patients: different authors have found different prognostic criteria on primary tumors; in our opinion, the lack of agreement implicates the weakness of each of these criteria.

Stage III

Patients with distant metastases have a very bad prognosis, and there is no concrete chance of cure for them. The period of life that may be expected depends upon the site of secondary deposits and the total tumor burden. Patients with distant metastases localized in the central nervous system have the worst prognosis, while those with superficial localizations usually have a relatively long survival. It is important to observe that so-called local recurrences after adequate surgery and in-transit metastases also carry a bad prognosis which is no different from the one related to metastases at a distance from the site of origin of the superficially located primary (Cascinelli et al. 1986a).

Screening of Asymptomatic Disease

The screening of asymptomatic disease is of paramount importance in the control of cutaneous melanoma. The improvement in prognosis that has been observed in the past 30 years must be ascribed to the excision of lesions that were diagnosed at an ever earlier phase. The success of a campaign against melanoma is related to the achievement of two fundamental goals: professional and public education. The second is not within the aims of this paper, but as far as health professionals are concerned, besides training aimed at recognizing "thin" melanoma, deep-seated prejudice must be removed. For many years it was assumed that the excision of a mole was dangerous: once touched by the scalpel, the mole would suddenly transform into a malignant disease and kill the patients. Although this concept is now rejected, there is unfortunately an important statement still current, "let's check this mole and excise it as soon as any modification occurs." We now know enough about the potential aggressiveness of an apparently innocent mole for this knowledge to be transferred to the nonspecialized medical community, thus enabling them to formulate a diagnosis of suspicion. We are firmly convinced that the decision whether or not a pigmented mole has to be excised must be taken at the first consultation.

The diagnosis of "thin melanoma" is certainly not easy. The recognition of a potentially dangerous mole is difficult because melanoma is a relatively infrequent disease (less than 10 cases per 100 000 all over the world except Oceania), and for this reason it is difficult for a general practitioner to achieve enough experience.

Diagnosis of Thin Melanoma

Definition

"Thin melanoma" is defined as a cutaneous melanoma in an early proliferative phase with a maximal tumor thickness of no more than 1 mm and with no clinical and histological evidence of spontaneous regression. Its aggressiveness is only potential: an adequate surgical excision always cures the patient. This melanoma has always been defined using different adjectives ("flat," "small," "early," "macular") but we think that "thin" is the most appropriate because it is most closely related to the most important prognostic factor.

Semiological Elements

Thin melanoma may arise on normal skin or in association with a benign melanocytic nevus. The onset within a benign nevus is not surprising and may be suggested by the clinical history and confirmed by histological examination: the patient states that a pigmented mole present for decades suddenly changed and histological examination shows the presence of a residual nevus. Thin melanoma may be diagnosed when at least 5 mm at the maximal diameter.

These lesions are usually flat, asymptomatic, observed on a careful examination of the skin, and the patient is usually unaware of them. The semiological characteristics that allow diagnosis are the following: (a) the shape, always asymmetrical; (b) the color brown or blackish, with an uneven distribution; (c) margins "knotted" and irregular, defining the lesion sharply from the surrounding skin. The simultaneous presence of these three characteristics, of the edges in particular, must lead to a diagnosis of suspected melanoma.

At a later stage, a clinical history may be of extraordinary importance because the patient is aware of the lesion and may be able to describe the evolution. The modifications that are usually described are: (a) increase of radial dimension: the surface doubles in a period of 3–8 months; (b) variations of the shape: the lesion which had been approximately regular becomes irregular due to the digitiform expansion of the margins; (c) color variations: the lesion usually becomes darker; (d) modification of the surface: it becomes rough and superficial desquamation or ulceration is frequently observed. In this phase the mole becomes symptomatic because of itching and modest pain. Clinical characteristics are similar to those previously described but more evident.

The signs which are usually considered pathognomonic, such as serous ooze or bleeding, appear late. Typical of this late phase are nodules, usually

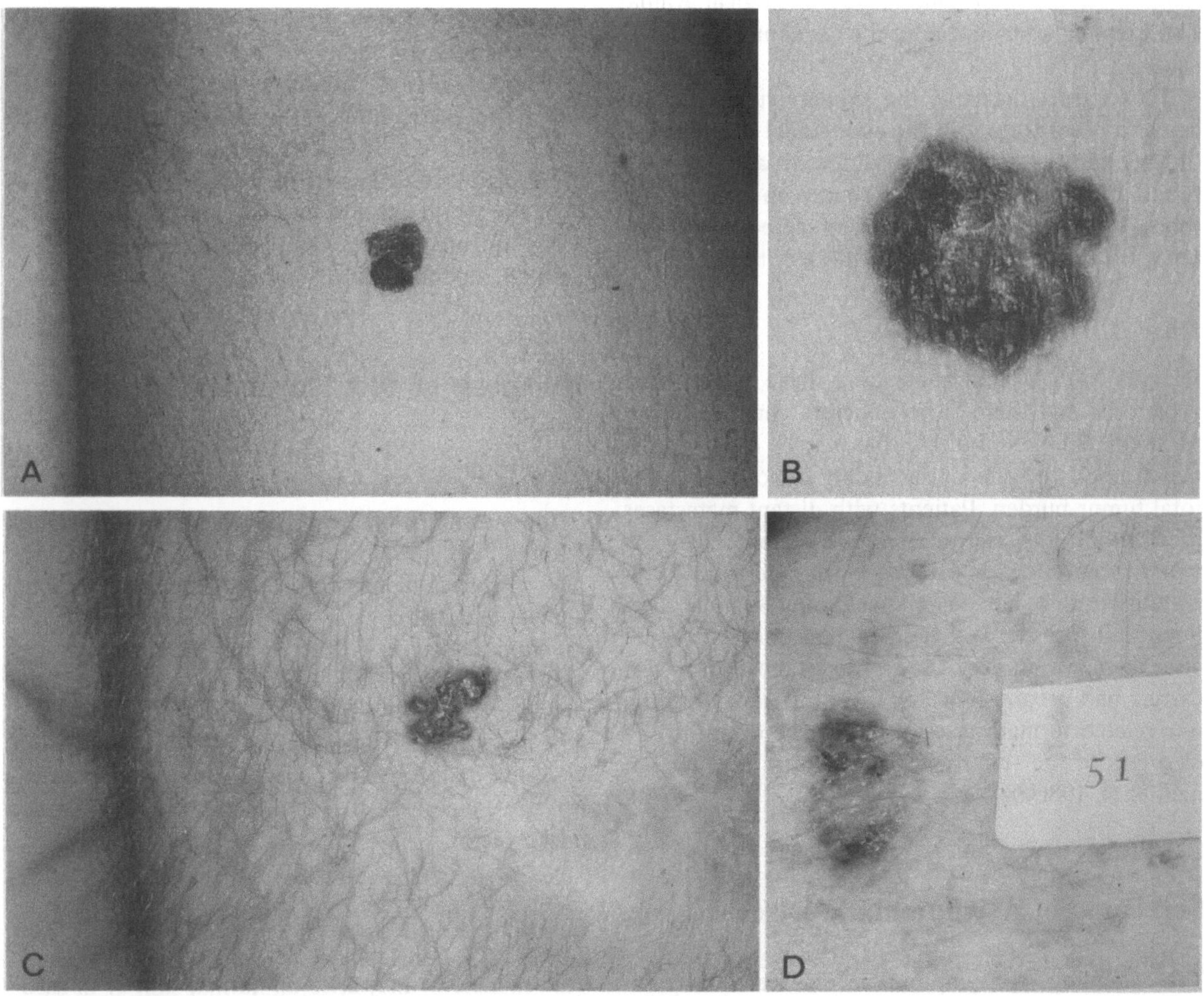

Fig. 1 A–H. Representative examples of different types of melanoma

not pigmented, that appear on the surface of the flat lesion. In this situation one cannot call the melanoma "thin" any longer.

Melanoma may arise on a benign pigmented mole as may be shown by the history (a nevus had been present at the site of origin of the melanoma for many years) and by the fact that an accurate histological examination reveals more or less wide areas with the structure of a nevus. It is impossible, however, to state what the relationship between the two lesions is. It is certain that by reducing the frequency of large melanomas we are more likely to observe a preexisting macular lesion, usually totally destroyed by melanoma of a large dimension. The evolution and the clinical aspect of a melanoma arising on a nevus are identical to those observed de novo in melanoma. Figure 1 shows the clinical characteristics of established melanoma.

Treatment

As with all solid tumors, melanoma requires surgical treatment as long as it is confined to the site of origin and not extended beyond regional nodes. Palliative surgical procedures may be planned in selected patients with advanced disease. For the sake of simplicity, the surgical indications will be described separately for primary melanoma, regional nodes, local recurrence and distant metastases.

Surgery of the Primary Tumor

It is generally thought that wide excision is the treatment of choice for primary cutaneous melanomas. As a general rule, the skin should be excised with a margin of 3–5 cm, in all directions, from the visible

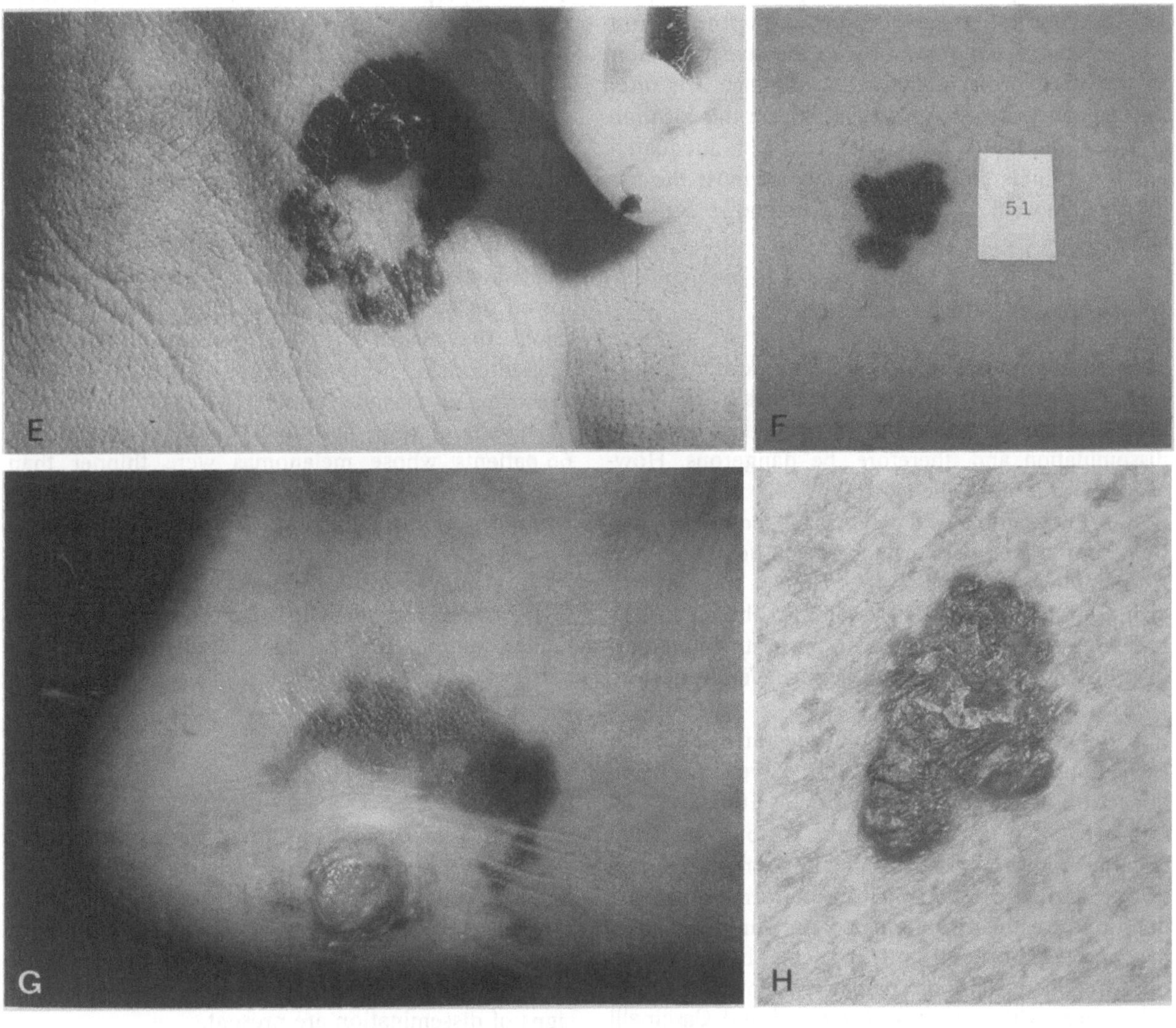

edge of the tumor together with a somewhat larger area of subcutaneous fat and muscle fascia. This wide excision alone controls the disease in most cases. Irrespective of whether or not an elective node dissection is performed, the rate of local recurrence in clinical stage I malignant melanoma of the limbs is around 2% (Veronesi et al. 1982; Cascinelli et al. 1980).

To meet the requirements for wide excision, amputation of the digit is needed when the site of origin is the distal part of fingers or toes. When malignant melanoma originates in the proximal half of digits, disarticulation is performed at the level of the corresponding tarsometatarsal or carpometacarpal joint. When an interdigital site (web space) is affected, the two contiguous metacarpals or metatarsals are disarticulated. Major radical amputations of the extremities (interscapulothoracic, interscapulomammothoracic amputations, hip and sacroiliac disarticulation), suggested by some authors in the 1950s with the aim of improving survival in patients with positive regional nodes, are no longer performed routinely. When melanomas arise on the face, the extent of the resection is usually reduced, since it is often difficult to excise a large area of skin in this location.

Three questions have not yet been adequately answered: (a) is biopsy dangerous; (b) must the fascia be removed; (c) is wide excision always necessary?

Biopsy

Most surgeons are afraid to perform incisional biopsies of a pigmented mole because it has been widely held that this procedure might result in tumor cell dissemination and, therefore, be dangerous. However, there is no evidence to support this assumption. A histopathological diagnosis is required before treatment of a primary melanoma can be carried out. If the mole is ulcerated, a direct smear, after superficial abrasion of the ulcer, can be obtained. This procedure is safe and yields an accurate cytological diagnosis in over 90% of the cases (Veronesi et al. 1978).

If the lesion is raised and not ulcerated, a limited excision may be performed and a frozen section done with diagnostic accuracy of close to 100% (Veronesi et al. 1978). If the lesion is not considered suitable for cytological examination or frozen section, a limited excision may be performed and the definitive treatment determined. In our experience, prognosis is not significantly worsened by this procedure provided excisional biopsy is followed by radical surgery within 4 weeks (Veronesi and Cascinelli 1979). The results of a prospective, randomized clinical trial carried out by the WHO Melanoma Programme showed no difference in survival between patients not previously biopsied and patients submitted to excisional biopsy of primary melanomas within 1 month of definitive treatment. This was true whether or not an elective regional node dissection was performed (Figs. 2, 3). Incisional biopsy is not recommended unless one intends to compare surgical treatment to nonsurgical procedures and needs histological confirmation of the diagnosis since it may be possible to miss a microscopic area of malignant transformation if the lesion is not completely excised and thoroughly examined.

Excision of Muscle Fascia

It is difficult to state whether or not muscle fascia should be included in the surgical specimen since the literature contains few data on this question. Olsen (1972) reported better results when muscle fascia was not removed, but her results have not been confirmed.

Extent of Excision

Breslow and Macht (1977) have questioned the need to perform a wide excision in all cases. These authors reviewed a series of malignant melanomas treated at George Washington University and followed up for at least 5 years. The researchers compared the results of wide excision versus more limited excision in three subsets of patients grouped according to maximal tumor thickness. The margins of resection were less than 1 cm in two of the 66 patients whose melanomas were thinner than 0.76 mm. None of these patients developed local recurrences or distant metastases during the follow-up period. The authors suggested a narrow excision for melanomas of less than 0.76 mm. Although this series is too small to be considered definitive, limited surgery may be considered in selected cases.

Surgery of Lymph Nodes

Cutaneous malignant melanoma spreads to three main lymph node chains: cervical, axillary, and ilioinguinal. Other superficial or deep lymph node groups are affected very rarely, at least initially. There is no controversy on the need to dissect nodal areas which are obviously involved when no other signs of dissemination are present.

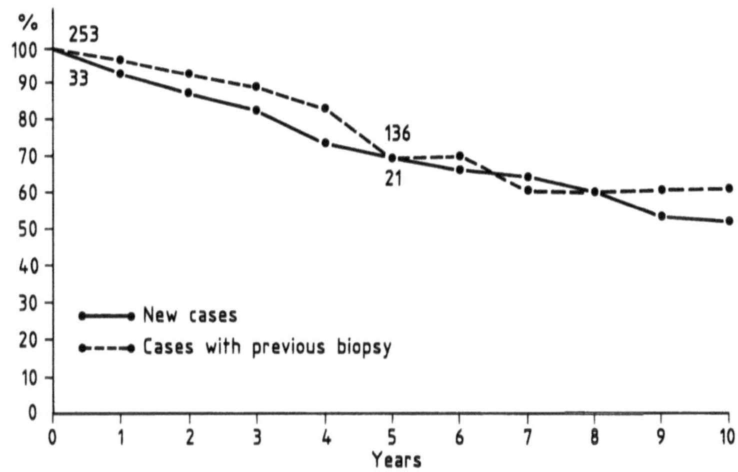

Fig. 2. Ten-year survival observed in 268 stage I patients submitted to excision of primary tumor and to possible lymph node dissection at the time of lymph node metastases. (From WHO Melanoma Program – Clinical Trial No. 1)

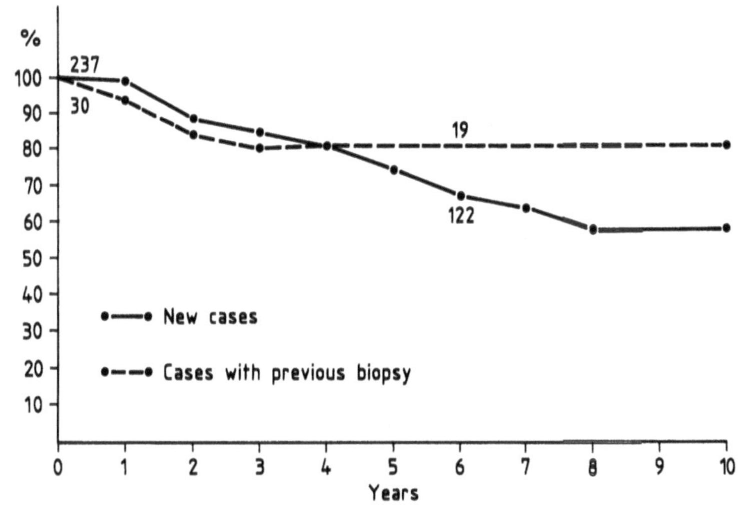

Fig. 3. Ten-year survival observed in 267 stage I patients submitted to elective regional lymph node dissection. (From WHO Melanoma Program – Clinical Trial No. 1)

Surgical techniques for lymph node dissection for melanoma are the same as those performed for other malignancies. When cervical nodes are affected, radical neck dissection is the operation of choice and should be combined with parotidectomy if the primary site is on the upper part of the face or temporal region. Axillary node dissection with en bloc removal of the pectoralis minor muscle is necessary if axillary nodes are involved. The role of internal mammary node dissection is not generally accepted. Inguino-femoral, external iliac, and obturator nodes must be removed when inguinal nodes are involved. A few years ago, Cohen et al. (1975) suggested laparotomy as a staging procedure. In five patients, they found occult para-aortic lymph node metastases, and in two of these patients there were occult liver metastases. However, the experience is too limited to recommend staging laparotomy as a routine procedure.

An unresolved question is whether or not lymph node dissection should be performed in continuity with resection of a primary melanoma. The question concerns mainly melanomas arising in the distal part of the extremities. The objective of an in-continuity procedure (even in lesions arising below the knee and the elbow) is to reduce the incidence of in-transit metastases. It was been reported (Fortner et al. 1975) that a 14% incidence of development of in-transit metastases after discontinuity lymph node dissection was reduced to 2% when en bloc dissections were performed.

The incidence of severe lymph edema of the limbs is reduced in in-continuity dissection according to Papachristou and Fortner (1977), who observed lymph edema of more than 2 cm in eight out of 36 patients treated by en bloc dissection and in 16 out of 45 patients treated by discontinuity dissection. Some authors (Southwick 1976) claim a higher 5-year survival rate, but this has not been confirmed by others (Veronesi et al. 1972).

In our experience, the incidence of in-transit metastases has not been affected by en bloc node dis-

Table 8. Frequencies of regional node metastases

Maximal thickness (mm)	Immediate dissection			Delayed dissection (if needed)		
	Patients (*n*)	N_{0+} (*n*)	(%)	Patients (*n*)	Dis-sected (*n*)	(%)
0 –0.9	16	–	–	16	–	–
1.0–1.9	35	5	14.3	35	5	14.3
2.0–2.9	44	6	13.6	25	14	56.0
3.0–3.9	26	3	11.5	41	13	31.7
>4	52	21	40.4	48	16	33.3
	173	35	20.2	165	48	29.1

$P = 0.0004$. $P = 0.0005$.

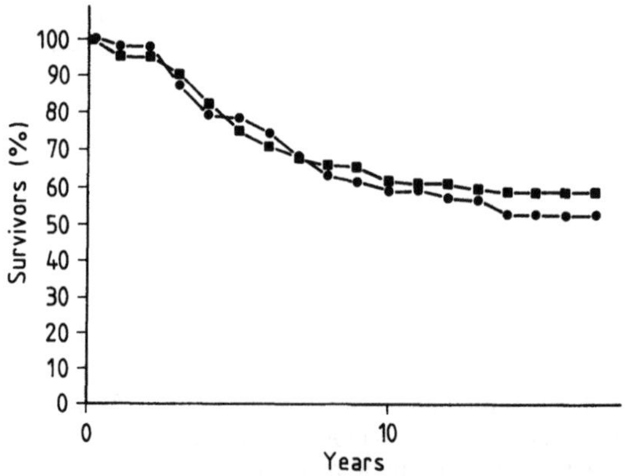

Fig. 4. Survival of 553 stage I patients with melanoma localized at extremities. *Squares*, excision only (286 patients; *diamonds*, excision plus regional lymph node dissection (267 patients)

section. In a series of 83 cases of stage II melanoma of the extremities, in-transit metastases appeared in four out of 52 patients treated by en bloc dissection and in one out of 31 treated by discontinuous lymph node dissection (Veronesi et al. 1972).

The most important problem in the surgical treatment of lymph nodes concerns dissection of clinically uninvolved regional lymph nodes. Should a surgeon perform an immediate elective node dissection as soon as the diagnosis of malignant melanoma is confirmed or should he wait for clinical evidence of node involvement before performing a regional lymph node dissection? The controversy dates back to the origin of surgical treatment of malignant melanoma, and the retrospective evaluation of results achieved with the two approaches has not provided convincing evidence as to the superiority of either approach. Even the new criteria for histopathological classification and staging which have been proposed in the past few years (Wanebo et al. 1975; Clark et al. 1969; Breslow 1975; Breslow et al. 1978; Balch and Milton 1984; Balch et al. 1984) have not clarified this issue. Although most authors agree that elective regional node dissection is not necessary for level I, level II, and level III melanomas thinner than 1 mm, these cases constitute the minority in most published series. The main argument in favor of performing elective regional node dissections for lesions greater than 1 mm in thickness is that the incidence of occult nodal metastases increases progressively with increasing levels of invasion and increasing tumor thickness. This has been true in our experience (Table 8), but no-one has yet demonstrated that immediate elective node dissection improves survival.

In order to evaluate the efficacy of elective regional node dissection objectively, in 1967 the WHO Melanoma Programme undertook a prospective, randomized clinical trial in patients with stage I melanoma of the extremities (Veronesi et al. 1977, 1980, 1982). The number of patients entered into the trial was large enough to permit evaluation of results, and the two groups of patients were fairly comparable. A total of 267 patients were submitted to wide excision of the primary lesion and immediate node dissection, and 286 to wide excision of the primary lesion only. Delayed node dissections were performed when clinically evident regional node metastases occurred. Figure 4 shows that the survival curves for the two groups are superimposable. Elective regional node dissection did not improve survival even when subgroups of patients were evaluated according to the presence or absence of a previous biopsy, sex, age, and site of origin (upper and lower extremity). As fas as the two main histological criteria of classification are concerned, the study (Veronesi et al. 1982) confirmed that the prognosis of stage I melanoma patients is related both to level of invasion and maximal tumor thickness. However, elective node dissection did not improve the survival of any subgroup, as shown in Tables 9 and 10 and Figs. 5 and 6.

The preliminary results of a prospective, randomized clinical trial at the Mayo Clinic (Sim et al. 1978) confirm that there is no difference in survival of patients with stage I melanoma, whether immediate (i.e., prophylactic), or delayed (i.e., therapeutic) node dissection is performed. These studies provide convincing evidence that prophylactic node dissection has not proven to be of value in the treatment of patients with stage I melanoma since it does not improve survival, and its usefulness as a staging procedure has not yet been determined since recent reports have not confirmed the efficacy of adjuvant chemotherapy or immunotherapy (Cascinelli et al. 1983b). Finally, it should not be forgotten that a radical lymph node dissection is not a minor surgical

Table 9. Five- and ten-year survival according to treatment and clinical findings

Criteria	Immediate dissection			Delayed dissection (if needed)			P
	Patients (n)	5 years (%)	10 years (%)	Patients (n)	5 years (%)	10 years (%)	
Sex							
Male	57	70.9	54.8	46	58.3	50.8	0.76
Female	210	74.2	63.2	240	74.4	65.0	0.38
Age							
⩽47	138	75.2	66.2	133	78.4	69.7	0.41
⩾48	129	71.6	55.1	153	66.3	56.7	0.50
Previous treatment							
Untreated	237	72.7	59.4	253	71.8	61.9	0.33
Biopsy	30	80.0	76.7	33	72.7	69.8	0.92
Site							
Upper limbs	52	67.0	55.4	43	78.8	73.9	0.31
Lower limbs	215	75.0	62.8	243	77.0	60.9	0.99
Maximal diameter (cm)							
⩽1.5	139	80.1	68.3	163	80.0	68.9	0.30
⩾1.5	98	61.9	46.3	90	56.5	48.5	0.86
Elevation (mm)							
1–5	139	82.4	69.3	159	77.5	67.3	0.80
⩾6	98	58.4	44.2	94	61.7	52.0	0.46
Satellite nodules							
Present	17	47.1	41.2	14	54.0	46.3	0.52
Absent	220	75.0	62.3	239	73.1	62.6	0.61

Table 10. Five- and ten-year survival according to type of treatment and Breslow clusters of thickness

Maximal thickness (mm)	Immediate dissection			Delayed dissection (if needed)			P
	Patients (n)	5 years (%)	10 years (%)	Patients (n)	5 years (%)	10 years (%)	
0–0.9	18	94.4	88.5	23	100	94.6	0.18
1–1.9	37	94.6	74.8	37	97.3	86.5	0.05
2–2.9	45	71.1	57.4	28	67.9	52.7	0.80
3–3.9	26	87.0	72.4	41	68.2	55.4	0.55
⩾4	55	50.7	38.4	52	48.6	44.0	0.75

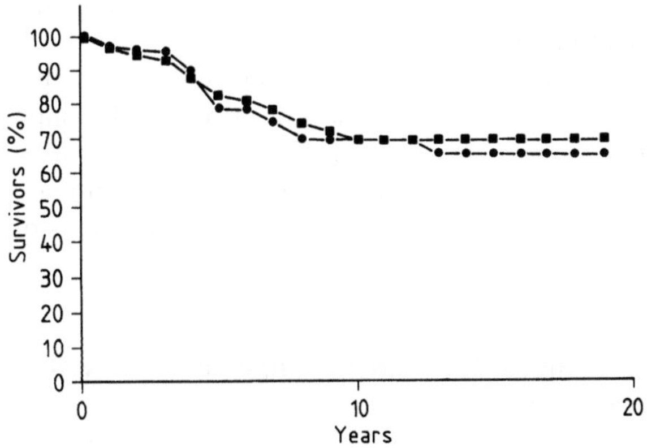

Fig. 5. Survival of 90 stage I patients according to treatment (Clark's level III). *Squares*, delayed dissection (50 patients); *diamonds*, immediate dissection (45 patients)

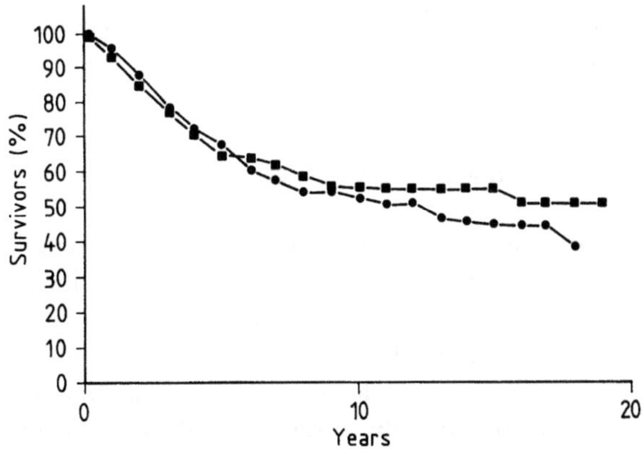

Fig. 6. Survival of 217 stage I patients according to treatment (Clark's level IV). *Squares*, delayed dissection (103 patients); *diamonds*, immediate dissection (114 patients)

procedure. The incidence of postoperative complications is not negligible. Groin dissections result in more complications than axillary or neck dissections. In a recent review, Papachristou and Fortner (1977) reported lymph edema of the lower extremities in 80% of patients. One may wonder whether the results obtained in the prospective study, which included only melanoma of the extremities, may be applicable to melanomas of the whole skin surface of the head and neck or trunk. In principle, there are no essential biological reasons for melanomas at other sites to behave differently. Moreover, in the trunk, lymphatic drainage is somewhat variable, and, in some cases, it is difficult to identify which lymph node group will be involved first. As far as face and scalp are concerned, there are a number of lymph node groups with so many connections that it is sometimes difficult to establish anatomical limits for regional lymph node dissection. In addition, radical cervical lymph node dissections (submandibular, superficial, and deep laterocervical and supraclavicular, in some instances associated with parotidectomy) involve such severe mutilation that one can hardly recommend this procedure in the absence of clinically detectable lymph node metastases.

In conclusion, we believe that elective regional node dissection is indicated in selected cases of clinical stage I malignant melanoma of the skin. The surgeon ought to perform it when the quarterly follow-up is dubious. The risk is that the patient, if not followed up closely, may return with nonresectable lymph node metastases. Other situations in which prophylactic node dissection may be considered are: (a) when malignant melanoma originates in the skin covering a lymph node basin, since the postoperative changes following excision of the primary melanoma may complicate the clinical evaluation of the lymph nodes; (b) when the primary melanoma is classified as level V, in which case, prophylactic dissection of regional lymph nodes seems to increase the chances of cure.

Surgery for Local Tumor Recurrence

Local recurrence of a malignant melanoma is generally defined as a relapse of the disease at the site of the primary tumor following its excision, or in a small area (usually 5 cm in diameter) around it. When melanoma recurs locally as a single cutaneous or subcutaneous nodule, surgery is indicated as the treatment of choice. The incidence is relatively low in clinical stage I (2% in our experience) (Cascinelli et al. 1980), but in stage II, it occurs more frequently. Fortner et al. (1972) reported on 30 cases of locally recurrent melanoma treated at Memorial Hospital. Of the 30 patients, 23 were initially treated elsewhere, in most instances with inadequate surgery. In the register of the WHO Melanoma Program, of 2006 surgically treated patients, 48 had local recurrences. It is interesting to note that 26 of these patients suffered a relapse during the first 3 years.

It is difficult to define strict guidelines for the surgical treatment of local recurrences. In the experience of the WHO Group and the Memorial Hospital (Fortner et al. 1975), treatment varied from simple excision, to wide excision and regional node dissection, and to major amputations. It seems reasonable to advocate wide excision of skin recurrences with margins similar to those usually applied to primary lesions. Regional lymph nodes, even if clinically uninvolved, may be dissected.

In selected cases with bulky recurrences in the extremities, or multiple in-transit metastases, or with involvement of nerves and/or major blood vessels, major amputative surgery, i.e., shoulder or interscapulothoracic amputation for upper extremities and hip disarticulation for lower limbs, may be indicated. Needless to say, every effort should be made to exclude the presence of distant metastases. Although in most cases this type of surgery is only palliative, the quality of palliation is generally good, and long-term survival may be observed.

Reductive Surgery for Distant Metastases

Surgery may be indicated in patients with symptomatic distant metastases. A not uncommon indication is bowel obstruction. In other cases, surgical excision of a single distant metastasis following a long disease-free interval after treatment of a primary lesion, e.g., a single lung or brain metastasis, may result in long-term survival, and such patients should be considered surgical candidates.

A debulking operation may be indicated in patients with superficial disease (superficial lymph nodes, subcutaneous metastases) before instituting chemotherapy or immunotherapy, even though there is no solid evidence that such reductive surgery is of definite value in such cases.

Treatment of "In-Transit" Regional Non-Nodal Metastases

The treatment of choice for the regional non-nodal metastases (Cascinelli et al. 1986a) of melanoma located at a limb is hyperthermic antiblastic perfusion:

the rate of complete regression after perfusion is 56% (Vaglini et al. 1986). Treatment is based upon three considerations: (a) neoplastic cells are more sensible to heat than normal cells; (b) the therapeutic efficacy of a chemotherapy dose ten times more than the normal one is much more remarkable; and (c) antineoplastic effect of heat and drugs is sinergic.

Therapy may be performed by previously isolating the external iliac tributary arterial and venous vessels of the limb: the axillary vessels are canulated for the upper limb, and the external iliac vessels are canulated for the lower limb. Blood circulation in the isolated limb is guaranteed by an external pump with an oxigenator and heating system. The most commonly used drug is melphalan which is administered at a dose of 1.5 mg/kg body weight. A temperature of 41 °C is reached and maintained for 1 h. Experimental bases for this therapeutic method were published by Cavaliere et al. in 1981, and a review of the world experience was published in 1986 by Krementz. Our experience of our institute has been published by Vaglini et al. (1982, 1983, 1985a, 1985b, 1987).

Acknowledgement. The present paper has been supported by the Associazione Italiana per la Ricerca sul Cancro and in cooperation with the Lega Italiana per la Lotta contro i Tumori – Sezione Milanese.

References

Ackerman LU, del Regato JA (1954) Cancer diagnosis treatment and prognosis. Mosby, St. Louis, pp 184–197

Ackerman AB, Mihara I (1985) Dysplasia, dysplastic melanocytes, dysplastic nevi, the dysplastic nevus syndrome and the relation between dysplastic nevi and malignant melanoma. Hum Pathol 161: 87–91

Anaise D, Steinz R, Nahum Ben Hur (1978) Solar radiation: a possible etiological factor in malignant melanoma in Israel (a retrospective study 1960–1972). Cancer 42: 299

Balch CM, Milton GW (eds) (1984) Cutaneous melanoma – clinical management and treatment results worldwide. Lippincott, Philadelphia

Balch CM, Milton GW, Cascinelli N, Sim F (1984) Elective lymph node dissection: pros and cons. In: Balch CM, Milton GW (eds) Cutaneous melanoma – clinical management and treatment results worldwide. Lippincott, Philadelphia, pp 131–157

Beral V, Ramcharan S, Faris R (1977) Malignant melanoma and oral contraceptive use among women in California. Br J Cancer 36: 804

Bodenham DC (1968) Study of 650 observed malignant melanomas in south-west region. Ann Coll Surg Engl 43: 218–239

Breslow A (1970) Thickness, cross-sectional areas and depth of invasion in the prognosis of cutaneous melanoma. Ann Surg 172: 902–908

Breslow A (1975) Tumor thickness, level of invasion, and node dissection in stage I cutaneous melanoma. Ann Surg 182: 572

Breslow A, Macht SD (1977) Optimal size of resection margin for thin cutaneous melanoma. Surg Gynecol Obstet 145: 691

Breslow A, Cascinelli N, van der Esch EP, Morabito A (1978) Stage I melanoma of the limbs: assessment of prognosis by levels of invasion and maximum thickness. Tumori 64: 273

Brocker EB, Kolde G, Steinhausen D, Peters A, Macher E (1984) The pattern of the mononuclear infiltrate as a prognostic parameter in flat superficial spreading melanomas. J Cancer Res Clin Oncol 107: 48–52

Cascinelli N (1983) La luce solare (radiazione ultravioletta): un fattore eziologico reale o immaginario del melanoma cutaneo? Argomenti Oncol 4: 85–98

Cascinelli N, van der Esch EP, Breslow A, Morabito A, Bufalino R (1980) Stage I melanoma of the skin: the problem of resection margins. Eur J Cancer 16: 1079–1085

Cascinelli N, Preda F, Vaglini M, Orefice S, Bufalino R, Morabito A, Nava M, Santinami M (1983a) Metastatic spread of stage I melanoma of the skin. Tumori 69: 449

Cascinelli N, Bajetta E, Vaglini M, Buzzoni R, Nava M (1983b) Present status and future perspectives of adjuvant treatment of cutaneous malignant melanoma. Pigment Cell 6: 187–198

Cascinelli N, Vaglini M, Nava M, Santinami M, Marolda R, Rovini D, Clemente C, Bufalino R, Morabito A (1984) Prognosis of skin melanoma with regional node metastases (stage II). J Surg Oncol 25: 240–247

Cascinelli N, Marubini E, Morabito A, Bufalino R (1985) Prognostic factors for stage I melanoma of the skin: a review. Stat Med 4: 265–278

Cascinelli N, Bufalino R, Marolda R, Belli F, Nava M, Galluzzo D, Santinami M, Levene A (1986a) Regional non-nodal metastases of cutaneous melanoma. Eur J Surg Oncol 12(2): 175–180

Cascinelli N, Vaglini M, Bufalino R, Morabito A (1986b) BANS – a cutaneous region with no prognostic significance in patients with melanoma. Cancer 57(3): 441–444

Cascinelli N, Santinami M, Urist MM, Holmstrom H (1987) Indications for management of primary. In: Veronesi U, Cascinelli N, Santinami M (eds) Cutaneous melanoma – status of knowledge and future perspective. Academic, London

Cavaliere R, Mondovi B, Moricca G (1981) Trattamento ipertermico dei tumori: basi biochimice, applicazioni sperimentali, risultati clinici. In: Bistolfi F (ed) L'ipertermia in terapia oncologica. Piccin, Padova

Clark WH Jr (1967) A classification of malignant melanoma in man correlated with histogenesis and biological behavior. In: Montagna W, Hu F (eds) Advances in biology of the skin. The pigmentary system, vol 8. Pergamon, London, pp 621–645

Clark WH Jr, From L, Bernardino EA, Mihm MC (1969) The histogenesis and biologic behaviour of primary human malignant melanomas of the skin. Cancer Res 29: 705–726

Clark WH Jr, Elder DE, Dupont Guerry IV, Epstein MN, Greene MH, van Horn M (1984) A study of tumor progression: the precursor lesions of superficial spreading and nodular melanoma. Hum Pathol 15: 1147–1165

Clemente C (1985) Immunohistochemical reactivity of the antimelanoma monoclonal antibody Mel-1. Tumori 71: 225–232

Clemente C, Pilotti S, Cattaneo M, Rilke F (1981) Valutazione statistica della diagnosi istopatologica intraoperatoria su sezioni al microtomo criostato. Pathologica 73: 561–578

Cochran AJ, Duan-Ren Wan (1985) S-100 protein as a marker for melanocytic and other tumours. Pathology 17: 340–345

Cohen MH, Schour L, Felix EL, Bernstein AD, Chretien PB, Rosenberg SA, Ketcham AS (1975) Staging laparotomy in the treatment of metastatic melanoma of lower extremities. Ann Surg 182: 710

Cook MG, Robertson I (1985) Melanocytic dysplasia and melanoma. Histopathology 9: 617–658

Cooper PH, Wanebo HJ, Hagar RW (1985) Regression in thin malignant melanoma, microscopic diagnosis and prognostic importance. Arch Dermatol 12(9): 1127–1131

Costa A, Silvestrini R, Cascinelli N, Attili A, Testori A (1985) Cell kinetics of human malignant melanoma: basic studies and potential clinical prospectives (Abstr 68). 1st International Conference on Skin Melanoma, Venice

Day CL, Harris TJ, Gorstein F, et al. (1981) Malignant melanoma: prognostic significance of "microscopic satellites" in the reticular dermis and subcutaneous fat. Ann Surg 194: 108–112

Day CL Jr, Mihm MC, Sober AJ, et al. (1982) Prognostic factors for melanoma patients with lesions 0.76–1.69 mm in thickness. An appraisal of "thin" level IV lesions. Ann Surg 195: 30–34

Elder DE (1985) The dysplastic nevus. Pathology 17: 291–297

Elwood JM, Gallagher RP, Hill GB, Pearson JCG (1985) Cutaneous melanoma in relation to intermittent and constant sun exposure – the Western Canada melanoma study. Int J Cancer 35: 427–433

Epstein JH, Epstein WL, Nakai T (1967) Production of melanomas from DMBA-induced "blue nevi" in hairless mice with ultraviolet light. JNCI 38: 19

Fortner JG, MacLean B, Mulcare RJ (1972) Treatment of recurrent malignant melanoma. In: McCarthy WH (ed) Melanoma and skin cancer. Blight, Sydney, p 453

Fortner JG, Schottenfeld D, MacLean BJ (1975) En bloc resection or primary melanoma with regional lymph node dissection. Arch Surg 110: 674

Friedman RJ, Heilman ER, Rigel DS, Kopf AW (1985) The dysplastic nevus. Clinical and pathologic features. Dermatol Clin 3(2): 239

Gatter KC, Ralfkiaer E, Skinner J, Brown D, Heryet A, Pulford KA, Hou-Jensen K, Mason DY (1985) An immunocytochemical study of malignant melanoma and its differential diagnosis from other malignant tumours. J Clin Pathol 38(12): 1353–1357

Green AC, O'Rourke MGE (1985) Cutaneous malignant melanoma in association with other skin cancers. JNCI 74: 977–980

Greene MH, Clark WH, Tucker MA, Elder DE, Kraemer KH, DuPont Guerry IV, et al. (1985) Current concepts. Acquired precursors of cutaneous malignant melanoma. The familial dysplastic nevus syndrome. N Engl J Med 312(2): 91–115

Gromet MA, Epstein WL, Blois MS (1978) The regressing thin malignant melanoma. A distinctive lesson with metastatic potential. Cancer 42: 2282–2292

Gupta SK, Rajwanshi AK, Das DK (1985) Fine needle aspiration cytology smear patterns of malignant melanoma. Acta Cytol (Baltimore) 29: 983–988

Holman CDJ, Mulroney CD, Armstrong BK (1980) Epidemiology of pre-invasive and invasive malignant melanoma in western Australia. Int J Cancer 25: 95

Holman CDJ, Armstrong BK, Heenan PJ (1986) Relationship of cutaneous malignant melanoma to individual sunlight-exposure habits. J Natl Cancer Inst 76: 403–414

Kelly JW, Sagebiel RW, Clyman S, Blois MS (1985) Thin level IV malignant melanoma. A subset in which level is the major prognostic indicator. Ann Surg 20: 98–103

Krementz ET (1986) Regional perfusion. Current sophistication, what next? Cancer 57: 416–432

Kripke ML (1979) Speculations on the role of ultraviolet radiation in the development of malignant melanoma. JNCI 63(3): 541

Lancaster HO, Nelson JI (1957) Sunlight as a cause of melanoma. A clinical survey. Aust Med J 1: 452

Lee JAH (1972) Sunlight and the etiology of malignant melanoma. In: McCarthy WH (ed) Melanoma and skin cancer. Blight, Sydney, pp 83–94

Lee JAH (1982) Melanoma and exposure to sunlight. Epidemiol Rev 4: 110–134

Magnus K (1977) Incidence of malignant melanoma of the skin in the five Nordic countries: significance of solar radiation. Int J Cancer 20: 477

McGovern VJ (1970) The classification of melanoma and its relationship with prognosis. Pathology 2: 85–98

McGovern VJ, Murad TQ (1985) Pathology of melanoma: an overview. In: Balch CM, Milton GW (eds) Cutaneous melanoma. Clinical management and treatment results worldwide. Lippincott, Philadelphia, pp 29–53

McGovern VJ, Shaw HM, Milton GW, McCarthy WH (1982) Ulceration and prognosis in cutaneous malignant melanoma. Histopathology 6: 399–407

McGovern VJ, Mihm MC, Bailly C, Booth JC, Clark WH Jr, Cochran AH, Hardy EG, Hicks JD, Levene A, Lewis MG, Little JH, Milton GW (1973) The classification of malignant melanoma and its histologic reporting. Cancer 32: 1446–1457

McGovern VJ, Cochran AJ, van der Esch EP, Little JH, MacLennan R (1986) The classification of malignant melanoma, its histological reporting and registration: a revision of the 1972 Sydney classification. Pathology 18: 12–21

Olsen G (1972) Surgical treatment of primary melanoma: some views of the sites and depth of excision. In: McCarthy WH (ed) Melanoma and skin cancer. Blight, Sydney, p 389

Papachristou D, Fortner JG (1977) Comparison of lymph-edema following in-continuity and discontinuity groin dissection. Ann Surg 185: 13

Pellegris G, Illeni MT, Vaglini M, Rovini D, Cascinelli N, Masserini C (1980) HLA antigens in malignant melanoma patients. Tumori 66: 51

Prade M, Sancho-Garnier H, Cesarini JP, et al. (1980) Difficulties encountered in the application of the Clark classification and Breslow thickness measurement in cutaneous malignant melanoma. Int J Cancer 26: 159–163

Privitera E, Ghidoni A, Raimondi E, Rovini D, Illeni MT, Cascinelli N (1985) Sister chromatid exchange and proliferation pattern in stimulated lymphocytes of cutaneous malignant melanoma patients. Cancer Genet Cytogenet 15: 37–45

Reed KM, Bronstein BR, Mihm MC Jr, Sober AJ (1986) Prognosis for polypoidal melanoma is determined by primary tumor thickness. Cancer 57: 1201–1203

Rigel DS, Friedman RJ, Kopf AW, Rogers GS, Heilman ER (1985) Precursors of malignant melanoma. Problems in computing the risk of malignant melanoma arising in dysplastic and congenital nevocytic nevi. Dermatol Clin 3(2): 361

Sagebiel RW, Chinn EK, Egbert BM (1984) Pigmented spindle cell nevus. Clinical and histologic review of 90 cases. Am J Surg Pathol 8(9): 645–653

Sim FH, Taylor WF, Ivins JC, Pritchard DJ, Soule EH (1978) A prospective randomized study of the efficacy of routine

elective lymphadenectomy in management of malignant melanoma. Preliminary results. Cancer 41: 948
Southwick HW (1976) Malignant melanoma: role of node dissection reappraised. Cancer 37: 202
Teppo L, Pukkala E, Hakama M (1980) Way of life and cancer incidence in Finland. Scand J Soc Med [Suppl] 19: 50
Vaglini M, Rovini D, Prada A, Nava M, Santinami M, Ammatuna M, Cascinelli N (1982) Le perfusioni ipertermico antiblastiche degli arti in circolazione extracorporea, meccanica e fisiopatologia. Arg Oncologia 3: 329–337
Vaglini M, Ammatuna M, Nava M, Prada A, Rovini D, Santinami M, Cascinelli N (1983) Regional perfusion at high temperature (42.5°–43°) in treatment of stage IIIA–IIIB melanoma patients. Tumori 69: 585–588
Vaglini M, Andreola S, Attili A, Belli F, Marolda R, Nava M, Prada A, Santinami M, Cascinelli N (1985a) Limb-salvage procedure in two patients with spindle cell carcinoma of the lower extremities using isolation perfusion. Tumori 71: 271–275
Vaglini M, Andreola S, Attili A, Belli F, Marolda R, Nava M, Prada A, Santinami M, Cascinelli N (1985b) Hyperthermic antiblastic perfusion in the treatment of cancer of the extremities. Tumori 71: 355–359
Vaglini M, Santinami M, Nava M, Belli F, Prada A, Ammatuna M, Cascinelli N (1986) Hyperthermic antiblastic perfusion in extracorporeal circulation: surgical technique and results in the treatment of extremities' tumor. The Journal of Extracorporeal Technology 18: 12–20
Vaglini M, Belli F, Marolda R, Prada A, Santinami M, Cascinelli N (1987) Hyperthermic antiblastic perfusion with DTIC in stage IIIA–IIIB melanoma of the extremities. Eur J Surg Oncol 13: 127–129
Van der Esch EP, Cascinelli N, Preda F, Morabito A, Bufalino R (1981) Stage I melanoma of the skin: evaluation of prognosis according to histologic characteristics. Cancer 48(7): 1668–1673
Van Duinen SG, Ruiter DJ, Hageman P, Vennegoor C, Dickersin R, Scheffer E, Rumke P (1984) Immunohistochemical and histochemical tools in the diagnosis of amelanotic melanoma. Cancer 53: 1566–1573
Veronesi U, Cascinelli N (1979) Surgical treatment of malignant melanoma of the skin. World J Surg 3: 279–288
Veronesi U, Cascinelli N, Balzarini GP, et al. (1972) Treatment of regional node metastases. In: McCarthy WH (ed) Melanoma and skin cancer. Blight, Sydney, p 417
Veronesi U, Adamus J, Bandiera DC, Brennhovd IO, Caceres E, Cascinelli N, Claudio F, et al. (1977) Inefficacy of immediate node dissection in stage I melanoma of the limbs. N Engl J Med 297: 627
Veronesi U, Bajetta E, Cascinelli N, Clemente C, Rilke F (1978) New trends in the treatment of malignant melanoma. In: Murphy GP (ed) International advances in surgical oncology, vol 1. Liss, New York, pp 113–156
Veronesi U, Adamus J, Bandiera DC, Brennhovd IO, Caceres E, Cascinelli N (1980) Stage I melanoma of the limbs. Immediate versus delayed node dissection. Tumori 66: 373–396
Veronesi U, Adamus J, Bandiera D, Brennhovd IO, Caceres E, Cascinelli N, et al. (1982) Delayed regional lymph node dissection in stage I melanoma of the skin of the lower extremities. Cancer 49(11): 2420–2430
Wanebo HJ, Fortner JG, Woodruff J, MacLean B, Binkowski E (1975) Selection of optimum surgical treatment of stage I melanoma by depth of microinvasion: use of the continued microstage technique (Clark-Breslow). Ann Surg 182: 302
Wards Hinds M, Laurence N, Kolonel (1980) Malignant melanoma of the skin in Hawaii, 1960–1977. Cancer 45: 811
Waterhouse J, Shanmugaratnam K, Muir C, Powell J (eds) (1982) Cancer incidence in five continents, vol 4. IARC Sci Publ 42

Cancer in Childhood – Solid Tumours

J. PLASCHKES

Introduction

Treatment of cancer in childhood has made enormous progress over the last 30 years. The strategies developed for leukaemia have also had a great impact on the management and treatment results of most solid tumours (Farber 1966). So far at least, somewhat paradoxically, the more effective other forms of treatment have become, the greater is the scope and role of surgery. *Ultimate surgical resection* still remains one of the most important prognostic factors and effective means of complete eradication of disease. The surgeon still has a central role in determining the outcome of children with solid tumours.

The improved results of treatment in children over the years have been far more spectacular than those achieved in adults. The reasons are not always obvious, but some of the different explanations are summarised in Table 1. Paediatric oncology groups were formed early on (see Appendix A), with cooperative studies now being the rule rather than the exception.

Table 1. Attributes of paediatric as opposed to adult tumours

Histology	- Embryonal and sarcomas, not carcinomas
Carcinogenic agents	- Not much in evidence
Genetic factors	- Important
Spontaneous regression	- Well known
Response to drugs	- Often good
Prognostic factors	- Relevant
Outcome	- > 50% Curable

Table 2. Relative incidence of pediatric malignancy in population < 15 years of age (about 100–150 per million/year)

	(%)
Leukaemia	20–30
CNS tumours	15–20
Lymphomas	10
Neuroblastoma	6– 8
Nephroblastoma	6– 7
Rhabdomyosarcoma	4– 5
Bone	4– 5
Germ cell tumours	4
Retinoblastoma	2– 3
Hepatoblastoma	1– 2
Histiocytosis	1– 2
Others	

It should also be noted that most paediatric tumours peak at a specific age so that, for instance, neuroblastoma, which peaks at about 2, is the most common tumour under the age of 1.

The main aim of this chapter is to provide the interested surgeon, whatever his surgical speciality, with up-to-date information to enable him to understand the principles involved in order to rationally treat children with malignant solid tumours within a multidisciplinary framework. Controversial issues are not avoided. *Surgical techniques* will only be mentioned if they differ from those used in adults.

A presentation system has been devised in which the *common specific paediatric tumours and their surgical implications* are initially discussed in more detail, followed by a brief mention of other tumours occurring in the same organ. Age is also considered, in that rarer adult-type carcinomas occurring in children, and those tumours most likely to occur in the 'pubertal' age or in neonates are each discussed separately. In this way, pride of place is given to the clinically significant tumours, yet "small print" examples can also be included.

No chemotherapy schedules or radiation dosages are given. The principal staging systems used appear separately (see Appendix B).

One cannot neglect to mention some of the more exciting discoveries being made in the basic sciences, in particular molecular biology. The discovery of oncogenes is already seeing clinical application (Brodeur et al. 1984).

General Aspects

Epidemiology and Aetiology

Incidence and Distribution

Death from cancer in children was, before the modern therapeutic era (apart from in the neonatal period), second only to mortality from trauma in most developed countries. The spectrum of malignancy is quite different and 100–200 times less frequent than in adults. The *incidence* of cancer up to the age of 15 is about 100–150 per 1 million population children/year (Table 2) (Young and Miller 1975; Draper et al. 1982). There are, with some exceptions, surprisingly small significant differences in various parts of the world.

Aetiology

Environmental factors and external *carcinogenic agents* are not of great significance in paediatric tumours. However, a recent interesting example is adenocarcinoma of the vagina and, rarely, cervix in young girls whose mothers were given diethyl stilboestrol during pregnancy (Herbst et al. 1971). Another is the occurrence of neuroblastoma in foetal hydantoin syndrome (Ehrenbard and Chaganti 1981). *The most potent carcinogenic agents may turn out to be some of the treatments themselves*, with the increasing appearance of second tumours in children cured of a primary (Meadows et al. 1985; Hawkins et al. 1987). It is estimated that by 1990 one in 1000 adults aged 20 will have been cured of a paediatric cancer. Surgery has no carcinogenic potential and, if it can help to minimise chemo- or radiotherapy, should always be considered from this point of view.

Genetic factors in the broadest sense are far more germane to the understanding of paediatric tumours. In general, solid tumours are more associated with deletions, and the leukaemias and lymphomas with translocations. Familial cancers have been known for some time. Different combinations such as retinoblastoma with osteosarcoma have also been recognised. An association between children with soft-tissue sarcomas and their mothers who have a higher incidence of breast cancer is intriguing (Birch et al. 1984).

The other clear genetic examples are the cancer malformation syndromes, e.g. the Beckwith-Wiedemann syndrome; Wilms' tumour, macroglossia, hemihypertrophy and visceromegaly (Beckwith 1983). There are many others. A strict distinction between environmental and genetic factors is somewhat arbitrary within the concept of *ecogenetics*, "The study of heritable variations in response to environmental agents" (Mulvihill 1985). Paediatric tumours are ideal models for these types of studies.

Prognostic Factors

The relevance of prognostic factors increases in proportion to the survival rate. With many of the toxic treatments achieving cure rates of well over 50%, it is important to identify the tumours that are "good actors" from the "bad ones", so as not to overtreat those with a good prognosis and maybe intensify the treatment of the poor ones. This state of affairs has already been achieved in many paediatric tumours and "customised" treatment is often the rule (see Fig. 1). For clinical purposes the practical prognostic variables are: site, histology, natural history, stage and markers.

Site

The resectability of a tumour is largely dependent on its site and size, and often the single most important prognostic factor in localised disease. There are, however, not infrequently in paediatric oncology, some paradoxical exceptions (see Rhabdomyosarcoma, Neuroblastoma, Germ Cell Tumours) with which the surgeon should be familiar and which could influence the choice and extent of the operative procedure.

Histology

Prognostically favourable and unfavourable histological variants have been identified in many children's tumours (see Wilms' Tumour, Rhabdomyosarcoma).

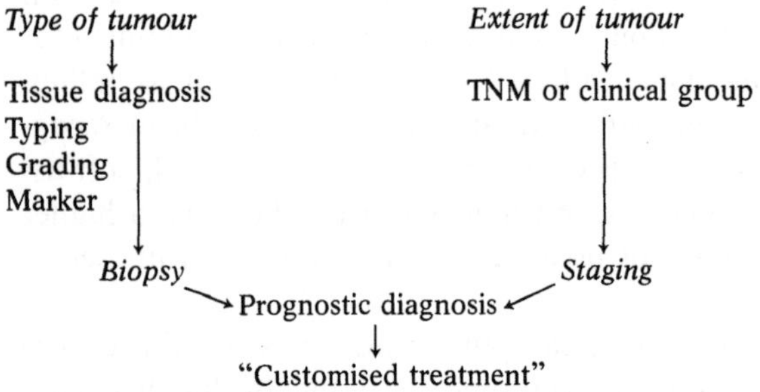

Fig. 1. Customised treatment

Natural History

Age

Age has clear prognostic significance. Children under the age of 1 often have a better prognosis. Neuroblastoma is the best example, congenital fibrosarcoma another. Brain tumours are the exception here. *Neonatal tumours* frequently behave better than the histology would suggest.

Staging

Surgery

Surgery is the most accurate, if not always the most appropriate means of staging. Assessing lymph node involvement (N), particularly abdominal and retroperitoneal, is quite inaccurate in children by any other means. Metastases (M) (lung, bones, liver) are more often appropriately assessed by the many new and sophisticated imaging techniques. Exact numbers and sites of lymph nodes are less crucial if there is effective chemotherapy. Appendix B gives details of some of the most used staging systems for the tumours commonly encountered in paediatric oncology.

Markers

Many markers – biochemical (enzyme and hormone markers), immunological (cell surface antigens and receptors), genetic (oncogene markers), etc. – are now being used prognostically in many paediatric tumours. Fresh untreated tumour tissue obtained at the initial biopsy is often required, and the surgeon must be aware of the importance of his contribution.

Biopsy

The main advantage of a "closed" biopsy (needle, fine needle, etc.) is that it can be done under local anaesthesia on an outpatient basis. In children this advantage cannot usually be utilised since the fear induced, even if disproportionate to the actual pain, makes some form of general anaesthesia desirable. Thus, with some exceptions (at very inaccessible sites), an open incisional or excisional biopsy is the method of choice. In paediatric oncology there is an increasing trend to more *conservative organ-preserving surgery* so that the location of the biopsy site is extremely important and must always lie in the region of the part to be excised later and should always be done by the surgeon likely to carry out the definitive operation. The concept of customised treatment according to the prognosis can be represented diagramatically (Fig. 1).

Surgery in Treatment

Definitive Operation

The main objective of curative surgical treatment is always total excision of all tumour. Fortunately, with the good response to chemotherapy in many paediatric tumours, it has become possible to reduce their size and make the surgery less "extensive" without jeopardising survival. More differentiated surgery can be performed *preserving organs and limbs*. Two sites are emminently suitable for this type of surgery – the limbs and the urogential tract. The type of surgery after pretreatment is known as "second look" or "delayed primary surgery" and is useful in the following situations:

1. Tumour too large for primary radical excision, e.g. hepatoblastoma
2. Tumour with risk of rupture because of size and consistency, e.g. large Wilms' tumour
3. Tumour invading or close to vital structure
4. Primary resection would involve major loss of function, e.g. limbs, bladder, head and neck region
5. Restaging

Table 3 shows the indications for second-look surgery. It represents only a simplified guide with much depending on surgical judgement. It should also be clear that many indications are relative to the efficacy and toxicity of the preoperative treatment and many change accordingly. This approach has been one of the most *fundamental changes* in the *surgical strategy* for paediatric solid tumours (Grosfeld et al. 1978).

Debulking

Reducing the bulk of a tumour to enhance other forms of treatment has lost much of its original appeal (see Neuroblastoma; Koop 1972) and is rarely practised except out of necessity (respiratory embarrassment, obstruction, compression of vital structures).

Metastatic Disease

Metastatic disease in the lungs can often be treated surgically very successfully. Children tolerate repeated or bilateral thoracotomies (simultaneous or sequential) very well (Baldy et al. 1984; Hazebrooek 1979).

Specific Paediatric Tumours

Abdomen and Retroperitoneum

Nephroblastoma Variants – Kidney

Nephroblastoma represents the gold standard of the advances achieved in paediatric oncology. From a survival rate of only about 20%–40% with surgery

Table 3. Indications for primary versus delayed surgery

Tumour	Primary surgery[a]	Delayed Surgery[a]
Brain	All	No established role
Retinoblastoma	Unilateral	Bilateral
Nephroblastoma	All stages	Very large and bilateral
Neuroblastoma	Stages I and II	Stages III and IV
Hepatoblastoma	Surgically easy	Surgically difficult
Rhabdomyosarcoma	Dependent on site and size	
Limb	Few	Majority
Head and neck	Superficial small lesions	Majority
Parameningeal	Usually no surgery	
Orbital	Usually no surgery	
Genitourinary	Small size, special sites	Majority
Others[a]		
Non-Rhabdo Soft-tissue sarcoma	Majority	Few
Ewing's sarcoma[a]	Small size	Majority
Osteosarcoma[a]	Unresponsive to chemotherapy	Majority
Non Hodgkin's lymphoma		
Abdominal	Localised	Disseminated
Mediastinal	Usually no surgery	

[a] See individual tumour section for details.

and radiotherapy alone in the 1940s, 90% can now be achieved in many instances with the progressive evolution of the first national and international trials (NWTS 1969, MRC 1970, SIOP 1971). Most (about 90%) of the tumours still fit the classical description by Wilms in 1899.

Histology. Histologically they consist of blastomatous, stromal and epithelial elements. The remainder are *variants* of nephroblastoma.

Prognostic Factors. In about 5%, *unfavourable prognostic entities* have been identified. One of these shows anaplasia (either focal or generalised).

Others with an unfavourable outcome are (a) *clear cell sarcoma* – often metastasing to bone (Marsden et al. 1980); (b) *rhabdoid tumour* (resembling rhabdomyoblasts but without any striations) – often metastasing to brain (Beckwith 1983). Both are now considered as separate entities. The tumours with especially *favourable* prognosis are *multicystic nephroblastoma* (see Fig. 2) and *"congenital" mesoblastic nephroma.* Both can usually be cured by surgery alone. About 7% of Wilms' tumours are bilateral. The prognosis is relatively good, that of the synchronous type being better than that of the metachronous. The histology need not be the same on each side. The bilateral forms, as well as some of the variants, can, to some extent, be explained by the nephroblastomatosis complex (Machin 1980). Association with *congenital malformations* have already been mentioned (Pendergrass 1976).

In siblings the risk of tumour of the simple type (unilateral, without malformations) is small.

Diagnosis. The discovery of a lump in the abdomen usually leads to diagnosis. *Haematuria* is a relatively rare presenting symptom occurring in only about one-third of cases, and a *varicocele* may indicate renal vein involvement. Extension into the vena cava is not uncommon and can nowadays be demonstrated as accurately on ultrasound as on venography. The prognosis with vena cava involvement in the NWTS trial is not particularly poor, as one might expect (d'Angio et al. 1981). Arteriography is unnecessary except in bilateral tumours where partial nephrectomy is envisaged. Cystoscopy is not practised by most surgeons since ureteric involvement and seeding is extremely rare (Stevens and Eckstein 1976).

Treatment. The treatment strategy should, with some exceptions, be primary surgical excision (no biopsy is usually necessary) followed by adjuvant chemotherapy with or without radiotherapy, depending on the stage and histology. Stage I favourable histology does not require radiotherapy. Unfavourable histology (all stages) requires additional radiotherapy. Radical lymph node dissection is not necessary as treatment, but generous sampling to detect occult spread must be done. The exceptions to primary surgery are unusually large (for the surgeon to decide): unilateral tumours and most bilateral ones. In all fairness it must be said that *many children in Europe are treated with preoperative therapy as a deliberate strategy according to SIOP protocols* and delayed surgery with equally good survival rates. The reason given for this strategy is the lower incidence of rupture in one of the trials (Lemerle et al. 1983).

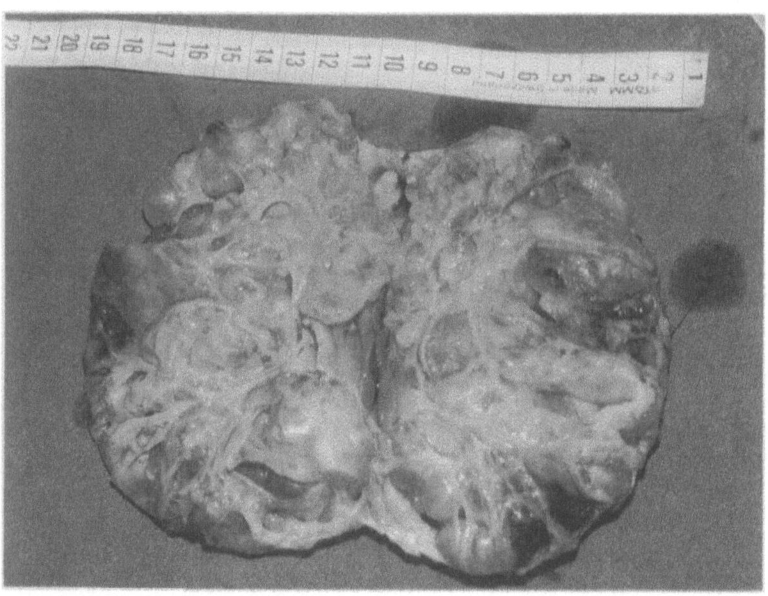

Fig. 2. Atypical rare multicystic Wilms' tumour with good prognosis

In *surgery* approach must be transabdominal through a large (transverse) incision. Although it is advisable to deal with the vascular pedicle of the side involved and also to inspect the contralateral kidney by complete exposure first, this is not essential if the size and location of the primary tumour makes it hazardous. Renal vein and vena caval involvement is common and must be recognised. It can often be dealt with adequately by clamping above the "thrombus" and sucking out the "floating" tumour. Bypass procedures are rarely needed. Adjacent structures which are involved should, in principle, be resected en bloc (e.g. colon, adrenal) but in some instances (liver, pancreas, etc.) it may be better to retreat and opt for chemotherapy first. There are no hard and fast rules for *bilateral tumours* and they should benefit from all three modalities in the sequence that seems most appropriate - each kidney being staged separately. Preoperative therapy is sensible in most bilateral cases to preserve as much kidney tissue as possible, and second- and even third-look operations are necessary. The results are more encouraging (over 50% survival) than one would at first expect from a bilateral tumour (d'Angio et al. 1981). Renal transplantation and bench surgery are rare options.

Local recurrence is a grave complication but all attempts, again using all three modalities of treatment to render the patient disease free should be made.

In cases of *metastatic disease* surgical metastasectomy in the lung has been practised successfully in many instances.

The late effects that have been seen are mainly growth disturbances (spine) due to radiotherapy and second tumours. The future lies in following up the many cured patients for these complications and refining and customising treatment to avoid them. It is unlikely that any new agents can improve the already extremely good results.

Other Kidney Tumours

Renal cell carcinoma can occur in children (Raney et al. 1983). About 80 cases have been described. The response to chemotherapy is being evaluated.

Other kidney tumours include rhabdomyosarcoma, angioliposarcoma.

Neuroblastoma - Adrenal Gland and Sympathetic Nervous System

Neuroblastoma has yielded least of all to the same treatment strategies used so successfully elsewhere. The apparently meagre successes owe more to the vagaries and idiosyncrasies of the natural history than to the often very aggressive attempts at treatment. Neuroblastoma can arise anywhere in the sympathetic ganglia or in the adrenal gland, and can penetrate the spinal canal - the so-called dumb-bell tumour - and even in the brain (Bousvaros et al. 1986). The unique features of the tumour are the ability to regress spontaneously and to mature into non-malignant forms, and the presence of very specific catecholamine metabolites as markers (Siegel et al. 1980).

Histology. The histological range extends from very undifferentiated tumours which are difficult to separate from other small round cell tumours to the typical rosettes and maturing ganglion cells (ganglioneuroma). Attempts have been made to link histological grade to prognosis (Shimada et al. 1984).

Prognostic Factors. One of the most important prognostic factors is age. Children under 1 year do much better - even those with multiple visceral liver and skin metastases (Pepper syndrome) defined as stage IVS (special) in the most widely used *Evan's staging system* (Evans et al. 1971). Lymph node involvement has prognostic significance (Ninane et al. 1982) and forms the rationale behind the newer staging systems POG/CCSG (Hayes et al. 1983). In Europe the TNM/UICC system is more favoured (Harmer et al. 1982).

Much has been made of the less favourable outcome if the tumour crosses the midline. This may make some sense if it arises in the adrenal (50%), but not if its origin is in the sympathetic chain or the midline coeliac or pelvic ganglia (15%) (Pellerin et al. 1982). In fact, those arising from the sympathetic chain in the neck (5%), mediastinum (29%) and pelvis (15%) have a better prognosis (Filler et al. 1972). They are more likely to be stage I or II tumours with 90% and 75% survival rates, respectively. Most tumours, however, unfortunately present as stage III (9%-10%) and IV (45%-56%) (Kinnier-Wilson and Draper 1974; Zucker and Margulis 1979) and have a very poor prognosis ($<50\%$ and $<5\%$ survival rates, respectively.

Other prognostic factors which have been identified are NMyc amplification - poor (Brodeur et al. 1984); high serum ferritin levels - poor (Mann et al. 1985); various ratios of catecholamine excretion, i.e. VMA/HVMA ratios of more than 1.5 - good; raised levels of cystathionine and homoserine in urine - poor (Siegel et al. 1980).

Diagnosis. The symptoms of neuroblastoma are notoriously protean and may be deduced from the widespread primary sites and metastases (particularly to the bone) as well as from the rare side effects of the catecholamines. Even more unusual ethereal symptoms are, for instance, opsoclonia (dancing eyes syndrome), ataxia and myoclonic jerks (myoclonic syndrome). Severe diarrhoea with potassium depletion is due to the rare VIP secretion (2%). Both these syndromes are often associated with the more mature ganglioneuroblastoma which has a better than average prognosis.

A range of highly specific *catecholamine products* in 24 h urine samples obviate the need for a biopsy if these are identified (Siegel et al. 1980). The spot test of Labrosse is notoriously inaccurate.

In *imaging* techniques, specks of calcifications are characteristic on plain X-ray and especially on CT, which is now the most relevant routine examination, specially for dumb-bell tumours and it has largely replaced the need for myelography. A highly specific scan with 2-meta-iodo-benzyl guanidine (MIBG) is extremely useful, especially for follow-up, and should replace other nuclear imaging methods (SIOP 1987).

Treatment. The role of *surgery* in stage I and II disease is clear, and total excision of the tumour without additional modalities is usually curative. In unresectable stage III and IV disease, great importance was attached to active debulking in the past, and this alone (Koop 1972) or followed by chemotherapy was supposed to have improved survival. Large series have not confirmed this. There followed a period of surgical nihilism which is now being replaced by very guarded optimism for second-look surgery, but the pendulum is still swinging (Wagner et al. 1983). After massive chemotherapy or radiotherapy the response rates are sometimes quite remarkable but have not effected cure. The normally very friable tumour becomes firm and fibrous. Although often intimately attached to vessels and other structures, it is possible to peel it away with meticulous dissection. The final word about the benefits of this have yet to come.

There is much debate about the need for *laminectomy in dumb-bell tumours* (Plaschkes 1981). Without neurological symptoms it is questionable as sole treatment. In established paralysis the symptoms do not often regress after laminectomy. Laminectomy should always be performed prior to attack on the extraspinal extension as the converse can precipitate paralysis.

Another surgical manoeuvre in stage IVS infants with massive liver involvement causing respiratory embarrassment is to extend the abdominal space temporarily with a Silastic patch (Schnaufer and Koop 1975).

Modern approaches using ^{131}I MIBG as treatment are disappointing (Zucker and Margulis 1979). More accurate targeting with monoclonal antibodies is the latest hope for the future. Screening of infants for catecholamines is an obvious way of improvement but has only been performed on a large scale in Japan (Natman 1987). Neuroblastoma is stimulating for imaginative and new approaches.

Other Tumours of the Sympathetic Chain and Adrenal

Phaeochromocytoma (Donath et al. 1965)
Neurofibroma
Adrenal cortical tumours

Hepatoblastoma – Liver

The most specific and common of the malignant liver tumours in children is known as "hepatoblastoma". It makes up about 60% of the total. It is usually uninodular and most often on the right side. It is rare after the age of 5, and there is a male preponderance of 3:2. No environmental factors have been implicated, but there is an association with several *malformations* such as *hemihypertrophy, organomegaly* (Beckwith-Wiedemann syndrome, De Soto's syndrome) and intestinal polyposis (Krush et al. 1988). Cases in siblings have been described.

Histology. Basically there are epithelial (resembling parenchymal liver cells) and mesenchymal elements (spindle cells, osteoid and even squamous cell differentiation), giving rise to the first-order distinction of (I) *pure epithelial;* (II) *mixed epithelial type.* The epithelial type is further divided into *foetal, embryonic and anaplastic variants* (Kasai and Watanabe 1970). The predominantly foetal tumour is said to have the best prognosis with over 80% survival by resection alone. The mixed mesenchymal tumours also appear to be more favourable than the more undifferentiated epithelial ones which metastasise readily (50%–100%) (Weinberg and Finegold 1983). There are no internationally recognised definitions and staging systems. A new preoperative staging system is being developed by SIOP.

Diagnosis and Treatment. The child with a liver tumour usually presents with an abdominal mass. Specific symptoms, such as jaundice, are uncommon. A CT scan and ultrasound are the most useful modalities in the differential diagnosis. On liver scans (technetium), malignant tumours are usually "cold".

Arteriography helps in planning surgery but should not be used as a criterion of resectability. Raised alpha-fetoprotein is found in over 80% of cases, and chorionic gonadotrophin, producing virilisation in males, only rarely.

Surgical resection offers the only chance of cure. About 50% of the tumours are very large and appear to be unresectable. In these, preoperative chemotherapy and/or radiotherapy have made resection easier or possible so that indications for delayed surgery should be more liberal. The pliability of ribs and liver in children makes a thoracic incision less necessary, but caval obstruction due to kinking occurs more readily. Liver clamps are easily applied in children. An internal caval or a general bypass is sometimes useful but not routine. Ultrasound fragmentation aspiration (Cavitron) can minimise blood loss in small children. The metabolic effects (hypoglycaemia, etc.) are usually less severe in children (healthy liver), and regeneration is extraordinarily rapid. Adjuvant chemotherapy should be given to the prognostically poorer groups. *The agents most commonly used are vincristine, actinomycin D and cyclophosphamide in combination (VAC), adriamycin, 5-fluorouracil 5FU* and *cis*-platinum (CDDP).

Hepatic artery ligation, hepatic arterial embolisation and intra-arterial chemotherapy have not been used extensively in children. A 70%–80% 3-year disease-free survival rate has been reported in resectable tumours and even 50% has been achieved in initially-unresectable tumours with preoperative radio- and chemotheapy (Vos et al. 1982; Douglas et al. 1985). The few controlled studies of the CCSG give similar results (Evans et al. 1982). A European cooperative study is being planned by SIOP. Recurrent disease is almost universally fatal. Distant metastases are uncommon (12.5%).

The future lies in cooperative studies and more interdisciplinary treatment with preoperative chemotherapy. Tolerance to chemotherapy is much better preoperatively than after major hepatic resection. New techniques with targeted irradiation using monoclonal antibodies are giving promising results (Wharam et al. 1987).

Hepatocellular Carcinoma

Hepatocellular carcinomas make up 35% of the rest of the malignant tumours. Association with cirrhosis is less frequent than in adults. The two peak ages of occurrence are 4 and 12 years. Chemotherapy and radiotherapy are known to be effective and have improved survival beyond the dismal 12% reported by Exelby et al. (1975).

Sarcomas

A variety of rare sarcomas have been described, but they account for only about 5% of all the malignant tumours (Perilongo et al. 1987). *Malignant mesenchymoma* is probably the best defined and an *undifferentiated sarcoma* has also been described. Although highly malignant, very active treatment can result in cure, as is shown in Fig. 3. This figure shows a huge undifferentiated liver sarcoma treated by debulking, then chemotherapy and finaly total resection. *Rhabdomyosarcoma of the biliary tract* is usually recognised late, and jaundice is common. Surgically it is highly inaccessable but may be operable after chemotherapy.

Benign Tumours

Some of the biologically benign tumours can achieve enormous size and can be lethal in small infants. Essentially they are: (a) mesenchymal hamartoma; (b) haemangioendothelioma; (c) cavernous haemangioma.

Central Nervous System

Brain

Tumours of the brain have only recently being given the attention they deserve due to their being the commonest of all solid tumours in children and the, as yet, generally poor outcome. Modern imaging together with better surgical techniques (microsurgery, ultrasound aspiration and laser surgery) have been a great stimulus to a more systematic and concerted effort of management.

The late effects of radiotherapy, particularly in young children, have prohibited optimal dosages. The obvious answer to the limitations of surgery and radiotherapy in the brain is chemotherapy. Initial attempts were disappointing and controversial, but lately more encouraging response rates are being achieved (van Eys et al. 1985; Allen et al. 1985). Many phase II studies such as the "8 in I" (eight drugs in 1 day) are currently at the forefront of paediatric oncology endeavours (Bleyer et al. 1983).

The five most common paediatric brain tumours are astrocytoma (30%), medulloblastoma (20%), ependymoma (10%), craniopharyngioma (10%) and optic glioma (5%). Except under the age of 2 years, infratentorial tumours make up 60% of the total. Spinal tumours are extremely rare (0.5%), as are metastases to the brain (Gilles et al. 1983).

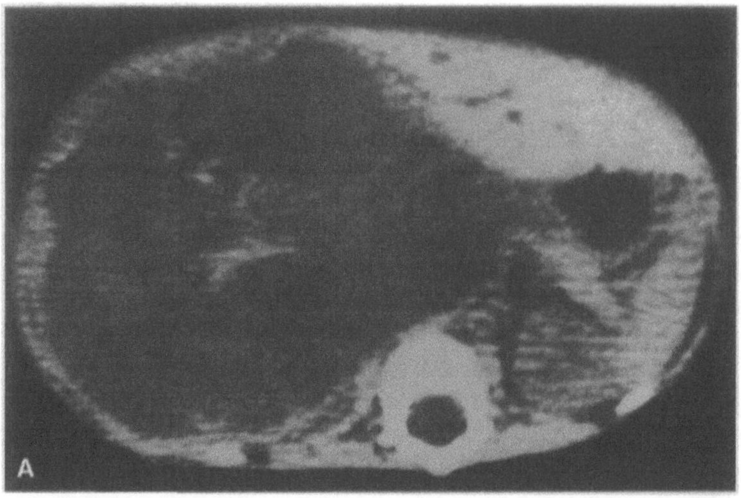

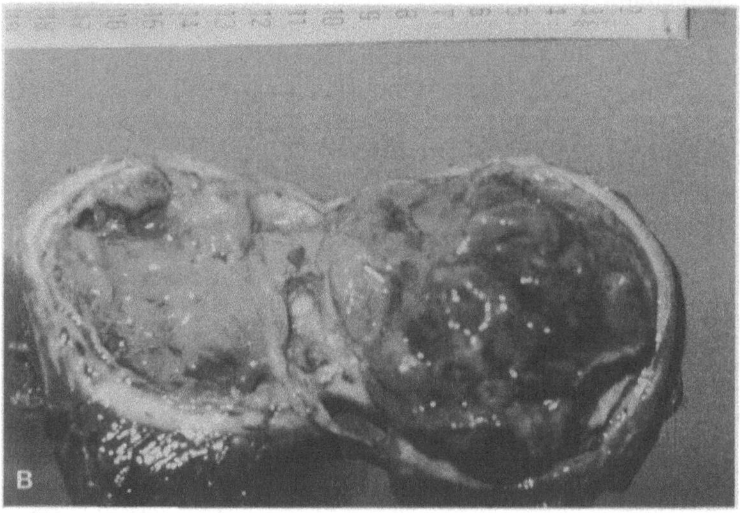

Fig. 3 A, B. Large apparently inoperable undifferentiated sarcoma of liver cured by debulking chemotherapy and delayed second-look complete resection. **A** CT. **B** Specimen after chemotherapy

Infratentorial Lesions

Medulloblastoma. The single most common specific paediatric brain tumour, medulloblastoma best exemplifies the difficulties with the traditional classification schemes and the need for new ideas. The term "medulloblastoma" was coined in 1927 by Cushing. Histologically it belongs to the "infamous" group of undifferentiated small round cell tumours. A desmoplastic variant with a better prognosis occurring in older patients has been recognised, and a grading system has also found some applications (Packer et al. 1984). Some authors now consider it as one of the primitive neuroepithelial tumours (PNET) (Rorke 1983).

Approximately 70% of cases of this tumour occur in the midline in the vermis cerebelli. Peak age distribution is between 2 and 4 years, and there is a male preponderence of nearly 2:1. There is a genetic variant associated with the basal cell nevus syndrome. Staging is not at all uniform. An intraoperative staging system has been devised (Chang et al. 1969).

Subarachnoid and intramedullary seeding is common. Spinal tap and myelography have, until recently, been the most accurate methods of detection. The significance of *single* tumour cells within the CSF is still under debate (Deutsch 1984).

Symptoms are mainly due to increased intracranial pressure from the almost inevitable hydrocephalus. Initially they may be very unspecific – morning headaches and personality and habit changes. Vomiting is often erroneously attributed to the other more common causes in children. Nowadays the mainstay of *diagnosis* is the CT scan with enhancement and nuclear magnetic resonance.

The principle of treatment is surgical exploration, using microsurgical techniques, and excision of as much tumour as possible and, since the tumour is very radiosensitive, followed by whole cranial and spinal irradiation with a boost to the posterior fossa (Choux and Lena 1982).

Preoperative stabilisation with an external ventricular shunt, steroids and anticonvulsants are important adjuncts. Operative mortality should not be more than 5%–10% and a 5-year survival rate in the order of 40%–60% (30%–40% over 10 years) can be achieved with standard treatment (Pichler et al. 1987). The first SIOP medulloblastoma trial (1975–1979) using concurrent chemotherapy and radiotherapy and CCNU as maintenance therapy showed no difference in outcome in a low-risk group with total or subtotal excision, but a statistically significant advantage in a high-risk group with partial excision. An early CCSG study showed no such difference.

A number of pilot studies with sandwich therapy between surgery and radiotherapy (GPO, Amsterdam; de Kraker et al. 1983) have led to the present SIOP medulloblastoma study started in 1984. The aim is to see if radiotherapy can safely be reduced using multiple chemotherapy in the low-risk group and also to evaluate chemotherapy in the high-risk group.

Medulloblastoma can also occur in the cerebellar hemispheres. Recurrences are usually fatal. Long follow-up is essential to detect and treat the many residual and late effects. The role of chemotherapy will certainly increase with more rational use of newer drugs.

Cerebellar Astrocytoma. This, the most common astrocytoma in childhood, occurs in the hemisphere. It is usually cystic with a good prognosis if it can be removed with its typical mural nodule. It is also known as "juvenile astrocytoma", "spongioblastoma" or "pilocytic astrocytoma". Hemangioblastoma should be considered in the differential diagnosis.

Ependymoma. This tumour occurs mainly (over 50%) in the floor or roof of the fourth ventricle and, although biologically benign, can invade the surrounding structures. Craniospinal radiation after surgery is usually given because of the high rate of seeding and recurrence. A 10-year survival rate of 44% has been reported (Cohen and Duffner 1984).

Brain Stem Gliomas. These are surgically very inaccessible so that one of the modern approaches is stereotactic biopsy and radioactive seeding (Godano et al. 1987).

Supratentorial Lesions

Astrocytoma. This is the most common supratentorial tumour and is usually more malignant than the one in the cerebellum, being grade III or IV. The most malignant type is also designated as "glioblastoma multiforme". The possibility of surgery depends on size and site, but it should be remembered that the children have a greater potential for recovery of function after an insult to the brain, even in the dominant hemisphere.

Tumours Around the Third Ventricle – Craniopharyngioma and *Optic Glioma* (Schulte 1987). These rarer and more esoteric tumours, i.e. pinealoma, germ cell tumours, oligodendrogliomas, are only mentioned for the sake of completeness.

Retinoblastoma – Eye

Retinoblastoma is a rare, probably congenital, tumour of the eye, usually diagnosed before the age of 3. A characteristic feature (already observed in the 1800s) is the high familial incidence. It fits very neatly after the tumours of the brain because it has histological similarities to medulloblastoma. Approximately 40% are hereditary, 30% of these being bilateral or multicentric (not necessarily simultaneous), but usually diagnosed within the 1st year; the other 10% are unilateral with a postulated germinal prezygotic mutation or from non-affected carriers. The remaining 55%–60% are non-hereditary and are always unilateral and solitary (Weller 1941). A similar tumour is found in the pineal gland (the third eye) and this has given rise to the concept of trilateral retinoblastoma (Bader et al. 1980). The familial incidence observed can, to a large extent, be explained by the two-hit mutation theory (Knudson 1978). A 13q14 deletion has been reported in 1.2% linked to esterase D deficiency at the same site.

Staging. The results of treatment, particularly as far as retaining vision are concerned, are very much dependent on the extent of disease, and a staging system with this aim in mind has been devised for this purpose (Elsworth 1969).

Diagnosis and Treatment. The most common symptom is leucokoria – "amaurotic cat's eye". Opthalmoscopy under anaesthesia is the main diagnostic tool if the intervening media are clear. A CT scan and ultrasonography of the bulbus are usually adjuncts. Alpha-fetoprotein and CEA may be raised. In sporadic and new hereditary cases the diagnosis is usually made when the tumour is large (stages IV–V). Fortunately, in bilateral cases one side is usually much less affected. Any involvement beyond the entry of the opthalmic artery inevitably implies subarachnoid spread and requires additional radio- or chemotherapy. In a high proportion of cases where sight cannot be saved in one eye, enucleation is the primary treatment. As much of the optic nerve as possible should be excised for examination of microscopic spread.

External beam radiotherapy is extremely effective and is the main treatment used in the less affected eye or in smaller lesions (stages I–III) in order to preserve vision. Exacting techniques are necessary to avoid cataract formation. *Cryotherapy* and *episcleral plaque irradiation* are used as adjuncts for small tumours anterior to the equator and *photocoagulation* for those posterior. Chemotherapy is, as would be expected from the histology, effective and used in disseminated and metastatic disease (Lemerle et al. 1978). Localised disease has an 80% overall survival rate with conventional treatment.

Intraocullar *recurrences* are in the order of 10%. Disseminated metastases rarely occur. *Second tumours* are not uncommon in retinoblastoma. Some can be attributed to radiation but others such as osteosarcoma, which is 500 times more common, are probably also genetically determined (Milé et al. 1982).

Pelvis

Germ Cell Tumours

The germ cell tumours, arising from the cells of the original pluripotential yolk sac or endodermal sinus and migrating to form the normal germ cells, have, because of their *varying differentiation* into *embryonal* and *extra-embryonal* structures and their *occurrence* at sites other than the gonads (mediastinum, brain, etc.), given rise to a confusing and inconsistent terminology. Adding to the disarray has been the term "teratoma", originally introduced by Virchow in 1869 to describe the purely *macroscopic* appearance of tumours containing *mature* elements of all three germ layers. However, these may dedifferentiate into, or at least contain, immature embryonal as well as malignant extra-embryonal elements (choriocarcinoma, yolk sac). The malignant potential of the undifferentiated (immature) embryonal elements is still not clear. Unhappily some terms are used differently in children and adults e.g. orchioblastoma.

A further stumbling block has been to try and make a clear distinction between the testis and ovary where, at the pluripotential level, there is not always one, e.g. dysgerminoma, seminoma and germinoma being the same tumour. Unexpectedly, the more mature tumours (teratomas) are often noted at birth and the most immature ones, e.g. germinoma, occur in adolescents or adults. Fortunately, one of the most consistent and useful markers – alfa-fetoprotein, has started to make understanding easier.

Table 4. Incidence and site of germ cell tumours over 20 years in the Manchester Children's Tumour Registry

Benign Teratoma	91	Ovary	54
Yolk sack tumours	50	Sacrococcygeal	39
Germinoma	23	Testis	38
Malignant teratoma	15	Central nervous system	24
Gonadoblastoma	1	Abdominal and pelvic	7
		Other genitourinary	6
		Thoracic	6
		Head and neck	6

The results of clinical practice, with an overall survival rate of only 20% in the past to over 75% in the last decade, have done better than the semantics (International Society of Pediatric Oncology 1987). The overall numbers of benign and malignant tumours from 180 cases registered in the Manchester children's tumour registry in over 20 years (Birch et al. 1987) are shown in Table 4. As far as the *malignant* ones are concerned the following generalisations can be made.

Yolk Sac Tumour – Endodermal Sinus Tumour

Histology. Yolk sac tumours (the most common tumours in children) show a typical histology with the characteristic Schiller-Duval bodies. The solid pattern has to be differentiated from the even more undifferentiated embryonal carcinoma (Hawkins 1987). The true malignancy of teratomas with immature or undifferentiated elements is difficult to estimate in children. They have been graded according to the amount of neuroglial tissue. No generally recognised classification or staging systems particularly applicable to children have been devised. The *staging* of both testicular and ovarian tumours usually take the age, size, lymph node involvement, histology, alphafetoprotein levels after surgery and peritoneal spread (in the ovary) into account. The normal values for alpha-fetoproteins are dependent on age as shown in Fig. 4.

Testis. Yolk sac tumours predominate in the testis, followed in frequency by teratomas. Under the age of 2, yolk sac tumours *rarely metastasise,* and surgery alone is usually curative. Prepubertal immature

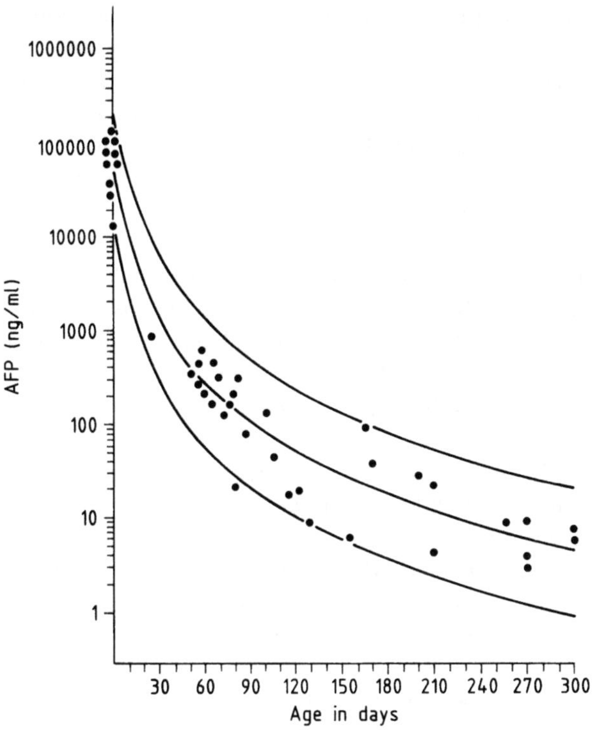

Fig. 4. Alpha-fetoprotein, levels according to age. (From Tschuctida et al. 1978)

teratomas are *rarely malignant*. Seminomas and stromal tumours are extremely unusual (Hawkins 1987; Harms et al. 1983).

Yolk sac tumours have been called a number of inappropriate names such as "orchioblastoma", "infantile adenocarcinoma", "infantile embryonal carcinoma" which should not be confused with the embryonal carcinomas of adults (Harms et al. 1983).

A painless swelling is noted early. It is not an error to make a frozen section biopsy after cross-clamping of the chord if there is any doubt about the diagnosis of malignancy (differential diagnosis – epididymitis), but usually orchiectomy is the rule.

Radical lymph node dissection is not necessary, but removal of bulky para-aortic disease is advisable and lymph node sampling helpful.

Multiagent chemotherapy (Green 1983) is extremely effective and, since the majority of cases have raised alfa-fetoprotein, should be given if this indicates residual (rate of fall to normal) or recurrent disease. Radiotherapy can control regional lymph node disease.

Ovary. Germinomas (dysgerminoma) and *teratomas* are the predominant tumours in the ovary. Teratomas in prepubertal girls are *more* likely to be malignant than in adults (Erikson and Gondas 1972).

Since bilateral and peritoneal involvement is common in the *ovary*, the treatment is more complicated, and chemotherapy is used extensively in all stages, and second-look operations for staging are important (Pinkerton et al. 1987; van Buningon 1987; Flamant et al. 1984).

Extragonadal Sites. Sacrococcygeal teratoma is the most common and primary resection together with the coccyx, essential in the neonatal early period. This resection is crucial to reduce the risk of malignancy which occurs more frequently if the tumour is removed later (Beddis et al. 1984). Careful monitoring of alpha-fetoprotein is necessary.

Retroperitoneal teratomas are often very large and diagnosed late. Preoperative therapy can be useful if surgery is difficult and biopsy shows malignant elements or alpha-fetoprotein is raised.

In pineal tumours radiotherapy rather than surgery is used because of the inaccessibility of the site.

Mediastinal germ cell tumours can be either benign or malignant. The ongoing trials of the GPO (MAKEI 83, 86), FPOG, CCSG and POG should help to clarify and further differentiate treatment.

Soft Tissue

Rhabdomyosarcoma

Rhabdomyosarcoma is the predominant soft-tissue tumour of childhood, 48% in the Kiel (FRG) children tumour registry series, 69% in the German CWS 81 trial series (Treuner et al. 1986). It can occur almost anywhere in the body and, in spite of its explicit name, even at sites where striated muscle is not usually found (bladder, bilary tract, etc.). In fact only about 30% show the characteristic striations by ordinary techniques. This implies origin from an undifferentiated mesenchymal cell, and to demonstrate the myogenic connection, special markers, such as desmin myosin etc., have to be found. Four main types are recognised and in children distributed as follows:

- Embryonal – 50%–60% including the botryoid subtype
- Alveolar – 30%–40%
- Undifferentiated
- Pleomorphic – very rare in children

Two unfavourable variants – monomorphous and anaplastic – were introduced by Palmer et al. (1982) from a detailed study of IRS I and II material. The European (SIOP) classification is different:

1. *Embryonal*
1.1 Dense
 1.1.1 Poorly differentiated
 1.1.2 Well differentiated
1.2 Loose
 1.2.1 Botryoid
 1.2.2 Non-botryoid
2. *Adult*

There is an association between congenital malformations, particularly of the brain, and also as an increased incidence of breast cancer in mothers of children with rhabdomyosarcoma (Birch et al. 1984) SBLA complex (sarcoma + breast and brain + lung and larynx + adrenocortical carcinoma). Familial cases have been described.

There are two peak occurrence age groups: one at 2–5 years and another at 12–16 years. In the lower age group pelvic and distal urogenital tumours predominate, the only other frequent site being the head and neck including the orbit. In the older group additional sites such as extremities, trunk, paratesticular, retroperitoneal and other sites make their appearance.

The natural prognosis and history is very much site- and histology-dependent (Gehan et al. 1981). The two are definitely interrelated because at sites where the prognosis is good, e.g. orbita, the histology is mainly embryonal, and where it is particularly bad, e.g. extremities, it is mainly alveolar. Both types are equally chemo- and radiosensitive. Size and stage of the tumour are important.

Diagnosis and Treatment. Usually an *open incisional biopsy* is best for an accurate diagnosis. If there is clinical suspicion of malignancy and the lesion is not too large (difficult to define in children), a frozen section and a wide *excisional* biopsy can be done. The main thrust of treatment, particularly in children, should be to preserve as much function as is consistent with cure.

Primary Versus Delayed Surgery. Classical radical cancer surgery as the sole treatment, still necessary in some other forms of non-responsive soft-tissue tumours, is definitely out, and multidisciplinary treatment is definitely in – the only questions being in which sequence, what agents and dosages? There are usually good answers from the various trials – SIOP (Flamant et al. 1985), Netherlands (de Kraker and Voûte 1986), Italy (Gasparini et al. 1983), France (Flamant and Hill 1984) and in particular from the IRS which accumulates over 200 patients a year – in that the most rational treatment is often determined according to the primary site of the tumours. Formal regional lymph node dissection is usually unnecessary in tumours that are chemosensitive and at sites other than the extremities, which are difficult to define and dissect. In the modern trials individual choice for the surgeon and the patient is possible (Hays 1986b).

The mainstay of chemotherapy has been VAC and adriamycin. Nowadays, in poor risk groups, cis-platinum and VP 16, as well as melphalan, are also used. The current SIOP trial (mixed mesenchymal tumours) is evaluating ifosfamide.

Radiotherapy is used extensively at those frequent sites inaccesible to surgery (Malpas et al. 1976). *Brachytherapy,* either in the form of *intraoperative radiation, interstitial seeds or after-loading,* could be used more extensively in children to reduce growth disturbances. An example is shown in Fig. 5.

Special Sites. There are three main sites for tumours of the *head and neck* (a) *parameningeal* in the strict sense (nasopharynx, paranasal sinuses and middle ear); (b) those arising in the *oropharynx, palate, maxillary sinus;* and (c) the *superficial ones of the scalp,* lips, eyelid and parotid gland etc. At least two modalities of treatment should be employed. Radiotherapy for local control and, usually, chemotherapy. Surgery remains in the background at many of these sites. The results are encouraging. Cure or long-term disease-free survival are being achieved in 80%–90% of the orbital tumours and lately even in the oral and superficial ones. In the parameningeal tumours, survival rates of 50%–70% can be achieved (Etcubanas et al. 1985).

In *pelvic* and *distal urogenital* tumours exact site of origin is important. There is a great deal of difference from the surgical point of view if the tumour arises in the bladder wall or in the prostate. Most recommendations are to begin treatment by chemotherapy followed by radiotherapy and, since local recurrence is not uncommon, to include surgery at the original site or in the case of residual disease.

It seems more logical to place surgery after chemotherapy and leave radiotherapy for residual disease. Elaborate and ingenious reconstruction techniques, such as bladder augmentation to avoid total exenteration, have been described. Cure and disease-free survival is in the order of 50%–70%. The vaginal and paratesticular tumours have the best prognosis (Hays 1986).

Results are not as good in the *trunk and extremities* (30%–40%) even with trimodality treatment as outlined above. Amputation does not improve the prognosis, and large compartmental resections are not necessary in chemosensitive tumours. The rules for marginal, wide resection, etc., with defined margins such as 3 cm also do not make much sense when faced with an infant no more than a few months old. More aggressive but rather toxic chemotherapy is being tried, which can be taken to the extreme of a bone marrow transplant.

Perineal and perianal and retroperitoneal sites are also prognostically poor groups.

Recurrences and metastatic disease have in general a poor prognosis.

Other Soft Tissue Sarcomas

Askin's Tumour (Askin et al. 1979). A tumour around the chest wall with similarities to Ewing's sarcoma, but with possibly a better prognosis, has been described and delineated (Barson et al. 1978).

Extraosseous Ewing's sarcoma. This has been known for some time and at various sites.

Both the above tumours may be related to the primitive neuroepithelial tumours (PNET).

The more common adult tumours, fibrosarcoma, synovial sarcoma, liposarcoma, malignant fibrous histiocytoma, lyomyosarcoma, are extremely rare in children. Fibrosarcoma, synovial sarcoma and liposarcoma (Castelberry et al. 1984) may have a better prognosis in young children.

Intermediate "Pubertal" Group

Bone

Ewing's Sarcoma

There is still no good term to replace the widely used eponym for the highly malignant round cell tumour occurring in bone rather than of bone, familiarised by Ewing in 1921 and occurring at a peak incidence between the ages of 10 and 15. There is a slight male preponderance, and the tumour is said to be extremely rare in blacks (Glass and Fraumeni 1970), although this has lately been disputed (Barnes 1985).

It is *localised* in the diaphysis and also occurs in flat bones (pelvis) and the axial skeleton (spine). It has several microscopic patterns including a large cell variant which is said to have a poorer prognosis (Kissane et al. 1983).

More significant poor *prognostic factors* are the size (>8 cm) and volume (>100 ml) of the tumour

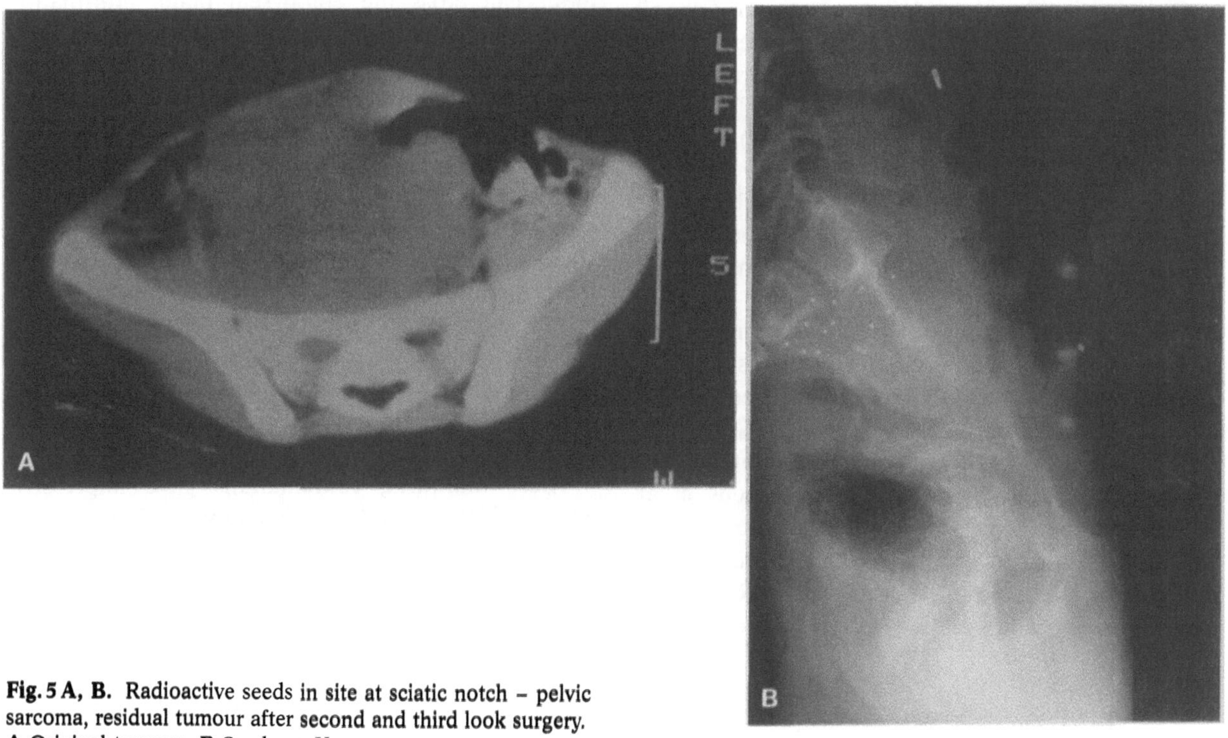

Fig. 5 A, B. Radioactive seeds in site at sciatic notch – pelvic sarcoma, residual tumour after second and third look surgery. **A** Original tumour. **B** Seeds on X-ray

(Jürgens et al. 1985), extraosseous extension (Mendenhall et al. 1983) and the presence of metastases at diagnosis (20%), half in the lungs and half in bone or bone marrow.

Diagnosis and Treatment

The *symptoms* are non-specific. The onion-peel periosteal reaction and moth-eaten appearance on X-ray are characteristic but not typical enough for a diagnosis. If there is a lot of extraosseous involvement, one need not violate the bone for biopsy at the site of the tumour, but for limb-saving operations it is extremely important to get safe upper and lower limits of the tumour by proven biopsy – so-called clearance biopsy. Standard treatment was for a long time radiotherapy to which adjuvant chemotherapy was later added because of the often generalised nature of the disease. With this treatment and consequent longer-term survival, local recurrence became more of a problem. Rebiopsy of an apparently complete remission has also shown viable cells at the centre (Jürgens et al. 1985). Radiation to the long bones of a child often leaves a functionless limb. Therefore the role of surgery is being successfully redefined. As far as *surgery* is concerned, a distinction was always made between *expendable* (ribs and other flat bones) and *none-expendable bones* (long bones). With limb-saving operations this *difference is no longer tenable.*

Our view is that the *modern treatment* for Ewing's sarcoma should be *preoperative chemotherapy plus local resection and reconstruction,* radiotherapy being reserved for situations where "reasonable" (Kilman et al. 1973) surgery is not possible (spine?) or resection incomplete, much the same as is now practised in osteosarcoma. A number of groups are beginning to use this approach (Marcove and Rosen 1980; Gnudi et al. 1983; Nesbit et al. 1981). Intensive four-drug chemotherapy (VAC + adriamycin) regimens are superior to the conventional three drugs (VAC) and newer drugs are also effective (Rosen et al. 1981). The results of long-term disease-free survival are very encouraging ranging from 50% to 80% (IESS, Milé et al. 1982; Milan, Gasparini et al. 1977; Villejuif, Zucker et al. 1983; CESS, Jürgens et al. 1985; Memorial Sloan Kettering Center, Rosen et al. 1981). The results of distal extremity lesions are superior to central lesions such as pelvis. *Recurrence and disseminated disease* are difficult to control because of resistant cells.

Osteosarcoma

The last few years have been marked by very heated controversies regarding osteosarcoma, particularly concerning the role of chemotherapy, and although the smoke is beginning to disperse and things becoming clearer, the flames still erupt occasionally. Osteosarcoma has also been the main stimulus for many ingenious attempts of avoiding amputation. Only a brief outline can be given here, with particular emphasis on those aspects *relevant to children and to limb-saving aspects.*

Osteosarcoma is a highly malignant spindle cell tumour producing osteoid in varying amounts. It is the most common *second tumour in children cured of cancers.* Some can be attributed to radiation. The genetic associations have already been mentioned (retinoblastoma) and may be the explanation for the others (Milé et al. 1982).

Several clinical and *pathological variants* are known. These are: (a) juxtacortical (parosteal and periosteal types); (b) central types; (c) teleangiectic; and (d) primary synchronus. The first two of these are reputed to have a better prognosis and the others a poorer one.

The most common sites are the metaphysis of the distal femur, proximal tibia and proximal humerus. The more peripheral lesions are also said to have a better prognosis (Marcove 1984). True "skip" lesions are much rarer than originally described, but the tumour can cross the epiphyseal plate, information which is surgically important. Bone pain is an early sign in children and must be taken seriously, and, as with most bone tumours, only a biopsy can establish the true nature.

The 5-year survival rate with radiotherapy alone, with or without amputation, is in the order of 20% (Goorin et al. 1985), so it is a little hard to understand why it took such a long time to accept chemotherapy as an integral part of management either in the adjuvant or preoperative setting. The first agent to show response was methotrexate. Other agents were soon found to be effective including bleomycin, adriamycin, vincristine, cyclophosphamide.

These multidrug combinations gave impressive (60%–90% 2-year relapse-free survival; Rosen et al. 1982), but the early enthusiasm waned when the rates had fallen to 40%–50% at 5 years. These figures began to approach the Mayo Clinic figures of 40% without chemotherapy. Additionally the extraordinarily good results of Rosen were not always reproducible by others and raised more doubts. Recently the French group at Villejuif, using the same type of protocol, have reconfirmed the results.

It took a brave randomised trial (Link et al. 1986) to finally settle the issue of adjuvant therapy. In Europe the initial results were not as convincing, the MRC (GB) and EORTC have collaborated in a number of trials. Prophylactic irradiation to the lungs did not improve survival significantly and methotrexate in normal dosage together with adriamycin were not effective (Burgers et al. 1985).

Currently in Europe EORTC, SIOP, MRC and UKCCSG have combined their efforts to find the most effective chemotherapy agents and schedules in three different studies (EOIS). There is another pilot study to judge the effect of i-fosfamide. The German COSS protocols use a complicated cross-over system determined by response, as originally described by Rosen (1982). The AIEOP also has its own protocols, and much surgical experience comes from the Rizzoli Institute (Campanacci et al. 1981).

Treatment – Limb-Saving Operations

Surgeons have on the whole accepted the idea of preoperative therapy more easily because the advantages outweigh the disadvantages – if the aim is to preserve the limb.

The advantages are:

1. The tumour becomes better defined, and safer margins are easier to determine.
2. There is time to make a really custom-made prosthesis and to plan properly.

The disadvantage is the generally poorer state of the patient and greater risk of infection because of immunosuppression. Many details can be found in the abstract and proceedings of annual meetings on limb-saving procedures (Kotz 1983; NIH 1984; Enneking 1985; Yamamuro 1987).

Some decisions about limb preservation are not purely medical but also a matter of philosophy, psychology, and ethics, e.g. is it worthwhile to attempt to save the lower limb in the case of a tumour of the tibia with its inherent risks when amputation and an external prosthesis might be less problematic? Limb saving in patients with disseminated disease seems justified because of the better quality of life.

There are several options for reconstruction – *endoprosthesis, autologous and allograft* and exceptionally a *rotation plasty,* as well as different methods of fixation (cement versus cement-less), just to mention a few. Our view is that *in children a truly custom-made endoprosthesis in all dimensions* (not only in length as in many of the modular kits used in adults) and which can be extended on growth offers by far the best potential, although the other options are not denied. It can be used in both extremities in growing children in over 75% of cases, and the results are very encouraging (Lewis 1986; Rao et al. 1983; Marcove and Abu Zair 1984). One of these used (most extensively) in Europe is the Stanmore endoprosthesis (Scales 1983). Technical considerations are unfortunately outside the scope of this short introduction, but an example is shown in Fig. 6.

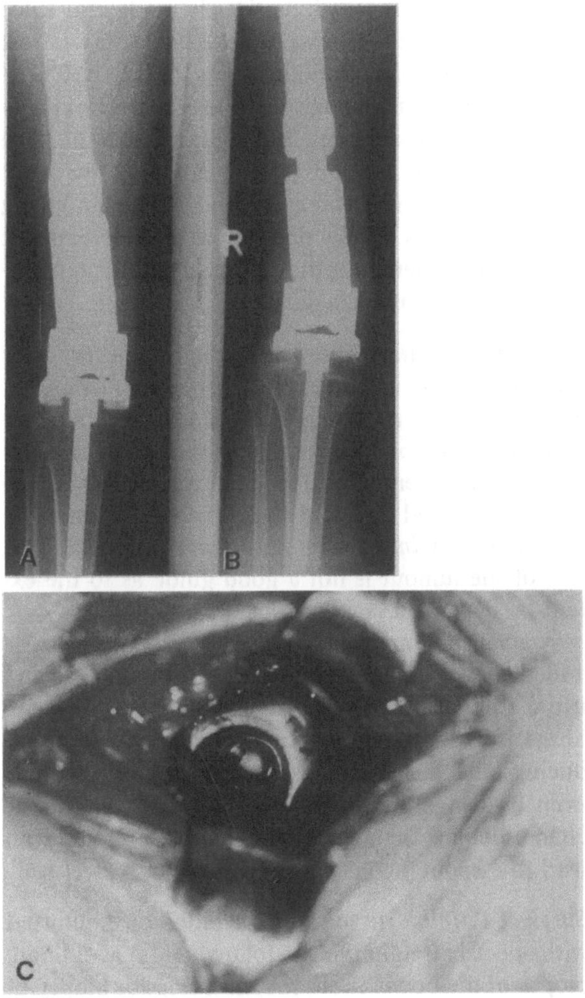

Fig. 6 A–C. "Growing" Stanmore custom-made distal femur endoprothesis **A** before extension; **B** after 2× extension; **C** port for introducing ball bearings to extend prosthesis

Lymphoma

The lymphomas are basically generalised diseases and not surgically curable except in rare instances. Interest to the surgeon is mainly in three aspects:

1. Problems associated with abdominal non-Hodgkin's lymphoma (NHL)
2. Staging in Hodgkin's disease
3. Biopsy

Non-Hodgkin's Lymphoma

The majority of children with NHL present with abdominal disease mainly localised in the ileocoecal region (Murphy 1980) and have B cell disease. About 50% of these are first seen by surgeons because of an acute abdomen. Most have generalised stage III or IV disease at diagnosis (Murphy 1980).

Surgical resection of bulky disease is still an important integral part of treatment (Exelby 1980), but equally essential is early intensive chemotherapy since B cell lymphoma is known to have one of the fastest doubling times of all tumours – less than 24 h (Hirt et al. 1984). Even in generalised disease survival rates of over 70% can be achieved, but children who still have residual disease 1 month after beginning treatment rarely survive (Anderson et al. 1983). Delay in giving chemotherapy is usually due to one of three reasons: deciding treatment priorities, surgical pitfalls and difficulties in differential diagnosis.

Treatment Priorities. There are no hard and fast rules for deciding the priorities of surgery and chemotherapy. If an acute abdomen is diagnosed *both* surgery and the need for chemotherapy should be considered as an emergency. The best way to make the right choice and to avoid the pitfalls is to treat the patient by an *interdisciplinary team approach.* The size of the tumour is not a good guide as to the extent or stage of disease.

A small tumour could be easily resected, but the added risk of an anastomosis would be unnecessary if the child also had, for instance, liver involvement. Large isolated tumours should be resected since reducing bulky disease improves the prognosis. It may even be dangerous to treat a very large tumour by chemotherapy first since the rapid regression can lead to a spontaneous perforation of the bowel wall.

Surgical Pitfalls. These can be avoided or minimised with special attention to the following: (a) avoiding a biopsy of the bowel itself, rather opting for biopsy of the lymph nodes or cytology of peritoneal fluid; and (b) realising that resection and anastomosis in generalised disease will delay chemotherapy and that under these circumstances the safest procedure – enterostomy versus anastomosis – is best.

Differential Diagnosis. The most common differential diagnostic problems include intussusception, enlarged Peyer's plaques, mesenteric adenitis, Crohn's disease and a carcinoid of the appendix.

The surgeon's correct initial decisions and actions are vital for overcoming an aggressive tumour which responds very well to modern treatment.

Mediastinal NHL is usually best left surgically alone. Even with compression of the airway, any indications for operations should be very strict because response to drugs is dramatic, sometimes within a few hours.

Hodgkin's Disease

Hodgkin's disease in children shows a different distribution but treatment is not essentially different from adults (Mauch et al. 1983; Fossati et al. 1984). However, because of the effects of radiotherapy on growth in younger children and of chemotherapy on fertility in the older ones, and the relatively high incidence of second tumours, the emphasis and strategies to try and avoid these problems are sometimes different in the different age groups (Donaldson and Kaplan 1982). There is still much controversy and variability as to the best way.

One such controversy of particular interest to surgeons is the need for *staging laparotomy* and splenectomy (Hays et al. 1984). Staging laparotomy is certainly the most precise way of determining the extent of disease and, when involved-field radiation was the primary form of therapy, had an important role in management. Partial splenectomy is sometimes done (West German Hodgkin's disease study; Schellong et al. 1986) to avoid the particular risk of sepsis in the young. Where chemotherapy has replaced (at an early stage) or is added to radiotherapy in late stage, exact localisation of disease loses its importance, and routine staging laparotomy becomes questionable. If done, however, an exact schedule of all sites should be used during laparotomy to avoid omissions. Liver biopsy should be at multiple sites (needle and superficial). Tantalum clips for marking should be used sparingly so as not to adversly affect future imaging. Displacing the gonads (ovaries) from the fields to radiation, usually to the midline (Baker et al. 1972), remains an important part of staging. Fertility is not affected by this manoeuvre (Le Floch et al. 1976), and it seems that it is unnecessary to put the ovaries back into the original normal position to maintain this fertility.

Rare "Adult" Tumours

Thyroid Carcinoma

Thyroid cancer is rare in children, and about 50% can be attributed to previous radiation. The classification and diagnostic work-up are similar to adults, but the prognosis of the papillary form is better (Halpern 1981; Winship and Rosvoll 1979). Treatment with radioactive agents is used much less frequently, and surgery is the mainstay of treatment. Radical neck dissection is usually not necessary.

Pancreatic Carcinoma

Pancreatic carcinoma occurs very rarely in children and is in some instances curable by surgery alone. It is likely that the good prognosis is due to the different origin of these tumours – acinar rather than ductal, or from non-functioning islet cells (Winship and Rosvoll 1979). Subtle but exact criteria for differentiating these tumours (Bienaymé and Gross 1976; Camprodon and Quintanilla 1984; Todani et al. 1988). An example of such a metastatic tumour cured by surgery alone is shown in Fig. 7.

Breast Carcinoma

Breast carcinoma can occur in children and adolescents, male as well as female (McDivitt and Stewart 1981). Once again it has been found that in some cases the prognosis is much better than in adults and is due to the subtle histological difference – the carcinomas in children are the so-called secretory types.

Carcinoid

In children a carcinoid often occurs in the appendix as localised disease. If resection is clean, no further treatment is necessary (Ryden et al. 1975).

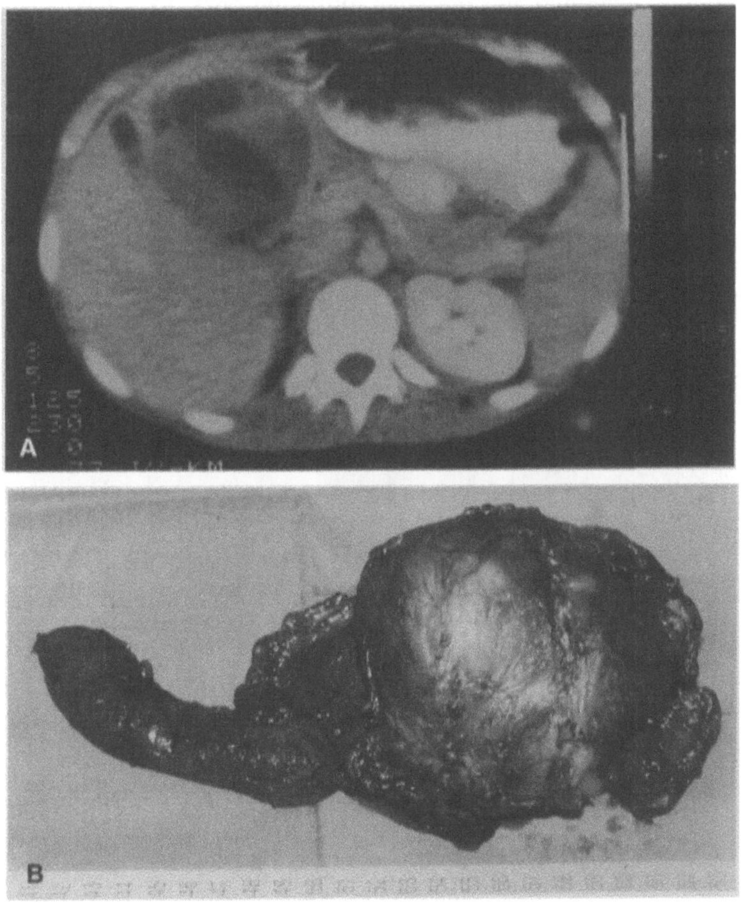

Fig. 7 A, B. Nonfunctioning islet cell carcinoma of pancreas with lymph node metastases cured by surgery alone. **A** CT-scan. **B** Specimen

Carcinoma of Colon

Carcinoma of the colon is virtually non-existant in children except in some familial polyposis cases, Gardner's syndrome and Peutz-Jeghers syndrome (Anderson and Bergdahl 1978; Rao et al. 1985).

Lung-Pulmoblastoma

Lung pulmoblastoma is a very rare tumour of both adults and children with a reputed poor prognosis (Ohtomo et al. 1983).

Neonatal Tumours

Neonatal tumours are extremely rare and varied in nature. In Britain the estimate was one malignant tumour per 27400 births (Barson 1978). Only 0.2% of all childhood malignancies are said to occur in the neonate (Children's Hospital of Los Angeles, Bader and Miller 1979). It is well recognised that many of the better known, more common neonatal tumours (e.g. neuroblastoma. sacrococcygeal teratoma, mesoblastic nephroma) and the rarer soft-tissue ones often behave in a more benign way than they would in the older age groups. There are no explanations for this except hypothetical ones (Bolande 1971). A example of congenital fibromatosis is shown in Fig. 8.

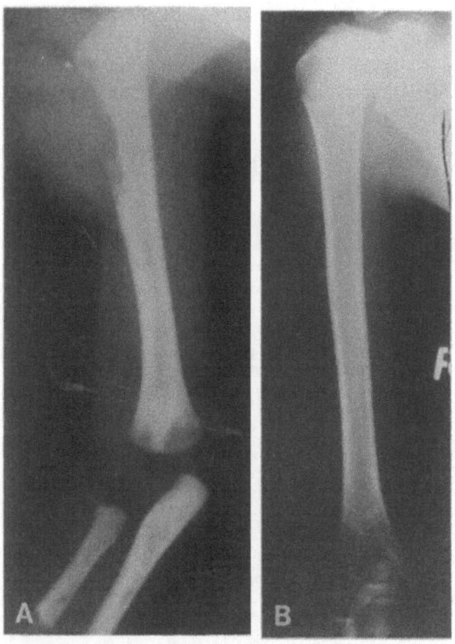

Fig. 8 A, B. Spontaneous regression of neonatal generalised fibromatosis involving bone **A** shortly after birth; **B** at age of 5 years

This now well-recognised entity was previously often diagnosed and treated as fibrosarcoma (Plaschkes 1974). There are often no exact criteria to delineate the "malignant" from the "benign". Surgery often remains the mainstay of treatment because of the special risks of radiotherapy (Littman and D'Angio 1981) and chemotherapy (Siegel and Meran 1981) in the neonate (Gale et al. 1982). With few exceptions, there is very little hard information in the literature on neonatal tumours on which to base one's decisions. For this reason, SIOP has a prospective neonatal tumour study underway.

Conclusions

In the preceding pages the necessity of a comprehensive multidisciplinary team approach to the management of children's solid tumours will have become apparent.

The importance of technical expertise and excellence in surgery may have been given short shrift in this attempt to give an overview in a very concise form. The contribution of the surgical organ specialists may have been overlooked in stressing the theoretical concepts. Nevertheless, in the final analysis, it is these as well which determine the success or failure of the treatment.

Because of the rarity of children's tumours, it is hardly forseeable in most situations, even if children are treated at special centres, that any one individual will be able to specialise solely in one particular tumour or organ as is possible in adults. Without going into the discussion as to who should do what (which in any case varies very much from one institution and country to another), it should have become apparent that there is certainly a need and room for a specialist in paediatric surgical oncology. Most of the tumours and many of the inherent problems are unique to children, and the surgeon dealing with them must have a broader overview of the subject to utilise his skill to the full and do justice to his patients. Only in this way can he remain flexible enough to deviate from strict rules and make progress.

It is unlikely that any new agents will make any significant inroads in those tumours with already high cure rates. Completely new approaches have a much better chance of success.

In the future, it will also become more and more important to carefully follow up the increasing numbers of cured children for complications and late effects of therapy. The surgeon must be involved in these activities.

All in all, with the good results, the skill and knowledge required in treating children with solid tumours and the many new challenges, paediatric surgical oncology is a very satisfying field of endeavour.

Appendix A

Abbreviations of Paediatric Oncological Groups and Trials

AIEOP	Italian Pediatric Oncology Group
CCSG	Children's Cancer Study Group, USA
CESS	Cooperative Ewing's Sarkoma-Studie
COSS	Cooperative Osteosarkoma-Studie, FRG and Austria
CWS	Cooperative Weichteil-Studie, (Cooperative Soft Tissue Study)
EIOS	European Intergroup Osteosarcoma Study
EORTC	European Organization for Research and Treatment of Cancer
ENSG	European Neuroblastoma Study Group
GPO	German Pediatric Oncology Group
IESS	Intergroup Ewing's Sarcoma Study, USA
IRS	Intergroup Rhabdomyosarcoma Study, USA
MAKEI	Maligne Keimzell Tumoren, of FRG (Malignant Germ Cell Tumours)
MRC	Medical Research Council, UK
NWTS	National Wilms' Tumour Study, USA
POG	Pediatric Oncology Group, USA
SFOP	French Pediatric Oncology Group
SIOP	International Society of Pediatric Oncology
UKCCSG	United Kingdom Children's Cancer Study Group

Appendix B

Staging Systems used in Paediatric Oncology

Table B 1. Nephroblastoma, NWTS and SIOP

Stage	Definition and comments
I	*Tumour limited to the kidney and completely excised* The renal capsule is intact. The tumour has not ruptured nor been punctured before its excision. No tumour is observed in the renal bed, and histological examination confirms that the capsule is intact.
II	*Tumour extends outside the kidney, but is completely excised* There is a local extension of the tumour, in particular: – Penetration of the tumour into the perirenal tissues beyond the false capsule of the tumour and "adhesions" that are confirmed histologically to be due to tumour. – Invasion of the para-aortic nodes, confirmed histologically; the pathologist must make a careful search of all the excised nodes for foci of tumour cells. – Invasion of the renal vessel walls outside the kidney or thrombosis caused by tumour in these vessels. Thrombosis which is apparently non-neoplastic may contain islands of tumour cells; thrombi must be examined vey carefully. – Invasion of the renal pelvis and ureter.
III	*Incomplete excision, without haematogenous metastases* This stage has been reached if one or several of the following conditions are present: – A tumour biopsy taken before or during surgey, tumour rupture before or during surgery. – Peritoneal metastases, as distinguished from the simple tumour adhesions of stage II. – Invasion of lymph nodes beyond the abdominal periaortic nodes. – Complete excision impossible (e.g. infiltration of the vena cava).
IV	*Haematogenous metastases* Involving lungs, liver, bones, brain, etc.
V	*Bilateral renal tumours*

Table B 2. Neuroblastoma, Evans et al. (1971)

Stage	Criteria
Stage I	Tumour limited to the organ or structure of origin
Stage II	Tumour with regional spread that does not cross the midline; ipsilateral lymph nodes may be involved
Stage III	Regional tumour crossing the midline; bilateral lymph nodes may be involved
Stage IV	Tumour with metastases to distant discontiguous sites such as lymph nodes, bone and bone marrow, organs and soft tissue
Stage IV-S	Localised primary tumour and disseminated disease limited to liver, skin and bone marrow

Table B 3. Neuroblastoma, POG (Hayes 1983)

Stage	Criteria
I	Localised tumour, completely resected without local invasion
IIA	Localised tumour, resected with residual microscopic tumour
IIB	Localised tumour, partially or not resected
IIIA[a]	Regional or systemic spread of disease, confined to regional lymph nodes, liver or skin without bone or bone-marrow involvement
IIIB	Same as IIIA, but with evidence of a single localised destructive lesion of bone. No bone marrow involvement
IIIC	Generalised tumour in bone and bone marrow or in bone marrow only

[a] Local regional nodes only.

Table B 4. Hepatoblastoma and hepatocellular carcinoma

Holton et al. (1975)	Evans et al. (1982)
1. Unicentric lobar lesion less than 6 cm in diameter, resectable	1. Tumour is completely resected by initial treatment
2. Unicentric lobar lesion more than 6 cm in diameter a. Margin clear b. Margin involved c. Multicentric, one lobe	2. a. Tumours rendered completely resectable by initial chemotherapy and irradiation b. Residual disease confined to one lobe
3. Multicentric, both lobes involved	3. a. Disease involving both lobes of the liver b. Regional lymph node involvement
4. a. Direct extension to adjacent viscera b. Distant spread	4. Distant metastases

Table B 5. Germ cell tumours

Stage	Brodeur (surgical)	Peckham (testis) (lymphography, CT)	FIGO (ovary) (surgical)
I	Localised disease completely resected	Disease confined to testis, markers negative	a. One ovary involved, no ascites b. Both ovaries involved, no ascites c. a. or b. with ascites
II	Microscopic residual disease, capsular invasion or microscopic lymph node involvement	Infradiaphragmatic node involvement	One or both ovaries involved and pelvic extension
III	Gross residual disease, gross node involvement; tumour in ascites or pleural fluid	Supra- and infradiaphragmatic node involvement	Intraperitoneal metastases outside pelvis or positive retroperitoneal nodes
IV	Disseminated disease	Extralymphatic involvement	Distant metastases

Table B 6. Soft tissue (rhabdomyosarcoma and others), SIOP, TNM

Clinical stage grouping				Postsurgical histopathological staging			
	TNM				pTNM		
Stage I	T1a, T1b	No, Nx	Mo	Stage I	pT1	pNo, pNx	pMo
Stage II	T2a, T2b	No, Nx	Mo	Stage II	pT2	pNo, pN1a, pNx	pMo
Stage III	Any T	N1	Mo		pT1	pN1a	pMo
Stage IV	Any T	Any N	M1	Stage III a	pT3a	pNo, pN1a, pNx	pMo
				Stage III b	Any pT	pN1b	pMo
					pT3b/c	Any pN	pMo
				Stage IV	Any pT	Any pN	pM1

Table B 7. Rhabdomyosarcoma, IRS

Group	Criteria
Group I	Localised disease, completely removed, regional nodes not involved I.1 Confined to muscle or organ of origin I.2 Contiguous involvement with infiltration outside the muscle or organ of origin, as through fascial planes Inclusion in this group includes both gross impression of complete removal and microscopic confirmation of complete removal
Group II	II.1 Grossly removed tumour with microscopic residual disease; no evidence of gross residual tumour; no evidence of regional node involvement II.2 Regional disease, completely removed (no microscopic residual disease) II.3 Regional disease with involved nodes, grossly removed, but with evidence of microscopic residual disease
Group III	Incomplete removal or biopsy with gross residual disease
Group IV	Distant metastatic disease present at onset

Table B 8. Rhabdomyosarcoma, GPO

Stage	Criteria
Stage I	Tumour completely removed, macroscopically and microscopically; no lymph nodes
Stage II	A Tumour macroscopically removed, but without microscopically free margins, negative regional lymph nodes B Tumour macroscopically removed, but without microscopically free margins, with positive regional lymph nodes
Stage III	Incomplete resection with macroscopical tumour residue, with or without positive regional lymph nodes
Stage IV	Metastatic disease present at diagnosis

References

Allen JC, Bloom HJG, Ertel I, Evans A, Hammond D, Jones H, Levin V, et al. (1986) Brain tumours in children: current cooperative and institutional chemotherapy trials in newly diagnosed and recurrent cases. Semin Oncol 13: 110–121

Anderson A, Bergdahl L (1978) Carcinoma of the colon in children. J Pediatr Surg 1: 967–981

Anderson JR, Wilson JF, Jenkin RDT, Meadows AT, Kersey J, Chilcote RR, Coccia P, et al. (1983) Childhood non-Hodgkin's lymphoma. The results of a randomized therapeutic trial comparing a 4-drug regimen (COMP) with a 10-drug regimen (LSA_2–1_2). N Engl J Med 308: 559–565

Askin FB, Rosai J, Sibley RK, Dehner LP, McAlister WH (1979) Malignant small cell tumours of the thoracopulmonary region in childhood. A distinctive clinical pathological entity of uncertain histogenesis. Cancer 43: 2438–2451

Bader JL, Miller RW (1979) US cancer incidence in the first year of life. Am J Dis Child 133: 157–159

Bader JL, Miller RW, Meadows AT, Zimmermann LE, Champion LAA, Voûte PA (1980) Trilateral retinoblastoma. Lancet 2: 582–583

Baker JW, Peckham MJ, Morgan RL, Smithes DW (1972) Preservation of ovarian function in patients requiring radiotherapy for para-aortic and pelvic Hodgkin's disease. Lancet 2: 1307–1308

Baldy O, Lemoine G, Zucker JM, Schweisguth O (1984) Pulmonary metastases in children. A study of 134 patients. J Pediatr Surg 19: 121–125

Barson AJ (1978) Congenital neoplasia (British Pediatraic Pathology Society's experience). Arch Dis Child 53: 436

Barson AJ, Ahmed A, Gibson AM, McDonald AM (1978) Chest wall sarcoma of childhood with a good prognosis. Arch Dis Child 53: 882:–889

Beckwith JB (1983) Wilms' tumour and other renal tumours in childhood. A selective review from the National Wilms's Tumour Study Pathology Centre. Hum Pathol 14: 481–492

Beddis JR, Noblett H, Mott MG (1984) Effective chemotherapy for metastatic sacrococcygeal teratoma. Med Pediatr Oncol 12: 231–234

Bienaymé J, Gross P (1976) Tumeurs malignes du pancreas chez l'enfant. Ann Chir Infant 17: 131–155

Barnes L, Verbin R, Goodman M et al. (1985) Diseases of bones and joints. In: Barnes L (ed) Surgical pathology of head and neck. Dekker, New York

Birch JH, Hartley AL, Marsden HB, Harns M, Swindell R (1984) Excess risk of breast cancer in mothers of children with soft tissue sarcoma. Br J Cancer 49: 325–331

Birch JM, Marsden HB, Blair V, Hartley AL (1987) An epidemiological study of germ cell tumours in children (Abstr). Meeting of the International Society of Pediatric Oncology, Jerusalem

Bleyer W, Millstein J, Balias F, Pendergrass T, Chard R, Hartmann J (1983) 8 drugs in one day. Chemotherapy for brain tumours – a new approach and rationale for preirradiation chemotherapy (Abstr). Med Pediatr Oncol 11: 213

Bolande RP (1971) Benignity of neonatal tumours and concept of cancer regression in early life. Am J Dis Child 122: 12–14

Bousvaros A, Kirks DH, Grossmann H (1986) Imaging in neuroblastoma. An overview. Pediatr Radiol 16: 89–106

Brodeur GM, Seeger Schwab, et al. (1984) Amplification of N Myc in untreated human neuroblastoma correlates with advanced stage disease. Science 224: 1121–1124

Bucalessi P, Veronesi U, Emanuelli H, Fossati-Bellani F (1976) Tumori infantili. Ambrosiono, Milano

Burgers JMB, Voûte PA, van Glabbeke M (1985) Adjuvant chemotherapy for osteosarcoma in limbs. Trial 20781 of the SIOP and EORTC radiotherapy/chemotherapy group. In: van Unnik W (ed) The management of bone and soft tissue sarcomas. Raven, New York

Campanacci M, Bacci G, Bentoni F, et al. (1981) The treatment of osteosarcoma of the extremities. Twenty years experience at the Instituto Ortopedico Rizzoli. Cancer 48: 1569–1581

Camprodon R, Quintanilla E (1984) Successful long term results with resection of pancreatic carcinoma in children. Favourable progress for an uncommon neoplasm. Surgery 95: 420–426

Castelberry RP, Kelly DR, Wilson ER, Cain WS, Solter MR (1984) Childhood liposarcoma. Cancer 54: 579–584

Chang CH, Houspian EM, Herbert CJ (1969) An operative

staging system and megavoltage radiotherapy technique for cerebellar medulloblastoma. Radiology 93: 1351

Choux M, Lena G (1982) Le medulloblastome. Neurochirurgie [Suppl 1] 28

Cohen ME, Duffner PK (1984) Brain tumours in children. Principles of diagnosis and treatment. Raven, New York

D'Angio GJ, Evans AE, Breslow E, et al. (1981) The treatment of Wilms' tumour. Results of the second National Wilms' Tumour Study. Cancer 47: 2302–2311

De Kraker J, Voûte PA (1986) The role of ifosfamide in pediatric soft tissue sarcoma (Abstr). 17th SIOP Annual Meeting, Venice

De Kraker J, Voûte PA, Burgers JM (1983) The sandwich scheme – a new approach in the treatment of medulloblastoma patients (Abstr). 13th International Congress of Chemotherapy, Vienna

Deutsch M (1984) The impact of myelography on the treatment results for medulloblastoma. Int J Pediatr Oncol Biol Phys 10: 999–1003

Donaldson SS, Kaplan HS (1982) Complications of treatment of Hodgkin's disease in children. Cancer Treat Rep 66: 977–989

Donath A, Kaeser H, Roos B, Ziegler W, Oetliker O, Colombo JP, Bettex M (1965) Le phéochromocytome familiale; discussion de la malignité et du héréditaire à propos d'un cas chez l'enfant à sécrétion particulière. Helv Paediatr Acta 20: 1–18

Douglas EC, Green AO, Wrenn E, Champion J, Sipp M, Pratt CB (1985) Effective cisplatin DDP based chemotherapy in the treatment of hepatoblastoma. Med Pediatr Oncol 13: 187–190

Draper GJ, Birch JM, Ittel JF, Wilson LM, Lack I, Marsden HB, Jones PHM, et al. (1982) Childhood cancer incidence. Survival and mortality. HMSO, London, no 37

Ehrenbard LT, Chaganti RSK (1981) Cancer in the fetal hydantoin syndrome. Lancet 2: 97

Elsworth RM (1969) The practical management of retinoblastoma. Trans Am Opthalmol Soc 67: 462–534

Enneking WF (1985) International symposium on limb salvage in musculoskeletal oncology, Orlando

Erikson RP, Gondas B (1972) Alternative explanation of the different behaviour of ovarian and testicular teratomas. Lancet 1: 1307–1308

Etcubanas E, Histu HO, Sklar M, Pratt C (1985) Influence of different treatment modalities on the curability of childhood rhabdomyosarcoma of the head and neck. Eur J Pediatr Haematol Oncol

Evans AE, d'Angio GJ, Randolph J (1971) A proposed staging system for children with neuroblastoma. Children's Cancer Study Group. Cancer 27: 374–378

Evans AE, Land VJ, Newton WA, Randolph JG, Sather HN, Tefft M (1982) Combination chemotherapy (vincristine, adriamycin, cyclophosphamide and 5 FU) in the treatment of children with malignant hepatoblastoma. Cancer 50: 821–826

Exelby PR (1980) Malignant lymphoma in children. World J Surg 4: 49–62

Exelby PR, Filler RM, Grossfeld JL (1975) Liver tumours in children in the particular reference to hepatoblastoma and hepatocellular carcinoma. J Pediatr Surg 10: 329–337

Farber S (1966) Chemotherapy in the treatment of leukemia and Wilms' tumour. JAMA 198: 826–836

Filler RM, Traggis NJ, Jaffe N, et al. (1972) Favourable outlook for children with mediastinal neuroblastoma. J Pediatr Surg 7: 136–138

Flamant F, Hill C (1984) The improvement in survival associated with combined chemotherapy in childhood rhabdomyosarcoma. A historical comparison of 345 patients treated at the same centre. Cancer 53: 2417–2421

Flamant F, Schwarz L, Delons E, Caillaud J, Hartmann M, Lemerle J (1984) Seminomatous non malignant cell tumours in children. Cancer 54: 1687–1691

Flamant F, Rodary CH, Voûte PA, Otten J (1985) Primary chemotheray in the treatment of rhabdomyosarcoma in children. Trial of the International Society of Pediatric Oncology SIOP (Preliminary results). Radiother Oncol 3: 187–297

Fossati-Bellani F, Kenda F, Lombardi F, Gianni C, Gasparini M, Pizetti P, Musumeci R, Bonnadonna G (1984) Childhood Hodgkin's disease. Treatment with ABVD chemotherapy and limited field irradiation (Abstr). 2nd International Conference on Malignant Lymphoma, Lugano

Gale GB, d'Angio GJ, et al. (1982) Cancer in neonates. The experience at the Children's Hospital of Philadelphia. Pediatrics 70: 409–413

Gasparini M, Barni S, La Hauda A, et al. (1977) Ten years experience with Ewing's sarcoma. Tumori 63: 77–89

Gasparini M, Lombardini F, Gianni C, Lavati C, Fossati-Bellani F (1983) Childhood rhabdomyosarcoma with meningeal extension. Results of chemotherapy including central nervous system prophylaxis. Am J Clin Oncol 6: 393

Gehan EA, Glover FN, Maurer HM, et al. (1981) Prognostic factors in children with rhabdomyosarcoma. NCI Monogr 56: 83

Gilles FH, Leviton A, Hedley-White T, et al. (1983) Childhood brain tumour update. Hum Pathol 14: 835–845

Glass AG, Fraumeni JR (1970) Epidemiology of bone cancer in children. JNCI 44: 187–199

Gnudi S, Picci P, Gherlinzoni F, Bacci G, Putti C (1983) Adjuvant chemotherapy for localised Ewing's sarcoma. Ten years experience in 121 cases at the Instituto Ortopedico Rizzoli. In: Spitzy KH, Karrer K (eds) Proceedings of the 13th International Congress of Chemotherapy, Vienna. 251: 19–22

Godano F, Fabrici B, Ricci RF (1987) Stereotactic surgery in the management of deep intracranial lesions in infancy and adolescents. Child Nerv Syst 3: 85–88

Goorin AM, Apelson HT, Frei E (1985) Osteosarcoma – fifteen years later. N Engl J Med 313: 1637–1642

Green DM (1983) The diagnosis and treatment of germ cell tumours in infants and children. Cancer Treat Rev 10: 265–288

Grosfeld JL, Ballantine RL, Bachner J (1978) Experience with second look operations in pediatric solid tumours. J Pediatr Surg 13: 275–286

Gutjahr P (1986) Krebs bei Kindern und Jugendlichen. Klinik und Praxis. Deutscher Ärzte Verlag, Cologne

Halpern S (1981) Thyroid carcinoma in childhood. Med Pediatr Oncol 9: 143–157

Harmer HM, et al. (1982) The TNM classification of pediatric tumours. UICC, Geneva

Harms D, Gottschalk J, Yänig U (1983) Pathologische Anatomie der Keimzelltumoren (besonders Hodentumoren bei Kindern). Klin Padiatr 195: 196–200

Hawkins E (1987) Pathology of germ cell tumours (Abstr). Meeting of the International Society of Pediatric Oncology, Jerusalem

Hawkins MM, et al. (1987) Incidence of second primary tumours among childhood cancer survivors. Br J Cancer 56: 339–347

Hays FA, Green AA, Histu HO, et al. (1983) Surgicopathological staging of neuroblastoma. Prognostic significance of regional lymphoid metastases. J Pediatr 102: 59

Hays DM (ed) (1986a) Pediatric surgical oncology. Grune and Stratton, Orlando
Hays DM (1986b) Rhabdomyosarcoma and other soft tissue tumours. In: Hays DM (ed) Pediatric surgical oncology. Grune and Stratton, Orlando
Hays DM, Ternberg JL, Clen TT, et al. (1984) Complication related to 234 staging laparotomies performed in the Intergroup Hodgkin's Disease in Childhood study. Surgery 96: 471-478
Hazebroock FW, Vos J, Voûte PA (1979) Experience of surgical resection of pulmonary metastases of osteosarcomas in children. Ned Tijdschr Geneeskd 123: 192-195
Herbst AL, Ulfelder H, Posckanzer DC (1971) Adenocarcinoma of the vagina. N Engl J Med 284: 878-881
Hirt A, Baumgartner C, Imbach P. Lüthy A, Wagner HP (1984) Differentiation and cytokinetic analyses of normal and neoplastic lymphoid cells in B and T cell malignancies of childhood. Br J Haematol 58: 241-248
Holton CP, Burrington JD, Hatch EI (1975) A multiple chemotherapeutic approach to the management of hepatoblastoma. A preliminary report. Cancer 35: 1083-1087
International Society of Pediatric Oncology (1987) Germ cell tumours. Meeting of the International Society of Pediatric Oncology, Jerusalem
Jones PG, Campbell PM (eds) (1976) Tumours of infancy and childhood. Blackwell, Oxford
Jürgens H, Gobel V, Michaelis J, Ramach W, Ritter J, Sauer R, Treuner J, et al. (1985) Die co-operative Ewing Sarkoma Studie, CESS 81 der GPO. Analyse nach 4 Jahren. Klin Paediatr 197: 225-232
Kasai M, Watanabe I (1970) Histological classification of liver cell carcinoma in infancy and childhood and its clinical evaluation. A study of 70 cases collected in Japan. Cancer 25: 557-563
Kilman JW, Clatworthy HW, Newton WA, et al. (1973) Reasonable surgery for rhabdomyosarcoma. Ann Surg 178: 346-357
Kinnier-Wilson LM, Draper GJ (1974) Neuroblastoma, its natural history and prognosis. A study of 487 cases. Br Med J 3: 301-307
Kissane JM, Askin FB, Foulkes M, Stratton LB, Shirely SF (1983) Ewing's sarcoma of bone: clinicopathologic aspects of 303 cases from the Intergroup Ewing's Sarcoma Study. Hum Pathol 14: 773-779
Knudson AG (1978) Retinoblastoma - a prototypic hereditary neoplasma. Semin Oncol 5: 57-60
Koop E (1972) The neuroblastoma. Progr Pediatr. Surg 14: 14
Kotz E (1983) Proceedings of the 2nd International Workshop in the Design and Application of Tumour Prosthesis for Bone and Joint Reconstruction. Vienna 5-8 Sept
Krush AT et al. (1988) Hepatoblastoma, pigmented ocular fundus and jaw lesions in Gardner syndrome. Am J Med Genet 29: 323-333
Le Floch O, Donaldson S, Kaplan H (1976) Pregnancy following oophoropexy and total modal irradiation in women with Hodgkin's disease. Cancer 38: 2263-2268
Lemerle J, Bloch-Michel E, Campinchi R, Chassagne D, Sarazzin D (1978) Chemotherapy as primary treatment in children with bilateral retinoblastoma. Proc Am Soc Clin Oncol 19: 416
Lemerle J, Voûte PA, Tournade MF, Rodary C, Delemarre JF (1983) Effectiveness of preoperative chemotherapy in Wilms' tumour. Results of an International Society of Paediatric Oncology (SIOP) clinical trial. J Clin Oncol 1 (10): 604-609
Lewis MM (1986) The use of an expandable and adjustable prosthesis in the treatment of childhood malignant bone tumours of the extremity. Cancer 57: 499-502
Link MP, Goorin AM, Miser AW, Green AA, Pratt CB (1986) The effect of adjuvant chemotherapy on relapse free survival in patients with osteosarcoma of the extremity. N Engl J Med 3/4: 1600-1606
Littman P, d'Angio GJ (1981) Radiation therapy in the neonate. Am J Pediatr Hematol Oncol 3: 279-285
Machin GA (1980) Persistent renal blastoma (nephroblastomatosis) as a frequent precursor of Wilms' tumour. A clinical and pathological review. Am J Pediatr Hematol Oncol 2: 253-261
Malpas JS, Freeman JE, Baxton A (1976) Radiotherapy and adjuvant chemotherapy for childhood rhabdomyosarcoma. Br Med J 1: 247-249
Mann HW, Evans AE, Siegel SE, et al. (1985) Prognostic importance of serum ferritin in patients in stage III and IV neuroblastoma. The CCSG experience. Cancer Res 45: 2843-2845
Marcove RC, Abu Zair K (1984) En bloc surgery for osteosarcoma, analysis and review of 90 cases. Bull NY Acad Med 60: 748-758
Marcove RC, Rosen G (1980) Radical en bloc excision for Ewing's sarcoma. Clin Orthop 153: 61-68
Marsden HB, Lennox EL, Lawler W, Kinnier-Wilson LM (1980) Bone metastases in childhood renal tumors. Br J Cancer 41: 875-879
Mauch PM, Weinstein H, Botnick L, Belli J, Cassady JD (1983) An evaluation of long term survival and treatment. Complications in children with Hodgkin's disease. Cancer 51: 925-932
McDivitt RW, Stewart FW (1981) Breast carcinoma in children. JAMA 195: 144-147
Meadows AT, Baum E, Fossati-Bellani F, Green D, Jenkin RDT, Marsden B, Nesbit M, et al. (1985) Second malignant neoplasms. An update from the Late Effects study group. J Clin Oncol 3: 532-538
Mendenhall CM, Marcus RB, Enneking WF, Springfield DS, Thar TL, Million RR (1983) The prognostic significance of soft tissue extension in Ewing's sarcoma. Cancer 51: 913-917
Milé V, Meadows AT, d'Angio GH (1982) Incidence of second malignant neoplasms in childhood: results of an international study. Lancet 2: 1326-1331
Mulvihill JJ (1985) Clinical ecogenetics. Cancer in families. N Engl J Med 312: 1569-1570
Murphy SB (1980) Classification, staging and end results of treatment of childhood non-Hodgkin's lymphomas: dissimilarities from lymphomas in adults. Semin Oncol 7: 332-339
Natman MG (1987) Screening for neuroblastoma. Lancet 2: 656-666
Nesbit M, Perez CA, Tefft M, Burgert EO, Vietti TJ, Kissane J, Pritchard DJ, Geman EA (1981) Multimodal therapy for the management of primary non metastatic Ewing's sarcoma of bone. An intergroup study. Natl Cancer Inst Monogr 56: 255-262
NIH (1984) Limb sparing treatment. Adult soft tissue and osteogenic sarcoma (Abstr). NIH Cancer development conference
Ninane J, Pritchard J, Morris-Jones PM, et al. (1982) Stage II neuroblastoma - adverse prognostic significance of lymph node involvement. Arch Dis Child 57: 438-441
Ohtomo K, Araki T, Yashiro N, Iio M (1983) Pulmonary blastoma in children. Radiology 147: 101-183

Packer RJ, Sutton LN, Rorke LB (1984) Prognostic importance of cellular differentiation in medulloblastoma in childhood. J Neurosurg 61 (2): 296–301
Palmer N, Sachs N, Foulkes M (1982) Histopathology and prognosis in rhabdomyosarcoma (IRSI). Proc Am Soc Clin Oncol 1: 170
Pellerin D, Nihoul-Fékété C, Revillon Y, Fernandes P (1982) Place of Surgery in Neuroblastoma Arch Franc Pediat 39: 13–16
Pendergrass TW (1976) Congenital anomalies in children with Wilms' tumour. Cancer 37: 403–408
Perilongo G et al. (1987) Undifferentiated (embryonal) sarcoma of the liver in childhood. Results of a retrospective Italian study. Tumor 73: 213–217
Pichler E, Kogelnik HD, Reinatz G, et al. (1987) Ergebnisse der Therapie des Medulloblastoms in den letzten 15 Jahren. Strahlentherapie 157: 508–515
Pinkerton R, McElwain T, Horwich A, Prilelardy J (1987) Cartoplatin VP 16 bleomycin in children with malignant germ cell tumours (Abstr). Meeting of the International Society of Pediatric Oncology, Jerusalem
Plaschkes J (1974) Congenital fibromatosis, localized and generalized forms. J Pediatr Surg 9: 95–101
Plaschkes J (1981) Congenital dumb-bell neuroblastoma with paraplegia – how to treat. Excerpta Med Int Congr Ser 57: 188–192
Raney RB, Palmer N, Sutow W, Baum E, Ayala A (1983) Renal cell Carcinoma in children. Med Pediatr Oncol 1: 91–98
Rao BN, Champion JE, Pratt CB, et al. (1983) Limb salvage procedures for children with osteosarcoma. An alternative to amputation. J Pediatr Surg 18: 901–908
Rao BN, Pratt CB, Fleming ID, Dilawari RA, Green AA, Austin B (1985) Colon Cancer in Children and Adolescents Cancer 55: 1322–1326
Rorke LB (1983) The cerebellar medulloblastoma and its relationship to primitive neuroectodermal tumours. J Exp Neuropathol Exp Neurol 42: 1–15
Rosen G, Caparos B, Nirnberg A, Marcove RC, Huvos AG, Kosloff C, Lane J, Murphy L (1981) Ewing's sarcoma – a ten years' experience with adjuvant chemotherapy. Cancer 41: 2204–2213
Rosen G, Caparros B, Huvos AC, et al. (1982) Preoperative chemotherapy of osteogenic sarcoma. Selection of postoperative adjuvant chemotherapy based on the response of primary tumour to preoperative chemotherapy. Cancer 49: 1221–1230
Ryden SE, Drake RM, Franciosi RA (1975) Carcinoid tumours of the appendix in children. Cancer 36: 1538–1542
Scales JJ (1983) Bone and joint replacement for the preservation of limbs. Br J Hosp Med 29: 220–232
Schellong J et al. (1986) Prediction of splenic involvement in children with Hodgkin's disease. A retrospective statistical analysis of 134 patients in the German therapy study DAL HD 78. Cancer 57: 2049–2056
Schnaufer L, Koop CE (1975) Silastic abdominal patch for temporary hepatomegaly in stage VS neuroblastoma. J Pediatr Surg 10: 73–75
Schulte FJ (1987) Pineal region tumours of childhood. Eur J Pediatr 146: 233–245
Schweisguth O (1979) Tumeurs solides de l'enfant. Flammarion, Paris
Shimada H, Chatten J, Newton WA, et al. (1984) Histopathologic factors in neuroblastic tumours. JNCI 73: 405–466
Siegel SE, Lang WE, Harlow PJ, et al. (1980) Patterns of urinary catecholamine metabolite excretion in neuroblastoma. In: Evans AE (ed) Advances in neuroblastoma research. Raven, New York
Siegel SE, Meran RG (1981) Problems in the chemotherapy of cancer in the neonate. Am J Pediatr Hematol Oncol 3: 287–299
SIOP (1987) The role of MIBG in therapy, diagnosis and monitoring of neuroblastoma. Proceedings of the 4th International Workshop on Pediatric Oncology. Med Pediatr Oncol 15: 155–227
Stevens PS, Eckstein HB (1976) Ureteral metastases from Wilms'. J Urol 115: 467–468
Todani T, Shimada K, Watanabe Y, Toki A, Fuji T, Uhushiwara N (1988) Frantz's tumour – a papillary and cystic tumour of the pancreas in girls. J Pediatr Surg 23: 116–121
Treuner J, Altmannsberger D, Niethammer D (1986) Soft tissue sarcomas. In: Riehm H (ed) Malignant neoplasma in childhood and adolescence. Karger, Basel
Tschuctida Y, Endo Y, Saido et al. (1978) Feto-protein levels according to age. J Pediatr Surg 13: 155–156
Van Buningon EN, Delemarre JFM, de Kraker J (1987) Germ cell tumours of the ovary. Results of the Amsterdam Group (Abstr). Meeting of the International Society of Pediatric Oncology, Jerusalem
Van Eys J, Cangir A, Coody D, Smith B (1985) Preoperative chemotherapy. MOPP regimen as primary chemotherapy for brain tumours. J Neurooncol 3: 237–243
Vos A, Voûte PA, Kraker I (1982) Influence of chemotherapy on radical excision of childhood hepatoblastoma (Abstr). 1st Congess of the European Society of Surgical Oncology, Amsterdam
Voûte PA, Barrett A, Bloom JB, Lemerle J, Niedhardt MK (eds) (1986) Cancer in children – clinical management. Springer, Berlin Heidelberg New York
Wagner HP, Käser H (1983) The role of surgery, radiotherapy and chemotherapy in the treatment of neuroblastoma. In: Rickham PP, Hecker WC, Prevot J (eds) Progress in Pediatric Surgery, Urban and Schwarzenberg, Munich
Weinberg ME, Finegold MJ (1983) Primary hepatic tumours of childhood. Hum Pathol 14: 512–537
Weller CV (1941) The inheritance of retinoblastoma and its relationship to practical eugenics. Cancer Res 1: 517
Wharam MD, Klein JL, Leichner PK, Order SE (1987) Preliminary experience with radioisotope labelled immunoglobulin for therapy of pediatric hepatoma (Abstr). 19th Meeting of the International Society of Pediatric Oncology, Jerusalem
Winship T, Rosvoll R (1961) Thyroid carcinoma in childhood. Final report on a 26 year study. Cancer 14: 734–743
Yamamuro K (1987) International symposium on limb salvage in musculoskeletal oncology, Kyoto
Young JL, Miller RW (1975) Incidence of malignant tumours in US children. J Pediatr 86: 254–258
Zucker JM, Margulis E (1979) Radiotherapy of postoperative minimal residual disease in neuroblastoma. Cancer Res 68: 423
Zucker JM, Henry-Amar M, Sarrazin D, Black R, Patte C, Schweisguth O (1983) Intensive systematic chemotherapy in localised Ewing's sarcoma in childhood. A historical trial. Cancer 52: 415–423

Soft-Tissue Sarcomas

A. KULAKOWSKI

Definition

Soft-tissue sarcomas (STS) are a malignant group of soft tissue tumours. STS originate mainly in the extraskeletal mesenchymal connective tissue and the mesodermal endothelium. They are characterised by similarities in their pathological appearance and common clinical behaviour. Most STS are highly malignant with a strong tendency to recur locally and a high rate of early distant blood-borne metastases.

Epidemiology

Despite the fact that about 50% of the body weight is composed of soft tissues, STS are rare tumours, comprising less than 1% of all human malignancies. The incidence rate is 1–2 per 100 000. They are frequent in children of less than 15 years of age, where they constitute 6.5% of all paediatric tumours. In adults they can occur at any age with a peak in the sixth decade of life, and more than 50% are in the extremities, 30% in the trunk and 15% in the head and neck. In children head and neck is the most common site. Incidence is about the same in both sexes.

Aetiology

Some promoting disease, environmental factors and genetic disorders may be risk factors, but the aetiology of STS remains unknown.

Promoting Disease

1. Viral infections
2. Long-standing lymphoedema (can induce lymphangiosarcoma, possibly after treatment for breast cancer)

Environmental Factors

1. Irradiation [malignant fibrous histocytoma (MFH) and others]
2. Foreign body, trauma, scars
3. Chemicals - vinyl chloride, thorotrast, herbicide, etc.

Genetic Disorders

1. Multiple neurofibromatosis (von Recklinghausen's disease, malignant schwannoma)
2. Werner's syndrome
3. Gardner's syndrome (fibromatosis and MFH)
4. Basal cell nevus syndrome

Histopathology

STS originate from the primitive mesenchyma that can develop into various stromal elements and connective tissues. STS are classified histologically according to the tissues they most resemble. Histological classification is extremely varied, sometimes controversial and frequently very difficult, despite the use of special staining, electron microscopic studies and tissue cultures. A common factor is the production of reticulin. The systems commonly used differentiate between the tissue or origin and its malignant transformation (Table 1).

An important and debated factor in histopathological diagnosis is the evaluation of the grade of malignancy. Any grading system is mainly based upon the number of mitoses, extension of necrosis, degree of cellularity, nuclear pleomorphism and new vascular formation. A significant prognostic value has been reported by stratifying sarcomas into three grades: I, low grade; II, moderate grade; III, high grade of malignancy.

Table 1. Histological types of STS (ICD-O Geneva 1978)

Histological type	ICD-O
Sarcoma, not otherwise specified (NOS)	M-8800/3
Fibrosarcoma NOS	M-8810/3
Malignant fibrohistiocytoma (MFH)	M-8830/3
Liposarcoma NOS	M-8850/3
Leiomyosarcoma NOS	M-8890/3
Rhabdomyosarcoma	M-8900/3
Malignant mesenchymoma	M-8990/3
Synovial sarcoma NOS	M-9040/3
Mesothelioma	M-9050/3
Angiosarcoma	M-9120/3
Extraskeletal osteosarcoma	M-9190/3
Extraskeletal chondrosarcoma	M-9221/3
Malignant schwannoma	M-9560/3
Alveolar soft-parts sarcoma	M-9581/3

Not included are: Kaposi's sarcoma, dermatofibrosarcoma, fibrosarcomas grade 1 (desmoid tumour) and sarcoma arising from the dura mater, brain or viscera. M, morphology.

Incidence and Characteristics of STS Types

Table 2 shows the epidemiological data on 329 adults with STS seen at the Marie Sklodowska-Curie (MSC) Memorial Institute of Oncology in Warsaw in the years 1950–1980. In stratifying STS by histotype we notice some specific behaviour.

Liposarcoma. This is most commonly located in the thigh. Subtypes are: lipoma-like (well-differentiated), myxoid type (intermediate grade), round cell and pleomorphic type (high-grade malignancy).

Fibrosarcoma. Fibromatosis, desmoid and dermatofibrosarcoma protuberans are grade I sarcomas and practically do not metastasise. They have a common location in the head and neck and trunk. High-grade fibrosarcomas have a very high metastatic rate, and many of these cases should often be included among malignant fibrous histocytomas.

Malignant Fibrous Histocytoma. MFH is a type which has been frequently recognised in recent years, in the past it was often confused with other types, or non-differentiated. The histocyte is a totipo-

Table 2. Incidence by histological type and anatomical location

Type	(%)	Location	(%)
Liposarcoma	9	Head and neck	8
Rhabdomyosarcoma	1	Trunk	10
Synovial sarcoma	19	Upper extremity	28
Neurofibrosarcoma	18	Lower extremity	54
Fibrosarcoma	15	(Thigh	25)
Angiosarcoma	5		
Leiomyosarcoma	3		
Malignant mesenchymoma	0.3		
Malignant fibrous histiocytoma	7		
Undifferentiated	14		
Others	8.7		

tent matrix of mesenchymal tissues, so that any STS on its way towards the dedifferentiation tends to coincide with malignant histocytoma. This pathological concept can explain its relative increase in current pathological reports. For the same reasons, MFH can occur at any site and is, usually, a deep-seated, large tumour with a high propensity to spread distant metastases.

Synovial Sarcoma. The common location is the distal part of the extremities (foot and hand) and the vicinity of the joints and tendons (knee, ankle) in young adults. Growth is monophasic or biphasic. According to the presence of several nodules, sometimes with calcifications, two histological features, epithelioid and synovial cell, are recognised. Lymph node metastases are possible (20%).

Rhabdomyosarcoma. In children the embryonal type has a common location in the head and neck (the orbit). The alveolar and pleomorphic types, in adults, affect the extremities and the pelvis.

Leiomyosarcoma. This can be present at any site and is a common retroperitoneal or visceral tumour with a high local recurrence rate, giving metastases to the lungs and also to the liver.

Malignant Schwannoma. This is included in the chapter of sarcomas despite the fact that it belongs to the neuroectodermal matrix: it usually occurs close to large nerves and the plexus (ischiatic nerve, supraclavicular region of the arm and forearm) and is frequently encountered as a degeneration of neurofibromas in von Recklinghausen's disease.

Natural History

Despite the clinical characteristics according to the different histotypes, the natural history of STS is characterised by two common principal features: local invasion and distant metastases, depending on the histological and clinical malignancy of the tumour. High-grade STS aggressively invade the surrounding local tissues along anatomical planes (nerve fibres, vascular bundles, fascial planes) and form pulmonary metastases early in the clinical course. Besides the infiltrating growth, they may also form satellite nodules or "jumping tumours" around the primary lesion. The expanding growth of sarcoma forms a pseudocapsule surrounding the tumour. The natural anatomical barriers (fasciae, adventitiae) prevent direct invasion. The recurrence rate depends on the radicality of excision. Blood-borne metastases almost always occur in the lungs during the first 12 months after treatment. Bones, intraperitoneal organs and CNS are less common sites of metastases, and nodal metastases are also uncommon.

Prognosis

The prognosis of STS depends on the histological grade and type, size and location of the tumour and the age and sex of the patient. The *grade* of tumour which reflects the histological malignancy is the most important recognised prognostic indicator. Pathologists use a three-degree scale, but for practical purposes one should know whether the tumour is well (grade I) or poorly differentiated (grade II or III) with 90% and 40% 5-year survival rates, respectively.

The *histological* types synovial sarcoma, rhabdomyosarcoma, leiomyosarcoma and malignant fibrohistocytoma generally have a worse prognosis (40%–50% 5-year survival) than liposarcoma or fibrosarcoma (80% 5-year survival), but, again, this fact depends on the grading because a high percentage of lipo- and fibrosarcoma are grade I sarcomas. The *size* of tumour is considered of some importance for treatment and prognosis. Tumours larger than 5 cm in diameter are classified with a worse prognosis than those of less than 5 cm. The correlation between tumour size and duration of clinical symptoms is a simple clinical indicator of tumour aggressivity. More recently this prognostic factor seems to have been less predictive of survival. There is, however, no doubt that the larger the lesion, the greater is the effort to perform radical conservative surgery. Similarly, location in the extremities and especially at a distant site permits a better surgical approach and better prognosis than when the tumour is situated at a proximal site or in the trunk, as in the case of retroperitoneal tumours which generally have a poor prognosis with a high recurrence rate. In the extremities the intracompartmental location is more favorable than extracompartmental. The age and sex of patients are less important, even though young people and the female sex seem to have a better prognosis. The appearance of a local recurrence or distant metastasis is obviously a bad prognostic factor.

Staging Systems

Many clinical classification and staging systems are based on clinical and pathological findings (Hermanek and Sobin 1987; Russel et al. 1977; AJC 1983) taking into account the most important or supposed prognostic factors. The staging work-up consists of the clinical assessment of the tumour, radiographical studies and pathological typing and grading. The UICC TNM classification (Hermanek and Sobin 1987) is based on the retrospective studies undertaken by the AJC and has the approval of other important committees (Tables 3 and 4).

In 1980 Enneking et al. proposed a different surgical staging of STS, based upon the new concept of compartment (Table 5). This classification considers the anatomical location of the tumour and simplifies the grading by combining grades I and II as G_1 (low grade) and grade III as G_2 (high grade). This is a surgical classification which is useful as a guide for planning the extent of surgery, defined as marginal excision, wide excision, radical or compartmental excision.

Table 3. Anatomic staging (TNM)

T – Primary tumours
- T1 Tumour less than 5 cm
- T2 Tumour 5 cm or greater
- T3 Tumour that grossly invades bone, major vessel or major nerves

N – Node involvement
- N0 No histologically verified metastases to lymph nodes
- N1 Histologically verified regional lymph node metastases

M – Distant metastases
- M0 No distant metastases
- M1 Distant metastases

G – Histopathology grade
- G1 Low grade
- G2 Moderate grade
- G3 High grade

Table 4. Stage grouping

Stage I					
	I a	G1	T1	N0	M0
	I b	G1	T2	N0	M0
Stage II					
	II a	G2	T1	N0	M0
	II b	G2	T2	N0	M0
Stage III					
–	III e	G3	T1	N0	M0
–	III b	G3	T2	N0	M0
–	III c	Any G	T1,2	N1	M0
Stage IV					
–	IV a	Any G	T3	Any N	M0
–	IV b	Any G	Any T	Any N	M1

Table 5. Staging based on compartment

Stage	G grade	T location	M
IA	G1 (low)	T1 (intracompartmental)	M0
B	G1 (low)	T2 (extracompartmental)	M0
IIA	G2 (high)	T1 (intracompartmental)	M0
B	G2 (high)	T2 (extracompartmental)	M0
III	Any G	Any	M1

T2 Including cases of local recurrence
M1 Including lymph node metastases

Screening Systems

Any soft tissue tumour should be accurately evaluated with clinical and radiological examinations and a pathological diagnosis should be confirmed before any treatment is undertaken. Up to the present time it has not been possible to detect or suspect asymptomatic STS.

Diagnosis

Diagnosis of STS is sometimes difficult. Important initial clinical symptoms are:

1. Painless mass in the soft tissue.
2. Slowly growing tumour with sudden acceleration in the growth.
3. The most frequent location is in the extremities and in the lower extremities more than in the upper: the adductor area or medial thigh more than other sites in the lower extremity.
4. Pain and paresthesia are late symptoms.

5. Paraneoplastic syndromes (hypoglycaemia in retroperitoneal STS) and tumour marker endocrine-like substances (extremely rare).

A complete history, physical examination and routine laboratory studies should be performed.

Radiographical Studies

1. Plan radiography or xeroradiography of the affected region may demonstrate a decreased radio-opacity or presence of calcifications.
2. High-resolution CT scans can precisely localise the lesion and delineate the proximity to nerves, vessels and bone. More recently, nuclear magnetic resonance (NMR) has provided better topographic images.
3. Arteriograms are useful for demonstrating pathological vascularity, the extent of the tumour and the possibility, or validity, of eventual regional infusion or perfusion therapies.
4. For lesions close to a skeletal structure, bone scintigraphy can document the possible infiltration of bone.
5. Chest films are required and should be completed by tomography and CT scan for any suspect lesion in order to detect lung metastases.

Biopsy

Any soft tissue mass suggestive of sarcoma should be biopsied before treatment, and a sample of tissue must be delivered to the pathologist. Frozen sections are usually possible.

Fine Needle Biopsy. This is not valuable for proper diagnosis.

Drill Biopsy or "Tru-Cut" Needle Biopsy. This can provide a valuable core of tumour tissue for examination and is a good compromise for reliable diagnosis and scarce invasivity and contamination.

Open Biopsy. This provides a wedge of tissue and is the most common bioptic procedure. The biopsy should be incisional and not excisional, with minimal contamination. The incision should be carefully planned so that it can be removed during the en bloc dissection: in the extremities it should be longitudinal and not transverse. Haematomas must be avoided at all cost and drainage should be avoided.

Once the diagnosis and staging of the sarcoma are concluded, the treatment strategy can be delineated.

Surgical Treatment of Locoregional Disease

The excision of the tumour should be done en bloc through the normal tissues (without visualisation of the tumour) with 2–3-cm margins, preferably with a group of muscles from one insertion to the other. The biopsy scar should be removed with wide margins of skin and subcutaneous tissues. Skin graft or rotation of musculocutaneous flap is sometimes necessary. When necessary, the amputation or disarticulation should be performed above the proximal insertions of the involved muscles. It is indicated when the tumour involves large joints, bone, major vessels and nerves, or as a palliative procedure.

Combined Treatment

Multimodality therapy seems to indicate real progress in the treatment of STS. The main treatments adjuvant to surgery are radiotherapy, chemotherapy or both.

Adjuvant Radiotherapy. Postoperative radiotherapy is indicated after marginal conservative surgery or when conservative surgery has been performed for recurrent disease. It seems to have very little effect when macroscopic residual disease remains. Megavoltage beams (4–20 MV) with modern radiotherapy techniques, such as cone down or shrinking fields, are essential to achieve the desired doses within the tumour. Doses of 50–70 Gy are given to the entire operative field with cone down techniques over a period of 6–8 weeks. Preoperative radiotherapy has been tried with some success, but has met with complications following surgery.

Adjuvant Chemotherapy. Since approximately 50% of patients have micrometastases at the time of diagnosis, the concept of adjuvant chemotherapy prior to or after surgery is a very attractive approach and should be studied in multicentre clinical trials. Up to now, although a few authors have documented successes with postoperative adjuvant chemotherapy, from the experience of others the role of this treatment seems to be questionable (Bramwell et al. 1985; Bramwell 1986; Das Gupta et al. 1982; Edmondson 1984; Rosenberg 1984).

On a theoretical basis, adjuvant chemotherapy is expected to play a role in the control of micrometastases. Single therapeutic agents are adriamycin (ADR), dacarbazine (DTIC), cyclophosphamide

(CPM), vincristine (VCR), methotrexate (MTX) and, more recently, ifosfamide (IFO). These drugs are more frequently used in combination (see Treatment of Metastatic Disease). Moreover, in order to obtain an improved local shrinkage of the primary lesions, intra-arterial regional infusion of chemotherapy has been employed, sometimes combined with preoperative radiotherapy. The drug used for intra-arterial chemotherapy has been ADR in all the reports (Azzarelli et al. 1983; Eibler 1984; Karakousis et al. 1980).

Treatment of Recurrence

The treatment of recurrence should be individualised. Recurrences in extremities are almost always treated by amputation or disarticulation, but various combination therapies (intra-arterial chemotherapy, radiotherapy and surgery) should be considered. The 5-year disease-free survival rate reflects the effectiveness of treatment. In about 80% of patients who develop local or systemic relapse, the recurrence occurs within 1 year of the treatment of the primary lesion.

Treatment of Metastatic Disease

The primary treatment of metastatic disease is chemotherapy: ADR alone or in combinations is commonly used for systemic chemotherapy. Survival depends on many factors of which the most important is tumour doubling time and performance status of the patient. The most commonly used combination is known as CYVADIC (Table 6). Other combinations are: ADR + DTIC, ADM + IFO, ADM + IFO + DTIC.

Lung metastases can also be treated by surgical resection. The best results can be obtained for solitary, peripheral lesions, particularly when they are discovered after an adequate disease-free interval (more than 1 year after primary treatment). Hilar nodal involvement, pleural or pericardial effusions are not suitable for surgical treatment. For other operable situations a bilateral resection by sternotomy is suggested. Clinical and radiological controls must therefore be very frequent in the first 12–18 months, including physical examination and chest X-ray every 2–3 months, radiography of the affected region, echography and/or CT scan for lesions of the retroperitoneum. After this period, if no signs of disease have appeared, the follow-ups can be performed every 4–6 months up to the 3rd year following the main treatment. Bone and brain metastases are treated by irradiation and/or systemic chemotherapy.

Table 6. CYVADIC scheme of treatment

Drug	Dose	Days 1–2–3
Cyclophosphamide	500 mg/m^2	X
Vincristine	2 mg/m^2	X
Adriamycin	50 mg/m^2	X
DTIC	400 mg/m^2	XXX

Disease-Free Periods and Survival

The experience of the MSC Institute of Oncology in Warsaw in 329 cases of STS treated only surgically between 1950 and 1980 (W. Ruka and J. Meyza, unpublished) showed different 5-year survival rates depending on the grade and histotype of the sarcomas: undifferentiated sarcoma – 23%, liposarcoma – 48%, synovial sarcoma – 35%, malignant schwannoma – 45%, fibrosarcoma – 45%, angiosarcoma – 33%, leiomyosarcoma – 42% and malignant fibrous histocytoma – 6%. The statistics of combined treatment (Lindberg et al. 1981; Suit et al. 1981) showed better survival rates of around 70%. The local recurrence rate in large series at the Memorial Sloan Kettering Cancer Center (Shin et al. 1975), University of Florida (Enneking et al. 1981), University of Göteborg (Markhede et al. 1982), M. D. Anderson Hospital (Lindberg et al. 1981), NCI, Massachusetts General Hospital (Suit et al. 1981; Tepper and Suit 1985) varied from 15% to 20% and in the case of distant metastases from 30% to 40%.

The 5-year survival rate varied in many institutions from 40% to 60% (Bramwell et al. 1985, 1987; Bramwell 1986; Edmondson 1984; Pinedo et al. 1984). The multicentre EORTC trials in advanced disease showed objective improvements of 37% treated with CYVADIC and ifosfamide (Schurette et al. 1986). An ongoing EORTC trial for adjuvant CYVADIC suggests that there is an advantage in the chemotherapy arm in relation to the local recurrence rate. Final results have not yet been published. Further multicentre randomised trials should be planned.

Rehabilitation

The limb-preserving combined procedures, surgery and radiotherapy and regional chemotherapy, improve the patients' quality of life. It is amazing how much musculature can be excised without appreciably affecting ordinary activity. This is due to the great amount of reserve in the musculature of the extremity and also the vigorous rehabilitation techniques which maximise the function of residual tissues.

Future Developments

Future developments in the field of STS depend on basic research, the improvement in diagnosis and modalities of treatment. In diagnosis, the recent technique of NMR has improved the anatomical staging by better tumour visualisation. In local treatment, surgery techniques are already well established, but performed well only in specialized centres. The role of radiotherapy and its optimalisation should be studied further. The new types of radiation (neutrons), optimal techniques (fields, doses) sequences (preoperative, postoperative) and the combination with other methods (regional chemotherapy, sensitisers) should be studied to improve local conservative treatment. The development of radiobiology can promote new ideas.

Chemotherapy in local and systemic treatment plays an important role. The search for more specific agents, optimal doses, timing and schedules should be studied. Not only laboratory research, but also randomised clinical trials, conducted on the basis of multicentre cooperation can improve the survival of patients with STS.

References

AJC, American Joint Committee on Cancer (1983) Manual for staging of cancer, 2nd edn. Lippincott, Philadelphia, pp 111–113

Azzarelli A, et al. (1983) Intra-arterial adriamycin followed by surgery for limb sarcomas. Preliminary report. Eur J Cancer Clin Oncol 19: 885–890

Bramwell VHC, (1986) Adjuvant chemotherapy for soft tissue sarcomas. In: Pinedo HM, Verweij J (eds) Clinical management of soft tissue sarcomas. Nijhoff, Boston, pp 89–101

Bramwell VHC, et al. (1985) Combined modality management of local and disseminated adult soft tissue sarcomas: a review of 257 cases seen over 10 years at the Christie Hospital and Holt Radium Institute, Manchester. Br J Cancer 51: 301–318

Bramwell VHC, et al. (1987) European experience of adjuvant chemotherapy for soft tissue sarcoma: interim report of a randomized trial of CYVADIC versus control. Proc of the Innisbrook International Symposium on Sarcomas. Oct 1987, Tarpon Springs, Florida, USA

Das Gupta TK, Patel MK, Chandhuri PK, et al. (1982) The role of chemotherapy as an adjuvant to surgery in the initial treatment of primary soft tissue sarcomas in adults. J Surg Oncol 19: 139–144

Edmondson JH (1984) Role of adjuvant chemotherapy in the management of patients with soft tissue sarcomas. Cancer Treat Rep 89–101

Eibler FR (1984) Soft tissue sarcomas of the extremity. Curr Probl Cancer 8: 3–41

Enneking WF, Spanier SS, Goodman MM (1980) Current concepts review: the surgical staging of musculoskeletal sarcoma. J Bone Joint Surg [Am] 62: 1027–1030

Enneking WF, Spanier SS, Malawer MM (1981) The effect of the anatomic setting on the results of surgical procedures for soft-part sarcomas of the thigh. Cancer 47: 1005–1022

Hermanek P, Sobin LH (1987) TNM classification of malignant tumours, 4th edn. Springer, Berlin Heidelberg New York

Karakousis CP, et al. (1980) Intraarterial adriamycin in the treatment of soft tissue sarcomas. J Surg Oncol 13: 21–27

Lindberg R, Martin R, Ramsdahl M, et al. (1981) Conservative surgery and postoperative radiotherapy in 300 adults with soft tissue sarcoma. Cancer 47: 2391–2397

Markhade G, Angervoll L, Stenner B (1981) A multivariant analysis of the prognosis after surgical treatment of malignant soft tissue tumors. Cancer 49: 1721–1733

Pinedo HM, et al. (1984) CYVADIC in advanced soft tissue sarcomas: a randomized study comparing two schedules. Cancer 53: 1825–1832

Rosenberg SA (1984) Prospective randomized trials demonstrating the efficacy of adjuvant chemotherapy in adult patients with soft tissue sarcomas. Cancer Treat Rep 68: 1067–1078

Russel WO, Cohen J, Enzinger F, Hajdu S, et al. (1977) A clinical and pathological staging system for soft tissue sarcomas. Cancer 40: 1562–1570

Schurette et al. (1986) Adriamycin and ifosfamide: a new effective combination in advanced soft tissue sarcomas: preliminary report of phase II study of the EORTC group. Proc Ann Meet Am Soc Clin Oncol 5: 145

Shin MM, et al. (1975) Ann Surg 182: 597–602

Suit HD, Proppe KH, Mankin HJ, et al. (1981) Preoperative radiation therapy for sarcoma of the soft tissue. Cancer 47: 2269–2274

Tepper JE, Suit HD (1985) Radiation therapy of soft tissue sarcomas. Cancer 55: 2273–2277

Bone Sarcomas

N. TRAPEZNIKOV

Introduction

Primary malignant bone tumours are neoplasms originating from tissues forming the bone constituents (bone, cartilage, marrow, etc.). They are relatively rare: bones are more frequently affected by metastases spread by tumours located in distant sites: breast, thyroid, prostate, kidney, lungs, etc.

Primary malignant bone tumours occur more often in the second decade of life, principally in the male (1.5–2.0 times more than in females) and average 1.0 (male) and 0.6–0.7 (female) cases per 100 000 of the population, with some epidemiological differences according to the histotypes. Bone sarcomas affect the long tubular bones of the lower limbs and the pelvic girdle, though they are also frequent in other parts of the bony skeleton.

Some factors stimulating the neoplastic growth are known (embryonal and postembryonal disorders, chemical cancerogenous substances, irradiation), but for most cases the aetiology and pathogenesis of bone tumours remains unclear. Some bone diseases, such as Paget's disease, fibrous dysplasia, osteocartilaginous exostosis, chronic osteomyelitis, can lead to the development of secondary bone tumours which are more frequently osteo- or chondrosarcomas.

Bone tumours are grouped by stages: for practical purposes it is reasonable to distinguish the local form of the disease from the disseminated type. There were about 60 classifications of bone tumours proposed during the 100 years leading to the working classification of bone tumours published by WHO in 1972. This is currently one of the most often employed, both for medical practice and for scientific activities (Table 1). This classification is reported because of its clear and rational schematicism, even though some tumours are now obsolete, mainly in the section on marrow tumours where the inclusion of Ewing's sarcoma is still debatable, and reticulosarcoma and lymphosarcoma can be better included among the lymphomas. As far as malignant bone lesions are concerned, with the exclusion of lymphomas and multiple myeloma which are of medical origin, the histotypes most frequently encountered are as follows: osteosarcoma (60%), chondrosarcoma (30%) and Ewing's sarcoma (10%), which together comprise more than 90% of all primary bone malignancies.

Osteogenic Sarcoma

Osteosarcoma is the main primary bone tumour and represents 60% of all primary bone sarcomas. It is found most frequently in the male, with a prevalence between the years of 10 and 20. It is located primarily in the metaphysis of the long tubular bones (distal femur, proximal tibia, proximal fibula, proximal humerus). More rarely, osteosarcoma arises from

Table 1. Histological typing of primary bone tumours and tumour-like lesions

Bone-forming tumours	
Benign	
	Osteoma
	Osteoid osteoma and osteoblastoma (benign osteoblastoma)
Malignant	
	Osteosarcoma (osteogenic sarcoma)
	Juxtacortical osteosarcoma (parosteal osteosarcoma)
Cartilage-forming tumours	
Benign	
	Chondroma
	Osteochondroma (osteocartilaginous exostosis)
	Chondroblastoma (benign chondroblastoma, epiphyseal chondroblastoma)
	Chondromyxoid fibroma
Malignant	
	Chondrosarcoma
	Juxtacortical chondrosarcoma
	Mesenchymal chondrosarcoma
Giant cell tumours	
Marrow tumours	
Malignant	
	Ewing's sarcoma
	Reticulosarcoma of the bone
	Lymphosarcoma of the bone
	Myeloma
Vascular tumours	
Benign	
	Haemangioma
	Lymphangioma
	Glomus tumour (glomangioma)
Intermediate	
	Haemagioendothelioma
	Haemangiopericytoma
Malignant	
	Angiosarcoma
Other connective tissue tumours	
Benign	
	Desmoplastic fibroma
	Lipoma
Malignant	
	Fibrosarcoma
	Liposarcoma
	Malignant mesenchyoma
	Undifferentiated sarcoma
Other tumours	
	Chordoma
	"Adamantoma" of long bones
	Neurilemmoma (schwannoma, neurinoma)
Unclassified tumours	
Tumour-like lesions	
	Solitary bone cyst (simple or unicameral cyst)
	Aneurysmal bone cyst
	Juxta-articular bone (intraosseous ganglion)
	Metaphyseal fibrous defect (non-ossifying fibroma)
	Eosinophilic granuloma
	Fibrous dysplasia
	"Myositis ossificans"
	"Brown tumour" or hyperparathyroidoma

Paget's disease or other chronic diseases, such as osteomyelitis, etc. Trauma as an aetiological factor has been denied by many investigators (Huvos 1979; Mirra et al. 1974).

Diagnosis is based on clinical and radiological data, as well as on pathological findings. The principle symptom of the disease is a dull pain which increases gradually and is more intense at night. The general status of the patient is not impaired at the first signs of the disease, but a slight swelling appears at the site of the pain. The lesion is most often discovered on palpation at the first medical visit. Where there is a large tumour, the skin is stretched and hot to the touch, and the subcutaneous veins are dilatated. A limp and functional limitation with flexion contraction in the neighbouring joint are frequently present. Pathological fractures occur in 5%–10% of the cases.

The radiological picture of osteosarcoma depends on its morphological tumour typing, the site and the rate of growth, but the osteolytic and osteoblastic components are predominant and usually concomitant. The osteolytic component is characterised by a large area of destruction with uneven damaged margins in the metaepiphyseal part of the bone. A typical feature of osteosarcoma is the detachment of the periosteum from the cortex border, thus forming a peculiar radiological image; the so-called Codman's triangle.

The osteoblastic component shows induration or eburnation of the bone structure. The tumour pressing against the periosteum leads to the formation of radial spicules, located perpendicularly to the bone surface: this is an early radiological finding which is highly specific for osteosarcoma. The inevitable companion of large osteosarcomas is osteoporosis, developing both from neutrophilic disorders and from bone inactivity as the result of severe pain (Fig. 1). The epiphyseal and articular cartilages serve as a barrier against tumour spread towards the joint; nevertheless, radiological imaging does not necessarily correspond to the extent of the spread. Scintigraphy and CT scans are helpful in determining the real osseous extent of the disease.

Up to the present time, we have no knowledge of any haematological finding or marker which is specific to osteosarcoma, even though alkaline phosphatase can be markedly elevated and, in these case, it should be used as a marker to predict a possible relapse of disease. A biopsy, performed with great care in order to prevent possible tumour cell dissemination, will confirm the clinico-radiological suspicions.

The histological appearance is characterised by direct production of atypical bone and ostoid matrix

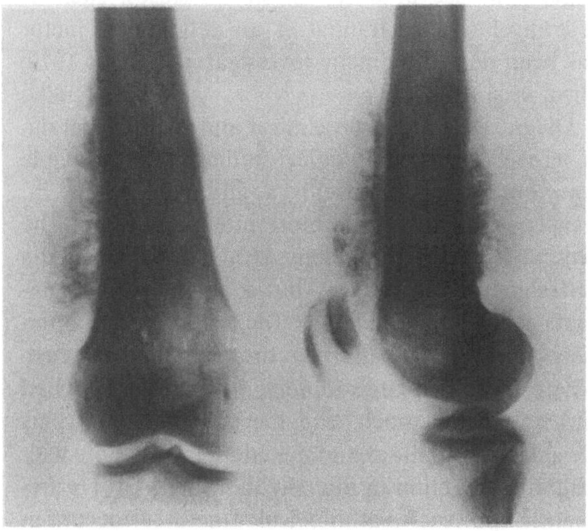

Fig. 1. Typical radiographic appearance of osteosarcoma of the distal femur

by the tumoral tissue itself. This is the predominant characteristic of this sarcoma, even though the osteoid element can be evidenced only by ultrastructural analysis or more specific techniques. The lesions are polymorphic, together with a marked osteoblastic tendency and the formation of a large mass of atypical tumour bone (osteoblastic type). Osteosarcoma can be characterised by a large amount of reactive cartilageneous (chondroblastic type) or fibrous (fibroblastic type) tissue. At other times the cells show a high degree of anaplasia and lose their capacity of producing bone substance completely (osteolytic and teleangiectic type). Between the two extremes there is a wide spectrum of manifestations with distinctly diverse cell elements and different degrees of atypia and polymorphism. Reactive osteogenesis occurs in the peripheral parts, usually close to the periosteum.

Prognosis of osteosarcoma is unfavourable – following surgical treatment alone, the survival rate is around 10%–12%. Haematogenic spread to the lungs occurs within the 1st year after diagnosis; lymphatic metastases are atypical, but not so rare.

In the treatment of primary non-metastatic osteosarcoma, surgery and chemotherapy are expected to provide radical tumour removal and the control of undetectable micrometastases. Radical tumour excision is carried out by amputation (exarticulation) of an extremity or with en bloc resection with endoprosthetic replacement. The latter procedure is always more feasible when operative neoadjuvant chemotherapy induces some grade of tumour regression.

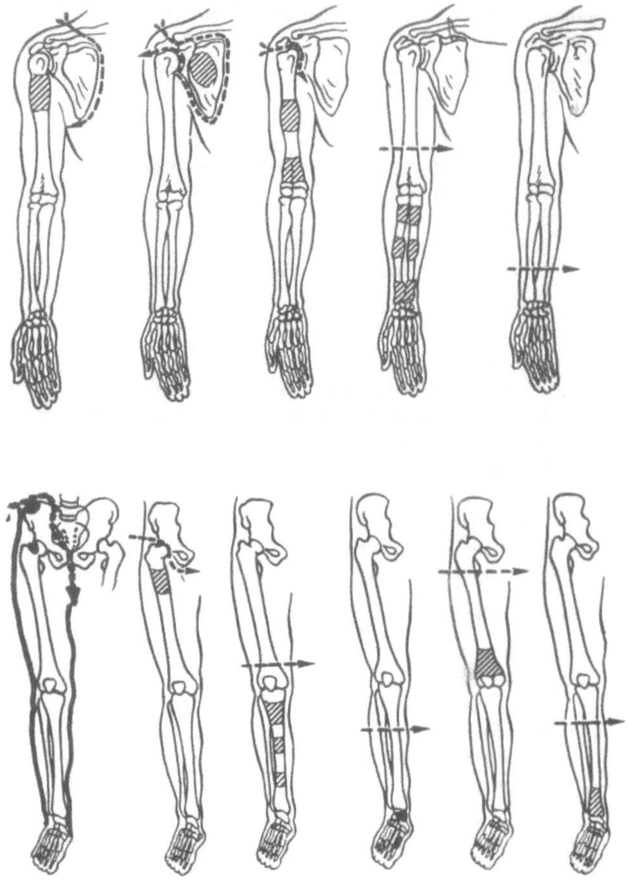

Fig. 2. Levels of amputation for bone sarcoma

The vital question when performing amputations is the choice of level at which to perform the amputation in relation to the site and spread of the tumour, the degree of soft-tissue involvement and the type of the endoprosthesis to be applied. The amputation should be performed at a level at which the function can best be preserved providing a hardy, painless and supportive stump. Amputation for osteosarcoma and other bone tumours should be performed beyond the affected part of the bone (Fig. 2). In exceptional cases, tumours located in the distal part of the femur can be treated with transmedullary amputation of the femur. In such cases high amputation is more advantageous for prosthetic replacement and is less traumatic than exarticulation.

In the past decade, together with the improvement in moveable endoprostheses (hip, knee, proximal humerus) and the better definition of surgical procedures, the possibility of performing en bloc resection has been made possible by the good response of the primary lesion to preoperative chemotherapies.

The preoperative regimen employed at our university in Moscow is as follows: intra-arterial adriamycin

Table 2. The most common chemotherapeutic regimens employed in the management of operable or advanced osteosarcoma

HDMTX	Methotrexate 8–12 mg/m^2 i.v. followed after 20–24 h by citrovorum factor 15 mg p.o. every 6 hours for 2–3 days. Some regimen schedules include vincristine (VCR) 1.4 mg/m^2 i.v. 30 min before HDMTX.
CDDP	*Cis*-platinum 120 mg/m^2 i.v. or 40 mg/m^2/daily for 3 days i.v. or, I arterial
ADM	Adriamycin 75 mg/m^2 i.v. or 30 mg/m^2/daily for 3 days i.v. or, I arterial
BCP	Bleomycin 18 mg/m^2/daily for 2 days i.v. Cyclophosphamide 600 mg/m^2/daily for 2 days i.v. Dactinomycin 0.6 mg/m^2/daily for 2 days i.v.

infusion at 30 mg/m^2 for 3 consecutive days, followed by radiotherapy at cumulative focus dose 35–36 Gy for 2 weeks (Trapeznikov 1983; Eilber et al. 1984). Other regimens, all employing different combinations of high-dose methotrexate (HDMTX) with good results, are: (a) HDMTX and adriamycin for two to three Courses (Rosen et al. 1982); (b) HDMTX – on average 8 g/M^2, four courses with a 1-week interval (Lejeune 1984); (c) HDMTX plus *cis*-platinum for two courses (Jaffe et al. 1985; Picci et al. 1985). Table 2 summarises the more common chemotherapeutic drugs and doses employed for osteosarcoma, either as pre-, postoperative, or advanced phases.

Following surgery, the indication for adjuvant treatment is a control of possible metastases which are frequently already present at the time of the first diagnosis and treatment. Adriamycin, HDMTX, *cis*-platinum and combined regimes [cyclophosphamide + adriamycin + melphalan + vincristine (Compadri I), with the addition od HDMTX and citrovorum rescue factor (Compadri II or Compadri III with increased adriamycin doses)] are effective regimens utilised as precautional treatment, even though ongoing phase II and phase III studies will probably verify the validity of other more simple regimens.

Nowadays, a different approach to adjuvant chemotherapy is related to the grade of tumour response (pathological necrosis) induced by preoperative chemotherapy. In marked regression, the schedule utilised as preoperative chemotherapy is recommended as adjuvant treatment. For non-responders a different regimen is given.

Having completed adjuvant chemotherapy, patients are followed up for 3–5 years. A radiological check of the thorax and the limb which has been operated on should be performed every 3 months for the first 3 years and every 4–6 months for the next 2 years. In the presence of metastases these checks should be performed every month for the 1st year and subsequently when indicated.

Recurrences following en bloc resections of long tubular bones occur in 3%–8% of cases. As a rule they require limb amputation or distarticulation. The policy of a multimodal approach significantly improves the end results: 3-year survival rates increased up to 50%–93% (Rosen et al. 1982; Jaffe et al. 1983) and 5-year survival up to 30%–50% (Trapeznikov et al. 1983; Cortes et al. 1979).

In the treatment of pulmonary metastases of osteosarcoma the main role belongs to chemotherapy (Winkler et al. 1983): HDMTX provides objective response in 40%, adriamycin in 30%, *cis*-platinum in 20%–60% of cases with remission extended up to 18 months. Combined chemotherapy obtains greater effects as an alternative to classical chemotherapies: bleomycin + cyclophosphamide + dacarbazine (DTIC) (BCD) can be employed with encouraging results. In selected cases, lung metastases can also be removed surgically, and this approach, frequently with repeated sternotomies or thoracotomies, has the theoretical and practical possibility of curing the patient in a few cases. This is a possibility which does not exist with other kinds of treatment for metastatic sarcomas and should be ratified in prospective protocols.

Chondrosarcoma

Chondrosarcoma occurs frequently, accounting for 20% of all primary malignant bone tumours. It is noted particularly in the middle aged and the elderly (fourth to sixth decades, incidence in the male is twice that of the female). In patients of less than 30 years of age, differentiated types occur more frequently. Chondrosarcoma may arise in any bone, developing from a cartilage as enchondral ossification. One out of three cases is localised in the pelvis, including the proximal femur. Other frequent sites are the knee area, scapular girdle, distant humerus, ribs and maxillofacial bones. In 10%–15% of patients chondrosarcoma develops as a secondary to chondromas, osteocartilaginous exostoses, dyschondroplasias (Ollier's disease) and deforming osteosis (Paget's disease).

The tumour has a lobate structure. On section the chondrosarcoma tissue looks like a bluey-white semitransparent mass with yellow necrosis foci, zones of haemorrhage and calcifications. Under microscopic examination it is characterised by different degrees of anaplasia. A determining feature in the diagnosis of the origin of cartilage tumour is the interstitial substance of chondroid character with area of necrosis and myxomatous transformation. Low-grade chondrosarcoma is characterised by a marked lobate structure. Interstitial substance prevails over, or is correlated with, the cell mass. Blood vessels are not present in the tumour. Cells are often associated in groups at the expense of cartilage capsulae. Mitoses are rare. Chondrosarcomas of moderate grade (II) are characterised by areas with a prevalent cellular component, in some places blood vessels and mitoses are present. Cells are small, hyperchromic, or giant and multinuclear; polymorphism is rarely noted. In grade II chondrosarcoma, there are areas with a greater prevalence of the cellular rather than the interstitial component. Cells are hyperchromic with marked polymorphism, they have a greater amount of mitoses.

Many cases show a change from well-differentiated to poorly differentiated chondrosarcoma. In mesenchymal chondrosarcoma two features are always present: zones of typical chondrosarcoma, which are usually low grade, and zones with cell elements resembling hemangiopericytoma. In "dedifferentiated" chondrosarcoma two features can also be distinguished: zones of differentiated chondrosarcoma and zones of spindle cell sarcoma resembling fibrosarcoma.

Typical symptoms of primary chondrosarcoma are swelling and pain which intensify with tumour growth. A long period of pain is characteristic before the diagnosis is made when a large, prominent and painful tumour is palpated. When the tumour is located close to the joint, movement is frequently difficult. The clinical course of chondrosarcoma depends on its morphological structure, the course of malignant tumours being typical: in anaplastic chondrosarcomas (most often occurring in patients of less than 30 years of age) prognosis is very short and does not exceed 1–3 months. Haematogenic metastasising is typical of grades II and III. Local recurrences are extremely frequent and are usually more malignant than primary tumours.

The most predictive prognostic factor for chondrosarcoma is the pathological grade (Azzarelli et al. 1986): favourable prognosis for grade I and poor for grades II and III. Moreover, tumour type is significant: secondary chondrosarcomas have a more favourable survival rate. The clinical suspicion of chondrosarcoma is based on comparing the clinical data of the course of the disease with the radiological picture; radiological findings are related to the tumour site and the malignant pattern. Central well-differentiated chondrosarcomas present as a single focus of abnormally round or oval shape, they are usually more radiopaque than the normal bone, with large and irregular intralesional calcifications and borders giving a picture of maculation. (Fig. 3). As opposed to osteosarcoma, in well-differentiated chondrosarcoma the bone spicules and periosteal visors are less frequent.

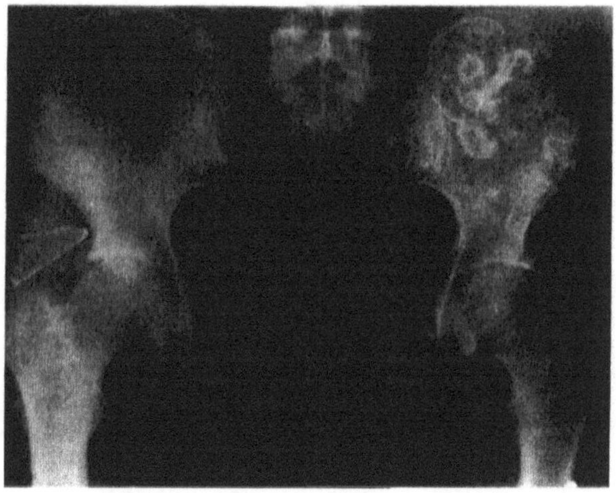

Fig. 3. Chondrosarcoma of the pelvis

In aggressive tumours (chondrosarcomas of moderate and high grade) the tumour spread greatly exceeds its visible diameter. Osteolytic areas are predominant and perilesional sclerosis is not so evident. Occurring prevalently in the metaphysis of the long tubular bones, the tumour spreads extensively to the diaphysis or the epiphysis, some more than the osteosarcomas. In some cases the tumour involves one-half or more of the length of the bone, or, destroying the cartilage plate, it spreads along the joint.

Peripheral chondrosarcoma has a relatively constant radiological picture: a calcified tumour with unclear margins spreading into the soft tissues close to the bone; the surface of the adjacent bone may be eroded and moderately selective. Periosteal reaction is manifested in periosteal visors, rough spicules and linear periostosis.

Chondrosarcoma is mostly chemo- and radio-resistant, therefore, surgery is the principle and perhaps only form of therapy to adopt. In small grade I and II chondrosarcomas, when located in easily removeable sites (upper flaring portion of the ilium bone, peroneum, scapula) resection can be performed. For lage lesions, when it is difficult to achieve radicality, an operation such as the hemipelvectomy, or forequarter amputation, is frequently needed. In patients with high-grade tumour types located in the trunk and girdles, such extensive mutilating surgery is less indicated; in fact, many patients die from metastases within 2 years after surgery. Nevertheless, it should be noted that many hind- or forequarter disarticulations are performed under emergency conditions. In some grade I–II cases palliative radiotherpy can be attempted. Chondrosarcomas located in the long tubular bones can be approached by en bloc resection and endoprosthetic replacement. Amputation and limb exarticulation are indicated for grade III tumours in the extremities.

Chondrosarcoma recurrences are treated on the same principles as primary tumours, with more aggressive or extended surgery up to enlarged hemipelvectomy or even hemocorporectomy. In recurrences occurring in the extremities following conservative surgery, limb amputation or distarticulation is required.

Rehabilitation attempts to eliminate or rectify cosmetic and functional defects by way of the correct prosthesis.

In endeavouring to improve the results of treatment, the trend is to differentiate the approach and the choice regarding the extent of surgery, bearing in mind the degree of tumour anaplasia, but it should be pointed out that grading of chondrosarcoma cannot always be evaluated by biopsy, though the clinico-radiological findings are of great importance in choosing the type and volume of surgical intervention.

The management of metastatic chondrosarcoma is difficult due to the above-mentioned poor tumour sensitivity to irradiation and to anti-tumour agents. For lung metastases, where possible, surgery is strongly recommended but should be performed only in cases where the primary tumour has been radically removed and in patients with a good performance status. Following surgery, chondrosarcoma patients should be followed up in the same way as for osteosarcoma.

Ewing's Sarcoma

Ewing's sarcoma makes up about 10% of all primary malignant bone tumours. It has a prediliction for young people of between 10 and 25 years of age, with a greater incidence in males. The tumour can affect any bone, but it is found mainly in the long tubular bones of the limbs and the trunk. The diaphysis of the tubular bones is frequently involved. Ewing's sarcoma can also occur in the distal bones (peroneum, ankle, distal humerus and bones of the forearm), which, as in the case of the other primary malignancies of the bones, are rare sites. The aetiology and predisposing factors are unknown.

Macroscopically, the tumour presents as a soft disintegrating mass, or a half-liquid mass of a pink-grey colour.

Microscopically, the tumour tissue consists of monomorphic cells, with a round or a slightly oval nucleus and a narrow rim of light-coloured cytoplasm with indistinct borders. Cells form almost solid fields, including cavities of a different size and form and contain more or less blood. Sometimes, the tumour cells form structures like pseudo-rosettes. Stromal fibrillar elements as well as mitoses are rarely seen. As with other bone sarcomas, the first symptoms of the disease are a non-specific, nagging, discontinuous pain which becomes more intense and continuous. As a rule, this is the moment when a solid tumour is diagnosed in the painful area. The clinical picture is nearly always typical: general weakness and overall indisposition, high temperature (up to 39°–40 °C), leukocytosis, and at diagnosis local hyperthermia and skin hyperaemia with subcutaneous phlebectasia are encountered. These clinical findings may decrease significantly and then reappear (cyclic disease course). An important biological feature of Ewing's sarcoma is its precocious metastatic spread to the lymph nodes and other bones, the vertebral column being the first target. Metastases to the lungs, liver and other organs are frequently observed in the advanced phase.

The prognosis is unfavourable. Without adequate therapy the 5-year survival rate is around 10%. The tumour localisation is of some significance. The survival rate is more favourable when the tumour is situated in the long tubular bones than when found in the flat bones. Competent chemotherapy increases the survival rate.

The radiological picture of Ewing's sarcoma is extremely polymorphic. When located in the diaphysis of the long tubular bones, osteoporosis can be observed in the early stages when the surrounding tissues are not involved, this gradually becomes more evident, giving the bone a "spotted" appearance. Extension into the bone marrow canal and the fibrillar cortical layer is typical of this tumour. Stratified periosteal bone apposition ("onion skin", Fig. 4) is one typical, but not specific, periosteal reaction in diaphyseal Ewing's sarcomas.

In the metaphyseal bone tumours, the main radiological image is that of microfocal destruction, periosteal reaction is noted more frequently than in a diaphyseal localisation. In pelvic and scapular bones, the periosteum is not so strong, and the tumour spreads rapidly beyound the bones invading the soft

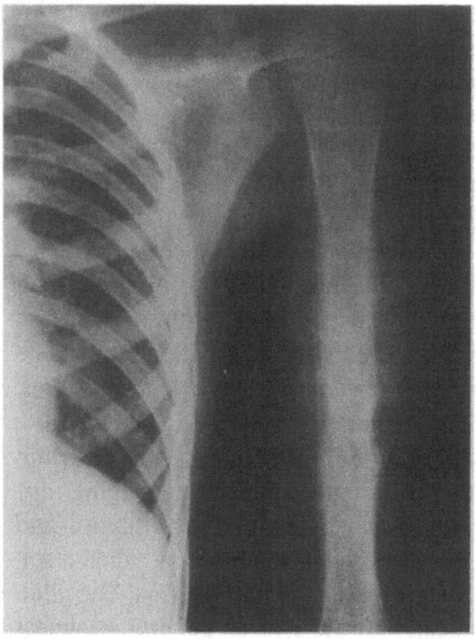

Fig. 4. Ewing's sarcoma of the humerus. Periosteal bone apposition causes the "onion skin" appearance

parts, and in this situation symptoms of periosteal bone formation are absent. The most evaluable and constant symptom for the diagnosis of Ewing's sarcoma is the presence of an extraosseous soft-tissue component, free of calcifications and providing good shapes of the iliac and body crest as falciform shadows. Ewing's sarcoma is highly sensitive to irradiation and some anti-tumour agents. Unlike in other malignant bone tumours, combined treatment modalities including radio- and chemotherapy with or without surgery, can control and cure Ewing's sarcoma. Surgery has no less an indication in the first-line treatment of local Ewing's sarcoma. Such an approach is related to the biological characteristics: tumour extension along the entire bone, high sensitivity to radio- and chemotherapy, early dissemination, independently of radical surgery. However, when indicated, surgical treatment (usually after chemo- and/or radiotherapy) comprises the removal of the affected bone entirely to prevent early recurrences. Surgery can be employed for lesions of the ribs, clavicula, fibula and scapula.

Similarly, radiotherapy for Ewing's sarcoma should be delivered to the entire affected bone, regardless of the tumour size. A single focal dose is 1.8–2.0 Gy, a cumulative focal dose averages 55–60 Gy. As irradiation sources, radioactive cobalt (telegamma unit) and sources of high energy (betatrons, linear X-ray accelerator) are used. In children radiation therapy on the metaphyses of the long bones (distal femur and proximal tibia) can result in considerable discrepancy in the length of the extremity and, for this reason, amputation should be considered, both from the oncological and the rehabilitative points of view.

Taking into account the possibility of early tumour dissemination, chemotherapy is applied in almost all cases along with local treatment. Among the most active anti-tumour agents for this malignant neoplasm are adriamycin, dactinomycin, vincristine and cyclophosphamide which are employed in various regimens. Nowadays, the need for chemotherapy for Ewing's sarcoma has been proved. Combined programmes with the above-mentioned drugs are used more frequently. Treatment is conducted in cycles for 1.5–2 years. The 3-years survival rate is around 40%–50% (Trapeznikov et al. 1983; Bacci et al. 1985).

After the first treatment, patients with Ewing's sarcoma are followed up in the same way as for osteosarcoma. Ewing's sarcoma recurs locally in 6%–25% of cases (Trapeznikov et al. 1983; Bacci et al. 1985). The same treatment methods as for the primary tumour are used, with the exclusion of radiotherapy if it has already been delivered. If conservative methods have no effect, surgical ablative intervention is indicated, the extent being related to the tumour site and size and general status of the patient. For lung metastases from Ewing's sarcoma combined radio- and chemotherapy has been tried with good results (Evans et al. 1984). The irradiation technique is related to the extent of metastatic disease. Large-field irradiation is utilised: its specific feature is one dose over the whole mass on one or both lungs and local irradiation. Single doses are from 1.5–2.0 Gy to 3.3 Gy, with an average cumulative focal dose of 13.2–20.0 Gy.

Acknowledgement. The author wishes to thank Dr. Alberto Azzarelli for his assistance in the preparation of the manuscript.

References

Azzarelli A, Gennari L, Quagliuoro V, et al. (1986) Chondrosarcoma – 55 unreported cases. Epidemiology, surgical treatment and prognostic factors. Eur J Surg Oncol 12: 165–168

Bacci G, Picci P, Gherlinzoni G, et al. (1985) Localized Ewing's sarcoma of bone: ten years' experience at the Instituto Ortopedico Rizzoli in 124 cases treated with multimodal therapy. Eur J Cancer Clin Oncol 21 (2): 163–173

Cortes EP, Holland J-F, Elidewell O (1979) Adjuvant-therapy of operable primary osteosarcoma – Cancer and leukemia

Group B experience. Recent Results Cancer Res 68: 16–24

Eilber FR, Morton DL, Echardt J, Grant T, Weisenburger T (1984) Limb salvage for skeletal and soft tissue sarcomas – multidisciplinary preoperative therapy. Cancer 53 (12): 2579–2584

Evans RG, Burgert ED, Gilchrist ES et al. (1984) Sequential half-body irradiation and combination chemotherapy as salvage treatment for failed Ewing's sarcoma: a pilot study. Int J Radiat Oncol Biol Phys 10: 2363

Huvos AG (1979) Bone tumors: diagnosis, treatment and prognosis. Saunders, Philadelphia, p 52

Jaffe N, Smith E, Abelson H, Frei E (1983) Osteogenic sarcoma: alterations in the pattern of pulmonary metastases with adjuvant chemotherapy. J Clin Oncol 1 (4): 251–254

Jaffe N, Robertson R, Ayahe A et al. (1985) Comparison of intraarterial cis-diamminodichloroplatinum II with high-dose methotrexate and citrovorum factor rescue in the treatment of primary osterosarcoma. J Clin Oncol 3: 1101

Lejeune FJ, Klastersky J, Burny F, Otten J (1984) Le traitement de l'ostéosarcome par la chimiotherapie pre- et postopératoire et la chirurgie non multilante. Rev Med Brux 5 (8): 551–558

Mirra JM, Bullaugh SG, Marcove RC et al. (1974) Malignant fibrous histiocytoma and osteosarcoma in association with bone infarcts. Report of four cases, two in caisson workers. J Bone Joint Surg 56 A: 932–940

Picci P, Bacci G, Campanacci M et al. (1985) Histologic evaluation of necrosis in osteosarcoma induced by chemotherapy: regional mapping of viable and nonviable tumor. Cancer 56: 1515

Rosen G, Caparros B, Huvos A, Kosloff C, Nirenberg A, Cacavio A, Marcove R, et al. (1982) Preoperative chemotherapy for osteogenic sarcoma: selection of postoperative adjuvant chemotherapy based on the response of the primary tumor to preoperative chemotherapy. Cancer 49: 1221–1230

Trapeznikov NN, Solovjev YN, Yeremina LA, Amiraslanov AT (1983) Bone sarcomas. Medicine UzSSR, Tashkent

Winkler K, Bezon G, Brandels H, et al. (1983) Neoadjuvant chemotherapy for osteogenic sarcoma: results of a cooperative German/Austrian study. Proc Am Soc Clin Oncol 2: 233

Surgery in Hematologic Malignancies

K. SOLHEIM

Surgery for Injuries and Surgical Disease in Patients with Hematologic Malignancies

Patients with hematologic malignancy may be injured or suffer a surgical disease necessitating an operation. The hematologic malignancy may then complicate the surgical procedure and prolong the postoperative course. This may be due to insufficiency in hemostasis, poor general condition, drug therapy, etc.

For instance, improved treatment of patients with acute leukemia has resulted in a dramatic increase in the number and duration of remissions. Diseases and injuries that require surgical treatment are therefore seen more frequently. Consequently, the surgeon faces more often the problem of when and if to operate on a patient with leukemia. Presumed high morbidity and lethality has caused a leaning toward conservative treatment. Surgical intervention has often been avoided, with possible serious consequences for the patient.

In one series of 322 patients with acute leukemia, 21 (6.5%) underwent surgical procedures, ten of which where emergencies (Nagler et al. 1985). The most frequent procedures were drainage of abscesses, skin grafts, Scribner shunts, splenectomy, and appendectomy. There were no wound infections or hemorrhagic complications.

The true incidence of surgical procedures in leukemic patients is unknown but appears to be increasing (Rasmussen and Freeman 1975; Lehman and Armitage 1980). This is directly related to aggressive chemotherapy and improvement in the median survival rate. Surgical procedures are more frequent in acute myeloid leukemia than in acute lymphocytic leukemia, both in adults and in children, with an overall complication rate of 2%–9% (Seligman et al. 1972; Bjornsson et al. 1974; Exelby et al. 1975).

Acute abdominal abnormalities have previously been reported to occur in 2%–9% of all patients with leukemia (Prolla and Kirsner 1964; Lehman and Armitage 1980). However, most series have included only patients with acute leukemia or only children (Prolla and Kirsner 1964; Sherman et al. 1973; Exelby et al. 1975). A more recent series offers a unique perspective since it involves only adult patients with both chronic and acute leukemia managed over a long period of time (Hawkins et al. 1985). This series of 755 patients over age 16 admitted for leukemia had a 4% overall incidence of acute abdominal abnormalities. An acute condition within the abdomen, based on signs of peritoneal irritation, occurred in 5.3% of those with acute leukemia and 2.6% of those with chronic leukemia. The sex distribution was equal, while patients with chronic leukemia tended to be older (mean age 55 years) than those with acute leukemia (mean age 45 years), a reflection of the overall later presentation of the former. Acute abdominal abnormalities tended to occur during periods of chemotherapy in patients with acute leukemia, i.e. during the initial presentation or relapse, rather than during remission. In contrast, abdominal abnormalities tended to develop randomly in patients with chronic leukemia during the course of their disease.

Five of the 22 patients with acute leukemia and two of the nine patients with chronic leukemia either died before operation could be attempted or were judged to be too ill to undergo exploration. The rest underwent abdominal exploration with a lethality within 30 days of operation of four of 17 patients with acute leukemia and of two of seven patients with chronic leukemia.

Acute abdomen usually developed in patients with acute leukemia who were at the peak of immunosuppression due to chemotherapy and it was usually related to the state of the primary disease, i.e., neutropenic enterocolitis, splenic rupture, and splenic abscess and its treatment. In comparison, abdominal conditions similar to those seen in an elderly population, such as mesenteric vascular disease and biliary tract disease, developed in patients with chronic leukemia. Regardless of the abdominal findings, postoperative length of survival and prognosis paralleled a course of uncomplicated leukemia, with a much shorter length of survival in patients with acute leukemia compared with those with chronic leukemia.

The most common acute abdominal pathologic finding is typhlitis, or neutropenic enterocolitis, which occurs exclusively in patients with acute leukemia during the nadir of white cell depression after chemotherapy (Kingry et al. 1973; Varki et al. 1979). The cause of typhlitis is poorly understood, but it may be related to loss of mucosal integrity due to leukemic infiltration or ulceration and secondary bacterial invasion (Varki et al. 1979). Physical examination and a high index of suspicion must be emphasized in the early diagnosis and treatment (Exelby et al. 1975; Varki et al. 1979; Hunter and Bjelland 1984; Hawkins et al. 1985). The treatment of neutropenic enterocolitis is surgical. Medical management with antibiotics, fluid support, granulocyte transfusions, and close observation as previously suggested is contraindicated once acute peritoneal signs occur (Freeman et al. 1981; Shaked et al. 1983; Gandy and Greenberg 1983). Surgical treatment should include resection of the involved segment with exteriorization of the bowel and distal mucous fistula, or primary anastomosis in selected patients without perforation or gross peritonitis (Hawkins et al. 1985). Gastrointestinal hemorrhage due to leukemic infiltration with secondary hemorrhagic necrosis of the gastrointestinal mucosa is common in patients with leukemia, occurring in up to 18% of such patients (Gandy and Greenberg 1983). Massive hemorrhage or abdominal findings that suggest perforation calls for surgical therapy.

Finally, there is a small group of patients with leukemia and acute abdomen but without abnormal findings at laparotomy. This "pseudoacute abdomen" has been postulated by Prolla and Kirsner (1964) to be due to autonomic dysfunction or vascular derangement of the bowel secondary to the leukemic state resulting in a functional obstruction. Others have reported normal findings at laparotomy in leukemic patients with acute abdomen and thrombocytopenia and they have suggested irritation due to petechial hemorrhage as a cause of the peritoneal irritation (Kornberg and Eldor 1983).

The decision to operate must be based on careful repeated physical examination looking for the persistance or worsening of abdominal symptoms and not on the results of diagnostic testing. Emergency abdominal surgery in patients with leukemia should be limited to the procedure necessary to correct the acute condition and can be expected to yield an operative lethality of 10%–15% (Exelby et al. 1975, Hawkins et al. 1985).

In patients with abdominal aortic aneurysm, about 4% harbor a malignancy at the time of diagnosis or treatment of the aneurysm (Szilagyi et al. 1967). However, only rarely is this a hematologic neoplasm. To my knowledge, only four such patients have been reported (Szilagyi et al. 1967; Giarelli et al. 1978; Berguer et al. 1978; Schwartz and Johnson 1986). Such patients should undergo careful evaluation, including CT scan, to assess infiltration of the aortic wall, to balance both the risks of aneurysm rupture and aneurysmectomy against the risks of palliative medical therapy and death from the hematologic malignancy.

Surgery for a Definite Local Manifestation of a Hematologic Malignancy or a Complication of such a Disease

Malignant lymphoma with primary presentation in the spleen is uncommon, constituting 1%–2% of all patients with malignant lymphoma (Ahmann et al. 1966; Long and Aisenberg 1974). The criteria used to define primary splenic malignant lymphoma have varied. Das Gupta et al. (1965) and Skarin et al. (1971) both advocated splenomegaly without significant lymphadenopathy. Even though malignant lymphoma may clinically appear to be confined to the spleen, careful pathologic staging often reveals disease in other sites (regional lymph nodes, bone marrow, or liver) (Spier et al. 1985). The prognosis of primary splenic lymphoma after splenectomy and adjuvant therapy does not appear at this time to be significantly different from that of nodal lymphomas (Spier et al. 1985).

Although lymphoma and leukemia frequently infiltrate various other organs in cases of advanced disease, they are only rarely the initial site of recognized involvement. For instance, lymphoma of the lower female genital tract is a rare but treatable malignancy, which must be distinguished microscopically from inflammatory lesions and nonlymphoid tumors arising in this site. In one series of 27 cases, the treatment was surgery and adjuvant therapy (Harris and Scully 1984). These patients typically present with vaginal bleeding and a subepithelial mass without obvious ulceration or other epithelial abnormality.

Surgery may also be indicated because of a complication to the hematologic malignancy. In most cases this will mean splenectomy due to splenomegali, hypersplenism, or spontaneous rupture of the spleen; the most frequent being hypersplenism (Wilson et al. 1985). Some patients often demonstrate both hypersplenism and symptomatic splenomegaly, and it may be difficult to decide which indication is the primary one. The spleen in such patients may reach an enormous size, the largest in one series being over 5 kg in weight, with a mean size of 1700 g (Wilson et al. 1985). Splenic infarcts are common and are usually the cause of splenic pain. It is not rare for pain to be referred to the left shoulder as well as being abdominal in nature. Pleuritic symptoms are also common. Early satiety, due to gastric compression and abdominal distension are also complaints of these patients with massive splenomegaly.

Splenic irradiation may be used with benefit preoperatively before splenectomy in patients with excessive splenomegaly and hypersplenism (Aabo and Walbom-Jørgensen 1985). To be justified, the splenectomy must be performed in a meticulous manner so as to minimize morbidity and lethality. In these cases a midline incision is to be preferred. These patients have no marrow reserve and will not tolerate postoperative complications. The bone marrow fibrosis in agnogenic myeloid metaplasia is not felt to be primary, but rather a secondary event in the development of this disease state (Wilson et al. 1985).

The fibroplasia that occurs in the marrow is one of the most confusing aspects of myeloproliferative disorders. There is no certainty as to whether it is the primary disorder triggering extramedullary hematopoiesis or whether it is secondary to marrow hyperproliferation with intramedullary destruction of myeloid cells. The fibrosis seen in other nonrelated marrow proliferative disorders is thought to be a secondary phenomenom. The extramedullary hematopoiesis may be an effect of this proliferative disease, not compensatory. It may even represent metastatic foci of disrupted marrow stroma. This is a particularly important concept for the surgeon considering splenectomy. Fear of eliminating a compensatory site of hematopoiesis has played a major role in restricting the performance of splenectomy in these patients (Wilson et al. 1985).

Thus, in hypersplenism, it is important to note that a cytopenia present in several of the myeloproliferative disorders may respond to splenectomy in spite of the presence of decreased cellular precursors in the bone marrow (Coon 1985). However, the decision to perform splenectomy should be based on well-defined and often strictly limited indications. Confining the discussion to selected entities usually considered to be associated with "secondary" hypersplenism, it must be stressed that the specificity of this terminology is debatable since, in several secondary hypersplenic conditions (e.g., hairy cell leukemia), altered cell structure may also play a role in the pathophysiologic mechanism of cytopenia.

Many patients with chronic lymphocytic leukemia live for 5–10 years with little or no treatment. However, a small fraction of them may develop hypersplenism or massive symptomatic splenomegaly which will not always react positively to splenectomy (Coon 1985). The utilization of splenectomy in the management of chronic granulocytic leukemia has also been controversial. Several recent non-randomized comparisons of operation versus no operation early in the chronic phase of chronic granulocytic leukemia as well as a recent prospective trial have shown that splenectomy does not prolong survival (Ihde et al. 1976; Baccarini et al. 1981, Medical Research Council 1983).

On rare occasions, patients with far-advanced Hodgkin's disease or non-Hodgkin's lymphoma will develop severe hypersplenism which is refractory to chemotherapy, or a cytopenia interferes with administration of adequate doses of chemotherapeutic agents. Splenectomy in such patients may achieve a very satisfactory cytologic response (Coon 1985; Mitchell and Morris 1985). Selected patients with hypersplenism due to agnogenic myeloid metaplasia may obtain palliative benefit from splenectomy, but operative morbidity and lethality are appreciable, and it is doubtful whether removal of the spleen affects prognosis (Coon and Liepman 1982).

Rarer indications for splenectomy due to complications of hematologic malignancies are infarction of the spleen, abscess of the spleen, and spontaneous rupture. Bauer et al. (1981) reviewed the 53 cases of spontaneous splenic rupture in patients with hematologic malignancies described in the English literature up to 1981. It is most common in acute leukemia, but has also been well documented in chronic leukemia. A correct preoperative diagnosis of splenic rupture was reported in only ten of the 53 cases reviewed. Nearly all patients experienced abdominal pain at the time of rupture, however, this pain was frequently confused clinically with that of biliary tract obstruction, aortic aneurysm, perforated viscus, pancreatitis, and angina pectoris. A total of 52% of the patients underwent laparotomy; 48% died without operation. Of those who underwent surgery, 78% survived the procedure and the immediate postoperative period. The survival rate of all patients was 38%. There was no correlation of the type of hematologic malignancy, occurrence or type of treatment, peripheral blood counts, or spleen size to survival. The most important factor in predicting survival was appropriate surgery. Splenectomy because of spontaneous rupture in a patient with longstanding splenomegaly and hypersplenism has led to the final diagnosis of hairy cell leukemia (von der Walde et al. 1981).

In multiple myeloma, surgery may be necessary to treat pathologic fractures or to prevent them by early internal fixation.

Surgery Aiming at Treatment of the Hematologic Malignancy Per Se

Although the spleen is often the site of secondary involvement by Hodgkin's disease and non-Hodgkin's lymphomas, lymphoid malignancies are uncommon as primary splenic tumors (Morgenstern et al. 1985). When lymphoma does involve the spleen, either as a primary or secondary process, the white pulp is involved first. There may be relatively diffuse involvement, particularly in the case of nodular lymphomas, or there may be large irregular tumor masses, as in the case of the diffuse large cell lymphomas. In contrast, malignant tumors of the true histiocytic origin, although uncommon as a group, frequently involve the spleen, and splenomegaly may be the only abnormal physical sign. Involvement is diffuse, and, unlike the usual lymphoma, tumor masses are not formed. Primary plasmocytoma of the spleen is exceedingly rare and is not macroscopically recognizable, but is easily identified histologically as a plasma cell neoplasm. The spleen may be involved as a primary, isolated site. Usually when the spleen is involved as a part of a generalized myelomatosis, there is no dominant tumor (Morgenstern et al. 1985).

Hairy cell leukemia, an uncommon type of leukemia – 2%–5% of the total, was first definitively described in 1958 under the name of "leukemic reticuloendotheliosis" (Bouroncle et al. 1958). The origin of the malignant cell of hairy cell leukemia has not yet been completely elucidated. Most investigators believe the hairy cell to be a B-lymphocytic cell. This origin will locate hairy cell leukemia in the group of lymphoproliferative disorders, perhaps near chronic lymphocytic leukemia and prolymphocytic leukemia. The therapy of choice in hairy cell leukemia is claimed to be quite different from that in other lymphoproliferative disorders. However, the therapy of choice in most centers is splenectomy. The conclusion of a retrospective multicenter analysis of 391 patients was that splenectomy in patients with definite splenomegaly and pancytopenia seems to be beneficial, while in patients without distinctly enlarged spleen other therapeutical modalities should be considered (Jansen and Hermans 1981). The therapeutic importance of surgery, however, may well be challenged by the recent therapeutic success of α interferon in the disease (Worman et al. 1985).

The most controversial issue concerning splenectomy in hematologic malignancies has been its indication in Hodgkin's disease. Glatstein et al. (1969) introduced explorative laparotomy with splenectomy and biopsy from the liver and retroperitoneal lymph nodes to obtain information about abdominal involvement. In an unexpectedly large number of patients, whose clinical manifestations indicated disease above the diaphragm only, abdominal involvement was found. This staging laparotomy has provided information about the spread and progression of the disease (Taylor et al. 1985).

However, during the past 10 years there has been an increasing challenge to the routine use of staging laparotomy and splenectomy for the following reasons:

1. Computed axial tomography has improved the accuracy of identifying tumor involvement of abdominal lymph nodes, as well as noduli in the liver and spleen.
2. Polychemotherapy has become much more widely used as a curative treatment in Hodgkin's disease.

For some stages and presentations of the disease, chemotherapy is more effective than irradiation. Chemotherapy can also be very effective for treating minimal or occult sites of Hodgkin's disease so that accuracy of staging is not always required.

3. Morbidity, and sometime lethality, has been associated with the laparotomy and splenectomy, the most serious being overwhelming postsplenectomy septicemia, especially in infants and children.
4. A few randomized trials have been performed attempting to determine the value of the laparotomy and splenectomy and have failed to demonstrate any increased survival (Askergren et al. 1980; Tubiana et al. 1981). At the Norwegian Radium Hospital, staging laparotomy has not been used for that reason during recent years (Foss Abrahamsen et al. 1980).

In conclusion, it must be emphasized that the value of staging laparotomy is diagnostic and not therapeutic, and the morbidity and rare lethality of staging laparotomy and splenectomy are acceptable only if less morbid and dangerous treatment programs can be selected because of greater diagnostic accuracy.

Overwhelming Postsplenectomy Septicemia

Since splenectomy is often considered in hematologic malignancies, it is appropriate in this review to stress that splenectomy is not an innocent procedure. It has been demonstrated beyond doubt that splenectomy, regardless of age or underlying disease, leads to an increased risk of infection (West and Grosfeld 1985). Such postsplenectomy infection usually takes a fulminant course with a very high lethality and is seen most often in infancy and early childhood and after splenectomy for hematologic diseases. This is why splenectomy should be avoided whenever possible as now recommended in trauma (Solheim and Høivik 1985). The indication for elective splenectomy in hematologic malignancies should be very strict, especially in children, e.g., in the surgical staging of Hodgkin's disease. Consequently, partial splenectomy has been recommended when staging laparotomy for Hodgkin's disease in children is contemplated (Holschneider et al. 1985). Current recommendations when splenectomy is indicated are prophylactic antibiotics and pneumococcal vaccination 2 weeks before splenectomy.

Conclusion

Surgery in hematologic malignancies may be indicated when the patient is injured or suffers a surgical disease. In such patients, an aggressive attitude is justified, as otherwise the diagnosis may be missed with fatal consequences, i.e., in acute abdomen. Operation may, in most cases, be expected to yield the same complication rates and results as in patients without malignancies. Surgery in complications of hematologic malignancies, or aiming at the malignancy per se, has a definite place, often supplemented by adjuvant therapy.

In all cases, a close cooperation between the surgeon, the oncologist, hematologist, and anesthestist is mandatory to achieve optimal results.

References

Aabo K, Walbom-Jørgensen S (1985) Spleen irradiation in chronic lymphocytic leukemia: palliation in patients unfit for splenectomy. Am J Hematol 19: 177–180

Ahmann DL, Kiely JM, Harrison EG Jr, et al. (1966) Malignant lymphoma of the spleen: a review of 49 cases in which the diagnosis was made at splenectomy. Cancer 19: 461–469

Askergren J, Björkholm M, Holm G, et al. (1980) Prognostic effect of early diagnostic splenectomy in Hodgkin's disease: a randomized trial. Br J Cancer 42: 284–291

Baccarini M, Corbelli G, Tura S, and the Italian Cooperative Study Group on Chronic Myoloid Leukemia (1981) Early splenectomy and polychemotherapy versus polychemotherapy alone in chronic myeloid leukemia. Leuk Res 5: 149–157

Bauer TW, Haskins GE, Armitage JO (1981) Splenic rupture in patients with hematological malignancies. Cancer 48: 2729–2733

Berguer R, Schneider J, Wilner HI (1978) Induced thrombosis of inoperable abdominal aortic aneurysm. Surgery 84: 425–429

Bjornsson S, Yates JW, Mittelman A, et al. (1974) Major surgery in acute leukemia. Cancer 34: 1272–1275

Bouroncle BA, Wiseman BK, Doan CA (1958) Leukaemic reticuloendotheliosis. Blood 13: 609–630

Coon WW (1985) Splenectomy for splenomegaly and secondary hypersplenism. World J Surg 9: 437–443

Coon WW, Liepman MK (1982) Splenectomy for agnogenic myeloid metaplasia. Surg Gynecol Obstet 154: 561–563

Das Gupta T, Coombes B, Brasfield RD (1965) Primary malignant neoplasms of the spleen. Surg Gynecol Obstet 120: 947–960

Exelby PR, Ghandchi A, Lansigan N (1975) Management of acute abdomen in children with leukemia. Cancer 35: 826–829

Foss Abrahamsen A, Høst H, Jørgensen OG (1980) Is staging laparotomy of therapeutic value in patients with supradiaphragmatic Hodgkin's disease, clinical stage IA–IIA? Scand J Haematol 25: 439–444

Freeman HJ, Rabeneck L, Owen D (1981) Survival after necro-

tizing enterocolitis of leukemia treated with oral vancomycin. Gastroenterology 81: 791–794
Gandy W, Greenberg B (1983) Successful medical management of neutropenic enterocolitis. Cancer 51: 1551–1555
Giarelli L, Melato M, Antonutto G, Milani S (1978) Lymphoma and aortic aneurysm rupture: an unusual complication. Haematologica (Pavia) 63: 586–590
Glatstein E, Guernsey JM, Rosenberg SA, Kaplan HS (1969) The value of laparotomy and splenectomy in the staging of Hodgkin's disease. Cancer 24: 709–718
Harris NL, Scully RE (1984) Malignant lymphoma and granulocytic sarcoma of the uterus and vagina. Cancer 53: 2530–2545
Hawkins JA, Mower WR, Nelson EW (1985) Acute abdominal conditions in patients with leukemia. Am J Surg 150: 739–742
Holschneider AM, Löhrs U, Haas R, Dickerhoff R, Gollmitzer W (1985) Selective hemisplenectomy for Hodgkin's disease. Prog Pediatr Surg 18: 162–168
Hunter TB, Bjelland JC (1984) Gastrointestinal complications of leukemia and its treatment. AJR 142: 513–518
Ihde DC, Canellos GP, Schwartz JH, DeVita VT (1976) Splenectomy in the chronic phase of chronic granulocytic leukemia. Ann Intern Med 84: 17–21
Jansen J, Hermans J (1981) Splenectomy in hairy cell leukemia: a retrospective multicenter study. Cancer 47: 2066–2076
Kingry RL, Hobson RW, Muir RW (1973) Cecal necrosis and perforation with systemic chemotherapy. Am Surg 39: 129–133
Kornberg A, Eldor A (1983) Acute surgical abdomen caused by thrombocytopenia in patients with acute leukemia and multiple myeloma. Isr J Med Sci 19: 1094–1096
Lehman JA, Armitage JO (1980) Surgical intervention in complications of acute leukemia. Postgrad Med 68: 89–92, 95
Long JC, Aisenberg AC (1974) Malignant lymphoma diagnosed at splenectomy and idiopathic splenomegaly: a clinicopathologic comparison. Cancer 33: 1054–1061
Medical Research Council's Working Party for Therapeutic Trials in Leukemia (1983) Randomized trial of splenectomy in Ph^1-positive chronic granulocytic leukemia, including an analysis of prognostic features. Br J Haematol 54: 415–430
Mitchell A, Morris PJ (1985) Splenectomy for malignant lymphomas. World J Surg 9: 444–448
Morgenstern L, Rosenberg J, Geller SA (1985) Tumors of the spleen. World J Surg 9: 468–476
Nagler A, Yoffe G, Argov S (1985) Surgery in acute leukemia. Curr Surg 42: 365–369
Prolla JC, Kirsner JB (1964) The gastrointestinal lesions and complications of the leukemias. Ann Intern. Med 61: 1084–1103
Rasmussen BL, Freeman JS (1975) Major surgery in leukemia. Am J Surg 130: 647–651
Schwartz JA, Johnson G Jr (1986) Chronic lymphocytic leukemia complicating abdominal aortic aneurysmectomy. J Vasc Surg 3: 159–161
Seligman BR, Rosner F, Ritz ND (1972) Major surgery in patients with acute leukemia. Am J Surg 124: 629–633
Shaked A, Shinar E, Freund H (1983) Neutropenic typhlitis. A plea for conservatism. Dis Colon Rectum 26: 351–352
Sherman NJ, Williams K, Woolley MM (1973) Surgical complications in the patients with leukemia. J Pediatr Surg 8: 235–244
Skarin AT, Davey FR, Moloney WC (1971) Lymphosarcoma of the spleen: results of diagnostic splenectomy in 11 patients. Arch Intern Med 127: 259–265
Solheim K, Høivik B (1985) Changing trends in the diagnosis and management of rupture of the spleen. Injury 16: 221–226
Spier CM, Kjeldsberg CR, Eyre HJ, Behm FG (1985) Malignant lymphoma with primary presentation in the spleen. Arch Pathol Lab Med 109: 1076–1080
Szilagyi DE, Elliot JP, Berguer R (1967) Coincidental malignancy and abdominal aortic aneurysm: problems of management. Arch Surg 95: 402–412
Taylor MA, Kaplan HS, Nelsen TS (1985) Staging laparotomy with splenectomy for Hodgkin's disease. The Stanford experience. World J Surg 9: 449–460
Tubiana M, Hayat M, Henry-Amar M, et al. (1981) Five year results of the EORTC randomized study of splenectomy and spleen irradiation in clinical stages I and II of Hodgkin's disease. Eur J Cancer 17: 355–363
Varki AP, Armitage JO, Feagler JR (1979) Typhlitis in acute leukemia. Successful treatment by early surgical intervention. Cancer 43: 695–697
Von der Walde J, Mashiah A, Berrebi A (1981) Spontaneous rupture of the spleen in hairy cell leukemia. Clin Oncol 7: 241–244
West KW, Grosfeld JL (1985) Postsplenectomy sepsis: historical background and current concepts. World J Surg 9: 477–483
Wilson RE, Rosenthal DS, Moloney WC, Osteen RT (1985) Splenectomy for myeloproliferative disorders. World J Surg 9: 431–436
Worman CP, Catovsky D, Bevan PC, et al. (1985) Interferon is effective in hairy-cell leukemia. Br J Haematol 60: 759–763

Metastatic Cancer from Unknown Primary Site

K. Lote

Introduction

No generally accepted definition of "cancer of unknown primary" (CUP) exists in the literature. A clinical definition is that when no primary site can be determined in a patient with metastatic cancer, after careful history taking and physical examination including pelvic, breast, and rectal examinations, urinalysis, and chest X-ray, the patient is considered to have CUP.

Incidence estimates are uncertain since the extent of clinical or postmortem investigations performed on these patients differs considerably in the literature. Also, the diagnosis is usually reclassified upon detection of a primary source, making retrospective incidence analysis difficult. Statistics from the Cancer Registry of Norway (1978) indicate that no primary source was identified in 5% of all cancer patients in Norway. Other authors report incidences of 3% (Holmes and Fouts 1970; Krementz et al. 1979) or 5%–10% of all cancer patients (Stewart et al. 1979; Scott Nystrom et al. 1979; Nissenblatt 1981). Abrams et al. (1950) did not locate the primary source in 2.6% of 1000 autopsied patients with carcinomas.

The prognosis of patients with CUP is grim. Median survivals of 3–7 months are reported (Moertel et al. 1972; Didolkar et al. 1977; Woods et al. 1980;

Nissenblatt 1981, Gaber et al. 1983; Neilan 1983; Snee and Vyramuthu 1985; Altman and Cadman 1986). Patients with disease confined to lymph nodes have the longest survival (Didolkar et al. 1977; Nissenblatt 1981).

Pathophysiology

Like the proverbial tip of the iceberg, clinical neoplastic disease is the end result of a prolonged and complex development where, over a period of years or even decades, a single or a few transformed cells grow into a detectable tumor (Schabel 1975). Systemic dissemination often occurs before the primary tumor is recognized clinically. In the CUP syndrome, the pattern of spread is often atypical for the neoplasm in question (Scott Nystrom et al. 1979).

Malignant cells usually metastasize to regional nodes (Sugarbaker 1980; Cady 1984) or to the first capillary bed encountered (Weiss et al. 1980), but may bypass regional nodes or the first capillary filter (Scanlon 1985). Rapidly growing tumors often disseminate early, and cells derived from metastases may possess increased metastatic capacity (Talmadge and Fidler 1982). A small tumor may produce multiple metastases which outgrow the primary tumor and manifest themselves at distant sites long before the primary can be clinically detected. In addition, host defence mechanisms against tumor growth and dissemination may be inadequate in patients developing CUP.

Philosophy of Management

All too often these patients are overinvestigated (Stewart et al. 1979; Scott Nystrom et al. 1979; Brewin 1981; Snee and Vyramuthu 1985). The clinician should only search for those relatively few disseminated neoplasms which are curable or treatable by surgery, radiotherapy, systemic cytotoxic or hormonal therapy; and perform such investigations of symptomatic organs as are necessary for planning palliative treatment. Investigations which can have no therapeutic consequences are not in the patient's interest; nor are they likely to detect the primary source (Tables 4 and 5).

Which Neoplasms are Treatable?

Every effort must be made to diagnose treatable neoplasms. Leukemias (Frei 1982), Hodgkin's disease (McVie and Somers 1985), non-Hodgkin's lymphomas (Rosenberg 1979; Coleman 1985), and testicular (Dahl 1985), ovarian (Scott 1983), or extragonadal (Hainsworth et al. 1982) germ cell cancer, as well as Ewing's tumor, osteosarcoma, and gestational choriocarcinoma (Frei 1982) may be curable by combinations of surgery, chemotherapy, or irradiation. Disseminated carcinomas of the breast (Henderson and Canellos 1980), ovary (Muggia et al. 1985), prostate (Kirk 1985), or small cell lung carcinoma (Spiro 1985) often respond to treatment.

Patients with resectable solitary metastases from renal carcinoma (Kjaer and Engelholm 1982) or colorectal carcinoma (Malt 1985) to the lung or liver may benefit from surgery provided the primary tumor is controlled. Regional lymphatic metastases from stage II malignant melanoma are also best treated by regional lymphadenectomy (Morton 1984).

What is the Probable Organ of Origin?

Table 1 summarizes data from eight reports concerning 1086 patients with CUP. The primary tumor was eventually detected in 423 patients, 39% of all cases. In decreasing order of frequency, the lung, pancreas, colon and rectum, liver, stomach, and kidney were the most probable sites of origin. Taken together,

Table 1. Location of the primary site in 423 out of 1086 patients with metastases from an initially unknown primary tumor. (Data from Moertel et al. 1972: Didolkar et al. 1977; Osteen et al. 1978; Stewart et al. 1979; Scott Nystrom et al. 1979; McMillan et al. 1982; Karsell et al. 1982; Gaber et al. 1983)

Primary site	(%)	Treatable when disseminated (%)
Lung	26(assuming none had SCLC)	
Pancreas	19	
Colon	8.5	
Liver	7.5	
Stomach	6.5	
Kidney	6	
Ovaries	5.5	5.5
Prostate	3.5	3.5
Lymphomas[a]	3.5	3.5
Breast	3	3
Thyroid[a]	1	1
Germ cell[a]	1	1
Others	9	
	100	17.5

[a] Potentially curable.
SCLC, small cell lung carcinoma

these six organs accounted for 73.5% of all primary sites. Common tumors like breast or prostatic carcinoma rarely caused CUP. Approximately two-thirds of all occult primaries were located below the diaphragm. Less than 10% were potentially curable by present systemic therapy. Assuming a similar distribution of primary sites in all 1086 patients, potentially valuable systemic treatment exists for at least 17.5% of the patients.

Diagnosis

Histopathology

Clinician-pathologist teamwork is absolutely essential in reaching a reliable diagnosis in the CUP syndrome. All original specimens should be carefully reviewed. Whenever considered necessary for the diagnosis of treatable neoplasms, new biopsies should be obtained in a preplanned manner to ensure a maximal informative yield of the biopsy procedure. Tissue may be obtained for hormone receptor determination, immunological and immunohistological study, or electron microscopy.

Although all are unspecific, some histopathological features may suggest a site of origin (Table 2). Detection of estrogen or progesterone receptors in tumor tissue favors a diagnosis of breast, ovarian, or uterine carcinoma (Nissenblatt 1981).

Electron microscopy (Olsen 1982), as well as new immunohistological methods (Gatter et al. 1984; Pinkus and Kurtin 1985; Kurtin and Pinkus 1985; Miettinen et al. 1985; Gown and Vogel 1985; Loeffel et al. 1985; Gatter et al. 1987) employing panels of monoclonal antibodies against tumor cell antigens (Table 3), can discriminate between carcinomas, non-Hodgkin's lymphomas, and melanoma. In patients with morphologically undifferentiated neoplasms, monoclonal antibodies facilitate the diagnosis of malignant lymphomas (Gatter et al. 1984; Gatter et al. 1987; Taylor 1985, Berg et al. 1985), mesenchymal tumors (Gatter et al. 1987), nonseminomatous germ cell (Bosman et al. 1980), or prostate (Ford et al. 1985; Tell et al. 1985) tumors. Immunohistochemical studies on fresh tissues are generally more sensitive than studies performed on formalin-fixed, paraffin-embedded tissues. Negative reactions are usually of less diagnostic value. Unexpected cross-reactions do occur, for example, antibody directed against cytokeratin may stain smooth muscle tumors, lymphomas may react with epithelial membrane antigen (Gatter et al. 1987), and adenocarcinomas may express S-100 protein (Herrera et al. 1988). Careful interpretation of immunohistochemical studies remains necessary.

Table 2. Histopathological features which may suggest the site of origin in patients presenting with metastases from an unknown primary tumor

Histopathological feature	Possible site of origin
Mucin production	Gastorintestinal tract, lungs, prostate
Papillary growth, psammomas	Ovary, thyroid gland
Clear cell carcinoma	Kidney, lung, ovary
Melanin production	Melanoma
Anaplastic small or large cell carcinoma	Lung, thyroid gland

Table 3. Antigens which can be detected in routinely processed formalin-fixed, paraffin-embedded tissue sections with the use of monoclonal antibodies and their diagnostic specificity in selected human tumors. A panel of monoclonal antibodies can discriminate between carcinomas, lymphomas, and melanoma. (Data from Gatter et al. 1984; Pinkus and Kurtin 1985; Kurtin and Pinkus 1985; Miettinen et al. 1985; Gown and Vogel 1985; Loeffel et al. 1985)

Antigen	Carcinomas	Non-Hodgkin's lymphoma	Hodgkin's disease	Melanoma
Epithelial membrane antigen (EMA)	+	–	–	–
Cytokeratins	+	–	–	–
Leukocyte common antigen (LCA)	–	+	(–/+)	–
S-100 proteins	–	–	–	+

Roentgenology

Contrast imaging of asymptomatic organs in the search for an occult primary tumor is of little value (Table 4) and may produce false positive results (Scott Nystrom et al. 1979). Nor are endoscopic investigations of asymptomatic organs helpful (Fitzpatrick and Kotalik 1974; McMillan et al. 1982; Gaber et al. 1983). In contrast, investigation of symptomatic organs may result in clinical information which proves valuable for patient management (Osteen et al. 1978; Gaber et al. 1983). Computed tomography of the body detected the primary site in one-third of patients with CUP (McMillan et al. 1982; Karsell et al. 1982) and is of value in selected patients.

Table 4. Diagnostic yield of roentgenological contrast procedures in the evaluation of asymptomatic organs in patients with metastases from an unknown primary tumor. (Data from Didolkar et al. 1977; Osteen et al. 1978; Stewart et al. 1979; Scott Nystrom et al. 1979; McMillan et al. 1982; Gaber et al. 1983)

Investigation	(*n*)	Positive (%)
Upper gastrointestinal series	582	8
Barium enema	542	6.5
Excretory urography	470	4

Table 5. Detection rate of the primary source and survival in 945 patients who presented with metastases to lymph nodes in the neck from an unknown primary

Author	Cases (*n*)	Primary detected (*n*)	(%)	Three-year survival (%)
Barrie et al. (1970)	123	38	31	30
Jesse et al. (1973)	210	37	18	48
Leipzig et al. (1981)	48	14	29	27
Spiro et al. (1983)	132	17	13	38
Fitzpatrick and Kotalik (1974)	233	38	16	28
Dickson and Vargas (1979)	199	35	18	21

Serum Tumor Markers

No serum marker is specific for any site of origin. Carcinoembryonic antigen (CEA) is of no value in detecting the organ of origin. Either or both of alpha-feto-protein (aFP) and beta human chorionic gonadotropin (beta-HCG) are elevated in 85%–90% of patients with testicular nonseminomatous germ cell tumors (Klee and Go 1982; Hainsworth and Greco 1983) and may also be increased in extragonadal germ cell tumors (Hainsworth et al. 1982). However, both serum markers may be elevated in patients with other neoplasms (Klee and Go 1982; Dahl 1985).

Serum acid phosphatases are elevated in 60%-80% of patients with metastatic prostatic carcinoma (Klee and Go 1982), but may also be increased in patients with bone metastases from other tumors (Yam 1974). Prostate-specific antigen is elevated in more than 95% of patients with untreated prostatic cancer but may also be elevated in benign prostatic hyperplasia (Stamey et al. 1987).

Serum or urine monoclonal immunoglobulins can be detected in 99% of patients with multiple myeloma (Kyle 1975) and in some patients with non-Hodgkin's lymphomas or plasmocytoma. However, a homogenous serum spike is also found in 1% of the normal population or in patients with various neoplasms (Bloch and Franklin 1982).

Clinical Presentation and Locoregional Treatment

Lymph Nodes in the Neck

Most lymph node metastases from an unknown source are found in the neck. Table 5 summarizes data from six reports. In 945 patients, the primary tumor was identified in only 179 patients, 19% of all cases. Of these 179 patients, 114 (64%) had a primary in the head and neck area. The nasopharynx (20%), base of tongue (10%), tonsils (9%), and hypopharynx (9%) were the most common head and neck sites identified. In 65/179 patients (36%) the primary was located below the clavicles, mostly in the lung.

Node location and tumor histology were prognostically important. Patients with metastases confined to cervical nodes had a better prognosis after radical local therapy. In contrast, almost all patients with supraclavicular nodes died within 2 years (Fitzpatrick and Kotalik 1974; Dickson and Vargas 1979). Patients with epidermoid carcinoma or melanoma (Santini et al. 1985) located in cervical nodes had better survival than patients with node metastases from adenocarcinoma (Jesse et al. 1973; Fitzpatrick and Kotalik 1974; Dickson and Vargas 1979). In only 19% of these 945 patients was the primary site identified clinically (Table 5). Endoscopies and blind biopsies of asymptomatic organs were unrewarding (Fitzpatrick and Kotalik 1974; Devine 1978). Nevertheless, the work-up should include careful visualization of the mucocutaneous surfaces in the head and neck area by clinical examination, and appropriate endoscopies, and chest X-ray examination. Patients with thyroid nodules or suspect histology may also need thyroid scintigraphy or sonography. Extensive investigation of asymptomatic organs below the clavicles should be avoided.

No absolute treatment recommendations suiting all patients can be given. Generally, cervical nodes containing epidermoid carcinoma, adenocarcinoma, or melanoma should be removed by neck dissection (Jesse et al. 1973; Devine 1978). A modified neck dissection is effective surgical neck treatment (Byers 1985).

With the exception of melanoma metastases, in which radiotherapy is of questionable value, larger (N2–3) nodes, multiple nodes, or nodes with histopathological evidence of extracapsular invasion should receive pre- or postoperative radiotherapy (Jesse et al. 1973; Devine 1978; Spiro et al. 1983; Byers 1985). Primary radiotherapy is recommended in undifferentiated or anaplastic carcinoma (Devine 1978). The fields of irradiation should include possible primary sites as well as palpable disease.

Axillary Lymph Nodes

Most females with CUP confined to axillary nodes have breast cancer (Copeland and McBride 1973). The diagnostic work-up of women with axillary metastases of an undetermined source should include mammography and, whenever possible, biopsy for hormone receptor determination. Axillary dissection for local control together with radiotherapy to the ipsilateral breast are advocated by Copeland and McBride and seem rational. Radiotherapy may be used as an adjuvant to or replacement for axillary dissection.

Inguinal Lymph Nodes

Zaren and Copeland (1978) reported 2232 patients with metastases to inguinal nodes. Only 22 patients had an unknown primary tumor. Superficial groin dissection of metastastic nodes is recommended. Radiotherapy is an alternative or supplementary local treatment.

Mediastinal and Retroperitoneal Nodes

In patients with CUP in retroperitoneal or mediastinal nodes, malignant lymphomas or primary or metastastic germ cell tumors must be excluded. Appropriate lymph node biopsy must be obtained, if necessary by thoracotomy or laparotomy. Patients with superior vena caval obstruction often benefit from radiation therapy.

Central Nervous System

The commonest sources for brain metastases are lung, breast, melanoma, and unknown sites (Vieth and Odom 1965). Neurosurgical resection of single lesions followed by radiotherapy; either local or whole brain irradiation may control devastating CNS manifestations. However, median life expectancy for patients with brain metastases is only 3–4 months (Hendrickson 1975).

Metastases to the spine presenting with symptoms and signs of cord compression represent a true therapeutic emergency. Immediate surgical decompression and/or radiotherapy may save such patients from paraparesis (Rodriguez and Dinapoli 1980).

Liver

Ultrasound or computed tomography supplemented by directed needle biopsy will usually reveal the extent and histological type of tumor. Of the curable malignancies, non-Hodgkins's lymphomas (Osborne et al. 1985) or small cell carcinoma of the lung (Spiro 1985) may occasionally present in the liver. A few patients with liver metastases from adenocarcinomas of the colon and rectum may be cured by liver resection provided the primary tumor can also be controlled (Adson et al. 1984; Malt 1985). Resectable patients therefore need roentgenological or endoscopic studies of the large bowel. Patients with incipient intestinal or biliary obstructions may need palliative surgery.

Lung

In at least 7% of patients dying with lung cancer, the primary is not discovered during life (Clary et al. 1983). No single roentgenological (Scott Nystrom et al. 1979) or bronchoscopic (Mohsenifar et al. 1978) criterion can unequivocably discriminate metastatic from primary carcinoma of the lung. Patients with lung tumors who are deemed operable or are candidates for radical radiotherapy must be investigated for the presence of extrathoracic primary or metastatic tumours. Neoplasms amenable to systemic treatment must be excluded.

Bone

In 5%–20% of patients with CUP, the clinical presentation is that of skeletal metastases (Holmes and Fouts 1970; Didolkar et al. 1977; Stewart et al. 1979). Carcinomas of the breast or prostate are infrequent sources of bone metastases in the CUP syndrome (Simon and Karluk 1982). Radiotherapy to bone lesions gives pain relief to 80% of symptomatic patients (Snee and Vyramuthu 1985). Fractures through metastatic sites in the femur need internal fixation followed by radiotherapy (Harrington 1982).

Table 6. Response rates and median survival in patients with CUP treated with various cytotoxic drugs

Author	Agents	Response rates (%)	Survival (months)
Moertel et al. (1972)	Mainly 5-FU	12	4
Didolkar et al. (1977)	5-FU, NM C, V, MTX	6	5
Woods et al. (1980)	CMF, DM	5, 36	2, 4.5
Shild et al. (1983)	FAC, 5-FU	0	3.5

5-FU, 5-fluorouracil; NM, nitrogen mustard; C, cyclophosphamide; V, vincristine; MTX, methotrexate; CMF, cyclophosphamide/methotrexate/5-FU; DM, doxorubicine/mitomycin C; FAC, 5-FU/doxorubicine/cyclophosphamide.

Chemotherapy

When specific treatable neoplasms are excluded, current chemotherapy in patients with CUP is disappointing. Complete responses are few, and side effects of treatment may be severe. Reported median survival in treated groups is no different from survival in untreated patients (Table 6). These results clearly indicate that cytotoxic therapy of patients with CUP at present is warranted only in clinical trials. No specific regime can be advocated. However, chemotherapy directed against germ cell tumors or lymphomas may be tried in patients in whom these diagnoses cannot be excluded.

Summary

Diagnostic investigations in patients with CUP should focus on early biopsy and optimal histopathological evaluation (Fig. 1). Further investigations are best restricted to those necessary to diagnose treatable neoplasms or plan symptomatic treatment. Patients with nodal regional metastases in the neck should undergo a thorough investigation of the head and neck area. Also, patients with metastases confined to regional lymph nodes should, whenever possible, receive radical local surgical and/or radiological treatment. In the majority of patients with CUP, only individual palliative surgical or radiological treatment is possible. Present-day chemotherapy is of uncertain value.

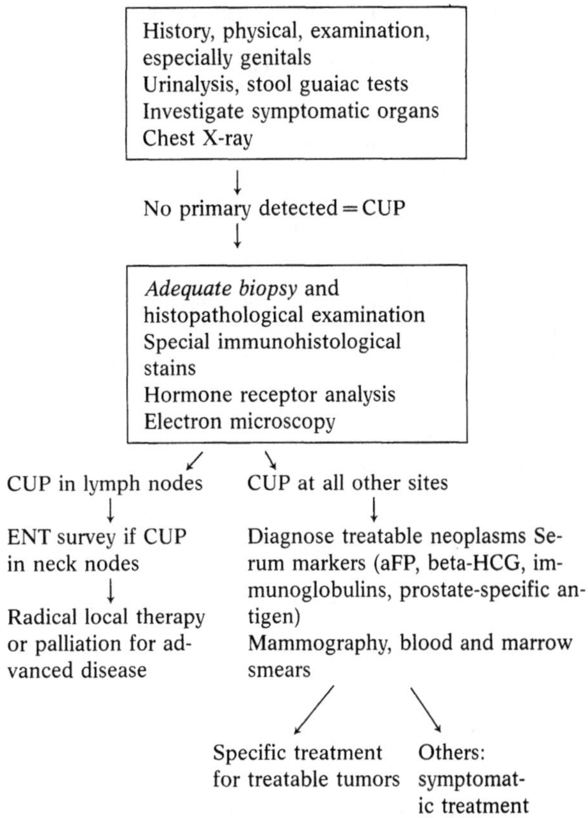

Fig. 1. Suggested general approach to patients with metastatic CUP. The message is: diagnose treatable neoplasms, but avoid overinvestigation!

References

Abrams HL, Spiro R, Goldstein N (1950) Metastases in carcinoma. Analysis of 1000 autopsied cases. Cancer 3: 74–85

Adson MA, van Heerden JA, Adson MH, Wagner JS, Ilstrup DM (1984) Resection of hepatic metastases from colorectal cancer. Arch Surg 119: 647–651

Altman E, Cadman E (1986) An analysis of 1539 patients with cancer of unknown primary site. Cancer 57: 120–124

Barrie JR, Knapper WH, Strong EW (1970) Cervical nodal metastases of unknown origin. Am J Surg 120: 466–470

Berg AR, Linder J, Anderson RW, et al. (1985) The undifferentiated malignant neoplasm. Identitification of lymphoma arising in skeletal muscle by immunohistochemical analysis. JAMA 254: 2625–2626

Bloch KJ, Frankin E (1982) Plasma cell dyscrasias and cryoglobulins. JAMA 248: 2670–2676

Bosman FT, Giard RWM, Kruseman ACN, Knijnenburg G, Spaander PJ (1980) Human chorionic gonadotrophin and alpha-fetoprotein in testicular germ cell tumours: a retrospective immunohistochemical study. Histopathology 4: 673–684

Brewin T (1981) The cancer patient – too many scans and X-rays? Lancet 1: 1098–1099

Byers RM (1985) Modified neck dissection. A study of 967 cases from 1970 to 1980. Am J Surg 150: 414–421

Cady B (1984) Lymph node metastasis. Indicators, but not governors of survival. Arch Surg 119: 1067–1072

Cancer Registry of Norway (1978) Incidence of cancer in Norway 1972–1976. Oslo
Clary CF, Michel RP, Wang NS, Hanson RE (1983) Metastatic carcinoma. The lung as the site for the clinically undiagnosed primary. Cancer 51: 362–366
Coleman M (1985) Chemotherapy for large-cell lymphoma: optimism and caution. Ann Intern Med 103: 140-142
Copeland EM, McBride CM (1973) Axillary metastases from an unknown primary site. Ann Surg 178: 25–27
Dahl O (1985) Testicular carcinoma. A curable malignancy. Acta Radiol [Oncol] 24: 3–15
Devine KD (1978) Cancer in the neck without obvious source. Mayo Clin Proc 53: 644–650
Dickson R, Vargas DR (1979) Occult primary of the head and neck. J Otolaryngol 8: 427–434
Didolkar MS, Fanous N, Elias EG, Moore RH (1977) Metastatic carcinomas from occult primary tumors. A study of 254 patients. Ann Surg 186: 625–630
Fitzpatrick PJ, Kotalik JF (1974) Cervical metastases from an unknown primary tumor. Radiology 110: 659–663
Ford TF, Butcher DN, Masters JRW, Parkinson MC (1985) Immunocytochemical localisation of prostate-specific antigen: specificity and application to clinical practice. Br J Urol 57: 50–55
Frei E III (1982) The National Cancer Chemotherapy Program. Science 217: 600–606
Gaber AO, Rice P, Eaton C, Pietrafitta JJ, Spatz E, Deckers PJ (1983) Metastatic malignant disease of unknown origin. Am J Surg 145: 493–497
Gatter KC, Alcock C, Heryet A, et al. (1984) The differential diagnosis of routinely processed anaplastic tumors using monoclonal antibodies. Am J Clin Pathol 82: 33–43
Gatter KC, Mason DY, Heyderman E, Isaacson PG (1987) Commentary: which antibodies for diagnostic pathology? Histopathology 11: 661–664
Gown AM, Vogel AM (1985) Monoclonal antibodies to human intermediate filament proteins. III. Analysis of tumors. Am J Clin Pathol 84: 413–424
Hainsworth JD, Greco A (1983) Testicular germ cell neoplasms. Am J Med 75: 817–832
Hainsworth JD, Einhorn LH, Williams SD, Stewart M, Greco FA (1982) Advanced extragonadal germ cell tumors: successful treatment with combination chemotherapy. Proc Am Soc Clin Oncol 1: C-413
Harrington KD (1982) New trends in the management of lower extremity metastases. Clin Orthop 169: 53–61
Henderson IC, Canellos GP (1980) Cancer of the breast. The past decade. N Engl J Med 302: 17–30, 302: 78–79
Hendrickson FR (1975) Radiation therapy of metastatic tumors. Semin Oncol 2: 43–46
Herrera GA, Turbat-Herrera EA, Lott RL (1988) S-100 protein expression by primary and metastatic adenocarcinomas. Am J Clin Pathol 89: 168–176
Holmes FF, Fouts TL (1970) Metastatic cancer of unknown primary site. Cancer 26: 816–820
Jesse RH, Perez CA, Fletcher G (1973) Cervical lymph node metastasis: unknown primary cancer. Cancer 31: 854–859
Karsell PR, Sheedy PF II, O'Connell MJ (1982) Computed tomography in search of cancer of unknown origin. JAMA 248: 340–343
Kirk D (1985) Prostatic carcinoma. Br Med J 290: 875–876
Kjaer M, Engelholm SA (1982) The clinical course and prognosis of patients with renal adenocarcinoma with solitary metastasis. Int J Radiat Oncol Biol Phys 8: 1691–1698
Klee GG, Go VLW (1982) Laboratory report. Serum tumor markers. Mayo Clin Proc 57: 129–132
Krementz ET, Cerise EJ, Foster DS, Morgan LR (1979) Metastases of undetermined source. Curr Probl Cancer 4: 4–37
Kurtin PJ, Pinkus GS (1985) Leukocyte common antigen – a diagnostic discriminant between hematopoietic and nonhematopoietic neoplasms in paraffin sections using monoclonal antibodies. Hum Pathol 16: 353–365
Kyle RA (1975) Multiple myeloma. Review of 869 cases. Mayo Clin Proc 50: 29–40
Leipzig B, Winter ML, Hokanson JA (1981) Cervical node metastases of unknown origin. Laryngoscope 91: 593–597
Loeffel SC, Gillespie Y, Mirmiran SA, et al. (1985) Cellular immunolocalization of S100 protein within fixed tissue sections by monoclonal antibodies. Arch Pathol Lab Med 109: 117–122
Malt RA (1985) Current concepts. Surgery for hepatic neoplasms. N Engl J Med 313: 1591–1596
McMillan JH, Levine E, Stephens RH (1982) Computed tomography in the evaluation of metastatic adenocarcinoma from an unknown primary site. Radiology 143: 143–146
McVie JG, Somers R (1985) Chemotherapy of Hodgkin's disease comes of age. Br Med J 290: 950–951
Miettinen M, Virtanen I, Talerman A (1985) Intermediate filament proteins in human testis and testicular germ cell tumors. Am J Pathol 120: 402–410
Moertel CG, Reitemeier RJ, Schutt AJ, Hahn RG (1972) Treatment of the patient with adenocarcinoma of unknown origin. Cancer 30: 1469–1472
Mohsenifar Z, Chopra SK, Simmons DH (1978) Diagnostic value of fiberoptic bronchoscopy in metastatic pulmonary tumors. Chest 74: 369–371
Morton DL (1984) Surgical treatment for malignant melanoma. Clin Oncol 3: 517–529
Muggia FM, Piccart MJ, Speyer JL (1985) Ovarian cancer: New therapeutic concepts, renewed optimism. Ann Intern Med 103: 795–797
Neilan BA (1983) Adenocarcinoma of unknown origin. CA 33: 237–241
Nissenblatt MJ (1981) The CUP syndrome (carcinoma unknown primary). Cancer Treat Rev 8: 211–224
Olsen EGJ (1982) Electron microscopy: an essential tool for a morphological diagnosis? Br Med J 284: 1897–1898
Osborne BM, Butler JJ, Guarda LA (1985) Primary lymphoma of the liver. Ten cases and a review of the literature. Cancer 56: 2902–2910
Osteen RT, Kopf G, Wilson RE (1978) In pursuit of the unknown primary. Am J Surg 135: 494–498
Pinkus GS, Kurtin PJ (1985) Epithelial membrane antigen – a diagnostic discriminant in surgical pathology: Immunohistochemical profile in epithelial, mesenchymal, and hematopoietic neoplasms using paraffin sections and monoclonal antibodies. Hum Pathol 16: 929–940
Rodriguez M, Dinapoli RP (1980) Spinal cord compression with special reference to metastatic epidural tumors. Mayo Clin Proc 55: 442–448
Rosenberg SA (1979) Non-Hodgkin's lymphoma – selection of treatment on the basis of histologic type. N Engl J Med 301: 355–358
Santini H, Byers RM, Wolf PF (1985) Melanoma metastatic to cervical and parotid nodes from an unknown primary site. Am J Surg 150: 510–512
Scanlon EF (1985) The process of metastasis. Cancer 55: 1163–1166
Schabel FM (1975) Concepts for systemic treatment of micrometastases. Cancer 35: 15–24
Scott JS (1983) Rays of hope for rare ovarian cancers. Br Med J 286: 824–825

Scott Nystrom J, Weiner JM, Meshnik WR, Bateman JR, Viola MV (1979) Identifying the primary site in metastatic cancer of unknown origin. Inadequacy of roentgenographic procedures. JAMA 241: 381–383

Shildt RA, Kennedy PS, Chen TT, Athens JW, O'Bryan RM, Balcerzak SP (1983) Management of patients with metastatic adenocarcinoma of unknown origin: A Southwest Oncology Group study. Cancer Treat Rep 67: 77–79

Simon MA, Karluk MB (1982) Skeletal metastases of unknown origin. Diagnostic strategy for orthopedic surgeons. Clin Orthop 166: 96–103

Snee MP, Vyramuthu N (1985) Metastatic carcinoma from unknown primary site: the experience of a large oncology centre. Br J Radiol 58: 1091–1095

Spiro RH, DeRose G, Strong EW (1983) Cervical node metastasis of occult origin. Am J Surg 146: 441–446

Spiro SG (1985) Chemotherapy of small cell lung cancer. Clin Oncol 4: 105–120

Stamey TA, Yang N, Hay AR, McNeal JE, Freiha FS, Redwine E (1987) Prostate-specific antigen as a serum marker for adenocarcinoma of the prostate. N Engl J Med 317: 909–916

Stewart JF, Tattersall MNH, Woods RL, Fox RM (1979) Unknown primary adenocarcinoma: incidence of overinvestigation and natural history. Br Med J 1: 1530–1533

Sugarbaker EV (1980) Patterns of metastasis in human malignancies. In: Marchalonis JJ, Hanna MG, Fidler IJ (eds) Cancer biology reviews, vol 2. Dekker, New York

Talmadge JE, Fidler IJ (1982) Enhanced metastatic potential of tumor cells harvested from spontaneous metastases of heterogeneous murine tumors. JNCI 69: 975–980

Taylor CR (1985) Monoclonal antibodies and routine paraffin sections. Arch Pathol Lab Med 109: 115–122

Tell DT, Khoury JM, Taylor HG, Veasey SP (1985) Atypical metastasis from prostate cancer. Clinical utility of the immunoperoxidase technique for prostate-specific antigen. JAMA 253: 3574–3575

Vieth R, Odom GL (1965) Intracranial metastases and their neurosurgical treatment. J Neurosurg 23: 375–383

Weiss L, Haydock K, Pickren JW, Lane WW (1980) Organ vascularity and metastatic frequency. Am J Pathol 101: 101–114

Woods RL, Fox RM, Tattersall MHN, Levo JA, Brodie GN (1980) Metastatic adenocarcinomas of unknown primary site. N Engl J Med 303: 87–89

Yam LT (1974) Clinical significance of the human acid phosphatases. Am J Med 56: 604–615

Zaren HA, Copeland EM (1978) Inguinal node metastases. Cancer 41: 919–923

Subject Index

A

B

C

D

E

F

G

H

I

J

K

L

M

N

O

P

Q

R

S

T

U

V

W

Y

MIX
Papier aus verantwortungsvollen Quellen
Paper from responsible sources
FSC® C105338

If you have any concerns about our products,
you can contact us on
ProductSafety@springernature.com

In case Publisher is established outside the EU,
the EU authorized representative is:
Springer Nature Customer Service Center GmbH
Europaplatz 3, 69115 Heidelberg, Germany

Printed by Libri Plureos GmbH
in Hamburg, Germany